Clarke's Analytical Forensic Toxicology

Edited by

Sue Jickells
Senior Lecturer,
Department of Forensic Science
& Drug Monitoring,
King's College London,
London,
UK

Adam Negrusz
Associate Professor of Forensic Sciences,
Assistant Director of Forensic Sciences,
and the Director of Animal Forensic
Toxicology Laboratory,
Department of Biopharmaceutical Sciences,
College of Pharmacy,
University of Illinois at Chicago,
USA

This book is adapted from contributions published in Volume 1 of *Clarke's Analysis of Drugs and Poisons* 3rd edition.

Consulting Editors:

Anthony C Moffat
Head of the Centre
for Pharmaceutical Analysis,
The School of Pharmacy,
University of London,
UK

M David Osselton
Director,
Centre for Forensic Sciences,
Bournemouth University,
UK

Brian Widdop
Consultant Toxicologist,
Medical Toxicology Unit,
Guy's Hospital,
London,
UK

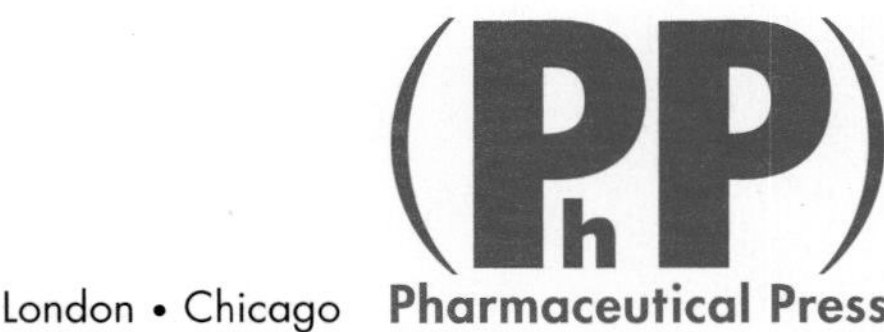

London • Chicago Pharmaceutical Press

Published by the Pharmaceutical Press
An imprint of RPS Publishing

1 Lambeth High Street, London SE1 7JN, UK
100 South Atkinson Road, Suite 200, Grayslake, IL 60030-7820, USA

(PhP) is a trade mark of RPS Publishing
RPS Publishing is the publishing organisation of the Royal Pharmaceutical Society of Great Britain

First published 2008

Typeset by J&L Composition Ltd, Filey, North Yorkshire
Printed in Great Britain by Cambridge University Press, Cambridge

ISBN 978 0 85369 705 3

A catalogue record for this book is available from the British Library.

Clarke's Analytical Forensic Toxicology

Contents

Preface *xii*
Contributors *xiv*
About the editors *xvi*
Abbreviations *xviii*

1 **Introduction to forensic toxicology** 1
A C Moffat, M D Osselton, B Widdop, S Jickells and A Negrusz
Introduction 1
Principles of forensic toxicology 2
Range of cases submitted 4
Case investigation 5
Classification of poisons 7
Samples 8
Sample analysis 8
Conclusions 10
References 10
Further reading 11

2 **Pharmacokinetics and metabolism** 13
O H Drummer
Introduction 13
Basic concepts of pharmacokinetics 13
Drug metabolism 22
Adverse drug interactions and pharmacogenetics 29
Drug concentration and pharmacological response 34
Postmortem redistribution 36
Interpretation 36
Further reading 41

3 **Drugs of abuse** 43
L A King, S D McDermott, S Jickells and A Negrusz
Introduction 43
Commonly abused drugs 44
Analysis of seized drugs 58

Clandestine laboratories 68
Analysis of the main drugs of abuse 68
Conclusion 77
References 77

4 **Other substances encountered in clinical and forensic toxicology** 79
R J Flanagan, M Kala, R Braithwaite and F A de Wolff
General introduction 79
Volatile substances 80
Pesticides 90
Metals and anions 101
Natural toxins 116
Summary 129
References 129

5 **Workplace drug testing** 135
M Peat
Introduction 135
Evolution of workplace testing in the USA 136
Regulatory process in the USA 136
Proposed changes to the *HHS Guidelines* 141
Adulterated and substituted specimens 143
Collection of specimens 145
Role of the medical review officer 146
References 150

6 **Alternative specimens** 153
P Kintz, V Spiehler and A Negrusz
Introduction 153
Hair analysis 153
Drugs in oral fluid 165
Detection of drugs in sweat 181
References 183
Further reading 189

7 **Postmortem toxicology** 191
G R Jones
Introduction 191
Specimens and other exhibits 191
Analytical toxicology 198
Interpretation of postmortem toxicology results 207
Summary 216
References 216
Further reading 217

8 **Clinical toxicology, therapeutic drug monitoring, *in utero* exposure to drugs of abuse** 219
D R A Uges, M Hallworth, C Moore and A Negrusz
Introduction 219
Clinical toxicology 219
Therapeutic drug monitoring 237
In utero exposure to drugs of abuse 256
References 260
Further reading 260

9 **Drug abuse in sport** 263
D A Cowan, E Houghton and S Jickells
Introduction 263
Rules 264
Reported analytical findings 267
Sampling 271
Analytical approach 273
Confirmatory methods 277
References 281

10 **Drug-facilitated sexual assault** 287
A Negrusz and R E Gaensslen
Introduction and basic terms 287
The extent of the problem 288
History and legislation 289
Drugs used to facilitate sexual assault 290
Specimens and analytical methods 296
Summary 297
References 297
Further reading 298

11 **Alcohol, drugs and driving** 299
B K Logan, R G Gullberg, A Negrusz and S Jickells
Introduction 299
Alcohol and driving 308
Drugs and driving 317
References 321

12 **Forensic chemistry and solid dosage form identification** 323
J Ramsey
Introduction 323
Dosage forms 324
Examination of unknown products 331
References 333

13 **Colour tests and thin-layer chromatography** 335
W Jeffery and C F Poole
Introduction 335
Colour tests 335
Thin layer chromatography 343
References 372
Further reading 372

14 **Immunoassays** 375
C Hand and D Baldwin
Introduction 375
Basic principles of immunoassay 377
Heterogeneous immunoassays 382
Homogeneous immunoassays 386
Automation of immunoassay 388
Analysis of alternative samples to urine 388
Quality control, calibration, standardisation and curve fitting 389
References 391

15 **Ultraviolet, visible and fluorescence spectrophotometry** 393
J Cordonnier and J Schaep
Introduction and theoretical background 393
UV and visible spectrophotometry 394
Instrumentation 399
Instrument performance checks 401
Sample preparation and presentation 402
Data processing and presentation of results 404
Interpretation of spectra and qualitative analysis 407
Quantitative analysis 410
Fluorescence spectrophotometry 411
Instrumentation 414
Instrument performance checks 415
Sample preparation and presentation 416
Data processing and presentation of results 416
Interpretation of spectra and qualitative analysis 417
Quantitative analysis 418
References 419
Collections of data 419
Further reading 420

16 **Infrared spectroscopy** 421
A Drake
(with 'Near infrared' by *R D Jee*)
Introduction 421
Instrumentation 425

Data processing 428
Instrument calibration 429
Sample preparation 431
Sample presentation 432
Interpretation of spectra 441
Qualitative analysis 442
Quantitative analysis 447
Collections of data 447
Near infrared 448
References 453
Further reading 454

17 Raman spectroscopy 455
D E Bugay and P A Martoglio Smith
Introduction and theory 455
Instrumentation 457
Coupled techniques 459
Data processing and presentation of results 459
System suitability tests 460
Sample preparation and sample presentation 461
Interpretation of spectra 462
Qualitative analysis 464
Quantitative analysis 466
Collections of data 467
References 468
Further reading 468

18 Gas chromatography 469
S Dawling, S Jickells and A Negrusz
Introduction 469
Gas chromatography columns 470
Inlet systems 483
Detector systems 493
Specimen preparation 498
Quantitative determinations 505
Optimising operation conditions to customise applications 506
Specific applications 508
References 510
Further reading 511

19 High-performance liquid chromatography 513
T Kupiec, M Slawson, F Pragst and M Herzler
Introduction 513
Practical aspects of HPLC theory 514
Hardware 515

Columns 522
Maintenance 525
Separation techniques 526
Quantitative analysis 528
Validation 530
New emerging trends 530
Systems for drug analysis 531
Selection of chromatographic systems 533
Analysis of drugs in pharmaceutical preparations 533
Analysis of drugs in biological fluids and tissues 534
References 536
Further reading 536

20 Capillary electrophoresis for drug analysis 539
D Perrett
Background to capillary electrophoresis 539
Theoretical outline 540
Modes of capillary electrophoresis 543
Instrumentation for capillary electrophoresis 545
Method development and optimisation 548
Analytical methods 550
General applications to drug assays 554
Conclusions and future directions 556
References 556
Further reading 556

21 Mass spectrometry 557
D Watson, S Jickells and A Negrusz
Introduction 557
Theory 559
Instrumentation 563
Coupled techniques 568
Data processing 572
System suitability tests 573
Sample preparation and presentation 574
Data interpretation 574
Mass spectrometry in qualitative analysis 579
Identification of drug metabolites 582
Some applications of mass spectrometry in quantitative analysis 583
Collections of data 584
References 585

22 **Emerging techniques** 587
M Sanchez-Felix
Introduction 587
Emerging techniques 587
Conclusion 602
References 603
Useful websites 605

23 **Quality control and assessment** 607
R K Bramley, D G Bullock and J R Garcia
Introduction 607
Quality assurance terminology 608
Quality systems 609
Customer requirement and/or specification 609
Procedures for sample selection, collection, preservation, packaging, identification, storage and transport 610
Validation of new methods 612
Measurement uncertainty 614
Equipment maintenance and calibration 615
Evaluation of materials and reagents 615
Sample and data handling in the laboratory 616
Sample disposal 616
Protocols for sample preparation, analyte recovery and analysis 616
In-process performance monitoring 616
Assessment, interpretation and reporting of results 618
External quality assessment arrangements 618
Corrective actions for noncompliance 619
Management of laboratory facilities 620
Avoidance of contamination 620
Competence standards, training programme and monitoring arrangements for the analyst 620
Assessment and accreditation 620
References 622
Further reading 622

Index 625

Preface

This text is aimed at master's students studying forensic science, forensic toxicology and analytical chemistry involving forensic toxicology, and at PhD students carrying out research in these areas. The driver for this student text has been the opportunity to make the wonderful resource that is *Clarke's Analysis of Drugs and Poisons* more readily accessible to students. As those familiar with the third edition of Clarke's will know, this is a resource *par excellence* in the field of toxicology, but out of the financial reach of most students. We hope that this text will redress this balance.

The early chapters of the text cover the main elements of forensic toxicology with an introduction to the subject in Chapter 1. An understanding of the importance of pharmacokinetics and metabolism is essential for forensic toxicology (Chapter 2). It is impossible to cover all significant substances encountered in toxicology in a text of this nature. The most important substances, such as drugs of abuse, are described in Chapter 3. Examples of other toxicologically significant substances are discussed in Chapter 4. Although blood, urine and tissues such as liver, lung, etc., are still widely used for forensic analysis, alternative matrices are of considerable interest (Chapter 6), particularly for drugs screening, for example in workplace drug testing (Chapter 5), roadside drug testing (Chapter 11), sports doping (Chapter 9) and drug monitoring in clinical settings (Chapter 8). For the purpose of clarity, the chapters on drugs in saliva and hair analysis from the third edition of *Clarke's* have been combined and a separate section on drugs in sweat added (Chapter 6). The subject of *in utero* exposure to drugs was not included in the third edition of *Clarke's* but is included in this text (Chapter 8) as it is a topic of increasing interest. Another topic of current interest not included in the third edition of *Clarke's* is drug-facilitated sexual assault (Chapter 10). Impairment of driving through ingestion of alcohol has been known for some time, but the aspect of impairment due to drugs is a more recently recognised phenomenon: both aspects form a major element in the casework of toxicology laboratories and are addressed in Chapter 11.

There are many situations in clinical and forensic toxicology when the solid form of a drug is encountered and it is advantageous to be able to identify the drug directly from this evidence without recourse to analysis (Chapter 12), although the suite of analytical techniques available to and used by toxicologists is extensive. Colour tests and TLC (Chapter 13) and immunoassays (Chapter 14) are typically used for screening purposes to direct the choice of analyses used for identification and quantification. Spectroscopic techniques such as UV, visible and fluorescence (Chapter 15) may be used as standalone techniques for screening or quantification, but are also often hyphenated with chromatographic techniques such as high performance liquid chromatography (HPLC) (Chapter 19) or capillary electrophoresis (CE) (Chapter 20). Gas chromatography (GC) (Chapter 18) is another important technique used in toxicology and, like HPLC and CE, is typically coupled with mass spectrometry (Chapter 21) to provide what is often considered to be the 'gold standard' technique for identification and quantification. Spectroscopic techniques such as infrared and near-infrared (Chapter 16) find uses in toxicology as does Raman spectroscopy (Chapter 17). Although a very important technique elsewhere in chemistry, nuclear magnetic resonance (NMR) spectroscopy is not widely used in toxicological analysis and hence is not covered in this text.

Being as certain as one can be of the correct answer is of fundamental importance in analytical chemistry and the field of toxicological analysis is no exception, particularly where someone's career may be affected by the outcome of drugs screening, as may be the case in workplace drug testing and sports doping testing, or when a person faces prosecution and possible conviction, for example, for causing death by dangerous driving due to impairment through alcohol or drugs, for suspected poisoning, or for supplying drugs of abuse. Analytical laboratories involved in toxicological analyses should employ suitable quality control (QC) and quality assurance (QA) procedures and this aspect is covered in Chapter 23. The material included in the third edition of *Clarke's* on emerging techniques has been revised and updated (Chapter 22).

In editing the third edition of *Clarke's* for student use we recognise that we have still produced a text of considerable depth and complexity. This is due in part to our reluctance to lose too much of the excellent information in *Clarke's* and also because we believe that this information provides an excellent introduction for students intent on a career in toxicology. We are indebted to the authors of chapters in the third edition of *Clarke's Analysis of Drugs and Poisons* who have co-operated with our edit of their original chapters and to Professor Anthony Moffat, Professor David Osselton and Professor Brian Widdop for putting our names forward to Pharmaceutical Press as possible editors of this student text.

S Jickells
A Negrusz
April 2008

Contributors

D Baldwin
Cozart Bioscience Limited, Abingdon, UK
R Braithwaite
Department of Forensic Science & Drug Monitoring, Kings College London, UK
R K Bramley
Forensic Science Service, Birmingham, UK
D E Bugay
SSCI Inc., An Aptuit Company, West Lafayette, IN, USA
D G Bullock
Wolfson EQA Laboratory, Birmingham, UK
J Cordonnier
Chemiphar n.v., Brugge, Belgium
D A Cowan
Drug Control Centre, King's College London, UK
S Dawling
Diagnostics Laboratories, Vanderbilt University Medical Centre, Nashville, TN, USA
F A de Wolff
Toxicology Laboratory, Leiden University Medical Center, Leiden, The Netherlands
A Drake
The Department of Pharmacy, King's College London, UK
O H Drummer
Victorian Institute of Forensic Medicine, Melbourne, Australia
R J Flanagan
Department of Clinical Biochemistry, King's College Hospital Foundation Trust, London, UK
J R Garcia
Pharmaceutical Division, BovisLendLease, USA
R E Gaensslen
Forensic Sciences, Department of Biopharmaceutical Sciences, College of Pharmacy, UIC, Chicago, IL, USA
R G Gullberg
Washington State Toxicology Laboratory, Seattle, WA, USA
M Hallworth
Department of Clinical Biochemistry, Royal Shrewsbury Hospital, Shrewsbury, UK
C Hand
Cozart Bioscience Limited, Abingdon, UK
M Herzler
Institute of Legal Medicine, Humboldt University, Berlin, Germany
E Houghton
HFL, Fordham, UK
R D Jee
The School of Pharmacy, University of London, UK
W Jeffery
Forensic Laboratory, Royal Canadian Mounted Police, Vancouver, BC, Canada
S Jickells
Department of Forensic Science & Drug Monitoring, King's College London, UK
G R Jones
Office of Chief Medical Examiner, Edmonton, AB, Canada
M Kala
Department of Forensic Toxicology, Institute of Forensic Research, Krakow, Poland
L A King
Formerly, Drugs Intelligence Unit, Forensic Science Service, London, UK
P Kintz
Institut de Médecine Légale, Strasbourg, France
T Kupiec
Analytical Research Laboratories, Oklahoma City, OK, USA

B K Logan
Washington State Toxicology Laboratory, Seattle, WA, USA
P A Martoglio Smith
SSCI Inc., An Aptuit Company, West Lafayette, IN, USA
S D McDermott
Forensic Science Laboratory, Dublin, Ireland
A C Moffat
Centre for Pharmaceutical Analysis, The School of Pharmacy, University of London, UK
C Moore
Immunalysis Corporation, Toxicology Research and Development, Pomona, CA, USA
A Negrusz
Forensic Sciences, Department of Biopharmaceutical Sciences, College of Pharmacy, UIC, Chicago, IL, USA
M D Osselton
Director, Centre for Forensic Sciences, Bournemouth University, UK
M Peat
Quest Diagnostics Inc., Houston, TX, USA
D Perrett
Department of Medicine, St Bartholomew's Hospital, London, UK
C F Poole
Department of Chemistry, Wayne State University, Detroit, MI, USA
F Pragst
Institute of Legal Medicine, Humboldt University, Berlin, Germany
J Ramsey
TicTac Communications Ltd, St George's Hospital Medical School, London, UK
M Sanchez-Felix
Eli Lilly, Minneapolis, MN, USA
J Schaep
Chemiphar n.v., Brugge, Belgium
M Slawson
Department of Pharmacology and Toxicology, University of Utah, UT, USA
V Spiehler
Newport Beach, CA, USA
D R A Uges
Laboratory for Clinical and Forensic Toxicology and Drug Analysis, University Hospital Groningen and University Centre of Pharmacy, Groningen, The Netherlands
D Watson
Institute of Pharmacy and Biomedical Sciences, University of Strathclyde, Glasgow, UK
B Widdop
Formerly, Medical Toxicology Unit, Guy's and St Thomas' Hospital Trust, London, UK

About the editors

Dr Sue Jickells obtained her BSc degree at Reading University, UK. She started her career as an analytical chemist in 1975 in the Somerset Public Analyst Service, carrying out analysis of foodstuffs, pesticides and animal feeds. This was followed by several years spent with Strathclyde Regional Chemist Department, Glasgow, Scotland, where she helped pioneer sampling techniques using trapping on Tenax to investigate environmental pollution incidents using GC-MS. After seven years in Bermuda at the Bermuda Biological Station, she returned to the UK in 1985 and obtained her MSc in Forensic Science a year later from King's College London, followed by a PhD from the University of Leeds in 1990. In her subsequent post at the UK Ministry of Agriculture and Fisheries and Foods Food Science Laboratory (now the Central Science Laboratory) she led an R&D team developing methods for the analysis of trace organic contaminants in foodstuffs. She was a UK representative and, subsequently, Consultant Expert, to the Council of Europe (CoE) Committee of Experts on Materials Coming into Contact with Foods developing analytical methods in support of CoE Resolutions on packaging materials, and a member of the European Committee for Standardisation (CEN) Technical Committee developing technical standards in support of EU Directives on packaging materials. In 1999 she joined King's College London where she is currently a Senior Lecturer in the Department of Forensic Science and Drug Monitoring, lecturing in analytical chemistry to MSc students in Forensic Science and Pharmaceutical Sciences. She is responsible for the chemistry modules of the MSc Forensic Science programme at KCL, including Forensic Toxicology and Drugs of Abuse. She has an active research programme in forensic science with a particular interest in the chemistry of fingerprints. She has published nearly 40 research articles and chapters in several books.

Adam Negrusz, PhD is an Associate Professor, Assistant Director of Forensic Sciences, and the Director of Animal Forensic Toxicology Laboratory, Department of Biopharmaceutical Sciences, College of Pharmacy, University of Illinois at Chicago. His research interests focus on drug-facilitated sexual assault, equine testing for illicit substances, and the development of state-of-the-art chromatographic methods for the determination of drugs in biological specimens including hair and postmortem samples, and forensic urine drug testing.

Dr Negrusz received a Masters degree in Pharmacy from Nicholas Copernicus Medical University in Krakow, Poland (1981), and a PhD in Pharmaceutical Sciences from the same university in Poland (1989). In 2001 he received a Doctor Habilitatus degree from Jagiellonian University, Krakow, Poland. Adam is a registered pharmacist (1981) and licensed toxicologist (1987) in Poland. After 8 years at the Department of Toxicology, Medical University in Krakow, he joined the University of Illinois at Chicago in 1990 where he developed various procedures, including the analysis of meconium, amniotic fluid and umbilical cord for cocaine and its metabolites. After completion of his postdoctoral training he worked for one year as a toxicologist at the Cook County Office of the Medical Examiner.

In 1993 he re-joined the University of Illinois and in 1995 became an Assistant Professor of Forensic Sciences. In 2002 he was promoted to the rank of Associate Professor with tenure.

Currently Adam is involved as a coordinator and lecturer in courses required to obtain a Master of Sciences degree in Forensic Sciences. He also teaches professional PharmD students. Overall, he has 27 years of experience in academic forensic toxicology and drug analysis which has resulted in the publication of nearly 50 research articles, several book chapters, nearly 60 abstracts presented at scientific meetings, over 30 professional analytical chemistry reports for sponsors, and many standard operating procedures (SOPs). He is a Fellow (Toxicology Section) of the American Academy of Forensic Sciences where he served for one year as a Section Chair, a member of the Society of Forensic Toxicologists (SOFT) and The International Association of Forensic Toxicologists (TIAFT), and an affiliate member of the Association of Official Racing Chemists, the Society of Hair Testing, and the Polish Society of Toxicology.

Abbreviations

1,4-BD	1,4-butanediol
2,4,5-T	2,4,5-trichlorophenoxyacetic acid
2,4-D	2,4-dichlorophenoxyacetic acid
5-HT	5-hydroxytryptamine (serotonin)
6-MAM	6-monoacetylmorphine
8-MOP	8-methoxypsoralen
AAS	androgenic-anabolic steroid
AAS	atomic absorption spectrophotometry
ACE	affinity CE
ACE	angiotensin-converting enzyme
AcCh	acetylcholine
AChE	acetylcholinesterase
ADC	analog-to-digital converter
ADD	attention deficit disorder
ADH	alcohol dehydrogenase
ADI	acceptable daily intake
AED	atomic emission detector
AEME	anhydroecgonine methyl ester
AES	atomic emission spectrometry/spectrometer
AFID	alkali flame ionisation detector
AHB	alpha-hydroxybutyric acid
APCI	atmospheric pressure chemical ionisation
ASP	amnesic shellfish poisoning
ASV	anodic stripping voltametry
ATR	attenuated total reflectance
AUC	area under the curve
BAC	blood alcohol (ethanol) concentration
BGE	background electrolyte
BHB	beta-hydroxybutyric acid
BMC	4-bromomethyl-7-methoxycoumarin
BOAA	β-*N*-oxalylamino-L-alanine
BPA	boronphenylalanine
BrAc	breath alcohol
BrAC	breath alcohol concentration
BSA	bovine serum albumin
BSTFA	*N,O*-bis(trimethylsilyl)trifluoroacetamide
BZE	benzoyl ecgonine
BZP	1-benzylpiperazine
CBD	cannabidiol

CBN	cannabinol
CCD	charged coupled device
CD	cyclodextrin
CE	capillary electrophoresis
CEC	capillary electrochromatography
CEDIA	cloned enzyme donor immunoassay
CFP	Ciguatera fish poisoning
CGE	capillary gel electrophoresis
ChE	pseudocholinesterase
CI	chemical ionisation
CIA	capillary ion analysis
cIEF	capillary isoelectric focusing
CIRMS	combustion isotope ratio MS
cITP	capillary isotachophoresis
CNS	central nervous system
COHb	carboxyhaemoglobin
COMT	catecholmethyltransferase
CRM	certified reference material
CSE	capillary sieving electrophoresis
CSF	cerebrospinal fluid
CSP	chiral stationary phase
CTX	ciguatoxins
CV	coefficient of variation
CZE	capillary zone electrophoresis
Da	Dalton
DAD	diode-array detection/detector
d.c.	direct current
DESI	desorption electrospray ionisation
DFSA	drug-facilitated sexual assault
DMS	dimethylpolysiloxane
DMSO	dimethyl sulfoxide
DNBC	3,5-dinitrobenzoyl chloride
DNS-Cl	dansyl chloride
DOB	4-bromo-2,5-dimethoxyamfetamine
DOC	4-chloro-2,5-dimethoxyamfetamine
DOI	4-iodo-2,5-dimethoxyamfetamine
DON	deoxynivalenol
DRIFT	diffuse reflectance IR Fourier transform (spectroscopy)
DSP	diarrhoetic shellfish poisoning
DUI	driving under the influence
DUIA	driving under the influence of alcohol
DUID	driving under the influence of drugs
EA	enzyme acceptor
EC	electrochemical
ECD	electron capture detection/detector
ED	enzyme donor
EDDP	2-ethylidene-1,5-dimethyl-3,3-diphenylpyrrolidine
EDTA	ethylenediaminetetraacetic acid
EI	electron impact
EK	electrokinetic

ESI	electrospray ionisation
EIA	enzyme immunoassay
EIPH	exercise-induced pulmonary haemorrhage
ELCD	electrolytic conductivity detection
ELISA	enzyme-linked immunoabsorbent assay
EM	extensive metaboliser
EMDP	2-ethyl-5-methyl-3,3-diphenyl-1-pyrrolidine
EME	ecgonine methyl ester
EMIT	enzyme multiplied immunoassay technique
EOF	electro-osmotic flow
EPO	erythropoietin
EQA	external quality assessment
ESI	electrospray ionisation
ETAAS	electrothermal atomic absorption spectrophotometry
Fab	antibody binding fragment
FAB	fast-atom bombardment
FAME	fatty acid methyl ester
Fc	crystalline fragment
FFAP	free fatty acid phase
FIA	flow injection analysis
FID	flame ionisation detection/detector
FL	fluorescence
FPIA	fluorescence polarisation immunoassay
FSH	follicle-stimulating hormone
FTIR	Fourier transform IR
FTIRD	Fourier transform IR detector
GABA	gamma-aminobutyric acid
GBL	gamma-butyrolactone
GC	gas chromatography
GFAAS	graphite furnace atomic absorption spectrophotometry
GHB	gamma-hydroxybutyric acid
GLC	gas–liquid chromatography
GLP	good laboratory practice
GST	glutathione *S*-transferase
HBOC	haemoglobin-based oxygen carrier
hCG, HCG	human chorionic gonadotropin
HD	hydrodynamic
HFBA	heptafluoropropionic anhydride
hGH	human growth hormone
HGN	horizontal gaze nystagmus
HIV	human immunodeficiency virus
HMG-IR2/L	Human Menopausal Gonadotropin 2nd International Reference Preparation per litre
HMMA	4-hydroxy-3-methoxymethamfetamine
HPLC	high-performance liquid chromatography
HPTLC	high-performance TLC
HRP	horseradish peroxidase
HS-SPME	headspace solid-phase microextraction
HTS	high-throughput screening
ICAT	isotope-coded affinity tagging

ICE	interaction CE
ICP-AES	inductively coupled plasma–atomic emission spectrophotometry
ICP-MS	inductively coupled plasma–mass spectrometry
ICP-OES	inductively coupled plasma–optical emission spectrometry
i.d.	internal diameter
IEF	isoelectric focusing
Ig	immunoglobulin
IGF-1	insulin-like growth factor 1
INR	International Normalised Ratio
IP	ion pair
IQC	internal quality control
IR	infrared
IRMA	immunoradiometric assay
IRMS	isotope ratio mass spectrometry
ITP	isotachophoresis
kDa	kilodalton
KIMS	kinetic interaction of microparticles in solution
KLH	keyhole limpet haemocyanin
LAMPA	lysergic acid *N*-(methylpropyl)amide
LC-MS	HPLC-MS
LCTF	liquid crystal tunable filter
LH	luteinising hormone
LIF	laser-induced fluorescence
LIMS	laboratory information management system
LLE	liquid–liquid extraction
LOD	limit of detection
LOQ	limit of quantification
LPG	liquefied petroleum gas
LSD	lysergide
MALDI	matrix-assisted laser desorption ionisation
MALDI-TOF-MS	matrix-assisted laser desorption ionisation–time of flight–mass spectrometry
MAM	monoacetyl morphine
MAO	monoamine oxidase inhibitor
mAU	(milli)absorbance unit
MBDB	*N*-methyl-1-(1,3-benzodioxol-5-yl)-2-butanamine
MBTFA	*N*-methylbis(trifluoroacetamide)
MCF	(1*R*,2*S*,5*R*)-(−)-methylchloroformate
MCPA	methylchlorophenoxyacetic acid
mCPP	*m*-chlorophenylpiperazine
MDA	methylenedioxyamfetamine
MDEA	methylenedioxyethylamfetamine
MDMA	methylenedioxymethylamfetamine
MDP2P	1-(3,4-methylenedioxyphenyl)-2-propanone
MDR	multidrug resistance
MECC/MEKC	micellar electrokinetic capillary chromatography
MEEKC	microemulsion electrokinetic capillary chromatography
MEL	maximum exposure limit
MGF	mechano growth factors
MRL	maximum residue limit

MRO	medical review officer
MS	mass spectrometry
MS/MS	tandem mass spectrometry
MSTFA	*N*-methyltrimethylsilyltrifluoroacetamide
MT	methyltransferase
MTBSTFA	*N*-methyl-*N*-(*t*-butyldimethylsilyl)trifluoroacetamide
NA	numerical aperture
NACE	non-aqueous capillary electrophoresis
NAD	nicotinamide–adenine dinucleotide
NADH	nicotine–adenine dinucleotide reduced form
NADP	nicotinamide–adenine dinucleotide phosphate
NAPQI	*N*-acetyl-*p*-benzoquinoneimine
NAT	*N*-acetyltransferase
NBD-F	4-fluoro-7-nitro-2,1,3-benzoxadiazole
NC-SPE	non-conditioned SPE
NICI	negative-ion chemical ionisation
NIOSH	National Institute for Occupational Safety and Health
NIR	near infrared
NIST	National Institute of Standards and Technology
NMDA	*N*-methyl-D-aspartate
NMR	nuclear magnetic resonance
NPD	nitrogen–phosphorus detection/detector
NSAID	nonsteroidal anti-inflammatory drug
NSB	nonspecific binding
NSP	neurotoxic shellfish poisoning
ODS	octadecyl silica
OES	Occupational Exposure Standard
OLST	one-leg-stand test
OP	organophosphorus
P-2-P	phenyl-2-propanone
P-III-P	procollagen type III
PC	phencyclohexene
PCA	principal component analysis
PCI	positive chemical ionisation
PCP	phencyclidine
PCR	polymerase chain reaction
PDA	photodiode array
PDH	glucose-6-phosphate dehydrogenase
PEEK	polyetheretherketone
PEG	poly(ethylene glycol)
PFDTD	perfluoro-5,8-dimethyl-3,6,9-trioxidodecane
PFK	perfluorokerosene
PFP	puffer fish poisoning
PFPA	pentafluoropropionic anhydride
PFTBA	perfluorotributylamine
P-gp	P-glycoprotein
PICI	positive ion chemical ionisation
PID	photoionisation detection/detector
PLOT	porous layer open tubular
PLS	partial least squares

PM	poor metaboliser
PMT	photomultiplier tube
PSI	pre-column separating inlet
PSP	paralytic shellfish poisoning
PSX	polysiloxane
PTFE	polytetrafluoroethylene
PTV	programmable temperature vaporising (sample inlet)
QC	quality control
QC&A	quality control and assessment
rhEPO	recombinant human erythropoietin
RI	refractive index
RI	retention index
RIA	radioimmunoassay
RMM	relative molecular mass
RP	reversed phase
RSD	relative standard deviation
SAR	structure–activity relationship
SARMs	selective androgen receptor modulators
SBW	spectral bandwidth
SCF	supercritical fluid
SCOT	support-coated open tubular
SDS	sodium dodecyl sulfate
SERMs	selective estrogen receptor modulators
SFE	supercritical fluid extraction
SIM	selected ion monitoring
SNP	single-nucleotide polymorphism
SNPA	*N*-succinimidyl-*p*-nitrophenylacetate
SOFT	Society of Forensic Toxicologists
SOP	standard operating procedure
SPE	solid-phase extraction
SPME	solid-phase microextraction
SSRI	selective serotonin reuptake inhibitor
STIP	systematic toxicological identification procedure
STX	saxitoxins
SULT	sulfotransferase
μTAS	micro total-analysis systems
TCD	thermal conductivity detection/detector
TCO_2	total carbon dioxide
TCRC	time-coupled time-resolved chromatography
TDC	time-to-digital converter
TDM	therapeutic drug monitoring
TFA	target factor analysis
TFAA	trifluoroacetic anhydride
TGS	triglycine sulfate
THC	tetrahydrocannabinol
THCA	11-carboxy-Δ^9–tetrahydrocannabinol
THC-COOH	Δ^9-tetrahydrocannabinol-9-carboxylic acid
THEED	tetrahydroxyethylenediamine
TIAFT	The International Association of Forensic Toxicologists
TIC	total ion current

TLC	thin layer chromatography
TMB	tetramethylbenzidine
TMCS	trimethylchlorosilane
TMS	trimethylsilyl
TMT	thiol methyltransferase
TOF	time of flight
TPC	*n*-trifluoroacetyl-1-propyl chloride
TPMT	thiopurine methyltransferase
TTAB	tetradecyltrimethyl ammonium bromide
TTX	tetrodotoxin
UDPGT	uridine diphosphate glucuronosyltransferase
UEM	ultra-extensive (= ultra-rapid) metaboliser
uHTS	ultra-high-throughput screening
UNODC	United Nations Office of Drugs and Crime
UV	ultraviolet
VSA	volatile substance abuse
VTEC	verotoxin-producing *E. coli*
WADA	World Anti Doping Agency
WATT	walk-and-turn test
WCOT	wall-coated open tubular
WHO	World Health Organization
XRD	X-ray diffraction
XRF	X-ray fluorescence
ZPP	zinc protoporphyrin

1

Introduction to forensic toxicology

A C Moffat, M D Osselton, B Widdop, S Jickells and A Negrusz

Introduction 1
Principles of forensic toxicology 2
Range of cases submitted 4
Case investigation 5
Classification of poisons 7
Samples 8
Sample analysis 8
Conclusions 10
References 10
Further reading 11

Introduction

The term 'forensic toxicology' covers any application of the science and study of poisons to the elucidation of questions that occur in judicial proceedings. The subject is usually associated with work for the police, the coroner and the criminal law courts. However, the analysis and identification of medicines and the maintenance of agricultural, industrial and public health legislation (to ensure clean air, pure water and safe food supplies) are also aspects of forensic toxicology, although usually associated with civil courts rather than criminal courts. Like the forensic toxicologist in criminal cases, analysts employed in these civil areas may at times find their work subject to severe public scrutiny in a law court, and both groups should be aware of the strengths and limitations of each other's methodology.

Accidental self-poisoning and attempted suicide cases are generally the responsibility of the clinical toxicologist or the hospital biochemist, who may work in conjunction with a poison control centre. A small proportion of these cases is referred to the forensic toxicologist, either because of an allegation of malicious poisoning or because the patient dies and a coroner's inquest is ordered.

The defining difference between the clinical toxicologist and the forensic toxicologist is the judicial element. As we shall see later in this book, the samples taken for analysis and the techniques used to detect and identify poisons are generally similar for both clinical and forensic toxicology. The clinical toxicologist is primarily concerned with the identification of drugs and poisons as an aid to the diagnosis and treatment of acute and chronic poisoning. If the patient dies, the analytical data obtained by the clinical toxicologist may well be sufficient for use by the pathologist and the coroner in determining the cause of death in cases where there are no suspicious circumstances. In other cases, including those where the patient recovers but claims to have been poisoned by a third party, it is usual for the investigation to be referred to a forensic toxicologist.

Although the above indicates that the forensic toxicologist is generally involved in cases of suspected poisoning, more recently other roles have developed in areas such as doping in sports, of both humans and animals, and workplace drug testing. The question to be answered in these areas is not 'Has this person been poisoned?', or at least not in the conventional sense where poisoning is taken to mean harm having been induced. Instead, such questions as 'Has a drug or poison been administered which might affect performance?' or 'Is this person taking an illegal substance?' may need to be investigated. Workplace drug testing and drug abuse in sport are discussed in more detail in Chapters 5 and 9 respectively.

In many jurisdictions the forensic toxicologist also deals with drink and drug driving offences, and these aspects are addressed in Chapter 11.

Forensic toxicology has evolved throughout the centuries and has now become a multidisciplinary and highly specialized 'tool' to investigate a wide range of scenarios involving the potential effects of drugs and chemicals on humans and animals. The first highly significant individual in the history of forensic toxicology was, without a doubt, Paracelsus (1493–1541). He was born in Switzerland and is considered one of the greatest men of the European Renaissance along with Nicholas Copernicus, Christopher Columbus, Martin Luther, Erasmus of Rotterdam, and Leonardo da Vinci. Paracelsus defined a poison for the first time. He wrote: *'All substances are poisons: there is none which is not a poison. The right dose differentiates a poison and a remedy'.* Today we know that the definition of a poison is much more complex, but Paracelsus's approach was proved to be correct. His statement has become famous and has been broadly cited in the literature throughout the years. Paracelsus was also a pioneer of what would be today called occupational medicine. Several chemists became interested in the properties of poisons over the years and their work led ultimately to the development of the first forensic analytical tests. For example, in the late 18th century, the German pharmaceutical chemist Carl Wilhelm Scheele (1742–1786) converted arsenic trioxide to arsine gas using nitric acid in the presence of zinc. In 1836, the English chemist James Marsh (1794–1846) modified and perfected Scheele's procedure and developed a test ('arsenic mirror') to detect this poison in biological specimens. At that time arsenic trioxide was a favourite poison and was impossible to detect. The symptoms of arsenic poisoning resemble those caused by the bacterial disease cholera. As a result, many murderers got away with their crimes. The metallic arsenic test developed by Marsh constituted a significant achievement in the toxicological investigation of murder.

The first complete work of international importance on the subject of forensic toxicology was written by Mathieu J. B. Orfila in 1813 (*Traité des poisons tires des règnes minéral végétal et animal, ou, Toxicologie générale, considérée sous les rapports de la physiologie, de la pathologie et de la médecine légale*; see Orfila 1818). It was an immediate success and won him the title of 'Father of Toxicology'. 'The Chemist,' said Orfila, 'horrified by the crime of homicidal poisoning, must aim to perfect the process necessary for establishing the case of poisoning in order to reveal the crime and to assist the magistrate to punish the guilty'. It is interesting to note that he realised the necessity of adequate proof of identification, emphasised the importance of what we now call quality assurance and anticipated the need for pharmaceutical, clinical, industrial and environmental toxicology. In 1850 the Belgian analytical chemist Jean Stas and the German scientist Friedrich Otto developed a complex system for the extraction of unknown poisons from biological specimens based on the chemical properties of the substances. This methodology was successfully applied for alkaloidal poisons such as colchicine and strychnine. With some modifications, the methodology developed by Stas and Otto is still used.

Principles of forensic toxicology

The objective of the forensic toxicologist is to attempt to provide answers to questions that may arise during criminal investigations or in subsequent court proceedings. The traditional question that must be answered is 'Has this person been poisoned?', together with the supplementary queries that follow if the result is affirmative, such as 'What is the identity of the poison?', 'How was it administered?', 'What are its effects?' and 'Was it a dangerous or lethal amount?'. Note that it is not the role of the forensic toxicologist to determine who administered the poison. That is typically the role of the police or the courts. Nor is it the role of the forensic toxicologist to confirm the cause of death. That is the role of the pathologist.

Chemical analyses are used to detect the presence of the poison, measure its concentration and relate this to its known toxicity or effects on the organism.

Generally, the forensic toxicologist is involved in the following situations:

Toxicological investigations

- to establish poisoning as the cause of death
- to investigate unlawful poisoning by a third party (e.g. in suspicious deaths; in cases of non-accidental child poisoning; in cases of drug-facilitated sexual assault (DFSA))
- to establish the presence of substances that may affect a person's behaviour or ability to make rational/reasoned judgement, e.g. DFSA and driving under the influence of drugs or alcohol.

Human and animal performance testing

- to investigate incidents of driving under the influence of drugs and alcohol
- to detect the use of performance-enhancing drugs in human and animal sports.

Forensic drug testing

- to detect non-compliance with policies governing the use of drugs in the workplace
- to provide evidence in cases where parents may be denied access to young children on the basis of a history of drug abuse and where continued abuse may endanger the child.

If the poison for which the forensic toxicologist has to test is not specified by name, the request to 'test for poisons' is a major problem. Given that all substances can be poisons, depending on the dose, in theory this means that an exceedingly broad range of substances with very different chemical natures may need to be tested for. Thankfully for the forensic toxicologist, in practice the number of substances encountered as poisons is considerably less than the total number of compounds that exist in the world. However, this still leaves a relatively large number of substances as poisons likely to be encountered, and there is always the possibility of an unexpected substance being involved in any particular case. By their very nature, most chemical methods of analysis employ some form of detection that relies on a specific interaction with some aspect of the physicochemical properties of the compound under test. There is no universal method of analysis for all substances, particularly where the requirement is to be able to detect, identify and quantify the substance, typically at low concentrations and in complex matrices such as organ tissues and blood. At least seven different analytical schemes are required to exclude even the most commonly encountered poisons (Fig. 1.1).

Forensic toxicology demands an overall analytical system designed to exclude or indicate the presence of any poison in each of the chemical groups shown in Fig. 1.1. Most of the numerous screening procedures reported in the literature are too limited to permit a confident negative report.

Apart from these analytical problems, the legal aspect of the work demands a scrupulous attention to detail. Failure to make full descriptive notes on the items received, a simple error in the date the analysis was performed or neglecting to check reagent purity can be presented as evidence of careless work by an astute lawyer. The lawyer may, with justification, explore the extent of the toxicologist's experience and knowledge, demand a detailed account of the

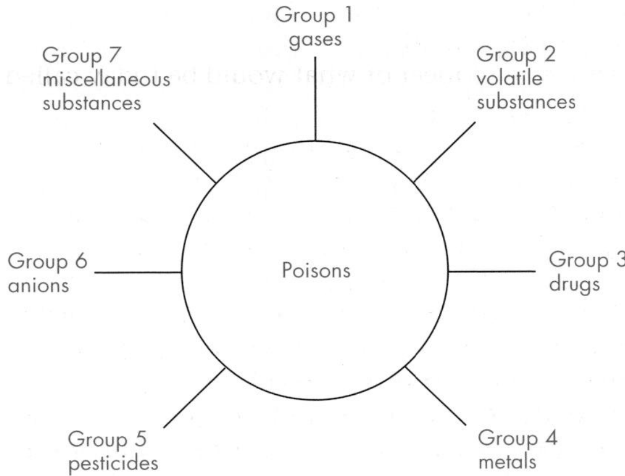

Figure 1.1 The seven major groups of poisons.

analytical methods and challenge the integrity of any opinion. The crucial evidence of identification and quantification of the poison may be faultless and the conclusions correct, but if the court's confidence in the forensic toxicologist as an unbiased scientific expert is destroyed, the case may be lost. A secure chain of custody of all the exhibits submitted also has to be proved. Aspects of sampling, avoidance of contamination, appropriate packaging of samples, chain of custody and recording sample information at all stages of the process are emphasised throughout this book. As will be seen in the various chapters, the types of body fluids, tissues and other samples of importance in forensic toxicology can vary depending on the analytes under consideration, the aim of the analysis and individual case circumstances. As will also be seen in the chapters that follow, the nature of the sample can also impact on the methods used for analysis and the interpretation of results.

Orfila was well acquainted with the aspects of forensic toxicology outlined above, and the guiding principles he established nearly 200 years ago are still applicable. These may be summarised as follows:

- all chemists who undertake this work must have toxicological experience
- the analyst must be given a complete case history that contains all the information available
- all the evidential material, suitably labelled and sealed in clean containers, must be submitted and examined
- all the known identification tests should be applied and adequate notes made at the time
- all the necessary reagents used for these tests should be pure, and blank tests should be performed to establish this fact
- all tests should be repeated, and compared with control samples to which the indicated poison has been added.

Strict adherence to these principles makes forensic toxicology one of the slowest and most expensive forms of analysis. However, this must be accepted not only to ensure justice for the poisoned victim and for the accused, but also to protect the integrity and reputation of the analyst and the laboratory he or she represents. A comparison of the principles listed above with the modern requirements of quality control and assurance may be made by reference to Chapter 23.

Range of cases submitted

The range of cases the forensic toxicologist is asked to deal with is typically very broad, although it may be restricted by the expertise and instrumental resources of a particular laboratory or the nature of the cases with which they are authorised to deal. For example, in the areas of workplace drug testing (Chapter 5) and drug abuse in sport (Chapter 9) much of the testing is carried out by laboratories with special expertise and that are devoted entirely to this type of work.

In the chapters that follow, a broad range of poisons and the techniques used for their analysis will be discussed, together with the types of samples encountered and the advantages and disadvantages that these sample types offer the toxicologist.

The forensic toxicologist is most often associated with the investigation of sickness or suspicious deaths where poisoning is suspected, whether it be self-administered or malicious. However, it should be remembered that in many incidents of suspicious death there may be no obvious indication of poisoning from the case history. For example, if an elderly person is found dead at home and the postmortem examination does not reveal an obvious medical cause of death, the coroner will request toxicological analysis even though no drugs or poisons were found near the body.

The forensic toxicologist will also receive samples from road traffic accidents to investigate whether alcohol and/or drugs may have been a contributing factor. Laws that govern the possession and use of narcotic and stimulant drugs, and legislation concerned with the influence of drink or drugs on driving skills, have increased the workload of many forensic laboratories; these cases can account for over 70% of the total workload submitted.

Modern analytical methods can give the forensic toxicologist the ability to answer questions that previously were considered either hopeless or not worth considering because the results were so often negative. Methods that are sensitive to nanogram amounts of drugs and poisons make it worthwhile to undertake an analysis, even when the plate, cup or container involved has apparently no food or drink left in it.

Drugs may be detected in blood at therapeutic concentrations, so it is possible to obtain clues to the clinical history of the deceased, the victim or the accused, even when they are unable or unwilling to provide this information for themselves. Thus, the discovery of drugs used in the treatment of epilepsy, diabetes, etc., in a blood sample taken from an unidentified body may start a new train of inquiries that leads to successful identification of the body. Similarly, allegations of doping prior to rape or robbery may be refuted or confirmed.

A newer form of forensic toxicology concerns the analytical checking of statements made by witnesses during the course of a police inquiry. Provided that a blood or urine sample is taken within about 12 h of an event, there is a good chance of checking the truth of statements such as 'I don't remember what happened because I was high on drugs at the time', 'I used to be an addict, but I haven't taken anything for over a year', 'I killed him in self-defence because after taking LSD he went berserk and attacked me with a knife', 'He spiked something into my drink, I don't remember much after that but I think he raped me'.

Stains can also be examined successfully for drugs and poisons. For example, if the victim notices a nasty taste and spits out the drink, the allegation that someone had tried to poison him or her can be investigated if the stain is submitted for analysis.

In most cases, the results obtained in the various types of cases mentioned above can be proved conclusively, that is the identity of the poison can be confirmed by more than one method and it can be quantified. Even when specific identification is not feasible, an opinion as to whether the suspect is most probably telling the truth or lying can be of value to the investigator.

Case investigation

Most cases that enter a forensic toxicology laboratory start with the suspicion that a drug or poison is present. A fatality might be an accident, suicide or murder, but a toxicological examination must be carried out to assist the investigating officer to decide which of these it might be. Often the investigating officer will not know whether or not any offence has been committed until the results of the toxicological analyses are available, so that forming the correct questions for him or her to ask is vital if accurate and useful answers are to be given.

Thus, details of the circumstances that lead to the conclusion that a criminal action might have taken place must be supplied to the toxicologist so that the analyses can be planned. Figure 1.2 indicates the type of information that should be supplied along with the samples submitted for toxicological analysis. Not all this information will be available or relevant to all cases, but as much information as possible should be obtained and submitted as it will assist the toxicologist to use the most directly useful methods of analysis and to interpret the results in the context of the case at a later stage. If possible, a personal consultation with the investigating officer should be arranged, either in person or by telephone. A few minutes talking with the investigating officer can save many hours, or even days, of analysis time.

All those involved in a toxicological investigation need to consider the circumstances of a case. Although the discussion here is focused on forensic toxicology and the role of the forensic toxicologist, it is rarely the forensic toxicologist who encounters the body, be it living or dead, involved in an investigation. In the case of a reported poisoning or a suspicious death, the police and/or paramedics may be the first persons to attend the scene. They need to be aware of associated samples or circumstances that may be of importance in a toxicological investigation. For example, is there a fuel heater in the room which may give rise to carbon monoxide poisoning? Are there any medicines, drugs, drug paraphernalia or other suspicious materials near the body? Is there an odour which

Victim's information

Name ....

Gender ....

Age ....

Weight or height ....

Nationality ....

Recent foreign travel? ....

Occupation (details of end-product of factory or firm) ....

Medical history

Did victim suffer from viral hepatitis or any other infectious disease? ....

Any recent illness or chronic disease? What drugs were prescribed? ....

Was victim an alcoholic, drug addict or smoker? ....

What poison is suspected? How much? (tablet bottles, syringes, etc., found near the body should be submitted) ....

Give names of any drugs or poisons to which victim or associates had access (apart from any mentioned above) ....

Timings

Date and time victim last seen to have been in normal health ....

Date and time of illness or death, and where victim found (e.g. at work, in bed, outdoors) ....

If these times are not known, when was the victim found? ....

Time and details of last meal ....

Treatment

Any medical attention given after the suspected poisoning or doping? ....

Time of hospital admission. Date and time discharged ....

Details of any treatment given (volume of stomach wash, time when blood/urine samples taken) ....

Hospital analysis: supplied/not done/not available ....

Tick any of the following symptoms that apply:

diarrhoea ☐	vomiting ☐	thirst ☐	blindness ☐	constipation ☐	cyanosis (blue tinge to skin) ☐
jaundice ☐	loss of weight ☐	shivering ☐	convulsions ☐	eye pupils dilated ☐	eye pupils constricted ☐
delirium ☐	coma ☐	sweating ☐	renal failure ☐		

Name of pathologist or doctor ....

Autopsy report sent: Yes/No

Date of autopsy and possible cause of death ....

Any further information that could be useful to the laboratory, such as victim pregnant, details of suspect (especially occupation and end-product of factory or firm, comments made by victim, witnesses or suspect) ....

Samples required

If victim alive:

Vomit, stomach aspirate or wash, blood and urine

If victim dead:

Stomach contents. All available (no preservative); enquire if stomach wash or vomit is available. If no contents, submit stomach

Blood	
Femoral vein	30 mL unpreserved and 5 mL preserved (for alcohol analysis); identify source; do not mix
Heart	All available from intact heart chambers; avoid body cavity samples; enquire if antemortem samples are available
Urine	All available, however small a volume (preserved); enquire if antemortem samples are available. If no urine, submit kidney and bile
Liver	250 g; gall bladder should not be included with this sample

If the suspected poison is a volatile substance, brain and lungs will be required. Bone and hair are needed if metal poisoning is suspected. Brain should always be submitted if the body is decomposed.

If in doubt, consult the laboratory.

Glass jars should be used whenever possible. Samples should be properly labelled and sealed. The label should include the name of the victim, signature of pathologist and the date. Antemortem samples should also specify time of sampling.

Figure 1.2 Information to be submitted with the exhibits in all cases in which there is suspicion of poisoning or doping.

may implicate a certain poison (e.g. the smell of almonds pointing to cyanide poisoning)? Has the incident taken place in a place of occupation and, if so, what operations was the victim carrying out at the time of the incident? Samples need to be taken and packaged appropriately and passed to the toxicologist, with suitable storage through this process. Failure to manage this stage correctly can ruin any subsequent analyses. The pathologist carrying out a postmortem examination will be experienced in knowing which samples should be taken for toxicological analysis, but caution should again be exercised to ensure that samples are placed in appropriate containers and stored correctly before and during transportation to the forensic toxicology laboratory.

Where clinical treatment has preceded a forensic investigation, case notes and any samples taken during clinical treatment should be requested via the consultant physician responsible for the patient.

Classification of poisons

Drugs and poisons can be classified alphabetically, pharmacologically (antidiabetic, anticonvulsant, etc.) or by chemical structure (barbiturates, phenothiazines, etc.). However, for analytical purposes it is more useful to classify poisons according to the method used for extraction. Five major groups are usually considered:

- gaseous and volatile substances isolated by distillation or, more usually, by sampling the headspace above the sample held in a closed container
- organic non-volatile substances isolated by solvent extraction (drugs and pesticides)
- metallic poisons isolated by ashing, by wet oxidation of the organic matter or by enzymatic hydrolysis of the tissue
- toxic anions isolated by dialysis
- miscellaneous poisons that require immunoassays or special extraction techniques, such as ion-exchange columns, formation of derivatives or ion-pairs, freeze-drying and continuous extraction with a polar solvent.

Some of these groups have been subdivided because they are too large or because alternative methods of extraction are available. For example, gases are considered separately from volatile substances. Pesticides are considered as a separate category from drugs, although both typically fall into the category 'organic non-volatile substances isolated by solvent extraction' and share similar methods of analysis. The seven groups so formed are illustrated in Figure 1.1 and were introduced earlier in the chapter.

Most analyses require several unit operations, namely:

- separation of the poison and its metabolites from the biological material
- concentration
- identification
- confirmation of identity
- quantification.

Not all these steps will be required for all tests and particularly not where rapid screening methods are applied. The most useful methods are those that combine two or more of these unit operations. Thus, colour tests (Chapter 13), which can be applied to the sample directly without the need for any isolation or purification processes, are indispensable in the initial stages of an analysis. Immunoassay techniques (Chapter 14) also eliminate the need for many separate operations and, like colour tests, can provide a tentative identification and approximate quantification of the poison. However, a disadvantage of both these methods is that a negative result eliminates only a few of the possible toxic substances. Consequently, additional colour tests or immunoassays are required before that particular group of poisons can be excluded. This type of sequential testing can be time consuming and judgement must be made depending on the quantity of tissue available for analysis.

A broad-spectrum screen, able to detect or eliminate most of the poisons in a group, usually requires a combination of three or more of the available techniques. For the drug and pesticide groups, the only combination potentially able to encompass all the required steps is mass spectrometry (MS) coupled with either gas chromatography (GC) or high-performance liquid chromatography (HPLC). However, a simple, direct solvent-extraction scheme is generally employed before MS analysis to eliminate endogenous substances that might otherwise reduce the efficiency of the system.

Screening strategies are discussed in Chapter 7 on postmortem toxicology. It should be recognised that strategies of this type have a far wider application than just postmortem investigations.

Samples

It is essential that the appropriate samples be collected as soon as possible, correctly and informatively labelled, and stored appropriately. Their acquisition, storage and transportation to the laboratory should be documented adequately (with timings where appropriate) to ensure a safe chain of custody. A list of suggested postmortem examination samples for routine toxicological screening is given in Figure 7.1 (Chapter 7) and those for particular anions and metals in Chapter 4. Specimens for investigating volatile substance abuse are discussed in Chapter 4; for workplace drug testing in Chapter 5; for clinical toxicology and therapeutic drug monitoring in Chapter 8; for drug abuse in sport in Chapter 9; and for drink and drug driving offences in Chapter 11.

Samples other than blood, urine, tissues and organs are finding increased uses in toxicological analysis. These samples are often referred to as alternative specimens and are discussed in detail in Chapter 6. Examples include oral fluid (saliva), which is of particular interest as a specimen for workplace drug testing (Chapter 5) and for suspected drug-driving offences (Chapter 11); hair which can be used to evaluate the history of drug use (Chapters 4 and 5); and sweat (Chapter 5).

The containers used for the samples may vary depending on the analysis to be performed, and it is vital that the correct types are used. For example, a fluoride oxalate sample tube for blood is useless if a fluoride estimation is required, and gamma-hydroxybutyrate may be destroyed by citrate. If containers are to be examined for fingerprints and/or for DNA, this should be carried out before any toxicological examinations. Containers to be used for sampling for various analytes, volumes or masses to be sampled and any special preservation to be applied are noted in the chapters for the various drugs and poisons covered.

Sample analysis

General methodology

The forensic toxicologist should remember Orfila's maxim 'The presence of a poison must be proved in the blood and organs before it can be considered as a cause of death'.

There are typically four main steps in any toxicological examination:

1. **Detection** – to detect any drugs or poisons in the samples submitted by means of screening procedures.
2. **Identification** – to identify conclusively any drugs, metabolites or poisons present by means of specific relevant physicochemical tests.
3. **Quantification** – to quantify accurately those drugs, metabolites or poisons present.
4. **Interpretation** – to interpret the analytical findings in (2) and (3) in the context of the case, the information given and the questions asked by the investigating officer.

Note the distinction above between detection and identification. In forensic toxicology, as with many other areas of chemistry, there is a clear difference between these two aspects. Colour tests, thin-layer chromatography, immunoassays and other screening tests are commonly applied in toxicology. These tests rely on detecting a particular interaction with a functionality of the compound being tested for. For colour tests (Chapter 13) this interaction is generally via a reaction with a functional group present in the chemical structure of a substance or group of substances. However, other substances that may be present may have this same functional group and hence give the same or a very similar interaction. Thin-layer chromatography (TLC) (Chapter 13) relies on the molecular interactions of analytes with a solvent or mixture of solvents and an inert medium called the stationary phase to enable separation from other substances present in the sample. However, some of the other substances present may have similar molecular interactions and hence may behave similarly to drugs and poisons such that complete separation is not achieved. If techniques such as GC and/or HPLC are not available and the analyst has to rely on TLC, at least two, and preferably three, non-correlating TLC systems should be employed in order to improve the discrimination of the analysis. The specificity of an immunoassay is only as good as the specificity of the antigen–antibody interaction. As we will see in the chapter on immunoassays (Chapter 14), for some drug assays an antibody with broad specificity for the drug class under test is often deliberately employed to minimise the number of tests that need to be carried out to detect members of a drug group. Thus, in the case of opiates, immunoassays may give a positive result in the presence of diamorphine (heroin), morphine or codeine. The reporting of a positive result for such an immunoassay without being certain which of these substances is present could have serious implications for the interpretation of cases in a court of law. Toxicologists typically refer to the results of these initial tests as presumptive, i.e. there is a strong indication that a particular substance or class of substances may be present but further tests are required to confirm the identity of the particular substance.

The detection of the drug or poison is the most difficult part, as the nature of the poison may not be known. Hence toxicologists employ screening tests for a wide range of drugs or poisons. General screening methods are usually more flexible than special methods and can therefore be applied to a wide variety of materials. They are essential for the investigation of unknown poisonings, and have some advantages even when the toxic agent is known or suspected.

Once a toxic agent has been detected, specific analytical procedures can be used to identify it conclusively. Most analytical procedures in toxicology rely on a combination of chromatography to separate out the substances in the sample and some form of spectroscopy to detect and/or identify the separated substances. The most commonly employed chromatographic techniques include TLC (Chapter 13), GC (Chapter 18), HPLC (Chapter 19) and capillary electrophoresis (CE) (Chapter 20). Spectroscopic techniques used include ultraviolet–visible and fluorescence UV-visible (Chapter 15), infrared (IR) and near infrared (NIR) (Chapter 16), Raman (Chapter 17) and MS (Chapter 21).

In toxicological analyses where a body fluid or tissue is being analysed, maximum efficiency is gained by coupling a chromatographic technique with a suitable detection technique (so called hyphenation) so that separation and detection can be carried out in-line, typically with automation of sample introduction to the analytical instrument and automated data collection. This also allows analysis to be carried out on a 24 h basis. Hyphenated techniques most commonly used are GC-MS, HPLC-UV or HPLC-fluorescence and HPLC-MS (generally abbreviated to LC-MS). As we will see in Chapter 18, GC can be combined with several other types of detector but the powerful combination offered by GC-MS analysis has made it the workhorse instrument in most modern analytical toxicology laboratories. LC-MS offers several advantages over GC-MS and is finding more and more uses in toxicology laboratories. CE-MS is still a developing technique and has yet to find routine use in many toxicology laboratories. However, the advantages that it offers in terms of relatively simple sample preparation and the simplicity of analysing certain types of analytes that are more difficult to analyse by GC or HPLC mean that its use is likely to increase in the future as the technology matures. Nuclear magnetic resonance (NMR) spectroscopy is the workhorse technique of most organic chemistry laboratories, enabling identification of a compound from an NMR spectrum. However, the relative insensitivity of NMR and the difficulty of interpreting a spectrum of a complex mixture has meant that NMR is not a technique used in most toxicology laboratories. LC-NMR instruments have been developed. At the present time these instruments are costly relative to GC-MS and LC-MS and considerably more complex to use, and thus they are not in routine use in most toxicology laboratories. As a result, NMR is not covered in this textbook. IR, NIR and Raman spectroscopies are covered because, although they are not used in combination with chromatographic techniques in most toxicology laboratories, they are used to identify bulk drugs.

Conclusions

As can be seen, the knowledge and skills required by the forensic toxicologist are extensive. The range of cases they may be required to investigate can be very variable. The potential outcomes if they make a mistake in analysis or interpretation are very serious. All this makes the job of a forensic toxicologist an exceedingly challenging one but also a very rewarding one.

In the chapters that follow, the areas of knowledge that a forensic toxicologist must have are covered first. The primary requirement is a knowledge of how drugs are administered and how they are distributed, metabolised and excreted from the body. This is detailed in Chapter 2.

As we have seen above, the forensic toxicologist must be familiar with a wide range of poisons (Chapters 3 and 4). This familiarity should include an understanding of how drugs and poisons affect the body and how to detect and quantify the types of substances that may be encountered.

The various judicially-related areas that the forensic toxicologist may have to address are discussed in Chapters 5, 7, 8, 9, 10 and 11. These cover workplace drug testing (Chapter 5), post-mortem toxicology (Chapter 7), *in utero* exposure to drugs of abuse (Chapter 8), drug abuse in sport (Chapter 9), toxicological investigation of drug-facilitated sexual assault (Chapter 10), and alcohol, drugs and driving (Chapter 11). Samples to be taken for analysis and related issues are discussed within these various chapters because there are special circumstances relating to this aspect for many of these particular areas. The issue of alternative specimens is covered in Chapter 6.

Although the emphasis of this text is on forensic toxicology, the forensic toxicologist should have some knowledge of the role of the clinical toxicologist and vice versa because their work often overlaps. Clinical toxicology, therapeutic drug monitoring and *in utero* exposure to drugs are discussed in Chapter 8.

Both the clinical toxicologist and the forensic toxicologist may be faced with the situation where they need to identify tablets, capsules, etc. This is covered in Chapter 12.

These chapters are followed by those on the analytical methodologies used in toxicological analysis. These methods include colour tests and thin-layer chromatography (Chapter 13), immunoassays (Chapter 14); UV, visible and fluorescence spectrophotometry (Chapter 15), infrared (including near-infrared spectroscopy) (Chapter 16), Raman spectroscopy (Chapter 17), gas chromatography (Chapter 18), high-performance liquid chromatography (Chapter 19), capillary electrophoresis (Chapter 20) and mass spectrometry (Chapter 21). Techniques which are not yet sufficiently developed and established to be employed routinely in forensic toxicology but which offer much promise for the future are discussed in Chapter 22. Chapter 23 covers one of the most important aspects of any forensic toxicology analysis: analytical quality control and assessment.

References

M. J. B. Orfila, translated by J. A. Waller, *Treatise on Mineral, Vegetable, and Animal Poisons, Considered as to Their Relations with Physiology, Pathology, and Medical Jurisprudence*, Volumes I and II, 2nd edn, London, E Cox and Son, 1818.

Further reading

R. C. Baselt, *Disposition of Toxic Drugs and Chemicals in Man*, 7th edn, Foster City, Biomedical Publications, 2004.

H. Brandenberger and R. A. A. Maes (eds), *Analytical Toxicology for Clinical, Forensic and Pharmaceutical Chemists*, Berlin, Walter de Gruyter, 1997.

A. S. Curry, *Poison Detection in Human Organs*, 3rd edn, Springfield, Charles C. Thomas, 1976.

R. C. Dart (ed.), *Ellenhorn's Medical Toxicology: Diagnosis and Treatment of Human Poisoning*, 3rd edn, Baltimore, Lippincott, Williams & Wilkins, 2003.

B. A. Goldberger, *Forensic Toxicology Methods*, Oxford, Taylor and Francis, 2002.

B. Levine (ed.), *Principles of Forensic Toxicology*, 2nd edn, Washington DC, American Association for Clinical Chemistry, 2003.

2

Pharmacokinetics and metabolism

O H Drummer

Introduction 13
Basic concepts of pharmacokinetics 13
Drug metabolism 22
Adverse drug interactions and pharmacogenetics 29
Drug concentration and pharmacological response 34
Postmortem redistribution 36
Interpretation 36
Further reading 41

Introduction

An important part of any investigation involving drugs or poisons is the interpretation of toxicological data. The onset, duration and intensity of action of a drug after administration are controlled by the rate at which the drug reaches its site of action, by the concentration of the drug and by the sensitivity of the individual to the drug. Hence, a good understanding of the basic concepts of pharmacokinetics and metabolism is essential to enable an informed comment to be made on the approximate amount and timing of the exposure, and a likely response to the substance(s) under question. These answers are always predicated on the amount of information available to the toxicologist (the route of administration, age, sex, presence of disease and whether exposure was acute or chronic are important factors).

These issues are explored in this chapter and relevant examples are given.

Basic concepts of pharmacokinetics

The disposition of a drug includes the following processes:

- absorption
- distribution
- metabolism
- excretion.

The processes of metabolism and excretion are often referred to as elimination because they function together to eliminate poisons from the body.

Pharmacokinetics describes the time course of the blood and tissue concentration profile, while pharmacodynamics refers to the relationship between dose and the intended pharmacological response.

The absorption phase relates to the entry of drug from the absorption site. This may be relatively slow, as from the gastrointestinal tract for oral absorption, or rapid if given intravenously.

During the absorption phase, drugs are distributed by the blood to all parts of the body. The uptake of drug into tissues is a time-dependent process and differs between tissues and from drug to drug. Shortly after entry into the tissues, drugs are subject to both metabolism and excretion from the body. These two processes are often the more important for toxicologists and are also often the most variable.

Most drugs given intravenously or orally produce blood (or plasma) concentration–time curves of the type shown in Figures 2.1A and 2.1B, respectively. Following intravenous administration, there is initially a rapid decrease in plasma drug concentration. Decline of plasma drug concentration is usually exponential. For some drugs, it is possible to distinguish two components (biexponential) following intravenous administration: the early phase (α-phase) in which distribution is the major process, and a second period with a slower decay, in which elimination predominates (β-phase). After oral administration, plasma concentrations initially increase while the drug is being absorbed and then decrease when elimination becomes the major process. The drug distribution phase is often not considered, since it tends to be more rapid than either the absorptive or elimination phases; however, in some situations it needs to be considered.

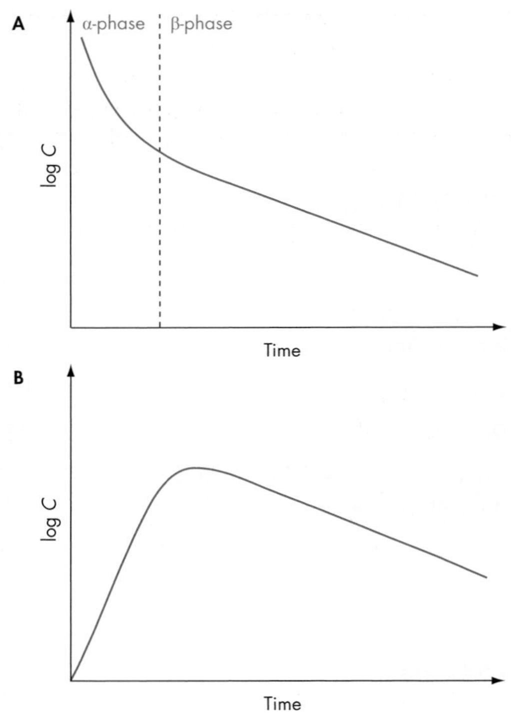

Figure 2.1 Typical semilogarithmic plots of plasma concentration (C) versus time for a drug given (A) by intravenous injection and (B) orally. The terminal rate of decline of plasma concentration is the same irrespective of the route of administration.

Absorption

Drug absorption is an important process in drug pharmacokinetics. The route of administration is an important factor in determining the rate and extent of absorption. Routes of administration can include oral, rectal, ocular, inhalation through the nose or mouth, absorption through the skin and other body surfaces, and injection into muscle or veins, etc. All of these routes have different rates and extents of absorption.

Most drugs are administered orally, and hence an understanding of the mechanism of absorption by this route is most important for the toxicologist.

Absorption from the gastrointestinal tract

Drugs are usually absorbed either by passive diffusion of the un-ionised drug or by active transport. Passive diffusion is by far the most common mechanism.

Absorption is possible throughout the gastrointestinal tract, from stomach to rectum, although the major site is the upper small intestine. This has high peristalsis, a high surface area (200 m^2), high blood flow and optimal pH (pH 5–7) for the absorption of most drugs, all of which result in a high absorption rate. Drug absorption tends to be much less rapid from other parts of the gastrointestinal tract.

Some drugs are absorbed to a small extent in the stomach, although these are largely acidic drugs that are un-ionised in the low pH (pH 1–3) environment in this organ. These drugs include aspirin, nonsteroidal anti-inflammatory drugs and some angiotensin-converting enzyme inhibitors.

Absorption also occurs if drugs are given rectally as suppositories. In this situation absorption is usually less efficient than following oral administration. For example, oxycodone suppositories require a higher dose to achieve the desired response than oxycodone by oral administration.

Absorption of ionised drugs and poisons also occurs. For example, paraquat is highly ionised but appears to be absorbed slowly from the gastrointestinal tract throughout its length and over a considerable period of time from the moment of ingestion.

Poisoning with orally active drugs can be treated effectively by the prompt administration of an oral adsorbent, such as activated charcoal, which prevents further absorption of the drug. This is only effective if given less than 2 h after ingestion of the drug, so that the drug has not passed too far down the gastrointestinal tract for the charcoal to gain contact with it.

Absorption from other sites

Absorption through the lungs occurs for substances that are smoked or inhaled, such as smoked cocaine, heroin, tetrahydrocannabinol (THC) from cannabis, drugs such as salbutamol from inhalers, and volatile substances that are abused such as butane and toluene. The lungs are an efficient organ for the transport of a drug from the air into the blood supply, such that the rate of absorption approaches that of intravenous injection.

Absorption of drugs through mucous membranes and skin is also common. This includes nasal insufflation of cocaine ('snorting'), sublingual and buccal absorption of buprenorphine and nitroglycerine-like vasodilators, as well as absorption of drugs through skin patches (e.g. oestrogens, fentanyl, nicotine, etc.). Less commonly, toxicologists also encounter the vaginal and ocular absorption of drugs. The rate of absorption can vary significantly from one site to another. Sublingual absorption is very rapid, with drug effects noticeable within minutes, while drugs are absorbed relatively slowly through the skin.

Drugs injected into the spinal canal and into muscle or surface tissues (intramuscular, intraperitoneal) usually exhibit relatively rapid absorption. However, absorption from an intramuscular injection can be slow if the site of injection is perfused poorly by the blood supply and if the site is very fatty.

Drugs that are administered to bypass the gastrointestinal tract will not be subject to first-pass metabolism (see the next section). These drugs, therefore, show higher bioavailability than the same drug delivered through the gastrointestinal tract.

First-pass metabolism and bioavailability

Drugs may be destroyed by the acid in the stomach or by enzymes in the gastrointestinal tract, or may hardly be absorbed at all because of their chemical nature. These factors reduce the drug's bioavailability.

Drugs absorbed after oral ingestion pass through the mesenteric circulation into the liver before they enter the systemic circulation. In this 'first-pass', drugs can be substantially metabolised by the liver before ever having a pharmacological effect. The proportion of the drug that reaches the systemic circulation after oral administration compared to that obtained after intravenous dosing is the oral (or absolute) bioavailability (F). This is measured by comparing the area under the curve (AUC) for the oral and intravenous doses from time zero to the time-point at which most or all of the drug is finally eliminated by the body. The formula is:

$$F = \frac{\text{AUC (oral route)}}{\text{AUC (intravenous route)}} \tag{2.1}$$

where AUC (the area under the plasma concentration–time curve) (see Fig. 2.1) represents the amount of drug that enters the systemic circulation from time zero to infinite time for each route of administration.

The relative bioavailabilities of drugs can be determined by comparing other routes of administration with oral or another reference route of administration, or between drug formulations.

The oral bioavailabilities of selected drugs are shown in Table 2.1. In general, drugs that are readily metabolised by liver enzymes have lower bioavailabilities than drugs that are not metabolised as readily by the liver. Some drugs are metabolised in the liver to active forms. While the effect of first-pass metabolism is to reduce the action of the parent drug, a drug that is administered orally and metabolised in the liver to active forms has a different profile of activity from that when the drug is given parenterally (not through the gastrointestinal system). For example, when cannabis is consumed orally (cookies), THC is converted in the liver to the 11-hydroxy metabolite, which is active and hence exerts a significant drug effect. When cannabis is smoked, first-pass metabolism of THC to the 11-hydroxy metabolite is markedly reduced and effects due to the metabolite are less. Some drugs which are activated by liver metabolism are administered as pro-drugs, with oral administration of the pro-drug preferred to other routes of administration to maximise the activity of the drug. An example is enalapril, which is converted into enalaprilic acid. The latter form is much more active than the parent drug. Drugs given rectally are subject to only a small degree of first-pass metabolism, since only about one-third of the blood supply from the lower part of the gastrointestinal system passes though the liver.

Enterohepatic circulation

Drugs and metabolites present in the liver are often also excreted into bile. These pass into the jejunum and may be reabsorbed or passed into the faeces. The process of biliary excretion and reabsorption may occur a number of times before a drug is completely eliminated by the body. This recycling of drugs is known as enterohepatic circulation.

Table 2.1 Bioavailabilities and volumes of distribution for selected drugs

Drug	Bioavailability (%)[a]	Volume of distribution (L/kg)	Clearance (mL/min/kg)
Alprazolam	90	0.7–1.3	1.2
Amitriptyline	–	6–10	–
Diazepam	100	0.5–2.6	0.5
Ethanol	50–80	0.4–5	N/A
Flunitrazepam	70	3.4–5.5	N/A
Imipramine	–	20–40	–
Morphine	15–60	3–5	21
Oxazepam	93	0.5–2	1.2
Pentobarbital	95	0.7–1.0	0.3–0.5
Temazepam	>80	0.8–1.4	1.2
Thioridazine	–	18	–
Tetrahydrocannabinol	6	9–11	14
Zaleplon	30	1.3	0.9
Zolpidem	70	0.5–0.7	0.25
Zopiclone	80	1.5	2.2–3.3

[a] Oral bioavailability compared with an intravenous injection.

N/A = not available.

Common examples include the glucuronide conjugates of drugs such as morphine. Enterohepatic circulation prolongs the persistence of a drug in the body and may lead to delayed toxicity. Drugs that undergo enterohepatic circulation may be detected in the faeces or in gastric contents (small amounts) after reflux or vomiting, or in unchanged forms, even if administered by a parenteral route. Basic drugs (e.g. amfetamine) may also appear in the gastric contents by passive diffusion across the gastric mucosa from the blood. It is therefore important that if gastric contents are analysed and small amounts of drug are detected, these are not automatically assumed to be from oral administration.

In the absence of urine, bile can be a useful body fluid for analysis (e.g. for opioids, benzodiazepines and colchicine).

Distribution of drugs into tissues

The uptake of drugs (distribution) into tissues depends on a number of factors. These include the blood flow to the tissues, the partition coefficient of the drug between blood and the tissue, the degree of ionisation of the drug at the pH of plasma, the molecular size of the drug and the extent of tissue and plasma protein binding. For example, the distribution of plasma protein-bound drugs such as the warfarin-type anticoagulants is restricted to plasma and extracellular fluid, whereas alcohol distributes equally into the total body water.

The approximate volumes of the body water compartments for a person of average weight are 25 L for intracellular water and 17 L for extracellular water (of which 3 L is plasma water). An intravenous dose of a drug distributed immediately and equally into the total body water (approximately 42 L) gives an initial plasma concentration (dose divided by 42) approximately two-fifths of that obtained if the same dose were distributed only into extracellular water (dose divided by 17). If the drug is extensively bound to tissue proteins, an even lower initial plasma concentration is obtained, and the volume term relating the dose to the plasma concentration can exceed the volume of the body. The approximate proportions of drugs with particular volumes of distribution in the plasma water are given in Table 2.2.

The instantaneous equilibrium of drug concentrations throughout the body does not necessarily require that the concentrations be equal throughout the body. In fact, drug concentrations in tissues are rarely equal to those in plasma. For example, the tissue : plasma concentration ratio is very low immediately after intravenous administration because it takes time for the drug to transfer from the blood to tissues. As time progresses, the amount of drug in the tissue compartment increases and, like that in the plasma compartment, eventually reaches a maximum. If the drug is stored actively in a particular tissue compartment, the ultimate concentration ratio between the tissue and plasma will be relatively high. Note also that the tissue : plasma concentration ratio depends not only on the processes of distribution but also to a large extent on the route of drug administration and on whether single or multiple doses are given.

Knowledge of how a particular drug or metabolite partitions between blood and tissues is important in interpreting analytical results, particularly where only one sample type (e.g. blood but not tissue) has been analysed.

Blood and plasma concentrations

Many drugs show differences in concentration between whole blood and plasma (or serum). This occurs because the uptake of drugs into red blood cells (erythrocytes) can be limited by the

Table 2.2 Proportion of a drug in the body water compartment

Volume of distribution (L/kg)	Proportion in water compartment (%)
0.1	40
0.15	27
0.6	6.7
1.0	4
10	0.4

physiochemical properties of the drug and its ability to move through cellular membranes. For example, THC is almost absent from red blood cells, and hence the plasma concentration is almost twice that of whole blood, assuming a haematocrit of 0.5. In contrast, chloroquine has a much higher red blood cell concentration than plasma concentration (plasma : whole blood ratio about 0.3). If this ratio is known, then the blood concentration can be estimated from a plasma concentration, or vice versa.

Toxicologists should be wary of performing this calculation for haemolysed specimens, since haemolysis liberates the contents of red blood cells into the plasma (serum), and thereby affects this equilibrium. This applies particularly to postmortem specimens.

Binding of drugs to plasma proteins

Many, if not most, drugs bind to proteins in plasma with sufficient affinity to prevent that portion of the drug being biologically active. For example, if a drug is 90% bound to plasma proteins, only 10% can exhibit biological activity.

The binding sites for drugs in plasma are predominantly albumin (which preferentially binds acidic drugs), although β-globulin and α_1-acid glycoprotein are also significant sites for some drugs (particularly basic ones).

The significance of the protein binding of drugs is that the 'free' or unbound fraction in plasma may be affected by illness and by the use of other drugs. In disease states (particularly kidney and liver dysfunction), protein binding can be reduced markedly, and often increases the apparent effects of drugs. Since binding sites are saturable, other drugs can compete with the binding and reduce the net binding of the drug. This can cause a net increase in drug action for some drug combinations and may need to be taken into account when interpreting results of an analysis.

Volume of distribution

The apparent volume of distribution (V_d) is the amount of drug in the body (A_p) divided by the plasma concentration (C_p) after distribution equilibrium has been established:

$$V_d = \frac{A_p}{C_p} \tag{2.2}$$

It can be difficult to determine V_d experimentally because elimination will typically start before distribution equilibrium is reached. An estimate of V_d can be obtained by calculating the concentration before elimination has occurred by extrapolating the concentration versus time curve for intravenous doses to time zero (C_0) and dividing this value into the dose delivered.

If oral doses are used the dose must be adjusted for the bioavailability (F):

$$V_d = \frac{FD_0}{C_0} \tag{2.3}$$

Drugs that are taken up into body fat or bind to cellular structures have a higher V_d and it is not uncommon for volumes of distribution to be over 1.0 L/kg. Morphine has a V_d of 3–5 L/kg. A range of 0.5 to 5 L/kg is seen for most of the amfetamines and many of the benzodiazepines. The highly lipid-soluble THC has a volume of distribution of about 10 L/kg. Drugs with high octanol–buffer partition coefficients, such as psychotropic drugs, generally have high volumes of distribution. Octanol–water coefficients for specific drugs are available (e.g. *Clarke's Analysis of Drugs and Poisons*, 3rd edition, 2004, Vol. II monographs).

The drug concentration in body fluids other than plasma may be used, e.g. whole blood, but different values for V_d are obtained for each; hence it is important to note which fluid is being used.

The value of the volume of distribution is determined mainly by the physiological processes of perfusion and protein binding, but it seldom has a true physiological meaning. For example, the volume of distribution of highly protein-bound furosemide (syn. frusemide), is of the order of 15 L, and that of ethanol is about 35 L; however, the value for digoxin, which is extensively distributed and bound in extravascular tissues, is of the order of 450 L.

After distribution equilibrium has been established, knowledge of the volume of distribution allows the amount of drug in the body (*D*) to be estimated from a single measured blood concentration (*C*):

$$D = V_d \times C \tag{2.4}$$

If the time elapsed since drug administration (*t*) is known, together with some pharmacokinetic data for the drug, then it should be possible to estimate the original dose (D_0) of the drug. Thus, for a drug given by intravenous injection:

$$D_0 = V_d C\, e^{k_{el} t} \tag{2.5}$$

where k_{el} is the elimination rate constant (see later).

However, if the drug is given orally, a much more complex relationship applies. It is necessary to know the bioavailability (*F*), and the absorption rate constant (k_a). Then the dose is given by the expression:

$$D_0 = \frac{V_d C(k_a - k_{el})}{F k_a (e^{-k_{el} t} - e^{-k_a t})} \tag{2.6}$$

If a drug were distributed instantaneously throughout the body, then the volume of distribution would be constant at all times and the decrease in plasma concentration could be attributed solely to elimination of the drug. However, in practice there are time-dependent changes in tissue concentration, which include absorption and distribution.

In a drug overdose, nonlinear pharmacokinetics may occur, that is the plasma concentration does not increase in proportion to the dose since one or more of the pharmacokinetic processes reaches saturation. Hence, calculation of dose from the volume of distribution can be substantially wrong and misleading. The recommendation is to use the volume of distribution only when an overdose has not been taken and there is a reasonable chance of equilibrium.

Elimination of drugs

Most drugs are eliminated from the body by metabolism in the liver and/or by excretion of the drug and its metabolites by the kidneys. Other mechanisms for drug metabolism and excretion also apply for some drugs and poisons. For example, volatile substances are partially removed by expiration, although other mechanisms (e.g. via faeces and sweat) also apply.

Two terms, clearance and half-life, are frequently used to quantify the rate and extent of drug removal from the body.

Clearance

Clearance is the sum of the elimination process of metabolism, renal excretion and other minor processes. Overall, the efficiency of elimination by an organ can be expressed as the proportion of drug entering the organ that is eliminated from the plasma in a single passage; this is called the extraction ratio.

The other major factor that controls the overall ability of an organ to remove drug from the body is the rate of delivery of the drug (i.e. blood flow) to the organ. Drug elimination can be represented as the product of this rate of delivery and the extraction ratio. This product gives the volume of plasma from which drug is completely removed per unit time and is given the name clearance (Cl). Clearances by different organs are additive. Although the reference fluid normally used is plasma, whole blood may also be used.

The concept of clearance has found particular application in clinical work as it offers a simple relationship between dose rate (dose divided by the time interval between doses, D/τ), and the average plasma concentration (C_{av}) of the drug:

$$C_{av} = \frac{D/\tau}{Cl} \tag{2.7}$$

Renal clearance is often measured with creatinine. Creatinine is a metabolic by-product of protein metabolism that is neither reabsorbed nor secreted by the tubules. Its concentration can therefore be used to measure the degree of concentration of urine from the glomerular filtrate.

The efficiency of an eliminating organ in removing a drug from plasma depends on the health of the organ. Thus, diseased kidneys operate less efficiently, and the net change in clearance is proportional to the extent of renal impairment.

Despite its clinical utility, the concept of clearance has certain limitations for the forensic toxicologist because it does not give an immediate indication of the persistence of a drug in the body. For example, although gentamicin and digoxin have similar clearances (about 100 mL/min), digoxin stays in the body much longer than gentamicin. This is because the volume of distribution of digoxin is several times that of gentamicin, and there is therefore a much greater volume of fluid from which the drug must be cleared before it is all eliminated. It is therefore of some advantage to the toxicologist to be able to relate clearance to the persistence of a drug in the body.

This can be done by expressing clearance as a fractional clearance; that is clearance divided by the volume of distribution. Fractional clearance (Cl/V_d) has the dimensions of reciprocal time and represents the proportion of drug removed from the body per unit time, so it is a first-order rate constant for drug elimination (k_{el}). This rate constant is given by the gradient of the terminal part of the concentration–time curve shown in Figure 2.2.

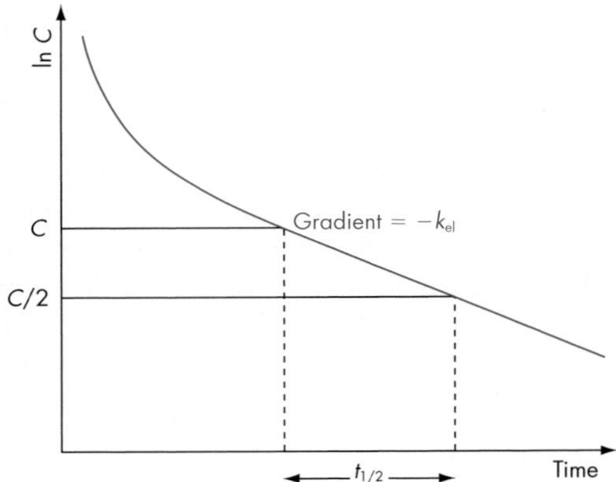

Figure 2.2 Plot of the natural logarithm of plasma drug concentration (ln C) versus time (t) after intravenous administration. The gradient of the linear part of the curve is equal to the elimination rate constant ($-k_{el}$).

Half-life

The elimination half-life of a drug ($t_{1/2}$) is the time required for plasma concentrations to decline by 50%, provided that elimination occurs by a first-order process (Fig. 2.2). It is related to the elimination rate constant (k_{el}) by the equation:

$$t_{1/2} = \frac{0.693}{k_{el}} \tag{2.8}$$

The half-life of a drug provides a measure of the rate of drug loss from the blood. If the dose is known, the half-life of a drug can be used together with information on the volume of distribution and bioavailability, where necessary, to estimate the time elapsed since administration. Conversely, if the elapsed time is known, the half-life can be used to estimate the drug dose, subject to the limitations discussed earlier. The half-life is a function of volume of distribution, clearance and the proportion of drug elimination in unit time. This last term depends on both the extent of its distribution and on the efficiency of its elimination. Thus, the half-life of a drug may differ between children and adults because of size and weight, even though the clearances are equivalent.

Zero-order processes are best described as a loss of drug per unit time. For example, ethanol elimination is often assumed to be zero order for concentrations over 0.02 g/100 mL and the rate of elimination is expressed as a loss of ethanol per unit time, that is 0.10–0.25 g/L/h (mean 0.18 g/L/h).

Excretion

Drugs and metabolites are excreted mainly by the kidneys into urine (Fig. 2.3). Renal clearance can result either from glomerular filtration or through tubular secretion. In some cases reabsorption occurs, which reverses the secretion process.

The drug or metabolite is brought to the kidneys with a total plasma flow for both kidneys of approximately 1400 mL/min. Plasma is filtered at the rate of 125 mL/min in the glomeruli, which are the principal sites of excretion. Filtration is passive and only the non-protein-bound drug in the plasma is eliminated by this pathway. A considerable amount of filtered drug may be reabsorbed into the plasma by diffusion back across the tubule wall (which is permeable to non-ionised, lipid-soluble species). The filtrate (125 mL/min) is gradually concentrated as it passes down the tubule to give a final production of urine of about 1 mL/min. About 575 mL/min of plasma circulates in intimate contact with the proximal and distal renal tubules.

The renal tubule may contribute to elimination by active secretion (tubular secretion), and in such cases protein-bound drug may also be eliminated from the plasma.

The extent of elimination by the kidneys can be extremely variable depending on which of the three processes of filtration, secretion or reabsorption predominates for the drug in question. Thus, procainamide is eliminated partly by metabolism and partly as unchanged drug through the kidney. Its renal clearance is of the order of 450 mL/min, which indicates a major involvement of tubular secretion. By contrast, digoxin has a renal clearance of about 120 mL/min, which could be explained by either filtration alone, or because secretion is balanced by reabsorption. In practice, it is known that filtration accounts for almost all of the renal clearance of digoxin. A further example is methaqualone, which has a renal clearance of about 1 mL/min, indicating extensive reabsorption of filtered drug.

One of the major physiological factors that determines the variability in the rate of drug excretion into the urine is the pH of the urine. Only non-ionised species are available for reabsorption by the tubules along the concentration gradient. Thus, acidic drugs (e.g. barbiturates, salicylates) are excreted more rapidly at high pH than basic drugs (e.g. amfetamines). Conversely, basic drugs are excreted more rapidly at low pH. For example, about 85% of a dose of aspirin is excreted as free salicylic acid in alkaline urine, but only about 5% is excreted when the urine is acidic. Conversely, about 75% of a dose of

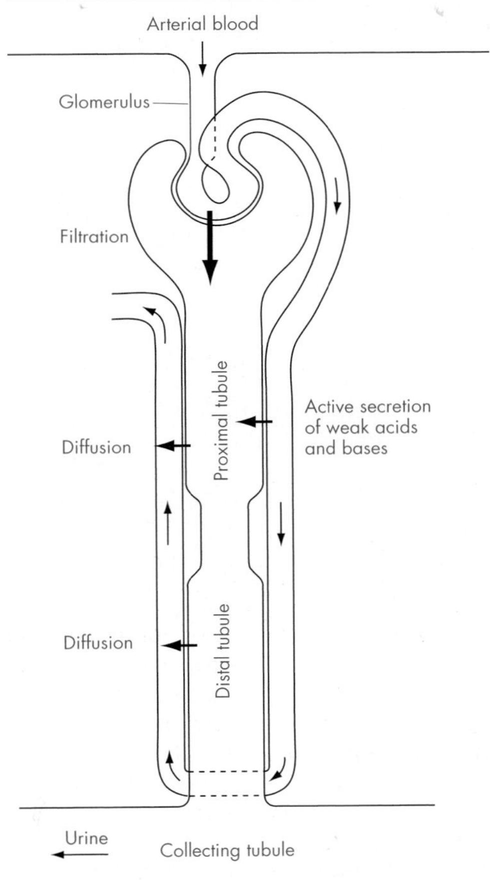

Figure 2.3 Drug elimination by the kidneys. Schematic diagram of a nephron to illustrate the sites of filtration, diffusion and active secretion of drugs.

amfetamine is excreted unchanged in acidic urine, but less than 5% if the urine is alkaline.

The effect of varying urinary pH has been used in the treatment of drug overdose by applying alkaline diuresis as an adjunct to the treatment of salicylate or phenobarbital poisoning. The success of the treatment is limited by the extent to which these drugs are distributed, and by the presence of alternative pathways of elimination. Unfortunately, a drug with a high volume of distribution has a relatively long half-life; hence, any increase in clearance does not make much difference to its pharmacological or toxicological effect.

Persons who abuse amfetamines have used the effect of urinary pH on excretion to advantage by simultaneously ingesting bicarbonate. This produces alkaline urine, which delays elimination of the amfetamine and therefore prolongs its stimulant effect. Conversely, substances that acidify urine have been taken to enhance the elimination of amfetamine-like stimulants in the hope of avoiding detection in routine dope-screening procedures. Exercise in itself can also decrease urinary pH and thus increase the renal clearance of basic drugs.

While the quantity of drug in a urine sample is the product of the renal clearance of the drug, the average plasma concentration of the drug during the interval that the urine was produced, and the duration of that interval, the calculation of a likely plasma concentration or even dose from urinary data is not advised, since urinary flow rate and the degree of metabolism must also be considered. Many drugs also show nonlinear pharmacokinetics, that is their excretion rate and degree of metabolism are dose dependent.

Chronic dosing

Drugs accumulate in plasma or tissues if more than one dose is administered and the interval between the doses is less than the time taken to eliminate the previous dose. Under these circumstances, a change in the shapes of the plasma concentration–time and the tissue concentration–time curves also occurs. In all cases, accumulation is controlled by the size of the dose, the dose interval and the terminal elimination phase for loss of drug from the body (k_{el}). The problems of drug accumulation are of particular interest to the toxicologist because the resultant high drug concentrations may lead to a progressive and insidious toxicity.

The extent to which a drug accumulates in multiple dosing can be estimated. After each successive dose, the maximum, minimum and average plasma concentrations will be higher than those for the previous dose. This is so in the early stages, but since drug elimination is often a first-order rate process, the total amount of drug in the body increases until the amount eliminated during a dose interval equals the amount taken in (total injected dose or the net absorbed dose after oral dosing). This is called *steady state*. The clearance (Cl) can be related to dose rate (D/τ) divided by steady state plasma concentration (C_{ss}).

$$\mathrm{Cl} = \frac{D}{\tau C_{ss}} \tag{2.9}$$

A good example of the importance of this concept is the use of methadone to treat opioid dependency. Methadone has a long pharmacokinetic half-life of about 24 h. At once-a-day dosing, the plasma concentrations of methadone accumulate for at least 5 days. Therefore, the effects of methadone increase during the first 5 days of therapy. If the dose consumed is too high, or dose increases are made during these 5 days, potentially life-threatening respiratory depression can set in.

Repeated dosing leading to possible accumulation should be taken into account when interpreting the results of a toxicological analysis.

Drug metabolism

Metabolism is an integral part of drug elimination. As well as facilitating excretion of a drug, it may also affect the pharmacological response of a drug by altering its potency and/or duration of action. With few exceptions, the metabolites of drugs are more polar (and water soluble) than the parent drug and are therefore more likely to be excreted from the body.

Metabolites may be pharmacologically inactive (e.g. salbutamol sulfate) or they may be active. This is the case with many drugs of toxicological interest. For example, glucuronidation of morphine on the 6-hydroxyl moiety yields an opioid with more activity than morphine itself. The hydroxylation of THC to the 11-hydroxy form yields an active cannabinoid. Hydroxylation and demethylation of the benzodiazepine diazepam gives the metabolites temazepam and oxazepam, both of which are also available as drugs. Similarly, amitriptyline, a tricyclic antidepressant, is demethylated to yield another antidepressant, nortriptyline. Heroin is deacetylated to 6-acetylmorphine and morphine, both potent opioids.

Active metabolites may also have different modes of action and different potencies; thus dealkylation of the antidepressant drug iproniazid gives the tuberculostatic drug isoniazid, while the anticonvulsants primidone and methylphenobarbital are both metabolised to phenobarbital, another anticonvulsant with a much longer duration of action. Clearly, the formation of active metabolites changes the profile of drug action.

Pathways of drug metabolism can be divided into two types: Phase I and Phase II.

- **Phase I** reactions include oxidation, hydroxylation, *N*- and *O*-dealkylation and sulfoxide formation as well as reduction and hydrolysis reactions.
- **Phase II** processes involve conjugation reactions, such as with glucuronic acid, as well as acetylation, methylation and conjugation with amino acids and sulfate. Phase II reactions remove or mask functional groups (e.g. amino, carboxyl, hydroxyl, sulfhydryl, etc.) on the drug or Phase I metabolite by the addition of an endogenous substrate.

Examples of Phase 1 reactions such as oxidation, hydroxylation and dealkylation can be seen in Figures 2.4 to 2.6. An example of sulfoxidation is shown in Fig. 2.8.

Examples of Phase II reactions such as conjugation with glucuronic acid and sulfate are indicated in Fig. 2.13 and 2.16.

Many drugs undergo a combination of Phase I and Phase II reactions. The major Phase II reaction is conjugation of glucuronic acid with the phenolic or alcoholic hydroxyl groups that are common products of Phase I reactions. Thus, chlorpromazine gives rise to at least 20 metabolites by its three major routes of metabolism (hydroxylation, *N*-demethylation and sulfoxidation). Fortunately, such complicated patterns of metabolism are not a major problem to the analyst since at most only one or two key metabolites are usually targeted during a toxicological analysis, these typically being major metabolites or those which are particularly diagnostic.

As noted previously, the liver is a major site of metabolism. Many of the critical pathways are catalysed by microsomal membrane-bound enzymes in the hepatocytes (parenchymal cells of the liver). For example, the cytochrome P450 mixed-function oxidase system (which catalyses oxidations) and glucuronyl transferase (the enzyme responsible for conjugation with glucuronic acid) are both located on microsomal membranes.

Metabolism can occur in tissues other than the liver. The major additional sites are the gastrointestinal tract, kidneys and lungs. Their contribution clearly depends on the route of administration. For example, many metabolic reactions occur in the gastrointestinal tract before an orally administered drug is absorbed, carried out by enzymes in the mucosal lining or by microflora. Most of these reactions involve reduction and hydrolysis because of the anaerobic environment. Plasma esterases cause extensive hydrolysis of drugs such as heroin, cocaine and procaine.

In postmortem cases, anaerobic bioconversion occurs by endogenous enzymes active in such situations or by invading gastrointestinal bacteria. The nitrobenzodiazepines nitrazepam, clonazepam and flunitrazepam are subject to reduction to their 7-amino metabolites.

Using drugs principally of forensic interest, a number of examples are given below to illustrate the variety of metabolic routes that can be followed in humans and the effects that these might have on disposition and pharmacological activity. The examples given are not intended to be exhaustive with regard to either the pathways or the drugs covered.

All the major oxidative mechanisms can be illustrated by considering the metabolism of the benzodiazepines, amfetamines, antidepressants and opioids.

Benzodiazepines and other sedatives

The benzodiazepines are one of the most widely prescribed groups of drugs and are frequently found in toxicological cases. They undergo extensive metabolism by *N*-dealkylation, hydroxylation and conjugation pathways (Fig. 2.4). Many of the metabolites of diazepam show pharmacological activity, including desmethyldiazepam (nordiazepam), 3-hydroxydiazepam (temazepam) and desmethyl-3-hydroxydiazepam (oxazepam).

Ring-substituted benzodiazepines based on the triazolam structure show much higher potency than the first-generation benzodiazepines based on chlordiazepoxide and diazepam (Fig. 2.5). These also include midazolam and alprazolam. For example, triazolam is one of the most potent members in active use, with daily doses starting at 0.125 mg. By comparison, a typical dose for diazepam is 5–10 mg, and for chlordiazepoxide it is 100 mg. Administrative doses (including overdose) need to be taken into account when developing methods of analyses for drugs and their metabolites. Methods with higher sensitivity need to be used for these higher-potency drugs because the metabolites are likely to be present at much lower levels in blood and urine.

Benzodiazepines that do not belong to these two classes are still likely to be metabolised by the same routes. The atypical benzodiazepine chlordiazepoxide is metabolised by demethyla-

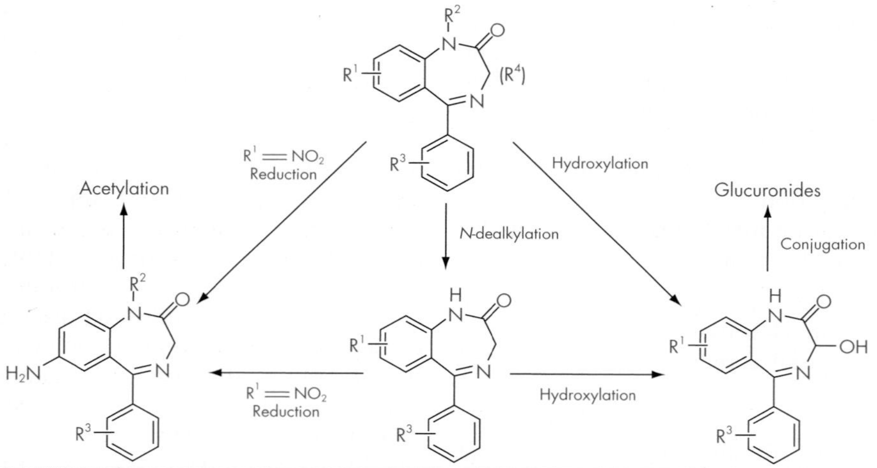

R^1	R^2	R^3	R^4	Drug
7-Chloro	Methyl	Hydrogen	Hydrogen	Diazepam
7-Chloro	Hydrogen	Hydrogen	Hydrogen	Nordiazepam
7-Chloro	Hydrogen	Hydrogen	Hydroxy	Oxazepam
7-Chloro	Methyl	Hydrogen	Hydroxy	Temazepam
7-Nitro	Hydrogen	2-Chloro	Hydrogen	Clonazepam
7-Nitro	Methyl	2-Fluoro	Hydrogen	Flunitrazepam
7-Nitro	Hydrogen	Hydrogen	Hydrogen	Nitrazepam
7-Chloro	Hydrogen	2-Chloro	Hydroxy	Lorazepam
7-Chloro	Diethylaminoethyl	2-Fluoro	Hydrogen	Flurazepam

Figure 2.4 Metabolic scheme for 1,4-benzodiazepines. [Note: For flunitrazepam, where *N*-dealkylation is followed by reduction, R^2 = H.]

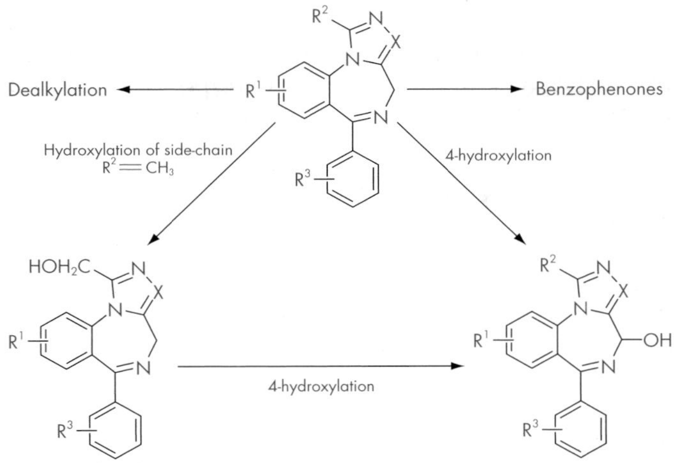

R^1	R^2	R^3	X	Drug
8-Chloro	Methyl	Hydrogen	Nitrogen	Alprazolam
8-Chloro	Methyl	2-Fluoro	Hydrogen	Midazolam
8-Chloro	Methyl	2-Chloro	Nitrogen	Triazolam
8-Chloro	Dimethylaminomethyl	Hydrogen	Nitrogen	Adinazolam
8-Chloro	Hydrogen	Hydrogen	Nitrogen	Estazolam

Figure 2.5 Metabolic scheme for diazolo- and triazolobenzodiazepines.

tion and deamination to desmethylchlordiazepoxide and demoxepam. Demoxepam is further metabolised to nordiazepam by hydrolysis and cleavage of the lactam ring.

The pharmacokinetic half-lives of benzodiazepines are used largely to determine their principal medical use. Benzodiazepines with a relatively short half-life are used predominantly as hypnotics and as supplements to preoperative anaesthesia, whereas the longer acting benzodiazepines (such as diazepam) are used as minor tranquillisers (anxiolytics).

The urine usually contains extensive metabolites of benzodiazepines, often with little parent drug present. It is essential to know the individual metabolites of target benzodiazepines when assessing the urine of persons exposed to this class of drug.

The clearance of benzodiazepines is decreased by liver disease, although the greatest effects occur with those drugs metabolised by the P450 system. Lorazepam and oxazepam, and other similar drugs metabolised by glucuronidation, are least affected. Kidney disease particularly affects benzodiazepines metabolised to active drugs and those that show a high degree of protein binding.

Advanced age has similar effects to liver and kidney disease because of the reduction in output of major organs and changes in the volume of distribution. Doses of sedatives are usually halved in the elderly (>65 years), although oxazepam, lorazepam and temazepam are least affected by age.

Amfetamines and other stimulants

The amfetamines are metabolised by a combination of hydroxylation of the ring and the side-chain carbon atom adjacent to the ring, and removal of the nitrogen (Fig. 2.6). Drugs with alkyl groups on the nitrogen are dealkylated (methamfetamine and methylenedioxymethylamfetamine (MDMA)) to other

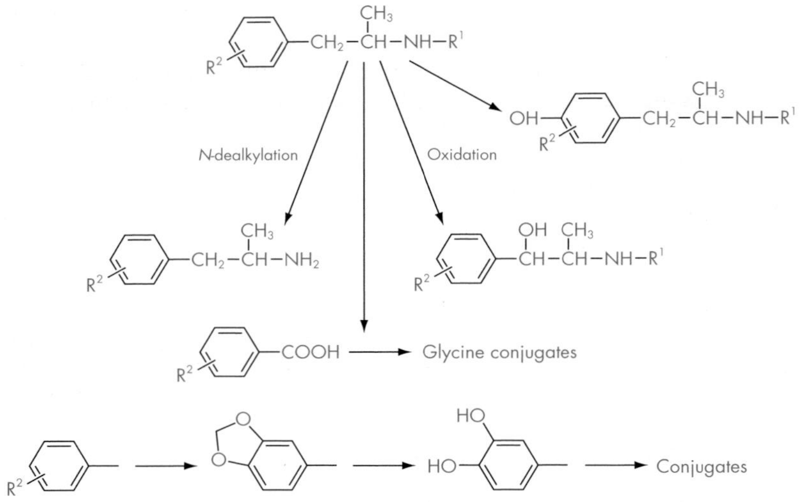

Figure 2.6 Major routes of amfetamine metabolism.

active amfetamines (amfetamine and methylenedioxyamfetamine (MDA), respectively; Fig. 2.6). Methylenedioxyethylamfetamine (MDEA) and MDMA are both metabolised to MDA as well as other metabolites. The methylenedioxyamfetamines are also transformed into dihydroxy compounds (catechols) following opening of the ring. These hydroxy metabolites can be either monomethylated or conjugated with sulfate esters or with glucuronic acid. The side chain of non-*N*-substituted amfetamines is oxidised to form benzoic acid derivatives (e.g. amfetamine), which are excreted as the glycine conjugate, or the sulfate or glucuronide conjugate. Amfetamine and methylamfetamine are also oxidised at the β-carbon to form the pharmacologically active ephedrine analogues.

A number of legal stimulant drugs are metabolised to methylamfetamine or amfetamine. These include benzfetamine, clobenzorex, fenethylline, fenproporex and mefenorex. The antiparkinsonian drug selegiline is metabolised to the weakly active *l*-isomer of methylamfetamine. Detection of the parent drug and possibly the conduct of chiral analyses are essential to determine the source of the amfetamine.

As expected from its different structure, cocaine undergoes substantially different routes of metabolism from the amfetamine class. Cocaine is hydrolysed rapidly by ubiquitous enzymes to the inactive benzoylecgonine. This is the main metabolite in both blood and urine. Other significant metabolites are ecgonine methyl ester (EME) and ecgonine (Fig. 2.7).

Anhydroecgonine methyl ester (AEME, also known as methylecgonidine) is a pyrolytic substance formed by smoking cocaine. Cocaethylene is also found as a metabolite in persons who co-consume alcohol. Metabolism of cocaine to norcocaine allows the oxidation of the nitrogen to *N*-hydroxynorcocaine. *N*-Nitrosonorcocaine and the *N*-oxide are also produced in small amounts.

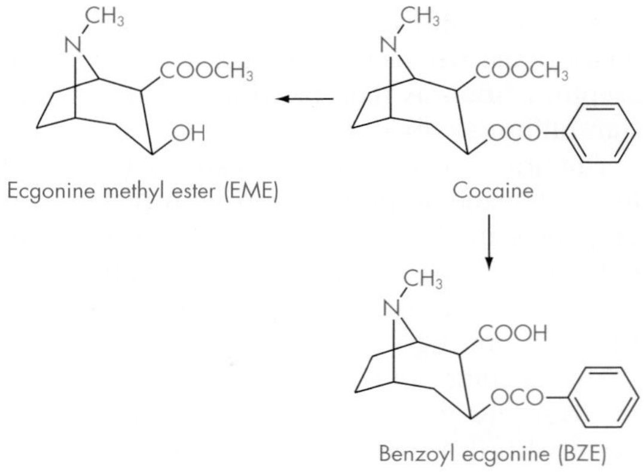

Figure 2.7 Main cocaine metabolic pathways.

Antidepressants

Modern antidepressants can be divided into several chemical classes. The traditional tricyclic antidepressants include amitriptyline, clomipramine, dosulepin (dothiepin), doxepin and imipramine. The newer generation of antidepressants include the selective serotonin reuptake inhibitors (SSRIs) citalopram, fluoxetine, fluvoxamine, paroxetine and sertraline. Other antidepressants include the monoamine oxidase inhibitor moclobemide, and other mixed-uptake inhibitors (mirtazapine, nefazodone and venlafaxine).

The tricyclic antidepressants are metabolised by three major pathways: *N*-oxidation, hydroxylation of the alicyclic ring and of the aromatic ring, and *N*-dealkylation of the dialkylamino group. The last route gives rise to the most important metabolites, since the *N*-demethylated metabolites are themselves pharmacologically active. Amitriptyline is metabolised to nortriptyline, and imipramine to desipramine; both metabolites are also available as therapeutic agents (Fig. 2.8).

When monitoring concentrations of tricyclic antidepressants for their therapeutic effect, it is important to determine both the parent drug and the desalkyl metabolites, as the latter may be present in a significant quantity. These can be summed to provide an estimate of therapeutic activity. The hydroxy metabolites predominate in the urine, and usually occur as glucuronide conjugates.

The other classes of antidepressants have varied chemical structures, and hence their fate is very much dependent on the drug concerned (Fig. 2.9).

Antipsychotic drugs

The first antipsychotic drugs were largely of the phenothiazine type represented by thioridazine and chlorpromazine. They undergo sulfoxidation to yield sulfoxides and sulfones. In addition,

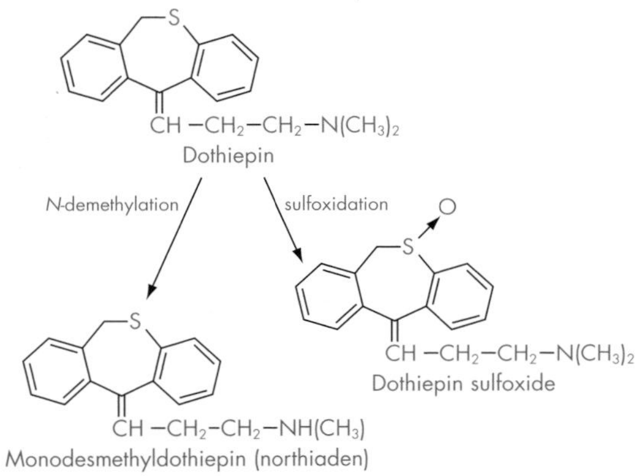

$$\text{CH}-\text{CH}_2-\text{CH}_2-\text{N(CH}_3)_2$$

Dothiepin

N-demethylation

sulfoxidation

$$\text{CH}-\text{CH}_2-\text{CH}_2-\text{NH(CH}_3)$$

Monodesmethyldothiepin (northiaden)

$$\text{CH}-\text{CH}_2-\text{CH}_2-\text{N(CH}_3)_2$$

Dothiepin sulfoxide

Figure 2.8 Major pathways of dosulepin (dothiepin) metabolism.

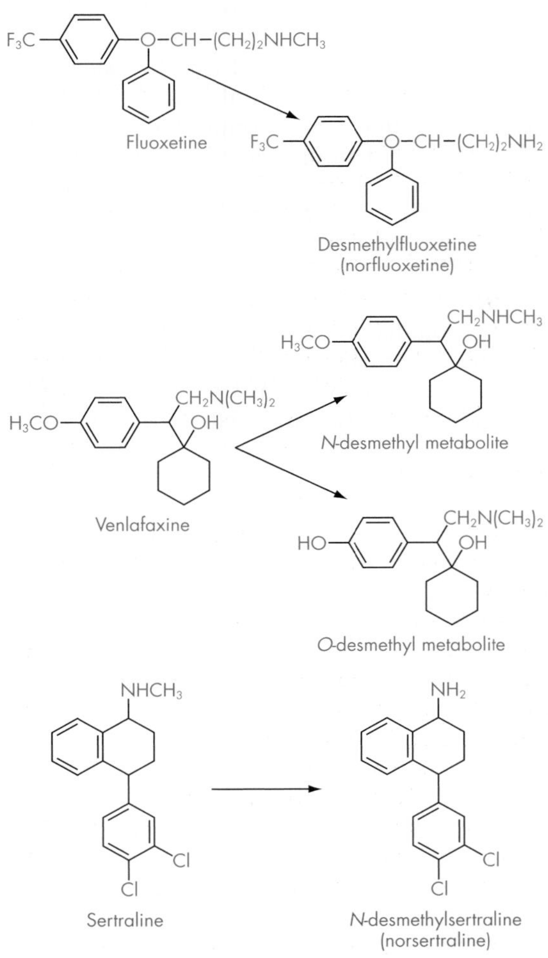

F_3C—C_6H_4—$O-CH-(CH_2)_2NHCH_3$

Fluoxetine

F_3C—C_6H_4—$O-CH-(CH_2)_2NH_2$

Desmethylfluoxetine (norfluoxetine)

H_3CO — $CH_2N(CH_3)_2$ — OH

Venlafaxine

H_3CO — CH_2NHCH_3 — OH

N-desmethyl metabolite

HO — $CH_2N(CH_3)_2$ — OH

O-desmethyl metabolite

$NHCH_3$ — Cl — Cl

Sertraline

NH_2 — Cl — Cl

N-desmethylsertraline (norsertraline)

Figure 2.9 Key metabolic pathways for selective serotonin reuptake inhibitors.

oxidation at the nitrogen, hydroxylation of one or both of the aromatic rings, *N*-dealkylation of the side-chain and fission of the side-chain may also occur. The phenolic metabolites are then conjugated with glucuronic acid or sulfate and excreted in both the urine and the bile.

The number of different metabolic routes that are possible results in a complex mixture of metabolites for many phenothiazines. For example, many of the drugs that contain an *N*,*N*-dialkylaminoalkyl side-chain (e.g. chlorpromazine) are metabolised extensively by *N*-oxidation, together with hydroxylation, sulfoxidation and *N*-dealkylation. Thioridazine is oxidised predominantly on the side-chain sulfur to active sulfoxide and sulfone metabolites (Fig. 2.10).

Haloperidol is metabolised by side-chain oxidation to a propionic acid derivative (Fig. 2.11) which is then conjugated, or by reduction of the keto group. Clozapine is metabolised to the active desmethyl form (norclozapine), which is often measured with the parent drug in therapeutic drug monitoring situations. Olanzapine is metabolised by *N*-demethylation and oxidation to a 2-hydroxymethyl metabolite, and *N*-glucuronidation. Risperidone is metabolised to the pharmacologically active 9-hydroxy metabolite. Inactive 7-hydroxy and *N*-dealkyl metabolites are also produced.

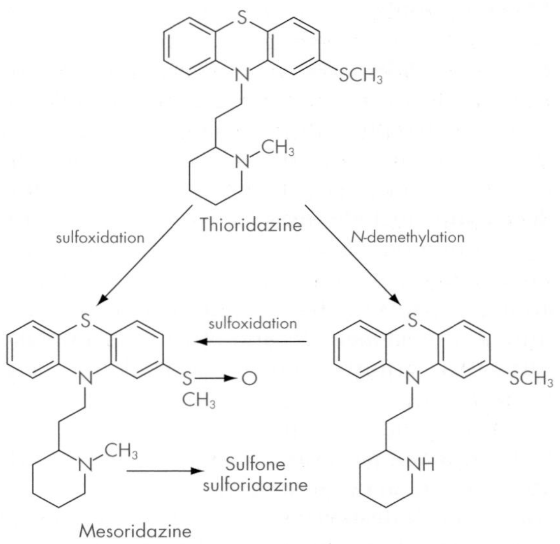

Figure 2.10 Thioridazine metabolic pathways.

Opiates and centrally active analgesics

The opiates include the analogues of morphine, such as codeine, ethylmorphine and diamorphine, as well as the synthetic opiates methadone, pethidine, dextropropoxyphene and the highly potent fentanyl derivatives. Depending on their structural features, the metabolism of opiates can vary widely.

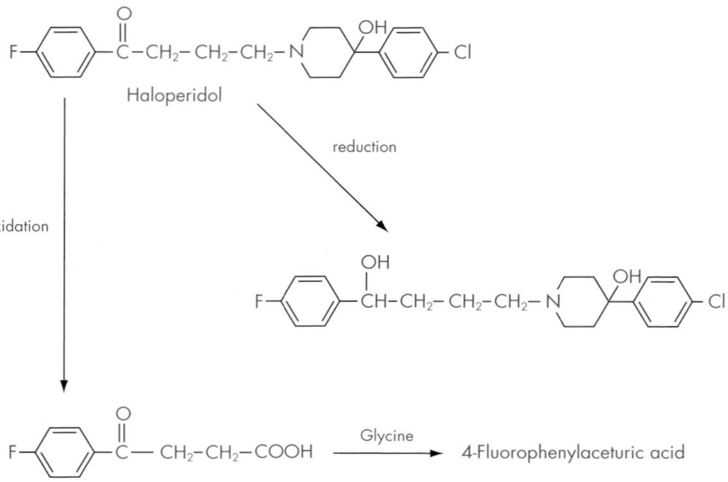

Figure 2.11 Haloperidol metabolic pathways.

The morphine analogues are metabolised by *O*-dealkylation or de-esterification and conjugation with glucuronic acid. Thus, diamorphine (heroin) is hydrolysed rapidly in the body to 6-acetylmorphine, which is further and more slowly hydrolysed to morphine. The morphine so formed is excreted largely as the 3- and the 6-glucuronides together with some free morphine. Codeine and ethylmorphine are conjugated and metabolised by *O*-dealkylation to morphine. Morphine is also metabolised to a minor extent by *N*-demethylation to normorphine (Fig. 2.12).

Oxycodone is subject to demethylation and conjugation (Fig. 2.13).

Methadone, dextropropoxyphene and pethidine are largely dealkylated. In the case of methadone a cyclisation product known as 2-ethylidene-1,5-dimethyl-3,3-diphenylpyrrolidine (EDDP) is formed (Fig. 12.14), as well as 2-ethyl-5-methyl-3,3-diphenyl-1-pyrrolidine (EMDP).

The non-opioid centrally active analgesic tramadol is metabolised to *N*- and *O*-demethylated products followed by sulfation and glucuronidation of the phenol. The *N*-desmethyl metabolite (known as M1) is active pharmacologically (Fig. 2.15).

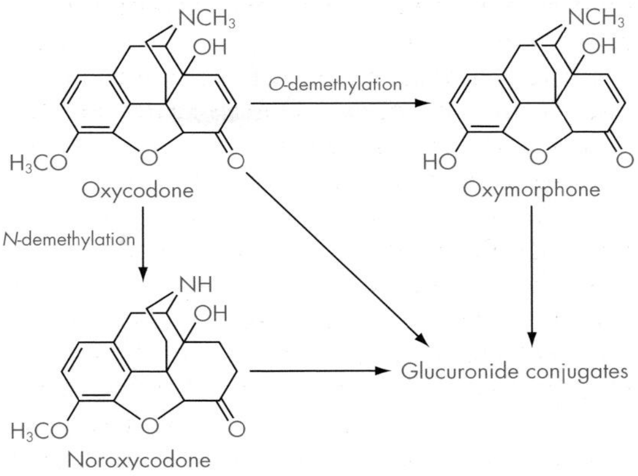

Figure 2.13 Oxycodone metabolism.

Adverse drug interactions and pharmacogenetics

Drug interactions

In the majority of cases in clinical and forensic toxicology, more than one drug is involved. Multidrug therapy and abuse is prevalent and this, together with the added problems of self-medication with over-the-counter drugs and the

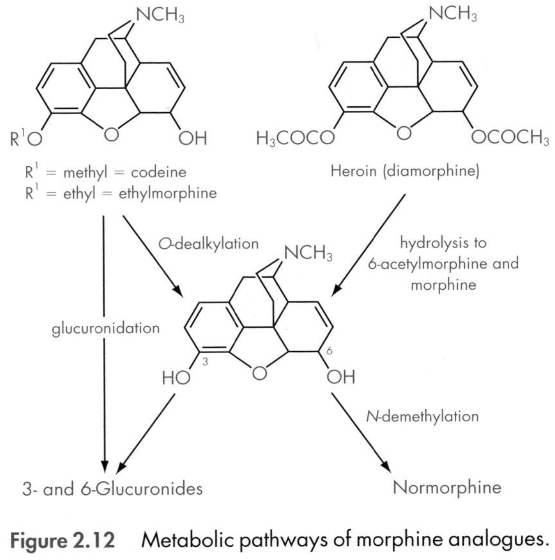

Figure 2.12 Metabolic pathways of morphine analogues.

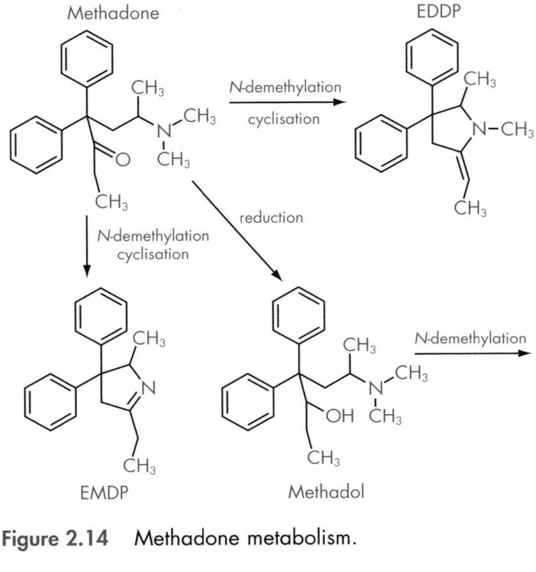

Figure 2.14 Methadone metabolism.

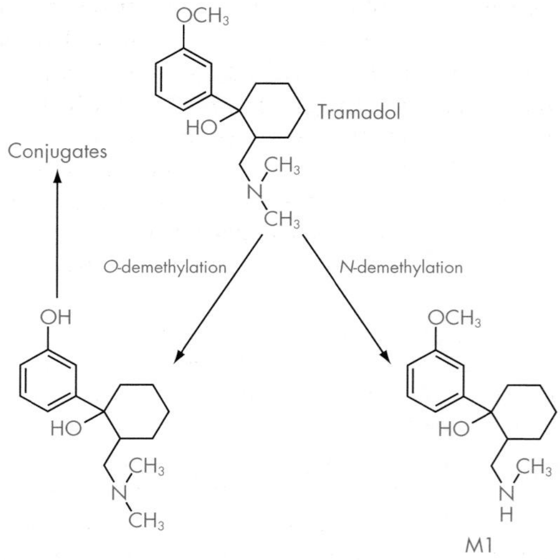

Figure 2.15 Tramadol metabolism.

widespread use of alcohol, makes interpretation of data even more complicated. Pharmacokinetic and other data available in the scientific literature often refer to drug concentrations and responses observed after administration of the drug alone. In practice, when these data are compared with analytical results that involve several drugs, it must be remembered that the clinical response is often a consequence of the combined actions of more than one drug. If the significance of the analytical results is to be assessed correctly, it is essential to consider the quantitative effects of any interactions that might occur between drugs taken in combination.

Drug interactions can be divided into two types:

- those that affect the drug concentration (i.e. alter the processes of absorption, distribution and elimination)
- those that affect the response (by changing its duration and severity).

The consequences of most drug combinations can be predicted with knowledge of the usual effects of drugs.

Drugs with opposite pharmacological activities (e.g. barbiturates and amfetamines) may have an antagonistic effect. Conversely, the additive effects or side-effects of two drugs with the same pharmacological action (e.g. central nervous system depressants) may prove fatal even though the individual drug concentrations are not toxic themselves. Further, a drug with a high affinity for tissue proteins might displace a second drug from binding sites, while a drug that changes urinary pH or that competes for the same active transport system in the proximal tubules of the kidney might inhibit renal excretion. Other important mechanisms for drug interactions include:

- interference with absorption of other drugs
- modification of rates and routes of metabolism
- changing the accessibility of receptors and tissue sites.

Metabolic effects

There are many examples of drugs that affect the metabolism or pharmacology of other drugs. For example, cimetidine (an anti-ulcer drug) and a number of the newer generation of antidepressants inhibit the metabolism of many of the benzodiazepines by a subtype of the cytochrome P450 enzymes, CYP3A. This occurs either by competitive inhibition of the enzyme(s) involved in their mutual metabolism or by inhibition of the enzyme(s). Cimetidine also inhibits the metabolism of opioids. Many of the newer selective serotonin reuptake inhibitors (SSRIs) (e.g. fluoxetine, paroxetine and sertraline), as well as some of the antifungal drugs (e.g. fluconazole) and antiviral drugs are relatively potent inhibitors of this enzyme.

Cimetidine (used in the treatment of gastric and duodenal ulcers) inhibits the metabolism of opioids that require microsomal cytochrome enzymes.

Monoamine oxidase inhibitors nialamide, phenelzine and tranylcypromine also inhibit P450 enzyme metabolism and have been shown to increase the effects of alcohol, amfetamines, barbiturates, pethidine and other opioids. The analgesic dextropropoxyphene may have similar activity.

A further variable is that drugs such as the barbiturates and the anticonvulsants phenobarbital and phenytoin enhance the production of the enzymes and therefore induce metabolism of drugs metabolised through this and related enzyme systems. In fact, barbiturates also induce their own metabolism, which results in a time-dependent increase in clearance as the liver produces more enzyme. If the presence of more than one drug is detected in a toxicological analysis, the possibility of metabolic effects must be considered.

Pharmacogenetics

From a toxicological perspective we are still at the early stages of understanding the impact of genetic polymorphisms in drug disposition. Nevertheless, we can anticipate that the impact of 'toxicogenomics' in toxicology will increase sharply over the coming years. Some of the known effects of pharmacogenetics on the toxicology of drugs are given below.

Cytochrome P450

Cytochrome P450 is a family of mixed-function oxidases that participate actively in the disposition of drugs from the body. The large number of isoforms suggests that, in addition to participating in the metabolism of xenobiotics, physiologically they participate in the maintenance of homeostasis in the body. There are 39 functional human genes that encode isoforms of cytochrome P450. Three subfamilies (1, 2 and 3) include 19 of these isoforms, the most relevant in xenobiotics metabolism. Polymorphisms have been observed in several isoforms (CYP2D6, CYP2C9, CYP2C19, CYP2E1 and CYP3A4). Genetic polymorphisms, related in particular to CYP2D6, are of relevance from a pharmacological and toxicological point of view. This is because there are drugs for which disposition from the body is regulated by this enzyme (opiates, beta-blockers, anti-arrhythmics and antidepressants), and because of other drugs that act as inhibitors of this enzyme (i.e. methadone, dextropropoxyphene) and thus enhance the toxicity of drugs that are substrates. Patients with mutations in CYP2D6 have impaired metabolism of drugs if the metabolism co-segregates with this enzyme; hence such drugs tend to accumulate in the body, with an enhanced risk of toxicity if the dose is not adjusted according to the genotype.

For example, the main metabolic pathway for codeine, dextromethorphan and ethylmorphine is the metabolism to morphine through *O*-dealkylation. Some 7% of caucasians are deficient in this enzyme and are unable to produce significant amounts of morphine. In these people, codeine and ethylmorphine appear to be far weaker analgesics than in those who are able to produce morphine. The same enzyme is involved in the bioconversion and activation of oxycodone to oxymorphone, hydrocodone to hydromorphone, risperidone to 9-hydroxyrisperidone and in the metabolism of olanzapine. The efficacy and toxicity of these drugs are therefore affected by this genetic difference.

P-Glycoprotein

P-Glycoprotein (P-gp) is an adenosine triphosphate (ATP)-dependent transporter that participates in the active transport of drugs and their metabolites. P-gps are encoded by members of a gene family referred as the multidrug resistance (MDR) genes for their role in MDR in cancer chemotherapy. Physiologically, P-gp seems to act as a barrier to entry and as an efflux mechanism for xenobiotics and cellular metabolites. It is located in the liver, intestine, kidney, blood–brain barrier and other barrier-epithelial tissues. P-gp influences the oral bioavailability of drugs, and an overlap of substrates with CYP3A has been observed. This observation is of relevance because as many as 50% of drugs are metabolised through this enzyme. Hence, at the intestinal level, the co-ordinated activity of P-gp and CYP3A may condition the absorption and pre-systemic disposition of many drugs. From a toxicological point of view, drug–drug interactions at the absorption level or at the biliary excretion levels may lead to accumulation of drugs and an enhanced toxicity.

Glucuronidation

Glucuronidation is an important conjugation reaction. It is considered as Phase II metabolism where metabolites from Phase I metabolism are conjugated. In the case of glucuronidation, metabolites are conjugated to glucuronic acid, making the resultant metabolite more water soluble. Two gene families encode for uridine diphosphate glucuronosyltransferase (UDPGT) isoforms: UGT1 and UGT2. Several polymorphic forms of isoforms encoded by UGT2 have been identified; none of them results in significant changes in the rate of glucuronidation of drugs and other xenobiotics. In UGT1, mutation of the isoform UGT1A1 leads to a partial or total impairment of bilirubin conjugation. This results in hyperbilirubinaemias associated with Gilbert syndrome.

There is currently considerable interest in the direct detection of glucuronide metabolites because they typically have a longer excretion time than the Phase I metabolites and hence may be detected a longer time after administration. This can be particularly useful in cases of drug-facilitated sexual assault where victims often present some time after the incident. When GC-MS was the primary tool for drugs analysis, glucuronide conjugates were hydrolysed back to the parent compound for analysis because glucuronides do not chromatograph well by GC. LC-MS enables direct analysis of glucuronides.

Glutathione *S*-transferases

Glutathione *S*-transferases (GSTs) participate in the activation and detoxification of many drugs and xenobiotics. There is a high prevalence in humans of genetic polymorphisms for several GSTs. Several studies have tried to associate such polymorphisms with an increased risk for the development of cancer of environmental origin, with conflicting results. Paracetamol toxicity is associated at high doses with a depletion of hepatic glutathione stores. Other drugs using this metabolic pathway may result in an enhanced hepatotoxicity at relatively normal doses because of competition for the same detoxification mechanism.

N-Acetylation

N-Acetylation is the oldest and probably the best-known polymorphism of drug-metabolising enzymes. In addition to polymorphisms that give rise to slow and rapid acetylator phenotypes, there are high inter-ethnic variations in the prevalence of such phenotypes in the population. A cytosolic *N*-acetyltransferase (NAT-2) is the polymorphic enzyme. Acetylation polymorphism regulates the metabolism of drugs with arylamine (e.g. isoniazid) and hydrazine (e.g. hydralazine) chemical structures as well as promutagenic/mutagenic heterocyclic arylamines from dietary or environmental origin.

Sulfation and methylation

Sulfation and methylation are important pathways in the metabolism of many drugs and xenobiotics. Sulfotransferases (SULT, SULT1 and SULT2) and methyltransferases (methyltransferase (MT), catecholmethyltransferase (COMT), thiopurine methyltransferase (TPMT) and thiolmethyltransferase (TMT)) catalyse such reactions. Several polymorphisms have been identified for these enzymes but, to date, their clinical significance is unclear.

The possible influence of genetic polymorphisms on drug metabolism should be taken into account in clinical treatment and interpretation of toxicological analyses, although information on these polymorphisms may well not be available for many toxicological investigations.

Altered physiological state

The role of altered physiological status on drug pharmacokinetics and drug actions is of particular importance in the area of adverse reactions to drugs.

Neonates and elderly people generally have a lower metabolic capacity compared to subjects between these extremes of age. The enhanced sensitivity of the very young to drugs occurs because the microsomal enzymes responsible for metabolism are not fully active until several months after birth.

Furthermore, very young children do not have the necessary plasma-binding proteins that help to compartmentalise drugs. Infants (over 1 year old) usually metabolise drugs at similar rates and by similar routes as adults, but they require lower doses to produce comparable effects because the drugs are distributed into a smaller volume. It is important that the known pharmacokinetics of a drug in question be examined when neonates, and even children generally, are a focus of an investigation relating to drug effects, since some drugs may behave differently than in adults.

In elderly subjects (over 65 years old) there appears to be a decreasing capacity for drug metabolism as a consequence of a gradual decline in overall physiology. This includes effects on volume of distribution, protein binding and both hepatic and renal clearance. The change in the pharmacokinetics is an explanation of the increased sensitivity to drug effects in the elderly. For example, doses of benzodiazepines are reduced in the elderly to avoid excessive sedation and adverse effects on cognition.

Diseases can affect all the processes by which a drug is absorbed, distributed and eliminated from the body. A drug may be absorbed poorly during gastrointestinal disturbance. The rate of uptake of drugs that rapidly cross tissue membranes may be altered in cardiovascular diseases that alter blood flow to critical organs such as the liver, kidney, lungs and heart. Diseases that fundamentally affect metabolic and excretory pathways of drugs also alter their pharmacokinetics.

Diseases that affect the liver or kidneys probably have the greatest effect on drug concentrations because normal functioning of these organs is essential for efficient metabolism and excretion. The liver has a large metabolic reserve. However, severe disease, such as cirrhosis or drug-induced necrosis, causes the pharmacokinetic terminal elimination half-life to increase dramatically, leading to increased concentrations of drugs in plasma or tissues.

Renal disease leads to a decreased ability to excrete drugs and/or their metabolites. A drug accumulates in the plasma or tissues if the interval between doses is such that not all of the previously administered drug is removed before the next dose. Even those drugs for which excretion into the urine does not normally appear to be an important route of elimination can carry a risk of increased toxicity during disease if significant drug accumulation takes place. This is especially true when potentially serious interactions may occur with the accumulated drug or metabolite. For example, metabolites can displace their parent drugs from binding sites on plasma and tissue proteins if their concentrations build up sufficiently.

Another example is the toxicity of benzodiazepines, which is increased in persons with significant respiratory diseases and in the elderly who have some form of age-related reduction in organ function.

Physiological status should be considered in the interpretation of toxicological findings (see later in this chapter)

Reactive metabolites

Toxic metabolites can occur in the same way that pharmacologically active and/or inactive metabolites are produced. For example, deacetylation of phenacetin yields *p*-phenetidine, the precursor of substances believed to be responsible for methaemoglobinaemia. Similarly, paraoxon, the oxygenated metabolite of parathion, is responsible for the severe toxicity observed after the ingestion of parathion.

Changes in the pathways of metabolism of a drug can also result in toxicity. In paracetamol intoxication (e.g. from drug overdose), the pathways responsible for sulfate and glucuronide conjugation become saturated and the concentrations of cysteine and mercapturic acid metabolites increase. When the production of these two metabolites increases sufficiently to deplete stores of glutathione, the active intermediate can no longer be conjugated and is thought to bind irreversibly to cellular macromolecules such as DNA, RNA and proteins, which results in a dose-related hepatic necrosis. It is believed that the toxic molecule arises from the oxidation of paracetamol to *N*-acetyl-*p*-benzoquinoneimine (Fig. 2.16).

Whatever the actual pathway, the administration of compounds that contain sulfhydryl

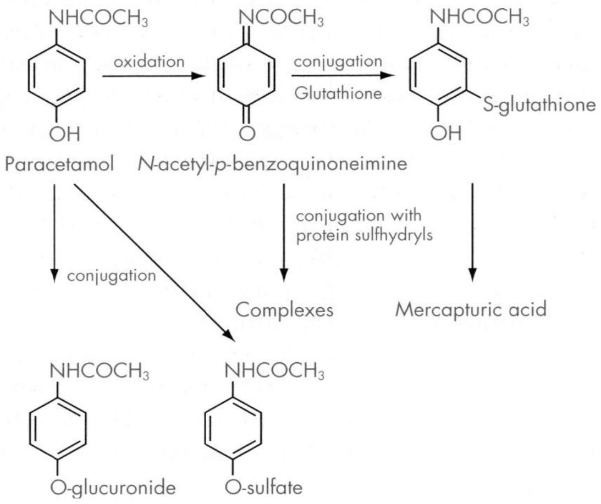

Figure 2.16 Paracetamol metabolism.

groups has been shown to be effective in treatment of paracetamol intoxication, presumably because they are able to bind to the electrophilic species in the same way as glutathione does.

Another example of drug toxicity induced by metabolism is that associated with acetylation. The rate of acetylation is controlled by an *N*-acetyltransferase that shows genetic polymorphism; about 60% of caucasians are classified as 'slow' acetylators. The extent of acetylation is related to the toxic effects of certain drugs. For example, the *N*-hydroxy metabolite of acetylated isoniazid is thought to cause isoniazid-related hepatotoxicity. This toxicity is more severe in 'rapid' acetylators than in 'slow' acetylators, but (as with paracetamol) some protection can be given by sulfhydryl compounds. There are diagnostic tests for acetylator status.

In contrast, 'slow' acetylators appear to show a greater incidence of systemic lupus erythematosus after the administration of hydrazine drugs than do 'rapid' acetylators, as this toxic reaction is related to the parent drug.

The possible role of reactive metabolites should be taken into account in toxicological investigations.

Drug concentration and pharmacological response

The relationship between drug action and the processes of absorption, distribution and elimination has been applied successfully in clinical pharmacology to optimise and individualise the therapy of many drugs. In clinical and forensic toxicology, similar relationships can be applied in the interpretation of analytical results.

For most drugs there is a correlation between the dose given, the concentration of drug in the blood and the duration and intensity of the biological effect. In general, as blood concentrations rise above those associated with a therapeutic effect, the frequency and severity of toxic side-effects increase. It should be stressed that this correlation is at best poor for most drugs, and there is considerable individual variability. Hence, any prediction of response from a drug concentration is poor.

The significance of toxicological data is assessed by attempting to explain the clinical or toxicological effects in terms of the drug concentrations found. Before this can be done the toxicologist must be satisfied that the clinical and analytical data are valid.

Validity of toxicological data

A number of physical factors affect the validity of toxicological findings. Paramount are the accuracy of the analytical tests conducted and the nature of the specimen used.

Blood and urine are the most commonly used specimens for analysis, although blood drug concentrations are generally considered to provide the best possible estimate of the likely pharmacological responses. Urine is an excretory fluid, and while it is useful for detection of drugs and metabolites, it does not necessarily provide an indication of the likely effect of a drug on the body.

In postmortem cases the origin of a blood sample must be stated and the sample should preferably be obtained from peripheral sites, such as the leg (femoral vein) or arm (subclavian vein), as blood from central parts of the body can have very different drug concentrations (see section on postmortem redistribution below).

When a toxic response to a drug (or drugs) is suspected, it is advantageous to measure the drug concentration in two or more independent samples; the value of a result from a single sample is limited unless the distribution of the drug is known. This could be from two peripheral blood samples or from a peripheral blood and a liver specimen.

Tissues that selectively take up a particular drug may have a much higher concentration than that found in blood. For example, 11-carboxytetrahydrocannabinol has high concentrations in fat; digoxin and other cardiac glycosides are taken up by cardiac muscle; biliary concentrations of drugs excreted from the liver as glucuronides (e.g. morphine) are usually considerably higher than their concentrations in blood.

In addition to being distributed unevenly throughout the body, a drug may not be distributed evenly within the separate parts of a single tissue (see section on blood and plasma concentrations above). In blood, drugs may tend to be concentrated either in the plasma or in the erythrocytes. Thus, it may prove to be of little value to examine a plasma sample in a case where the drug involved is known to be concentrated in the red blood cells (e.g. acetazolamide).

Pharmacological response

Even when it has been established that the measured drug concentration in the blood accurately represents the concentration of drug at the receptor site, it must also be established that the clinical response is a primary consequence of the presence of the drug. For example, drugs with an irreversible biochemical effect, such as reserpine and some monoamine oxidase inhibitors, still have clinical effects long after drug administration has stopped, and when plasma concentrations of the drug are negligible. Similarly, unless the time of ingestion is known with reasonable accuracy, it is almost impossible to relate drug concentrations with the secondary and potentially fatal responses to substances such as paracetamol (liver damage) and paraquat (lung necrosis). Incorporation of drugs or chemicals into endogenous metabolic cycles may result in a toxicity (lethal synthesis) that is not related to blood concentrations of the drug. Finally, interpretation is made difficult or impossible when underlying disease alters the pharmacological action of the drug, or when a patient has died from complications associated with inhalation of vomit.

Active metabolites

A number of drugs have been modified such that metabolism is required to produce an active species. This is often done to facilitate oral absorption or to reduce toxicity, although for some drugs the active form was not established until after clinical use. Examples include diamorphine, which is hydrolysed to morphine; the esters of many angiotensin-converting enzyme (ACE) inhibitors (e.g. enalapril, quinapril), which are hydrolysed to potent di-acid forms; azathioprine, which is metabolised to mercaptopurine; and zidovudine which is metabolised to zidovudine triphosphate.

When an active metabolite makes an important contribution to the overall pharmacological response, the interpretation of toxicological data is further complicated. Toxicological situations that involve such metabolites (e.g. oxazepam, nortriptyline, desipramine and phenobarbital, derived from diazepam, amitriptyline, imipramine and methylphenobarbital, respectively) can be misinterpreted if only the parent drugs are assayed. The concentrations of active metabolites must be taken into account. Although it is unclear what is the best way to evaluate the contribution of metabolites, the individual concentrations of drug and metabolites are often added together to provide an estimate of the total amount of active drug species present in the sample. This assumes that their relative pharmacological activities are equal, which is not generally true.

Postmortem redistribution

The unequal distribution of drugs in tissues leads to changes in the blood concentration of drugs after death. This is called postmortem redistribution and occurs primarily by diffusion of drug from neighbouring tissue sites and from organs, such as from stomach contents. This process is particularly significant for drugs with high lipid solubility, since these drugs tend to show concentration differences in tissues and blood. Such drugs, e.g. dextropropoxyphene, digoxin, tricyclic antidepressants and phenothiazines, can show increases in excess of 5-fold. Blood collected from the heart and other thoracic or abdominal sites may be similarly affected, and should be avoided wherever possible. Examples of drugs particularly subject to this process include:

- amfetamines
- barbiturates
- cocaine
- chloroquine
- digoxin
- methadone
- phenothiazines
- dextropropoxyphene
- propranolol
- pethidine
- tricyclic antidepressants.

The collection of peripheral blood, e.g. femoral or subclavian, reduces the extent of changes, although some increase in blood concentration can still occur.

Unequal drug distribution can also occur in the liver due to diffusion from intestinal contents or from incomplete circulation and distribution within the liver.

How postmortem redistribution may affect interpretation of results is discussed further in Chapter 7.

Interpretation

What are therapeutic, toxic and fatal concentrations?

The term 'therapeutic' as used in this text refers to concentrations of drugs normally expected following recommended doses of the substance. Clearly, the term 'therapeutic' has no application for some substances, e.g. illicit drugs and poisons such as organophosphates. A toxic concentration occurs when the dose of substance causes or has the potential to cause serious adverse reactions, while a fatal concentration relates to levels that are associated with fatal poisonings.

Large collections of data are available in various texts and in databases concerning the potentially therapeutic, toxic and fatal concentrations of drugs and poisons. These can be an aid to establishing a likely response to a drug when interpreting a toxicological result. Unfortunately, the use of such data is subject to many restrictions and limitations. These are detailed below.

Reliable assessments of the significance of any analytical finding can be made only by comparing the results with information on drug concentrations and associated clinical responses that have been reported in other related cases. In particular, it is essential that a distinction is made between acute and chronic use since repeated use of a drug may give rise to much higher blood concentrations than a single dose. This causes pharmacokinetic accumulation. For example, methadone has a half-life of about 24 h, resulting in significant accumulation of the drug in the blood and tissues for at least 5 days of dosing.

Persons often develop a tolerance to drugs with repeated administration compared to their first use; hence some background knowledge on the use of drugs will assist in determining if this is a likely event. This is relevant in understanding the effects of many opioids: a potentially toxic concentration in a single dose may be easily tolerated with repeated use.

Furthermore, it is essential that when toxicity to a drug is suspected the possible involvement of other drugs also is considered. Databases may not indicate whether a poisoning was due to that agent alone or in combination with other substances. Common examples here include the presence of ethanol in cases involving other central nervous system (CNS) depressant drugs, e.g. opioids, benzodiazepines. The use of cocaine or amfetamine in combination with diamorphine (heroin) is more toxic than one drug alone.

The route of drug administration, together with the nature of the dosage form, determines the rate and extent of absorption. Administration by inhalation, intravenous or intramuscular injection leads to a high bioavailability and quick and often intense response, while oral administration produces lower concentrations of longer duration. Thus, a fatal drug dose given intravenously is often much smaller than a fatal dose given by mouth because the injected drug is able to reach the site of action very rapidly.

If proprietary preparations are given by the recommended route, it may be possible to make predictions of the dose from blood concentrations because comparable data are usually available. When illicit drugs or preparations are involved, prediction of blood concentration is much more difficult. Particular examples of variable and unpredicted doses include use of volatile substances through inhalation (abuse), and the smoking of cannabis, diamorphine or cocaine. In all of these cases the degree of inhalation together with the technique used greatly affects the amount of drug actually absorbed.

An important source of variable absorption is through oral dosing, since this route is probably the most common. Most of the variability in absorption is related to any first-pass metabolism that occurs for drugs with low oral bioavailability. A number of factors can influence bioavailability. These include the motility of the stomach and bowel, pH and (for a small number of drugs) activity of gut enzymes that metabolise the drug before it is even absorbed. This issue also applies in situations when coexisting natural disease or injuries may affect the nature of the response to the drug, or when the very young or the elderly are being treated with drugs.

The combined effect of all of these factors is to make the task of interpreting analytical results even more difficult. Pharmacokinetic and toxicological data must be used circumspectly when a specific case is being examined because there is always the possibility of misinterpretation if consideration is not given to the special circumstances of the case.

Several drugs, including salicylate (in overdose), alcohol, and possibly some hydrazines and other drugs which are metabolised by acetylation, have saturable elimination kinetics. With these drugs, capacity-limited elimination is complicated further by their low therapeutic index. A good example is phenytoin. A 50% increase in the dose of phenytoin can result in a 600% increase in the steady-state blood concentration, and thus expose the patient to potential toxicity.

When repeated doses of a drug are given, tolerance to the drug may arise if they affect its own disposition or response. Enzyme activities can be enhanced, which leads to an increased capacity for metabolism (e.g. patients on chronic therapy with barbiturates metabolise the drugs more rapidly than patients who have not previously taken the drugs). Alternatively, the receptor sensitivity may be modified so that the effect of a particular concentration of a drug is reduced after chronic use (e.g. the sedative effects of benzodiazepines).

Increasing tolerance results in a progressively decreasing drug effect, and the need for an increased dose; habituation and addiction may be the final clinical outcome. Thus, addicts can tolerate doses of morphine that might be considered toxic or even fatal in non-addicts. Similarly, rapidly developing tolerance to the sedative effects of phenobarbital is a common feature of prolonged therapy with the drug. Epileptic patients treated with phenobarbital are often free from any adverse effects despite having blood drug concentrations normally associated with serious toxicity in patients not accustomed to taking the drug.

Tolerance invariably extends the upper limit of the therapeutic range of drugs, and there is a more marked overlap between concentrations associated with different clinical responses. When tolerance is suspected, some of the problems of interpreting data can best be resolved by reference to previous results from the same patient (e.g. results of a therapeutic drug monitoring programme). Unfortunately, in most forensic cases such background information is not available, and in these instances blood concentrations alone are of little value. A more reliable interpretation of analytical data can only be made by comparison of blood concentrations with those measured in urine, bile or liver (where concentrations can be much higher in addicts), and/or by measuring the relative amounts of unchanged drug and its metabolite(s).

Use of pharmacokinetics to predict time and dose

Estimations of the time since last administration and of the dose are frequently required, yet these questions can be extremely difficult to answer from pharmacokinetic data. The reasons derive from factors discussed in previous sections: the large individual variability, possible effects of disease states and injuries, possible effects of other drugs, single or multiple ingestions and assumptions made on the route of administration.

Estimating the time after administration

In any situation requiring the formation of an opinion, it is important to establish the known relevant facts. In this case, it will be essential to determine the likely route of ingestion from the circumstances and clinical or pathological data, the physiological state of the person and their relevant personal characteristics (weight, age and sex), and the likely minimum and maximum time boundaries.

One of the most useful tests to indicate time in fatal poisonings is the measurement of gastric contents and, if possible, bowel contents. This test is easy to perform but must include the whole contents to be useful and must show a mass amount, i.e. milligrams of drug found in the contents. The presence of substantial drug relevant to the dosage form probably indicates oral consumption and, if present in the gastric contents, relatively recent ingestion, i.e. a few hours before death.

Care is needed to avoid over-interpreting these data, since coma and certain other physiological states can lead to reduced gut motility which substantially delays gastric emptying time and drug absorption from the bowel. Furthermore, most drugs are excreted into bile and may be present in measurable amounts in gastric and bowel contents even following intravenous injection. For example, morphine has biliary concentrations some 20–100-fold over those in blood. As a result, submilligram amounts of morphine and morphine conjugates may be excreted into the bowel.

Another measure to establish recency of drug use is the absence of significant amounts of the drug in urine. This is a useful test in cases of diamorphine overdose when death has occurred soon after injection (presence of morphine in blood) and little or no morphine is present in urine (<1 mg/L of total morphine). This indicates that death occurred within several minutes of injection. It is important to realise that the absence of the drug in urine also indicates that there was no use of this drug in the day or two prior to the most recent dose. If a dose was administered in this period, the drug will be present in urine even in a rapid death. Despite these limitations, this test can be useful in a significant number of diamorphine deaths.

When a drug has a relatively rapid rate of metabolism, the relationship between time and drug or metabolite concentrations can help to indicate whether the drug was taken recently or in the more distant past. Diamorphine is rapidly metabolised to morphine via 6-acetylmorphine. Following intravenous injection, neither diamorphine nor 6-acetylmorphine can be detected in postmortem tissues if the survival time is prolonged. Thus, even if only traces of 6-acetylmorphine are detected in a postmortem sample of blood, this indicates intravenous use of diamorphine in the very recent past, or the use of massive doses. No matter how rapidly death occurs, diamorphine itself is rarely detected because of the hydrolytic action of the plasma esterases.

Cannabis provides a similar example. The detection of Δ^9-tetrahydrocannabinol in blood (>2 ng/mL) indicates very recent use of the drug (within 8 h). Further, the concentrations of 11-nor-Δ^9-tetrahydrocannabinol-9-carboxylic acid and its glucuronide increase with time, the ratio of the acid to Δ^9-tetrahydrocannabinol increasing to over 50 after about 3 h. This metabolite can be present in blood for several days, whereas the pharmacological effects only persist for some few hours. If acute use of cannabis is known, then pharmacokinetic modelling can be used to estimate time of ingestion.

Concentration ratios of drug : metabolite or metabolite : metabolite can provide an estimate of the time since ingestion. Unless a drug is very rapidly metabolised (as is the case with diamorphine, cocaine and cannabis), only very low blood concentrations of metabolites are present a short time after a single dose. Consequently, a relatively high drug : metabolite ratio can be expected in cases of very rapid death following acute overdose. Conversely, the presence of significant amounts of metabolite indicate sufficient time has existed for metabolism to occur.

As well as relating drug and metabolite concentrations in the same biological sample, the concentration of the drug in one tissue can be related to a concentration in another. For example, if a fatality occurs shortly after the oral ingestion of a drug, then the liver : blood concentration ratio is higher than if death had occurred after a more prolonged period. In fact, liver concentrations can be more reliable measures of toxicity than blood for compounds subject to significant postmortem redistribution (see above and also Chapter 7), e.g. tricyclic antidepressants, dextropropoxyphene and phenothiazines.

Frequently one may need to estimate a likely dose taken some hours previously to a measured drug concentration. This can be calculated if a reasonable estimate of half-life is available from the equation:

$$C_x = C_t e^{0.693\Delta T/\text{half-life}} \tag{2.10}$$

where C_x is the concentration required at ΔT hours before the measured concentration C_t.

This equation only works if the blood concentration versus time curve is in the elimination part of the pharmacokinetic curve relevant to the half-life of first-order elimination, and if the half-life has not been affected by disease, injuries or saturable metabolism. It is advised that a range of likely half-life data be used to indicate a likely range of blood concentrations. This will give a much more realistic estimate than a point calculation.

For alcohol, this equation does not apply since ethanol elimination is for the most part zero-order, or more accurately obeys Michaelis–Menten kinetics. Michaelis–Menten kinetics is defined by the term:

$$C_t = \frac{K_m R}{(V_{max} - R)} \tag{2.11}$$

where K_m is a constant equal to the plasma concentration at which the rate is one-half of the maximum, R is the rate of metabolism and V_{max} is the maximum rate of metabolism. In practice, the rate of elimination over most of the blood ethanol concentration (BAC) range can be regarded as 0.015 g/100 mL per h, with a common range of 0.010–0.020 g/100 mL per h. Back calculation can be made based on a linear model using the point estimate and the likely extremes (see Chapter 11).

With very high-strength alcoholic beverages, absorption of ethanol is retarded and may take up to 2 hours. Some alcoholics will be able to eliminate alcohol faster than 0.020 g/100 mL per h, and in some individuals at very high BAC microsomal metabolism of alcohol may also occur; this is rarely beyond 0.025 g/100 mL per h, however.

Estimating the dose

The estimation of dose is often helpful to confirm other pieces of evidence or to indicate the possibility of an accidental or suicidal death. As indicated previously, many assumptions need to be made if any realistic calculation is to be performed. Of particular importance is the knowledge whether a single dose has occurred or multiple doses, the overall health of the person and the time elapsed since the last dose.

Measurement of a blood concentration may not always allow the differentiation of multiple therapeutic doses from large accidental or suicidal doses. Thus, long-half-life drugs, such as thioridazine, may show a marked overlap in blood concentrations following multiple doses with those seen in fatal poisonings.

In the same way that drug and metabolite concentrations can be linked to time, they can also be related to dose regimens. Thus, steady-state drug : metabolite concentration ratios are sometimes used to check drug compliance. Also, since the extent of drug metabolism tends to decrease with increasing dose, the ratio of unchanged drug to metabolite will increase with increasing dose. Examination of the relative concentrations of parent drug and its major metabolite(s) in blood, or in other tissues as necessary, can provide useful information on the likely size of the dose administered. Thus, an amitriptyline : nortriptyline concentration ratio of less than 2 is consistent with steady-state drug concentrations following administration of therapeutic doses, while a ratio greater than 2 is more consistent with the ingestion of larger, potentially toxic doses.

When a drug is extensively metabolised, large acute doses can result in metabolic profiles significantly different from those seen after therapeutic doses. Thus, following administration of normal single doses of phenylbutazone, the ratio of the blood concentrations of its major metabolites oxyphenbutazone and 3′-hydroxyphenylbutazone may be as high as 10 : 1. In overdose, the pattern of metabolism can be reversed, giving ratios as low as 1:5.

Similarly, the metabolic profile of diazepam in urine changes dramatically with dose, and the ratio of nordiazepam : oxazepam concentrations may provide useful information regarding the relative size of an ingested dose of the drug. When doses are low, demethylation of diazepam appears to be more important than hydroxylation, while hydroxylation becomes more important at higher doses.

Once tissue drug concentrations or drug : metabolite concentration ratios have established whether an overdose was administered, the actual amount of drug ingested may be estimated. Ideally, the dose should be determined by measuring the total amount of drug remaining in the body (including any unabsorbed drug in the gastrointestinal tract), adding to this the amount that has been metabolised and/or excreted. For obvious reasons, this is rarely possible. A compromise is usually made by estimating the minimum amount of drug ingested. This can be attempted in a number of ways.

Analytical results may be compared with previously recorded data in fatal cases for which drug doses are known. The next best method is the direct comparison of peripheral blood concentrations with clinical data, i.e. blood concentrations following the administration of therapeutic doses. Finally, drug doses can be estimated using pharmacokinetic data.

The half-life of the drug ($t_{1/2}$) and a reasonable estimate of the time elapsed between administration and sampling (t), together with the blood concentration at the time of sampling (C_t), allow the calculation of a theoretical drug concentration at time zero (C_0), which for intravenous administration is

$$\ln C_0 = \ln C_t + 0.693t/t_{1/2} \tag{2.12}$$

This concentration can be used to estimate the dose if the volume of distribution of the drug (V_d) is known (see section on volume of distribution), or it may be compared with clinical data as described above.

This pharmacokinetic approach probably gives a better estimate of the actual dose administered since it takes some account of the amount of drug eliminated. However, pharmacokinetic equations should be interpreted with great caution, especially if relatively accurate survival times are not available and if the kinetic characteristics of the drug following administration of large acute doses are significantly different from those observed following therapeutic doses. In reality, elimination rates of drugs following overdose are invariably slower than with normal doses due to saturation of normal metabolic and excretory mechanisms, or even drug-induced reduction in physiological state. If these formulae are applied, the use of a range of likely pharmacokinetic parameters to estimate a possible range of doses is advised, rather than relying on a point estimate.

Some of these problems can be overcome in a clinical situation if sufficient samples are available to characterise the terminal elimination kinetics of a drug taken in overdose. Such an approach is not possible with postmortem samples and considerably more care needs to be taken when estimating the dose (see Chapter 7).

Identifying the route of administration

The rate at which a drug reaches its site of action is a critical factor governing the duration and the severity of the pharmacological response. If analytical findings are to be interpreted correctly, the route by which a drug is given should, therefore, always be considered. In a case of criminal poisoning it may be essential to establish the route of drug administration in order to corroborate evidence.

In some cases, simple facts give a clear indication of the route. Thus, residual drug in the stomach contents or gastrointestinal tract may point to oral ingestion, a needle mark in the arm suggests intravenous injection, and high concentrations in muscle tissue may point to intramuscular injection. However, in the majority of cases it is not reasonably possible to determine with any certainty the route of administration from toxicological data.

When there is no direct evidence to indicate how the drug entered the body, drug : metabolite concentration ratios can be particularly helpful because rates and pathways of metabolism can vary markedly with the route of administration. Thus, drug : metabolite concentration ratios in the blood are high if a drug is given intravenously, because the drug is not subject to first-pass metabolism. A common example is diazepam. If this drug is given intravenously during emergency procedures, little if any nordiazepam is found in blood, whereas oral dosing always produces significant amount of metabolite.

Concentration ratios can be low where the drug is given by mouth because of first-pass metabolism by the liver. Thus, more than 90% of orally administered fluphenazine is oxidised in the liver before it even reaches the systemic circulation.

The route-dependent variability of drug disposition into tissues may also provide useful information relating to the route of administration. Because of the physiological processes involved, substantially smaller amounts of an intravenously administered drug are partitioned into the liver than when the same drug is given orally. If death results rapidly following a large overdose by intravenous injection, the liver-to-blood drug concentration ratio would therefore be lower than that observed had the drug been given by mouth. Thus, liver : blood ratios of 2.5 and 5.0 have been observed in pentobarbital fatalities involving intravenous and oral administration, respectively, and ratios of 1.3 and 4.2 have been found for intravenous and oral fatalities involving morphine.

Further reading

R. C. Baselt, *Disposition of Toxic Drugs and Chemicals in Man*, 6th edn, Foster City, Biomedical Publications, 2004.

M. J. Ellenhorn, *Medical Toxicology*, 2nd edn, Baltimore, Williams & Wilkins, 1997.

R. E. Ferner, *Forensic Pharmacology*, Oxford, Oxford University Press, 1996.

I. Freckleton and H. Selby, *Expert Evidence*, 5 volumes, Sydney, LBC Information Services, 1993.

M. Gibaldi, *Biopharmaceutics and Clinical Pharmacokinetics*, 4th edn, Philadelphia, Lea & Febiger, 1991.

J. P. Griffin *et al.*, *A Manual of Adverse Drug Interactions*, 4th edn, London, Wright, 1988.

S. Karch, *Drug Abuse Handbook*, 2nd edn, Boca Raton, CRC Press, 2006.

Y. Kwon, *Essential Pharmacokinetics, Pharmacodynamics and Drug Metabolism for Industrial Scientists*, Dordrecht, Kluwer Academic, 2001.

B. Levine, *Principles of Forensic Toxicology*, 2nd edn, Washington DC, AACC Press, 2003.

H. Levy *et al.*, *Metabolic Drug Interactions*, London, Lippincott Williams & Wilkins, 2000.

B. R. Olin (ed.), *Drug Interaction Facts*, 2nd edn, St Louis, J. B. Lippincott, 1990.

G. M. Pacifici and O. Pelkonen (eds), *Interindividual Variability in Human Drug Metabolism: Variability in Drug Metabolism*, London, Taylor & Francis, 2001.

H. P. Rang *et al.*, *Pharmacology*, 6th edn, Edinburgh, Churchill Livingstone, 2007.

W. A. Ritschel and G. L. Kearns, *Handbook of Basic Pharmacokinetics*, 6th edn, Washington DC, American Pharmaceutical Association, 2004.

J. E. Riviere, *Comparative Pharmacokinetics. Principles, Techniques and Applications*, Ames IA, Iowa State University Press, 1999.

L. Shargel *et al.*, *Applied Biopharmaceutics and Pharmacokinetics*, 5th edn, Maidenhead, McGraw-Hill Medical, 2004.

A. Siegel *et al.*, *Encyclopedia of Forensic Science*, London, Academic Press, 2000.

K. Baxter, *Stockley's Drug Interactions*, 8th edn, London, Pharmaceutical Press, 2007.

G. Williams and O. I. Aruoma, *Molecular Drug Metabolism and Toxicology*, London, OICA International, 2000.

T. F. Woolf, *Handbook of Drug Metabolism*, New York, Dekker, 1999.

3

Drugs of abuse

L A King, S D McDermott, S Jickells and A Negrusz

Introduction 43
Commonly abused drugs 44
Analysis of seized drugs. 58
Clandestine laboratories 68
Analysis of the main drugs of abuse. 68
Conclusion 77
References 77

Introduction

Definitions

One definition of the term 'drug of abuse' is any substance that, because of some desirable effect, is used for some purpose other than that intended. The intended use of the substance could be for a therapeutic effect, e.g. as with opiates such as morphine and diamorphine which are used clinically to alleviate severe pain. Some persons find the effect opiates produce pleasurable and hence take the drug (abuse it) for non-therapeutic purposes. Another example of substances being used for a purpose other than that intended is the deliberate inhalation of solvents used in various commercial products. Toluene and xylene are used as solvents in some types of adhesives. Inhalation of the adhesive vapours produces a euphoric effect and hence these types of adhesives are abused, giving rise to the term 'glue-sniffing'.

Another definition of the term 'drug of abuse' is 'any substance the possession or supply of which is restricted by law because of its potential harmful effect on the user'. Such drugs are known as controlled or scheduled substances. They comprise both licit materials (i.e. those manufactured under licence such as morphine, amfetamine, benzodiazepines), the illicit products of clandestine factories (e.g. methamfetamine, methylenedioxymethamfetamine (MDMA), lysergide (LSD), heroin) and some natural products (e.g. cannabis, 'magic mushrooms'). Although many plant-based drugs have been self-administered for thousands of years (e.g. coca leaf, cannabis (marijuana and hashish), opium, peyote cactus), the imposition of criminal sanctions is mostly a product of the 20th century. Many of the drugs currently abused were once not only on open sale but often promoted as beneficial substances by the food and pharmaceutical industries. A pattern developed whereby initial 'misuse' of pharmaceutical products, such as diamorphine, cocaine and amfetamine, led to increasing legal restrictions and the consequent rise of an illicit industry. Nowadays, nearly all serious drug abuse involves illicit products. Most abused drugs fall into just a few pharmacological groups, such as central nervous system (CNS) stimulants, narcotic analgesics, hallucinogens and hypnotics. The most prevalent drugs are still the plant-derived or semisynthetic substances (e.g. cannabis, cocaine and diamorphine), but the view of the United Nations (UN) Office of Drugs and Crime (UNODC) is that wholly synthetic drugs (e.g. amfetamine, methamfetamine, MDMA and related designer drugs) are likely to pose a more significant social problem in the future.

This limited definition of drug abuse excludes those pharmaceutical products that may be misused in the sense that they could lead to accidental or deliberate overdose (e.g. paracetamol and aspirin) or that could contribute to vehicle accidents (e.g. antihistamines) or are banned by sporting organisations (e.g. diuretics). Also excluded are drugs such as alcohol, tobacco and caffeine, which either are foodstuffs, with or without nutritional value, or the use of which is considered socially acceptable in many countries. It also excludes the types of substances involved in glue sniffing as they are typically not controlled substances. According to the World Health Organization (WHO), scheduled drugs are 'abused' rather than 'misused'. Drugs of abuse may or may not lead to physical or psychological 'dependence', a term used by the WHO in preference to 'addiction'.

Legislation

The international laws that cover drugs of abuse are set out in three UN treaties. Substances are listed in the various schedules to the UN Single Convention on Narcotic Drugs (1961), referred to as UN 1961, and the UN Convention on Psychotropic Substances (1971), referred to as UN 1971. Together with the provisions of the UN Convention Against Illicit Traffic in Narcotic Drugs and Psychotropic Substances (1988), these treaties are implemented in domestic law by all signatories, and have been extended considerably in some countries. In the UK the primary legislation is the Misuse of Drugs Act (MDA) (1971) and the Misuse of Drugs Regulations 2001; in the USA it is the Controlled Substances Act (CSA) (1970) and each country, in effect, has its own set of regulations to govern the sale and supply of controlled substances.

Table 3.1 shows the control status of the more common drugs of abuse under international, US and UK legislation. In international and US law, the scheduling of a substance is based on a pharmacological risk assessment. Pragmatic decisions by many countries, and now by the UN itself, to include stereoisomers of 'UN 1971' substances, for example, mean that some scheduled drugs may have little or no abuse potential. In the UK, the criteria for control have been based on a looser concept of propensity to constitute a social problem.

Commonly abused drugs

Amfetamine and methamfetamine

Amfetamine and methamfetamine are indirect sympathomimetic agents giving rise to release of norepinephrine (noradrenaline) and inhibition of monoamine oxidase. Effects via this action result in hypertension, tachycardia, and inhibition of gut motility. It was this last effect that led to their medical use in treating obesity. However, they are also CNS stimulants and their effect on the CNS soon led to these drugs being abused.

Amfetamine (α-methylphenethylamine) and methamfetamine (*N*-methyl-α-methylphenethylamine) (Fig. 3.1) in free-base form are both liquids. Amfetamine is normally produced as amfetamine sulfate, hyddrochloride or phosphate and is more commonly abused in Europe than is methamfetamine. Methamfetamine is normally produced as methamfetamine hydrochloride and is more popular in North America and Japan than is amfetamine.

Street-level amfetamine and methamfetamine are normally submitted to the laboratory as white to off-white powders with relatively low purity (e.g. $<20\%$) but may sometimes occur in tablet form (Fig. 3.1).

Synthesis of amfetamine and methamfetamine

Many methods are available for the illicit synthesis of amfetamine, but the Leuckart reaction has been the most popular. This method is simple, rapid, gives a good yield and does not involve any particularly hazardous chemicals or procedures. It may be considered as a three-step reaction that involves the condensation of

Table 3.1 The control status under international, US and UK legislation of the more common drugs of abuse[a,b]

Drug	UN 1961	UN 1971	USA	UK
Amfetamine	–	(+)2	(+)2	(+)B2
Anabolic steroids	–	–	(+)3	(+)C4
Barbiturates	–	(+)3	(+)3	(+)B3
Benzodiazepines[c]	–	(+)4	(+)4	(+)C4
Cannabinol and cannabinol derivatives†	–	(+)1	(+)1	(+)C1
Cannabis (herbal, resin)	(+)1	–	(+)1	(+)C1
Cocaine	(+)1	–	(+)2	(+)A2
Diamorphine (heroin)	(+)1	–	(+)1	(+)A2
Gamma-hydroxybutyric acid	–	(+)4	(+)1‡	(+)C4
Lysergide	–	(+)1	(+)1	(+)A1
MDMA	–	(+)1	(+)1	(+)A1
Methamfetamine	–	(+)2	(+)2	(+)A2
Phencyclidine	–	(+)2	(+)1	(+)A2
Psilocin/psilocybine	–	(+)1	(+)1	(+)A1

[a] Listed substances are shown as (+) with the appropriate UN Schedule number, or Class in the case of the UK Misuse of Drugs Act and Schedule in the UK Misuse of Drugs Regulations, or the Schedule in the US CSA.

[b] Although legislations vary in detail, the salts, stereoisomers and preparations of most scheduled drugs are also controlled, as are the esters and ethers, where appropriate, of those substances originally listed under UN 1961 Schedule 1.

[c] Flunitrazepam, one of the benzodiazepines, is listed in Schedule 3 of the UN 1971 Convention.

† In the UK Dronabinol is in Schedule 2.

‡ When medically prescribed in the USA, where it is approved for the treatment of narcolepsy, GHB is classified under Schedule III.

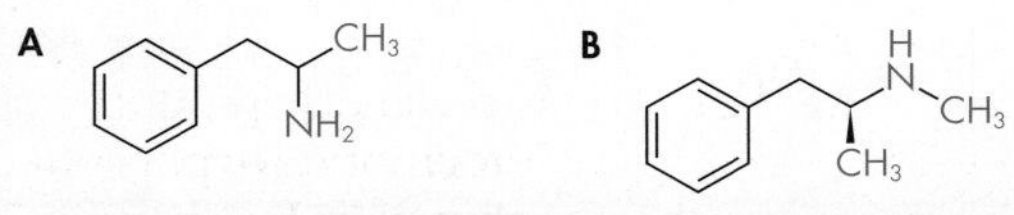

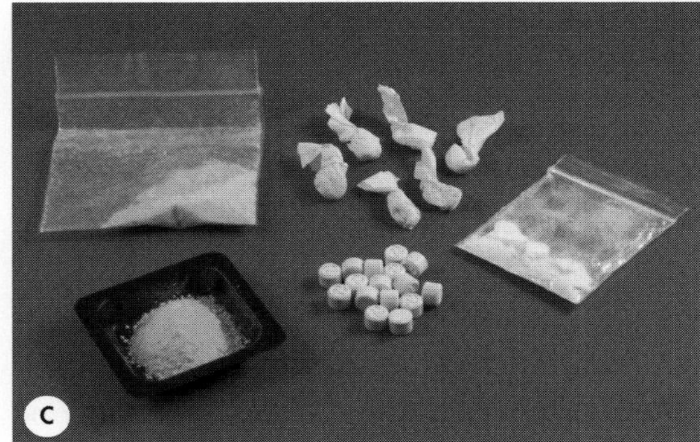

Figure 3.1 (A) Amfetamine and (B) methamfetamine and (C) examples of forms in which these drugs occur.

phenyl-2-propanone (P-2-P) with formamide followed by a hydrolysis of the *N*-formylamfetamine and finally purification by steam distillation (Fig. 3.2).

Methamfetamine can be made by the Leuckart reaction using either methylamine and formic acid or *N*-methylformamide in the condensation step (Fig. 3.2).

Common adulterants for amfetamine include caffeine to increase the stimulant effect and/or to mask low levels of the drug, and sugars (e.g. lactose) used as a diluent.

Amfetamine and methamfetamine have isomeric (enantiomeric) forms. Studies have shown that the *d*-isomer has a more potent effect on the CNS system than the *l*-isomer and that the *d*-isomer is eliminated from the body slightly faster than the *l*-isomer.

Cannabis, cannabis resin and cannabinoids

Herbal cannabis (marijuana) means all parts of the plant *Cannabis sativa* L., but excludes the seeds and mature woody stalk material. *Cannabis sativa* L., which can be grown in all parts of the world, is an annual plant and attains a height of

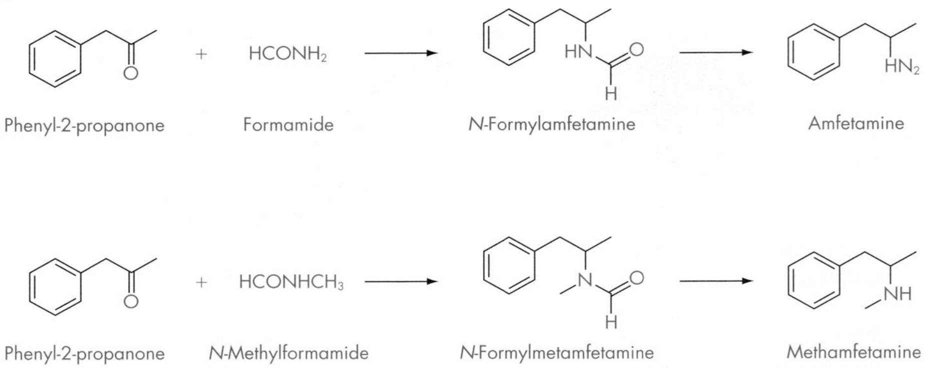

Phenyl-2-propanone + $HCONH_2$ (Formamide) → *N*-Formylamfetamine → Amfetamine (HN_2)

Phenyl-2-propanone + $HCONHCH_3$ (*N*-Methylformamide) → *N*-Formylmetamfetamine → Methamfetamine (NH)

Figure 3.2 Leuckart reaction for the synthesis of amfetamine and methamfetamine.

1 to 5 m (Fig. 3.3). In tropical climates it grows readily outside, but in temperate climates such as the UK cultivation is typically carried out indoors to provide year-round supplies and to ensure good flowering. When it is planted for the production of hemp fibre and hemp oil, the stalks are crowded and without foliage except near the top of the plant. The varieties grown for commercial hemp production are typically selected to be low in cannabinoids – the active substances. The wild-growing plant, in contrast, has numerous branches (Fig. 3.3). The resin of the plant occurs mainly in the flowering area, the leaves and the stem, particularly at the top of the plant. The greatest amount of resin is found in the flowering part. Up to the time of flowering, male and female plants produce resin nearly equally, but after shedding their pollen the male plants soon die. Female plants are selected for illicit cannabis production.

The leaves of *Cannabis sativa* L. are compound and consist of 5 to 11 separate leaflets, each characteristically hair covered, veined and with serrated edges (Fig. 3.3). Under microscopic examination, features characteristic for cannabis may be seen for herbal cannabis and cannabis resin:

- cystolithic hairs
- glandular hairs.

The cystolithic hairs contain a deposit of calcium carbonate at their base (Fig. 3.4). These hairs are mostly single cells. The glandular hairs

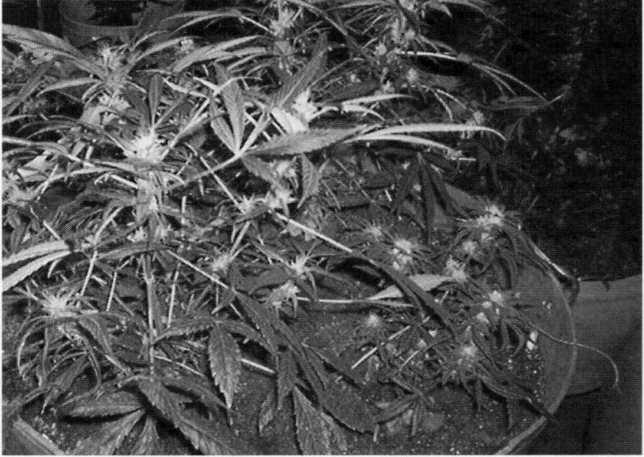

Figure 3.3 Cannabis plants in cultivation. Note the characteristic leaves and the flowering tops which contain the highest proportion of THC. (Photograph: US Drug Enforcement Administration.)

(trichomes) are most important since they contain and secrete the resin. They are short and may be unicellular or multicellular. The larger glandular hairs have a multicellular stalk with heads that contain 8 to 16 cells (Fig. 3.4).

Cannabis herbal material (Fig. 3.5B) may be encountered in blocks of dried flowering tops and dried leaves. Cannabis resin (hashish) is a compressed solid made from the resinous parts of the plant (Fig. 3.5A). It is usually produced in 250 g blocks. Herbal cannabis imported into Europe may originate from West Africa, the Caribbean or South East Asia, but cannabis resin derives largely from either North Africa or Afghanistan. Cannabis has a characteristic odour

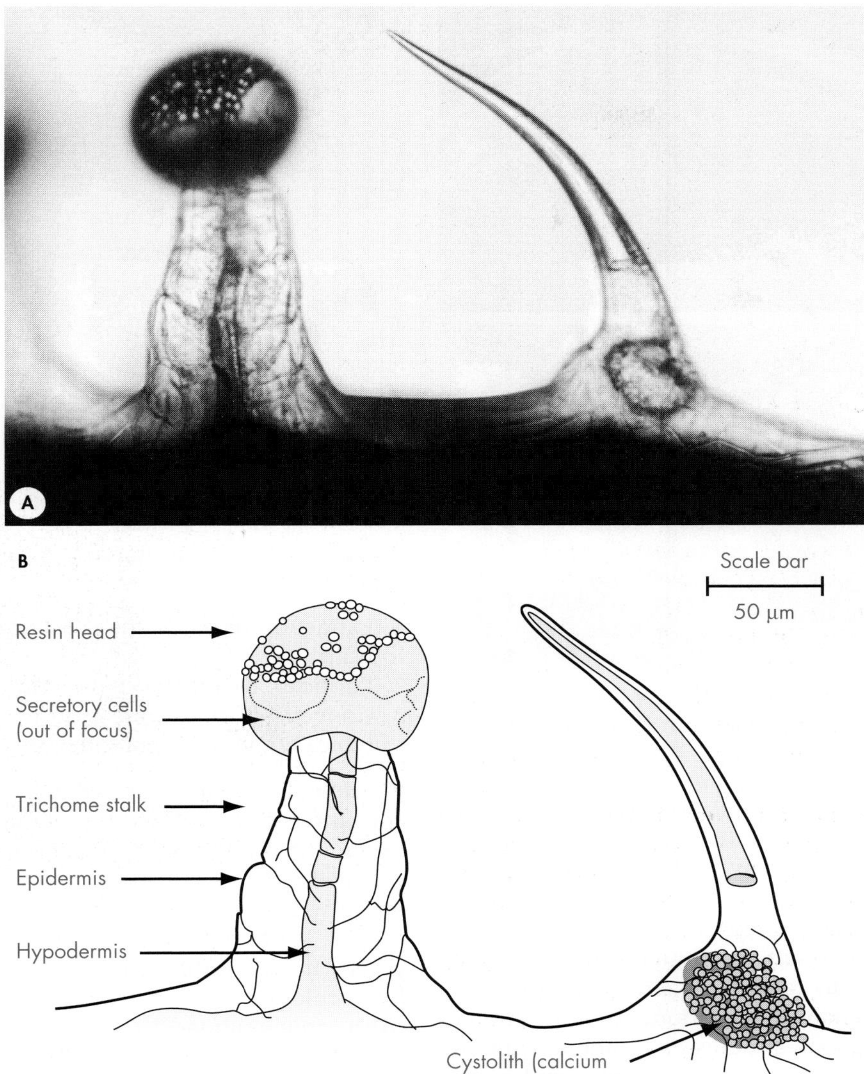

Figure 3.4 (A) Photograph and (B) diagram of a glandular stalked trichome (left) and cystolithic non-glandular trichome (right). (Photo from *The Medicinal Uses of Cannabis and Cannabinoids* p. 26; courtesy of David Potter.)

which can aid in identification of the material. Cannabis and cannabis resin are normally mixed with tobacco and smoked, but can be ingested. The average 'joint' contains around 200 mg of herbal cannabis or cannabis resin. Cannabis oil (hash oil) is an extract of cannabis or cannabis resin and can contain up to 60% of cannabinoids.

The main psychoactive compound in cannabis and cannabis resin is Δ^9-tetrahydrocannabinol (Δ^9-THC) (Fig. 3.6A). Cannabinol (CBN) (Fig. 3.6B) and cannabidiol (CBD) (Fig. 3.6C) are among the other main components. Cannabinol is the major breakdown product of Δ^9-THC and cannabinol is a precursor to Δ^9-THC. The interaction with the active components in cannabis is

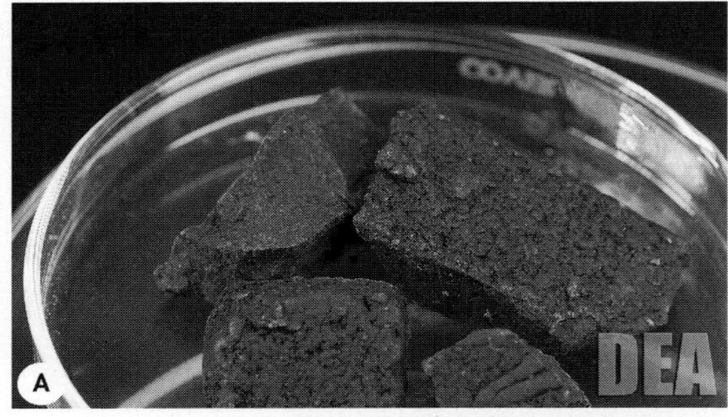

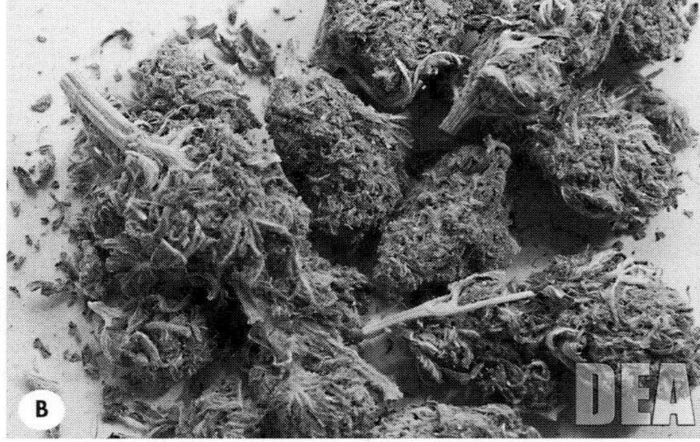

Figure 3.5 (A) Cannabis resin (hashish); (B) herbal cannabis – dried flowering tops. (Photograph: US Drug Enforcement Administration.)

via specific cannabinoid receptors (CB1 receptors in brain, lung, and kidney, and CB2 receptors in the immune system and in haematopoietic cells). These receptors are members of the G-protein-coupled receptors. Binding of THC to the receptor results in inhibition of adenylate cyclase and in calcium channel inhibition and potassium channel activation. Administration of cannabis initially produces a feeling of euphoria and heightened sensory awareness and distortion of time, sound and colour which is followed by a feeling of relaxation.

Cocaine

Cocaine is a naturally occurring alkaloid found in certain varieties of plants of the genus *Erythroxylum*. Coca cultivation is distributed throughout the central and northern Andean Ridge, with approximately 60% in Peru, 30% in Bolivia and the remainder in Columbia, Ecuador, Venezuela, Brazil, Argentina and Panama.

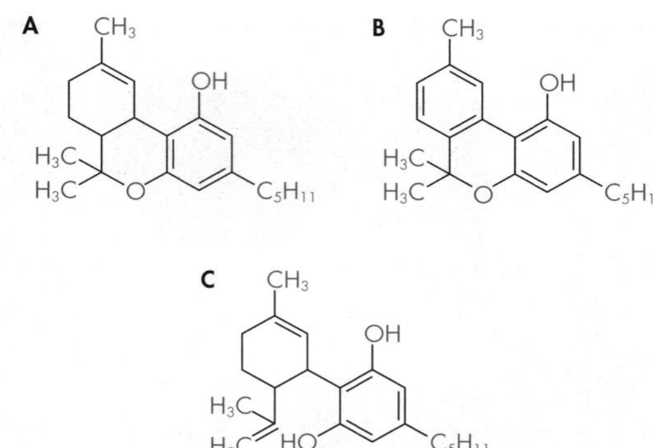

Figure 3.6 (A) Δ^9-Tetrahydrocannabinol; (B) cannabinol; (C) cannabidiol.

Cocaine production

Production of illicit natural cocaine involves three steps:

1. Extraction of crude coca paste from the coca leaf.
2. Purification of the coca paste to cocaine base.
3. Conversion of cocaine base to cocaine salt, typically the hydrochloride salt.

Cocaine (Fig. 3.7) in its salt form is normally encountered as a white or off-white powder (see Figure 3.8a). At 'street' level it is normally supplied in paper wrappers, plastic bags or heat-sealed wraps. The base form of cocaine – 'crack cocaine' – has become more prevalent in recent years. It is readily prepared from cocaine hydrochloride using baking soda and water. It has a more granular texture than the salt form, often occurring as 'rocks' (Fig. 3.8b) which have a slightly waxy appearance.

Cocaine often occurs in high purity. In the UK, examples with purities ranging from 40% to 80% are not uncommon. It is also commonplace for

Figure 3.7 Cocaine.

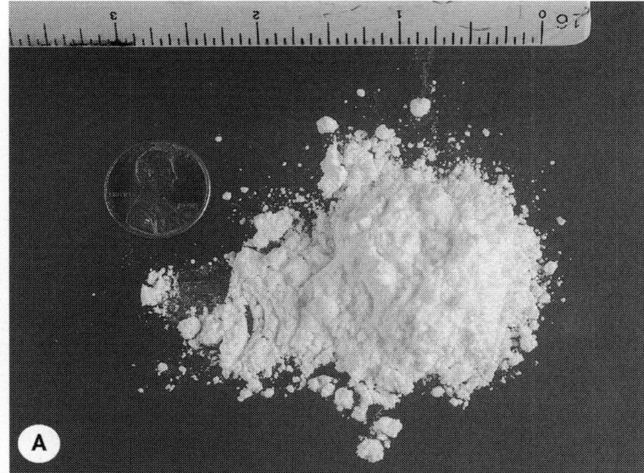

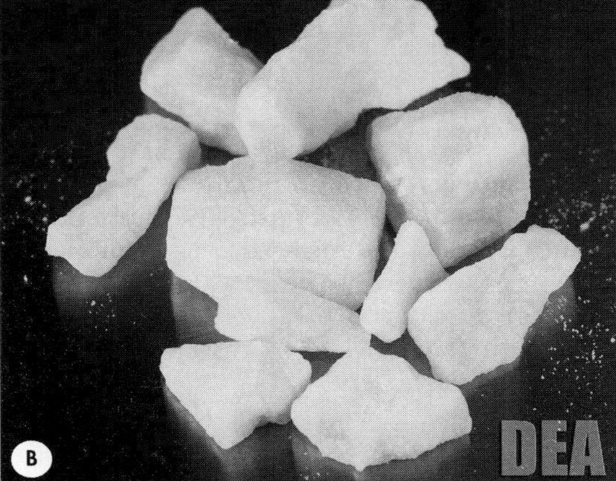

Figure 3.8 (A) Cocaine hydrochloride; (B) crack cocaine. (Photograph: US Drug Enforcement Administration.)

cocaine to be 'cut' with other substances. Cutting agents include sugars such as glucose, mannitol and lactose, caffeine to increase the stimulant properties and/or to mask a reduced drug content, and analgesics such as lidocaine, procaine or benzocaine to mimic the analgesic properties of cocaine.

Cocaine is a local anaesthetic, a vasoconstrictor and a powerful psychostimulant. It is this last action that gives rise to abuse of the drug. Cocaine binds to the dopamine reuptake transporter in the central nervous system, thereby increasing the concentration of dopamine and norepinephrine in the synapses. The result is a feeling of euphoria, garrulousness, and a heightened sense of awareness and pleasure. This is followed by reduced euphoria and anxiousness.

Heroin

Street-level heroin (diamorphine, diacetylmorphine, Fig. 3.9A) is normally encountered in the laboratory in paper or plastic packs that typically contain 100 to 200 mg of brown (or sometimes white) powder (Fig. 3.10A). The street-level purity varies depending on availability and other factors, but values of 40–60% are common in the UK. Bulk shipments of heroin may be packaged as rectangular blocks or in other configurations (Fig. 3.10B)

Cutting agents for heroin include sugars, paracetamol (acetaminophen) and caffeine.

Production of heroin

The raw material for the production of heroin is opium, a naturally occurring product of the plant *Papaver somniferum* L. (opium poppy). The green seed heads are cut to release a milky latex which contains morphine. This latex dries on the seed head to form a gum, which is then collected and bulked as raw opium. The raw opium is treated to extract the morphine (Fig. 3.9B) and the extract is then acetylated with acetic anhydride to produce diamorphine. Opium contains other alkaloids and natural substances which can be carried through to the final product.

Sometimes known as 'Chinese heroin', heroin from South East Asia is a white powder that consists of diamorphine hydrochloride and minor amounts of other opium alkaloids, but

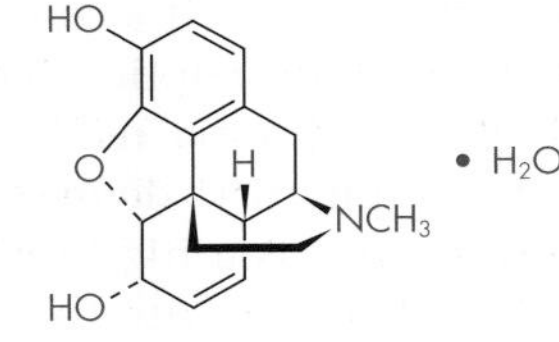

Figure 3.9 (A) Diacetylmorphine (heroin); (B) morphine.

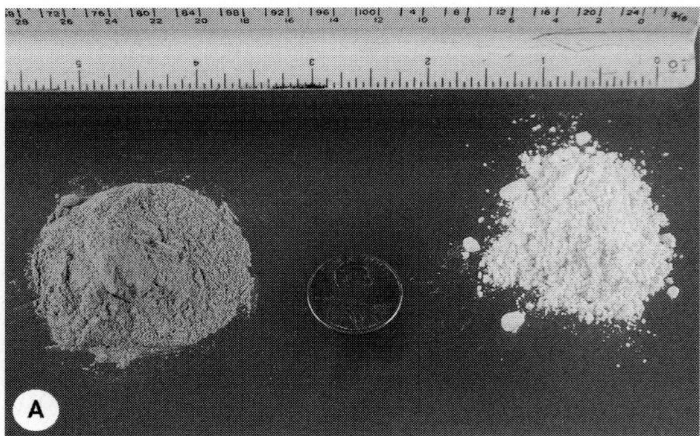

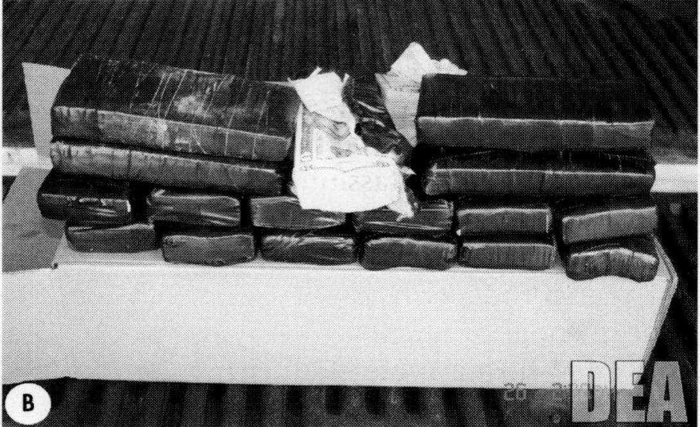

Figure 3.10 Heroin. (A) Examples of heroin powder showing the variety of colour of the material. (B) Compressed form typically used for importation (the blocks shown are wrapped in plastic and overwrapped with tape). (Photograph: US Drug Enforcement Administration.)

adulterants are unusual. This material is ideally suited to injection. Heroin from South West Asia is a much cruder product. Typically seen as a brown powder that contains diamorphine base, it has variable amounts of other opium-derived alkaloids (e.g. monoacetylmorphine, noscapine, papaverine and acetylcodeine) as well as adulterants such as caffeine and paracetamol. It is believed that these cutting agents are added to heroin either at the time of manufacture or during transit.

'Profiling' of heroin is carried out to provide intelligence information. This typically involves identifying and quantifying the various alkaloids together with the active drug and the adulterants.

The action of heroin is via interaction with G protein-coupled opioid receptors in the brain, the brainstem and the spinal chord. Heroin is rapidly metabolised to morphine. Like morphine, heroin is an agonist primarily for the mu (μ) opioid receptor but with some agonist action against kappa (κ) and delta (Δ) receptors. Binding to the receptor closes Ca^{2+} channels on presynaptic nerve terminals, thereby reducing neurotransmitter release. It also opens K^+ channels inhibiting postsynaptic neurons. Effects include analgesia, euphoria, reduction in anxiety, constipation, respiratory depression and pin-point pupils. Heroin is a highly addictive drug. Prolonged use also gives rise to drug tolerance, resulting in higher levels of drug intake required to gain the same pleasurable effects.

Lysergide

Lysergide (Fig. 3.11A), or LSD as it is more commonly known, is one of the most potent hallucinogenic substances known. Its properties were first discovered in the 1930s and its popularity as a drug of abuse was very high during the 1960s and 1970s, when it was associated with the 'hippy' movement.

Synthesis of LSD

LSD can be produced by several different methods, the majority of which use lysergic acid

Figure 3.11 (A) LSD; (B) lysergic acid.

as the starting material. Lysergic acid (Fig. 3.11B) itself is also produced in clandestine laboratories using, most commonly, ergometrine or ergotamine tartrate as the starting material. Reflux of ergotamine with potassium hydroxide solution and hydrazine in an alcohol–water mixture produces lysergic acid.

The methods used for the production of LSD yield a crude product, which is cleaned up and converted into a more stable form (e.g. tartrate salt).

In the past, LSD was encountered in a variety of substrates, including powder in gelatine capsules, gelatine squares, sugar cubes and microdots. Nowadays, LSD is encountered mostly in paper-dose form. The paper dosages are produced by soaking pre-printed paper in a solution of LSD. These sheets are then perforated into squares (typically 5 mm × 5 mm) with each square ('tab') containing approximately 50 μg of LSD.

The designs on the paper can vary from one design per square to one large design that covers many squares (Fig. 3.12).

LSD is an exceedingly potent drug, with doses of about 25–50 μg producing psychological effects such as alterations in perception such that colours, sound, sense of time, etc. appear distorted. LSD acts on various 5-hydroxytryptamine (5-HT; serotonin) receptor subtypes and is thought to act as a 5-HT agonist in the CNS.

Methylenedioxymethamfetamine

Methylenedioxymethamfetamine (MDMA) (Fig. 3.13A) is the prototypical member of a large series of phenethylamine designer drugs and has become one of the main drugs of abuse in many countries in Northern Europe. Clandestine production is centred largely in Europe. A number of homologous compounds with broadly similar effects, such as methylenedioxyamfetamine (MDA) (Fig. 3.13B), MDEA (Fig. 3.13C) and *N*-methyl-1-(1,3-benzodioxol-5-yl)-2-butanamine (MBDB) have also appeared, but have proved less popular. These substances are collectively known as the 'ecstasy' drugs.

MDMA is the most common drug encountered in 'ecstasy' tablets. The tablets are typically 10 mm in diameter, either flat or biconvex, and weigh approximately 200–300 mg. The MDMA content varies, but is generally in the range 30–100 mg per tablet. The tablets normally carry a characteristic logo or imprint. These designs are not restricted to MDMA tablets but may be found on amfetamine and other illicit products. In other words, the logo and other physical characteristics provide no reliable information on the drug content. Many hundreds of different impressions have been found, several examples of which are shown in Figure 3.14.

The main pharmacological effect of MDMA is an increase in secretion and inhibition of re-uptake of serotonin, dopamine and norepinephrine in the brain. MDMA causes euphoria, a feeling of empathy, increased energy and tactile sensation. In some cases MDMA can cause mild stimulation and severe stimulation similar to that of cocaine. MDMA can impair judgement, resulting in dangerous behaviour. The short-term health risks associated with taking MDMA include hypertension, hyperthermia and dehydration, while the main long-term effect includes severe depression due to permanent disruption of serotonin production in the CNS.

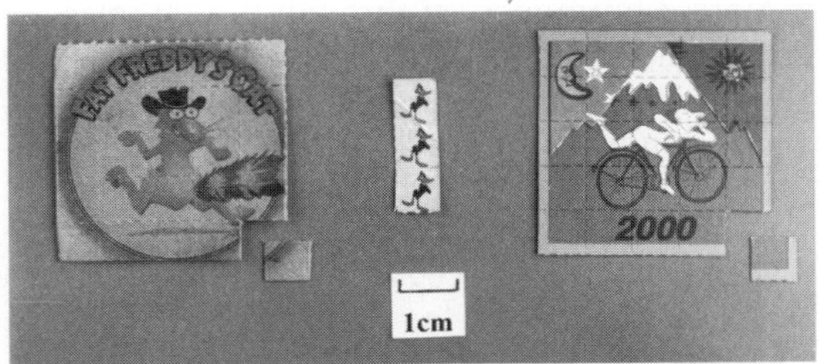

Figure 3.12 Examples of LSD paper squares.

Synthesis of MDMA

Several methods of synthesis can be employed, including:

- an amine displacement method using safrole as the starting material
- a pathway via the intermediate 1-(3,4-methylenedioxyphenyl)-2-propanone (MDP2P) with isosafrole or a nitrostyrene as the starting material (Fig. 3.15).

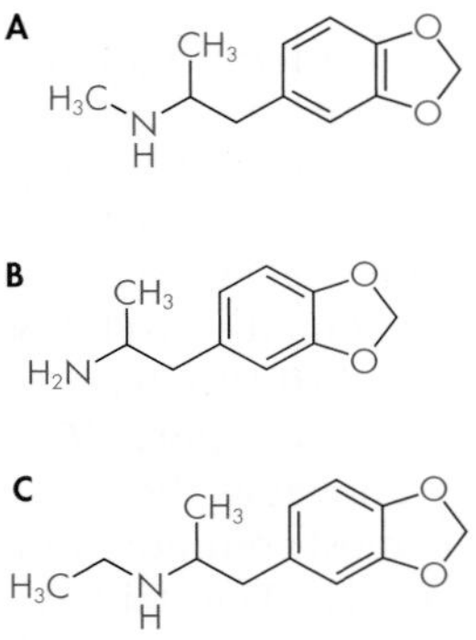

Figure 3.13 (A) Methylenedioxymethamfetamine (MDMA); (B) methylenedioxyamfetamine (MDA); methylenedioxyethylamfetamine (MDEA).

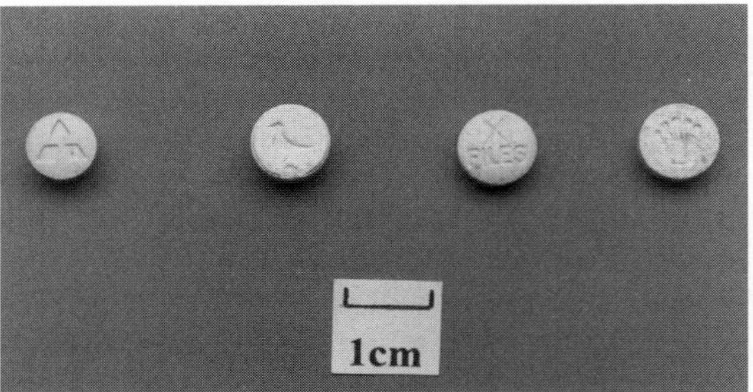

Figure 3.14 Examples of ecstasy tablets showing the different impressions and shapes of illicitly produced tablets. Tablets may be coloured.

Identifying reaction intermediates and by-products can help identify the synthetic route.

Anabolic steroids

Anabolic steroids may be abused by 'body builders' and athletes. In the UK, 48 steroids are listed specifically and generic legislation covers certain derivatives of 17-hydroxyandrostan-3-one or 17-hydroxyestran-3-one. Methanedienone, nandrolone, oxymetholone, stanozolol, and testosterone and its esters account for most cases of abuse (Fig. 3.16). Further nonsteroidal anabolic compounds are also controlled, such as human chorionic gonadotropin (HCG), clenbuterol, nonhuman chorionic gonadotropin, somatotropin, somatrem and somatropin. Certain anabolic steroids are scheduled in the US CSA, but these drugs are not listed in the UN Conventions. A large number of the anabolic steroids encountered in seizures are found in counterfeited packaging and the drug content may differ qualitatively or quantitatively from information on the product label. This mislabelling can be particularly frustrating to the forensic chemist trying to identify the particular steroid in the product. Formulations may be either as tablets (Fig. 3.17) or as steroid esters dissolved in vegetable oil and suitable for injection. The oils may be extracted using hexane–methanol (Chiong *et al.* 1992) with the methanol layer being used for analysis. More recently, scientists involved in doping in sports have noted the use of so-called 'prohormones'. An example is the use of androstenedione, which has been marketed to body builders in dietary supplements and claimed to have an anabolic effect. The majority of studies have not demonstrated an anabolic effect in men taking this substance. However, it has been shown that androstenedione taken by women caused a marked increase in blood testosterone and well above the normal physiological levels of testosterone in females (Kicman *et al.* 2003). This has obvious health implications for women if they take these supplements with potential virilising and other effects. Serum concentrations of oestrogen in men can increase with androstenedione administration, giving rise to an increased risk of gynaecomastia. Boldione is another prohormone marketed in dietary supplements. It is converted to boldenone in the body, an anabolic steroid used in veterinary medicine which is abused by body builders. Androstenedione, boldione and boldenone are included in the World Anti-Doping Agency prohibited list (WADA 2008).

Steroid hormones act through the cytoplasmic steroid hormone receptors which are a part of the nuclear receptor family. Sex hormone receptors include androgen, oestrogen and progesterone receptors. Together with glucocorticoid and mineralocorticoid receptors, they constitute so-called type I receptors. Anabolic steroids produce the following physiological effects: increase in protein synthesis, muscle mass, strength, appetite and bone growth. Anabolic

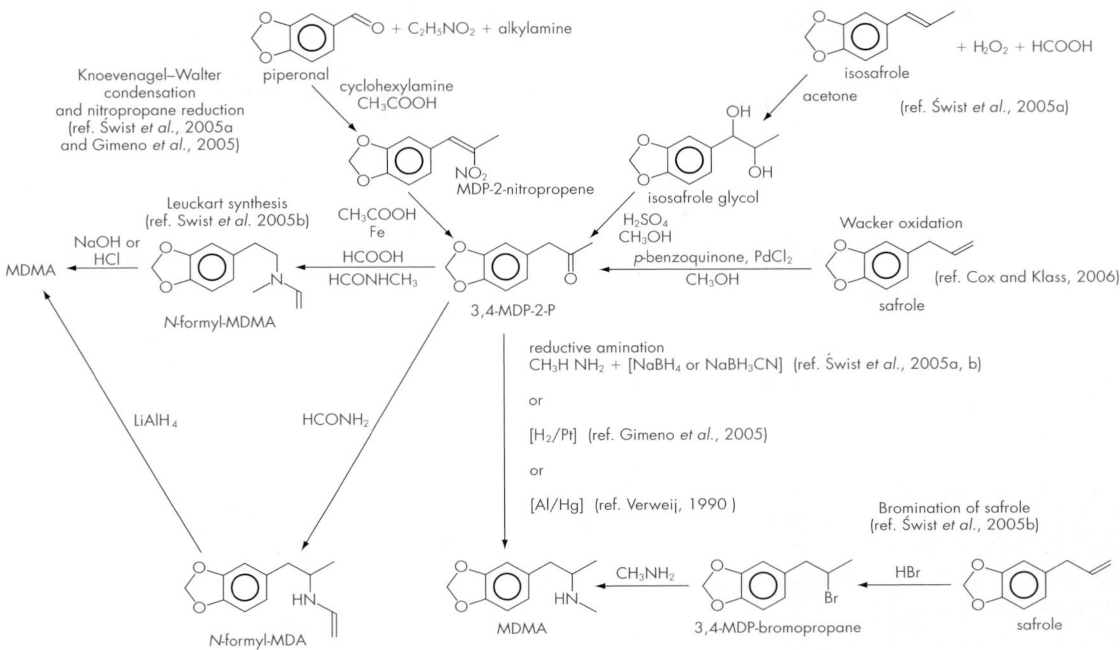

Figure 3.15 Schematic of the main reaction routes used for the synthesis of MDMA. Other routes and variations are possible.

steroids may produce various side-effects such as elevated cholesterol levels, acne, high blood pressure, liver damage and damage to the left ventricle of the heart.

Benzodiazepines

Thirty-four benzodiazepines are listed in Schedule 4 of the UN 1971 Convention. Most are now rarely prescribed and abuse is restricted largely to pharmaceutical preparations that contain diazepam, flunitrazepam, nitrazepam, flurazepam and temazepam (Fig. 3.18). In the US, lorazepam and alprazolam are the benzodiazepines which are typically abused.

Illicit synthesis of benzodiazepines is rare. Instead, the main source of supply is the pharmaceutical product, with persons obtaining prescriptions from several doctors or forging prescriptions, or pharmaceutical supplies being diverted into the illegal market.

Benzodiazepines may be abused in their own right but are commonly abused in conjunction with other drugs, particularly opiates (e.g. diamorphine, methadone) or with alcohol. In some countries, abuse of flunitrazepam has become widespread. This drug has also gained notoriety for its association with 'date rape' or drug-facilitated sexual assault (see Chapter 10). For these reasons, flunitrazepam was moved to Schedule 3 of the UN 1971 Convention and is therefore subject to more stringent controls. Flunitrazepam is banned from use in the US.

Benzodiazepines express their pharmacological activity by binding to the so-called $GABA_A$ receptor which mediates the effect of gamma-aminobutyric acid (GABA), the inhibitory neurotransmitter in the brain. After binding to the receptor, the benzodiazepine locks the $GABA_A$ receptor into a conformation in which the neurotransmitter GABA has higher affinity for the receptor. This increases the frequency of opening of the associated chloride ion channel and causes hyperpolarization of the membrane.

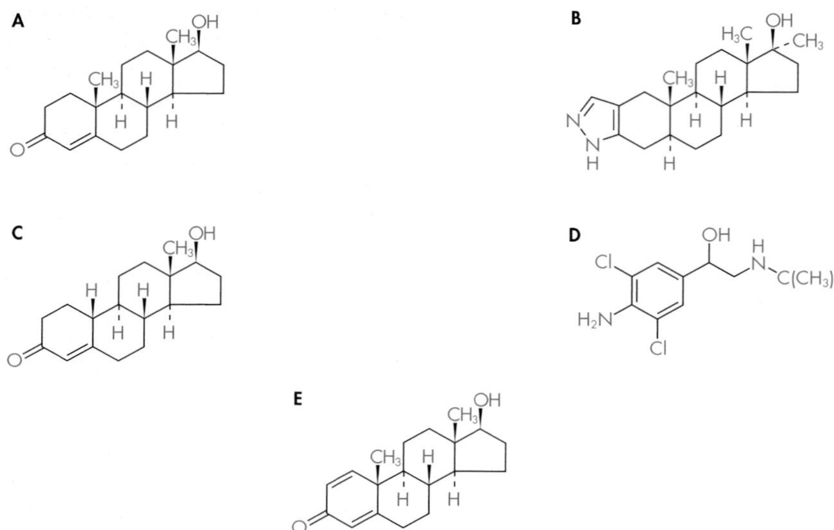

Figure 3.16 Some anabolic steroids which are abused: (A) testosterone, (B) stanozolol, (C) nandrolone, (D) clenbuterol, (E) boldenone.

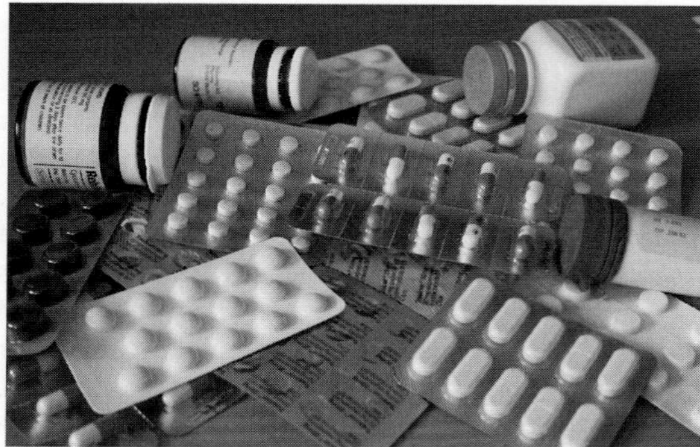

Figure 3.17 Examples of some of the various forms in which anabolic steroids may be encountered. (Photograph courtesy of the Drug Control Centre, King's College London.)

As a result, the inhibitory effect of the available GABA is increased, leading to sedation and other symptoms. In addition, benzodiazepines cause hypnotic, anticonvulsant, muscle relaxant and amnesic effects. All the above pharmacological properties make benzodiazepines useful in treating anxiety, insomnia, agitation, seizures and muscle spasms.

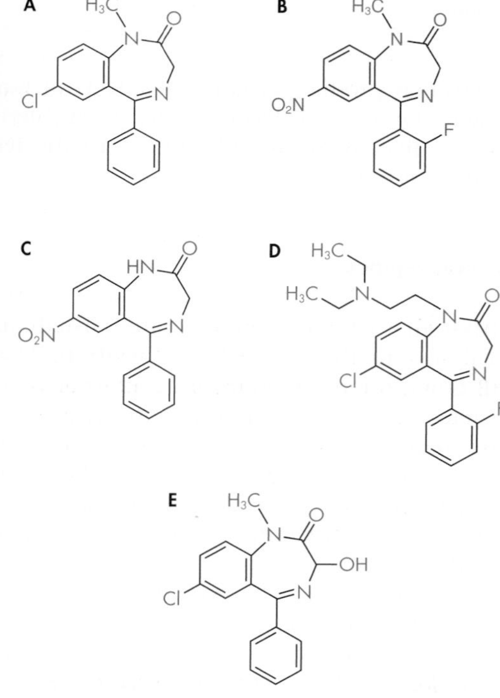

Figure 3.18 (A) Diazepam; (B) flunitrazepam; (C) nitrazepam; (D) flurazepam; (E) temazepam.

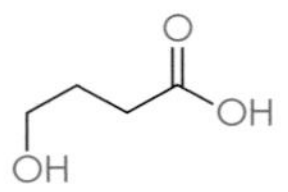

Figure 3.19 Gamma-hydroxybutyric acid (GHB).

Gamma-hydroxybutyric acid and analogues

Gamma-hydroxybutyric acid (GHB) (Fig. 3.19) is a substance endogenously present in the brain. It was originally developed as an anaesthetic drug and is still used for that purpose in some countries. It acts as a CNS depressant and hypnotic and is chemically related to the brain neurotransmitter GABA. It is believed that GHB acts via a so-called 'GHB-receptor' as well as the $GABA_A$ receptor. Synonyms for GHB include sodium oxybate, gamma-OH, Somotomax, 'GBH' and 'liquid ecstasy'.

The effects of GHB have been likened to those produced by alcohol and there are claims that it has anabolic properties. It has gained notoriety for its use in drug-facilitated sexual assault (see Chapter 10). GHB is manufactured easily by adding aqueous sodium hydroxide to gamma-butyrolactone (GBL) to leave a weakly alkaline solution. Not only is the precursor GBL widely used as an industrial solvent, but it can also be ingested directly to produce the same effects as GHB. Although it occurs as a white powder in pure form, illicit GHB is normally sold in solution as a clear liquid in 30 mL opaque plastic bottles. The typical dose is around 10 mL, equivalent to about 1 g or more of GHB. The sodium and potassium salts of GHB are hygroscopic, so GHB is almost never found as a powder or in tablets. GHB is readily soluble and the fact that it is available in liquid form and is odourless and more or less tasteless makes it relatively simple for someone to spike into another person's drink without their notice.

Khat

Catha edulis is a flowering evergreen shrub cultivated in East Africa and the Arabian Peninsula. The leaves and fresh shoots are commonly known as khat, qat or chat. Khat can be used by chewing the leaves or by brewing them as a 'tea'; daily consumption can be up to several hundred grams. It is typically imported into Europe and the US with the stems tied into bundles (Fig. 3.20). Khat has stimulant effects similar to those of amfetamine. Alcoholic extracts (tinctures) of khat have been noted, especially in 'Herbal High' sales outlets and at music festivals.

The active components of khat, cathinone ((S)-2-amino-1-phenyl-1-propanone) and cathine ((+)-norpseudoephedrine) (Fig. 3.21), are usually present at around 0.3–2.0%. Both substances are close chemical relatives of synthetic drugs such as amfetamine and methcathinone. Khat must be used fresh as the more active cathinone begins to deteriorate rapidly after harvesting.

Since cathinone and cathine are closely related to synthetic drugs such as amfetamine, their mechanism of pharmacological activity is similar (see Amfetamine and Methamfetamine and MDMA above). Receptors for 5HT were shown to have an affinity to cathinone, suggesting that the chemical is responsible for feelings of euphoria associated with chewing khat.

Both cathine and cathinone are scheduled under the UN 1971 Convention, but khat itself is only specifically listed in a few jurisdictions. In the US, khat is controlled, but in the UK it is currently not because its use is relatively restricted, being more or less confined to a particular ethnic grouping for whom it has an

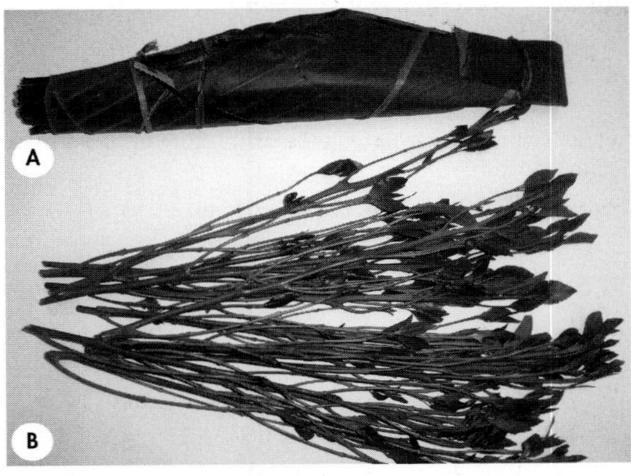

Figure 3.20 (A) Bundles of khat as typically traded and (B) showing leaves, which are chewed.

important social function, rather in the way that tea and coffee do in other populations. Use has not graduated beyond that community to become an abuse problem.

Psilocybe mushrooms

The hallucinogenic substances psilocin and its phosphate ester psilocybin (Fig. 3.22) occur in a number of fungi, particularly those of the genus *Psilocybe*. These are small, brown/grey mushrooms that grow wild over large areas, although they are commonly cultivated under controlled conditions for abuse purposes.

After ingestion, psilocybin is rapidly converted in the body to psilocin, which then acts as an agonist at the 5-HT_{2A} serotonin receptor in the brain where its effect is similar to that of 5-HT. Psilocin is also a 5-HT_{1A} and 5-$HT_{2A/2C}$ agonist.

The control for psilocybin varies between jurisdictions. Until recently in the UK, cultivation and possession of *Psilocybe* was not considered an offence, only the deliberate drying or processing of the mushroom constituted the preparation of a controlled drug. This situation has now changed, with cultivation and possession of *Psilocybe* considered an offence. In the US cultivation and possession of non-dried material are offences.

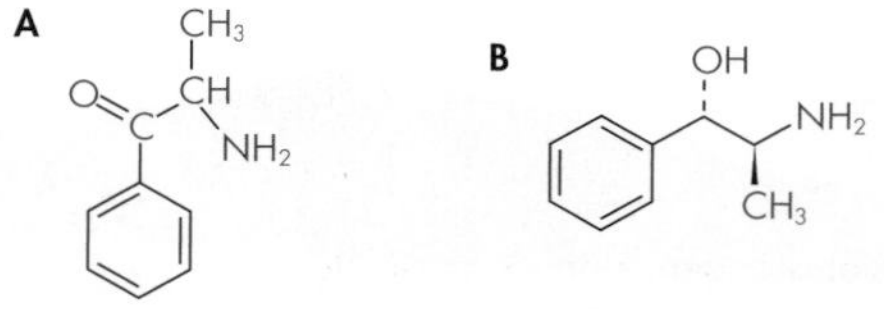

Figure 3.21 (A) Cathinone; (B) cathine.

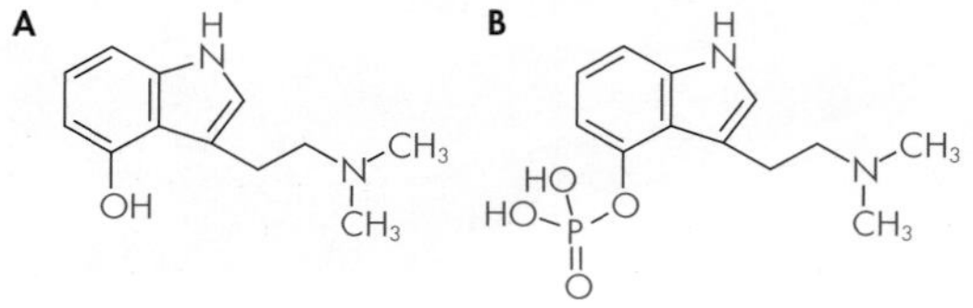

Figure 3.22 (A) Psilocin and (B) psilocybin.

'Designer drugs'

Although a few ring-substituted phenethylamines, such as 4-bromo-2,5-dimethoxyamfetamine (DOB), have been subject to limited abuse since at least the 1960s, it was not until the 1980s that the phenomenon of so-called designer drugs was fully recognised.

Starting in the late 1980s, a large series of designer drugs began to appear, all of which were based on the phenethylamine nucleus. Just as with the production of the major illicit phenethylamines (e.g. MDMA), much of this synthetic activity takes place in Europe.

Table 3.2 lists a number of designer drugs that have appeared in Europe and the US since the mid-1990s. This list, which may not necessarily be complete, shows that the phenethylamines comprise the largest group. Ring-substituted compounds were more common than *N*-substituted homologues without ring-substitution. The substances shown in Table 3.2 have appeared both as powders and as tablets, often manufactured, packaged or marked in such a way that they may appear to the user to be amfetamine or MDMA. Considerable scope exists to develop further series of phenethylamine-related 'designer drugs'. Thus, ring-substituted analogues of cathinone and methcathinone might have MDMA-like activity, while 1-phenylethylamine could also be the parent of novel psychoactive derivatives. Misuse of aryl-substituted piperazines, such as 1-benzylpiperazine (BZP) and *m*-chlorophenylpiperazine (mCPP), has recently increased. mCPP is typically found in combination with MDMA.

Phencyclidine

Phencyclidine (PCP) (street names: Angel Dust, Crystal, Keeler Weed) was synthesised in the early 1900s and tested during World War I as a surgical anaesthetic (Fig. 3.23). It was then patented by Parke-Davis in 1957 under the name Sernyl but was quickly discontinued for human use owing to the side-effects such as delirium, paranoia, hallucinations and euphoria subsequently leading to addiction, and its very long half-life (in plasma 7–46 hours). It was

Table 3.2 Designer drugs reported in Europe and the USA since the mid-1990s[a]

Drug/compound	Acronym	UN/UK
Ring-substituted phenethylamines		
3,4-Methylenedioxyamfetamine	MDA	+/+
3,4-Methylenedioxymethamfetamine	MDMA	+/+
3,4-Methylenedioxyethamfetamine	MDEA	+/+
4-Bromo-2,5-dimethoxyamfetamine	DOB (Bromo-STP)	+/+
4-Methoxyamfetamine	PMA	+/+
N-Hydroxy-MDA	N-OH MDA	+/+
3,4-Methylenedioxypropylamfetamine	MDPA	−/+
N-Methyl-1-(1,3-benzodioxol-5-yl)-2-butanamine	MBDB	−/+
1-(1,3-Benzodioxol-5-yl)-2-butanamine	BDB	−/+
4-Bromo-2,5-dimethoxyphenethylamine	2C-B	+/+
3,4-Methylenedioxydimethamfetamine	MDDM	−/+
2,5-Dimethoxy-4-(*n*)-propylthiophenethylamine	2C-T-7	−/+
4-Allyloxy-3,5-dimethoxyphenethylamine	AL	−/+
3,5-Dimethoxy-4-methylallyloxyphenethylamine	MAL	−/+
N-Hydroxy-MDMA	FLEA	−/+
2,5-Dimethoxy-4-chloroamfetamine	DOC	−/+
4-Methylthioamfetamine	4-MTA	+/+
2,5-Dimethoxy-4-ethylthiophenethylamine	2C-T-2	−/+
4-Methoxy-*N*-methylamfetamine	Me-MA	−/+
6-Chloro-MDMA	–	−/+
N-(4-Ethylthio-2,5-dimethoxyphenethyl)hydroxylamine	HOT-2	−/+
2,5-Dimethoxy-4-iodophenethylamine	2C-I	−/+
4-Methoxy-*N*-ethylamfetamine	–	−/+
***N*-Substituted amfetamines without ring substitution** Control status depends on exact structure		
N-Hydroxyamfetamine	N-OHA	−/+
N,*N*-Dimethylamfetamine	–	−/−
N-Acetylamfetamine	–	−/−
Di-(1-phenylisopropyl)amine	DIPA	−/−
Tryptamines		
N,*N*-Dimethyl-5-methoxytryptamine	5-MeO-DMT	−/+
N,*N*-Di-(*n*)-propyltryptamine	DPT	−/+
4-Acetoxy-*N*,*N*-di-isopropyltryptamine	–	−/−
α-Methyltryptamine	α-MT	−/−
Other phenylalkylamines and miscellaneous Control status depends on exact structure		
1-Phenylethylamine	1-PEA	−/−
N-Methyl-1-phenylethylamine	N-Me-PEA	−/−
4-Methyl-1-phenylethylamine	4-Me-PEA	−/−
1-Phenyl-3-butanamine	–	−/−
N-Benzylpiperazine	BZP	−/−
1-(3-Chlorophenyl) piperazine	mCPP	−/−
Methcathinone	–	+/+

[a] Those substances listed in UN 1971 or that are controlled in the UK by the Misuse of Drugs Act (1971) are shown by (+). In the USA, unscheduled substances may still be deemed to be controlled by virtue of the Controlled Substances Analogue Enforcement Act (1986). The above list is far from exhaustive – many other 'new psychoactive substances' have been reported in Europe in recent years. Further information on some of these can be found in L. A. King and R. Sedefov, Early-warning system on new psychoactive substances, Lisbon, EMCDDA, 2007; ISBN 978-92-9168-281-2.

subsequently manufactured as a veterinary anaesthetic but was discontinued again. In the early 1960s PCP was replaced by ketamine, which is still in use. PCP is an antagonist of the *N*-methyl-D-aspartate (NMDA) ionotropic receptor in the CNS causing an inhibition of de-polarization of neurons and subsequent interferences with cognitive and other functions of the brain. The natural agonist for this receptor is glutamate, which is believed to be a major excitatory neurotransmitter in the brain. In its pure form PCP is a white crystalline powder that readily dissolves in water. Owing to the presence of impurities, the colour of PCP can range from white to dark brown. It is smoked (cigarettes dipped in PCP solution), or taken orally. In the US PCP is currently in Schedule II and is covered as a mandatory drug by the workplace drug testing programmes.

Mescaline

Mescaline (Fig. 3.24) occurs naturally in three major species of cacti: peyote (*Lophophora williamsii*), Peruvian torch cactus (*Echinopsis peruviana*), and San Pedro cactus (*Echinopsis pachanoi*). The drug was first isolated and identified in 1897 by German scientist Arthur Heffter who performed for the first time a controlled mescaline self-administration. The drug was subsequently synthesised in the early 1900s. Similarly to LSD, psilocin or tryptamine, mescaline acts through a G protein-coupled type 5-HT receptor, specifically the 5-HT_{2A} receptor. The drug causes hallucinations, euphoria and many other symptoms. The pharmacologically active dose of pure mescaline in humans is 300–500 mg. In the US mescaline is listed in Schedule I.

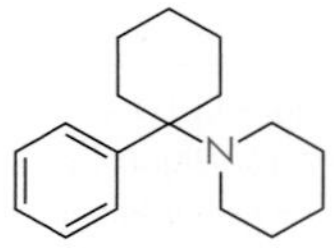

Figure 3.23 Phencyclidine (PCP).

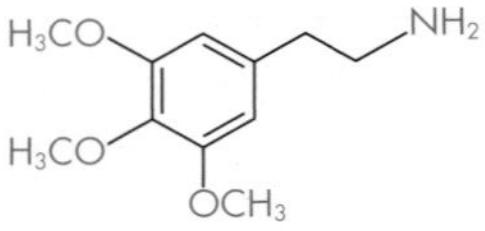

Figure 3.24 Mescaline.

Analysis of seized drugs

Items suspected of containing drugs occur in four principal forms: powders; tablets and capsules; living plants or dried vegetable matter; and liquids. Examples of each have been shown above. Apart from situations in which the analyst has made extracts from clothing or other matrices, drugs encountered in liquid form could include solvents, aqueous solutions (e.g. GHB), injection solutions, alcoholic solutions (e.g. cocaine in liquor) and hash oil, many of which have a characteristic appearance or packaging. Powders are unlikely to show any clear visual clues to their identity and are often presented in paper or plastic wrapping, although when they are imported in bulk the type of packaging and appearance may be characteristic, particularly to the experienced analyst.

Although the analytical approach to each may differ, there are six basic components, not all of which will be needed in every case:

- physical examination
- sampling
- screening
- qualitative analysis
- quantitative analysis
- profiling and/or comparison.

The particular techniques used depend on the available equipment, staff skills and objectives of the analysis, but there are certain minimum criteria that need to be satisfied, particularly when the results are presented as evidence in court. Figure 3.25 outlines the major steps for the analysis of an unknown substance.

Physical examination

A natural starting point in any analytical procedure is the physical examination of the item in

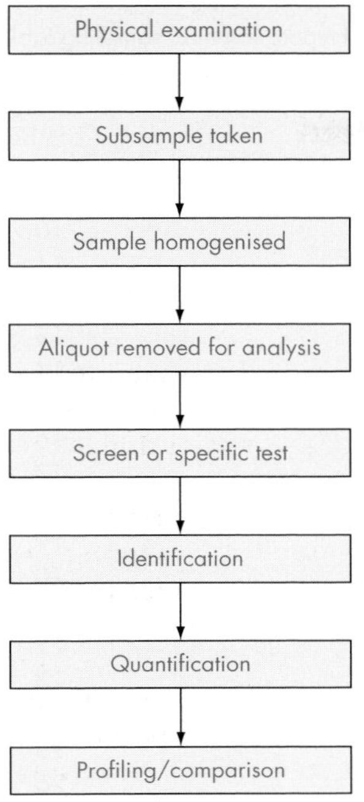

Figure 3.25 Flowchart for the examination of an unknown substance.

question. This may involve making a sketch or taking a photograph of the item. It invariably involves either taking some physical measurements, such as length or diameter, and/or a record of the number of items (e.g. number of tablets or the mass of the item in question). It may involve taking detailed notes on the type of wrapping material present. On many occasions, details such as these can become significant. Wrapping materials themselves can provide important evidence. For example, it may be possible to link seizures using physical fits, chemical composition of the packaging material, specific characteristics of a plastic polymer and marks produced during manufacture.

While the physical appearance of a suspect material can sometimes give an early indication of the possible drug(s) present, it is only after chemical analysis that the full picture can emerge.

Sampling

Drugs submitted to forensic science laboratories can vary enormously in the manner of presentation. One exhibit might be a quantity of ecstasy tablets that are well made and essentially clean to handle, and the next might be packs of diamorphine or cocaine that had been concealed internally by a drug user. The initial approach to each scenario depends on such matters as:

- health and safety
- linking of packaging material
- fingerprint analysis
- other evidence (e.g. DNA).

It is also true that, because of time constraints and costs, not all of the items submitted will be analysed and therefore a sampling policy must be established. The number of items tested is determined by a number of factors, such as the number of items seized, their physical appearance and the need to satisfy a court of law.

Exhibits of controlled substances may be received by forensic laboratories in large numbers, particularly where trafficking shipments have been intercepted (Fig. 3.26), and a representative sampling plan must be established. The benefits of a sampling plan are to:

- reduce the number of analytical determinations
- reduce the overall workload
- decrease exposure to controlled substances
- reduce handling of biologically contaminated evidence.

With any sampling plan, an initial visual examination of all the units in the population is conducted. If all the units are the same in appearance, the population can be considered homogeneous and a sampling plan can be implemented (Clarke and Clark 1990; Frank *et al.* 1991; Tzidony and Ravreby 1992; Colon *et al.* 1993; Aitken 1999). The most frequently used sampling procedures are as follows:

1. Take a sample (n) equal to the square root of the population size (N), that is $n = \sqrt{N}$ (e.g. from a population of 400 take a sample of 20).
2. Take a sample equal to 10% of the population size, that is $n = 0.1N$ (e.g. from a population of 400 take a sample of 40).

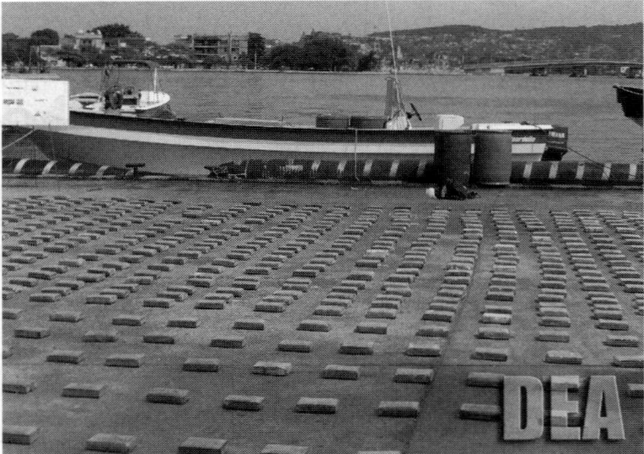

Figure 3.26 Example of a large-scale drug seizure illustrating the potential workload that can arise for a drug laboratory and why a sampling plan may be necessary. (Photograph: US Drug Enforcement Administration.)

Table 3.3 Hypergeometric sampling table[a] (UN 1998)

Total number of items in exhibit	Number of items to be tested
10–12	9
13	10
14	11
15–16	12
17	13
18	14
19–24	15
25–26	16
27	17
28–35	18
36–37	19
38–46	20
47–48	21
49–58	22
59–77	23
78–88	24
89–118	25
119–178	26
179–298	27
299–1600	28
>1600	29

[a] This table was constructed based on a 95% probability that 90% of the exhibit contains the identified compound.

Although experience has shown that the square-root method produces reliable results, it does not provide a statistical foundation to the sampling problem.

Another popular method of sampling is to use a hypergeometric distribution. This procedure involves statistical tables that can be used to determine how many samples should be taken for analysis. Table 3.3 is an example of such a table. If after testing these samples are positive, an inference can be made for the whole population. For example, if 1000 suspect tablets are seized and sent to the laboratory, if 28 tablets are tested and if the tests are positive for MDMA, there is a 95% probability that 90% of the tablets contain MDMA.

In relation to sampling from single items, it is important that a correct sampling procedure be put in place. The principal reason for a sampling procedure is to produce a correct and meaningful chemical analysis. Most methods – qualitative and quantitative – used in forensic science laboratories for the examination of drugs require very small aliquots of the material, so it is vital that these small aliquots be entirely representative of the bulk from which they are drawn.

Because of various legal requirements it may not always be possible to render a sample into a homogeneous state before sampling. This could be the case if the sample has to be tested separately by another laboratory or if the sample in its original 'heterogeneous' state is an important piece of physical evidence.

As a rule, however, items should be in a homogeneous state prior to sampling, which is especially important in quantitative analysis. This may involve a simple grinding of a small amount of powder (or tablet) in a mortar and pestle, or may involve taking numerous samples from a larger quantity of powder and grinding them together.

Screening tests

Colour and/or spot tests give a valuable indication of the content of any particular item tested, but it is stressed that positive results to colour tests are only presumptive indications of the possible presence of the drug. They must be followed up by other tests which offer confirmation of the presence of a drug. Colour tests have the advantage that they are rapid and inexpensive and unskilled operators can use them as field tests, with the obvious need for follow-up analyses in the laboratory. For example, they could be used at customs to give an indication as to whether a suspicious substance is likely to be a controlled drug or not. One of the most important and widely used colour tests is the Marquis reagent test. Opiates, including heroin, give a purple colour in response to the test. Amfetamine and methamfetamine give an orange-red colour. Other useful tests are the Van Urk test for LSD and the cobalt thiocyanate test for cocaine. Details of these and other useful colour tests are given in Chapter 13.

Another important screen is thin-layer chromatography (TLC; see Chapter 13). It has many advantages as an analytical and/or screening tool. It is quick, easy to use, has a low cost, is relatively sensitive and can give a good degree of discrimination. A wide variety of solvent systems are available (Moffat *et al.* 2004, and Table 3.4 below) but the following solvent systems are suitable for many drugs:

- methanol–strong ammonia solution (100:1.5 v/v)
- cyclohexane–toluene–diethylamine (75:15:10 v/v).

Visualisation of many of the drugs may be achieved by a variety of methods (see Chapter 13); however, spraying with acidified potassium iodoplatinate reagent is suitable for many drugs.

A variety of immunoassay-based test kits are available for screening for drugs. These have the advantage of avoiding the use of hazardous chemicals, are simple to use and offer a quick test result with good drug specificity, but can be expensive on a per test basis compared with some of the simpler colour tests.

Qualitative analysis

Gas chromatography and mass spectrometry

Using capillary gas chromatography (GC) (operated under a suitable temperature programme), coupled to a mass spectrometer (GC-MS) (see Chapter 21) the drug components of most samples can be separated and identified. The reduced capital outlay now required for such instruments means that it is not uncommon for laboratories to have several instruments working with automatic samplers enabling GC-MS analysis on a 24-hour basis. The use of GC-MS has become the routine method of identification of most drugs. A general GC-MS screen method can be used to separate and/or identify most of the drugs encountered in exhibits. Figure 3.27 shows the separation achieved of a mixture of the main drugs described here using a general screen method. There are literally dozens of GC methods available for the analysis of drugs of abuse and interested readers should consult Moffat *et. al.* (2004) for further details.

Identification of the various components of a suspect mixture can be made with a search of commercial libraries, but it is important to run a standard of the specific drug being tested (e.g. standard diamorphine). This obviously needs to give a retention time and mass-spectral match.

High-performance liquid chromatography

High-performance liquid chromatography (HPLC; see Chapter 19) is a simple and reliable method of analysis for most drugs. Operated correctly, it is both accurate and precise and thus lends itself to quantitative analysis. It is especially useful for compounds that are thermally labile. HPLC has some advantages over GC because of the variety and combinations of mobile phases that can be chosen. There is also a choice of detectors available for specific applications. HPLC can, however, involve significantly more method development than GC, which is capable of resolving a greater number of substances.

No single system is suitable for the optimum separation of all the different drug types, so different systems are used to give optimum separations for specific analysis. The system that is best for the separation of heroin–acetylcodeine–noscapine–papaverine (Huizer 1983) is not the same as the one that separates cocaine from its impurities and processing by-products (Moore and Casale 1994).

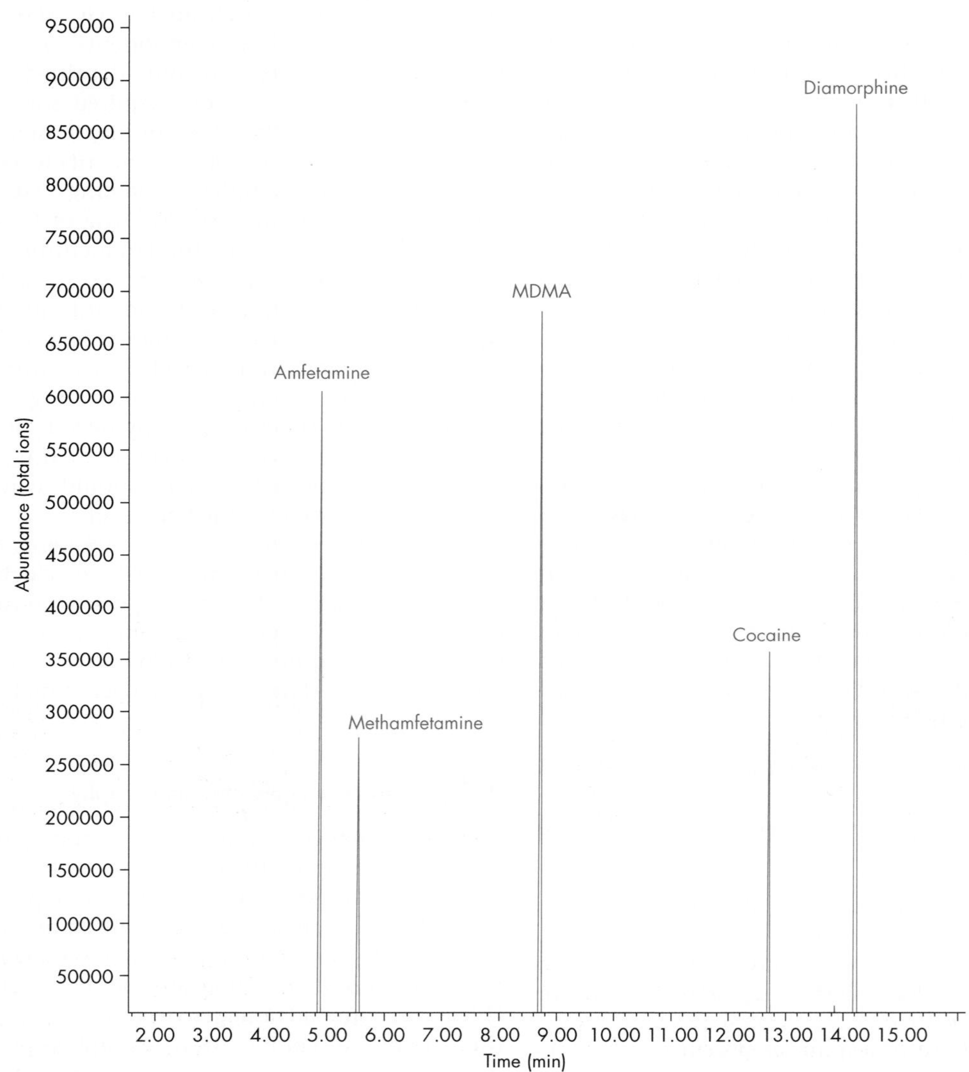

Figure 3.27 Gas chromatographic separation on an HP Ultra-1 (cross-linked methylsiloxane) capillary column (12.5 m × 0.2 mm × 0.33 μm phase thickness). He carrier gas at 1 mL/min; 50:1 split ratio; temperature programme 60°C for 2 min, then 15°C/min to 180°C, then 25°C/min to 290°C and hold 3 min. Mass spectrometer operated in electron-impact mode, scanning from 40 to 550 amu (S. D. McDermott, unpublished information.)

A general screen method can be used for the separation of heroin, cocaine, amfetamine and methamfetamine (Fig. 3.28). The reader is referred to Moffat *et al.* (2004) for further details of HPLC systems that can be used for the analysis of drugs of abuse.

Using the chromatographic conditions shown in Figure 3.28, methamfetamine and MDMA co-elute. However, by changing the relative proportions of the acetonitrile–triethylammonium phosphate buffer mobile phase and reducing the flow rate, amfetamine, methamfetamine,

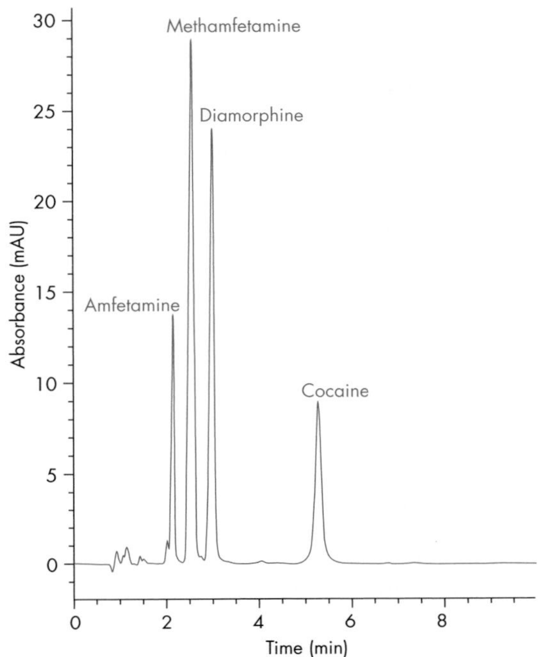

Figure 3.28 HPLC analysis of amfetamine, methamfetamine, diamorphine and cocaine on Spherisorb ODS-1 (150 mm × 4.6 mm) at 30°C. Mobile phase: acetonitrile–triethylammonium phosphate buffer (pH 2.5) (50:50 v/v) at 1.5 mL/min. Note that methamfetamine and MDMA co-elute on this system.

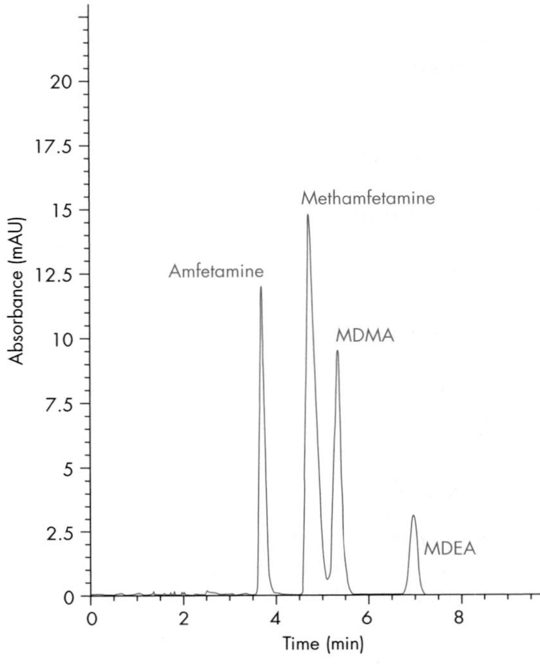

Figure 3.29 HPLC analysis of amfetamine, methamfetamine, MDMA and MDEA on Spherisorb ODS-1 (150 mm × 4.6 mm) at 30°C. Mobile phase: acetonitrile–triethylammonium phosphate buffer (pH 2.5) (20:80 v/v) at 1.0 mL/min. Note that methamfetamine and MDMA are resolved on this system.

MDMA and MDEA can be separated (Fig. 3.29). This illustrates the versatility of HPLC – separations can be made between compounds that co-elute by altering the elution system.

A system such as the above could be used for screening purposes, but identification of substances necessitates a spectroscopic method, such as MS or infrared (IR) spectroscopy.

Fourier transform infrared spectroscopy

Most modern laboratories are now equipped with Fourier transform IR (FTIR) spectrophotometers (see Chapter 16), which have many advantages over traditional IR instruments. They are faster and can work with smaller samples (when coupled with a microscope, tiny samples can be analysed). The difficulty with IR analysis of drug samples is the presence of other material that interferes with the spectrum. These interfering compounds could be other drugs that occur naturally in the samples (or from the synthetic process) or adulterants, such as caffeine and paracetamol (acetaminophen). IR analysis can, however, give valuable information on chemicals that are not suitable for GC-MS analysis.

Another popular technique is GC-FTIR, because the speed of scanning of the FTIR instrument means it can be used to obtain a spectrum of compounds that have been separated by GC. Like GC-MS, this can provide confirmation of drug identity.

In practice, neither spectra nor pure reference samples may be available for comparison for the more unusual substances which can occur in drug samples. In such situations, nuclear magnetic resonance (NMR) spectroscopy may be the method of choice.

Quantitative analysis

For most controlled drugs there are no minimum quantities below which an offence does not occur. The quantitative analysis of drugs is therefore not carried out routinely on all exhibits. The main reason for determining the purity and/or drug content of powders and tablets is to enable a court to establish a monetary value of the seizure, or when sentencing structures are based on equivalent pure-drug content. In some countries, the death sentence can result if a person is convicted of possession and/or supply of more than a specified quantity of a substance. Hence an accurate identification and quantification of the controlled substance is crucial because it literally can mean life or death. In some situations, information on drug purity is used for intelligence purposes, such as to assess trends in the illicit drug market or for use in drug comparison and profiling, and so quantification of active drug is required.

The powder having already been identified as, for example, diamorphine, quantitative analysis may be carried out on a GC or HPLC instrument. In performing quantitative analysis, it is always desirable to include an internal standard in the analysis (see Chapter 19). This has the advantages of being easy to use, giving increased accuracy and no need for measuring the injection volume, enabling the easier determination of reproducibility and of serving as a possible monitor for the GC or HPLC system's performance.

Important factors to consider when selecting an internal standard are that the substance chosen must be absent from the sample, must be readily available (and not too costly), must be pure, should not react with the analyte or sample matrix, should show good chromatographic behaviour and should be soluble in the solvent used. Internal standards chemically related to the compound being analysed are preferable as they behave similarly. Straight-chain hydrocarbons are often used for GC as internal standards because they elute as a homologous series and hence can provide accurate relative retention time data, although it should be recognised that they are typically rather dissimilar chemically to the compound being analysed.

In a general approach to quantification by GC, the conditions given for qualitative analysis can be used. A standard calibration line is established by preparing up to five standard solutions of the drug to be quantified. A range from 1 mg/mL to 5 mg/mL is typically prepared using a solvent that contains the internal standard. A concentration of internal standard of 0.5 mg/mL or 1 mg/mL is normally adequate. A test sample is prepared so that it has a concentration between 1 mg/mL and 5 mg/mL (i.e. within the range of the calibration set). If, after analysis, the test sample is found to be outside the range of the calibration standards, a second sample is prepared based on the information from the first sample, for example taking a smaller or larger sample mass, adding more or less solvent for extraction, and so on. Extrapolation of the calibration line beyond the actual concentration range analysed to determine the concentration of drug in the sample is poor scientific practice and is not acceptable for legal purposes.

In general, it is suggested that at least two samples of the powder to be tested are taken for quantitative analysis and an average of these used as the true result. The amount of the drug in the test sample can then usually be calculated using the data-analysis function of the instrument.

Both GC and HPLC are used extensively for quantitative analysis and it is useful, for a given drug, to compare the results obtained by one method with those from the other. Use of both techniques is particularly useful when establishing and validating a new method because samples can be analysed by the established method and the new method to check that they give the same results. Ideally, a certified reference material (CRM) with a known and agreed result can be used for quality control (QC) purposes.

This can be analysed alongside seized samples. If the CRM material gives the expected result, this gives a greater degree of confidence in the results for the seized samples. CRMs can be expensive and are not available for many drugs or adulterants. Laboratories can set up their own 'in-house' reference materials for QC purposes.

Profiling and comparison

A more detailed analysis of drug samples can be used to provide 'collective' information. This is generally called profiling when it involves the chemical analysis of powders, but is known as characterisation when the physical properties of tablets and other dosage forms are measured (see also Chapter 12). Chemical profiling has been the technique used most widely and is often based on the chromatographic separation of impurities and precursors (as in the case of amfetamine and methamfetamine) or other naturally occurring components and adulterants (e.g. diamorphine, cocaine, cannabis resin). Detection may range from GC with flame-ionisation (see Chapter 18) to isotope-ratio MS. Non-separation methods, for example using IR, Raman, X-ray fluorescence (XRF) spectroscopy or X-ray diffraction (XRD) spectroscopy, have only limited scope for identifying individual components in a drug sample because other substances present will also be detected by these techniques, giving rise to spectra which are difficult to interpret.

Drug profiling may be used for two quite separate purposes. In the first case, it can establish connections between a number of exhibits suspected to be linked as part of a local distribution chain. This is known as comparison or tactical profiling, and may be carried out as a routine requirement in forensic casework. There is a second stage (intelligence or strategic profiling) in which answers to wider questions may be sought. These depend on the drug concerned, but include:

- estimating the number of different profile-types in circulation and relating them to the number of active laboratories and the period for which they have been in operation
- determining the extent of importation by comparing the profiles of police and customs seizures
- identifying the route of synthesis and types of precursors used
- creating large-scale maps of drug distribution and identifying the country or region of origin.

Figure 3.30 illustrates how analysis can be used to identify region of origin. Ehleringer *et al.* (2000) used isotope ratio mass spectrometry (IRMS) (Fig. 3.31) to determine the carbon ($\delta^{13}C$) and nitrogen ($\delta^{15}N$) isotope-ratio signatures of 200 samples of coca leaves from the five primary coca growing regions of Bolivia, Columbia and Peru. They then combined these data with information on the trace alkaloids truxilline and trimethoxycocaine and $\delta^{13}C$ and $\delta^{15}N$ ratios in cocaine samples extracted from the coca leaves. This enabled them to predict correctly the country of origin of 96% of the coca samples (Fig. 3.30).

Tablet comparisons using general physical features, gross drug content and microscopic examination of defects and punch marks (so-called ballistic analysis) can be of some value, but they suffer because at any one time a large fraction of illicit tablets in circulation may be almost identical. Such small differences as may exist could simply reflect inherent differences in the punches and dies of a multiple-stage tableting machine. This is illustrated by the Mitsubishi logo (Fig. 3.14), which was found on over half of all tablets seized in Europe in the late 1990s. A similar pattern was also found in the UK for amfetamine in the early 1990s, when nearly half of all samples belonged to one profile type. In these circumstances, any connection between two separate seizures of otherwise identical tablets or powders may be purely fortuitous.

This, in turn, raises other problems with profiling. It is necessary to maintain a database of profiles such that the significance of any 'match' or 'non-match' can be assessed critically. However, for a situation in which profiles may

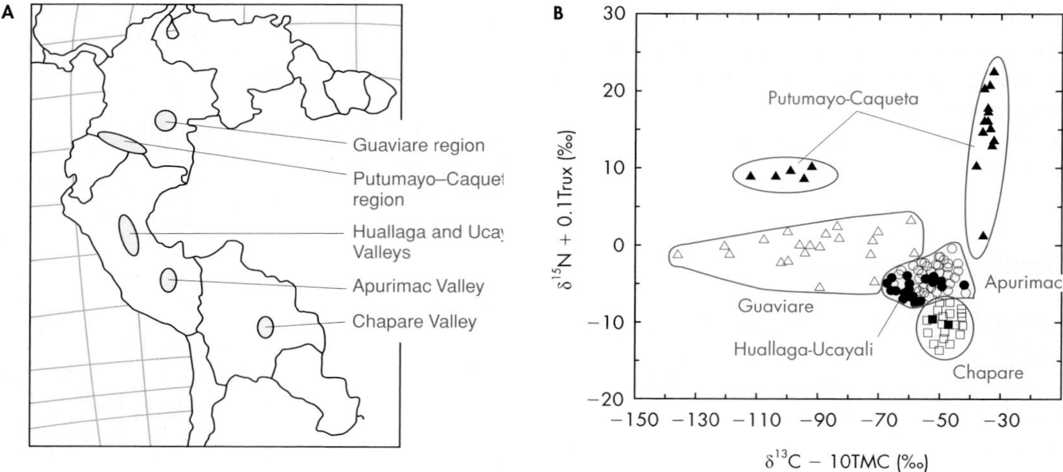

Figure 3.30 Isotope ratio mass spectrometry has been used to identify the geographic origin of illicit cocaine. (A) Regions producing illicit cocaine. (B) Identification of cocaine-growing regions based on a combined model derived from carbon- and nitrogen-isotope ratios as well as abundance of minor alkaloid components: squares, Bolivia; triangles, Colombia; circles, Peru. Regions within a country are distinguished by solid and open symbols. Trux, truxilline; TMC, trimethoxycocaine. Isotope ratios are expressed as $(R_{sample}/R_{standard} - 1) \times 1000$ ppt, where R is the molar ratio of heavy-to-light stable isotope; standards for carbon and nitrogen are PDB and air, respectively. (Reprinted by permission from Macmillan Publishers Ltd (Nature Publishing Group) from Ehleringer J, Casale J, Lott M and Ford V, Tracing the geographical origin of cocaine. *Nature* **408** 311–312; copyright (16 Nov. 2000).

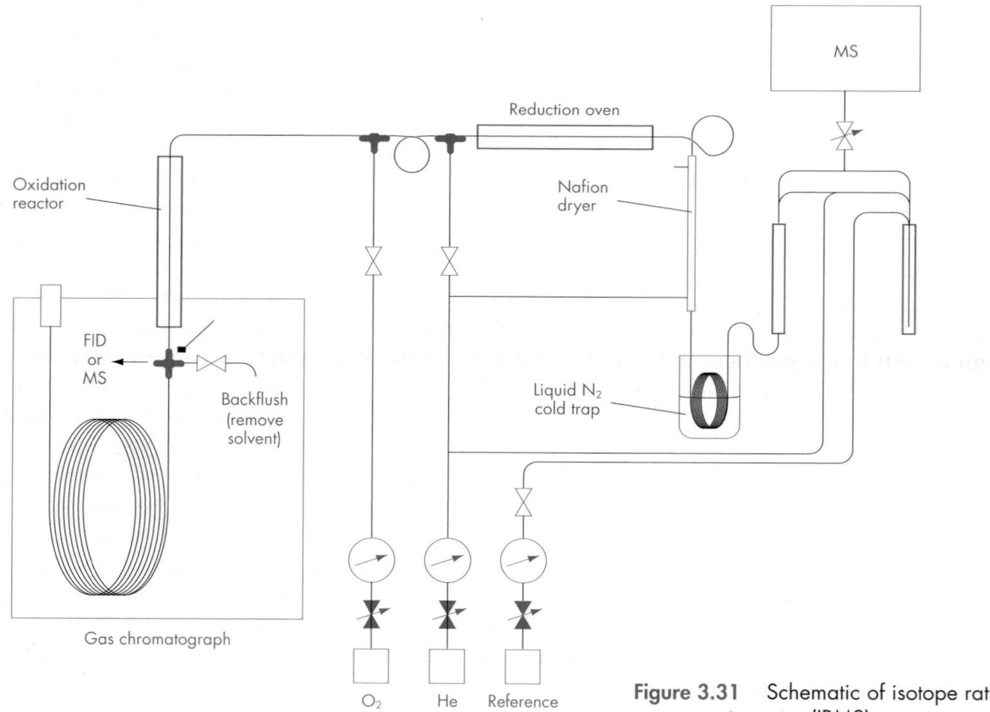

Figure 3.31 Schematic of isotope ratio mass spectrometer (IRMS).

change with time, what constitutes a 'current' database is not always clear. In the case of determination of country of origin, authentic samples are required to provide a statistical 'training set', yet such samples may be difficult to obtain and their true provenance uncertain.

A general approach to the analysis of unknown substances

A general approach to the analysis of unknown substances is outlined in Fig. 3.25. A different approach is required depending on whether the exhibit is a powder, vegetable matter, tablet/capsule or liquid.

Powders

When a powder is submitted for analysis, the most likely drugs to be present include diamorphine, cocaine, amfetamine, methamfetamine and 'ecstacy'. For crack cocaine, the sample may appear as 'rocks' rather than powder (Fig. 3.8). The initial examination involves describing and/or detailing the packaging material. If there are multiple packs present, a subsample of the drug sample may be removed for analysis. The powder must be weighed before analysis.

The powder is then homogenised and an aliquot is taken for analysis. A screen (colour test, immunoassay test kit, TLC, HPLC, GC) will indicate the drug(s) present. Identification of the drug can be achieved using GC-MS or FTIR. GC-MS has an advantage over FTIR because of retention time and a mass-spectral comparison with a known standard. Identification of the other components in the powder can be achieved using a range of analytical techniques, including FTIR, XRF, XRD and NMR spectroscopies and others.

The drug content can be quantified by GC or HPLC through the preparation of a calibration line using a range of concentrations of the drug in question (see section on quantitative analysis above). In some circumstances, comparison may be required between powders to establish links in a specific case or for intelligence purposes (see section on profiling and comparison above), and GC and HPLC can be employed to examine some of the minor ingredients of the powder.

Vegetable material

Vegetable material includes cannabis plants, herbal cannabis, cannabis resin, khat, psilocybe mushrooms and, occasionally, coca leaves. A physical examination includes a description of the material followed by a measurement of the mass of material or the height of the plant. A subsample of the sample population may be chosen and an aliquot taken for analysis. Homogenisation may be necessary, depending on the material. The physical appearance generally gives a very good idea of the drug present (e.g. cannabis plant or psilocybe mushrooms). It is therefore possible to go directly to a specific test rather than use a screening technique. Identification can be carried out by a combination of microscopic and chemical techniques.

The drug content can be quantified by GC or HPLC and comparison and/or profiling carried out by chemical and physical means.

Tablets and capsules

Tablet and/or capsules submitted to the laboratory include ecstasy (MDMA, MDEA, etc.), ketamine, benzodiazepines, steroids, LSD squares and others. An initial examination includes a description of any markings or logos, counting of the items, colour, shape and physical dimensions of the tablet or capsule, and a measurement of mass. Measurement of mass may include the total mass of sample submitted and for individual tablets. In the case of large-scale seizures, the individual mass of a portion of the tablets may be determined. An examination of a tablet or capsule identification database, such as TICTAC (see Chapter 12), may give an indication of the drug present. Subsampling followed by homogenisation gives essentially a powder sample, so the procedure for analysis of powder samples may then be followed.

For comparison and/or profiling a physical comparison of the logo or mark may be the most informative piece of information available, although, as noted above, it is not uncommon for the different drug samples carrying the same logo to be in circulation at the same time.

Liquids and others

Liquids and other samples include GHB, steroid oils, cocaine liquor, amyl nitrite and others. A physical examination may give an indication of the drug likely to be present. The physical measurements to be noted include the volume, colour, odour and general appearance of the liquid. A subsample may be taken and an aliquot removed for analysis. It may be necessary to extract the drug from the liquid into an organic solvent prior to analysis. The physical examination may allow the analyst to proceed to the identification stage; otherwise a screen may be used to indicate the presence of a certain drug. Identification, quantification and comparison and/or profiling can be carried out along the lines described for powders.

Clandestine laboratories

As a result of the increase in abuse of synthetic drugs, clandestine laboratories have become an increased part of forensic investigation. The investigation of such sites is very interesting as they reveal (*in situ*) the synthetic processes, intermediates and often notes and chemical equations that describe the various reactions. These laboratories, however, are also very hazardous sites to investigate. The use of the word 'laboratory' disguises the more usual scenario of a garage, shed or kitchen.

Forensic scientists frequently become involved in the initial stages of a clandestine laboratory investigation in an advisory capacity. Information may come to light about certain chemicals being used at the premises, and the scientist has the responsibility of formulating an opinion as to whether a controlled substance is being produced. The police can then act on the basis of this opinion.

Many countries have specially trained police and scientists to deal with the specific problems that clandestine laboratories pose. These problems could be in the form of hazardous chemicals (acids, bases, solvents and reagents); the drug itself, possibly in large quantity; fire and explosion potentials; and the possibility of booby traps. Presence of the final product in the laboratory can be particularly hazardous for drugs such as amphetamine and methamfetamine which are relatively volatile and which are absorbed via inhalation. For drugs in powder form (e.g. amfetamines and cocaine), investigation of the scene may cause finely powdered material to be dispersed into the atmosphere where it could be inhaled, and so precautions must be taken to minimise this risk.

Ultimately, if the seizure results in a court case, the testimony in these cases can be technically demanding for the scientist. In many situations, only a small amount (or none) of the final product (i.e. the controlled substance) may be found. In such instances, detailed explanations of the synthetic routes may be required. An explanation of the role of each of the chemicals found at the scene could be required. The scientist must also be aware of alternative explanations for the presence of the chemicals, as this is the likely defence in such cases. In many instances, the precursor chemicals themselves are controlled.

Analysis of the main drugs of abuse

It is not the intention of this section to give extensive details for the analysis of drugs of abuse. There are a plethora of methods available, with each laboratory adopting its own procedures depending on the aim of the analysis, the apparatus and/or equipment available, legal aspects, the number of analyses to be performed and possibly other details associated with the specific drugs' seizure. Rather, an indication will be given of spot tests which can be used to indicate the presence or absence of a particular drug class, conditions which can be used if TLC analysis is required, an indication whether GC or HPLC is more appropriate and other factors that may need to be taken into consideration. Further details of analytical methods can be found in Moffat *et al.* (2004).

Where GC analysis is applicable, separations for most drugs can be carried out on a capillary column with a dimethylpolysiloxane stationary phase (e.g. HP-1) (Moffat *et al.* 2004). The main variations between GC methods lie in the dimensions of the columns used and the temperature programme applied. For some drugs, derivatization is recommended.

For HPLC, a wide variety of stationary mobile phase combinations are applied (Moffat *et al.* 2004), with both normal and reversed-phase systems in use (see Chapter 19).

Information on TLC analysis for the various drugs is summarised in Table 3.4. Further details can be found in Moffat *et al.* (2004).

Table 3.4 Conditions for TLC analysis of the major classes of abused drugs[a]

Drug class	TLC system[a]	Stationary phase[a]	Mobile phase[a]	Visualisation	R_f values[a]
Amfetamines	TA	Silica gel G, 250 μmm	MeOH–25% ammonia (100:1.5 v/v)	Acidified iodoplatinate	Amfetamine: 0.43 Methamfetamine: 0.31
	TB	thick impregnated with 0.1 M KOH in MeOH and dried	Cyclohexane–toluene–diethylamine (75:15:10 v/v)		Amfetamine: 0.15 Methamfetamine: 0.28
Cannabis	TAH	Silica gel G, 250 μm thick	Hexane–diethyl ether (80:20 v/v)	Fast Blue B	THC: 0.50 (red colour) CBD: 0.60 (orange colour) CBN: 0.45 (purple colour)
Cocaine	TA TB			Acidified iodoplatinate	Cocaine: 0.65 Cocaine: 0.47
Heroin	TA TB			Acidified iodoplatinate	Diacetylmorphine: 0.47 Diacetylmorphine: 0.15
LSD	TAI	Silica gel G, 250 μm thick	Acetone	Van Urk's and heat 5 min/100°C. UV 254 and 365 nm	LSD: 0.58 (blue fluorescence) LAMPA: 0.49
MDMA	TA TB			Acidified iodoplatinate	MDMA: 0.31 MDMA: 0.23
Anabolic steroids	TP	Silica gel G, 250 μm thick	Methylene chloride–diethyl ether–methanol–water (77:15:8:1.2 v/v)	Sulfuric acid–ethanol reagent and heat 10 min/105°C	Fluoxymesterone: 0.51 Nandrolone: 0.87 Testosterone: 0.60 Methyltestosterone: 0.70
	TQ		Dichloromethane–methanol–water (95:5:0.2 v/v)	Or heat 15 min/120°C, spray *p*-toluenesulfonic acid solution and heat 10 min/120°C	Fluoxymesterone: 0.09 Nandrolone: 0.48 Testosterone: 0.07 Methyltestosterone: 0.16
Benzodiazepines	TA			Acidified iodoplatinate	Diazepam: 0.75 Flunitrazepam: 0.63 Nitrazepam: 0.68 Flurazepam: 0.62
	TB				Diazepam: 0.23 Flunitrazepam: 0.10 Nitrazepam: 0.00 Flurazepam: 0.30
Khat	TE	Silica gel G, 250 μm thick	Ethyl acetate–methanol–strong ammonia solution (85:10:5 v/v)	UV 254 nm and 0.5% ninhydrin	Cathinone: 0.46 (orange colour) Cathine: 0.25 (purple colour)
Psilocybin	TA			Van Urk's reagent	Psilocybin: 0.05 (blue colour) Psilocin: 0.39 (blue colour)
	TAN	Silica gel G, 250 μm thick	Butanol–acetic acid–water (2:1:1 v/v)	Van Urk's reagent	Psilocybin: 0.34 (blue colour) Psilocin: 0.59 (blue colour)

[a] See *Clarke's Analysis of Drugs and Poisons*, Vol. 1 (Moffat *et al.* 2004) for further details of TLC conditions and visualisation reagents.

Analysis of amfetamine and methamfetamine

As many of the street-level samples submitted to the laboratory are relatively low in purity (5%), pre-concentration of samples may be required for the analysis to be successful. Typically, 100 mg of sample is added to 1 mL of sodium hydroxide solution (0.5 M) and extracted with 1 mL diethyl ether, which is decanted and evaporated to dryness in an airflow without heat. A few drops of methanol can then be added to solubilise the drug.

Colour test

The Marquis test gives an orange colour for both amfetamine and methamfetamine.

Separation and/or identification

It is common practice with primary amines to prepare derivatives such as *N*-methylbis(trifluoroacetamide) (MBTFA) or trifluoroacetic anhydride (TFAA) derivatives for GC analysis. It is good practice to analyse both derivatised and underivatised samples, since *N*-hydroxyamines may give the same product as the parent amines.

Using a concentrated and/or base-extracted sample, the *m/z* 134 and *m/z* 148 molecular ion peaks for amfetamine and methamfetamine, respectively, can be achieved readily in an underivatised sample. As can be seen from the mass spectra (Fig. 3.32), the molecular ions for both drugs are of very low abundance and there are few other characteristic high-mass ions in the spectra. The only abundant ions are *m/z* 44 and 58 for amfetamine and methamfetamine, respectively, which are of low mass. This can cause problems for confirmation of the presence of the drug in a sample and hence it is more common to derivatise these substances to produce a mass spectrum which has more ions for matching against the standard substance similarly derivatised (Fig. 3.32).

Both amfetamine and methamfetamine have one asymmetric carbon atom that results in a pair of enantiomers in each case (Fig. 3.33). Depending on the synthetic route, *l*-, *d*- and *dl*-amfetamine or methamfetamine could be encountered in samples submitted to the laboratory for analysis. These optical isomers differ in their pharmacological activity and are subject to different regulatory measures in certain countries. In those countries in which the specific optical isomer needs to be identified, chiral

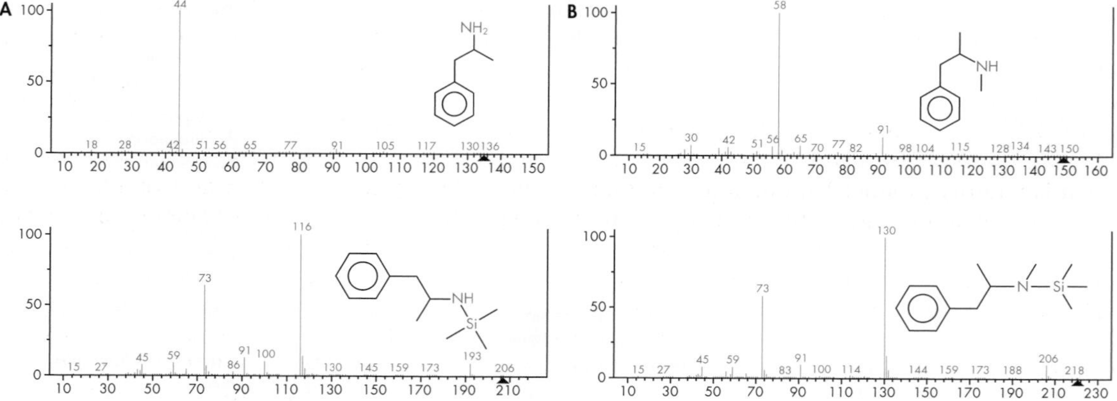

Figure 3.32 Mass spectra of (A) amfetamine and (B) methamfetamine (upper panels) and their trimethylsilyl (TMS) derivatives (lower panels). The spectra for the nonderivatised drugs show low-mass ions only, in contrast to the TMS derivatives which produce higher mass ions and more characteristic mass spectra. (Courtesy of NIST/EPA/NIH Mass Spectral Library.)

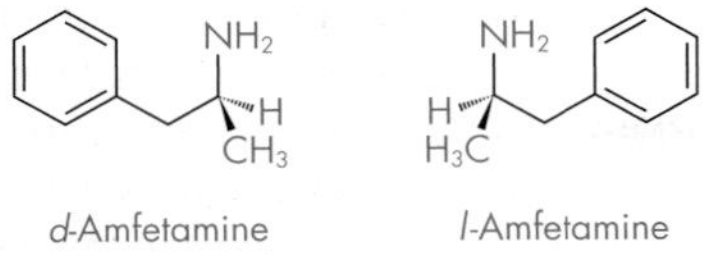

Figure 3.33 *l* and *d* Isomers of amfetamine.

analysis can be undertaken by derivatisation/GC, by the use of chiral columns (GC and HPLC) and, more recently, by the use of capillary electrophoresis (LeBelle *et al.* 1995; Sellers *et al.* 1996; Fanali *et al.* 1998; see Chapter 20).

Quantitative analysis and profiling of amfetamine and methamfetamine

Amfetamine and methamfetamine can be quantified by HPLC or GC. Normally, if GC is used, the samples are base-extracted into an organic solvent and either run directly or derivatised and then run. Using HPLC there is no need to extract; the sample can be dissolved in a suitable solvent, filtered if necessary and injected. In many cases HPLC is the preferred method for quantitative analysis of amfetamine and methamfetamine.

Amfetamine produced illicitly often contains impurities that result from the manufacturing process. The presence of these impurities can be used to compare and distinguish samples of amfetamine, since material used in the same manufacturing batch would almost certainly have the same number and relative amount of identical impurities. Samples from the same illicit laboratory produced at different times may show strong similarities, whereas samples from unrelated laboratories are expected to show major qualitative and quantitative differences.

Basic extracts into organic solvents are subjected to GC or GC-MS analysis. Samples are compared by visual inspection of the GC trace and by quantitative comparisons.

Methamfetamine impurity profiling is also carried out by GC analysis with the impurities also giving information on the synthetic route (Seta *et al.* 1994).

The purpose of comparison and/or profiling is to identify dealer–user links, establish possible sources (i.e. the clandestine laboratory) and build up databases to allow interpretation in comparison casework.

Analysis of cannabis, cannabis resin and cannabis oil

Colour test

The presence of cannabinoids in suspect material can be indicated by the Duquenois–Levine test. A sample of cannabis, cannabis resin or cannabis oil (3–5 mg) is first extracted with petroleum ether (0.5 mL). The solvent is removed and the extract is evaporated to dryness. The addition of Duquenois reagent (five drops) followed by concentrated hydrochloric acid (five drops) yields a purple colour after a few minutes. The addition of chloroform (0.5 mL) should result in the purple colour moving into the chloroform layer, which can be taken as good evidence for the presence of cannabinoids. Extracts can also be analysed by TLC (see Table 3.4).

Microscopic examination of cannabis and cannabis resin

As discussed earlier, the cannabis plant is characterised by cystolithic and glandular hairs, with the cystolithic hairs containing a deposit of calcium carbonate.

To carry out the microscopic test, place a small portion of the dry material (cannabis herbal material or cannabis resin) on a microscope slide. Identify the cystolithic and glandular hairs (Fig. 3.4). Add a few drops of Duquenois reagent (Moffat *et al.* 2004) followed by a few drops of concentrated hydrochloric acid. The cystolithic hairs contain a deposit of calcium carbonate at their base, from which a characteristic effervescence is observed. The heads at the end of the glandular hairs show as a red–purple colour.

An alternative method is to add a few drops of chloral hydrate solution to the dry material, which is particularly useful if more detailed information on the structure of the plant tissue is needed, since it removes coloured materials such as chlorophyll.

Quantitative analysis and comparison of cannabis, cannabis resin and cannabis oil

As already stated, cannabis resin is normally produced in 250 g blocks. Frequently, these blocks carry an impression, such as a number, a letter or a symbol. Comparison can be made between different blocks on the basis of similar impressions, but unrelated blocks frequently have the same impression so caution must be exercised not to assume automatically that similar impressions equals the same source. The street-level deal of cannabis resin is about 3 g (normally in the range 1–10 g), possibly wrapped in tinfoil or plastic. It may be possible to link a smaller piece of cannabis resin to its original block through a physical fit between the smaller and bigger piece.

GC or HPLC may be used to obtain a chemical profile of the cannabis, cannabis resin or cannabis oil. The THC content can be calculated and comparison made on that basis. Note that variations can occur in the THC content of a single block of cannabis resin, as the THC content decreases with age and storage conditions. The outside material in a block of cannabis resin can differ from that in the centre, with a lower THC content on the outside. This highlights the need for a careful sampling plan with consideration as to how subsamples should be taken from a larger sample.

Analysis of cocaine

Colour test

Cobalt thiocyanate test or modified cobalt thiocyanate test (Scott test) that gives a blue colour indicates the presence of cocaine.

Odour test

A 5% methanolic solution of sodium hydroxide added to the test sample and warmed gives a characteristic odour for the presence of cocaine (although other compounds may give a similar odour).

In addition to GC and HPLC, IR spectroscopy is routinely used in cocaine cases if a distinction is to be made between cocaine as a salt (e.g. cocaine hydrochloride) and cocaine in base form. The cocaine base is known as crack and, unlike cocaine hydrochloride, can be consumed by smoking.

The differences in the IR spectra are shown in Fig. 3.34. Differences at 1736 cm^{-1} and 1709 cm^{-1} for the base and 1729 cm^{-1} and 1711 cm^{-1} for the hydrochloride are explained by the effect of the hydrochloride ion on the C=O stretching bands (Elsherbini 1998).

A simple laboratory test also exists for the determination of the chemical form of cocaine (Logan *et al.* 1989). This utilises a series of liquid/liquid extractions with testing of the organic or aqueous phases using the cobalt thiocyanate test. The base form of the drug partitions into the hexane used in the test but not into the aqueous phase, while the reverse is true for the salt form of cocaine.

Quantitative analysis and profiling of cocaine samples

Quantitative analysis of cocaine samples may be carried out by GC or HPLC. The unsophisticated nature of the cocaine manufacturing process means that a multitude of trace-level alkaloid impurities are present in illicit cocaine. Many of these impurities are naturally-occurring alkaloids that originate from the coca leaf and are carried through the manufacturing process; they include *cis-* and *trans-*cinnamoylcocaine, tropacocaine, truxillines and hydroxycocaines. In addition, cocaine is also contaminated with a variety of manufacturing by-products, which include hydrolysis products, such as benzoylecgonine, ecgonine methyl ester, ecgonine and benzoic acids. The relative amount of these compounds can be used to compare cocaine samples (Moore and Casale 1998). Oxidation by-products also arise and include *N*-norcocaine and *N*-norecgonine methyl ester.

In addition to the above, solvent residues may be detected by NMR spectroscopy or headspace GC. The solvents detected include acetone, methyl ethyl ketone, benzene, toluene and diethyl ether (Cole 1998).

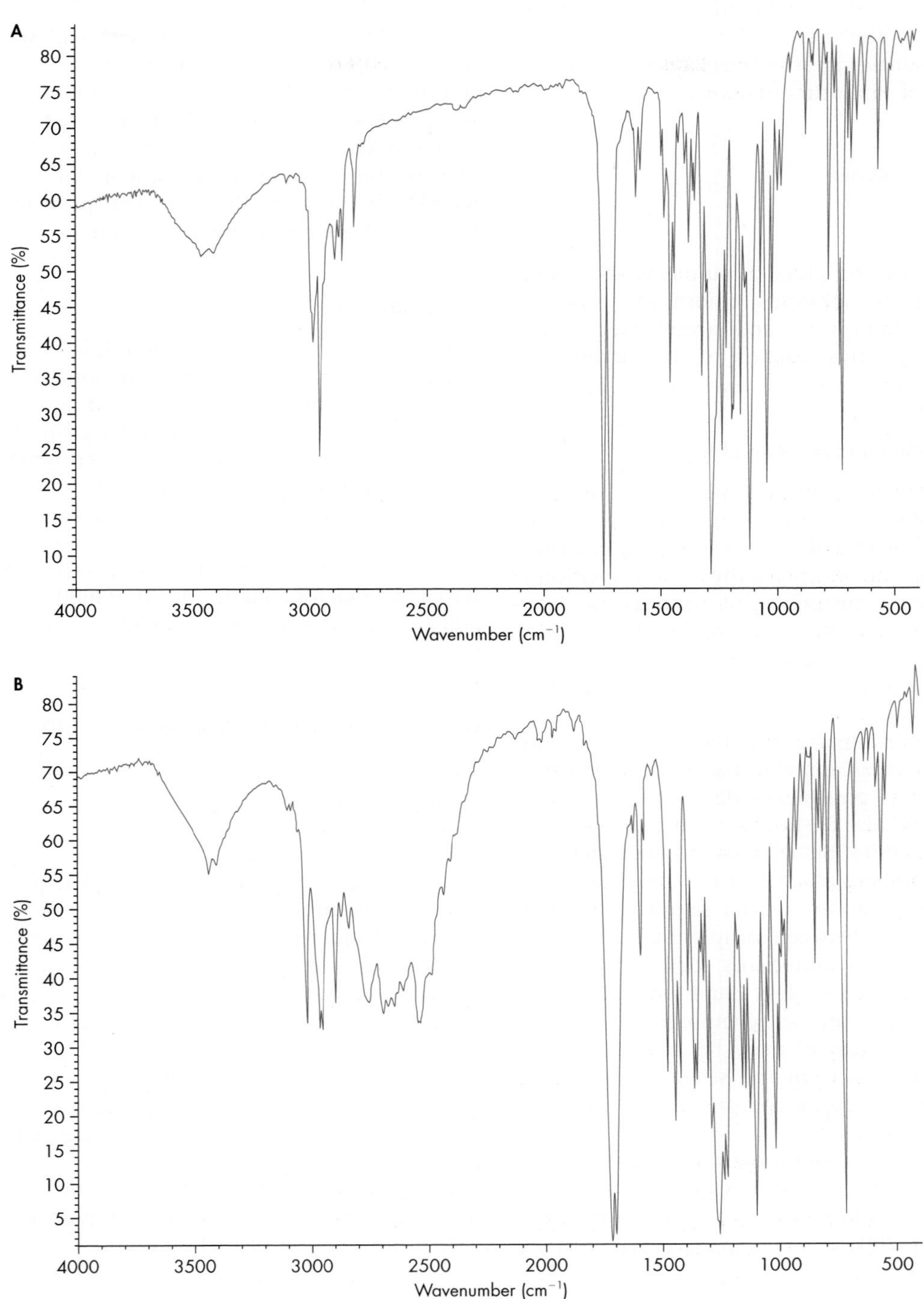

Figure 3.34 Infrared spectra of (A) cocaine base and (B) cocaine hydrochloride.

A comparison of cocaine samples can be achieved by a combination of qualitative analysis for the presence or absence of certain trace impurities and by quantitative analysis of the cocaine and other ingredients.

Analysis of heroin

Colour test

Marquis reagent gives a purple–violet colour. Other opiate alkaloids (morphine, codeine, monoacetylmorphine and acetylcodeine) give the same positive reaction to the Marquis test and the same colour.

Quantification and profiling of heroin

Heroin may be quantified by either GC or HPLC. One problem associated with GC analysis is that diamorphine may hydrolyse to 6-*O*-monoacetylmorphine, and another is the transacetylation of the common cutting agent paracetamol (acetaminophen) by diamorphine in the injection port of the GC column. The use of fresh samples and of chloroform as the solvent can avoid these problems.

By examining the amount of diamorphine, papaverine, noscapine and acetylcodeine in the samples it is possible to discriminate between samples and also to show a link between samples (Seta *et al.* 1994; Besacier and Chaudron-Thozet 1999; Stromberg *et al.* 2000). It may further be possible to examine heroin samples and show potential links between samples by the presence (and amount) of adulterants, such as caffeine, or by the presence of less common adulterants, such as diazepam or phenobarbital. In large seizures, differences may be found between various samples from the seizure, which indicates that the seizure comprises more than one batch of heroin.

In addition to examining the relative ratios of the main components, it is possible to analyse for solvent residues by headspace GC (Cole 1998; Dams *et al.* 2001).

Analysis of LSD

The only analogue of LSD to receive widespread interest is lysergic acid *N*-(methylpropyl)amide (LAMPA), and any analytical technique should be capable of separating LAMPA from LSD.

The presence of LSD may be signalled early by placing the suspect paper under long-wavelength ultraviolet (UV) light. The presence of LSD is indicated by a blue fluorescence.

Colour test

Van Urk's reagent gives a purple colour.

Some difficulty may be encountered in obtaining an unequivocal identification of LSD because of its low dosage (50 µg or less). However, if the sample is concentrated, a satisfactory analysis can be achieved.

Place a suspect LSD square in a glass vial and cover with methanol. After soaking (or sonicating) for 10–20 min, the methanol can be transferred to a vial for analysis. Another method is to add concentrated ammonia (about two drops) to the methanol.

Quantitative analysis and comparison of LSD

HPLC is the method of choice for quantitative analysis of LSD using a solvent mixture of methanol and water (1:1) (McDonald *et al.* 1984).

In some instances, a comparison is requested between one square of LSD and a large sheet of perforated squares. This can be an easy matter if the design on the large sheet spreads over the whole sheet and the 'missing' square fits neatly into the pattern (Fig. 3.12). In other instances the design may be on every individual square (or there may be no design). In such cases, it is necessary to examine the colour, design and/or dimensions of the squares and the perforation pattern.

Chemical comparisons can also be undertaken, but squares from the same large sheet can vary in the amount of LSD on each.

In addition to chromatographic separation, LSD can be discriminated from other ergot alkaloids by the MS fragmentation pattern. For example, the presence in the LSD spectrum of a m/z 100 fragment nearly as intense as the m/z 111 fragment serves to differentiate LSD from other disubstituted amides (Clarke 1989).

Analysis of MDMA

Colour test

The Marquis test gives a blue–black colour with MDMA.

Qualitative analysis.

Base extraction into an organic solvent and/or derivatisation prior to GC-MS analysis is common in the separation and identification of MDMA, although GC analysis can also be carried out without derivatisation.

Quantitative analysis, profiling and/or comparison of MDMA

To perform a quantitative analysis on 'ecstasy' tablets, these must first be ground to produce a homogeneous powder and the MDMA content determined by either GC (either directly or base extracted) or HPLC.

Chemical profiling of tablets that contain MDMA involves the examination and/or quantification of the drug and the main adulterants present, such as caffeine, sugars and binding agents. In addition to the main ingredients, many trace-level impurities from the synthetic process may be present and can be used for comparison (Bohn *et al.* 1993; Renton *et al.* 1993).

As already mentioned in this chapter, tablet comparisons can also be made using (so-called) ballistic analysis. This uses general physical features and microscopic examination of defects and punch marks for comparison. The difficulty is that a large fraction of illicit tablets in circulation may be almost identical at any one time.

Anabolic steroids

Colour test

Steroids can be visualised with sulfuric acid–ethanol reagent; *p*-toluenesulfonic acid–ethanol reagent or naphthol–sulfuric acid. Sulfuric acid in ethanol reacts with steroids to give fluorescent derivatives. *p*-Toluenesulfonic acid gives a variety of colours depending on the particular steroid, including yellow-orange and pink-violet. Naphthol–sulfuric acid gives a wide variety of colours ranging from red through to violet (Moffat *et al.* 2004).

Separation and/or identification of anabolic steroids

Both GC-MS and LC-MS methods are available for analysis. Steroids do not chromatograph well by GC unless derivatised and hence it is common practice to form, for example, silyl derivatives.

Analysis of benzodiazepines

Colour test

In the Zimmerman test, reddish purple or pink colour indicates the possible presence of some of the benzodiazepines.

Analysis of gamma-hydroxybutyrate

The legal distinction between GHB (gamma-hydroxybutyrate) and gamma-butyrolactone (GBL), coupled with the potential for GBL to undergo interconversion with GHB, raises important issues in the analytical approach to GHB analysis. The potential exists for aqueous-based GBL products to undergo conversion to GHB in the time between manufacture and consumption. Some of the factors that affect this interconversion have been explored by Ciolino *et al.* (2001).

Colour test

Cobalt nitrate 1% that gives a pink-to-violet colour is indicative of GHB. Other tests for GHB and GBL can be found in Moffat *et al.* (2004).

Separation and/or identification of GHB and analogues

GC analysis of GHB samples result in conversion of GHB to GBL, which necessitates the need for derivatisation prior to analysis. Test samples are taken to dryness under a stream of dry air. Samples are then derivatised with bis(trimethylsilyl)trifluoroacetamide–trimethyl chlorosilane (BSTFA : TMCS) (99 : 1) in the presence of pyridine and incubated at 70°C for 30 min. GHB is detected as the di-trimethylsilyl (TMS) derivative, whereas GBL does not form a silyl derivative.

HPLC can be used without derivatisation.

Analysis of khat

Approximately 5–6 g of plant material is cut into small pieces. Methanol (15–20 mL) is added and the mixture sonicated for 15 min. The green methanolic solution is filtered or decanted and condensed to near dryness. Approximately 20 mL of 0.2 M sulfuric acid is added and the solution acquires a reddish hue. A chloroform extract removes the neutral organic compounds. The aqueous layer (red layer) is basified with saturated sodium bicarbonate solution. Methylene chloride (20 mL) is added to extract the cathinone and cathine. A stream of air is used to reduce the volume to approximately 1 mL.

Colour test

Cathinone gives no reaction with Marquis reagent, but does produce a slow-forming yellow–orange colour with Chen's reagent.

Separation and/or identification

Both GC and HPLC methods are available for analysis.

Psilocybe mushrooms

A small quantity (approximately 1 g) of the dried mushrooms is sonicated with methanol (approximately 5 mL) for 10 min. The liquid is removed and reduced in volume at room temperature in an airflow. Psilocybin can be converted into psilocin by heating. This conversion can also occur if the mushrooms are not dried prior to or when they arrive in the laboratory.

Colour test

With Ehrlich reagent, a violet colour is indicative of psilocybin and psilocin.

Separation and/or identification

Direct injection of a solvent extract of psilocybe mushroom onto a GC column converts psilocybin into psilocin by thermal dephosphorylation, and only psilocin is detected. Thus, prior derivatisation is necessary if psilocybin is to be detected.

To eliminate sugars that may interfere with derivatisation, 1 ml of acetone is added to the methanolic solution and the mixture allowed to stand for 30 min and then filtered. The filtered solution is then taken to dryness in a stream of air. Pyridine (15 μL), TMS (15 μL) and BSTFA (100 μL) are added and the solution heated at 100°C for 30 min.

Psilocin is converted to psilocin di-TMS and psilocybin to psilocybin tri-TMS.

'Designer drugs'

The approach to the analysis of these compounds, especially the phenethylamine-related 'designer drugs', could be in line with the general procedure outlined for powders and with specific reference to the analytical procedures employed to analyse MDMA or amfetamine.

Conclusion

Many other compounds not discussed in detail above are encountered in the laboratory as 'drugs of abuse', such as opium, phencyclidine and its analogues, tryptamines, barbiturates, methadone, morphine, dihydrocodeine, ephedrine, ketamine and alkyl nitrites. Many of these are encountered rarely. However, the general approach to the analysis of an unknown substance outlined above should pose no difficulty to the identification of any of these drugs. Analytical information and background information on many of the drugs can be found in Moffat *et al.* (2004) and in some of the general texts in the area (Klein *et al.* 1989; Redda *et al.* 1989; Gough 1991; Shulgin and Shulgin 1992; CND Analytical 1994; United Nations 1994; Cole and Caddy 1995; Weaver and Yeung 1995; Karch 1996, Karch 1998; Ciolino *et al.* 2001).

References

C. G. G. Aitken, Sampling – How big a sample?, *J. Forensic Sci.*, 1999, **44**, 750–760.

F. Besacier and H. Chaudron-Thozet, Chemical profiling of illicit heroin samples, *Forensic Sci. Rev.*, 1999, **11**, 105–119.

M. Bohn *et al.*, Synthetic markers in illegally manufactured 3,4–methylenedioxyamfetamine and 3,4–methylenedioxymethamfetamine, *Int. J. Leg. Med.*, 1993, **106**, 19–23.

L. A. Ciolino *et al.*, The chemical interconversion of GHB and GBL: forensic issues and implications, *J. Forensic Sci.*, 2001, **46**, 1315–1323.

C. C. Clarke, The differentiation of lysergic acid diethylamide (LSD) from *N*-methyl, *N*-propyl and *N*-butyl amides of lysergic acid, *J. Forensic Sci.*, 1989, **34**, 532–546.

A. B. Clarke and C. C. Clark, Sampling of multi-unit drug exhibits, *J. Forensic Sci.*, 1990, **35**, 713–719.

CND Analytical, *Forensic and Analytical Chemistry of Clandestine Phenethylamines*, Auburn, CND Analytical Inc., 1994. (Other monographs in the series are devoted to analytical profiles of hallucinogens, designer drugs related to MDA, benzodiazepines, anabolic steroids, precursors and essential chemicals, methylaminorex and related designer analogues.)

M. D. Cole, Occluded solvent analysis as a basis for heroin and cocaine sample differentiation, *Forensic Sci. Rev.*, 1998, **10**, 113–120.

M. D. Cole and B. Caddy, *The Analysis of Drugs of Abuse: An Instruction Manual*, New York, Ellis Horwood, 1995.

M. Colon *et al.* Representative sampling of street drug exhibits, *J. Forensic Sci.*, 1993, **38**, 641–648.

M. Cox and G. Klass, Synthesis by-products from the Wacker oxidation of safrole in methanol using *p*-benzoquinone and palladium chloride. *Forensic Sci. Int.*, 2006, **164**, 138–147.

R. Dams *et al.*, Heroin impurity profiling: trends throughout a decade of experimenting, *Forensic Sci. Int.*, 2001, **123**, 81–88.

J. R. Ehleringer *et al.*, Tracing the geographical origin of cocaine, *Nature*, 2000, **408**, 311–312.

S. H. Elsherbini, Cocaine base identification and quantification, *Forensic Sci. Rev.*, 1998, **10**, 1–12.

S. Fanali *et al.*, New strategies for chiral analysis of drugs by capillary electrophoresis, *Forensic Sci. Int.*, 1998, **92**, 137–155.

R. S. Frank *et al.*, Representative sampling of drug seizures in multiple containers, *J. Forensic Sci.*, 1991, **36**, 350–357.

P. Gimeno *et al.*, A study of impurities in intermediates and 3,4-T. A. Gough (ed.), *The Analysis of Drugs of Abuse*, New York, Wiley, 1991.

T. A. Gough (ed.) *The Analyis of Drugs of Abuse*, New York, Wiley, 1991.

H. Huizer, Analytical studies on illicit heroin. II Comparison of samples, *J. Forensic Sci.*, 1983, **28**, 40–48.

S. B. Karch, *The Pathology of Drug Abuse*, 2nd edn, New York, CRC Press, 1996.

S. B. Karch, *Drug Abuse Handbook*, London, CRC Press, 1998.

M. Klein *et al.*, *Clandestinely Produced Drugs, Analogues and Precursors: Problems and Solutions*, Washington, DC, United States Department of Justice Drug Enforcement Administration, 1989.

A. T. Kicman *et al.*, The effect of androstenedione ingestion on plasma testosterone in young women; a dietary supplement with potential health risks. *Clin. Chem.* 2003, **49**, 167–169.

M. J. LeBelle *et al.*, Chiral identification and determination of ephedrine, pseudoephedrine, methamfetamine and methcathinone by gas chromatography and nuclear magnetic resonance, *Forensic Sci. Int.*, 1995, **71**, 215–223.

B. K. Logan *et al.*, A simple laboratory test for the determination of the chemical form of cocaine, *J. Forensic Sci.*, 1989, **34**, 678–681.

P. A. McDonald *et al.*, An analytical study of illicit lysergide, *J. Forensic Sci.*, 1984, **29**, 120–130.

A. C. Moffat *et al.*, *Clarke's Analysis of Drugs and Poisons*, 3rd edn, London, Pharmaceutical Press, 2004.

J. M. Moore and J. F. Casale, In depth chromatographic analyses of illicit cocaine and its precursor, coca leaves, *J. Chromatogr. A*, 1994, **674**, 165–205.

J. M. Moore and J. F. Casale, Cocaine profiling methodology – recent advances, *Forensic Sci. Rev.*, 1998, **10**, 13–45.

K. K. Redda *et al.*, *Cocaine, Marijuana, Designer Drugs, Chemistry, Pharmacology and Behaviour*, Boca Raton, CRC Press, 1989.

R. J. Renton *et al.*, A study of the precursors, intermediates and reaction by-products in the synthesis of 3,4-methoxymethylamfetamine and its application to forensic drug analysis, *Forensic Sci. Int.*, 1993, **60**, 189–202.

J. K. Sellers *et al.*, High performance liquid chromatographic analysis of enantiomeric composition of abused drugs, *Forensic Sci. Rev.*, 1996, **8**, 91–108.

S. Seta *et al.* (eds), Impurity profiling analysis of illicit drugs, *Forensic Sci. Int.* (special issue), 1994, **69**, 1–102.

A. Shulgin and A. Shulgin, *PIHKAL: A Chemical Love Story*, Berkeley, Transform Press, 1992.

L. Stromberg *et al.*, Heroin impurity profiling. A harmonisation study for retrospective comparisons, *Forensic Sci. Int.*, 2000, **114**, 67–88.

M. Swist *et al.*, Determination of synthesis route of 1-(3,4-methylenedioxyphenyl)-2-propane (MDP-2-P) based on impurity profiles of MDMA. *Forensic Sci. Int.*, 2005a, **155**, 141–157.

M. Swist *et al.*, Determination of synthesis method of ectasy based on the basic impurities. *Forensic Sci. Int.*, 2005b, **152**, 175–184.

D. Tzidony and M. Ravreby, A statistical approach to drug sampling: a case study, *J. Forensic Sci.*, 1992, **37**, 1541–1549.

United Nations, *Rapid Testing Methods of Drugs of Abuse*, New York, UNO, 1994. (Other monographs in the series are devoted to analysis of specific drugs, clandestine manufacture, staff skill requirements and basic equipment for narcotic laboratories.)

A. M. A. Verweig, Clandestine manufacture of 3,4-methylenedioxymethylamphetamine (MDMA) by low pressure reductive amination. A mass spectrometric study of some reaction mixtures. *Forensic Sci. Int.*, 1990, **45**, 91–96.

WADA 2008, *The World Anti-Doping Code, The 2008 Prohibited List*, International Standard, World Anti-Doping Agency, Sept. 2007 (http://www.wada-ama.org).

K. Weaver and E. Yeung, *An Analyst's Guide to the Investigation of Clandestine Laboratories*, Ontario, Drug Analysis Service, 1995. (Other monographs circulated by the Clandestine Laboratory Investigating Chemists Association Inc. are devoted to the synthesis and analysis of amfetamine, methylamfetamine, MDMA, their analogues and precursors, phencyclidine and fentanyl analogues, methcathinone and lysergide.)

4

Other substances encountered in clinical and forensic toxicology

R J Flanagan, M Kala, R Braithwaite and F A de Wolff

General introduction . . . 79
Volatile substances . . . 80
Pesticides . . . 90
Metals and anions . . . 101
Natural toxins . . . 116
Summary . . . 129
References . . . 129

General introduction

Although pharmaceuticals, drugs of abuse and ethanol (alcohol) are the most common poisons encountered in clinical and forensic toxicology, the possibility of poisoning with a wide range of other compounds has to be taken into account. These include pesticides, volatile substances, metals and anions, and natural toxins.

In some cases there may be useful history regarding ingestion or exposure to particular substances present in the home, workplace or local environment which can help. The clinical toxicologist needs to be familiar with the signs and symptoms of poisoning arising from acute or chronic poisoning with the above substances in order that the appropriate diagnostic tests are carried out so that effective clinical treatment can be applied. Similarly, the pathologist also needs to be aware of the recent history of the deceased, including recent admission to hospital or symptoms suggestive of poisoning. The general practitioner also needs to be familiar with signs of poisoning because patients may present with symptoms, not realising that they have been exposed to poisons whether it be accidentally or maliciously.

Thus, in most instances, the toxicologist will be provided with some recent history of a case giving them an indication that a substance may be present which is not likely to be picked up in the usual 'routine' tests most applied to samples. This then enables the toxicologist to apply additional analyses to the sample which are targeted to the types of substances suspected to be present. Applying these additional tests may confirm or rule out recent ingestion or exposure.

The 'routine' screens for alcohol and other drugs, particularly drugs of abuse, should still be applied because the finding of alcohol and/or other drugs may be pertinent to the case. For instance, if a worker in a factory suffers suspected exposure to solvents, the findings of high levels of alcohol in the bloodstream or urine may put a different complexion on an investigation of the incident.

In many instances, paraphernalia found alongside a victim of poisoning or the location and circumstances may give guidance about possible substances present. For example, in cases of accidental or deliberate poisonings with pesticide, containers may be close by. If the containers are labelled then this information should be recorded and passed to all those dealing with the incident who need this information, e.g. the clinical toxicologist where clinical treatment is still possible, the pathologist in the case of postmortem examination and the forensic toxicologist where poisoning has resulted in death. It is not uncommon for pesticides to be stored in unmarked soft drink containers. Any containers near the victim indicating possible traces of substances which might be implicated should be retained for analysis. In cases of volatile substance abuse, paraphernalia may include containers of adhesives, cigarette lighter refills, gas canisters, and aerosols. In workplace incidents, nearby containers, vats, gas lines, spilled liquids, etc. should be assessed for their possible contribution to poisoning.

Vomit or gastric contents can sometimes provide useful clues and should be considered by the clinical toxicologist to guide diagnosis and, when available, may also be analysed by the forensic toxicologist in the case of unexpected death.

The circumstances of poisoning should also be considered. If the victim is recovered from the sea in an area known to be inhabited by jellyfish and shows signs of rashes and wheals on the skin, clinical treatment should focus on jellyfish poisoning. If someone comes to an Accident and Emergency department complaining of vomiting and severe gastric upset who has recently eaten a meal of fungi collected from the wild, poisoning from fungi should be considered.

If information of the kind outlined above is not available and the more 'routine' investigations fail to identify substances that may indicate the cause of death, the toxicologist should then consider applying analyses for these less commonly encountered substances. This is the most difficult situation because the amount of sample may be limited, particularly in the case of children; methods of analysis may not be available in a local laboratory where particular poisons are not commonly encountered, plus there is the aspect of time and cost, although this latter aspect is generally not an issue in cases of a suspicious death.

The above discussion emphasises the fundamental principle that in all toxicological investigations it is important to obtain as much information as possible about a case. This includes:

- the recent history of the patient or deceased
- signs and symptoms on admission/death that might suggest poisoning
- laboratory investigations (including biomedical tests and toxicological investigations)
- postmortem examinations (in cases of death).

The sections that follow give an overview of some of the various classes of substances that may be encountered. It is not possible to discuss every substance in detail. Hence discussion is focused on those substances that are the most commonly encountered in their class. The reader is directed to *Clarke's Analysis of Drugs and Poisons* (Moffat *et al.* 2004) for further details, including details of analysis and body fluids, and concentrations of various substances encountered in clinical and forensic toxicology.

Volatile substances

If anaesthesia is excluded, acute poisoning with volatile substances usually follows the deliberate inhalation of a gas or solvent vapour by a person who wishes to become intoxicated ('glue sniffing', solvent abuse, inhalant abuse, volatile substance abuse (VSA)). VSA has been defined as 'The deliberate inhalation of a volatile substance (gas, aerosol propellants, solvents in glue and other solvents) to achieve a change in mental state' (Field-Smith *et al.* 2007). Solvents from adhesives (notably toluene), certain print-correcting fluids and thinners, hydrocarbons such as those found in cigarette lighter refills, halocarbon aerosol propellants and fire extinguishers, and anaesthetic gases are among the products and/or compounds that may be abused in this way (Table 4.1).

Those who ingest, or even more rarely inject, solvents or solvent-containing products, and the victims of clinical, domestic and industrial accidents, may also be poisoned by volatile

Table 4.1 Some products and/or compounds that may be abused by inhalation[a,b]

Type	Product	Major volatile components
Adhesives	Balsa wood cement	Ethyl acetate
	Contact adhesives	Butanone, hexane[c], toluene and esters
	Cycle tyre repair cement	Toluene and xylenes[d]
	PVC cement	Acetone, butanone, cyclohexanone, trichloroethylene
	Woodworking adhesives	Xylenes[d]
Aerosols	Air freshener	Purified LPG[e], DME and/or fluorocarbons[f]
	Deodorants, antiperspirants	Purified LPG[e], DME and/or fluorocarbons[f]
	Fly spray	Purified LPG[e], DME and/or fluorocarbons[f]
	Hair lacquer	Purified LPG[e], DME and/or fluorocarbons[f]
	Paint	Purified LPG[e], DME and/or fluorocarbons[f] and esters
Anaesthetics and/or analgesics	Inhalational	Nitrous oxide, cyclopropane[g], diethyl ether[g], halothane, enflurane, desflurane, isoflurane, methoxyflurane[g], sevoflurane, xenon
	Topical	Ethyl chloride, fluorocarbons[f]
Cigarette lighter refills		Purified LPG[e]
Commercial dry cleaning and degreasing agents		Carbon tetrachloride[g], dichloromethane, 1,1,2-trichlorotrifluoroethane (FC-113), 1,1-dichloro-1-fluoroethane (FC-141b), methanol, propylene dichloride[g], 1,1,1-trichloroethane[g], tetrachloroethylene, toluene, trichloroethylene
Domestic spot removers and dry cleaners; surgical plaster/chewing gum remover		Carbon tetrachloride[g], dichloromethane, 1,1,1-trichloroethane[g], tetrachloroethylene, trichloroethylene
Dust removers ('air brushes')		DME, fluorocarbons[f]
Fire extinguishers		Bromochlorodifluoromethane (FC-12B1, BCF)[g], trichlorofluoromethane (FC-11)[g], dichlorodifluoromethane (FC-12)[g]
Hydrocarbon fuels and/or solvents		Acetylene, 'butane'[e], petrol (gasoline)[h], petroleum ethers[i], 'propane'[i]
Industrial and/or laboratory solvents		Chloroform[g], methyl acetate, MIBK, MTBE
Injected oxidant (drag racing, blow torches)		Nitrous oxide
Paint and/or paint thinners		Acetone, butanone, esters, hexane[c], toluene, trichloroethylene, xylenes[d]
Paint stripper		Dichloromethane, methanol, toluene
Typewriter correction fluids and/or thinners (some)		1,1,1-Trichloroethane[g]
Vasodilators		Butyl nitrite, isobutyl nitrite ('butyl nitrite'), isopentyl nitrite (isoamyl nitrite, 'amyl nitrite')[k]
Whipped cream dispenser bulbs and/or cylinders		Nitrous oxide

Continued

Table 4.1 *(Continued)*

[a] The composition of some products varies with time and country of origin.

[b] DME, dimethyl ether; LPG, liquefied petroleum gas; MIBK, methyl isobutyl ketone; MTBE, methyl *tert*-butyl ether; PVC, poly(vinylchloride).

[c] Commercial 'hexane' mixture of hexane and heptane with small amounts of higher aliphatic hydrocarbons.

[d] Mainly *meta*-xylene (1,3-dimethylbenzene).

[e] LPG (butane, isobutane, propane; if unpurified also butenes, propenes, sulfur compounds, etc.).

[f] Nowadays often 1,1,1,2-tetrafluoroethane (FC-134a), but chlorodifluoromethane (FC-22), 1,1-difluoroethane (FC-152a), difluoromethane (FC-32), pentafluoroethane (FC-125), perfluoropropane (FC-218) and 1,1,1-trifluoroethane (FC-143a) might also be encountered.

[g] Rarely used for this purpose nowadays.

[h] Mixture of aliphatic and aromatic hydrocarbons with boiling range 40–200°C.

[i] Mixtures of pentanes, hexanes, etc., with specified boiling ranges (e.g. 40–60°C).

[j] Propane, butanes, etc.

[k] Commercial 'amyl nitrite' is mainly isopentyl nitrite but other nitrites are also present.

substances. In addition, chloroform, diethyl ether and other volatiles are still used occasionally in the course of crimes such as rape and murder. Another volatile compound, chlorobutanol (chlorbutol), sometimes employed as a sedative, a plasticiser and a preservative, has been used in doping greyhounds. Isobutyl and isopentyl ('amyl') nitrites may also be inhaled to experience their vasodilator properties, sometimes by male homosexuals.

Solvents and other abusable volatiles can produce dose-related central nervous system (CNS) effects similar to those of other sedative and hypnotic agents. Small doses can rapidly lead to euphoria and other behavioural disturbances that are similar to those caused by ethanol, and may also induce more profound effects such as delusions and hallucinations. Heightened sexual (self-) gratification may also be a feature, sometimes in association with partial asphyxia. Once exposure ceases, rapid recovery normally ensues – this process may take only a few minutes if a relatively volatile substance has been inhaled. Rapid recovery after exposure may be a factor in the continuing popularity of VSA among secondary school children (13–18 years of age, or thereabouts) in some countries. On the other hand, psychological dependence is common in chronic users, although withdrawal symptoms are rarely severe. VSA has now been reported from most parts of the world, mainly among adolescents, individuals who live in remote communities and those with occupational access to abusable volatiles (Flanagan and Ives 1994; Kozel *et al.* 1995). The prevalence of inhalant abuse has been increasing in the USA in recent years (Brouette and Anton 2001). In the UK, deaths due to VSA fell to their lowest annual total recorded in 2005 (Field-Smith *et al.* 2007); of the 45 deaths recorded, butane from all sources accounted for 80% of VSA deaths.

The major risk associated with VSA is that of sudden death. In a long-term monitoring study carried out in the UK, with findings reported annually (Field-Smith *et al.*, 2007), most sudden VSA-related deaths were attributed to 'direct toxicity', but deaths also occurred from 'indirect' causes such as inhalation of vomit, asphyxia associated with use of a plastic bag, and trauma. These 'indirect' deaths were frequently associated with abuse of products that contain toluene, usually adhesives (glue). The deaths that were attributed to 'direct toxicity' were predominantly associated with abuse of liquefied petroleum gas (LPG) cigarette lighter refills. In a US study utilising data from the Toxic Exposure Surveillance System of the American Association of Poison Control Systems (1996–2001), petrol (gasoline) was identified as the most commonly abused substance and was responsible for the highest proportion of deaths (45%) associated with VSA (Spiller 2004). Chronic toxicity from exposure to volatile substances has also been described both in abusers and after occupational use of certain compounds. Chronic toxicity, such as lead poisoning from abuse of leaded petrol, may be especially prevalent in developing countries or societies (ethnic populations).

Role of the analytical toxicology laboratory

The analytical toxicology laboratory may be asked to perform analyses for solvents and other volatile compounds in biological samples and related specimens to:

- assist in the diagnosis of acute poisoning, including the investigation of deaths in which poisoning by volatile compounds (including anaesthetic agents) is a possibility
- confirm a suspicion of chronic VSA in the face of denial from the patient and/or a person responsible for the care of the patient, such as a parent or guardian
- aid investigation of rape or other assault, or other offence such as driving a motor vehicle or operating machinery, that may have been committed under the influence of volatile substances or in which volatile substances may have been administered to a victim
- help investigate fire or explosion for which VSA might have been a contributory factor
- assess occupational or environmental exposure to anaesthetic or solvent vapour. However, other techniques, such as ambient or expired air monitoring or, in some instances, the measurement of urinary metabolite excretion, may be more appropriate in this context.

The analysis of volatile substances presents particular problems. Firstly, collection, storage and transport of biological samples must be controlled as far as practicable to minimise loss of analyte – quantitative work is futile if very volatile compounds, such as propane, are encountered unless precautions are taken to prevent loss of analyte from the sample prior to the analysis. Secondly, many of the compounds of interest occur commonly in laboratories carrying out the analysis and so precautions must be implemented against contamination and interference. Thirdly, many volatile compounds are excreted unchanged via the lungs, so that blood (and/or other tissues in fatalities), and not urine, is usually the sample of choice. Finally, the interpretation of results can be difficult, especially if legitimate exposure to solvent vapour is a possibility.

A diagnosis of VSA should be based on a combination of circumstantial, clinical and analytical evidence, rather than on any one factor alone. It is especially important to consider all circumstantial evidence in cases of possible VSA-related sudden death, since suicide or even homicide cannot be excluded simply on the basis of the toxicological examination. There have been a number of reports of the use of inhalational anaesthetics for suicidal purposes, for example, and in one example in the UK a serial homosexual rapist murdered his victims and disposed of the bodies by setting fire to them in garden sheds in circumstances that suggested that the victim had caused the fire accidentally while indulging in VSA (Scott 1996). The possibility of VSA should also be considered in individuals who give very high readings on evidential breath-alcohol instruments. A result of 333 μg alcohol in 100 mL breath was recorded in one instance after alcohol ingestion and butane inhalation; a contemporary specimen for blood ethanol measurement was not available for analysis (Brooke 1999).

Sample collection, transport and storage

If the analyte is very volatile (e.g. propane, butane) and a quantitative analysis is required, a blood sample should be collected directly into the vial in which the analysis will be carried out. Many other volatile compounds are relatively stable in blood and other tissues if simple precautions are taken. In the case of blood, the container used for the sample should be glass, preferably with a cap lined with metal foil. Plastic containers should be avoided because some plastics such as poly(ethylene) and poly(propylene) are permeable to volatile organic compounds. Attention should be given to the types of tubes used for sample collection. Gross contamination with volatile aromatic compounds (ethylbenzene, toluene, xylene) and butanol was found in blood collected into certain types of blood-collection tubes (Dyne *et al.* 1996). Contamination with butan-1-ol or 2-methylpropan-2-ol occurs commonly in blood collected into tubes coated with EDTA. Carbon disulfide has been detected in blood collected in tubes sealed with soft-rubber stoppers (Weller and Wolf 1989). Volatile substances by their very nature volatilise readily from samples. Volatilisation is a concentration- and temperature-driven process and hence the greater the air space above a sample and the higher the temperature, the more readily will the substance volatilise. Thus sample tubes should be as full as possible and should only be opened when required for analysis and then only when cold (4°C). An anticoagulant (sodium ethylenediaminetetraacetic acid (EDTA) or lithium heparin) should be used. Specimen storage between 2°C and 8°C (i.e. normal refrigerator temperature) is recommended and 1% (w/v) sodium fluoride should be added to minimise enzymic activity.

If a necropsy is to be performed, tissues (brain, lung, liver, kidney and subcutaneous fat) should be obtained in addition to standard toxicological specimens (femoral blood, urine, stomach contents and vitreous humour). Tissues should be stored before analysis in the same way as for blood but no preservative should be added. To avoid cross-contamination, products implicated in the incident (and stomach contents if ingestion is suspected) should be packed, transported and stored entirely separately from (other) biological specimens even when stored in refrigerators or freezers. Investigation of deaths that occurred during or shortly after anaesthesia should include the analysis of the inhalation anaesthetic(s), in order to exclude an error in administration. Clinical therapies and poor procedures during sample collection can also give rise to volatile compounds. For example, halothane or chlorobutanol may be used in therapy or inadvertently added to the sample as a preservative. Use of aerosol disinfectant preparations when collecting specimens may contaminate the sample if an aerosol propellant is used. Contamination of blood samples with ethanol or propan-2-ol may occur if an alcohol-soaked swab is used to cleanse skin prior to venepuncture.

Analytical methods

Static headspace gas chromatography (GC) often provides a convenient and easily automated mode of analysis for blood and other biological specimens that may be obtained without using special apparatus to collect the sample. Many analyses can be accomplished using flame ionisation detection (FID) and/or electron capture detection (ECD). Nitrous oxide and most halogenated compounds respond on the ECD, although the thermal conductivity detector (TCD) may be used as an alternative if nitrous oxide poisoning is suspected. Use of expired air collected into either a Tedlar bag or via a special device (Dyne *et al.* 1997; Fig. 4.1) with subsequent GC or GC-mass spectrometry (MS) analysis can facilitate the analysis of a number of compounds. Direct MS of expired air can also detect many compounds several days post exposure. However, the use of these techniques is limited by the need to take breath directly from the patient and the specialist equipment required (Ramsey 1984). Vapour-phase infrared (IR) spectrophotometry may be useful in the analysis of abused products or ambient atmospheres. High-performance liquid chromatography (HPLC) is useful in the analysis of polar metabolites of certain solvents.

A Schematic

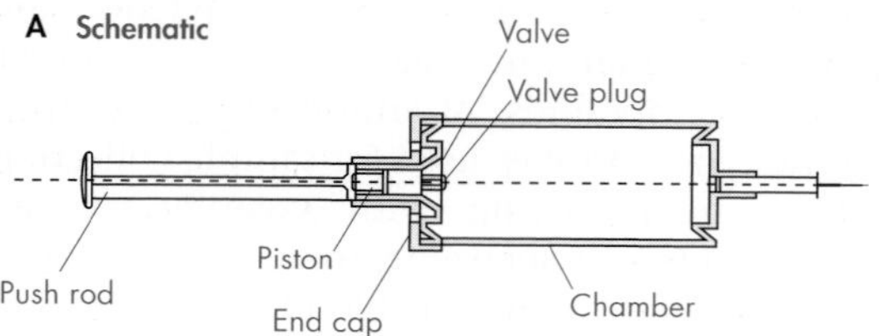

B Components

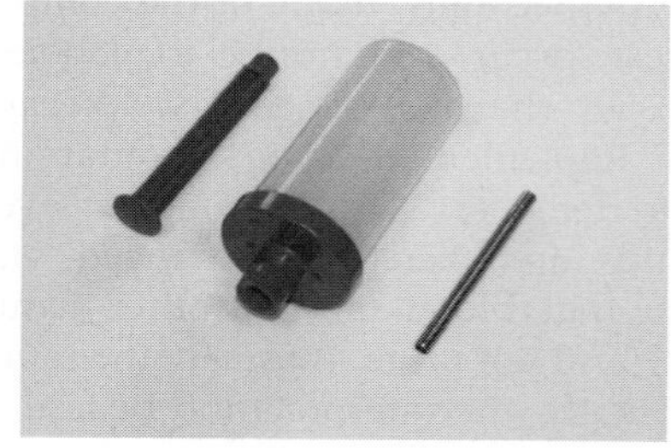

Figure 4.1 Device for capturing breath samples for solvent analysis. (Reprinted from D. Dyne *et al.*, A novel device for capturing breath samples for solvent analysis, *Sci. Total Environ.*, 1997, **199**, 83–89 with permission from Elsevier; illustrations courtesy of Dr J. Crocker, Health & Safety Laboratory, Broad Lane, Sheffield.)

Packed GC columns have been used extensively in conjunction with headspace sample preparation. Disadvantages include the poor resolution of some very volatile substances, a long total analysis time and variation in the peak shape given by alcohols between different batches of column packing.

GC separation using capillary columns offers superior resolution to the use of packed columns. However, the most commonly used columns such as a 30 m × 0.2 mm i.d. column with a chemically bonded stationary phase of dimethylpolysiloxane (DMS) 0.1 μm film thickness are unsuitable because volatile substances elute rapidly and resolution is poor. This difficulty can be overcome by the use of wide-bore capillary columns e.g. 60 m × 0.53 mm i.d. 5 μm film thickness DMS combined with large-volume injection. An alternative for the analysis of volatile substances is a porous layer open tubular (PLOT) column. These phases give good retention and thus resolution of compounds of similar relative formula mass, but peak shapes of polar compounds are poor and it is difficult to screen for compounds of widely different volatility in one analysis.

The use of a capillary column together with two different detectors (FID and ECD) confers a high degree of selectivity, particularly for low formula-mass compounds for which there are relatively few alternative structures. If more rigorous identification is required, GC combined with MS or Fourier transform IR spectrometry (FTIR) may be used. However, GC-MS can be difficult at high sensitivity when the fragments produced are less than *m/z* 40, particularly if the instrument is used for purposes other than solvent analyses. In particular, the available sensitivity and spectra of the low-molecular-weight alkanes renders them very difficult to confirm by GC-MS. Inertial spray MS allows the introduction of biological fluids directly into the mass spectrometer without prior chromatographic analysis and has been used in the analysis of halothane in blood during anaesthesia. A derivatisation method for toluene and ethylbenzene involving the use of chlorine gas prior to GC-MS has been described (El-Haj *et al.* 2000).

GC-FTIR may be more appropriate than GC-MS in the analysis of volatiles, but sensitivity is poor, particularly compared with ECD. Moreover, the apparatus is expensive and not widely available. In addition, interference, particularly from water and carbon dioxide in the case of biological specimens, can be troublesome. 'Purge and trap' and multiple headspace extraction offer ways to increase sensitivity and, although not needed for most clinical and forensic applications, 'purge and trap' has been used in conjunction with GC-FTIR and FID in forensic casework. Pulse heating has also been employed in the analysis of volatiles in biological specimens. This method involves the use of a Curie point pyrolyser employing a ferromagnetic alloy that can accurately attain temperatures in the range 150 to 1040°C very rapidly (4 s or so). Advantages of this technique include the use of a small sample volume (0.5–5 μL), short extraction time and lack of matrix effects. Headspace solid-phase microextraction (HS-SPME) has also been used in the analysis of volatile compounds in biological samples.

Chiral GC methods are available and have been applied to the enantiomer separation of anaesthetics such as enflurane and isoflurane because they have different anaesthetic potencies and side-effects.

Analysis of Products

Aerosols and fuel gases can be analysed after releasing a portion of the product into a headspace vial, and then transferring a few microlitres of the vapour to another vial for analysis. Liquids can be analysed in the same way, except that it is often possible to withdraw a portion (5–50 μL) of the headspace directly from the container. In this latter case, however, the result may not be representative of the composition of the liquid as a whole. Adhesives and other liquid or semi-liquid products can be analysed by headspace GC.

Quantitative analysis

Quantitative assays should involve analysis of standard solutions with addition of an appropriate internal standard.

For liquid and solid analytes, calibration solutions are prepared by adding a known volume of the liquid analyte to a volumetric flask that contains 'volatile-free' blood and ascertaining the exact amount added by weighing. Solid analytes are weighed in directly. After allowing time for equilibration, appropriate dilutions are performed, taking care to minimise loss of analyte by handling reagents and glassware at 4°C and storing samples and standards at 4°C with minimal headspace. Portions of the standards are transferred to headspace vials for analysis, as described above,

Calibration mixtures for gaseous analytes are prepared directly into headspace vials. Details of sample preparation can be found in Moffat *et al.* (2004).

Calibration graphs of peak height or area ratio to the internal standard are usually used to measure analyte concentrations in a sample, although absolute calibration in terms of amount of analyte injected should be possible, especially if an automated headspace analyser is employed. Such apparatus not only permits unattended operation, but also gives much better reproducibility in quantitative work.

Pharmacokinetics and the interpretation of results

In the UK, Maximum Exposure Limit (MEL) or Occupational Exposure Standard (OES) provide information on the relative toxicities of different compounds after chronic exposure to relatively low concentrations of vapour (some examples of MEL/OES limits are shown in Table 4.2). Inhaled compounds may rapidly attain high concentrations in well-perfused organs (brain, heart), while concentrations in muscle and adipose tissue may be very low. Should death occur, this situation is 'frozen' to an extent, but if exposure continues the compound accumulates in less accessible (poorly perfused) tissues, only to be slowly released once exposure ceases. Thus, the plasma concentrations of some compounds may fall mono-exponentially, while others may exhibit two (or more) separate rates of decline (half-lives).

The solubility of a volatile compound in blood is an important influence on the rate of absorption, tissue distribution and elimination of the compound. The partition coefficients of a number of compounds between air, blood and various tissues have been measured *in vitro* using animal tissues, and some *in vivo* distribution data have been obtained from postmortem tissue measurements in humans (Table 4.2). However, these data must be used with caution since there are many difficulties inherent in such measurements (sampling variations, analyte stability, external calibration, etc.). Published data on the plasma half-lives of volatile substances (such as that in Table 4.2) are not easily comparable, either because too few samples were taken or the analytical methods used did not have sufficient sensitivity to measure the final half-life accurately.

Many volatile substances, including butane, dimethyl ether, most fluorocarbon refrigerants and/or aerosol propellants, isobutane, nitrous oxide, propane, tetrachloroethylene and 1,1,1-trichloroethane, are eliminated largely unchanged in exhaled air. Others are partly eliminated in exhaled air and also metabolised in the liver and elsewhere, the metabolites being eliminated in exhaled air or in urine, or incorporated into intermediary metabolism. After ingestion, extensive hepatic metabolism can reduce systemic availability ('first-pass' metabolism) of certain compounds. Table 4.3 gives some examples in which blood or urinary metabolite measurements have been used to assess exposure to solvents and other volatile compounds.

Interpretation of qualitative results

As can be seen from Table 4.3 some volatile substances give rise to volatile metabolites which may themselves be substances associated with volatile substance abuse or accidental exposure, and this possibility must be considered when a volatile substance is detected. For example, acetone is a metabolite of propan-2-ol and ethanol is a metabolite of ethyl acetate. Detection of a volatile compound in blood does not always indicate VSA or occupational/environmental

Table 4.2 Physical properties and pharmacokinetic data of some volatile compounds (data summarized from Fiserova–Bergerova 1983; Pihlainen and Ojanperä 1998; Baselt 2002)

Compound	MEL/OES[a] (mg/m³)	Vapour pressure (20°C)[b] (mmHg)	Proportion absorbed dose (%)			Half-life[c] (h)	Brain:blood distribution ratio (deaths)	Partition coefficient (blood:gas) (37°C)
			Inhaled dose absorbed (%)	Eliminated unchanged (%)	Metabolised (%)			
Acetone	1210	183	–	–	–	3–5[d]	–	243–300
Benzene	16	75	46	12	80	9–24	3–6	6–9
Butane	1450	(1554)	30–45	–	–	–	–	–
Carbon tetrachloride	13	90	–	50?	50?	48	–	1.6
Chloroform	9.9	157	–	20–70 (8 h)	>30	–	4	8
Enflurane	383	172	90+	>80 (5 days)	2.5	36	1.4[f]	1.9
Halothane	82	244	90+	60–80 (24 h)	<20	2–3	2–3	2.57
Nitrous oxide	183	(39 800)	–	>99	–	–	1.1	0.47
Propane	1750[e]	(6 269)	–	–	–	–	–	–
Toluene	191	22	53	<20	80	7.5	1–2	8–16
1,1,1-Trichloroethane	555	98	–	60–80 (1 week)	2	10–12	2	1–3
Trichloroethylene	550	58	50–65	16	>80	30–38	2	9.0
'Xylene'	220	6	64	5	>90	20–30	–	42.1

[a] UK maximum exposure limit/occupational exposure standard (8 h time-weighted average; Health and Safety Executive 2002).

[b] Figures in parentheses indicate compound gas at 20°C.

[c] Terminal phase plasma half-life.

[d] Longer after high doses.

[e] As components of liquefied petroleum gas (LPG).

[f] Experimental: 37°C.

Table 4.3 Metabolites of some solvents and other volatile substances that may be measured to assess exposure

Compound	Formula weight	Parent compound	Body fluid[a]	'Normal'[b]	'High'[c]	Comment
Acetaldehyde	44.1	Ethanol	Blood	0.2 mg/L	[Not known]	
Acetone	58.1	Propan-2-ol	Blood Urine Urine	10 mg/L 10 mg/L –	 80 mg/L 10 mg/L	Blood/urine acetone concentrations can rise to 2 g/L in ketosis. Propan-2-ol is also an acetone metabolite
Carbon monoxide	28.0	Dichloromethane	Blood	<5% HbCO	>20% HbCO	CO blood half-life 13 h breathing air, atmospheric pressure (CO half-life 5 h after inhalation of CO). Blood HbCO is a useful indicator of chronic exposure
Cyanide ion	26.0	Acetonitrile, acrylonitrile, other organonitriles	Blood	0.2 mg/L (non-smokers)	2 mg/L	Cyanide metabolised to thiocyanate; both compounds may accumulate during chronic exposure
Ethanol	46.1	Ethyl acetate	Blood	0.1 g/L	0.8 g/L	0.8 g/L legal UK driving limit
Hippurate	179.2	Toluene	Urine	0.2 g/L	2 g/L	Not ideal indicator of toluene exposure as there are other (dietary, pharmaceutical) sources of benzyl alcohol/benzoate and hence hippurate
Methanol	32.0	Methyl acetate, methyl formate	Urine	–	30 mg/L	
2-Methylphenol (*ortho*-cresol)	108.1	Toluene	Urine	–	3 mg/L	Hippurate and other methylphenols are additional toluene metabolites
trans,trans-Muconate	142.1	Benzene	Urine	–	2 mg/L	Phenol and *S*-phenylmercapturic are acid additional benzene metabolites
Nitrite ion	46.0	Butyl nitrite, isopentyl nitrite, other organonitrites	Plasma Urine	2.5 mg/L –	[Not known] 1.0 mg/L	
Oxalate	90.0	Ethylene glycol	Urine	2.5 mg/L	4 mg/L	Glycolate and glyoxylate are also plasma and urinary ethylene glycol metabolites
Tolurates (methylhippurates)	193.2	Xylenes	Urine	0.01 mg/L	1.5 g/L	

Table 4.3 (*Continued*)

Compound	Formula weight	Parent compound	Body fluid[a]	'Normal'[b]	'High'[c]	Comment
Trifluoroacetate	114.0	Halothane and some other fluorinated anaesthetics	Urine	–	2.5 mg/L	
Trichloroacetate	163.4	Trichloroethylene	Urine	–	100 mg/L	Metabolite of 2,2,2-trichloroethanol
2,2,2-Trichloroethanol	149.4	Trichloroethylene	Plasma	10 mg/L	50 mg/L	Also a metabolite of chloral hydrate, dichloralphenazone, and triclofos

[a] Urinary excretion often expressed as a ratio to creatinine.
[b] Upper limit of normally expected or 'nontoxic' concentration.
[c] Lower limit of concentration associated with toxicity/occupational exposure action limit.

exposure to solvent vapour. Some medical conditions can give rise to volatile substances in blood. Acetone and some of its homologues may occur in high concentrations in ketotic patients. Large amounts of acetone and butanone may also occur in blood and urine of children with acetoacetylcoenzyme A thiolase deficiency for example, and may indicate the diagnosis.

Possible contamination via sampling procedures or clinical treatments (as discussed under sample collection, transport and storage) should be considered when evaluating data, although it should be recognised that such problems are best avoided by the use of sampling procedures and equipment designed to eliminate the possibility of contamination.

It is well known that ethanol may be both produced and metabolised by microbial action in biological specimens as may other low-molecular-weight alcohols such as propanols and butanols, so this possibility must be evaluated if these substances are detected. 'Congener alcohols', such as methanol, propan-1-ol, butan-1-ol, butan-2-ol, 2-methylpropan-1-ol, 2-methylbutan-1-ol, and 3-methylbutan-1-ol (and ketone metabolites of secondary alcohols) may arise from the ingestion of alcoholic drinks (Bonte 2000). Butyraldehyde, dimethyl disulfide, isovaleraldehyde and valeraldehyde may arise from putrefaction. Small amounts of hexanal may arise from degradation of fatty acids in blood on long-term storage, even at −5 to −20°C. This compound may co-elute with toluene on some GC systems and hence give rise to a false positive for toluene, particularly if GC-FID is use for analysis rather than GC-MS.

The likelihood of detecting exposure to volatile substances by headspace GC of blood is influenced by the dose and duration of exposure, the time of sampling in relation to the time elapsed since exposure, and the precautions taken in the collection and storage of the specimen. In a suspected VSA- or anaesthetic-related fatality, analysis of tissues (especially fatty tissues such as brain) may prove useful since high concentrations of volatile compounds may be present even if very little is detectable in blood.

Analysis of metabolites in urine may extend the time after which exposure may be detected but, of the compounds commonly abused, only toluene, the xylenes and some chlorinated solvents, notably trichloroethylene, have suitable metabolites (Table 4.3). The alkyl nitrites that can be abused by inhalation (isobutyl nitrite, isopentyl nitrite) are extremely unstable and break down rapidly *in vivo* to the corresponding alcohols and usually also contain other isomers (butyl nitrite, pentyl nitrite). Any products submitted for analysis usually also contain the corresponding alcohols as well as the nitrites. The profound methaemoglobinaemia that often arises after ingestion of these compounds can be detected easily.

Interpretation of quantitative results

In very general terms, soon after acute exposure, blood concentrations of volatile substances of 5–10 mg/L and above may be associated with clinical features of toxicity. In other words, pharmacologically effective concentrations of volatile substances are similar to those of inhalational anaesthetics and are thus an order of magnitude lower than those observed in poisoning with relatively water-soluble compounds, such as ethanol.

There may be a large overlap in the blood concentrations of volatile compounds attained after workplace exposure and as a result of deliberate inhalation of vapour. This has been demonstrated for toluene (Meredith *et al.* 1989; Miyazaki *et al.* 1990). Aside from individual differences in tolerance and possible loss of toluene from the sample prior to analysis, sample contamination, etc., the lack of a strong correlation between blood concentrations and clinical features of poisoning is probably due to rapid initial tissue distribution. Urinary excretion of 2-methylphenol provides a selective measure of toluene exposure for use in occupational and/or environmental monitoring (Table 4.3).

Pesticides

The term 'pesticide' encompasses a wide variety of substances used to destroy unwanted life forms. More than a thousand pesticides are available and widely used in the world today. In addition, several hundred compounds that are no longer manufactured or marketed for crop protection use still remain in people's houses. Both sources play an important role in clinical and forensic toxicology as causes of suicidal, homicidal and accidental poisonings.

Pesticides are applied in agriculture for crop protection and pest control, and in human and animal hygiene. The Compendium of Pesticide Common Names, a website (http://www.alanwood.net/pesticides/) listing information on pesticides, lists twenty-three classes based on their field of use. Examples include insecticides, herbicides, rodenticides, fungicides, nematocides, molluscicides and acaricides. Most pesticides have common names agreed by the International Organization for Standardization (ISO). These common names are used throughout this chapter for convenience and brevity, but their equivalent systematic chemical names can be ascertained easily according to the rules of the International Union of Pure and Applied Chemistry (IUPAC) and the Chemical Abstracts Service Registry Number (CAS RN; O'Neil *et al.* 2006; Tomlin 2006). Pesticides are also referred to in terms of chemical class. For example, substances used as insecticides include organophosphorus (OP) compounds, carbamates, chlorinated hydrocarbons, pyrethroids, organotin compounds and heterocyclic compounds. Some chemical classes have several uses. For example, OP compounds can be used as acaricides, insecticides, nematocides, fungicides, herbicides and rodenticides. Often the type of chemical is also indicated by a stem in the common name (e.g. 'uron' for ureas, and 'carb' for carbamates). Commercial formulations can be mixtures of pesticides from different classes, thus complicating the issue even further.

The major classes of pesticides are shown in Table 4.4 together with the major chemical groups associated with these classes and examples of substances. It should be recognised that the information contained in this table is a very simplistic overview of all the classes, associated chemical groups and substances that fall within the category of pesticides, and that a far wider variety of chemicals could be encountered in clinical and forensic toxicology. Structures of various pesticides are given in Figure 4.2. Table 4.5 shows data on pesticide poisonings in various countries. While the data in Table 4.5 should not be taken as applicable to all countries, it does illustrate the fact that the majority of pesticide poisonings arise from a few chemical groups including OP compounds, carbamates and herbicides such as paraquat and 2,4-D. It also shows that a wide variety of pesticides from other chemical groups also feature in poisonings. Hence the clinician must be ready to spot symptoms of poisoning by a wide variety of pesticides and the toxicologist should have analytical methodologies in place to identify these poisons. The data also show that certain pesticides are more commonly encountered in some locations than others, presumably reflecting the agricultural crops grown in an area, the infestations which affect those crops, the preference for certain pesticides together with other factors such as pesticide availability, cost, legal restrictions, etc.

Pesticide toxicity

The large variety of chemical compounds that show pesticide properties means that there is a very wide range of toxicity in humans. It is believed that an oral dose of only several drops (100 mg) of terbufos, an OP compound, is fatal to most adults, whereas another

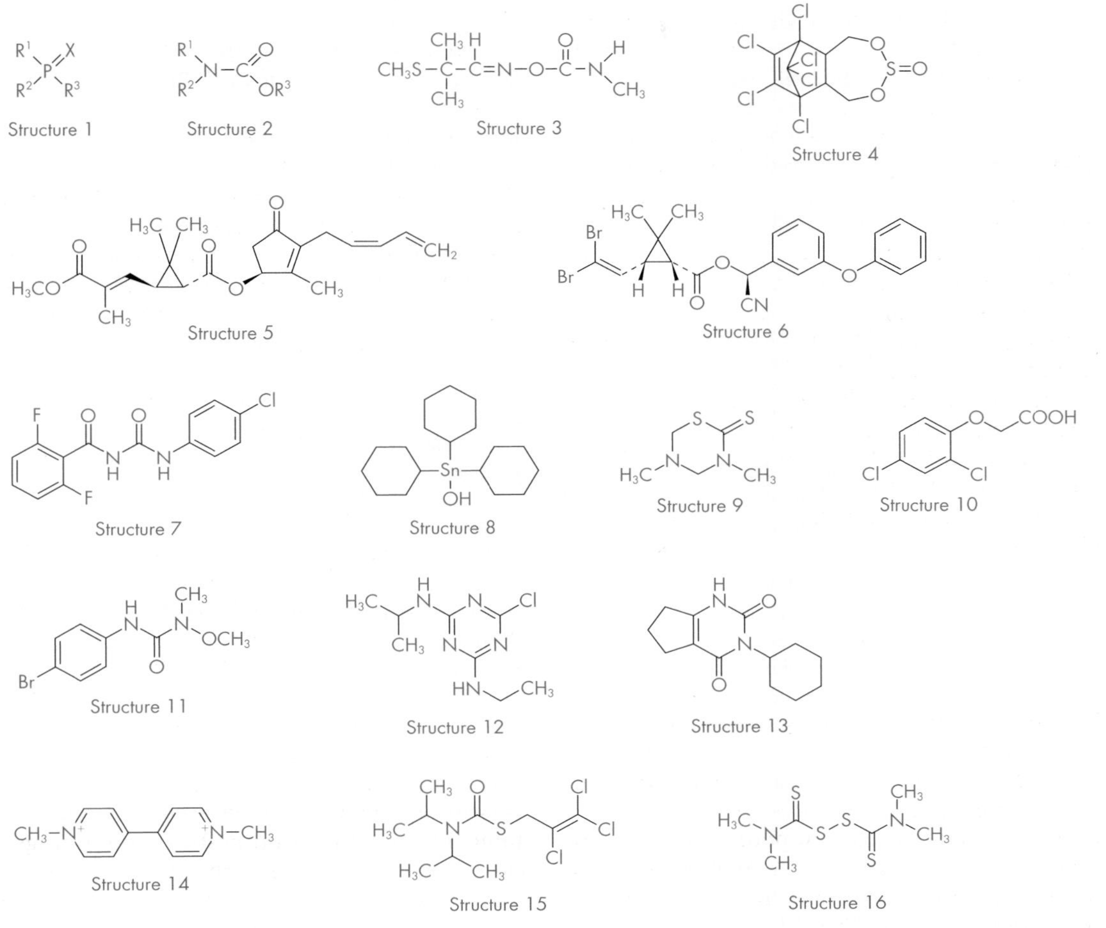

Structure 1

Structure 2

Structure 3

Structure 4

Structure 5

Structure 6

Structure 7

Structure 8

Structure 9

Structure 10

Structure 11

Structure 12

Structure 13

Structure 14

Structure 15

Structure 16

Figure 4.2 Structures of pesticides: **1**, general structure for organophosphates (see Table 4.4) where R^1 = alkyl, *O*-alkyl or *S*-alkyl, R^2 = *O*-alkyl, R^3 = alkyl, aryl, *O*-alkyl, *O*-aryl, *S*-alkyl, *S*-aryl, amine, X = O or S; **2**, general structure for carbamates where R^1 = methyl, R^2 = H or methyl, and R^3 = aryl, heterocyclic or oxime groups; **3**, aldicarb (an oxime carbamate insecticide, acaricide and nematocide); **4**, endosulfan (a chlorinated cyclodiene insecticide and an organochlorine acaricide); **5**, pyrethrin II (a natural pyrethroid insecticide); **6**, deltamethrin (a synthetic pyrethroid insecticide); **7**, diflubenzuron (a substituted urea insecticide); **8**, cyhexatin (an organotin acaricide); **9**, dazomet (a cyclic dithiocarbamate herbicide and fungicide); **10**, 2,4-D (a chlorinated phenoxyacetic acid herbicide); **11**, metobromuron (a substituted urea herbicide); **12**, atrazine (a triazine herbicide); **13**, lenacil (a uracil herbicide); **14**, paraquat (a quaternary ammonium herbicide); **15**, tri-allate (a thiocarbamate herbicide); **16**, thiram (a dithiocarbamate fungicide).

Table 4.4 Major classes of pesticides; associated chemical groups and examples of substances in use

Classification	Chemical groups	Examples
Insecticides	Organophosphorus compounds	Diazinon, dichlorvos (structure1 in Fig. 4.2 shows the general structure of organophosphorus compounds)
	Carbamates	Aldicarb (structure 3 in Fig. 4.2), pirimicarb
	Chlorinated hydrocarbons	Dichlorodiphenyltrichlorethane (DDT), lindane, endosulfan (structure 4 in Fig. 4.2)
	Pyrethroids (natural and synthetic)	Pyrethrin II (structure 5 in Fig. 4.2), deltamethrin (structure 6 in Fig. 4.2), cypermethrin
	Substituted ureas	Diflubenzuron (structure 7 in Fig. 4.2)
	Organotin compounds	
	Heterocyclic compounds	Dazomet (structure 9 in Fig. 4.2), dieldrin
Herbicides	Chlorinated phenoxy acids	2,4-Dichlorophenoxyacetic acid (2,4-D) (structure 10 in Fig. 4.2), (2,4,5-trichlorophenoxy)acetic acid (2,4,5-T)
	Substituted ureas	Metobromuron (structure 11 in Fig. 4.2), methabenzthiazuron
	Triazines	Atrazine (structure 12 in Fig. 4.2), simazine
	Uracils	Lenacil (structure 13 in Fig. 4.2), bromacil
	Quaternary ammonium compounds	Paraquat (structure 14 in Fig. 4.2), diquat
	Carbamates and thiocarbamates and carbanilates	Carboxazole (a carbamate), tri-allate (a thiocarbamate, structure 15 in Fig. 4.2), propham (a carbanilate)
	Carboxylic acids and esters	Dicamba
	Amides	Cyprazole
	Anilide and choroacetanilide compounds	Alachlor
	Organophosphorus compounds	Glyphosate
	Organoarsenic compounds	Sodium arsenate
Fungicides	Benzimidazoles	Carbendazim, thiabendazole
	Dithiocarbamates	Thiram (structure 16 in Fig. 4.2), disulfiram
	Acylalanines	Metalaxyl
	Organophosphorus compounds	Pyrazophos
	Dithiocarbamate complexes with manganese, nickel and zinc	
	Organic and inorganic compounds of tin, copper and mercury	Tributyltin oxide, mercury salts, phenylmercury salts, Bordeaux mixture
Rodenticides	Phosphines	(derived by the reaction of moisture with e.g. zinc phosphide)
	Inorganic rodenticides	Thallium sulphate, sodium arsenite
	Coumarin anticoagulants	Warfarin, brodifacoum, difenacoum
Acaricides	Organotin compounds	Cyhexatin (structure 8 in Fig. 4.2)
	Organophosphate compounds	Dichlorvos
Molluscicides		Niclosamide, tributyltin oxide, calcium arsenate, metaldehyde, thidicarb
Nematocides	Carbamates	Benomyl
	Organophosphorus compounds	Phorate, chlorpyrifos

Table 4.5 Pesticide poisonings reported by various countries

Country	Years	No. of poisoning cases	Pesticide class	Substance[a]
Matto Grosso do Sul, Brazil[b]	1992–2002	1026	Organophosphorus insecticides	Chlorpyrifos (3.1%), Dimethoate (1.3%), Malathion (5.9%), Methamidophos (16.7%), Monochrotophos (7.9%)
			Carbamate insecticides	Aldrin (4.6%), Carbofuran (9.3%),
			Organochlorine insecticides	DDT or lindane (0.8%), Endosulfan (1.7%)
			Pyrethroid insecticides	Cypermethrin (3.8%)
			Insecticides not classified	(45%)
		165	Organophosphorus herbicides	2,4-D (11.5%), Glyphosate (28.5%), Other organophosphorus herbicides (18.8%)
			Herbicides other	2,4-D + picloram (27.2%), Paraquat (3.6%), Picloram (2.4%), Trifuralin (10.3%)
		17	Fungicides	No information given
		23	Other classes	No information given
South India[c]	2002	643	Organophosphorus compounds	Acephate (1.3%), Chlorpyrifos (10.9%), Dimethoate (0.1%), Ethion (0.3%), Malathion (0.5%), Methyl parathion (0.5%), Mevinphos (0.1%), Monocrotophos (24.8%), Phorate (2.0%), Phosalone (0.2%), Profenofos (0.2%), Quinalphos (7.5%), Traizophos (0.6%), Unknown anticholinesterases (13.9%)
			Organochlorine compounds	Endosulfan (13.3%), Endrin (7.1%)
			Carbamate compounds	Indoxicarb (0.7%), Methomyl (0.3%),
			Pyrethroid insecticides	Cypermethrin (5.6%), Fenvalerate (0.2%)
			Other compounds	Spinosad (0.4%), Imidacloprid (0.8%), Unidentified pesticides (8.0%)

Continued

Table 4.5 *(Continued)*

Country	Years	No. of poisoning cases	Pesticide class	Substance[a]
Sri Lanka[d]	1998–1999	239	Organophosphosphorus insecticides	31%
			Carbamate insecticides	8.4%
			Organochlorine insecticides	Endosulfan (5.9%)
			Pyrethroid insecticides	2.1%
			Herbicides	Paraquat (13.4%)
			Herbicides other	7.9%
			Sulfur	0.8%
			Unidentified	29.7%

[a] Figures in brackets indicate percentage of cases for each substance. N.B. Figures are total for accidental and intentional poisonings.

[b] M.C.P. Recena, D.X. Pires, E.D. Caldas, Acute poisoning with pesticides in the state of Mato Grosso do Sul, Brazil. *Sci. Tot. Environ.*, 2006, **357**, 88–95.

[c] C. S. Rao, V. Venkateswarlu, T. Surender, M. Eddleston, N.A. Buckley, Pesticide poisoning in south India: opportunities for prevention and improved medical management. *Trop. Med. Int. Health.*, 2005, **10**, 581–588.

[d] W. van der Hoek, and F. Konradsen, Risk factors for actute pesticide poisoning in Sri Lanka. *Trop. Med. Int. Health.*, 2005, **10**,589–596.

pesticide (amitrole) is nontoxic in humans even when several hundred grams are ingested. Even within a particular class of pesticide the lethal dose may vary considerably. Moreover, the metabolites of many pesticides (e.g. oxygen analogues of phosphorothionates) are much more toxic than the parent compounds.

Commercially available preparations usually contain an active substance mixed with filler (solids) or dissolved in an organic solvent (liquids). Although certain pesticides are unlikely to cause acute toxicity, the vehicle in which they are formulated (toluene, xylenes, butan-1-ol, cyclohexanone, farbasol and solvent naphtha) may itself be toxic and, in some cases, can be the main causative agent for the symptoms observed. This needs to be taken into consideration in clinical treatment and in forensic toxicology both in terms of the analytical methods applied to samples and the interpretation of results.

The World Health Organization (WHO) has classified pesticides into five groups based on their hazard. In the WHO classification, hazard is considered as 'the acute risk to health (that is, the risk of single or multiple exposures over a relatively short period of time) that might be encountered accidentally by any person handling the product in accordance with the directions for handling by the manufacturer or in accordance with the rules laid down for storage and transportation by competent international bodies' (the *WHO Recommended Classification of Pesticides by Hazard and Guidelines to Classification* 2006). Classification is based on acute oral and dermal toxicity to the rat (LD_{50}) and the estimated lethal doses related to a 70 kg person (see Table 4.6). It must be borne in mind that extrapolation of toxicity values from a test animal such as a rat to humans is a best estimate and may carry a high error factor for some substances. Realistic human lethal doses of pesticides can be estimated only on the basis of well-documented cases of poisoning.

The immense variety of chemical compounds with pesticidal properties means that the identification of an unknown substance is complex, particularly where no information is available about the likely identity of the pesticide. In clinical and forensic toxicology, unless specific information is available indicating that a particular pesticide should be targeted in analysis (e.g. a body found with a labelled pesticide product alongside), a broader screening procedure should be employed to identify active pesticide components. Some colour tests can be very useful preliminary indicators of the class of compound and can confirm the constituents of a proprietary formulation. The ammonium molybdate test is used for phosphorus and phosphides in stomach contents and nonbiological materials (Flanagan *et al.* 1995). The furfuraldehyde test is used for carbamates in the same matrices (Flanagan *et al.* 1995). The phosphorus test can be used to detect OP compounds; although the limited sensitivity of the test means that it is not able to detect OP compounds in blood and the sodium dithionite test is used for diquat and paraquat (Tompsett 1970).

While colour tests are useful to indicate preliminary classes, they are generally restricted to stomach contents and nonbiological materials and will only detect a rather restricted range of

Table 4.6 WHO hazard classification (WHO 2006)

Class	Description	Oral LD_{50} for the rat (mg/kg body mass)	
		Solids	Liquids
Ia	Extremely hazardous	<5	<20
Ib	Highly hazardous	5–50	20–200
II	Moderately hazardous	50–500	200–2000
III	Slightly hazardous	>501	>2001
T.5	Product unlikely to present acute hazard in normal use		

vomiting, and muscular weakness. Severe poisoning leads to coma, flaccid paralysis, breathing difficulties, cyanosis and cardiac arrhythmias. Atropine and pralidoxime are effective antidotes in severe cases. In acute clinical poisoning, diagnostic tests for depressed cholinesterase activity are most crucial. Detecting, identifying and quantifying the particular agent responsible has less bearing on immediate treatment, although some of the lipophilic diethyl phosphothiolates can be sequestered in the tissues for several days and patients who appear to have recovered may suffer a recurrence of toxic effects. Identification of the agent involved can alert clinicians to this possibility.

Two types of cholinesterases exist in the body. Acetylcholinesterase (AChE), which is also known as true cholinesterase, is found in red cells, nerve endings, lungs and brain tissues. Its main function is to hydrolyse AcCh at cholinergic nerve endings. The second type is usually known as pseudocholinesterase (ChE) and occurs in the plasma in addition to other body tissues. The exact physiological function of ChE is unknown, but it has the ability to hydrolyse a variety of esters in addition to cholinesterase. Depression of ChE can also be caused by non-pesticide chemicals, liver diseases and other factors (physiological, pharmacological or genetic). Measurement of red-cell AChE is therefore a more specific indicator of cholinesterase inhibition caused by OP or carbamate pesticides. Moreover, the repression of red-cell AChE activity can be demonstrated for up to 2–6 weeks after exposure, whereas that of plasma ChE returns to normal much more quickly. Nevertheless, in practice, plasma ChE activity is a useful indicator of exposure, since if normal values are found this effectively excludes acute poisoning by these substances.

Some carbamate herbicides and fungicides, such as the dithiocarbamates, do not inhibit cholinesterases to any significant degree and are relatively nontoxic in humans. Postmortem specimens for AChE assay must be kept in cold storage and analysed as soon as possible to minimise the effects of spontaneous reactivation of the enzyme.

Carbamates

In terms of toxicity, carbamate pesticides have a similar action to that of the OP compounds in causing a decrease in cholinesterase activity, but the binding to the active site of the cholinesterase enzyme is reversible. Consequently, although the symptoms are practically identical to those of OP poisoning, they have a shorter duration.

Carbamates can be divided into various subclasses, characterised by their different thermal stabilities. *N*-Methylcarbamates give thermal decomposition products, mainly substituted phenols. When analysed by GC-MS, these products give rise to mass spectra with abundant molecular ions. The compounds from other subclasses of carbamates are more thermally stable. GC-MS analysis of these more stable compounds results in mass spectra where the molecular ions are of low intensity but, together with diagnostic fragments, enable identification to be made. In LC-MS methods, the carbamates do not present a serious problem in terms of analysis. Positive-ion detection with a soft-ionisation technique is the method of choice (Niessen 1999). Lacassie *et al.* (2001) have reviewed methods of analysis of various classes of pesticides for use in clinical and forensic toxicology, including LC-MS methods for carbamates.

Chlorinated hydrocarbons

Chlorinated hydrocarbons are neurotoxins that also damage the liver and kidneys. Major clinical features of poisoning are headache, disorientation, paraesthesia and convulsions.

Chlorinated hydrocarbons may be analysed intact using chromatography with a dual FID-NPD (nitrogen–phosphorus detection) system, but greater sensitivity can be achieved using electron capture detection (ECD). The methods applied in clinical and forensic cases do not need to be highly sensitive, because most compounds that belong to this class are only slightly toxic and severe symptoms of poisoning are observed only after ingestion of large quantities (several grams). Moreover, the symptoms often result from the solvents in which the chlorinated hydrocarbons are formulated. A useful reference for the determination of chlorinated hydrocarbons in human serum using GC after SPE is Brock *et al.* (1996).

Pyrethrins and pyrethroids

The term 'pyrethrins' is used collectively for the six insecticidal constituents present in extracts of the flowers of *Pyrethrum cinerariaefolium* and other species. Pyrethrins comprise esters of the natural stereoisomers of chrysanthemic acid (pyrethrin I, cinerin I and jasmolin I) and the corresponding esters of pyrethric acid (pyrethrin II, cinerin II and jasmolin II). Their low photochemical stability has led to the manufacture of synthetic analogues (pyrethroids), which are highly toxic to insects. In recent years pyrethroids have been manufactured and used in large quantities.

Pyrethrins and pyrethroids have relatively low toxicity to humans, but exposure to these compounds by inhalation can cause localised reactions to the upper and lower respiratory tract, which leads to oral and laryngeal oedema, coughing, shortness of breath and chest pain. In acutely exposed sensitised patients a serious asthmatic-type reaction can be triggered that can prove fatal within a few minutes.

GC-FID and GC-MS are appropriate detection systems for pyrethrins and they can be analysed either without derivatisation or after methylation (Bissacot and Vassilieff 1997; Fernández-Gutierrez *et al.* 1998). Some pyrethroids such as cyfluthrine, cypermethrin and permethrin are halogen-containing and therefore GC-ECD provides a sensitive and selective method of detection for these substances.

Nitrophenols and nitrocreosols

Dinitrophenol, dinitrocreosol and dinoseb stimulate oxidative metabolism in the mitochondria and cause profuse sweating, headache, tachycardia and fever.

Dinitrocreosol can be measured in blood specimens by colorimetry (Smith *et al.* 1978).

Chlorinated phenoxy acids

Chlorinated phenoxy acids are corrosive chemicals that damage the skin, eyes and respiratory and gastrointestinal tract. Ingestion of large doses causes vomiting, abdominal pain, diarrhoea, metabolic acidosis, pulmonary oedema and coma. Alkalinisation of the urine to increase the excretion of 2,4-dichlorophenoxyacetic acid (2,4-D) and other chlorophenoxy compounds has proved an effective therapy.

Substituted phenoxy acids occur in commercial products as salts or esters. Conversion of salts by extraction and derivatisation to the corresponding methyl esters improves their chromatographic properties. The presence of isooctyl (2,2,4-trimethylpentyl) esters of chlorinated phenoxy acid herbicides can be indicated by using mass spectrometry.

Triazines

Ingestion of about 100 g of atrazine can lead to coma, circulatory collapse, metabolic acidosis and gastric bleeding. This may be followed by renal failure, hepatic necrosis and a disseminated intravascular coagulopathy which may prove fatal. Haemodialysis is recommended for severe cases.

Triazines contain several nitrogen atoms (e.g. atrazine, structure 12, Fig. 4.2), making GC-NPD a good choice for analysis. Most triazines, which are readily amenable to GC-MS, exhibit highly characteristic mass spectra of the parent compounds and yield the important degradation products, hydroxy- and des-alkyl triazines. By using LC-MS with atmospheric pressure chemical ionisation (APCI) and electrospray, and optimising the in-source parameters, the protonated triazine molecule can be seen without fragmentation (Niessen 1999).

Quaternary ammonium compounds

Ingestion of concentrated paraquat formulations causes burning of the mouth, oesophagus and stomach, and after massive absorption patients die of multiple organ failure. Absorption of smaller amounts can lead to renal damage followed by a progressive pulmonary fibrosis that causes death from respiratory failure, in some cases after 2 to 3 weeks of ingestion. Treatments to reduce absorption or increase elimination have not been effective. A strongly positive urine test with the dithionite test (see below) in a sample collected more than 4 hours after ingestion indicates a poor prognosis. Measurement of the plasma paraquat concentration is a more accurate prognostic guide. Diquat is also an irritant poison that causes vomiting, diarrhoea and epigastric pain. In severe cases, liver and renal failure, convulsions and coma may ensue, but diquat ingestion does not lead to progressive pulmonary fibrosis.

Paraquat and diquat are not extractable by conventional LLE. The diene or monoene products of reduction of paraquat and diquat by sodium borohydride can be extracted by diethyl ether from alkaline solution for chromatography. Very limited data are available for the mass spectral characterisation of these compounds using electron impact ionisation. Colorimetric determination of paraquat and diquat after reduction with sodium dithionite under alkaline conditions is probably the most widely used technique. Both of the bipyridylium reduction products have absorbance maxima at 396 and 379 nm. Using an ion-pairing extraction technique, a lower limit of measurement of 50 μg/L can be achieved (Jarvie and Stewart 1979). Radioimmunoassay and fluorescence polarisation immunoassay methods for the determination of paraquat in serum are very sensitive and require only small sample volumes, but they are not widely available. Paraquat can also be determined in serum by HPLC-UV. Diquat may be analysed in biological specimens by most of the procedures described for paraquat. Specific HPLC procedures for paraquat and/or diquat have also been described (Ameno *et al.* 1995; Arys *et al.* 2000; Ito *et al.* 2005) and a capillary electrophoresis–MS method has recently been developed for the analysis of paraquat and diquat in serum (Vinner *et al.* 2001). An LC-MS/MS method is available for the analysis of paraquat and diquat in whole blood and urine following SPE clean-up (Lee *et al.* 2004).

Phosphides

Hydrogen phosphide (IUPAC name phosphane; commonly known as phosphine) is widely used as an insecticide and rodenticide (agricultural fumigant) and is usually generated by the action of water on metallic phosphides (aluminium, magnesium or zinc). Inhaled phosphine is readily absorbed by the lungs. Following the ingestion of metallic phosphides, phosphine is generated in the stomach and the gas acts on the gastrointestinal system and CNS. In severe cases abdominal pain, vomiting, convulsions and coma develop rapidly and death usually ensues within 2 hours.

The ammonium molybdate test and commercially available detector tubes (Guale *et al.* 1994) may be used as qualitative and quantitative procedures for stomach contents and nonbiological materials. Phosphine can also be determined in biological samples by using GC and NPD detection (Chan *et al.* 1983).

Coumarin anticoagulants

Accidental and intentional ingestion of 4-hydroxycoumarin rodenticides (Fig. 4.3) can lead to serious poisoning manifested by bleeding in multiple organ sites. Treatment consists of supplements of vitamin K (mild cases) and, for serious cases, infusions of fresh frozen plasma or purified clotting factors until the prothrombin time returns to the normal range.

Warfarin and the superwarfarin anticoagulant rodenticides (brodifacoum, bromadiolone, coumatetralyl and difenacoum; Fig. 4.3) can be analysed either intact or after derivatisation, by either GC or GC-MS methods, these being the most sensitive and selective. Five of the 4-hydroxycoumarin anticoagulants (brodifacoum, bromadiolone, coumatetralyl, difenacoum and warfarin) can also be resolved and determined in serum by HPLC with fluorimetric detection (Felice *et al.* 1991).

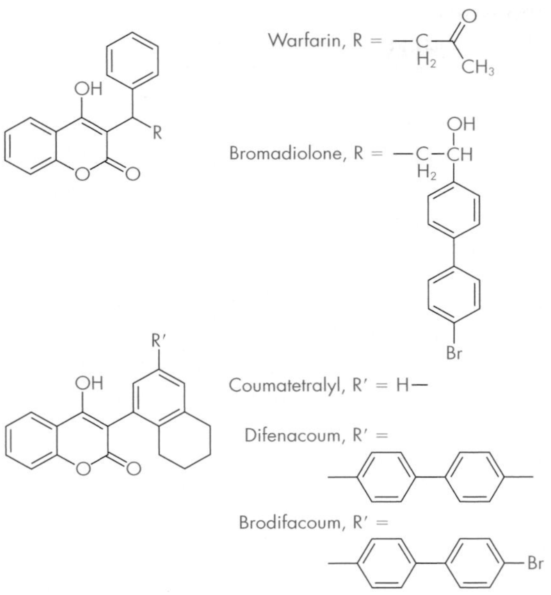

Figure 4.3 Chemical structures of the 4-hydroxycoumarin anticoagulant rodenticides.

Organic and inorganic metallic compounds

A wide range of organic and inorganic metallic compounds are found in agricultural use. Inorganic and organometallic compounds are used as acaricides (organotin), herbicides (organoarsenic), fungicides (dithiocarbamate compounds of nickel and dithiocarbamate complexes with manganese and zinc, organic and inorganic compounds of copper and mercury) and rodenticides (magnesium, aluminium and zinc phosphides, and thallium sulfate). For some compounds, exposure to the organic form results in more serious toxicity and the features of poisoning may be quite different from those of the inorganic compound. Metallic compounds and their associated clinical symptoms are discussed below under metals and anions together with the methods used for their analysis.

Metals and anions

Metals and anions form an important, but disparate, group of poisons that present many difficulties in their systematic chemical analysis (Yeoman 1985; Baldwin and Marshall 1999). Acute poisoning with these agents is rare in developed countries, but remains common in many underdeveloped parts of the world. Chronic poisoning, as a result of industrial or environmental exposure, occurs in many countries.

The toxicity of metallic poisons may be influenced by the chemical nature of the compound ingested (valence state, solubility, inorganic or organic compound) and the route of administration. Inhalation of vapours (e.g. arsine, hydrogen cyanide and mercury phosphine) can cause acute toxicity, including rapid death. The signs and symptoms of acute poisoning may differ from those associated with chronic toxicity. Some metallic (e.g. arsenic) and anionic (e.g. cyanide) substances undergo extensive metabolism after ingestion. These factors have a significant bearing on analytical investigations applied to biological materials and their interpretation. It is important in individual cases, therefore, to know whether poisoning resulted from acute, chronic or acute-on-chronic exposure. Of equal importance is the time of specimen collection in relation to the alleged time of ingestion or exposure.

The wide range of metallic or anionic poisons that might be involved in any case of suspected poisoning means that great care is required in the collection of appropriate specimens and the selection of toxicological and other tests. There is no simple systematic way to investigate cases for which the history is uncertain and the identity of the poison unknown. The investigation is often led by a process of elimination of the more likely causes of poisoning (e.g. pharmaceuticals and illicit drugs), and then a careful examination of the detailed history of the patient or deceased, in particular any access to compounds associated with industrial and agricultural use.

Considerable advances in analytical techniques for measuring metals in biological fluids have been made since the early 1980s, particularly in electrothermal atomic absorption spectrometry (ETAAS), inductively coupled plasma–mass spectrometry (ICP-MS) and ICP coupled with atomic emission spectrometry (ICP-AES). Table 4.7 summarises methods for analysis of metallic elements.

Metals

Aluminium

Aluminium is the most abundant metal in the earth's crust, but its role in biology and medicine became understood only relatively recently (Martin 1986). The normal intake of aluminium from food and beverages is up to 100 mg per day, but its absorption from the gut is relatively poor and depends on the speciation of the element and the presence of other substances (e.g. phosphate) in the diet. A number of over-the-counter antacid preparations that contain aluminium hydroxide are used widely which can increase the daily intake by several grams. Incidences of acute aluminium poisoning are relatively uncommon in the normal population. However, those exposed to aluminium through occupation and patients undergoing certain types of clinical treatment may be at risk. It has been established that excessive exposure in patients undergoing dialysis can cause 'dialysis dementia', a type of encephalopathy that can be rapidly progressive and lead to death within a few months (Alfrey *et al.* 1976). Use of aluminium sulfate as a flocculating agent in domestic water supplies is the major source of the metal in these patients, particularly if the water used for dialysis is not purified. The large quantities of oral aluminium salts that may be given to some renal patients to reduce the intestinal absorption of phosphate may also cause toxicity. Plasma aluminium concentra-

Table 4.7 Commonly employed methods of analysis for metallic elements

Element	Commonly used methods of analysis
Aluminium	ETAAS, ICP-AES, ICP-MS
Antimony	ETAAS, ICP-MS
Arsenic	ETAAS (after acid digestion and hydride generation), ICP-MS, Reinsch test (stomach contents or 'scene residues'). Gutzeit test (stomach contents, water, food and other materials), spectrophotometric methods
Barium	ETAAS, ICP-MS
Beryllium	ETAAS, ICP-MS
Bismuth	ETAAS (direct or after hydride generation), ICP-MS
Cadmium	ETAAS (with Zeeman background correction), ICP–MS, AAS (with specialised sample introduction to maximise sensitivity)
Copper	Colorimetric analysis or by flame AAS
	ETAAS, ICP–AES or ICP–MS for urine (generally only of value in the investigation of chronic copper-related liver disease)
Iron	Colorimetric assay, ETAAS, ICP-MS
Lead	AAS (with specialised sample introduction to maximise sensitivity), ETAAS, ICP-MS
Lithium	Flame photometry, colorimetric assays, ion-selective electrodes, flame AAS and ETAAS, ICP-MS
Mercury	'Cold vapour' AAS
Selenium	Most earlier methods for measuring selenium in blood were based on fluorimetry. Techniques recently described include liquid chromatography (LC) and GC, ETAAS by direct analysis or after hydride generation and ICP–MS, which can also measure selenium in tissues[a]
Thallium	Spectrophotometry at 550 nm using rhodamine 'B' dye, AAS, ETAAS, ICP-MS

[a] T. M. T. Sheehan and D. J. Halls, Measurement of selenium in clinical speciments, *Ann. Clin Biochem.*, 1999, **36**, 301–305.

tions should be monitored routinely in *all* patients in end-stage renal failure who receive dialysis therapy to ensure that absorption of aluminium is kept to an absolute minimum. In addition, regular testing is needed of water supplied to patients who have home dialysis. De Wolff *et al.* (2002) reported blood and tissue aluminium concentrations in four patients who had died as a result of the use of dialysate contaminated with aluminium, which indicates that this is an ongoing problem despite controls being in place and good general awareness of the requirements. Concern has developed as to the harmful effects of occupational exposure to aluminium. Where occupational exposure involves inhalation of fine particles or dusts, aluminium may be stored in the lung tissue and leach out very slowly over many months. As a result, plasma and urine aluminium concentrations can remain elevated for several weeks or months. There is also evidence of a dose-dependent association between increased aluminium body-burden and CNS effects in these workers (Akila *et al.* 1999), and thresholds for these effects in aluminium welders have been proposed (108–160 μg/L in urine and 7–10 μg/L in plasma) (Riihimäki *et al.* 2000). In situations of acute or chronic occupational or environmental exposure to aluminium, measurement of blood (plasma) and/or urine aluminium is an effective way to assess the degree of exposure.

Where renal function is normal, aluminium is excreted rapidly from the body and there is little possibility of accumulation. The reference value for urine aluminium in non-exposed healthy adults is <15 μg/L.

Antimony

Various salts of antimony (e.g. tartar emetic, antimony potassium tartrate) have a long history of use as medicines (McCallum 1999) and continue to be used to treat tropical parasitic diseases such as schistosomiasis (bilharziasis) and leishmaniasis. Antimony compounds are also used industrially in the manufacture of lead batteries, semiconductors, paints, ceramics and pewterware. Other modern industrial compounds include antimony oxychloride ($Sb_6O_6Cl_4$), widely used as a fire retardant on fabrics and mattresses. The fatal dose of antimony in the form of tartar emetic is about 1 g in an adult, but there is much interindividual variability. The signs and symptoms of acute antimony poisoning include metallic taste, dysphagia, epigastric pain, violent vomiting, diarrhoea, abdominal pain and circulatory collapse. These symptoms are almost indistinguishable from those of acute arsenic poisoning, but larger doses are required. Similarly, the effects of exposure to stibine (SbH_3) are similar to those of arsine (AsH_3). Chronic effects of occupational antimony exposure include 'antimony spots' on the skin and pneumoconiosis. Reference values for antimony in body fluids and tissues are <1 μg/L. However, there is limited information on the concentrations of antimony in blood, urine and tissues in cases of antimony poisoning or in body fluids of patients who receive antimony-containing drugs. Values of up to 150 μg/L have been reported in urine of occupationally exposed workers (Smith *et al.* 1995).

Arsenic

Arsenic is widely distributed in the environment, particularly in rocks, sediments and some water supplies. Organic forms of arsenic (e.g. arsenobetaine, arsenocholine) occur naturally in seaweed, fish and shellfish, but are mostly nontoxic (Le *et al.* 1994; Francesconi *et al.* 2002). Arsenic is metabolised in the liver to mono- and dimethylated species as a means of detoxification. Different forms of arsenic have widely differing human toxicity. These forms are also handled by the body in different ways, which causes problems in their determination and in the interpretation of laboratory findings, particularly when the source of arsenic is unknown. Arsenic has three common valence or oxidation states: 0 (metalloid), 3^+ (arsenite) and 5^+ (arsenate). The trivalent inorganic salts of arsenic (e.g. sodium arsenite, $NaAsO_2$) are the most toxic and may cause serious toxicity or death after acute ingestion of relatively small doses (<200 mg). Inhalation of arsine gas (AsH_3) may cause massive haemolysis, renal failure and rapid death, as in industrial accidents. The signs and symptoms of chronic arsenic poisoning (arsenic oxide) are quite complex and include weight loss, malaise, hyperpigmentation of the skin, transverse white lines on the nails, liver damage, changes in the blood, peripheral neuropathy and increased risk of skin and liver cancer. Acute poisoning is characterised by bloody diarrhoea, vomiting, excruciating abdominal pain, circulatory collapse and coma. Skin and respiratory cancer is another major feature of chronic arsenic exposure; huge populations are affected in parts of India, Bangladesh and Vietnam because of the consumption of contaminated well-water supplies (Piamphongsant 1999; Ahsan *et al.* 2000; Chowdhury *et al.* 2000; Smith *et al.* 2000; Berg *et al.* 2001). The main sources of the problem are wells sunk into land that contains rocks with a high content of arsenic salts, with subsequent contamination of the underground aquifers. Ingestion of seafood can give rise to elevated levels of arsenic and consideration should be given to this possibility when interpreting analytical results. Measurement of urine arsenic helps in the assessment of acute or chronic exposure (Apostoli *et al.* 1999). Hair analysis has also been used in the diagnosis and evaluation of chronic arsenic poisoning, particularly suspected homicides. However, there can be problems distinguishing external contamination from ingested arsenic (Hindmarsh 2002).

Normal values for arsenic are <10 μg/L in blood and urine but elevated values can be seen after ingestion of seafood and where there is occupational exposure, and elevated levels of arsenic potentially arising from these sources should be taken into account when assessing measured arsenic concentrations. In cases of acute inorganic arsenic poisoning, concentrations above 500 μg/L may be seen in blood and urine.

Barium

The inorganic compounds of barium are widely used as pigments and glazes in industry and in the manufacture of paint, glass and ceramics. The insoluble sulfate salt is widely used as radiographic contrast medium. Most (insoluble) barium salts are relatively nontoxic. However, pneumoconiosis related to the inhalation of barium dusts (baritosis) has been recognised in the mining industry. By contrast, the soluble salts of barium, particularly the carbonate and chloride, are extremely toxic if ingested orally or given intravenously. The oral fatal dose of soluble barium salts may be as little as 0.8 g. Signs and symptoms of barium poisoning may show within 1 to 2 hours of ingestion and include abdominal pain, diarrhoea, vomiting and a tingling around the mouth. Severe hypokalaemia may also develop from a shift of extracellular potassium into muscle. This may cause cardiac rhythm disturbances, which require close monitoring, and the administration of potassium chloride intravenously to correct the hypokalaemia. Other useful investigations in cases of acute barium poisoning include radiography of the abdomen for the presence of radio-opaque material in the gut. Careful monitoring of serum potassium concentrations in any case of suspected barium poisoning is of vital importance.

Reference concentrations of barium in plasma are <1 μg/L. Urine excretion is <20 μg/24 h. In nonfatal cases of barium poisoning, plasma barium concentrations of up to 8 mg/L have been reported (Boehnert *et al.* 1985).

Beryllium

Beryllium is used in the manufacture of corrosion-resistant and high-strength alloys. Such products are commonly used in the nuclear, aerospace and weapons industries. Beryllium–copper alloys are also used in diverse products such as springs, gears, electrical contacts and other engine components. Beryllium itself is a highly toxic element and is associated with a characteristic occupational disease (Kolanz 2001). The major target organ is the lung, where it causes granulomatous disease (berylliosis) and an increased risk of lung cancer. Other organ systems may also be affected, including the lymphatics, liver, heart, kidney, skin and bone (Stiefel *et al.* 1980). Most of an absorbed dose of beryllium is excreted in urine over a period of several days, but lung deposits may leach beryllium so slowly that urine excretion continues for several years.

Normal values for beryllium in urine are generally accepted as <1 μg/L.

Bismuth

Bismuth, a heavy metal, produces toxicity that can sometimes mimic that associated with lead and mercury. For this reason, it can be useful to include bismuth in any heavy-metal screening procedure undertaken in patients with unexplained neurological symptoms. Bismuth salts have been used in medicine for more than a century, such as in the treatment of gastrointestinal disorders, and are available in over-the-counter preparations. Some inorganic salts of bismuth are relatively insoluble in water and cause minimal toxicity, whereas other compounds, particularly lipid-soluble organic compounds, are known to accumulate in the body after excessive dosing and can cause severe neurotoxicity. Water-soluble compounds of bismuth are more likely to cause renal damage, including acute renal failure. A number of deaths have been reported after acute and chronic overdose with various bismuth medicinal products. Measurement of urinary bismuth concentrations may be useful diagnostically or after treatment of poisoning using oral chelating agents, which can greatly increase urinary clearance of bismuth.

Reference values for bismuth in blood and urine are low (<1 μg/L). Acceptable 'therapeutic concentrations' in blood are generally up to 50 μg/L. Concentrations >100 μg/L are generally associated with toxicity and concentrations >1000 μg/L may be found in patients with severe neurological symptoms such as encephalopathy.

Cadmium

Cadmium and its salts and alloys are used in the manufacture of nickel–cadmium batteries, pigments and special alloys. Many of the risks associated with occupational and environmental exposure to cadmium have been known for many years. These include emphysema from the acute inhalation of cadmium fumes and, more long term, renal impairment (Jarup *et al.* 1988). Water supplies contaminated with industrial cadmium in Japan led to accumulation of the metal in rice and other dietary sources with subsequent human poisoning on a vast scale. Those affected developed renal damage, skeletal deformities caused by disturbances of calcium and phosphate metabolism, and severe back and leg pain (Friberg *et al.* 1971). This painful condition became known as itai-itai (ouch-ouch) disease. For those not occupationally exposed, the major source of cadmium remains the diet, although it is absorbed poorly from the gut. Inhalation of tobacco smoke is another source of cadmium exposure, as the bioavailability of cadmium via the lung is very high and heavy smokers may have blood cadmium concentrations at the limit of current occupational guidance values. Following absorption, cadmium is stored mainly in the liver and kidney, where it is bound to metallothionein and stays in the body for decades. The most important toxic effect is on the kidney, with proximal renal tubular necrosis; this can be detected by a characteristic increase in the excretion of low-molecular-weight proteins. Individuals who have a long history of excessive occupational cadmium exposure can have a high body burden, which persists into old age (Mason *et al.* 1999). Elevated blood and urine cadmium concentrations may be observed many years after the cessation of exposure in such individuals. Blood cadmium concentrations in non-smokers are <2 μg/L and in smokers <6 μg/L. Urine concentrations are generally below 1 μg/L in both smokers and non-smokers. Cadmium-induced renal tubule impairment is generally related to urine cadmium concentrations >15 μg/L.

Copper

Copper is an essential trace element with a recommended intake of 2.5–3.0 mg per day in adults (Piscator 1979; Aggett 1999). Wilson's disease (hepatolenticular degeneration) is a genetically inherited disorder of copper metabolism in which there is an inability to transport and excrete copper from the liver into bile (Aggett 1999). This leads to 'copper overload' and associated liver and neurological damage that can cause death unless treated early. There is some evidence that excess environmental exposure to copper in drinking water or diet (from copper cooking pots) may lead to copper-related liver disease in babies and young children (e.g.

Indian childhood cirrhosis; Sethi *et al.* 1993; Von Mühlendahl and Lange 1994; Müller *et al.* 1996). Copper toxicity has also been found in patients who undergo dialysis with defective copper-containing dialysis membranes (O'Donohue *et al.* 1993). Occupational exposure to copper compounds is relatively rare. The main risk is associated with copper fumes in smelting furnaces, which lead to respiratory illness and metal-fume fever. Copper-related liver and respiratory disease has also been reported in vineyard workers who spray copper-containing fungicides (Bordeaux mixture). Acute copper poisoning may sometimes be seen in cases of accidental and suicidal ingestion of copper salts and solutions, particularly water-soluble salts, such as the sulfate, chloride or acetate. The signs and symptoms of acute (oral) copper poisoning are metallic taste, abdominal pain, vomiting, diarrhoea and gastrointestinal bleeding. In severe cases this can lead to hypotension, shock, cardiac failure and death (Walsh *et al.* 1977; Gulliver 1991).

The reference range for plasma copper is wide and depends on age, pregnancy and any underlying disease state. In healthy adults the reference range is 0.7–1.6 mg/L. The urinary excretion of in healthy adults is <50 μg/day. Significantly raised values are associated with patients with hepatobiliary disease (50–100 μg/day) or Wilson's disease (>100 μg/day).

Iron

Iron is widespread in nature and is found in rocks and minerals and in a wide variety of foodstuffs. It is essential to the functioning of the body. Accidental or suicidal ingestion of iron preparations in adults is rare, but poisoning is commonly seen in young children after the accidental ingestion of iron tablets. Over-the-counter products contain various iron salts (sulfate, fumarate, gluconate) and many are slow-release preparations The amount of elemental iron in a particular brand of tablet can range from 35 to 105 mg, which makes assessment of the actual dose of iron ingested very difficult. Serious toxicity after acute ingestion is generally seen at doses of more than 60 mg elemental iron/kg body mass. Fatalities are common when the ingested dose of iron is above 200 mg/kg body mass. The clinical presentation of iron poisoning and its time course can be quite complex, particularly when dealing with young children or babies. Reference ranges for serum iron are dependent on age and sex, with typical values in the range of 0.6–2.2 mg/L for men and 0.3–1.9 mg/L for women. A serum iron concentration above 5 mg/L on initial presentation is an indication of potentially serious toxicity and the need to consider active intervention, e.g. chelation therapy. Serum ion concentrations of 2.8–25.5 mg/L have been reported in children who survived the ingestion of up to 10 g of ferrous sulfate (Baselt 2002).

Lead

The toxic effects of (inorganic) lead have been known since ancient times, but this metal still presents significant health problems (Tong *et al.* 2000). Lead compounds have been used as cosmetics and components of medicines (Bayly *et al.* 1995; Hardy *et al.* 1998; Fisher and Le Couteur 2000; Moor and Adler 2000). Acute lead poisoning is relatively uncommon, however, and most symptomatic cases result from chronic ingestion, or inhalation of lead fumes or dusts during occupational exposure, or use of lead-containing 'traditional' medicines and ingestion of paint (pica) in children (Carton *et al.* 1987; Braithwaite and Brown 1988). Recognition of exposure to lead from leaded fuels has led to the withdrawal of these products in most developed countries. In adults, barely 10% of ingested lead is absorbed from the gastrointestinal tract but in children this proportion may be much higher. However, the bioavailability of ingested lead may be influenced substantially by the individual's diet and nutritional status (e.g. iron and calcium deficiency). Lead absorbed by inhalation has a much greater bioavailability, but this may depend on factors such as respiratory rate, particle size, the atmospheric concentration of lead and the duration of exposure. The clinical diagnosis of lead poisoning can be difficult when there is no clear history of exposure, since many of the signs and symptoms of lead poisoning are relatively nonspecific, e.g. tiredness, abdominal pain, anorexia. Laboratory investigations, therefore, play an essential part in the diagnosis and management of lead poisoning and also in the assessment of occupational and environmental lead exposure. By measuring lead isotope ratios in biological specimens it is possible to correlate these with the likely sources of exposure that might be found in a chemical incident or poisoning from an unusual source of lead (Delves and Campbell 1988, 1993).

The best-understood toxic effect of lead is its influence on haemoglobin synthesis leading to anaemia. Lead inhibits the enzyme ferrochelatase, which is involved in iron transport in the bone marrow and catalyses the introduction of ferrous iron (Fe^{2+}) into the porphyrin ring to form haem (Sakai 2000). (This is the last stage of haemoglobin synthesis.) Chronic lead exposure leads to the incorporation of zinc (rather than iron) into the porphyrin ring to produce erythrocyte zinc protoporphyrin (ZPP). The assay of ZPP is relatively simple and is used as an inexpensive screening test for chronic lead exposure (Solé *et al.* 2000). Monitoring the reduction in blood haemoglobin and the elevation in erythrocyte ZPP helps to assess chronic lead poisoning (Braithwaite and Brown 1988).

About 95% of the lead in blood is associated with the erythrocytes and has a half-life of a few months. Constant exposure results in the accumulation of lead in blood and tissues until a 'steady-state' is reached. Provided the degree and type of exposure are relatively constant, blood lead concentrations in environmentally, as well as in some occupationally, exposed individuals may be stable over long periods of time. Although lead can be found in most tissues of the body, over 90% of the body burden is deposited in the skeleton as insoluble lead phosphate. Following chronic exposure over many years, as occurs in some industrial workers, tissue stores such as bone become saturated. This effectively causes a much slower apparent elimination of lead from the circulation, so that, on cessation of exposure, the blood lead concentration may decline relatively slowly, with an elimination half-life of up to 1 year. Lead is poorly excreted from the body, the most important route being via the kidney. Normal urinary output of lead is less than 10 μg/day (50 nmol/day), but this can be increased greatly by chelation therapy.

Extensive studies have demonstrated the harmful effect of lead exposure on child development, behaviour and intelligence (Needlemann and Gatsonis 1990) and many countries have adopted occupational restrictions for blood lead concentrations to protect workers including young children and the developing fetus in pregnant women.

Normal urinary output of lead is <10 μg/day. A maximum blood lead concentration of 100 μg/L has been recommended in adults and children (Bellinger *et al.* 1992) but recent evidence suggests that there may be intellectual impairment in children with blood lead concentrations below this value (Canfield *et al.* 2003). Somewhat higher levels may be acceptable in adults who are occupationally exposed to lead, but careful monitoring of exposure is essential.

Lithium

Lithium salts are used in the prophylaxis of manic-depressive (bipolar) psychiatric disorders. These are usually prepared from lithium carbonate or citrate, and most are in the form of sustained-release preparations. The drug is well absorbed from the gut, with peak plasma lithium concentrations observed within 2 h for instant-release preparations and 2.5–5 h for sustained-release formulations. Lithium is not bound to plasma proteins and is eliminated only via the kidney. Plasma concentrations can accumulate to toxic levels if renal impairment develops. It is recommended that patients who receive therapy with lithium have regular monitoring to maintain plasma lithium concentrations in the therapeutic range. Nevertheless, overdosage with lithium, either acute, acute on chronic, or chronic is relatively common (Bailey and McGuigan 2000). Signs and symptoms of toxicity include ataxia, tremor, dysarthria, slurred speech, drowsiness and coma. The toxicity of lithium is exacerbated in cases in which there has been sodium depletion, through vomiting, and may sometimes be associated with the concurrent use of diuretic drugs. The therapeutic and toxic range in terms of plasma and serum values are rather close. Recommended therapeutic concentrations of lithium in plasma or serum are 0.6–1.2 mmol/L and may be associated with side-effects such as gastrointestinal upset, polyuria, thirst and fatigue. Signs and symptoms of toxicity are generally associated with values >1.5 mmol/L, and values >2 mmol/L require urgent medical attention.

Mercury

Mercury has been used in the manufacture of thermometers and a range of other scientific instruments for hundreds of years, but this use has now declined. Mercury and its compounds have also been used widely in the chemical industry and in the manufacture of drugs and pesticides. Mercury-containing dental amalgam fillings are still used in many countries.

The toxicity of mercury and its compounds is influenced greatly by the chemical form and valence state. The most toxic form of inorganic mercury is its divalent (Hg^{2+}) salt, particularly mercuric chloride, which was used as a disinfectant in earlier times. The fatal (oral) dose of mercuric chloride is less than 1 g, which led to its popularity as a homicidal and suicidal poison. There is significant toxicity associated with inhalation of (elemental) mercury vapour, which has a very high vapour pressure at normal room temperature. Broken mercury thermometers can constitute a serious risk in children through inhalation of vapour, particularly in a home environment such as a bedroom (Velzeboer *et al.* 1997). Organic forms of mercury, such as methyl mercury, are strongly neurotoxic and, being relatively lipid-soluble, can accumulate in fatty tissues of the body such as the brain. Large-scale environmental disasters have occurred, such as that involving the Minimata Bay area in Japan where hundreds of people died or became incapacitated. This was caused by the factory discharge of industrial waste that contained mercury, which settled into the sediments of the bay and river and was methylated by microorganisms. The methyl mercury became incorporated into the fish diet on which the residents of Minimata largely existed, and this resulted in so-called Minimata disease. Mercury poisoning may also be seen after the use of traditional medicines and cosmetics (Weldon *et al.* 2000).

The signs and symptoms of acute and chronic mercury poisoning mainly involve the CNS, kidney or skin. Characteristic symptoms in children include acrodynia ('pink disease'), which include signs such as pink hands and feet (Velzeboer *et al.* 1997). Mercury species may be retained in the body for a long time after the cessation of exposure, and blood elimination and urine excretion rates show long half-lives. Mercury may be excreted in the urine for 6–12 months after cessation of exposure, which makes urine measurements an attractive way to assess historical exposure, and analysis of hair can be useful in environmental studies or unusual clinical cases. Mercury from the diet (particularly fish) contributes to the concentration of mercury found in blood, but is usually well within normal limits. However, populations who consume unusually large quantities of certain fish (e.g. swordfish) or of whale meat may accumulate high concentrations of (methyl) mercury (Kales and Goldman 2002). There is some evidence that such exposure presents a serious risk in pregnancy and early child development. Reference values for mercury in non-exposed populations in blood and urine are <4 μg/L and <5 μg/L, respectively.

Selenium

Selenium is now firmly established as an essential trace element, although historically it was associated only with toxicity as a result of occupational or environmental exposure (Glover 1970; Yang *et al.* 1983). Selenium is present in the earth's crust in relatively small quantities, but some rocks may contain levels of up to 1.5 ppm. Selenium is also found in coal, and the combustion of fossil fuels is an important source of its occurrence as pollution in the environment. Most of the earliest reports of selenium toxicity are associated with poisoning in grazing livestock and the cause of 'alkali disease' and 'blind staggers'. The sources of selenium in such cases are particular plants that concentrate selenium when growing in selenium-rich soils. There are many industrial uses of selenium, such as the manufacture of semiconductors, glass and ceramics. Selenium compounds are also used as anti-dandruff agents in shampoos and as gun-blueing compounds, which contain selenous acid. Many nutritional supplements now contain selenium compounds, sometimes in relatively high concentrations, which may cause toxicity if ingested in excess (Clark *et al.* 1996). Selenium is a metalloid and is in group 6 of the periodic table. Common oxidation states of selenium are 2^+ (selenide), 4^+ (selenite) and 6^+ (selenate). There are also a number of important organoselenium compounds in which selenium is able to substitute for sulfur (e.g. selenocysteine and selenomethionine).

Recent years have seen a large increase in our understanding of the essential biological role of selenium, and important selenoproteins and glutathione peroxidases (GSHPx) are found in most tissues of the body (Thompson 1998). Selenium has been shown to have an important role in thyroid function, fertility (particularly sperm motility), mood regulation, immunity to infectious disease and as a cellular 'antioxidant', acting in association with vitamins E and C (Reilly 1993; Rayman 2000). Deficiency of selenium is associated with a number of disorders, such as Keshan disease (China), and, more recently with an increased risk of cancer. Selenium can also have a protective role in ameliorating human exposure to mercury (Hansen 1988). In cases of occupational exposure, selenium is associated with signs and symptoms such as skin irritation, garlic breath, metallic taste, painful nail beds and pulmonary oedema.

Acute poisoning has occurred after ingestion or inhalation of selenium compounds. A number of fatalities that involved selenium are well described (Köppel *et al.* 1986; Matoba *et al.* 1986; Schellmann *et al.* 1986; Quadrani *et al.* 2000). Reference ranges for selenium in whole blood and plasma vary from country to country because of differences in dietary sources of selenium. In the UK, adult plasma reference ranges are generally between 70 and 130 μg/L. In cases of acute poisoning, very high concentrations of selenium may be detected in whole blood, plasma and urine. Blood selenium values <1000 μg/L indicate minimal toxicity, whereas values >2000 μg/L predict serious complications (Gasmi *et al.* 1997).

Thallium

Most thallium compounds are colourless, tasteless and odourless. The water-soluble salts of thallium include the sulfate, acetate and carbonate, all of which are highly toxic. Modern industrial uses of thallium salts include the manufacture of imitation jewellery and optical lenses, and in producing special alloys for seawater batteries. Thallium salts were also introduced as rodenticides and insecticides in the 1920s. Their use has been discontinued in many countries owing to their high toxicity, but they continue to be applied in some countries. The fatal oral dose of thallium in adults is less than 2 g.

The clinical picture of thallium poisoning is highly complex, and poisoning may be difficult to diagnose in its early stages. Initial signs and symptoms of acute thallium poisoning include fever, gastrointestinal upset and convulsions. Neurological symptoms may develop later and include both peripheral and central neurological changes. Cardiovascular changes, such as an increase in blood pressure and tachycardia, may develop after 1 to 2 weeks. The most characteristic signs associated with thallium toxicity are dermatological changes, which may take up to 3 weeks to develop, and include an initial black pigmentation of the hair (visible under a microscope) followed by loss of body hair, which can result in total alopecia. Nail growth may also be impaired with the development of white transverse lines, similar to those seen with arsenic poisoning. In particularly severe cases of thallium poisoning, extremely high levels of thallium in blood, plasma and urine may be recorded within the first few days after ingestion. Measurement of thallium excretion in urine is useful in cases for which oral antidotal therapy with Berlin (Prussian) blue (potassium ferric hexacyanoferrate) is instituted. This dye forms an insoluble complex with thallium in the gut, which leads to enhanced faecal excretion. Reference values for thallium in blood and urine are <1 μg/L. Concentrations in excess of 100 μg/L in blood and 200 μg/L in urine are associated with toxicity.

Analysis for metals

A wide variety of methods are available for the analysis of metallic elements at trace levels in biological matrices, including colorimetric and fluorimetric assays, electrochemical detection (anodic stripping voltammetry), flame atomic absorption spectrophotometry (AAS), electrothermal AAS (ETAAS) (also referred to as graphite furnace AAS (GFAAS)), inductively coupled plasma emission spectrometry (ICP-AES) (also referred to as ICP-optical emission spectrometry (ICP-OES)), and ICP-mass spectrometry (ICP-MS). AAS and ETAAS offer good sensitivity but the nature of the instrumentation means that only one element can be analysed at a time. This presents difficulties when specimen volumes are limited and the measurement of several elements is required because a certain volume of sample is required for the analysis of each element. If a large number of elements have to be analysed for, there may be insufficient sample available. Alternative technologies have been developed, such as anodic stripping voltammetry (ASV), but this needs careful specimen preparation (digestion) before specimens can be run. ICP-AES and ICP-MS offer the significant advantage of multi-element analysis with some instruments capable of analysing up to 75 elements simultaneously. This advantage comes at a significant cost in terms of instrument purchase and running costs relative to AAS and ETAAS but the multi-element capability makes screening for metals much quicker. ICP-MS is now the 'gold standard' for high sensitivity multi-element analysis (see Chapter 21). It is possible to analyse a small volume of sample for many elements simultaneously. In addition, it is possible to derive information on the relative isotopic abundance of some elements (e.g. lead), which can be used to link a biological sample to a suspect source material or scene residue. Heavier elements that are difficult to determine using ETAAS (e.g. platinum, uranium) are determined easily using ICP-MS. AAS, ICP-AES and ICP-MS can be linked to hydride-generation systems to analyse elements that form gaseous hydrides (such as arsenic and antimony); ICP-MS and -AES can also be connected to liquid chromatographic systems to study metal speciation in biological fluids and tissues. Interferences, including isobaric and polyatomic interferences, occur with ICP-MS which can give rise to problems in analysis for some elements, but newer instrument design and software capabilities have significantly reduced this problem. Nevertheless, the instrument operator must be aware of possible interferences.

The high sensitivity of methods such as AAS, ETAAS, ICP-AES and ICP-MS means that strict precautions must be observed in sample collection and preparation and in the choice of sample containers. Aluminium is a particular case in point because it is ubiquitous in the environment and can readily contaminate samples.

Colorimetric assays are also commercially available for the analysis of serum zinc, magnesium and copper, and are suitable for use on modern clinical laboratory equipment.

Some screening tests that are simple to apply and that can be used to identify some metallic elements in stomach contents and scene residues are available. One such test is the Reinsch test, which can detect arsenic, antimony, bismuth and mercury. The test involves the use of copper foil, with inspection of the foil to determine its appearance after the test is applied. Interpretation can be difficult and is not entirely specific. However, the test may at least indicate that one or more of the above metals is present or otherwise and direct further, more specific, analyses.

The Gutzeit test is a colorimetric test for the qualitative and semi-quantitative analysis of arsenic in urine, stomach contents, tissues, scene residues and contaminated water. It involves the reduction of inorganic arsenic to arsine gas, which then reacts with a solution of silver diethyldithiocarbamate to give a red complex. A specially designed Gutzeit apparatus can be purchased from commercial sources, and a detailed description of the test can be found in Flanagan *et al.* (1995). The sensitivity for arsenic is approximately 0.5 mg/L. A later modification of the basic technique has been applied to arsenic and other hydride-forming elements, such as antimony and selenium, with measurement by AAS giving better sensitivity (Crawford and Tavares 1974; Kneip *et al.* 1977). Several convenient colorimetric methods can be applied to determine thallium in urine, stomach contents and suspect preparations. One of these methods (Flanagan *et al.* 1995) is based on measuring the absorbance of a chloroform-extractable pink–red thallium–dithizone complex from an alkaline solution that contains potassium, sodium and cyanide ions to mask interference from other metal ions. It indicates the presence of thallium in urine at concentrations of 1 g/L or more. However, the method is not specific and AAS, ETAAS, ICP-MS or ICP-AES are more reliable techniques.

Anions

Borates

Boric acid has for many years been used as a common household antiseptic for external use. Sodium borate (borax) is used in cleaning agents, wood preservatives and fungicides. Compounds of boron have relatively low toxicity. However, a number of cases of acute and chronic boron poisoning have been reported in children and adults. Signs and symptoms have generally included diarrhoea and vomiting, and seizures in more severe cases.

ICP-MS has been used to measure the concentration of boron in blood and tissues in patients who receive treatment with boron-containing drugs such as boronphenylalanine (BPA) as part of boron neutron capture therapy of certain cancers (Morten and Delves 1999). Plasma boron concentrations ranging from 200 to 1600 mg/L have been reported in children in fatal cases of acute poisoning with borates. Survival has also been reported in cases of adult poisoning despite admission boron concentrations in excess of 1000 mg/L.

Bromide

Bromide salts (e.g. of ammonium, potassium and sodium) were first introduced into medicine in the 19th century and were used extensively as anticonvulsants and sedatives. However, with the exception of organic bromides such as carbromal (a sedative), their use is now limited. Methyl bromide (a fumigant) releases bromide ion as a metabolite. Absorption of bromide ion takes place rapidly from the stomach and proximal small intestines by passive diffusion. Bromide ions behave like chloride ions and are distributed mainly in extracellular fluid. The most important route of elimination is via the kidney. Their elimination half-life is relatively long, being of the order of 10 days after acute dosing, or several weeks following the cessation of chronic intake, particularly in cases of bromide intoxication. Bromide poisoning may cause neurological symptoms (e.g. tremor, ataxia, autonomic disturbance, cognitive impairment) and clinical diagnosis can be difficult if the use of bromide salts is not suspected. 'Normal' reference values for bromide are <5 mg/L in plasma. Concentrations in cases of bromide intoxication show markedly elevated levels in excess of 1000 mg/L. 'Therapeutic' concentrations in adult epileptics are of the order of 750–1000 mg/L.

Chlorate

Sodium chlorate ($NaClO_3$) is an effective, inexpensive, nonselective herbicide. Potassium chlorate is used in the manufacture of matches and some explosives. Both compounds are powerful oxidising agents. Serious and sometimes fatal poisoning can occur after the ingestion of 15 g or more of sodium or potassium chlorate. Early signs and symptoms of chlorate poisoning include nausea, vomiting and abdominal pain. Systemic absorption leads to substantial oxidation of haemoglobin to form methaemoglobin, which may cause cyanosis, dyspnoea and coma; intravascular haemolysis and severe metabolic acidosis may also occur (Ellenhorn 1997).

Cyanide

Severe or fatal cyanide poisoning is relatively rare and mostly involves suicidal ingestion. Hydrogen cyanide (HCN; prussic acid) is a highly toxic volatile liquid. Fumes of hydrogen cyanide are given off when cyanide salts are mixed with acids or produced in the stomach following oral ingestion. Although HCN has a characteristic almond-like odour, about 50% of the population are unable to smell it. Soluble salts of cyanide include potassium and sodium cyanide, which are used industrially in electroplating and metal processing and as laboratory reagents. Less soluble salts of cyanide include silver and gold cyanide, and mercuric cyanide, which also release HCN on contact with strong acids. HCN may also be formed as a combustion product in fires from nitrogen-containing materials such as wool and silk or synthetic polymers such as polyurethanes, polyamides and polyamides (Baud *et al.* 1991; Barillo *et al.* 1994, Chaturvedi *et al.* 2001). Less common sources of cyanide include the accidental or intentional ingestion of cyanogenic plants or their seeds.

The signs and symptoms of cyanide toxicity appear rapidly after inhalation of HCN or ingestion of cyanide salts; the estimated fatal doses are approximately 100 mg HCN or 300 mg potassium cyanide (Ellenhorn *et al.* 1997). Early neurological signs include headache, dizziness, anxiety and confusion. In severe cases there may be a rapid loss of consciousness, respiratory failure and convulsions that lead to cardiorespiratory arrest and death. Cyanide is metabolised rapidly in the liver by an enzyme (rhodanase) to thiocyanate (SCN), which is largely nontoxic. As a consequence, blood cyanide concentrations decline rapidly after exposure or ingestion, with an estimated elimination half-life of 1–2 h. A number of antidotes are useful in the treatment of cyanide poisoning (e.g. cobalt EDTA and hydroxocobalamin). In postmortem cases after suicidal ingestion of cyanide salts, elevated levels of cyanide may occur in blood samples taken from the heart or other central sites owing to postmortem diffusion of unadsorbed cyanide from the stomach. Hence blood samples should be taken from peripheral sites such as the femoral vein. It should also be noted that bacteria and fungi can break down or generate cyanide in the body or in specimens. Precautions should, therefore, be taken to collect blood into anticoagulated tubes that contain sodium fluoride to prevent/minimise microbial growth in the sample. Where there is evidence of putrefaction in the body before sampling, this should be taken into account when interpreting data on cyanide levels. Quantitative analysis of cyanide in stomach contents can be helpful when the route of ingestion is uncertain. In cases of fire, inhalation of smoke and fumes can result in concentrations of cyanide of up to 1 mg/L in blood, both in antemortem and in postmortem specimens. Reference values for cyanide in blood are <0.05 mg/L. Minor signs and symptoms of toxicity are associated with blood concentrations up to 1 mg/L, and severe symptoms with higher concentrations, up to 20 mg/L, on admission to hospital after suicidal ingestion or industrial exposure (Singh *et al.* 1989).

Fluoride

Fluoride is present in variable amounts in the soil and natural water supplies. It is also found in almost all plant and animal food products, and is regarded as an essential trace element. Fluoride salts may also be added to domestic water supplies as a prophylaxis against dental caries, generally at a concentration of 1 mg/L where the 'natural' water content is low. Fluoride compounds are available in tablet form to prevent dental decay in infants and children. They are also prescribed in the treatment of osteoporosis and other bone disorders. Inorganic salts of fluoride have widespread use in industry, for example in smelting aluminium, and are also applied as insecticides and rodenticides. Fluoride is an effective enzyme inhibitor that has found extensive use in the preservation of biological specimens. The highly corrosive hydrofluoric acid is also used industrially.

Both acute and chronic poisoning caused by the ingestion of fluoride compounds have been well documented. Signs and symptoms of acute fluoride poisoning include nausea, vomiting, diarrhoea, abdominal pain and paraesthesia. Reference ranges for serum, blood and urine vary widely, depending on dietary intake, access to fluoridated water and the use of fluoridated dental products. Reference ranges of 6–42 μg/L in serum, 20–60 μg/L in blood and 0.2–3.2 mg/L in urine have been reported. In fatalities, fluoride concentrations of 2.6–56 mg/L in blood and 17–320 mg/L in urine have been measured.

Hypochlorites

Hypochlorites, such as sodium and calcium hypochlorite, are used as disinfectants. Domestic products contain relatively low concentrations, whereas industrial products are much more concentrated and produce greater toxicity if ingested. Hypochlorite poisoning produces characteristic symptoms and qualitative tests are generally not used for diagnosis, although they may be used to confirm diagnosis or in the investigation of fatalities.

Nitrites and nitrates

Sodium nitrate finds uses in artificial fertilisers, food preservatives, explosives (as do the potassium salts). Sodium nitrite is also used as a food preservative and in the manufacture of explosives and as a cleaner in dentistry. Nitrite has the additional property of causing vasodilation, which has led to its application in treating angina pectoris. This vasodilatory effect of alkyl nitrites (e.g. amyl, butyl and isobutyl nitrites) has led to abuse of these drugs for the 'rush' they provide and, reportedly, heightened sexual arousal, disinhibition and muscle relaxation. Ingestion of these substances, which are supplied to be inhaled, can be fatal. Organic nitrates (e.g. glyceryl trinitrate, isosorbide mononitrate and dinitrate) release nitrite ion when ingested and are also used as vasodilators.

Symptoms of nitrate and/or nitrite poisoning include nausea, vomiting, diarrhoea, abdominal pain, confusion and coma. Nitrite in the body combines with haemoglobin to produce methaemoglobin which reduces the capacity of the blood to carry oxygen (methaemoglobinaemia). Unborn babies and those up to 3–4 months old are particularly susceptible to methaemoglobinaemia because they are deficient in methaemoglobin reductase, the enzyme that converts methaemoglobin to haemoglobin, and because their stomachs are less acidic than those of adults and hence are more likely to permit growth of nitrate-reducing bacteria. Thus, if nitrates are ingested by babies they are more likely to be converted to nitrites with resultant methaemoglobinaemia, which gives rise to the so-called 'blue-baby' syndrome because the skin appears blue. To minimise problems arising from high nitrate levels, levels in water in most developed countries are closely controlled, with maximum levels imposed. Public water supplies are treated to reduce nitrate levels but this may not be the case for water drawn from wells or other untreated sources. Methaemoglobin measurement is the most useful test in the diagnosis and clinical management of poisoning cases. Methaemoglobin causes blood to turn brown. This can be exploited in colour tests where the addition of two drops of potassium cyanide solution to 1 mL of blood gives an immediate colour change from brown to red in the presence of methaemoglobin.

Several other medical conditions can give rise to contraindications for nitrate and nitrite intake. These include persons with congenital NADPH-methaemoglobin reductase deficiency and those with glucose-6-phosphate dehydrogenase deficiency. Plasma nitrite and nitrate concentrations in unexposed subjects are about 0.2 mg/L and 1.2 mg/L, respectively. In a fatal suicide, nitrite concentrations were 0.5 mg/L in blood. Survival has been reported in two men who accidentally ingested about 1 g of sodium nitrite.

Oxalate

Oxalic acid and a number of its salts may be used as cleaning or bleaching agents and in the manufacture of explosives. Oxalic acid is also present in certain plants (e.g. rhubarb leaves), which can cause toxicity if ingested in error. Oxalate is also an important active metabolite in ethylene glycol poisoning and may appear in urine as calcium oxalate crystals. Signs and symptoms of oxalate ingestion include local tissue damage, shock, convulsions and renal damage. There may also be a marked fall in plasma calcium concentration that requires active treatment. Hyperoxaluria is caused by a genetically-induced enzyme deficiency and can lead to renal failure followed by oxalosis if not treated. Patients are advised to minimise intake of oxalates. Patients with hyperoxaluria may excrete much higher oxalate concentrations in urine. Reference values for plasma oxalate of up to 2.4 mg/L have been reported in healthy subjects. A plasma oxalate value of 3.7 mg/L has been seen in an individual who survived oxalate poisoning, but concentrations of between 18 and 100 mg/L were seen in three fatalities.

Phosphine and phosphides

Phosphine (hydrogen phosphide; PH_3) is a highly toxic colourless gas with a strong garlic or fishy smell, and is used in a number of industrial processes (e.g. the production of acetylene gas and manufacture of semiconductors). It is also generated by the action of moisture on phosphides. Aluminium phosphide is used extensively as a cheap and effective grain fumigant and rodenticide in developing countries. Aluminium phosphide poisoning has a high mortality and the 1990s saw a dramatic increase in the number of poisoning cases and deaths caused by suicidal ingestion, particularly in India (Christophers *et al.* 2002). Poisoning cases have also occurred in France (Anger *et al.* 2000), Turkey (Bayazit *et al.* 2000) and Germany (Popp *et al.* 2002). Signs and symptoms of poisoning include headache, nausea, vomiting and hypotension, which may progress to hepatic and renal failure (Guale *et al.* 1994; Sing *et al.* 1996; Lakshmi 2002; Popp *et al.* 2002). Methaemoglobin formation has also been reported (Lakshmi 2002).

Sulfide

Many organic and inorganic sulfide compounds are used in industry, but the most common cause of sulfide poisoning is by inhalation of hydrogen sulfide gas, particularly in industrial or waste disposal sites, including sewers. The gas has a characteristic foul odour of rotten-eggs and has a very low odour threshold (0.03 ppm). However, very high sulfide concentrations may cause paralysis of the olfactory nerves (Guidotti 1994). Hydrogen sulfide occurs naturally in volcanic gases and hot springs. Hydrogen sulfide is unstable and is metabolised rapidly in the body so that it may be difficult to detect in biological samples from cases of suspected poisoning. In cases of suspected acute or chronic exposure to hydrogen sulfide, blood specimens must be collected as soon as possible because of its rapid metabolism. It is metabolised into thiosulfate and so measurement of blood or urine thiosulfate concentration may be the most viable approach to the investigation of acute or chronic sulfide poisoning. Reference values for sulfide concentrations in biological fluids are <10 μg/L but have been reported to be considerably higher in poisoning incidents. Sulfide concentrations ranged from 30 to 130 μg/L in blood taken from workers 0.5–2 h after accidental exposure to hydrogen sulfide from a sulfate pulp mill. Postmortem results after industrial accidents have shown blood sulfide concentrations of 0.9–3.8 mg/L.

Analytical methods for anions

The systematic analysis of anions in body fluids presents a major analytical challenge. Historically, the main approach was the analysis of stomach contents and scene residues using classic colorimetric methods of analysis (Yeoman 1985). Many anions are unstable and undergo rapid breakdown in the stomach and gut after absorption. The analysis of metabolites and various hydrolysis products in blood or urine using modern methods is not well described. In some cases, the investigation of poisoning caused by anions that are oxidising agents (e.g. chlorates) is best carried out by measurement of changes in blood chemistry, such as the formation of oxidised haemoglobin (methaemoglobin).

The development of analytical techniques such as ion chromatography to separate and measure anions in biological fluids is in its infancy. A number of methods have been developed for use by the water industry. Classic analytical chemical methods (colour tests) may still be applicable for cases in which stomach contents or scene residues are available. ETAAS and ICP-MS have been used for the quantitative determination of boron, and ICP-MS has also been used for the quantitative determination of bromide ions and phosphorus (from aluminium phosphide). Ion-selective electrodes are also available for various anions. The reader is referred to Moffat (2004) for details of the various analytical methods available for anions.

Specimen collection and analysis

In cases of suspected poisoning admitted to hospital, specimens of blood and, where possible, urine should be taken. When blood specimens are received in the laboratory and analyses are not required immediately, it is useful to separate off plasma or serum from red cells, prior to deep freezing. However, for toxins that have a significant distribution into the red cells (e.g. lead, cadmium, mercury and cyanide), it is essential to conserve samples of anticoagulated whole blood. In postmortem examinations it is important to undertake a more systematic specimen collection and great care is required in the selection of sampling sites, method of collection and use of appropriate specimen containers. Where an industrial accident has occurred there may be access to 'scene residues' or materials used in a chemical process. Analysis of these materials can yield valuable clues when the precise nature of the chemical agent is unknown. However, prior to transportation to the laboratory, separate packaging from any biological specimens is advisable to avoid the risk of contamination.

Vomit, stomach aspirate and washout fluid are now rarely available from cases of acute poisoning admitted to hospital. Stomach washout procedures (except in rare cases) have been replaced by the administration of oral activated charcoal in most developed countries. In fatal cases, the whole stomach and its contents can be removed at postmortem examination. When dealing with the initial examination of stomach contents, or vomitus, it is helpful to note any unusual smell, colour or other appearance, such as the presence of fresh or altered blood (e.g. vomit with the appearance of ground coffee indicates bleeding in the upper gastrointestinal tract). Great care should be taken when dealing with cases that involve the oral ingestion of cyanide salts, as the contents of the stomach may represent a serious hazard and risk of secondary poisoning (a fume cupboard, or safety cabinet, *must* be used in these circumstances). Earlier techniques used to examine stomach contents, such as isolation of poisons by dialysis or steam distillation, are now obsolete, particularly since the development of more sensitive and specific analytical techniques.

Venous blood should be collected in all cases of suspected poisoning; for metallic poisons and anions, such as cyanide, a potassium ethylenediaminetetraacetic acid (K-EDTA) container is the most appropriate. A wide range of blood-collection tubes are available commercially; to avoid the possibility of contamination, the use of products certified as suitable for trace-element analyses is strongly recommended, particularly when dealing with environmental or subclinical exposure to agents such as lead, cadmium and aluminium. Blood-collection tubes that contain gel separation barriers should not be used. When blood specimens are received in the laboratory in an unusual container, it may be useful to request a 'blank' container that can be analysed for the presence of any contaminating substance. It is equally important to ensure that reliable blood-specimen containers are used for postmortem examinations. These can be supplied to the pathologist ahead of any postmortem examination as part of standard specimen-collection kits.

An early specimen of urine with no preservatives added should be collected, with care taken to ensure that the sample is not contaminated during the collection process. If patients are undergoing chelation therapy it can be useful to collect sequential 24-hour urine specimens into acid-washed plastic urine containers.

Hair analysis for trace elements has often been used for diagnostic purposes in cases where an individual complains of symptoms for which no cause can be found by routine medical or pathological investigations. However, experience and published studies show that the results can be misleading (Taylor 1986; Seidel *et al.* 2001). Hair analysis has more application in surveys of population exposure and in investigations of suspicious deaths, such as those that involve arsenic or mercury. The long persistence of metals in hair samples compared to their relatively short duration in blood or urine specimens is a major advantage in this context. Analysis of hair sections can also yield a chronological record of when doses were administered.

Specimens such as tissues, skin and bone may sometimes be collected at postmortem examination as part of the investigation of complex medicolegal cases.

Lung tissue should be collected from postmortem examination in cases of beryllium-related deaths as this is a target organ for this element.

All those involved in selecting and submitting samples for analysis should consider the possibility of metals and anions being present so that suitable samples, packaging and storage are employed at the start. This is particularly important for volatile substances, where attention should be paid to ensuring that loss due to volatilisation from the sample or sorption into sample containers is minimised. Similarly, for metals and anions, precautions must be taken to prevent contamination with these substances. Some types of sample containers can leach metallic elements (e.g. some gel-containing blood tubes may be contaminated with barium) and solutions added to prevent microbial growth may contain metals and/or anions if they are not prepared from standards and solvents (including water) of suitable purity. Glass containers should never be used to collect specimens for aluminium analysis.

Natural toxins

The term 'natural toxins' usually refers to potentially toxic organic compounds of natural origin, in contrast to mineral poisons and synthetic drugs. Sources of these toxins range from simple microorganisms to highly developed vertebrates, and their chemical structures are correspondingly diverse. Exposure to natural toxins may lead to acute as well as long-term symptoms that affect almost any organ system. The highly varied chemical, biological and clinical nature of this class of poisons means that the contribution of the analytical toxicologist to the diagnosis, therapy and follow-up of 'naturally-poisoned' patients is limited.

An extensive number of substances that comply with the definition of natural toxins have been used for therapeutic purposes. Classic examples are ergotamine, salicylic acid and the cardiac glycosides such as digoxin, and penicillin. More recent examples are ciclosporin and botulinum toxin (which is being used in the treatment of blepharospasms). Most of these substances are not discussed in this chapter. Similarly, commonly abused substances of natural origin, such as cannabis, cocaine and morphine, are covered elsewhere in this book.

The diversity in chemical composition of natural toxins prevents an arrangement according to chemical structures. Accordingly, a biological classification has been chosen. Substances are discussed that originate from:

- bacteria
- fungi
- higher plants
- invertebrates
- vertebrates.

Bacteria

The impact of pathogenic bacteria on human health mostly, if not always, results from their ability to produce microbial toxins. For this chapter, a selection has been made of three common potent bacterial toxins: tetanus toxin, botulinum toxin and verotoxin. The former two are related neurotoxic proteins produced by several *Clostridia* strains; verotoxin is produced by certain *Escherichia coli* strains. Bacteria may also be the source of toxins previously attributed to other organisms, such as tetrodotoxin (TTX), which is found in puffer fish, but most probably produced by commensal microorganisms. For reasons of convention, TTX is discussed in the section on fish poisoning. The same holds for those freshwater cyanobacteria that produce saxitoxins, which are described in the section on mollusc poisoning.

Clostridium spp.

Botulinum and tetanus neurotoxins are produced by strictly anaerobic bacteria belonging to the genus *Clostridium* and cause the neuroparalytic syndromes of botulism and tetanus. The botulinum toxins consist of at least four peptides with molecular sizes that range from 150 to 900 kDa. The tetanus toxin has two disulfide-linked peptide chains of molecular size 50 kDa and 100 kDa. The clostridial neurotoxins are the most potent toxins known, with a mouse-lethal dose of 0.3 ng/kg and a reported LD_{50} in unvaccinated humans of <2.5 ng/kg for tetanus toxin. Botulinum toxins are food poisons, whereas the tetanus toxin is not. Tetanus follows the contamination of necrotic wounds with spores of *C. tetani*. Tetanus is rare in countries with immunisation programmes, but it has a high case fatality rate of 24%. An estimated

800 000 newborns die from neonatal tetanus worldwide each year. Treatment with antitoxin and intravenous administration of penicillin soon after infection may reduce mortality.

Classic food-borne botulism occurs after ingestion of food contaminated by preformed toxin of *C. botulinum*. The clinical presentations are stereotypical. Within 12–36 h of ingestion, the patient develops diplopia and ptosis, followed by a descending pattern of weakness that affects the upper and then the lower limbs, and respiratory paralysis in severe cases. There is no specific treatment for botulism; recovery is not uncommon but it requires the regeneration of new motor endplates, which takes weeks. Laboratory proof of botulism requires the detection of the toxin in the patient's blood or stools. If still available, the suspected food should also be tested for the toxin. A number of immunoassay methods have been reported for the detection of botulinum toxins including radioimmunoassay (RIA) and enzyme-linked immunosorbent assay (ELISA). A promising new method for the detection of bacterial spores and toxins uses a biosensor based on electrochemiluminescence (Gatto-Menking *et al.* 1995). A mouse bioassay is also available for detection of botulism toxins and, more recently, matrix-assisted laser desorption ionisation–time of flight mass spectrometry (MALDI-TOF-MS) and LC-ESI-MS/MS have been used for detection and quantification of the botulinum toxins (Barr *et al.* 2005). Generally applicable analytical methods for the identification and quantification of tetanus toxin have not been reported (Cherington *et al.* 1995) but an ESI-MS/MS method has recently been reported for detecting tetanus toxin in bacterial cultures (vanBaar *et al.* 2002).

Escherichia coli

Several strains of the common intestinal bacterium *E. coli* may cause diarrhoeal disease in man. One such strain, which occurs naturally in the gut of cattle and other animals, produces verotoxin (or verocytotoxin), a potent cytotoxin. This *E. coli* strain, usually referred to as verotoxin-producing *E. coli* (VTEC), is geographically widespread and is associated with life-threatening human diseases that range from bloody diarrhoea to the haemolytic-uraemic syndrome and thrombocytopenic purpura. Young children, especially those from urban areas, are a particularly vulnerable group because of their age and immunological naivety to farmhouse infections. The chemical nature of verotoxin has not yet been elucidated. VTEC strains are characterised through polymerase chain reaction (PCR) and deoxyribonucleic acid (DNA) hybridisation, and by a Vero-cell cytotoxicity assay (Leung *et al.* 2001). ELISA methods have also been developed for the detection of verotoxin.

Other *E. coli* strains (O157:H7) and other bacterial species produce Shiga toxins, which may produce disease in humans after consumption of undercooked contaminated beef. In humans these toxins may cause haemorrhagic colitis and haemolytic uraemic syndrome. Enzyme immunoassays are available that detect Shiga toxins in diarrhoeal stool samples from humans, and in contaminated beef (Atalla *et al.* 2000; Hyatt *et al.* 2001).

Fungi

Given the large number of fungal species, remarkably, only a very few species are deadly poisonous after ingestion. A more insidious risk for humans comes from various fungi that produce toxins in foods. Of particular importance are the fungal species that produce mycotoxins.

Mycotoxins is the name given to a group of potentially toxic substances produced by certain fungal species that grow on food crops pre- or post-harvest. Mycotoxins which have given rise to most concerns in terms of risk to health include aflatoxins, ochratoxins, deoxynivalenol, fumonosins, tricothecenes and ergot alkaloids. The fungal species associated with the production of these toxins include *Aspergillus* spp., *Fusarium* (*Gibberella zeae*) spp., *Penicillium verruculosum* and *Claviceps purpurea*. Mycotoxins are often present in foods at low levels. Consumption of these foods generally does not give rise to acute, and hence readily detectable, symptoms of poisoning, although some cases of acute exposure have been reported. Instead, chronic exposure to mycotoxins is more likely. Mycotoxins are linked with producing neurotoxic, carcinogenic or teratogenic effects together with suppression of the immune system.

Aflatoxins are produced by *Aspergillus* spp., mainly *A. flavus*, *A. parasiticus* and *A. nomius* that are found as contaminants in both human foodstuffs and animal feed, particularly in maize, groundnuts and other nuts such as pistachios. Exposure to the toxins occurs through consumption of contaminated food and also during the handling and processing of aflatoxin-contaminated crops. Aflatoxins have been detected in human milk, urine and blood samples. It has also been shown that ingestion of contaminated feed by cattle can produce milk contaminated with aflatoxin metabolites and that these substances pass to cheese and other dairy products during manufacture. Aflatoxin-B_1 is a very potent human carcinogen that reacts with DNA once it has been bioactivated to the epoxide and is thought to cause hepatocellular carcinoma.

Ochratoxin-A (Fig. 4.4) is a widespread mycotoxin produced mainly by the fungi *A. ochraceus* and *Penicillium verruculosum* during the storage of cereals, cereal products, herbs, spices and other plant-derived products like coffee. It has been found primarily in northern temperate barley- and wheat-growing areas. Consumption of mouldy pig feed may result in detectable levels of ochratoxin-A in pork-derived products. Since ochratoxin-A is hydrolysed rapidly by ruminal flora, it is unlikely to be found in milk or meat from cattle. When ingested by humans, ochratoxin-A is very persistent, with an elimination half-life of about 35 days attributed to very strong binding to plasma proteins.

Deoxynivalenol (DON) is a mycotoxin belonging to the trichothecene type of toxins produced by *Fusarium graminearum* (*Gibberella zeae*) and *F. culmorum*. These fungi grow on cereal crops, mainly wheat and maize. As wheat and maize products form a considerable part of the diet in many regions, the toxicity and the content of DON is an important issue in food safety control. DON can affect the immune system, and both suppression and activation have been reported, but the toxin is not considered to be mutagenic or carcinogenic. Outbreaks of human disease related to trichothecenes have been reported. Consumption of mouldy wheat or maize results within 5–30 minutes in nausea, vomiting, abdominal pain, diarrhoea, dizziness and headache.

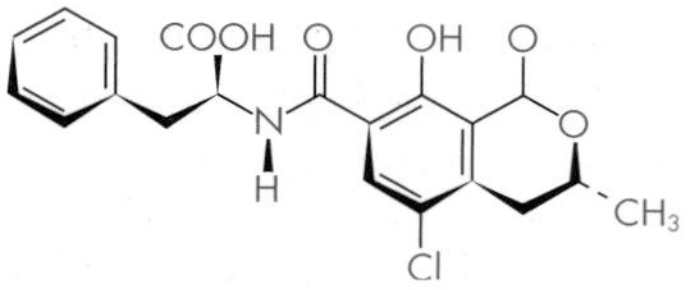

Zearalenone is a benzoxacyclotetradecin derivative produced in *F. graminearum* (*Gibberella zeae*) and related species, and is primarily associated with maize (*Zea mais*). It is among the most widely distributed mycotoxins. Toxic effects in humans are extremely difficult to assess as, in cases of contaminated cereals, several mycotoxins are present simultaneously. Endocrine-disrupting effects occur in animals, but these were not reported in two outbreaks in which both DON and zearalenone were involved (IARC 1993).

A number of analytical methods have been described for the analysis of aflatoxins in foodstuffs. HPLC with fluorescence detection is considered to be the method of choice, with pre- or post-column detection with bromine or iodine for the B and G aflatoxins, or trifluoroacetic anhydride for the M aflatoxins to improve sensitivity. More recently, LC-MS/MS methods have been developed. Immunoassay methods are available and TLC can also be used and is particularly useful as a screening procedure. Several analytical procedures have been proposed for the identification and measurement of ochratoxin-A in food products, as reviewed by Van Egmond (1991), Valenta (1998) and Gilbert and Vargas (2003).

Poisoning by ergot alkaloids produced by the mould *Claviceps purpurea* is usually referred to as *ergotism*, and is probably the oldest recorded food-borne disease of fungal origin. *Cl. purpurea* grows on food grain, particularly rye, during wet seasons. Symptoms of ergotism include erythema, diarrhoea, vomiting, a burning sensation of the limbs and, eventually, gangrene. CNS effects are convulsions, catalepsy, dullness or maniacal excitement. These symptoms can be explained by the pharmacological properties of

COOH O OH O
N
H
O
CH_3
Cl

Figure 4.4 Ochratoxin-A.

the ergot alkaloids, which may cause an alpha-adrenergic blockade, as well as serotonin (5-hydroxytryptamine; 5-HT) antagonism. The ergot alkaloids ergotamine (the best known, Fig. 4.5) and ergometrine, or ergonovine, have been used for centuries as therapeutic agents to stimulate uterine contractions and in the treatment of migraine attacks. Overdose with these agents, and intoxication with ergot alkaloids from other sources, can be treated symptomatically with potent vasodilator drugs, such as sodium nitroprusside, and by maintaining adequate circulation.

The method of choice for analysis of ergot alkaloids in serum is HPLC with fluorescence detection after liquid–solid extraction. More recently a number of LC-ESI-MS/MS methods have been developed. The structural chemistry and a comparison of the available analytical techniques for ergot alkaloids have been reviewed extensively by Flieger *et al.* (1997).

Hallucinogenic mushrooms

A number of basidiomycetes contain hallucinogenic principles, the most well-known examples being the *Amanita muscaria* and the *Psilocybe* types. The fly agaric *Am. muscaria* is the European archetypical 'mother of all mushrooms' in legends and fairy tales, with a red hood and white spots. It is indigenous to the northern hemisphere, but is also found in some parts of South Africa, South America, Australia and New Zealand. The most important toxin in *Am. muscaria* is *not* muscarine (which does occur in trace amounts), but ibotenic acid and its decarboxylation product muscimol (Fig. 4.6). Poisoning with *Am. muscaria* usually results from deliberate ingestion to obtain a psychoactive response and symptoms occur within 20–180 minutes. Muscimol is a gamma-aminobutyric acid (GABA)-receptor agonist. It causes CNS depression that results in drowsiness and dizziness, followed by elation, increased motor activity, tremor, agitation and hallucinations. There are no specific antidotes and recovery is complete upon awakening.

A modification of the ion-interaction HPLC method of Gennaro *et al.* (1997) for ibotenic acid and muscimol was applied to urine and serum from two dogs who were found to have ingested *Am. muscaria* (Rossmeisl *et al.* 2005). Tsujikawa and colleagues determined ibotenic acid and muscimol in *Amanita* mushrooms by GC-MS (Tsujikawa *et al.* 2006) and by LC-MS/MS (Tsujikawa *et al.* 2007).

Toxins from *Am. phalloides* and related *Agaricales* are among the most lethal natural substances. In countries where the consumption of wild mushrooms is popular, as in Middle and Eastern Europe and some Mediterranean countries, hundreds of fatalities are reported every summer and autumn. The toxic principles are cyclic polypeptides: the phallotoxins are bicyclic heptapeptides, the virotoxins are monocyclic heptapeptides and the amatoxins are bicyclic octapeptides (Fig. 4.7). The most important biochemical effect of the amatoxins is an irreversible inhibition of ribonucleic acid (RNA) polymerase-II; the phallotoxins stimulate the polymerisation of G-actin and stabilise the F-actin filaments (De Wolff and Pennings 1995; Vetter 1998).

Symptoms of *Am. phalloides* poisoning can roughly be divided in three phases, the first appearing over 6 h after mushroom consumption and characterised by violent emesis and cholera-like diarrhoea. This phase is ascribed to the action of the phalloidins, and can usually be treated successfully with fluid and electrolyte replacement. The second phase occurs after

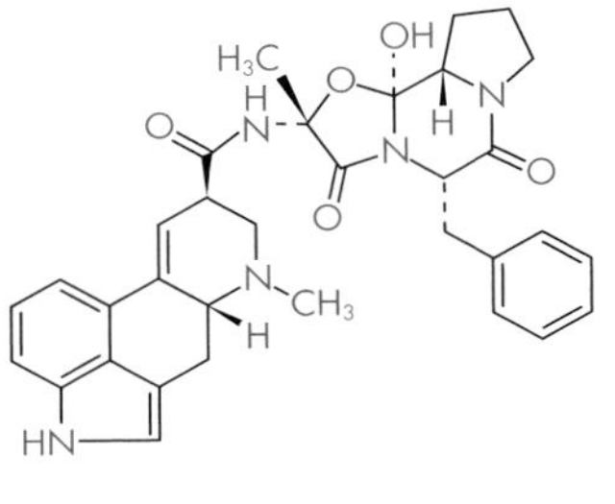

Figure 4.5 Ergotamine.

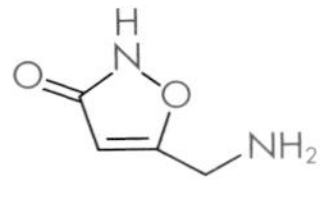

Figure 4.6 Muscimol.

the juice of this plant and exposure to sunlight. The best-known psoralen from hogweed is 8-methoxypsoralen (8-MOP), which is also used in the therapy of psoriasis in combination with UV-A irradiation (De Wolff and Thomas 1986) (Fig. 4.10). Psoralens can be measured in biological matrices with HPLC.

Lathyrus sativus

Lathyrus sativus contains the excitatory amino acid β-*N*-oxalylamino-L-alanine (BOAA), which is the cause of a neurodegenerative disorder, lathyrism, that occurs in many parts of the world. Lathyrism is characterised by spastic paresis of the lower limbs and, in a more advanced stage, by loss of control of the bladder and rectum, and by impotence. Human consumption of 400 g of *L. sativus* daily for a prolonged period leads to symptoms. Young males form the most sensitive part of the population. Treatment is limited to reduction of muscular spasm, with some success. For a review on lathyrism, see Spencer (1995).

Blighia sapida

Jamaican vomiting sickness affects mainly young children and is a form of toxic hepatitis associated with ingestion of the arilli of the unripe fruit of the ackee tree, *Blighia sapida*. The ackee tree was imported into the West Indies but is native to West Africa, and deaths among children have been reported there. The disease presents with severe vomiting and hypoglycaemia followed by neurological symptoms, which include convulsions, coma and death. The toxin responsible is hypoglycin, L(*S*)-2-amino-3-(2-methylidenecyclopropyl)propionic acid. Seeds of the common sycamore (*Acer pseudoplatanus*) and of the lychee fruit (*Litchi sinensis*) also contain hypoglycin. Most of the metabolic effects of hypoglycin are caused by its metabolite, methylenecyclopropylacetyl-coenzyme-A (MCPA-CoA). Sherratt (1995) has reviewed the biochemical mechanism of hypoglycin in detail.

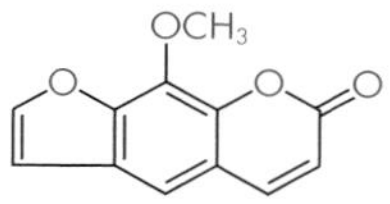

OCH_3

Figure 4.10 8-Methoxypsoralen.

No methods are available that detect hypoglycin in body fluids to confirm a suspected intoxication. However, hypoglycin exposure may be confirmed indirectly by measuring dicarboxylic acids in urine (ethylmalonic, glutaric and adipic acids) by GC with flame-ionisation detection after derivatisation with bis(trimethylsilyl)trifluoroacetamide (Meda *et al.* 1999).

Invertebrates

Many species of animals without backbones produce venoms or contain toxins that may be harmful to humans, either externally by stinging or after ingestion. As with plants, the number of invertebrates that can cause poisoning is vast and hence only a few examples will be given. Emphasis is on mollusc species that usually cause human food poisoning by transmitting accumulated toxins produced by protozoal organisms. Analytical toxicology may be instrumental in the prevention and management of these food-borne diseases. Animals often reported to cause envenomation (representatives of the Cnidaria and Arthropoda) are also mentioned briefly.

Molluscs

Mollusc poisoning or 'shellfish poisoning' is caused by the consumption of bivalve molluscs that accumulate toxins of protozoal or algal origin. Toxins from algal sources are also referred to as phycotoxins, analogous to the mycotoxins from fungal sources (see above). Mollusc poisoning caused by algal toxins is usually classified according to the symptoms they cause in humans:

- paralytic shellfish poisoning (saxitoxins)
- diarrhoetic shellfish poisoning (okadaic acid)
- neurotoxic shellfish poisoning (brevetoxin)
- amnestic shellfish poisoning (domoic acid)
- intoxication with venoms (the conotoxins) from snails belonging to the genus *Conus* is another form of mollusc poisoning.

Paralytic shellfish poisoning (PSP) is caused by saxitoxins (STX; Fig. 4.11) produced by marine 'red tide' dinoflagellates and freshwater

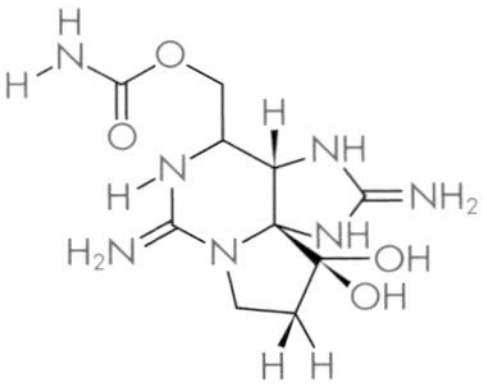

Figure 4.11 Saxitoxin.

blue–green algae such as *Alexandrium* spp., *Gymnodinium catenatu* and *Pyrodinium bahamense*. STX are potent agents that can block sodium channels in nerves and muscles at the extracellular side of the channel, which leads to conductivity disturbances and paralysis. About 1600 cases of poisoning are estimated to occur every year. In severe cases, the neurological symptoms spread to the extremities and respiratory muscles and, without ventilatory support, patients die between 2 and 12 hours after ingestion. Lawrence *et al.* (1996) described a fast and reliable analytical method to detect STX in molluscs, based on HPLC with fluorescence detection after pre-chromatographic oxidation. LC-MS methods are now available.

The major causative agent of *diarrhoetic shellfish poisoning (DSP)* is okadaic acid (Fig. 4.12), which is produced primarily by 'red tide' dinoflagellates belonging to the genera *Dinophysis* and *Prorocentrum*. DSP toxins are lipophilic and accumulate in the digestive gland of mussels. Okadaic acid is a potent inhibitor of protein phosphatases 1 and 2A. In humans, consumption of contaminated molluscs leads almost exclusively to gastrointestinal symptoms: diarrhoea, nausea, vomiting and abdominal pain, which appear between 30 minutes and a few hours after the meal and can be caused by as little as 40 µg of toxin. Treatment is supportive and recovery is complete after a few days. An LC-MS/MS method has been developed for the detection and quantification of okadaic acid in mussels (McNabb *et al.* 2005). The method is applicable for the detection of other algal toxins including domoic acid.

Neurotoxic shellfish poisoning (NSP) is caused by a toxin produced by another 'red tide' dinoflagellate, *Gymnodinium breve*, which has been observed on the west coast of Florida, in the Gulf of Mexico, Japan and New Zealand. The active principle is the lipid-soluble polyether brevetoxin (Fig. 4.13), which has a molecular weight of around 900 and is one of the most potent neurotoxins known. In humans, ingestion of brevetoxin-contaminated shellfish can result in gastroenteritis with neurological symptoms. Within 3 hours, nausea and vomiting, paraesthesias, reversal of hot/cold sensation, throat tightness and ataxia may occur. There is no paralysis. There is complete recovery from these symptoms within 2 days without specific treatment. No human deaths have been reported with brevetoxin poisoning. ELISA methods have been developed to detect brevetoxins in shellfish (Quilliam 1999, Naar *et al.* 2002) and the toxins may also be detected with the HPLC-MS/MS method for ciguatoxin (CTX) described by Lewis *et al.* (1999) and the LC-MS method of Nozawa *et al.* (2003).

Amnesic shellfish poisoning (ASP) was identified as a marine toxin disease in 1987 in Canada, when more than 150 people were affected by the consumption of cultured blue mussels, which resulted in the deaths of three patients. The toxin responsible is the tricarboxylic acid, domoic acid, which is formed by certain species of the diatom genus *Pseudonitzschia*. Domoic acid (Fig. 4.14) is a neurotoxic agent. Acute symptoms include vomiting and diarrhoea and, in some cases, are followed by confusion, memory loss, disorientation, coma or death. A large number of different analytical methods

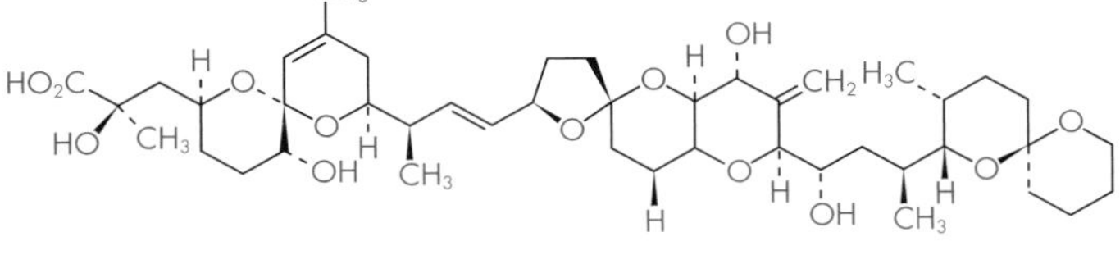

Figure 4.12 Okadaic acid.

Vertebrates

Fish

Poisoning by the consumption of fish flesh (ichthyosarcotoxism) usually occurs in warm climates, but is also observed in moderate climate zones when hygiene measures are ignored. Tetrodotoxic and ciguatoxic fish poisoning are caused by ingestion of fish that accumulate toxin-producing organisms, such as bacteria or protozoa, without being affected themselves. Scombroid poisoning is an example of a toxin produced by improper storage after death, and other fish produce poisonous stings. For a review, see Mebs (2002).

Ciguatera fish poisoning

Ciguatera fish poisoning (CFP) is caused by two groups of toxins, of which the principal one includes the lipid-soluble ciguatoxins (CTXs) (Fig. 4.15) and gambierol, produced by the epiphytic dinoflagellate *Gambierdiscus toxicus*. The other group comprises the water-soluble maitotoxin. CTXs are a group of heat-stable, lipid-soluble, highly oxygenated cyclic polyether molecules, which appear in the food chain through coral reef-fishes that have become toxic through their diet. CTX-containing dinoflagellates live on solid surfaces of macroalgae and are consumed during fish grazing. The mechanism of CTX toxicity is through its direct effects on excitable membranes. Consumption of contaminated fish leads to gastrointestinal disturbances (nausea, vomiting and diarrhoea) within a few hours, followed by neurological symptoms. The latter include paraesthesias, tooth pain and reversal of hot/cold temperature sensation. The third symptom is pathognomonic for CFP. Paraesthesia and weakness may persist for months after the acute illness.

CFP is the most common cause of poisoning with marine toxins. Of those who live in or visit subtropical and tropical areas, an estimated 10 000 to 50 000 people per year suffer from ciguatera. The fatality rate, however, is probably less than 1%.

There is no specific therapy for CFP. Prevention of consumption of contaminated fish is essential. Analysis is difficult because of the low toxin level in fish and the complex structure of the CTX group of toxins. A method based on HPLC and tandem electrospray MS offers the required sensitivity (less than parts per billion; Lewis *et al.* 1999) and other LC-MS methods are available (Hamilton *et al.* 2002). A membrane immuno-bead assay appears to be a simple, rapid, sensitive and specific detection method for CTX and its related polyethers, but further validation of this test is required; for a review, see Quilliam (1999). A commercially available immunoassay-based test kit based is available but is not yet validated.

Puffer fish poisoning

Puffer fish poisoning (PFP), or tetrodotoxin (TTX) (Fig 4.16) intoxication, causes gastroenteritis with severe neurological manifestations similar to those of PSP or saxitoxin intoxication. TTX intoxication constitutes a public health problem in subtropical and tropical regions. It is not limited to Japan, where consumption of

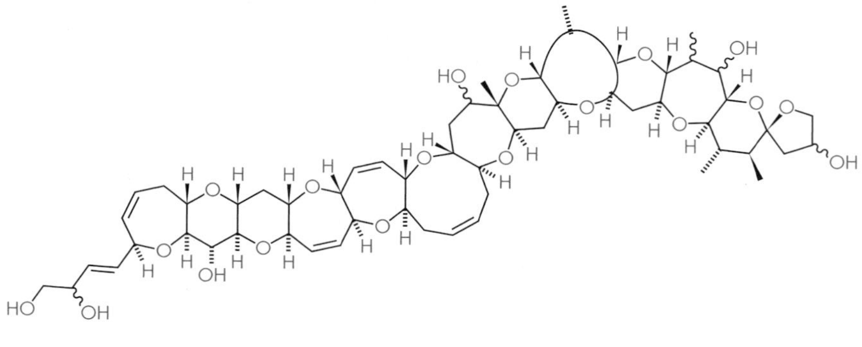

Figure 4.15 Ciguatoxin.

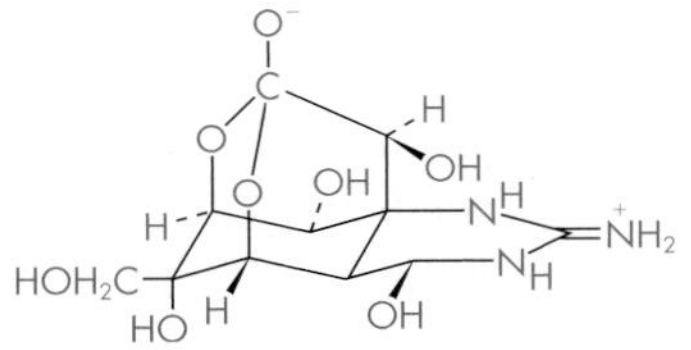

Figure 4.16 Tetrodotoxin.

Fugu – a local puffer fish – is popular. Fugu is harmless if prepared by a qualified chef who discards the organs in which TTX accumulates – the ovaries, roe, liver, intestines and skin. TTX can also be found in Tetraodontiformes, but these can usually be distinguished by their peculiar morphology and their ability to inflate themselves when in danger. TTX is produced by bacteria which colonise the gut and skin mucosal layers of the fish. The toxin is sequestered in the gonads and the liver of fish and, in some species, in muscle. Other marine organisms, like the Japanese ivory shell, the trumpet shell and the blue-ringed octopus, may also contain TTX. The toxin is also found in the skin of certain frogs.

TTX is one of the most potent of the natural toxins; the lethal ingested dose for humans is 5–30 mg/kg wet tissue. The symptoms of TTX poisoning are comparable to those of PSP (see above), except for marked hypotension, and are apparent within 5–30 minutes after consumption. They include gastroenteric effects, paraesthesias, motor paralysis, hypotension and respiratory paralysis. In Japan the mortality rate is reported to be about 60%. Therapy consists of supportive measures, such as artificial ventilation and management of hypotension. Bioassays for PSP and PFP have been reported. In addition, an HPLC method with fluorimetric detection has been described (Yotsu *et al.* 1989) for measurement of TTX and its analogues in puffer fish liver. A test kit for TTX has been developed and is currently undergoing testing in the US by the Center for Food Safety and Applied Nutrition in association with the Food and Drug Administration to evaluate its applicability for testing for the rapid detection of adulteration of food.

Scombroid fish

Scombrotoxin poisoning is the most commonly reported fish poisoning and occurs in many parts of the world. Scombrotoxin is formed in improperly stored fish, and its name derives from the type of fish in which it was described originally. Scombroid fish (Scombridae) are dark-fleshed migratory species, such as mackerel and tuna. Cases of poisoning have also been described after ingestion of non-scombroid species, such as herring, sardines and salmon. Scombrotoxin is generally thought to be identical to histamine. The flesh of scombroid fish has a high histidine content, which is readily decarboxylated to histamine by enteric bacteria (*Proteus morgani*, *P. vulgaris*, *Clostridium* spp., *Escherichia coli*, *Salmonella* spp. and *Shigella* spp.) when stored for as little as 2–3 hours at temperatures above 20°C. However, other amines such as saurine may also be involved. Prolonged cooking does not effectively destroy scombrotoxin and therefore it may also be present in canned products.

Clinical manifestations of the disease occur rapidly (10–30 min) after ingestion, and include acute gastrointestinal symptoms (vomiting, cramps, diarrhoea) associated with erythema, urticarial patches and oedema. The disease is distressing, but seldom, if ever, fatal and recovery is spontaneous within 24 hours. Treatment with intravenous cimetidine resolves most symptoms very quickly. In suspect fish samples, histamine concentrations can be measured with standard methods for the analysis of histamine in food (Grant 1997; Trevino 1998; Clark *et al.* 1999). The Association of Official Analytical Chemists (AOAC) official method for histidine utilises ion exchange clean-up, derivatisation with *o*-phthaldialdehyde and fluorimetric measurement. Several immunoassay test kits are available for determining histamine in fish and have been compared by Rogers and Staruszkiewicz (2000).

Stonefish and weeverfish

Several species of fish with venom-containing spines have been reported to cause fatalities. The stonefishes *Synanceja horrida*, *S. trachynis* and *S. verrucosa*, belonging to the family Scorpaenidae, are located in temperate and tropical seas that extend across South Africa, Japan, the Pacific and

Indian Oceans, Australia and New Zealand. Their venoms contain cholinesterase, alkaline phosphatase and phosphodiesterase. Stonefish stings are severely painful and patients may suffer collapse, cyanosis or pulmonary oedema.

Weeverfishes (*Trachinus draco*, *T. vipera*, *T. radiatus* and *T. araneus*) occur in European coastal waters. Their venom contains 5-HT, a kinin-like substance, epinephrine (adrenaline) and histamine, as well as several enzymes. Weeverfish sting causes an intense burning pain and death can occur rapidly through severe pulmonary oedema.

Amphibians

Of the amphibians, the toads are of major interest to the toxicologist because a number of species produce noxious substances in their dermal glands. These compounds include amines, peptides, proteins, steroids and both water-soluble and lipid-soluble alkaloids. With the exception of the last, these substances are produced by the toad itself rather than bioaccumulated. The genus *Bufo* exudes the alkaloid bufotenine (*N*,*N*-dimethyl-5-hydroxytryptamine; Fig. 4.17), and there have been reports of attempts to gain psychedelic effects by licking the toad or smoking its venom, although Lyttle *et al.* (1996) point out that the psychedelic effects of bufotenine cannot be confirmed by objective studies. Bufotenine is also a product of the 5-HT degradation pathway, and its presence in urine has been suggested as a diagnostic indicator of psychiatric disorders (Takeda *et al.* 1995): these workers devised a three-dimensional HPLC method with electrochemical detection to measure bufotenine in urine. An ESI-LC-MS method for the determination of bufotenine and other potentially hallucinogenic *N*-dimethylated indoleamines in human urine has also been described by Forsstrom *et al.* (2001).

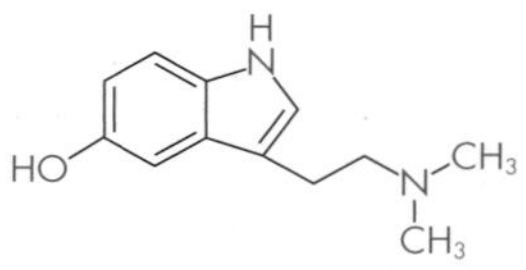

HO, H, N, N, CH_3, CH_3

Figure 4.17 Bufotenine.

Reptiles

Gila monsters

These venomous lizards belong to the genus *Helodermatidae* (*Heloderma suspectum*, the Gila monster, and *H. horridum*, the Mexican bearded lizard and their subspecies) and are indigenous to the south-western US and Mexico. They have venom glands on the mandible and deliver the venom along grooved teeth into a bite. The venom contains hyaluronidase and proteases, in addition to gilatoxin, a 35 kDa glycoprotein with serine protease and kallikrein-like activity. The bite can lead to anaphylactoid syndrome.

Snakes

Three main families of poisonous snakes exist – the Elapidae (cobras), the Viperidae (vipers) and the Crotalidae (pit vipers). The elapids comprise about half the world's species of venomous snakes and include the cobras and the mambas. Genera of the elapid family are found in Asia, the Pacific, the Americas and Africa. The true vipers, Viperidae, of which the common viper is the best known, inhabit Europe, Asia and Africa. The pit vipers, Crotalidae, are mainly found in North, Central and South America and include the rattlesnake genera *Crotalus* and *Sistrurus*. An estimated 30 000 lethal cases of snakebite occur annually in Asia and 1000 in Africa and South America (WHO 1995).

The symptoms of snakebites in humans vary greatly depending on the species, but in general consist of local pain, oedema, blistering and necrosis. Systemic effects of neurotoxic species include blurred vision, ptosis and respiratory paralysis. Haemostatic toxins, such as the haemorrhagins, cause spontaneous bleeding in the gingival sulci, nose, skin and gastrointestinal tract. Fatalities result from cerebral haemorrhage or massive retroperitoneal bleeding. Renal lesions include glomerulopathy, vasculopathy, tubular necrosis and interstitial nephritis, and often accompany snakebites with haematotoxic and neurotoxic venoms.

The only specific and effective treatment for systemic and severe local envenomation is the administration of antivenom, a hyperimmune immunoglobulin (Warrell and Fenner 1993;

Moroz 1998). For administration of the proper antivenom, the species that has bitten the patient must be known, and panacea antivenom is not and will not be available. Purification and characterisation of snake venoms is important not only for the elucidation of their mechanism of action but also for the preparation of these antivenoms. A future development in reducing snakebite fatalities may be active immunisation of populations at risk (Chippaux and Goyffon 1998).

Summary

As can be seen from the above, the number of poisonous substances that could be encountered by the clinician dealing with emergency medicine and by the forensic toxicologist is vast. It is not possible to screen for all these substances and so the toxicologist must rely on clinical records where available or other information which may provide clues as to the type of substances to be analysed for. The clinician and pathologist must be familiar with the symptoms that are characteristic for the various substances so that they can guide the toxicologist in their analyses.

References

R. A. Abuknesha and A. Maragkou, A highly sensitive and specific enzyme immunoassay for detection of β-amanitin in biological fluids, *Anal. Bioanal. Chem.*, 2004, **379**, 853–860.

P. J. Aggett, An overview of the metabolism of copper, *Eur. J. Med. Res.*, 1999, **4**, 214–216.

H. Ahsan *et al.*, Association between drinking water and urinary arsenic levels and skin lesion in Bangladesh, *J. Occup. Environ. Med.*, 2000, **42**, 1195–1201.

R. Akila *et al.*, Decrements in cognitive performance in metal inert gas welders exposed to aluminium, *Occup. Environ. Med.*, 1999, **56**, 632–639.

L. Alder *et al.*, Residue analysis of 500 high priority pesticides: better by GC-MS or LC-MS/MS? *Mass Spectrom. Rev*, 2006, **25**, 838–865.

A. C. Alfrey *et al.*, The dialysis encephalopathy syndrome. Possible aluminium intoxication, *N. Engl. J. Med.*, 1976, **294**, 184–188.

K. Ameno *et al.*, Simultaneous quantitation of diquat and its two metabolites in serum and urine by ion-paired HPLC, *J. Liq. Chromatogr.*, 1995, **18**, 2115–2121.

F. Anger *et al.*, Fatal aluminium phosphide poisoning, *J. Anal. Toxicol.*, 2000, **24**, 90–92.

P. J. Aplin and T. Eliseo, Ingestion of castor oil plant seeds, *Med. J. Aust.*, 1997, **167**, 260–261.

P. Apostoli *et al.*, Biological monitoring of occupational exposure to inorganic arsenic, *Occup. Environ. Med.*, 1999, **56**, 825–832.

K. Arys *et al.*, Quantitative determination of paraquat in a fatal intoxication by HPLC-DAD following chemical reduction with sodium borohydride, *J. Anal. Toxicol.*, 2000, **24**, 116–121.

H. N. Atalla *et al.*, Use of a Shiga toxin (Stx)-enzyme-linked immunosorbent assay and immunoblot for detection and isolation of Stx-producing *Escherichia coli* from naturally contaminated beef, *J. Food Prot.*, 2000, **63**, 1167–1172.

B. Bailey and M. McGuigan, Lithium poisoning from a poison control centre perspective, *Ther. Drug Monit.*, 2000, **22**, 650–655.

D. R. Baldwin and W. J. Marshall, Heavy metal poisoning and its laboratory investigation, *Ann. Clin. Biochem.*, 1999, **36**, 267–300.

G. A. Balint, Experimentally induced contributions to the therapy of ricin intoxication, *Tokushima J. Exp. Med.*, 1978, **25**, 91–98.

D. J. Barillo *et al.*, Cyanide poisoning in victims of fire: analysis of 364 cases and review of the literature, *J. Burn Case Rehabil.*, 1994, **15**, 46–57.

J. R. Barr *et al.*, 2005 Botulinum neurotoxin detection and differentiation by mass spectrometry. http://www.cdc.gov/ncidod/EID/vol11no10/04-1279.htm (accessed 19.01.08).

R. C. Baselt, *Disposition of Toxic Drugs and Chemicals in Man*, 6th edn, Foster City, Biomedical Publications, 2002, pp. 542–543.

R. C. Baselt, *Disposition of Toxic Drugs and Chemicals in Man*, 7th edn, Foster City, Biomedical Publications, 2004.

F. J. Baud *et al.*, Elevated blood cyanide concentrations in victims of smoke inhalation, *N. Engl. J. Med.*, 1991, **325**, 1761–1766.

A. K. Bayazit *et al.*, A child with hepatic and renal failure caused by aluminium phosphide, *Nephron*, 2000, **86**, 517.

G. R. Bayly *et al.*, Lead poisoning from Asian traditional remedies in the West Midlands – report of a series of 5 cases, *Hum. Exp. Toxicol.*, 1995, **14**, 24–28.

D. C. Bellinger *et al.*, Low-level lead exposure, intelligence and academic achievement: a long-term follow-up study, *Pediatrics*, 1992, **90**, 855–861.

[Comment in: *Pediatrics*, 1992, **90**, 995–997; *Pediatrics*, 1993, **91**, 855–856.]

M. Berg *et al.*, Arsenic contamination of groundwater and drinking water in Vietnam: a human health threat, *Environ. Sci. Technol.*, 2001, **35**, 2621–2626.

D. Z. Bissacot and I. Vassilieff, I. HPLC determination of flumethrin, deltamethrin, cypermethrin, and cyhalothrin residues in the milk and blood of lactating dairy cows, *J. Anal. Toxicol.*, 1997, **21**, 397–402.

M. Boehnert, Soluble barium salts, *Clin. Toxicol. Rev.*, 1988, **10**, 1–2.

W. Bonte, Congener analysis, in *Encyclopedia of Forensic Sciences, Volume I*, J. A. Siegel *et al.* (eds), London, Academic Press, 2000, pp. 93–102.

R. A. Braithwaite and S. S. Brown, Clinical and subclinical lead poisoning: a laboratory perspective, *Hum. Toxicol.*, 1988, **7**, 503–513.

J. W. Brock *et al.*, An improved analysis for chlorinated pesticides and polychlorinated biphenyls (PCBs) in human and bovine sera using solid-phase extraction, *J. Anal. Toxicol.*, 1996, **20**, 528–536.

C. Brooke, Ten times the limit: drink-driver who sniffed butane gas is told she could have died, *Daily Mail*, 14 April 1999, p. 37.

T. Brouette and R. Anton, Clinical review of inhalants, *Am. J. Addict.*, 2001, **10**, 79–94.

J. W. Burnett *et al.*, Coelenterate venom research 1991–1995: clinical, chemical and immunological aspects, *Toxicon*, 1996, **34**, 1377–1383.

R. Butera *et al.*, Diagnostic accuracy of urinary amanitin in suspected mushroom poisoning: a pilot study, *J. Toxicol. Clin. Toxicol.*, **42**, 901–9112.

R. L. Canfield *et al.*, Intellectual impairment in children with blood lead concentrations below 10 microg per deciliter, *N. Engl. J. Med*, 2003, **348**(16), 1517–1526.

J. A. Carton *et al.*, Acute and sub-acute lead poisoning clinical findings and comparative study of diagnostic tests, *Arch. Int. Med.*, 1987, **147**, 697–703.

L. T. Chan *et al.*, Phosphine analysis in postmortem specimens following ingestion of aluminium phosphide, *J. Anal. Toxicol.*, 1983, **7**, 165–167.

A. K. Chaturvedi *et al.*, Blood carbon monoxide and hydrogen cyanide concentrations in fatalities of fire and non-fire associated civil aviation accidents, 1991–1998, *Forensic Sci. Int.*, 2001, **121**, 183–188.

M. Cherington *et al.*, Microbial toxins, in *Handbook of Clinical Neurology: Intoxications of the Nervous System, Part II*, F. A. De Wolff (ed.), Amsterdam, Elsevier Science, 1995, 209–250.

J.-P. Chippaux and M. Goyffon, Venoms, antivenoms and immunotherapy, *Toxicon*, 1998, **36**, 823–846.

U. K. Chowdhury *et al.*, Groundwater arsenic contamination in Bangladesh and West Bengal, India, *Environ. Health Perspect.*, 2000, **108**, 393–397.

A. J. Christophers *et al.*, Dangerous bodies: a case of fatal aluminium phosphide poisoning, *Med. J. Aust.*, 2002, **176**, 403.

R. F. Clark *et al.*, Selenium poisoning from a nutritional supplement, *JAMA*, 1996, **275**, 1087–1088.

R. F. Clark *et al.*, A review of selected seafood poisonings, *Undersea Hyperb. Med.*, 1999, **26**, 175–184.

G. M. Crawford and O. Tavares, Simple hydrogen sulfide trap for the Gutzeit arsenic determination, *Anal. Chem.*, 1974, **46**, 1149.

H. T. Delves and M. J. Campbell, Measurement of total lead concentrations and of lead isotope ratios in whole blood by use of inductively coupled plasma source mass spectrometry, *J. Anal. Atomic Spectrom.*, 1988, **3**, 343–348.

H. T. Delves and M. J. Campbell, Identification and apportionment of sources of lead in human tissue, *Environ. Geochem. Health*, 1993, **15**, 75–84.

F. A. De Wolff and T. V. Thomas, Clinical pharmacokinetics of methoxsalen and other psoralens, *Clin. Pharmacokinet.*, 1986, **11**, 62–75.

F. A. De Wolff and E. J. M. Pennings, Mushrooms and hallucinogens: neurotoxicological aspects, in *Handbook of Clinical Neurology: Intoxications of the Nervous System, Part II*, F. A. De Wolff (ed.), Amsterdam, Elsevier Science, 1995, pp. 35–60.

F. A. de Wolff *et al.*, Subacute fatal aluminium poisoning in dialyzed patients: post-mortem toxicological findings, *Forensic Sci. Int.*, 2002, **128**, 41–43.

D. Dyne *et al.*, Toluene, 1-butanol, ethylbenzene and xylene from Sarstedt Monovette serum gel blood collection tubes, *Ann. Clin. Biochem.*, 1996, **35**, 355–356.

D. Dyne *et al.*, A novel device for capturing breath samples for solvent analysis, *Sci. Total Environ.*, 1997, **199**, 83–89.

B. M. El-Haj *et al.*, A GC-MS method for the detection of toluene and ethylbenzene in volatile substance abuse, *J. Anal. Toxicol.*, 2000, **24**, 390–394.

M. J. Ellenhorn, Chlorate, in *Ellenhorn's Medical Toxicology*, 2nd edn, M. J. Ellenhorn *et al.* (eds), Baltimore, Williams and Wilkins, 1997, pp. 1642–1643.

M. J. Ellenhorn *et al.*, Cyanide poisoning, in *Ellenhorn's Medical Toxicology*, 2nd edn, M. J. Ellenhorn *et al.* (eds), Baltimore, Williams and Wilkins, 1997, pp. 1476–1484.

J. Felice *et al.*, Multicomponent determination of 4-hydroxycoumarin anticoagulant rodenticides in blood serum by liquid chromatography with fluorescence detection, *J. Anal. Toxicol.*, 1991, **15**, 126–128.

A. Fernández-Gutierrez *et al.*, Determination of endosulfan and some pyrethroids in water by micro liquid–liquid extraction and GC-MS, *Fresenius J. Anal. Chem.*, 1998, **5**, 568–572.

M. E. Field-Smith *et al.*, Trends in death associated with abuse of volatile substances 1971–2005, St. George's, University of London, Division of Community Health Sciences, 2007. http://www.vsareport.org (accessed 19.01.08).

M. Filigenzi *et al.*, Determination of alpha-amanitin in serum and liver by multistage linear ion trap mass spectrometry, *J. Agric. Food Chem.*, 2007, **55**, 2784–2790.

V. Fiserova–Bergerova, *Modelling of Inhalation Exposure to Vapours: Uptake, Distribution and Elimination, Volumes I and II*, Boca Raton, CRC Press, 1983.

A. A. Fisher and D. G. Le Couteur, Lead poisoning from complementary and alternative medicine in multiple sclerosis, *J. Neurol. Neurosurg. Psychiatry*, 2000, **69**, 687–689.

R. J. Flanagan and R. J. Ives, Volatile substance abuse, *Bull. Narc.*, 1994, **46**, 49–78.

R. J. Flanagan *et al.*, *Basic Analytical Toxicology*, Geneva, World Health Organization, 1995.

M. Flieger *et al.*, Ergot alkaloids – sources, structures and analytical methods, *Folia Microbiol. (Praha)*, 1997, **42**, 3–29.

T. Forsstrom *et al.*, Determination of potentially hallucinogenic *N*-dimethylated indoleamines in human urine by HPLC/ESI-MS-MS, *Scand. J. Clin. Lab. Invest.*, 2001, **61**, 547–556.

K. A. Francesconi *et al.*, Arsenic metabolites in human urine after ingestion of an arsenosugar, *Clin. Chem.*, 2002, **48**, 92–101.

L. Friberg *et al.*, *Cadmium in the Environment*, Cleveland, CRC Press, 1971.

Y. Gaillard and G. Pepin, Poisoning by plant material: review of human cases and analytical determination of main toxins by high-performance liquid chromatography–(tandem) mass spectrometry, *J. Chromatogr. B*, 1999, **733**, 181–229.

A. Gasmi *et al.*, Acute selenium poisoning, *Vet. Hum. Toxicol.*, 1997, **39**, 304–308.

D. L. Gatto-Menking *et al.*, Sensitive detection of biotoxoids and bacterial spores using an immunomagnetic electrochemiluminescence sensor, *Biosens. Bioelectron.*, 1995, **10**, 501–507.

M. C. Gennaro *et al.*, Hallucinogenic species in amanita muscaria. Determination of muscimol and ibotenic acid by ion-interaction HPLC, *J. Liq. Chromatogr. Relat. Technol.*, 1997, **20**, 413.

J. Gilbert and E. A. Vargas, Advances in sampling and analysis for aflatoxins in food and animal feed, *J. Toxicol. Toxin Rev.*, 2003, **22**, 381–422.

J. R. Glover, Selenium and its industrial toxicology, *Ind. Med.*, 1970, **39**, 50–54.

A. Godal *et al.*, Radioimmunoassays of abrin and ricin in blood, *J. Toxicol. Environ. Health*, 1981, **8**, 409–417.

I. C. Grant, Ichthyosarcotoxism: poisoning by edible fish, *J. Accid. Emerg. Med.*, 1997, **14**, 246–251.

F. G. Guale *et al.*, Laboratory diagnosis of zinc phosphide poisoning, *Vet. Hum. Toxicol.*, 1994, **36**, 517–519.

T. L. Guidotti, Occupational exposure to hydrogen sulphide in the sour gas industry; some unresolved issues, *Int. Arch. Occup. Environ. Health*, 1994, **66**, 153–160.

J. M. Gulliver, A fatal copper sulfate poisoning, *J. Anal. Toxicol.*, 1991, **15**, 341–391.

B. Hamilton, *et al.*, Multiple ciguatoxins present in Indian Ocean reef fish. *Toxicon* 2002, **40**, 1347–1353.

J. C. Hansen, Has selenium a beneficial role in human exposure to inorganic mercury? *Med. Hypotheses*, 1988, **25**, 45–53.

A. D. Hardy *et al.*, Composition of eye cosmetics (Kohls) used in Oman, *J. Ethnopharmacol.*, 1998, **60**, 223–234.

F. Hasler *et al.*, Determination of psilocin and 4-hydroxyindole-3-acetic acid in plasma by HPLC-ECD and pharmacokinetic profiles of oral and intravenous psilocybin in man, *Pharm. Acta Helv.*, 1997, **72**, 175–184.

G. M. Hawdon and K. D. Winkel, Spider bite. A rational approach, *Aust. Fam. Physician*, 1997, **26**, 1380–1385.

T. J. Hindmarsh, Caveats in hair analysis in chronic arsenic poisoning, *Clin. Biochem.*, 2002, **35**, 1–11.

D. R. Hyatt *et al.*, Usefulness of a commercially available enzyme immunoassay for Shiga-like toxins I and II as a presumptive test for the detection of *Escherichia coli* O157:H7 in cattle feces, *J. Vet. Diagn. Invest.*, 2001, **13**, 71–73.

IARC, Toxins derived from *Fusarium graminearum*, *F. culmorum* and *F. crookwellense*: zearalenone, deoxynivalenol, nivalenol and fusarenone X, *IARC Monogr. Eval. Carcinog. Risks Hum.*, 1993, **56**, 397–444.

M. Ito *et al.*, Rapid analysis method for paraquat and diquat in the serum using ion-pair high-performance liquid chromatography. *Biol Pharm Bull.* 2005, **28**, 725–728.

L. Jarup *et al.*, Health effects of cadmium exposure – a review of the literature and risk estimate, *Scand. J. Work Environ. Health*, 1988, **24**(Suppl. 1), 7–51.

D. R. Jarvie and M. J. Stewart, The rapid extraction of paraquat from plasma using an ion-pairing technique, *Clin. Chim. Acta*, 1979, **94**, 241–251.

S. N. Kales and R. H. Goldman, Mercury exposure: current concepts, controversies, and a clinic's experience, *J. Occup. Environ. Med.*, 2002, **44**, 143–154.

T. Kamata *et al.*, Liquid chromatography–mass spectrometric and liquid chromatography–tandem mass spectrometric determination of hallucinogenic indoles psilocin and psilocybin in "magic mushroom" samples, *J Forensic Sci.*, 2005, **50**, 336–340.

T. J. Kneip *et al.*, Arsenic selenium and antimony in urine and air analytical method by hydride generation and atomic absorption spectroscopy, *Health Lab. Sci.*, 1977, **14**, 53–58.

B. Knight, Ricin – a potent homicidal poison, *BMJ*, 1979, **1**, 350–351.

M. E. Kolanz, Introduction to beryllium: uses, regulatory history and disease, *Appl. Occup. Environ. Hyg.*, 2001, **16**, 559–567.

C. Köppel *et al.*, Fatal poisoning with selenium dioxide, *Clin. Toxicol.*, 1986, **24**, 21–35.

N. Kozel *et al.* (eds), *Epidemiology of Inhalant Abuse: An International Perspective*, NIDA Research Monograph 148, Rockville, National Institute on Drug Abuse, 1995.

E. Lacassie *et al.*, Sensitive and specific multiresidue methods for the determination of pesticide of various classes in clinical and forensic toxicology, *Forensic Sci. Int.*, 2001, **121**, 116–125.

B. Lakshmi, Methemoglobin formation with aluminium phosphide poisoning, *Am. J. Emerg. Med.*, 2002, **20**, 1–3.

J. F. Lawrence *et al.*, Determination of decarbamoyl saxitoxin and its analogues in shellfish by prechromatographic oxidation and liquid chromatography with fluorescence detection, *J. AOAC Int.*, 1996, **79**, 1111–1115.

X-C. Le *et al.*, Human urinary arsenic excretion after one-time ingestion of seaweed, crab and shrimp, *Clin. Chem.*, 1994, **40**, 617–624.

X. P. Lee XP *et al.*, Determination of paraquat and diquat in human body fluids by high-performance liquid chromatography/tandem mass spectrometry. *J. Mass Spectrom.*, 2004, **39**, 1147–52.

P. H. M. Leung *et al.*, The prevalence and characterization of verotoxin-producing *Escherichia coli* isolated from cattle and pigs in an abattoir in Hong Kong, *Epidemiol. Infect.*, 2001, **126**, 173–179.

R. J. Lewis *et al.*, HPLC/tandem electrospray mass spectrometry for the determination of sub-ppb levels of Pacific and Caribbean ciguatoxins in crude extracts of fish, *Anal. Chem.*, 1999, **71**, 247–250.

T. Lyttle *et al.*, Bufo toads and bufotenine: fact and fiction surrounding an alleged psychedelic, *J. Psychoactive Drugs*, 1996, **28**, 267–290.

B. R. Martin, The chemistry of aluminium as related to biology and medicine, *Clin. Chem.*, 1986, **32**, 1797–1806.

H. J. Mason *et al.*, Follow up of workers previously exposed to silver solder containing cadmium, *Occup. Environ. Med.*, 1999, **56**, 553–558.

R. Matoba *et al.*, An autopsy case of acute selenium (selenious acid) poisoning and selenium levels in human tissues, *Forensic Sci. Int.*, 1986, **31**, 87–92.

H. H. Maurer, Liquid chromatography–mass spectrometry in forensic and clinical toxicology, *J. Chromatogr. B Biomed. Sci. Appl.*, 1998, **713**, 3–25.

R. I. McCallum, *Antimony in Medical History*, Durham, Pentland Press, 1999.

P. McNabb *et al.*, Multiresidue method for determination of algal toxins in shellfish: single-laboratory validation and interlaboratory study, *J AOAC Int.*, 2005, **88**, 761–772.

D. Mebs, *Venomous and Poisonous Animals*, Stuttgart, Medpharm Scientific Publishers (CRC), 2002.

H. A. Meda *et al.*, Epidemic of fatal encephalopathy in preschool children in Burkina Faso and consumption of unripe ackee (*Blighia sapida*) fruit, *Lancet*, 1999, **353**, 536–540.

T. J. Meredith *et al.*, Diagnosis and treatment of acute poisoning with volatile substances, *Hum. Toxicol.*, 1989, **8**, 277–286.

T. Miyazaki *et al.*, Correlation between 'on admission' blood toluene concentrations and the presence or absence of signs and symptoms in solvent abusers, *Forensic Sci. Int.*, 1990, **44**, 169–177.

A. C. Moffat, M. D. Osselton and B. Widdop (eds), *Clarke's Analysis of Drugs and Posions*, 3rd edn, London, Pharmaceutical Press, 2004.

C. Moor and R. Adler, Herbal vitamins: lead toxicity and developmental delay, *Pediatrics*, 2000, **106**, 600–602.

C. Moroz, *Vipera palaestinae* antivenin, *Public Health Rev.*, 1998, **26**, 233–236.

J. A. Morten and H. T. Delves, Measurement of total boron and ^{10}B concentration and the detection and measurement of elevated ^{10}B levels in biological samples by inductively coupled plasma mass spectrometry using the determination of ^{10}B:^{11}B ratios, *J. Anal. Atomic Spectrom.*, 1999, **14**, 1545–1556.

T. Müller *et al.*, Endemic Tyrolean infantile cirrhosis: an ecogenetic disorder, *Lancet*, 1996, **347**, 877–880.

J. Naar *et al.*, A competitive ELISA to detect brevetoxins from *Karenia brevis* (formerly *Gymnodinium breve*) in seawater, shellfish, and mammalian body fluid, *Environ. Health Perspect.*, 2002, **110**, 179–185.

H. I. Needlemann and C. A. Gatsonis, Low level lead exposure and IQ of children. A meta-analysis of modern studies, *JAMA*, 1990, **263**, 673–678.

W. M. Niessen, *Liquid Chromatography–Mass Spectrometry*, 2nd edn, New York, Marcel Dekker, 1999.

NIOSH, *Pocket Guide to Chemical Hazards*, Washington DC, Department of Health and Human Services (NIOSH) Publication No. 2005–140, 2005. Available on-line at http://www.cdc.gov/niosh/npg/ (accessed 19.01.08).

A. Nozawa *et al.*, Implication of brevetoxin B1 and PbTx-3 in neurotoxic shellfish poisoning in New Zealand by isolation and quantitative determination with liquid chromatography-tandem mass spectrometry, *Toxicol*, 2003, **42**, 91–103.

J. W. O'Donohue *et al.*, Micronodular cirrhosis and acute liver failure due to chronic copper self-intoxication, *Eur. J. Gastroenterol. Hepatol.*, 1993, **5**, 561–562.

I. Ojanperä *et al.* Identification limits for volatile organic compounds in the blood by purge-and-trap GC-FTIR, *J. Anal. Toxicol.*, 1998, **22**, 290–295

M. J. O'Neil *et al.* (eds), *Merck Index*, 14th edn, New York, Merck Research Laboratories Division of Merck & Co., Inc., 2006.

T. Piamphongsant, Chronic environmental arsenic poisoning, *Int. J. Dermatol.*, 1999, **38**, 401–410.

T. Piek and R. S. Leeuwin, Neurotoxic arthropod venoms, in *Handbook of Clinical Neurology: Intoxications of the Nervous System, Part II*, F. A. De Wolff (ed.), Amsterdam, Elsevier Science, 1995, pp. 193–207.

K. Pihlainen and I. Ojanperä, Analytical toxicology of fluorinated inhalation anaesthetics, *Foresic Sci. Int.* 1998, **97**, 117–133.

M. Piscator, Copper, in *Handbook on the Toxicology of Metals*, L. Friberg *et al.* (eds), Amsterdam, Elsevier Biomedical Press, 1979, pp. 411–420.

W. Popp *et al.*, Phosphine poisoning in a German office, *Lancet*, 2002, **359**, 1574.

D. A. Quadrani *et al.*, A fatal case of Gun Blue ingestion in a toddler, *Vet. Hum. Toxicol.*, 2000, **42**, 96–98.

M. A. Quilliam, Phycotoxins, *J. AOAC Int.*, 1999, **82**, 773–781.

J. D. Ramsey, Detection of solvent abuse by direct mass spectrometry on expired air, in *Drug Determination in Therapeutic and Forensic Contexts*, E. Reid and I. D. Wilson (eds), New York, Plenum, 1984, pp. 357–362.

M. Rayman, The importance of selenium to human health, *Lancet*, 2000, **356**, 233–241.

C. Reilly, Selenium in health and disease: a review, *Aust. J. Nutr. Diet.*, 1993, **50**, 136–144.

P. L. Rogers and W. F. Staruszkiewicz, Histamine test kit comparison, *J. Aquatic Food Product Technol.*, 2000, **9**, 5–17.

V. Riihimäki *et al.*, Body burden of aluminum in relation to central nervous system, *Scand J Work Environ Health*, 2000, **26**, 118–130.

J. H. Rossmeisl, Jr., *et al.*, *Amanita muscaria* toxicosis in two dogs, *J. Vet. Emerg. Crit. Care*, 2006, **16**, 208–214.

K. Saito *et al.*, Determination of psilocin in magic mushrooms and rat plasma by liquid chromatography with fluorimetry and electrospray ionization mass spectrometry, *Anal. Chim. Acta*, 2004, **527**, 149–156.

T. Sakai, Biomarkers of lead exposure, *Ind. Health*, 2000, **38**, 127–142.

B. Schellmann *et al.*, Acute fatal selenium poisoning – toxicological and occupational medical aspects, *Arch. Toxicol.*, 1986, **59**, 61–63.

R. Scott, Life for man who nearly got away with murder: plain evil of pervert who set fire to his victims' bodies, *Daily Mail*, 29 February 1996, p. 38.

S. Seidel *et al.*, Assessment of commercial laboratories performing hair mineral analysis, *JAMA*, 2001, **285**, 67–72.

S. Sethi *et al.*, Role of copper in Indian childhood cirrhosis, *Ann. Trop. Pediatr.*, 1993, **13**, 3–6.

H. S. A. Sherratt, Jamaican vomiting sickness, in *Handbook of Clinical Neurology: Intoxications of the Nervous System, Part II*, F. A. De Wolff (ed.), Amsterdam, Elsevier Science, 1995, pp. 79–113.

S. Sing *et al.*, Aluminium phosphide ingestion – a clinicopathological study, *Clin. Toxicol.*, 1996, **34**, 703–706.

B. M. Singh *et al.*, The metabolic effects of fatal cyanide poisoning, *Postgrad. Med. J.*, 1989, **65**, 923–925.

D. L. Smith *et al.*, *Criteria for a Recommended Standard-Occupational Exposure to Dinitro-ortho-cresol*, US Dept of HEW (NIOSH) Pub No. 78–131, Washington DC, NIOSH, 1978.

M. M. Smith *et al.*, Determination of antimony in urine by solvent extraction and electrothermal atomisation atomic absorption spectrometry for biological monitoring of occupational exposure. *J. Anal. Atomic Spectrom.*, 1995, **10**, 349–352.

A. H. Smith *et al.*, Contamination of drinking water by arsenic in Bangladesh: a public health emergency, *Bull. WHO*, 2000, **78**, 1093–1103.

E. Solé *et al.*, Zinc-protoporphyrin determination as a screening test for lead-exposure in childhood, *Bull. Environ. Contam. Toxicol.*, 2000, **65**, 285–292.

P. S. Spencer, Lathyrism, in *Handbook of Clinical Neurology: Intoxications of the Nervous System, Part II*, F. A. De Wolff (ed.), Amsterdam, Elsevier Science, 1995, pp. 1–20.

H. A. Spiller, Epidemiology of volatile substance abuse (VSA) cases reported to US poison centers, *Am. J. Drug Alcohol Abuse*, 2004, **30**, 155–165.

T. Stiefel *et al.*, Toxicokinetic and toxicodynamic studies of beryllium, *Arch. Toxicol.*, 1980, **45**, 81–92.

R. Stienstra *et al.*, Psilocybin poisoning resulting from eating mushrooms, *Ned. Tijdschr. Geneeskd.*, 1981, **125**, 833–835.

N. Takeda *et al.*, Bufotenine reconsidered as a diagnostic indicator of psychiatric disorders, *Neuroreport*, 1995, **6**, 2378–2380.

A. Taylor, Usefulness of measurements of trace elements in hair, *Ann. Clin. Biochem.*, 1986, **23**, 364–378.

C. D. Thompson, Selenium speciation in human body fluids, *Analyst*, 1998, **123**, 827–831.

C. Tomlin (ed.), *The Pesticide Manual*, 14th edn, London, British Crop Protection Council, 2006.

S. Tong *et al.*, Environmental lead exposure: a public health problem of global dimensions, *Bull. WHO*, 2000, **78**, 1068–1077.

S. L. Tompsett, Paraquat poisoning, *Acta Pharm. Toxicol.*, 1970, **28**, 346–358.

E. R. Tor *et al.*, Rapid determination of domoic acid in serum and urine by liquid chromatography-electrospray tandem mass spectrometry, *J. Agric. Food Chem.*, 2003, **51**, 1791–1796.

S. Trevino, Fish and shellfish poisoning, *Clin. Lab. Sci.*, 1998, **11**, 309–314.

K. Tsujikawa, *et al.*, Analysis of hallucinogenic constituents in Amanita mushrooms circulated in Japan, *Forensic Sci. Int.*, 2006, **164**, 172–178.

K. Tsujikawa, *et al.*, Determination of muscimol and ibotenic acid in Amanita mushrooms by high-performance liquid chromatography and liquid chromatography-tandem mass spectrometry, *J. Chromatogr. B*, 2007, **852**, 430–435.

H. Valenta, Chromatographic methods for the determination of ochratoxin A in animal and human tissues and fluids, *J. Chromatogr. A*, 1998, **815**, 75–92.

B. L. vanBaar *et al.*, Characterization of tetanus toxin, neat and in culture supernatant, by electrospray mass spectrometry. *Anal. Biochem.*, 2002, **301**, 278–289.

H. P. Van Egmond, Methods for determining ochratoxin A and other nephrotoxic mycotoxins, *IARC Sci. Publ.*, 1991, **115**, 57–70.

S. C. J. M. Velzeboer *et al.*, A hypertensive toddler, *Lancet*, 1997, **349**, 1810.

J. Vetter, Toxins of *Amanita phalloides*, *Toxicon*, 1998, **36**, 13–24.

E. Vinner *et al.*, Separation and quantification of paraquat and diquat in serum and urine by capillary electrophoresis. *Biomed. Chromatogr.*, 2001, **15**, 342–347.

K. E. Von Mühlendahl and H. Lange, Copper and childhood cirrhosis, *Lancet*, 1994, **344**, 1515–1516.

F. M. Walsh *et al.*, Acute copper intoxication, *Am. J. Dis. Child.*, 1977, **131**, 149–151.

D. A. Warrell and P. J. Fenner, Venomous bites and stings, *Br. Med. Bull.*, 1993, **49**, 423–439.

M. M. Weldon *et al.*, Mercury poisoning associated with a Mexican beauty cream, *West J. Med.*, 2000, **173**, 15–18.

J.-P. Weller and M. Wolf, Mass-spectroscopy and headspace-GC, *Beitr. Gericht. Med.*, 1989, **47**, 525–532.

WHO, Poisonous animal bites and stings, *WHO Weekly Epidemiol. Rec.*, 1995, **70**, 315–316.

WHO, *Recommended Classification of Pesticides by Hazard*, Geneva, World Health Organization, 2006.

G. Yang *et al.*, Endemic selenium intoxication of humans in China, *Am. J. Clin. Nutr.*, 1983, **37**, 872–881.

B. Yeoman, Metals and anions, in *Clarke's Isolation and Identification of Drugs*, 2nd edn, A. C. Moffat (ed.), London, Pharmaceutical Press, 1985, pp. 55–69.

M. Yotsu *et al.*, An improved tetrodotoxin analyzer, *Agric. Biol. Chem.*, 1989, **53**, 893–895.

5

Workplace drug testing

M Peat

Introduction 135

Evolution of workplace testing in the USA 136

Regulatory process in the USA 136

Proposed changes to the *HHS Guidelines* 141

Adulterated and substituted specimens 143

Collection of specimens 145

Role of the medical review officer 146

References 150

Introduction

Workplace drug testing began in the USA during the 1980s as a result of accidents in the railroad industry, and the political environment of the 'war on drugs' and the 'crack' epidemic. It is now an accepted practice, with between 30 and 40 million such tests being carried out in the USA annually. In Europe, Australia and other industrialised countries, workplace drug testing has gained increasing acceptance over the past decade. For example, in the UK, workplace testing was established about 15 years ago and now has an estimated annual turnover of £12 million. European laboratories have followed the American lead in setting up careful protocols for sample collection, analysis and medical review of results. There are potentially serious financial repercussions, not to mention damage to a laboratory's reputation, if an individual is refused a job or made redundant because of a positive test result but they subsequently prove that the test was faulty. There are differences between the USA and other countries both in criteria for the minimum concentration of a drug or metabolite in a urine specimen that constitutes a positive result, and in the selection of target drugs. Moreover, in the UK in particular, the ethos is that testing should be part of a package of measures that includes formulation of company policy, education of the workforce as regards the dangers of drug misuse, and treatment and/or rehabilitation programmes. Another major difference is that very little legislation has yet been enacted in Europe to govern the principles and practices of workplace testing. Instead, the European Guidelines drawn up by representatives of the leading European laboratories are designed to establish good laboratory practice and at the same time take account of the individual requirements of national custom and legislation. The European Guidelines relate to collection of samples, laboratory analyses and interpretation of the results.

The discussion which follows is based largely on the workplace testing system in operation in the USA because this is the most highly developed system. While threshold values applied for various drugs and test specimens may differ from country to country, as may the exact nature of workplace test schemes, the principles of the US system are applicable for all test schemes.

Evolution of workplace testing in the USA

The major milestones were:

- a major railroad accident in which there were several fatalities. The National Transportation Safety Board determined that cannabis (marijuana) use by one of the engineers was a causal factor in the accident
- the introduction of 'crack' cocaine and the deaths of high-profile sports and entertainment figures from cocaine use
- the declaration of a 'war on drugs' and a change of the US Government's policy to focus on reducing the supply of drugs
- in 1986 President Reagan issued an Executive Order (Federal Register 1986) that required those federal employees in safety- and security-sensitive positions to be drug tested. This Order also led to the publication by the Department of Health and Human Services (HHS) of the *Mandatory Guidelines for Drug Testing of Federal Employees* (Federal Register 1988a), which became known as the *National Institute on Drug Abuse (NIDA) Guidelines* (or today as the *Substance Abuse and Mental Health Services Administration (SAMHSA) Guidelines*). These were modified in 1994 (Federal Register 1994) to change the cut-offs for cannabis detection, and in 1998 (Federal Register 1998) to change the cut-offs for opiate detection. SAMHSA currently has responsibility for the *Guidelines*.

This confluence of events set the stage for the introduction of drug-testing programmes to the non-federal workplace. Their introduction focused on the expected improvement in safety and public health, and on the economic savings to be expected from decreased absenteeism, staff turnover rate and reduced health care costs. A limited number of major corporations were already performing pre-employment testing and claimed improvements in the factors listed, although they generally had not published their data. As the decade progressed, a number of studies (see Peat (1995) for earlier references and American Management Association (2001) for a more recent study) were published, the majority of which showed that some benefits were to be expected.

In the USA, the *HHS Guidelines* and the Department of Transport (DOT) *Code of Federal Regulations CFR Part 40* are the two major sets of rules that govern the practice of drug testing in the federal workplace and in that regulated by the DOT. Similar rules for testing are performed under the auspices of the Nuclear Regulatory Commission (NRC) and the Department of Defense (DOD). In April of 2004 a revised HHS document was released expanding the kinds of specimens that may be tested under federal agency workplace drug testing programmes, including hair, oral fluid and sweat (Federal Register 2004/Notices).

As stated previously, although there is far less regulation of workplace drug testing in other countries, the standards for acceptable practice are similar to those of the USA and cover specimen collection, laboratory analysis and medical review of results.

The question that underlies these drug-testing programmes is 'Have they been effective in reducing drug use in the workplace and/or in the general population?' For the USA, there are data (Quest Diagnostics 2005) that suggest a reduction in the number of positives throughout the 1990s, and that this reduction correlates with a reduction in the admitted use of illicit drugs (SAMHSA 2000). In all probability, numerous factors are responsible for the reduction in drug use, including targeted education programmes and supply reduction programmes, in addition to workplace drug testing.

Regulatory process in the USA

The HSS Guidelines consist of a number of parts. These cover issues such as:

- drugs to be tested
- specimen collection procedures
- laboratory personnel
- testing procedures
- quality assurance and quality control
- reporting and review of results.

As for all laboratories carrying out workplace drug testing, it is important that they can demonstrate their competence so that if they find a positive result, it truly is positive, and that if quantitative results are reported, they are accurate both in terms of the identity of the substance reported and the concentration. The HSS Guidelines also cover aspects such as laboratory performance testing, the certification process and inspections, and procedures that a laboratory should implement to demonstrate competency.

These sections of the *HHS Guidelines* have become models for other accreditation programmes, particularly those of the College of American Pathologists (CAP) and the American Board of Forensic Toxicology (ABFT; American Academy of Forensic Sciences and the Society of Forensic Toxicologists 2006). Each of the important sections is discussed in more detail below and, where applicable, discussed in the light of today's practices in the USA and Europe.

The HHS Guidelines (Federal Register 1988a) consist of a number of sub-parts, two of which relate directly to laboratory testing; these are sub-part B (Scientific and Technical Requirements) and sub-part C (Certification of Laboratories Engaged in Urine Drug Testing for Federal Agencies). Within sub-part B are included sections on drugs to be tested, specimen collection procedures, laboratory personnel, testing procedures, quality assurance and quality control, and reporting and review of results. Sub-part C includes sections on performance testing, the certification process and inspections.

Drugs to be tested

The HHS Guidelines clearly define the drugs that can be tested for under the regulatory programmes and the cut-offs (or thresholds) to be used for both the initial testing by immunoassay and confirmation testing by GC-MS. These two procedures are the only ones allowed for under the *HHS Guidelines*.

Table 5.1 includes details of the drugs tested and the cut-offs used in the USA, and those proposed for testing in the European Union (EU; European Workplace Drug Testing Society 2002) and the UK (London Toxicology Group 2001). There are two points to be made regarding Table 5.1.

Table 5.1 Initial testing cut-offs (μg/L) for those drugs and/or drug classes included in regulatory programmes in urine

Drug or drug class	USA HHS	Proposed EU	Proposed UK
Amfetamines	1000	300	300
Cannabis	50	50	50
Cocaine	300	300	300
Opiates	2000	300	300
Phencyclidine	25	Not tested	25

- When the HHS and European programmes are compared, significant differences are found between the cut-offs used for the opiates and amfetamines. Initially, the HHS included a cut-off of 300 ng/mL for opiates, but this was raised to 2000 ng/mL in 1998 to resolve some of the issues associated with the medical review of opiate positives following poppy seed ingestion and prescription codeine use. On the other hand, the cut-off for amfetamines has remained at 1000 ng/mL since 1989. That proposed by the European programmes is more realistic, considering the increasing use of the so-called 'designer amfetamines' throughout the 1990s. The 2004 proposed HHS document lowers amfetamine screening concentration to 500 ng/mL, with methamfetamine being the target analyte. Methylenedioxymethylamfetamine (MDMA) was also added to the initial testing at the concentration of 500 ng/mL. The proposed confirmation includes MDMA, methylenedioxyamfetamine (MDA) and methylenedioxyethylamfetamine (MDEA), with the threshold value for all three at 250 ng/mL. Cocaine metabolite concentration in initial screening was also lowered to 150 ng/mL.
- Phencyclidine (PCP) has always been included in the *HHS Guidelines*, even though it is not widely used in the USA. It is even less widely used in Europe and therefore its omission from the EU proposal is not surprising.

The majority of testing in the USA is performed in the nonregulated workplace, and although a large number of these programmes follow the federal guidelines, a number include drugs or drug classes other than the five listed in Table 5.1 or test these five drugs or drug classes at different cut-offs. Table 5.2 lists the other drugs or drug classes that are tested and the differing cut-offs used.

It can be seen that laboratories that perform workplace drug testing in the USA need to be prepared to offer a variety of tests and cut-offs if they are to satisfy fully the demands of the marketplace.

Table 5.2 Initial testing cut-offs (μg/L) for those drugs and/or drug classes included in non-regulatory programmes in urine

Drug or drug class	USA
Amfetamines	300 or 500
Barbiturates	100 or 200
Benzodiazepines	100, 200 or 300
Cannabis	20, 25 or 100
Cocaine	150
Methadone	100 or 300
Methaqualone	100 or 300
Opiates	300
Propoxyphene	100 or 300

The current *HHS Guidelines* require that all confirmations be performed by GC-MS using the cut-offs listed in Table 5.3. There are a number of points to be made regarding Table 5.3.

- Previous *HHS Guidelines* did not require certified laboratories to confirm the presence of MDMA, MDA and MDEA, whereas both European proposals do. In addition, the UK proposal suggests cut-offs for the confirmation of ephedrine and pseudoephedrine. The proposal of the *HHS Guidelines* (2004) require the inclusion of MDMA, MDA and MDEA.
- The proposed *HHS Guidelines* from 2004 require that a laboratory report methamfetamine as positive only if its concentration is 250 ng/mL or greater, and if that of amfetamine is ⩾100 ng/mL. The necessity to report amfetamine together with methamfetamine was introduced in the early 1990s after discovering a so called 'methamfetamine artefact'. In 1990 several specimens were reported as positive for methamfetamine when the specimen contained large amounts of pseudoephedrine or ephedrine. It was discovered subsequently (Hornbeck *et al.* 1993) that

Table 5.3 Confirmation cut-offs (μg/L) for those drugs and/or drug classes included in regulatory programmes in urine

Drug or drug class	Drugs tested	US HHS	Proposed EU	Proposed UK
Amfetamines	Amfetamine	500 (250)[a]	200	200
	Methamfetamine	500[b] (250)[a]	200	200
	MDMA[a], MDA[a], MDEA[a]		200	200
	Pseudoephedrine			200
	Ephedrine			200
Cocaine	Benzoylecgonine	150	150	150
Cannabis	THCA	15	15	15
Opiates	Morphine	2000	200	300
	Codeine	2000	200	300
	MAM	10	10	10
	Dihydrocodeine			300
Phencyclidine	PCP	25	Not tested	25

[a] HHS 2004 (proposed).

[b] To be reported positive for methamfetamine, urine also has to contain at least 200 ng/mL of amfetamine.

these hydroxylated sympathomimetics could convert to methamfetamine in either the extraction or chromatographic stages of the analysis. None of these specimens contained amfetamine when tested, and therefore the introduction of the reporting rule prevented the reporting of 'false-positive' methamfetamine results. Today, the vast majority of laboratories use a pre-oxidation step with periodate (Paul *et al.* 1994; Klette *et al.* 2000) to prevent the possibility of this happening.

- As with the initial testing cut-offs, there is a difference in the thresholds used for opiate confirmations. The HHS cut-off is 2000 ng/mL for morphine and codeine, whereas the European values are 200 ng/mL (EU) and 300 ng/mL (UK). There is also a difference across the three regions in the opiates to be tested. All require morphine and monoacetylmorphine (MAM) under certain circumstances; the HHS and proposed UK guidelines also require codeine, and the UK 1-dihydrocodeine. The *HHS Guidelines* require that certified laboratories analyse the specimen for MAM (with a cut-off of 10 ng/mL) if the morphine concentration equals or exceeds 2000 ng/mL.
- Cannabis (marijuana) use is confirmed by quantifying the major urinary metabolite of Δ^9-tetrahydrocannabinol (THC), 11-carboxy-Δ^9-tetrahydrocannabinol (THCA). The cut-off value for this confirmation is 15 ng/mL which has also been adopted by the European programmes.

Table 5.4 details the other drugs that may have to be confirmed in nonregulated programmes and the different cut-offs that may be used for the five drug classes tested for in the regulated programme.

Although several compounds are listed under some of the drug classes, this does not imply that all these tests are performed on every nonregulated specimen with a positive initial testing result.

Table 5.4 Confirmation cut-offs (μg/L) for those drugs and/or drug classes included in non-regulatory programmes in urine

Drug or drug class	Drugs tested	USA
Amfetamines	Amfetamine	300 or 500
	Methamfetamine	300 or 500
	MDMA, MDA	300 or 500
Barbiturates	Amobarbital	100 or 200
	Butalbital	100 or 200
	Pentobarbital	100 or 200
	Phenobarbital	100 or 200 (or higher)
	Secobarbital	100 or 200
Benzodiazepines	α-Hydroxyalprazolam	100 (or lower)
	Nordiazepam	100
	Oxazepam	100, 200 or 300
	Temazepam	100, 200 or 300
Cocaine	Benzoylecgonine	100 or 150
Cannabis	THCA	10 or 15
Methadone	Methadone	100 or 300
Methaqualone	Methaqualone	100 or 300
Opiates	Morphine	300
	Codeine	300
	Hydrocodone	300
	Hydromorphone	300
	MAM	10
Propoxyphene	Propoxyphene	100 or 300

Lysergide testing

Over the years there has been discussion regarding the usefulness of incorporating lysergide (LSD) into workplace drug testing programmes. There are many reasons for its exclusion, one of the major ones being that, demographically, those included in workplace drug-testing programmes are not in the age group expected to be users. Nevertheless, certain populations, such as inductees into the US military, are being tested using cut-offs for screening and confirmation of less than 1 ng/mL for LSD. A second major reason is the analytical challenge presented. Today, both enzyme and microparticle immunoassays are available for screening urine specimens, and LSD can be confirmed using tandem mass spectrometry. However, there has been concern regarding testing for unchanged LSD, and work published by Klette *et al.* (2000) and Poch *et al.* (2000) shows clearly that the 2-oxo-3-hydroxy LSD metabolite is the preferred target analyte.

Testing procedures

As already indicated, the *HHS Guidelines* mandate the use of immunoassay as the initial test and GC-MS as the confirmatory procedure. These are also the testing procedures generally used for nonregulated testing, although some laboratories may be using GC-MS/MS technology or liquid chromatography–mass spectrometry (LC-MS, or LC-MS/MS) for the confirmation of the nonregulated analytes.

The immunoassay methods have to have been approved by the Food and Drug Administration (FDA), which in the USA has regulatory authority for approval of diagnostic reagents. Although workplace drug testing is not being performed for diagnostic purposes, it was believed that requiring FDA approval would bring at least some standardisation to the reagents used. However, no regulations were introduced that required the immunoassay kits to use antibodies directed towards certain members of a drug class, and if the kits used for regulated and nonregulated testing are compared there is some variation in the target antigen (Liu 1995).

Nearly all drug testing laboratories use either reagents based on enzymes (e.g. enzyme multiplied immunoassay technique (EMIT) or cloned enzyme donor immunoassay (CEDIA)), microparticles (kinetic interaction of microparticles in solution; KIMS) or fluorescence polarisation (TDx). Given the difference in target antigens and calibrators, different detection rates on specimens that contain the same drug(s) and/or metabolites might be expected. For example, the CEDIA and EMIT assays for amfetamine have been shown to have almost 100% cross-reactivity for *d*-amfetamine, whereas the KIMS assay has little cross-reactivity to *d*-methamfetamine. In fact, the latter was designed to comply with the Reporting Rule issued by HHS for methamfetamine positives, and therefore is effective in detecting 'real-life' specimens that contain methamfetamine and its metabolite, amfetamine. Conversely, if a proficiency-testing specimen contained only methamfetamine it would give a negative result. Similar dichotomies exist in examining the benzodiazepines, for which the detection of the more traditional members of the group is not a problem, but the assays vary widely in their ability to detect some of the later members, such as lorazepam and flunitrazepam metabolites (Drummer 1998). Even when the procedures are targeted towards the same antigen and use the same calibrators, there can be variation in their ability to detect positive specimens. For example, immunoassays that have greater specificity towards the target urinary metabolite of THC, THCA, may not be as efficient as those that are more widely cross-reacting to the THC metabolites in detecting urine specimens from cannabis users, particularly when cut-offs are used.

One of the major concerns in the past few years has been the ability of the amfetamine assays to detect MDMA, MDA and MDEA. Some of the manufacturers have introduced special kits, whereas others have relied on the inherent cross-reactivity of their existing amfetamine assay. From existing data (Zhao *et al.* 2001), it appears that either approach is satisfactory, with the most variation being seen in specimens with concentrations close to the cut-off. In an attempt to resolve this problem, the draft proposals (SAMHSA 2002) from HHS on the new guidelines require that '*d*-methamfetamine be the target analyte and the test kit must cross-react with MDMA, MDA and MDEA (approximately 50 to 150% cross-reactivity)'. Whether this requirement can be satisfied, given the vagaries of immunoassays, remains to be seen.

Some of the issues that surround initial testing by immunoassay have been discussed already. Far fewer issues relate to confirmation testing by GC-MS. Numerous GC-MS procedures have been published for the identification and quantification of the drugs and their metabolites in urine specimens. Over the past decade numerous procedures based on mass spectrometry, particularly ones involving tandem mass spectrometry (MS-MS), have also been published for their detection and quantification in hair, oral fluid and other specimens. The use of these technologies is likely to raise issues similar to those that were debated two decades or so ago, when GC-MS was mandated for confirmation of drugs and metabolites in urine. Some of these issues are set out and discussed below:

- How reliable is the use of ion ratios and how many ions should be monitored? Experience has certainly shown that the monitoring of three ions for the analyte and two for the deuterated internal standard, and the use of a 20% range for ion ratios, result in satisfactory positive identification of the analyte.
- How diagnostic are the ions? Most toxicologists believe that using ions of higher mass is more appropriate than using ones of lower mass. For example, using *m/z* 91 for amfetamine is not recommended. On the other hand, there are a number of assays in use today that routinely use isotopes for identification and ratio purposes. Perhaps the best example is the confirmation of PCP, for which large numbers of laboratories use *m/z* 242 and its carbon isotope, *m/z* 243. This has become an accepted practice for this drug because, apart from *m/z* 205, there are no other diagnostic ions. Another example of a drug class for which isotopes may be used, with less justification, is the benzodiazepines (halogen isotope ratios are used).
- What is an acceptable chromatographic peak shape? Two integral parts of the *HHS Guidelines* are the need for proficiency testing (the *Guidelines* use the term performance testing) and regular inspections of the certified laboratories. In all proficiency testing programmes the participating laboratories are periodically provided with samples containing specified drugs and/or their metabolites, but the actual quantity of the substance is known only to the agency. The laboratory analyses the samples as part of its normal routine, and reports the results out to the agency. The laboratory is then provided with a report specifying how closely its results correspond to the accepted value, and if necessary, can then take appropriate action to improve performance. By participating in proficiency testing programmes the laboratory can prove to the accreditation body and to its customers that all analytical procedures are appropriately validated. In the USA the performance testing and inspection programmes are the major components of the National Laboratory Certification Program (NLCP). The inspection requirement is that each accredited laboratory be inspected at 6-monthly intervals. There are allowances within the *HHS Guidelines* for other inspections, specifically special inspections that can be performed at the direction of HHS and outside of the normal cycle. A number of accepted practices have evolved as a result of the inspections. Two examples are the detailed quality-control requirements and the definition of acceptable peak shape. The acceptance criteria for these practices, and others, are not included in the *HHS Guidelines* themselves, but are included in the *Resource Manual* for the NLCP (SAMHSA 2002). Within this manual, an acceptable chromatographic peak shape has been defined as having greater than 90% resolution (separation from other peaks) and symmetry.
- What are the limits of detection and quantification and how are they determined? The definition of these criteria has also evolved since 1988. Initially, the majority of certified laboratories used the traditional definitions based on the analysis of drug-free specimens and, although this is still acceptable, the favoured definitions are now ones based on serial dilutions and satisfying quantitative and ion-ratio criteria.

Although it is straightforward to define these criteria for GC-MS analysis of urine specimens, it is difficult to imagine the same criteria being applied to MS-MS technology, particularly if chemical ionisation or electrospray is used.

Proposed changes to the *HHS Guidelines*

As mentioned, in April 2004 HHS proposed the expansion of the *Guidelines* to include specimens other than urine and to lower the cut-offs in urine. The three new specimens being considered are hair, oral fluid and sweat (Tables 5.5 and 5.6). Today, each of these specimens is being used outside of the federally regulated workplaces for workplace and/or criminal justice testing (see Chapter 6 for a discussion of hair, oral fluid and sweat as alternative test specimens).

Hair

It is proposed that hair testing be included in the Federal Workplace Drug Testing Programs. It is well known that drugs and their metabolites may be incorporated into hair by several different pathways such as passive diffusion from the bloodstream, and secretions of the apocrine sweat and sebaceous glands. The amount of drug incorporated into hair can be influenced by several factors such as drug dose, length of exposure, chemical properties of the drug, environmental contamination and hair colour.

Oral fluid

- It will be permissible (proposed 2004 *HHS Guidelines*) to test initially all specimens for MAM using a 4 ng/mL cut-off.
- For a specimen to be positive for methamfetamine it must contain amfetamine at a concentration equal to or greater than the limit of detection for the same reason as described previously.

Table 5.5 Proposed initial testing cut-offs for alternative specimens

Drug or drug class	Hair (pg/mg)	Oral fluid (µg/L)	Sweat (ng/patch)
Amfetamines	500	50	25
Cocaine	500	20	25
Cannabis	1	4	4
Opiates	200	40	25
Phencyclidine	300	10	20

Sweat

- According to the 2004 HHS proposals, laboratories are permitted to test initially all specimens for MAM at 25 ng/patch.
- As for oral fluid, for a specimen to be positive for methamfetamine it must contain amfetamine at a concentration equal to or greater than the limit of detection.

Clearly, there will be a dramatic increase in the complexity of the analyses needed to test these alternative specimens for workplace drug testing, and in the proficiency testing and inspection programmes involved in certifying laboratories to do such testing.

Although no mention has yet been made regarding the specimen volume to be collected, it is important to realise that the current urine testing programme requires the collection of at least 45 mL which is divided into two samples: A and B. Sample A is the specimen analysed by the testing laboratory. Sample B is considered to be the donor's and can only be opened at the request of the donor. It is sealed and stored under suitable conditions and the A sample is analysed. If the A sample is found to be positive, the donor may request analysis of the B sample. The bottle is normally opened for re-test purposes by a second certified laboratory. Given the sensitivity of current technology available for testing urine specimens, there are no concerns regarding specimen availability during this process. However, that may not be the case for the alternative specimens, for which the minimum specimen sizes are recommended to be: hair, 100 mg; oral fluid, 2 mL (1.5 mL for the primary specimen and 0.5 mL for the split specimen); and sweat, one FDA-approved patch worn for 7–14 days.

The implementation of these proposed guidelines will require laboratories to be proficient in the use of more sensitive immunoassays (particularly enzyme-linked immunosorbent assay (ELISA)) and tandem mass spectrometry (probably with an LC interface).

Included in Table 5.7 is a comparison of hair, oral fluid and sweat as specimens for drug detection (also see Chapter 6).

Table 5.6 Confirmation cut-offs for alternative specimens

Drug or drug class	Drugs tested	Hair (pg/mg)	Oral fluid (μg/L)	Sweat (ng/patch)
Amfetamines	Amfetamine	300	50	25
	Methamfetamine[a]	300	50	25
	MDMA	300	50	25
	MDA	300	50	25
	MDEA	300	50	25
Cocaine	Benzoylecgonine	50[b]		
	Cocaine	500[b]		
	Cocaine or benzoylecgonine		8	25
Cannabis	THCA	0.05		
	THC		2	1
Opiates	Morphine	200	40	
	Codeine	200	40	
	Morphine, codeine or MAM			25
	MAM	200[c,d]	4	
Phencyclidine	PCP	300	10	20

[a] For a specimen to be positive for methamfetamine it must contain amfetamine at a concentration equal to or greater than 50 pg/mg. (See Chapter 6, p. 160).

[b] For a specimen to be positive for cocaine, both cocaine and benzoylecgonine must confirm positive and the ratio of metabolite to parent cocaine must be equal to or greater than 0.05.

[c] It will be permissible to test initially all specimens for MAM using a 200 pg/mg cut-off.

[d] If the specimen confirms positive for MAM, it must also contain morphine at a concentration equal to or greater than 200 pg/mg.

Adulterated and substituted specimens

Over the past decade increasing attention has been paid to attempts to 'beat the drug test'. There have always been donors who have attempted this through diuresis, through substitution of the specimen (with clean urine or another fluid) or through deliberate adulteration of the collected specimen. The DOT first issued guidance on this in 1992 and recommended that laboratories identify adulterants in a 'forensically acceptable manner'. A 'dilute urine specimen' was defined as one that contained less than 20 mg/dL creatinine and had a relative density (specific gravity) of less than 1.003. At that time regulations allowed an observed urine collection on a donor producing dilute urine at their next scheduled collection, and at the request of the employer. In practice this was hardly ever done. Collection guidelines also required the collector to perform an observed collection if there were suspicious circumstances during collection or if the urine temperature was out of range (the acceptable range being 32.2 to 37.7°C).

In recent years use has been made of the internet to sell products that are supposedly designed to beat the drug test. Whereas a number of these include the instructions to drink copious amounts of water before taking the test (i.e. diuresis), others are designed specifically to oxidise the THCA metabolite of cannabis and thereby reduce the ability of the laboratory to confirm cannabis use. Some examples of substances sold to prevent detection of a sample likely to test positive include nitrite, chromate (Cr^{VI}), halogens and peroxide.

Table 5.7 Comparison of hair, oral fluid and sweat as specimens for drug detection

Specimen	Detection window	Advantages	Disadvantages
Hair	Months – dependent to some extent upon the drug	Can be used as a long-term measure of drug use Relatively noninvasive collection Can obtain a second specimen for re-testing (if necessary) Relatively resistant to adulteration	Not a suitable specimen for detecting recent drug use May be an invasive collection if head hair is unavailable Requires sensitive immunoassays and MS-MS technology Deposition of drug and/or metabolite in hair is reported to be dependent upon hair colour Potential environmental contamination
Oral fluid	Hours or days – dependent to some extent upon the drug	Relatively noninvasive collection An 'observed' collection and therefore resistant to adulteration and substitution For some drugs correlates to free drug concentration in plasma	Short detection window for some drugs Requires sensitive immunoassays and MS-MS technology Collection methods can dilute the specimen, which makes drug detection more difficult After cannabis use, THC in the buccal cavity is the detected material; THCA is not detected
Sweat	Up to weeks – dependent to some extent upon the drug	Cumulative measure of drug use Monitor drug use for a period of weeks with a sweat patch	Requires sensitive immunoassays and MS-MS technology High inter-subject variability For workplace drug-testing, application of a sweat patch for several days is impractical

Although accurate data are difficult to obtain, a relatively recent estimate shows that at least 0.05% of the specimens tested for federally mandated purposes are adulterated (Kadehjian 2001). If so, this would be similar to the positive rate for some drugs, for example the amfetamines and PCP.

The recently published *CFR Part 40* (Federal Register 2000) requires certified laboratories to detect adulterated and substituted specimens. The HHS has issued detailed proposed rules (2004) for such testing, which include definitions and the testing and quality control procedures to be used. Steps that the medical review officer (MRO) can use for review of these non-negative specimens are also included.

The definitions for a dilute, substituted and adulterated specimen are as follows:

- dilute: creatinine less than 20 mg/dL and relative density less than 1.003, except when the definition of a substituted specimen is met

- substituted: creatinine less than 2 mg/dL and relative density less than 1.002 or equal to or greater than 1.020.
- adulterated:
  - nitrite is greater than or equal to 500 μg/mL
  - pH is less than 3 or greater than or equal to 11
  - specimen contains an exogenous substance (i.e. a substance that is not a normal constituent of urine)
  - specimen contains an endogenous substance at a concentration greater than that considered to be a normal physiological concentration.

The other definition included in the rules is for an invalid drug test, which, among others, includes one in which the laboratory has failed to identify the adulterant.

These rules are interesting for a number of reasons. Firstly, a workplace drug-testing laboratory now has to perform tests that, historically, have not been performed in toxicology laboratories. Secondly, the toxicologist and/or MRO may be called upon to defend these specimen validity testing procedures and their results when legally challenged, for example in an arbitration hearing. Defending a non-negative result may present new challenges in terms of the interpretation of the data. Thirdly, they expand the duties of the laboratory to include the identification of new and existing adulterants, which is a major analytical challenge. Finally, they are the first such rules to prescribe quality-control protocols for diluted, adulterated or substituted specimens.

According to the SAMHSA rules, in addition to performing creatinine tests on all specimens, a certified laboratory has to perform pH testing on all specimens, validity tests for substances that are commonly known as oxidising adulterants, and additional validity tests when one of three further conditions are observed (SAMHSA 2002).

This brief overview of some of the newer requirements and of the expansion of the programmes to include alternative specimens demonstrates that the range and complexity of workplace drug testing has increased dramatically and will continue to do so.

Collection of specimens

The proper collection, packaging and transportation of urine specimens is a crucial part of a drug-testing programme. Although this is the most frequently challenged aspect of the process in any legal proceeding, it is also the least regulated one.

It has been accepted practice, and is now a requirement, in most workplace drug testing programmes and certainly in the industries regulated by the DOT, that a urine specimen be collected and split into two portions (sometimes referred to as bottles A and B). Under DOT regulations, during the collection process the collector is required to monitor the temperature of the urine (within 4 minutes of the collection), ensure that the donor does not substitute or adulterate the specimen, and to complete the necessary chain-of-custody documents. This process includes the following major steps:

- preparation of the collection area, for example adding a blue dye to the toilet water and taping of the taps
- confirmation of the donor's identity using photographic evidence and requesting him or her to remove outer clothing and to empty pockets
- having the donor randomly select a collection container and two bottles, which should be wrapped separately (only the collection container should be taken into the toilet enclosure)
- checking the temperature of the sample within 4 minutes of voiding and noting the result on the chain-of-custody form. The collector has then to ensure that there is at least 45 mL of urine in the container and that the specimen has no unusual odour, colour or physical properties (e.g. excessive frothing) that may indicate attempted adulteration
- pouring at least 30 mL into bottle A and 15 mL into bottle B in the presence of the donor, and immediately closing the bottles and applying tamper-evident seals across the lids or caps of the bottles
- ensuring that the donor initials the seals and completes his or her section of the chain-of-custody form. The collector then

completes the remaining sections of the form
- preparing the specimen bottles for shipment to the laboratory.

Although these are the recommended steps for the completion of a regulated chain of custody, it is also the general procedure used to collect all urine specimens. The steps most often challenged are that the collector did not complete the process in the presence of the donor and that more than one specimen was being collected at the same time (i.e. there were multiple specimens and chains of custody in various stages of collection.)

Completion of the chain-of-custody form is an important part of this process

Almost all drug testing programmes in the USA have provisions for 'shy bladder syndrome'. In this situation the donor fails to provide an adequate urine volume after remaining at the collection site for up to 3 hours and being provided with 1.25 L of liquid. The donor is deemed to have a 'shy bladder' and is required to undergo a medical examination. If there is a reasonable medical explanation, the test is cancelled. If the donor requires a negative test for employment, specimens other than urine may be used, for example hair or oral fluid.

In the regulated industries, observed collections have to be performed by same-sex collectors and can currently only be performed in five special cases:

- when the specimen temperature is out of range at the collection site. In this case there has to be an immediate observed collection
- where the collector has identified an apparent tampering with the specimen at the collection site, for example the addition of bleach to the urine. Again, there has to be an immediate observed collection
- if the previous specimen has been declared invalid by the laboratory and when there is no obvious medical explanation for this. The most obvious example of this is where the laboratory has proof of adulteration, but cannot specifically identify the adulterant
- when the MRO has cancelled the test because the Bottle B specimen was unavailable or had been adulterated and was so identified by the laboratory performing the re-confirmation
- in return-to-work and follow-up tests, for which the employer can, in certain circumstances, decide to conduct observed collections.

These general guidelines are also followed outside the regulated industries, although some employers and some sectors may have more rigorous ones. For example, the US military requires observed collections for all specimens.

Despite these safeguards, donors are still able to adulterate urine specimens by adding oxidising agents after voiding. The amount of such material added is extremely small (a vial of it can be hidden easily in a shoe or sock) and, if it is liquid, the volume is insufficient to alter the temperature of the specimen. Alternative specimens to urine have advantages that their collection can be considered noninvasive and can be observed. For example, collection of oral fluid is usually performed using a pad or swab and the donor can do this themselves in the presence of the collector. Collection of hair is also 'observed', although some questions remain as to the invasive nature of this process, particularly when non-head hair has to be collected.

Role of the medical review officer

In workplace drug testing, the outcome of a positive result may be that an individual's employment contract is terminated or that they are not offered employment. These are critical decisions and the person making these decisions needs to be qualified to do so for their judgement to be considered acceptable. It is debatable whether the laboratory carrying out the testing has personnel suitably qualified to interpret the results in the full medical context and to make decisions based on the outcome of the tests. The medical history of the individual may be important in the context of interpreting the results and there may also be issues regarding bias of the test laboratory if a dispute arises over the results. Hence it is considered good practice in many jurisdictions for someone not associated with the test laboratory to make decisions whether a result is positive or not. In the USA, this role is carried out by an MRO.

The concept of MRO was introduced in the *HHS Guidelines*. Their initial role was to receive the testing results from the laboratory, contact the donor to determine whether a positive drug result could have arisen from the legal use of a drug and, if not, to verify the result as positive and contact the employer. Where the legal use of a medication explained the result, the MRO would report the result as negative and communicate this to the employer.

Increasingly, MROs serve as gatekeepers for drug-testing results and as administrators of functions ancillary to the process, such as the collection and storage of all documentation. Given the breadth of these tasks and the extent of drug testing in the USA, some physicians practice full time as MROs. Many others act as MROs in the course of their duties as occupational health physicians and corporate medical directors.

Before the introduction of the federal programmes, the laboratory toxicologists had filled the interpretative role, and few issues had arisen. However, within the federal programmes, which introduced random and post-accident testing to a large percentage of the workforce, there was a need for additional safeguards. It was anticipated that MROs would serve as the final quality-assurance check on the laboratory result and, indeed, they have done so. For example, some vigilant MROs who could not rationalise the laboratory result with the donor's demographics and medical history first raised the phenomenon of the conversion of ephedrine and pseudoephedrine to methamfetamine. They questioned the findings and requested the re-tests in which the second laboratory could not confirm the findings. Another reason for their introduction was a purely legal one; in the USA only licensed physicians can access prescription records, and it was obvious that this could be essential to determine the legitimacy of a donor's claim.

When the MRO receives a positive result, he or she has to contact and interview the donor, obtain prescription records (if necessary) and then verify the laboratory result as positive or negative before reporting the result to the employer. These reviews are generally straightforward; for example, there is no legal reason for a donor to test positive for PCP, whereas a large majority of specimens that test positive for codeine do so because of prescription use or, in countries such as the UK, as a result of the extensive use of codeine in over-the-counter medicines. In other areas questions arise, particularly in the interpretation of methamfetamine and morphine positives; these are discussed in more detail later in the chapter.

The MRO is also responsible for reviewing non-negative results from donors. These include adulterated, substituted and invalid specimens. Before 2000 when the new regulation was issued (Federal Register 2000), MROs had very little role in the review of substituted and adulterated specimens; they simply received the results from the laboratory, reviewed the paperwork and reported them to the employer. There was no requirement to contact the donor and no ability for the donor to request a re-test. The new regulations changed that and incorporated a requirement for the MRO to contact the donor to determine whether there was a medical reason for the laboratory findings, although this would be extremely unlikely, and allowed the donor to request a re-test. These particular re-tests were to be performed using the same criteria for defining a specimen as substituted or adulterated as used in the initial set of tests. For example, if a specimen was determined to be substituted, with creatinine readings of 4.8 and 4.7 mg/dL and with relative density readings of 1.001 on bottle A while bottle B had a creatinine reading of 5.1 mg/dL and a relative density of 1.001, the re-test specimen would be reported as 'Failed to Confirm: Substituted Specimen'. Some of the relevant interpretative issues associated with adulterated and substituted specimens are discussed later in the chapter.

Interpretation of amfetamine positive results

This particular drug-testing result has caused, and continues to cause, confusion among the MRO community. Some of this stems from the reporting rule for methamfetamine. This rule requires that for methamfetamine to be reported as positive there must be at least 200 ng/mL of amfetamine present, in addition to at least 500 ng/mL of methamfetamine. If both amines are present in concentrations greater than 500 ng/mL by GC-MS, both are reported as positive and there is no confusion. Difficulty arises when the amfetamine concentration determined by the laboratory is between 200 and 500 ng/mL (i.e. less than the amfetamine confirmation cut-off), but the methamfetamine concentration is above 500 ng/mL. In this situation, the MRO receives only a methamfetamine-positive result, rather than one that indicates that both methamfetamine and amfetamine are positive. Once the MRO understands that the laboratory must comply with this reporting rule, the confusion disappears.

The second area of confusion is in the differentiation of *d*-and *l*-methamfetamine. *l*-Methamfetamine is found in the USA in Vicks Inhaler (an over-the-counter decongestant product) and, although its use can result in the detection of methamfetamine and amfetamine in urine, the concentrations are generally low (Fitzgerald *et al.* 1988). Moreover, given the low cross-reactivities of immunoassays to the *l*-isomers of methamfetamine and amfetamine, a positive result is unlikely following normal use. However, a methamfetamine user may still claim that the positive arises because of his or her use of Vicks Inhaler and, in such cases, the MRO can request a GC-MS separation of the isomers. These are usually qualitative analyses and reported as *x*% of the *d*-isomer and *y*% of the *l*-isomer. Where the *l*-isomer is greater than 80%, the MRO reports the result as negative.

Although some drugs can metabolise to methamfetamine and amfetamine (e.g. benzphetamine and selegeline), these are available only on prescription in the USA and the interpretation of positive amfetamine results is relatively straightforward. In other countries, this may not be the case. Cody (2002) recently reviewed the issue of precursor medications.

Interpretation of opiate positive results

This is another area that has caused confusion in the MRO community. From 1989 to 1998 the cut-off used for the opiates was 300 ng/mL, both in the initial testing and in the confirmation of codeine and morphine by GC-MS. During this period there was no requirement that a certified laboratory should be able to confirm the presence of the characteristic metabolite of diamorphine, MAM, although several did so routinely. In 1998 the cut-offs were raised to 2000 ng/mL and the laboratories were required to confirm the presence of MAM if the morphine concentration exceeded 2000 ng/mL. The GC-MS cut-off for MAM was set at 10 ng/mL. The major reason for raising the opiate cut-offs was associated with MRO reviews of opiate-positive samples. Use of the 300 ng/mL cut-off criterion resulted in a large number of positive results that derived from either poppy-seed ingestion or therapeutic doses of codeine, and which were subsequently verified as negative by the MROs.

Where there was a prescription for codeine, the MRO's review presented no problems. However, in the absence of a prescription for codeine (or morphine) the MRO was required to observe 'clinical signs of opiate use' before reporting a verified opiate-positive result back to the employer. This requirement remains for some results, even within the new *CFR Part 40*, unless the specimen has tested positive for MAM, which is conclusive evidence of diamorphine use.

Under the new *CFR Part 40*, if the morphine concentration is greater than 15 000 ng/mL the donor has the responsibility for providing evidence that the presence of morphine was the result of a legitimate use of a drug, and not the illicit use of diamorphine or morphine. There are certainly no reports that indicate such urinary morphine concentrations from poppy-seed ingestion, even under extreme conditions (Selavka 1991), so if the donor cannot provide this evidence the MRO verifies the result as a positive.

Passive exposure

Passive exposure is an issue that still causes confusion in interpretation of results. It essentially deals with the passive inhalation of marijuana or hashish smoke and the unwitting ingestion of cocaine or marijuana. Although passive exposure to crack (free-base cocaine) smoke has been claimed as an excuse for a positive urine benzoylecgonine, there is no evidence that this is valid. In two studies that investigated this (Baselt *et al.* 1991; Cone *et al.* 1995), no urine specimens gave immunoassay readings above 300 ng/mL.

However, unwitting ingestion of cocaine may result in positive urine specimens with the cut-offs currently used. There is no doubt that an individual who ingests a drink fortified with cocaine can test positive. In one study (Baselt and Chang 1987) in which a volunteer consumed 25 mg cocaine hydrochloride, urine benzoylecgonine concentrations were greater than 300 ng/mL for 48 hours. The question most often raised is the use of decocainised coca teas. As with decaffeinated coffee, these teas contain small amounts of cocaine; one study found an average of 4.8 mg per tea bag (Jackson *et al.* 1991). After the ingestion of one cup of this tea, immunoassay results were positive for 21–26 hours. Obviously, the more regular the use, the more likely these specimens are to be positive and to be so for longer periods. In regulated industries, these samples would be validated as positives as these are not legitimate uses of cocaine. Outside these industries, more flexibility may be applied in interpreting the result.

Passive inhalation of cannabis smoke continues to be an excuse offered by donors for their positive results. There is no doubt that environmental exposure to cannabis smoke can occur through passive inhalation, but the question is, does it produce measurable concentrations in urine and if so for what time? In a number of early studies (Perez-Reyse *et al.* 1982; Law *et al.* 1984; Morland *et al.* 1985) there was evidence for the presence of THCA in urine after passive exposure, but the concentrations measured were orders of magnitude lower than the cut-offs in use in workplace drug testing. In a more extreme study by Cone *et al.* (1987) volunteers were exposed to 4 and 16 cannabis cigarettes for 1 hour for six consecutive days. After exposure to four cigarettes, few urine specimens were positive, while after 16 cigarettes many more specimens were positive with a maximum THCA concentration of 87 ng/mL reported by GC-MS. The authors stressed, however, that these were extreme conditions, in that exposure was in a nonventilated, tightly sealed, small room and that it occurred for multiple days. In fact, the smoke was of such intensity that goggles were required by a number of the volunteers. It is generally accepted that social exposure to cannabis smoke (at parties, in outdoor arenas) will not result in a positive urine specimen.

Interpretation of adulterated and substituted specimens

As noted earlier in this chapter, it is not uncommon for persons being tested to try to adulterate their sample in some way. This may be by substituting an alternative specimen or by addition of substances that will interfere in some way with analysis of the sample, that will change the nature of the sample such that it is not detected, or that dilutes the sample, thereby reducing the concentration of the drug.

Nearly all the adulterants that are used today to oxidise THCA are classified in the recently issued *HHS Guidelines* as exogenous substances not expected to be present in urine. One exception to this is nitrite, which can occur in urine as a result of bacterial infection, the ingestion of certain foodstuffs and the use of some medications. In one study (Urry *et al.* 1998) that considered these sources and the presence of nitrite in normal urine, the highest urinary concentration was approximately 130 μg/mL; the cut-off used today is 500 μg/mL, almost four times this concentration. Some of the other adulterants include chromium(VI), peroxide, iodine and bleach; none of these should be detected as a result of normal physiology and metabolism. However, a donor may claim that their presence is the result of workplace exposure or the ingestion of vitamins or herbal material, and the person interpreting the results needs to be prepared to refute these claims.

The interpretation of substituted specimens has already caused discussion; some investigators believe that the criteria of less than 5 mg/dL creatinine and less than 1.002 relative density are too high for some individuals and some occupations. To date they have produced no data to support this belief. Before establishing the criteria, HHS performed an extensive literature review on what might be expected to be normal ranges for creatinine and relative density in both healthy individuals and those with certain diseases that may lead to polyuria (Cook *et al.* 2000). Following this review, it was decided that the criteria of creatinine less than 5 mg/dL and a relative density of less than 1.002 or greater than 1.020 were sound ones for establishing a specimen as substituted.

Recently, Barbanel *et al.* (2002) reviewed over 800 000 urine specimens. In this population both creatinine and relative density measurements were taken from over 13 000 specimens, and none of these satisfied the criteria for a substituted specimen. These authors also examined the medical records of patients who satisfied one of the criteria and reported that these were either neonatal, moribund or so severely ill that essentially none could have been in the working population.

Further information has been provided by a study in which 12 volunteers (5 men and 7 women) consumed 2.5 L of water over a 6-hour period and urine specimens were collected for the measurement of creatinine and specific gravity; none of the 500 specimens collected was identified as substituted using the criteria (Edgell *et al.* 2002). In 2003 the Federal Aviation Authority sponsored a symposium to investigate whether 'substituted' specimens can be produced under normal conditions. It was reported that certain individuals had been shown to excrete urine with a creatinine of less than 5 mg/dL. This observation resulted in the differences in the procedures used to test federal employees and those covered under the DOT requirements.

References

American Academy of Forensic Sciences and the Society of Forensic Toxicologists, *Forensic Toxicology Laboratory Guidelines*, Colorado Springs, CO, American Academy of Forensic Sciences, 1991.

American Management Association, AMA Survey: Medical Testing, 2001 (see http://www.amanet.org/research/archives.htm).

C. Barbanel *et al.*, Confirmation of the Department of Transportation criteria for a substituted urine specimen, *J. Occup. Environ. Med.*, 2002, **44**, 407–417.

R. Baselt and J. Chang, Urinary excretion of cocaine and benzoylecgonine following oral ingestion in a single subject, *J. Anal. Toxicol.*, 1987, **11**, 81–82.

R. Baselt *et al.*, Passive inhalation of cocaine, *Clin. Chem.*, 1991, **37**, 2160–2161.

J. Cody, Precursor medications as a source of methamphetamine and/or amphetamine positive drug testing results, *J. Occup. Environ. Med.*, 2002, **44**, 435–450.

J. Cook *et al.*, The characterization of human urine for specimen validity determination – workplace drug testing: a review, *J. Anal. Toxicol.*, 2000, **24**, 579–588.

E. Cone *et al.*, Passive inhalation of marijuana smoke – urinalysis and room air levels of delta-9-tetrahydrocannabinol, *J. Anal. Toxicol.*, 1987, **11**, 89–96.

E. Cone *et al.*, Passive inhalation of cocaine, *J. Anal. Toxicol.*, 1995, **19**, 399–411.

Department of Transport, Omnibus Transportation Employee Testing Act, US Senate Public Law, 1991, 102–143.

O. Drummer, Methods for the measurement of benzodiazepines in biological samples: review, *J. Chromatogr. B*, 1998, **713**, 201–225.

K. Edgell *et al.*, The defined HHS/DOT substituted urine criteria validated through a controlled hydration study, *J. Anal. Toxicol.*, 2002, **26**, 419–423.

European Workplace Drug Testing Society, 2002: www.ewdts.org.

Federal Register, Executive Order 12564, Drug-free federal workplace, Federal Register, 1986, **51**, 32889–32983.

Federal Register, Mandatory guidelines for federal workplace drug testing programmes, Federal Register, 1988a, **53**, 11970–11989.

Federal Register, Mandatory guidelines for federal workplace drug testing programmes, Federal Register, 1994, **59**, 29908–29931.

Federal Register, Changes to the testing cut-off levels for opiates for federal workplace drug testing programmes, Federal Register, 1998, **60**, 57587.

Federal Register, Procedures for transportation workplace drug and alcohol programmes: Final rule, 49 CFR Part 40, Federal Register, 2000, **65**, 79462–75579.

Federal Register, Vol. 69, No. 71 (April 13, 2004) Notices.

R. Fitzgerald *et al.*, A resolution of methamphetamine stereoisomers in urine drug testing: urinary excretion of *R*-(−)-methamphetamine following use of nasal inhalers, *J. Anal. Toxicol.*, 1988, **12**, 255–259.

C. Hornbeck *et al.*, Detection of a GC/MS artifact peak as methamphetamine, *J. Anal. Toxicol.*, 1993, **17**, 257–263.

G. Jackson *et al.*, Urinary excretion of benzoylecgonine following ingestion of health Inca tea, *Forensic Sci. Int.*, 1991, **49**, 57–64.

L. Kadehjian, Urine specimen adulteration: attempts to thwart drug testing, Substance Abuse Specialties, Inc., Newsletters and Information, 2001. http://www.sas-i.com/news_info/story_02.html (accessed 19.01.08).

K. Klette *et al.*, Metabolism of lysergic acid diethylamide (LSD) to 2-oxo-3-hydroxy LSD (O-H-LSD) in human liver microsomes and cryoprocessed human hepatocytes, *J. Anal. Toxicol.*, 2000, **24**, 550–556.

B. Law *et al.*, Passive inhalation of cannabis smoke, *J. Pharm. Pharmacol.*, 1984, **36**, 578–581.

R. Liu, Evaluation of commercial immunoassay kits for effective workplace drug testing, in *Handbook of Workplace Drug Testing*, R. Liu and B. Goldberger (eds), Washington DC, AACC Press, 1995.

London Toxicology Group, 2001: www.ltg.uk.net.

J. Morland *et al.*, Cannabinoids in blood and urine after passive inhalation of cannabis smoke, *J. Forensic Sci.*, 1985, **30**, 997–1002.

B. Paul *et al.*, Amphetamine as an artifact of methamphetamine during periodate degradation of interfering ephedrine, pseudoephedrine and phenylpropanolamine: an improved procedure for accurate quantitation of amphetamine in urine, *J. Anal. Toxicol.*, 1994, **18**, 331–336.

M. Peat, Financial viability of screening for drugs of abuse, *Clin. Chem.*, 1995, **41**, 805–808.

M. Perez-Reyse *et al.*, Passive inhalation of marijuana smoke and urinary excretion of cannabinoids, *Clin. Pharmacol. Ther.*, 1982, **31**, 617–624.

K. Poch *et al.*, The quantitation of 2-oxo-3-hydroxy LSD (O-H-LSD) in human urine specimens, a metabolite of LSD: comparative analysis using liquid chromatography–selected ion mass spectrometry and liquid chromatography–ion trap mass spectrometry, *J. Anal. Toxicol.*, 2000, **24**, 170–179.

Quest Diagnostics, 2002, Drug Testing Index: www.questdiagnostics.com (accessed 19.01.08).

SAMHSA, Summary of findings from the 1999 National Household Survey on Drug Abuse, SAMHSA, DHHS Publication Number (SMA) 00–3446, 2000.

SAMHSA, 2002: www.samhsa.gov (accessed 19.01.08).

C. Selavka, Poppy seed ingestion as a contribution factor to opiate-positive urinalysis results: the pacific perspective, *J. Forensic Sci.*, 1991, **36**, 685–696.

F. Urry *et al.*, Nitrite adulteration of workplace urine drug-testing specimens I. Sources and associated concentrations of nitrite in urine and distinction between natural sources and adulteration, *J. Anal. Toxicol.*, 1998, **22**, 89–95.

H. Zhao *et al.*, Profiles of urine samples taken from ecstasy users at rave parties: analysis by immunoassay, HPLC and GC-MSD, *J. Anal. Toxicol.*, 2001, **25**, 258–269.

along the hair shaft correlated with the time of drug use. Today, gas chromatography coupled with mass spectrometry (GC-MS) is the method of choice for hair analysis, a technology routinely used to document repetitive drug exposure in forensic science, traffic medicine, occupational medicine, clinical toxicology and, more recently, sports.

The major practical advantage of hair testing compared with urine or blood testing for drugs is that it has a larger surveillance window (weeks to months, depending on the length of the hair shaft, against 2–4 days for most drugs in urine and blood). For practical purposes, the two tests complement each other. Urinalysis and blood analysis provide short-term information of an individual's drug use, whereas long-term histories are accessible through hair analysis. While analysis of urine and blood specimens often cannot distinguish between chronic use or single exposure, hair analysis can make the distinction.

Biology of hair

Hair is a product of differentiated organs in the skin of mammals. It differs in individuals only in colour, quantity and texture. Hair is primarily protein (65–95%, keratin essentially), together with water (15–35%) and lipids (1–9%). The mineral content of hair ranges from 0.25% to 0.95%. The total number of hair follicles in adults is estimated to be about 5 million, with 1 million found on the head (Harkey and Henderson 1989). Hair follicles are embedded in the epidermal epithelium of the skin, approximately 3–4 mm below the skin's surface.

Hair growth

A hair shaft begins in cells located in a germination centre, called the matrix, located in the base of the follicle (Fig. 6.1). Hair does not grow continually, but in cycles, alternating between periods of growth and quiescence. A follicle that is actively producing hair is said to be in the *anagen* phase. Hair is produced during 4–8 years for head hair (<12 months for non-head hair) at a rate of approximately 0.22–0.52 mm/day or 0.6–1.42 cm/month (Saitoh *et al.* 1969) for head hair (growth rate depends on hair type and anatomical location). After this period, the follicle enters a relatively short transition period of about 2 weeks, known as the *catagen* phase, during which cell division stops and the follicle begins to degenerate. Following the transition phase, the hair follicle enters a resting or quiescent period, known as the *telogen* phase (10 weeks), during which the hair shaft stops growing completely and hair growth begins to shut down. Factors such as race, disease states, nutritional deficiencies and age are known to influence both the rate of growth and the length of the quiescent period. On the scalp of an adult, approximately 85% of the hair is in the growing phase and the remaining 15% is in a resting stage.

Types of hair

Pubic hair, arm hair and axillary (armpit) hair have been suggested as an alternative sources for drug detection when scalp hair is not available. Various studies have found differences in concentrations between pubic or axillary hair and scalp hair. Comparisons of methadone, cocaine, morphine and phenobarbital concentrations show the highest values to be in the axillary hair, followed by pubic hair and scalp hair. In contrast, in another study the highest morphine concentrations were found in pubic

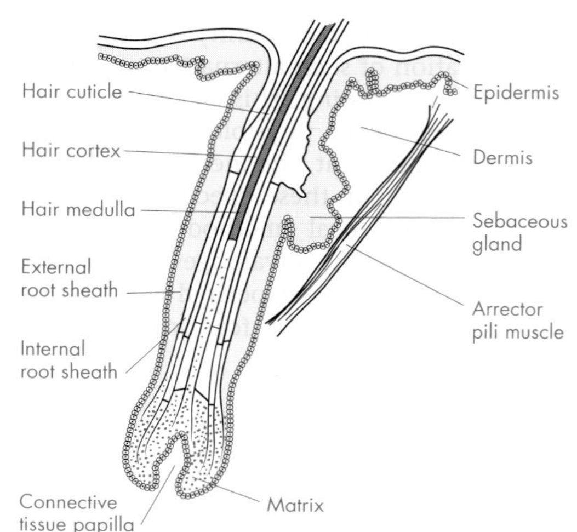

Figure 6.1 Cross-section through hair follicle.

hair (0.80–1.34 ng/mg), followed by head hair (0.62–27.10 ng/mg) and axillary hair (0.40–24.20 ng/mg). The significant differences of the drug concentrations in these studies are explained by a better blood circulation, a greater number of apocrine glands, a totally different telogen : anagen ratio and a different growth rate of the hair (axillary hair 0.40 mm/day, pubic hair 0.30 mm/day).

Beard hair grows at about 0.27 mm/day and is considered a suitable alternative, as it can be collected on a daily basis with an electric shaver and can be used to evaluate the incorporation rate of drugs (Mangin 1996).

Mechanisms of drug incorporation into hair

It is generally accepted that drugs can enter into hair by two processes: adsorption from the external environment and incorporation into the growing hair shaft from blood that supplies the hair follicle. Drugs can enter the hair from exposure to chemicals in aerosols, smoke or secretions from sweat and sebaceous glands. Sweat is known to contain drugs present in blood. As hair is very porous and can increase its mass up to 18% by absorbing liquids, drugs may be transferred easily into hair via sweat. Chemicals present in air (smoke, vapours, etc.) can be deposited onto hair (Fig. 6.2).

Drugs appear to be incorporated into the hair by at least three mechanisms:

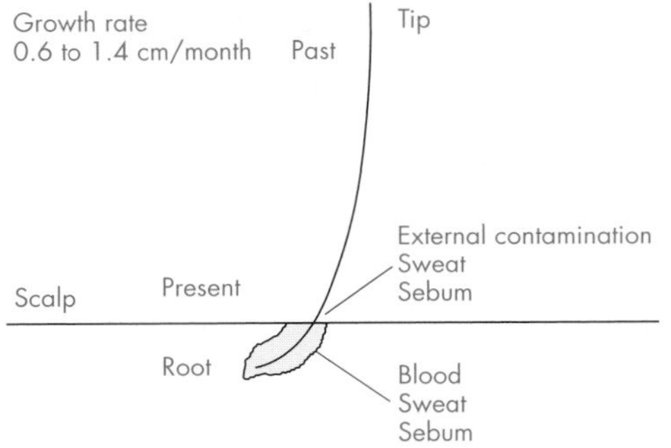

Figure 6.2 Possible model of drug incorporation into hair.

- from the blood during hair formation
- from sweat and sebum
- from the external environment.

This model is more able than a passive model (transfer from the blood into the growing cells of the hair follicle) to explain several experimental findings such as:

- drug and metabolite ratios in blood are quite different from those found in hair
- drug and metabolite concentrations in hair differ markedly in individuals who receive the same dose.

Evidence for the transfer of the drug via sweat and sebum is that drugs and metabolites are present in sweat and sebum at high concentrations and persist in these secretions for longer than they do in blood. The parent drug can be found in sweat long after it has disappeared from the blood (Henderson 1993; Cone 1996).

The exact mechanism by which chemicals are bound into hair is not known. It has been suggested that passive diffusion may be augmented by drug binding to intracellular components of the hair cells, such as the hair pigment melanin. For example, codeine concentrations in hair after oral administration are dependent on melanin content (Kronstrand *et al.* 1999). However, this is probably not the only mechanism, since drugs are trapped in the hair of albino animals which lack melanin. Another proposed mechanism is the binding of drugs with sulfhydryl-containing amino acids present in hair. There is an abundance of amino acids, such as cystine, in hair; these form cross-linking S—S bonds to stabilise the protein fibre network. Drugs that diffuse into hair cells could be bound in this way.

The course of the appearance of drugs in hair has been evaluated in beard hair. Variable time lags between the administration and appearance in hair were observed in all cases: 1 day for codeine to 8 days for morphine and codeine (Mangin 1996). This time lag probably results from the growth time necessary for the hair shaft to emerge from the bulb area in the follicle to a sufficient height above the skin surface for collection. Various studies have demonstrated that, after the same dosage, black hair incorporates much more drug than blond hair (Henderson *et al.* 1998; Höld *et al.* 1999). This has resulted in discussions about a possible genetic variability of drug deposition in hair, and is still under evaluation.

Specimen collection and procedures

Collection procedures for hair analysis for drugs have not been standardised. In most published studies, the samples are obtained from random locations on the scalp. Hair is best collected from the area at the back of the head, called the vertex posterior. Compared with other areas of the head, this area has less variability in hair growth rate, the number of hairs in the growing phase is more constant, and the hair is less subject to age- and sex-related influences. Hair strands are cut as close as possible from the scalp, and their location on the scalp is noted. Once collected, hair samples may be stored at ambient temperature in aluminium foil, an envelope or a plastic tube. The sample size taken varies considerably between laboratories and depends on the drug to be analysed and the test methodology. For example, when fentanyl or buprenorphine are investigated, a 100 mg sample is recommended. Sample sizes reported in the literature range from a single hair to 200 mg, cut as close to the scalp as possible. When sectional analysis is performed, the hair is cut into segments of about 1, 2 or 3 cm, which corresponds to about 1, 2 or 3 months' growth.

Stability of drugs in hair

The presence of opiates was detected in five hair shafts (about 7.5 cm in length) from the Victorian poet John Keats 167 years after his death (Baumgartner *et al.* 1989). It is believed he took laudanum (opium) to control the pain of tuberculosis. The scalps of eight Chilean and Peruvian mummies dating from 2000 BC to AD 1500 also tested positive for benzoylecgonine (Cartmell *et al.* 1991). All these studies indicate that drug incorporation is very stable in hair and that modern medical technology can assist other disciplines. Clearly, organic substances are able to survive in hair for thousands of years under favourable conditions (ambient temperature, dry atmosphere).

Decontamination procedures

Contaminants of hair would be a problem if they were drugs of abuse or their metabolites, or if they interfered with the analysis and interpretation of the test results. It is unlikely that anyone would intentionally or accidentally apply anything to their hair that contained a drug of abuse. The most crucial issue facing hair analysis is to avoid technical and evidentiary false-positives. Technical false-positives are caused by errors in the collection, processing and analysis of specimens, while evidentiary false-positives are caused by passive exposure to the drug.

Approaches to prevent evidentiary false-positives through external contamination of the hair specimens have been described by Baumgartner and Hill (1992). Most, but not all, laboratories use a wash step; however, there is no consensus or uniformity in the washing procedures. Among the agents used in washing are detergents (such as shampoo), surgical scrubbing solutions, surfactants (such as 0.1% sodium dodecyl sulfate), phosphate buffer and organic solvents (such as acetone, diethyl ether, methanol, ethanol, dichloromethane, hexane or pentane) of various volumes for various contact times. Generally, a single washing step is used, although a second identical wash is sometimes performed. If external contamination is found by analysing the wash solution, the washout kinetics of repeated washing can demonstrate that contamination is removed rapidly. According to Baumgartner and Hill (1992), the concentration of drug in the hair after washing should exceed the concentration in the last wash by at least ten times. It has also been proposed that hair should be washed three times with phosphate prior to analysis, to remove any possible external contamination, and that the total concentration of any drug present in the three phosphate washes should be greater than 3.9 times the concentration in the final wash.

Detection of drug metabolite(s) in hair that cannot be explained by hydrolysis or environmental exposure unequivocally establishes that internal drug exposure has occurred (Cone *et al.*

1991). Cocaethylene and norcocaine would appear to meet these criteria, as these metabolites are only formed when cocaine is metabolised. As these metabolites are not found in illicit cocaine samples, they would not be present in hair as a result of environmental contamination, and thus their presence in hair could be considered a marker of cocaine exposure. This procedure can be extended to other drugs. However, there is still great controversy about the potential risk of external contamination, particularly for crack, cannabis and heroin when smoked, as several authors have demonstrated that it is not possible to remove these drugs fully using wash procedures (Blank and Kidwell 1995; Kidwell and Blank 1996). In conclusion, although it is highly recommended to include a decontamination step, there is no consensus as to which procedure performs best, so each laboratory must validate its own technique.

Effects of cosmetic treatments

An important issue of concern for drug analysis in hair is the change in the drug concentration induced by the cosmetic treatment of hair. Hair is subjected continuously to natural factors, such as sunlight, weather, water, pollution, etc., which affect and damage the cuticle, but hair cosmetic treatments have been shown to enhance that damage. Particular attention has been focused on the effects of repeated shampooing, permanent waving, relaxing and dyeing of hair. Repeated shampooing was found to have no significant action on the drug content of hair (Baumgartner and Hill 1992). After cosmetic treatments, drug concentrations decline dramatically by 50–80% from their original concentration. The products used for cosmetic treatments, such as bleaching, permanent waving, dyeing or relaxing, contain strong bases. These reagents may cause hair damage and affect drug content (by loss), or could affect drug stability (Cirimele *et al.* 1995a).

Drug solubilisation

To determine the amount of a drug that remains in hair after washing, it is necessary to solubilise the drugs in the hair. Solubilisation must be such that the analytes are not altered or lost. Care is necessary to prevent the conversion of cocaine to benzoylecgonine or 6-monoacetylmorphine (6-MAM) to morphine, for example.

The hair sample can be pulverised in a ball-mill prior to testing, cut into segments or the entire hair dissolved. The preparation techniques are generally based on one of the following procedures:

- incubation in an aqueous buffer and analysis using immunological techniques, mostly RIA
- incubation in an acidic or basic solution followed by liquid–liquid extraction or solid-phase extraction and analysis with chromatographic techniques, mostly GC-MS
- incubation in an organic solvent (generally methanol with or without hydrochloric acid), liquid–liquid extraction or solid-phase extraction and analysis with chromatographic techniques, mostly GC-MS
- digestion in an enzymatic solution, liquid–liquid extraction or solid-phase extraction and analysis with chromatographic techniques, mostly GC-MS.

The protein matrix is destroyed completely by incubating the hair sample in sodium hydroxide. The parameters to be determined are the molarity of sodium hydroxide, the time of incubation and the temperature of incubation. The alkaline hydrolysis of hair is not suitable for the extraction of chemically unstable compounds such as cocaine, 6-MAM, benzodiazepines or esters of anabolic steroids, which are hydrolysed under strong alkaline treatment. Several authors have proposed acid hydrolysis to enable the extraction of cocaine or 6-MAM from hair. The samples can be incubated in 0.1 M hydrochloric acid overnight at room temperature, at 45°C or at 56°C, or in 0.6 M hydrochloric acid for 30 min at 120°C. The organic solvent incubation method is the simplest. It involves placing hair samples in methanol or in ethanol and then in an ultrasound bath at 45°C for several hours. GC-MS analysis can be carried out directly following evaporation of the organic solvent. With this method, it is possible to detect diacetylmorphine in the hair of heroin addicts.

In addition to chemical hydrolysis and direct extraction of hair with organic solvents, various types of enzymatic digestion of keratin matrix have been proposed. Hair samples can be treated with pronase solution, glucuronidase arylsulfatase or proteinase K. The enzymes act on the keratin without altering the chemical structure of the analytes present in the hair. This is particularly important when the substances being analysed are chemically unstable, such as heroin or cocaine (Sachs and Kintz 1998).

An interesting extraction procedure has been developed using supercritical fluid extraction with carbon dioxide. Adding polar modifiers like water, methanol or triethylamine leads to a subcritical fluid with high extractive properties. The high speed of the extraction (30 min) and the potential to connect on-line with GC-MS are advantages that have to be balanced against the high instrumental costs compared with solid-phase or liquid–liquid extraction. However, only small amounts of non-halogenated organic solvents are needed, which keeps environmental pollution low (Edder *et al.* 1994).

Drug analysis

The first publication to deal with the analysis of morphine in hair to determine the history of opiate abuse reported the use of RIA (Baumgartner *et al.* 1979). This article was followed by a great number of procedures, most of which used RIA and/or GC-MS. Chromatographic procedures are a powerful tool for the identification and quantification of drugs in hair, owing to their separation ability and their detection sensitivity and specificity, particularly when coupled with MS. Proposed cut-off concentrations and expected concentrations for drugs of abuse in hair are presented in Table 6.1.

Immunological methods

Immunoassays are used as screening tests because of their sensitivity, speed and convenience. The procedure must be compatible with the screening test used (i.e. detergents or hair-digestion products must not interfere with the assay). Neutralisation, in case of chemical hydrolysis, is always necessary. The destruction of the organic protein matrix of hair must be done under conditions sufficiently mild not to damage the entrapped analyte or the protein antibodies subsequently added for the immunoassay. Quantification by immunoassay is difficult to achieve, as the specificity of most kits is directed to a group of drugs and drug metabolites rather than to a single substance.

Table 6.1 Proposed cut-off concentrations (when tested by GC-MS) and expected concentrations for drugs of abuse in hair

Drug	GC-MS cut-off concentration	Expected concentrations
Heroin	0.2 ng/mg of 6-acetylmorphine	0.5–100 ng/mg; in most cases <15 ng/mg
Cocaine	0.5 ng/mg of cocaine	0.5–100 ng/mg; in most cases <50 ng/mg; in crack abusers >300 ng/mg is possible
Amfetamine, MDMA	0.3 ng/mg for both drugs	0.5–50.0 ng/mg
Cannabis	0.05 ng/mg for THC	THC: 0.05–10 ng/mg; in most cases <3 ng/mg
	0.05 pg/mg for THC-COOH	THC-COOH: 0.5–50 pg/mg; in most cases <5 pg/mg

MDMA, methylenedioxymethamfetamine; THC, tetrahydrocannabinol; THC-COOH, 11-nor-Δ^9-THC carboxylic acid.

Radioimmunoassay

RIA is the most common screening test for hair. Kits, generally designed for urine, can be used without any modification at pH values above 7. Calibration curves are obtained either from the controlled urine samples in the kit or from extracts of drug-free hair samples spiked with the drugs. Duplicate determinations are recommended. The RIA results should be confirmed by GC-MS. In the absence of a second independent method, RIA detection must be interpreted with caution. However, even the high sensitivity of GC-MS is sometimes not sufficient to detect drugs, especially when starting with a small quantity of hair. For these reasons, it may be necessary to carry out immunological analysis of drugs in hair using RIA reagents that are specific for the selective estimation of drugs such as fentanyl, lysergic acid diethylamide (lysergide, LSD) or buprenorphine.

Enzyme multiplied immunoassay technique

The enzyme multiplied immunoassay technique (EMIT), based on spectroscopic measurement, is subject to interferences by colour and turbidity, and therefore should not be used to analyse hair samples.

Fluorescence polarisation immunoassay

First reported in 1987 (Franceschin *et al.* 1987), fluorescence polarisation immunoassay (FPIA) results appear to correlate with those from GC-MS analyses. FPIA can therefore be used to screen hair samples, but the results must always be confirmed.

Chromatographic methods

Chromatographic methods have been used as screening and confirmatory tests. Moreover, they allow quantification of the drugs and drug metabolites.

Thin-layer chromatography

Klug (1980) reported a thin-layer chromatography (TLC) method to detect morphine in the hair of drug abusers. Detection and quantification were made by fluorimetry. A high-performance TLC method was used to determine morphine in human hair with quantification by densitometry (Jeger *et al.* 1991).

High-performance liquid chromatography

High-performance liquid chromatography (HPLC) methods have been used to detect morphine, haloperidol, beta-blockers and buprenorphine. Different kinds of detectors were used, including ultraviolet (UV), fluorimetry and coulometry. The latter two detectors have sufficient sensitivity to enable the detection of low drug concentrations (Sachs and Kintz 1998). Very few articles present data using LC-MS, except for buprenorphine, diuretics and corticosteroids.

Gas chromatography

Gas chromatography (GC) coupled to flame ionisation or nitrogen detection is less useful for the analysis of drugs in hair as the large number of interfering substances (exogenous and endogenous compounds) makes the interpretation of chromatograms very difficult. GC-MS is the most powerful tool for the detection of drugs in hair. Moeller (1992) presented a screening procedure for the simultaneous analysis of amfetamines, cocaine, benzoylecgonine, codeine, morphine and 11-nor-Δ^9-tetrahydrocannabinol-9-carboxylic acid THC-COOH). Kauert and Röhrich (1996) presented a screening procedure based on methanolic incubation, which was suitable for the opiates, cocaine, amfetamines, methadone and cannabis.

Other methods

Capillary zone electrophoresis (CZE) has been proposed for the quantitative determination of cocaine and morphine in hair taken from cocaine and heroin users (Tagliaro *et al.* 1997). Infrared microscopy can delineate passive exposure from the drug user by analysing only the central core of the unextracted hair shaft with either cross-sectionally microtomed or laterally microtomed hair. Infrared spectra can be obtained from the medulla, cortex and cuticle of the single hair with a nominal spatial resolution of 10 μm. Fourier transform infrared microscopy was presented as more sensitive than classic GC-MS procedures by Kalasinsky *et al.* (1994). Fluorescence microscopy was used to detect organic substances in hair, and was presented as a good alternative to chromatographic procedures (Pötsch and Leithoff 1992).

to hide that drugs have been used, whereas intermittent drug use may be difficult to detect if urine or blood tests alone are undertaken, even when the tests are repeated.

Determination of gestational drug exposure

Maternal drug abuse is a health hazard for the fetus, and the effects of cocaine, PCP, nicotine and other compounds are well documented. In 1987, Parton first reported the quantification of fetal cocaine exposure by the RIA of hair obtained from 15 babies. Other studies have demonstrated placental transfer of maternal haloperidol and the presence of nicotine, morphine, amfetamine and benzodiazepines in neonatal hair (Klein *et al.* 2000). It has been suggested that fetal accumulation of cocaine and its metabolites follows a linear pattern within clinically used doses (Forman 1992) and that a dose-dependent transfer of maternal nicotine to the baby exists (Kintz *et al.* 1993). Analysis of new-born hair may overcome the disadvantages of currently used methods to verify drug abuse, such as maternal self-reported drug history, maternal urinalysis (risk of false-negatives) and analysis of the urine or the meconium of the baby at the time of delivery (risk of false-negative information during the preceding 1–3 days).

Applications in forensic science

Numerous forensic applications have been described in the literature. In these, hair analysis has been used to document differentiation between a drug dealer and a drug consumer, chronic poisoning, crime under the influence of drugs, child sedation and abuse, suspicious death, child custody, abuse of drugs in jail, body identification, survey of drug addicts, chemical submission, obtaining a driving licence and doping control (Moeller *et al.* 1993; Sachs 1996).

More than 450 articles concerning hair analysis have been published and report applications in forensic toxicology, clinical toxicology, occupational medicine and doping control. The major practical advantage of hair for testing drugs, compared with urine or blood, is its larger detection window, which is weeks to months, depending on the length of hair shaft analysed, against a few days for urine. In practice, detection windows offered by urine and hair testing are complementary: urine analysis provides short-term information on an individual's drug use, whereas long-term histories are accessible through hair analysis. Although there is reasonable agreement that the qualitative results from hair analysis are valid, the interpretation of the results is still under debate because of some unresolved questions, such as the influence of external contamination or cosmetic treatment, and possible genetic differences.

Specific problems associated with doping control using hair

Although hair is not yet a valid specimen for the International Olympic Committee (IOC), it is accepted in most courts of justice. Some conflicting results have been observed, all of which involve athletes who tested positive in urine at accredited IOC laboratories and negative in hair in forensic certified laboratories.

Much experience has been acquired in the detection of opiates and cocaine in hair. In contrast, there is a serious lack of suitable references to interpret the analytical findings for doping agents. In hair, doping agent concentrations, such as anabolic steroids, corticosteroids, or β_2-agonists, are in the pg/mg range, whereas cocaine, amfetamines or opiates are generally found in the range of several ng/mg. The Society of Hair Testing has suggested that a consensus on hair testing for the presence of doping agents should be carried out (Sachs and Kintz 2000).

More research is required before all of the scientific questions associated with hair-drug testing can be satisfied. There is still a lack of consensus among the active investigators on how to interpret the analysis of drugs in hair. Among the unanswered questions, five are of critical importance:

1. What is the minimal amount of drug detectable in hair after administration?
2. What is the relationship between the amount of the drug used and the concentration of the drug or its metabolites in hair?

3. What is the influence of hair colour?
4. What is the influence of genetic differences in hair testing?
5. What is the influence of cosmetic treatments?

Several answers were proposed recently by Kintz *et al.* (1999, 2000a) on these specific topics.

Conclusions

It appears that the value of hair analysis in the identification of drug users is steadily gaining recognition. This may be seen from its growing use in pre-employment screening, forensic sciences and clinical applications. Hair analysis may be a useful adjunct to conventional drug testing in toxicology. Specimens can be obtained more easily with less embarrassment, and hair can provide a more accurate history of drug use.

Although there are still controversies on how to interpret the results, particularly concerning external contamination, cosmetic treatments, genetic considerations and drug incorporation, pure analytical work in hair analysis has reached a sort of plateau, with almost all the analytical problems solved. Although GC-MS is the method of choice in practice, GC-MS/MS or LC-MS are today used in several laboratories, even for routine cases, particularly to target low dosage compounds, such as THC-COOH, fentanyl, flunitrazepam or buprenorphine. Electrophoretic and/or electrokinetic analytical strategies, chiral separation or the application of ion mobility spectrometry constitute the latest new developments in the analytical tools reported to document the presence of drugs in hair. Quality assurance is a major issue of drug testing in hair. Since 1990, the National Institute of Standards and Technology (Gaithersburg, MD, USA) has developed interlaboratory comparisons, recently followed by the Society of Hair Testing (Strasbourg, France). In 2004 during the annual meeting of the Society of Hair Testing in Sevilla, Spain, a consensus was reached by the representatives from several European countries and the US and Canada, and subsequently the document entitled 'Recommendations for Hair Testing in Forensic Cases' was published. As indicated before, in April 2004 the US Department of Health and Human Services, Substance Abuse and Mental Health Services Administration (SAMHSA) issued *Proposed Revisions to Mandatory Guidelines* including hair (but also saliva and sweat) as the alternative specimens for workplace drug testing.

Drugs in oral fluid

Introduction

Definitions

Saliva is the secretion product of the saliva glands of the head and mouth. However, the fluids found in the oral cavity are a mixture of predominately saliva, with smaller amounts of gingival crevicular fluid, cellular debris and blood. For this reason, the New York Academy of Sciences meeting on saliva testing in 1993 agreed to use the word saliva for glandular secretions collected directly from the saliva glands (most often the parotid glands), and oral fluid for fluid collected by placing absorbants in the oral cavity or by expectoration (Malamud 1993).

Advantages

The advantages of oral fluid drug testing are mainly twofold. In principle, oral fluid drug concentrations can be related to plasma free-drug concentrations and the pharmacological effects of drugs. Second, saliva or oral-fluid collection is noninvasive and simple and can be done on-site under observation.

Saliva drug concentrations are related to blood or plasma concentrations of the unbound, non-ionised parent drug or its lipophilic metabolites (Haeckel and Hanecke 1996). Since it is the free lipophilic drug and drug metabolites that cross cell membranes, such as the blood–brain barrier, and cause physiological effects, free drug in the plasma, and its reflection in saliva, can be correlated with drug effects. The presence and concentration of drugs in saliva therefore provide much of the same information as the determination of drug presence and drug concentrations in blood or plasma. Saliva drug concentrations can be used to determine pharmacokinetic parameters. However, saliva or oral fluid collection is much easier than venepuncture.

The collection of saliva or oral fluid is simple and noninvasive. It can be carried out by the specimen donors themselves by having the donor place a cotton swab or absorptive material attached to a stick into their mouth for a few minutes. The oral fluid absorbed on the material is processed for testing. Saliva can be collected at the site of the incident in accident or crime investigation. If necessary, saliva flow can be stimulated with citrate hard candy or citrate salts or by chewing on gum or rubber to ensure an adequate sample volume. Some researchers believe that the lower pH due to use of citrates may significantly influence partitioning of some drugs and therefore should not be recommended (see Henderson–Hasselbalch equation). As oral fluid collection is noninvasive and can be done by the donors themselves in most situations, it is more acceptable to most people than providing urine, blood or hair (Fendrich *et al.* 2001) and can be carried out while the donor is under observation by the collector. An exception may be when the donor is unconscious or so sedated as to be unable to follow instructions. Finally, it is difficult to adulterate or substitute oral fluid specimens in an attempt to avoid detection of drug use, as any adulterating substances held in the mouth are dissipated, swallowed or spat out during the 10-minute observation period before collection of the specimen (Jehanli *et al.* 2001).

A simple noninvasive collection finds many applications in toxicology. For example, investigation of the involvement of drugs in impaired driving is facilitated by a roadside test for drugs in saliva, such as currently exists for alcohol in breath. The feasibility of detecting drugs in saliva samples obtained from impaired drivers was first investigated by Peel *et al.* (1984). They found that the presence of drugs in saliva correlated well with officers' judgements of driving while intoxicated. This was confirmed in a comparison of saliva testing to urinalysis in an arrestee population (Yacoubian *et al.* 2001) and in drugged drivers (Steinmeyer *et al.* 2001). The greatest advantage of saliva in roadside testing is the possibility of having the sample collected by the donor under observation shortly after the time of the incident.

Disadvantages

Like any biofluid from human subjects, oral fluid may transmit infectious agents and should be handled with the appropriate universal precautions for human biological fluids. Saliva contains mucopolysaccharides and mucoproteins that make it less fluid and less easily poured or pipetted than urine. Some drugs, medical conditions or anxiety can inhibit saliva secretion and cause dry mouth; therefore, oral fluid may not be available from all individuals at all times. Finally, because saliva drug concentrations depend on plasma drug concentrations, drugs that have a short plasma half-life and are cleared rapidly from the body are detectable in saliva for only a short time. This is a potential disadvantage over the detection of drugs in the hair, sweat or urine. Saliva and blood have the shortest detection window. Drugs or their long-lived metabolites are detectable in urine and sweat for several days to a week after use. Drugs are detectable in hair for months or even years after use, depending on the length of the hair. In general, drugs are detectable in the plasma and saliva from the time that the drug enters the general circulation until approximately four half-lives after administration.

Anatomy and physiology of saliva

The saliva glands

The human saliva glands produce between 0.5 and 1.5 L of saliva daily. During resting conditions, most mixed saliva is supplied by the submandibular glands (70%) with a lesser amount (25%) from the parotid glands and the remaining (5%) from the sublingual and other minor glands (Baum 1993). During stimulation, the parotid saliva output increases to about half of the total. Saliva is composed of 99% water, 0.3% protein (largely amylase) and 0.3% mucins. The parotid gland produces mostly serous fluid. The submandibular and sublingual glands excrete both serous fluid and mucins. The saliva glands, like the liver, kidney and brain, are well supplied with arterial blood.

Saliva glands comprise two regions, the acinar region (which contains the cells capable of secretion) and the ductal region lined with water-impermeable cells that carry the secretions to the outlets in the mouth (Turner 1993). Similarly, saliva formation occurs in two steps. Water and exocrine proteins are secreted by the secretory cells in the acinar region. The fluid collected in the acinar lumen is isotonic with plasma. As the fluid travels down the saliva ducts, sodium and chloride are reabsorbed, while potassium and bicarbonate are secreted. Therefore, when saliva moves rapidly through the ducts, less time is available for sodium reabsorption than otherwise and the pH of the saliva is higher (Dawes and Jenkins 1964; see later). When the fluid reaches the mouth it is hypotonic to plasma.

Saliva glands are activated by the autonomic nerves. Generally, sympathetic stimulation via noradrenaline (norepinephrine) causes low levels of fluid and high concentrations of protein, while parasympathetic stimulation via acetylcholine induces large amounts of fluid secretion.

Movement of drugs into saliva

Excretion and diffusion

Some drugs, such as digoxin, steroids and hormones, are actively excreted into saliva by the acinar cells. Most drugs enter saliva by simple diffusion across the phospholipid bilayer of the acinar cells or through the cell membranes of the ductal cells in the tubules. Diffusion across cell membranes requires that the molecules be lipid-soluble, non-ionised and unbound. For this reason, the concentrations of drugs in saliva represent the free, non-ionised fraction in the blood plasma.

Henderson–Hasselbalch equation

At equilibrium, the drug and lipophilic metabolite concentrations in saliva are a function of the drug's pK_a, plasma and saliva pH, and the fraction of drug bound to saliva and plasma protein, as shown by the form of the Henderson–Hasselbalch equation for saliva:

S/P, the saliva to plasma ratio, for basic drugs is

$$S/P = \frac{[1 + 10^{(pK_d - pH_s)}]}{[1 + 10^{(pK_d - pH_p)}]} + \frac{f_p}{f_s} \tag{6.1}$$

S/P for acidic drugs is

$$S/P = \frac{[1 + 10^{(pH_s - pK_a)}]}{[1 + 10^{(pH_p - pK_a)}]} + \frac{f_p}{f_s} \tag{6.2}$$

where S is the drug concentration in saliva, P is the drug concentration in plasma, pK_d is the log of the ionisation constant for basic drugs, pK_a is the log ionisation constant for acidic drugs, pH_s is the pH of saliva, pH_p is the pH of the plasma, f_p is the fraction of drug protein bound in plasma and f_s is the fraction protein bound in saliva.

The pH that governs this equilibrium is the pH of the saliva in the acinar lumen and in the duct at the moment of secretion. When the fluid enters the mouth, carbon dioxide is lost and the pH increases. Dawes and Jenkins (1964) demonstrated that saliva pH is inversely proportional to flow rate and the reabsorption of sodium in the salivary tubules. At faster flow rates, less sodium is reabsorbed in the tubules on the way from the saliva glands to the saliva outlets in the mouth, and the pH rises. For this reason, unstimulated saliva has a low pH (at low flow rates it is between 6.0 and 7.0, and fairly constant) and stimulated saliva has a higher pH (it can reach as high as 8.0).

Since human saliva normally has a lower pH than human plasma, the saliva : plasma ratios for acid drugs are generally less than unity and the saliva : plasma ratios for basic drugs are greater than unity, which provides an amplification of basic drug levels in saliva. For drugs that have a pK_a between 5.5 and 8.5, the saliva : plasma ratio can vary between stimulated and unstimulated saliva. This is true of many drugs of abuse. For this reason, it is more conservative to use a cut-off value for drugs of abuse in saliva rather than to determine the absolute concentration. The most common example given is that of cocaine, which has a pK_a of 8.6 (Schramm *et al.* 1992; Haeckel 1993). As the saliva pH varies from 5.0 to 7.8, the saliva : plasma ratio for cocaine varies from 273 to 0.44. The theoretical ranges of saliva : plasma ratios over a saliva pH range of 6.4 to 7.6 have been calculated for cocaine, amfetamine, methamfetamine, 6-MAM, morphine, codeine, methadone and diazepam and compared with published saliva : plasma ratios (Spiehler *et al.* 2000).

The protein binding of drugs is mainly to albumin or α-acid glycoprotein in plasma. Saliva mucoproteins have very little binding capacity for drugs. Oral fluids may contain albumin from the gingival crevicular fluid.

Oral deposition

The deposition into mouth tissues of drugs taken by smoking, snorting or oral routes of administration is an additional source of drugs in oral fluid. For example, Jenkins *et al.* (1995) showed that the saliva : plasma ratio for smoked heroin was 100–400 times that of heroin administered intravenously. After heroin was smoked, heroin was detected in oral fluid for up to 24 hours, compared to up to 30 minutes after heroin was intravenously administered.

O'Neal *et al.* (2000) reported codeine saliva : plasma ratios of 75–2580 in the first 15 to 30 minutes after dosing and of 13–344 for several hours after oral administration of liquid codeine phosphate, despite efforts at decontamination by having the subjects brush their teeth and vigorously rinse their mouth prior to saliva collection.

Similarly, Jenkins *et al.* (1995) reported that after cocaine was smoked the saliva : plasma ratio was 300–500 times that found after cocaine was administered intravenously. The pyrolysis product of cocaine, anhydroecgonine methyl ester (AEME), was detected in oral fluid collected after smoking cocaine, but not in plasma. Similarly, cannabinoids found in oral fluid result almost totally from oral deposition of cannabinoids from smoked marijuana rather than from secretions or diffusion into saliva (Ohlsson *et al.* 1986).

The formation of oral mucosal depots of drug, which are rapidly absorbed into the blood circulation, is used for drug administration. Sublingual or buccal absorption of drugs such as nitroglycerin, buprenorphine or fentanyl has the advantage of very rapid delivery that bypasses the liver and gastrointestinal first-pass metabolism. Drugs administered by this route also produce large concentrations of the parent drug in oral fluid, but with a short detection window as the drugs are absorbed rapidly.

Collection of saliva

The greatest advantage of saliva is the possibility that the sample can be collected from the donor under observation. In addition, in on-site testing, such as close to the patient or roadside testing, the specimen can be collected shortly after the time of the incident. Saliva collection is noninvasive and can be done by the donors themselves in most situations. An exception may be when the donor is unconscious or so sedated as to be unable to follow instructions. Oral fluid has been collected from donors by spitting, draining, absorption and suction. A number of devices are available for saliva and oral fluid collection.

Collection devices

Peel *et al.* (1984) asked 'driving-while-intoxicated' suspects to spit into a test tube with or without sour candy stimulus, and a similar approach was taken by Cone (1993) at the Addiction Research Center in their many controlled-administration drug studies. The Salivette collector (Sarstedt, Germany; Fig. 6.3) employs a dental cotton (polyester) roll, which is chewed by the donor for 30–45 seconds with or without citric acid stimulation. After being soaked with oral fluid, the cotton roll is placed in a container that fits into a centrifuge tube. During centrifugation the saliva passes from the cotton roll into the lower part of the tube. Cellular particles are retained at the bottom of the tube. The cotton roll reliably absorbs 1–1.5 mL of oral fluid. The disadvantage of the cotton roll is that it may adsorb analyte molecules or give off compounds that interfere in the hormone and drug assays (Hold *et al.* 1995).

Modern oral-fluid collection devices generally use an absorbent material on a stick similar to that employed for saliva alcohol tests. For example, the Epitope (now Intercept) saliva-

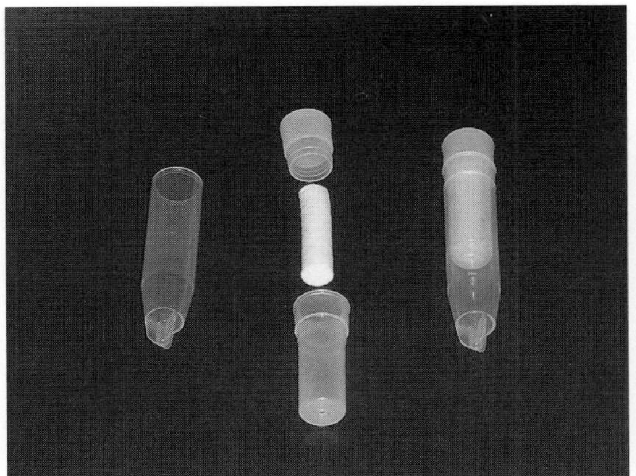

Figure 6.3 The Salivette collection device.

sampling device (Fig. 6.4) consists of an absorbent paper pad impregnated with buffered salts on a plastic rod. The pad is placed in the mouth for 2–5 minutes. After collection, the paper is placed in a tube with preservative liquid and shipped to the laboratory for analysis. The Intercept pad is estimated to absorb approximately 0.4 mL of oral fluid, which is diluted 1:3 by 0.8 mL preservative fluid. The Cozart RapiScan collector (Cozart BioScience, Abingdon, UK) uses a detachable absorbent cotton pad on an indicator handle (Fig. 6.5). After the indicator has turned from white to blue, which indicates that 1 mL of saliva has been collected on the pad, the pad can be detached and kept in a test tube that contains preservative buffer until analysis. The Finger collector (Avitar, Canton, MA, USA; Fig. 6.6) uses a proprietary dental absorbent (AccuSorb foam), which absorbs saliva when placed in the mouth for a few minutes. Saliva is expressed from the absorbent using finger pressure. The DrugWipe saliva test (Securitec, Munich, Germany; Fig. 6.7) attempts to wipe the tongue with a wiping pin and transfer the oral fluid collected by washing it onto a test strip (Frontline urine test strip, Boehringer Mannheim GmbH, Germany) developed to test surfaces for traces of drugs (Kintz *et al.* 1998). Pichini *et al.* (2002) reported that the DrugWipe wiping pin holds at most 2 μL of fluid and that placing 2 μL saliva on the collection pin produced the best accuracy, but that wiping the tongue with the pin produced an inadequate sample for reliable results.

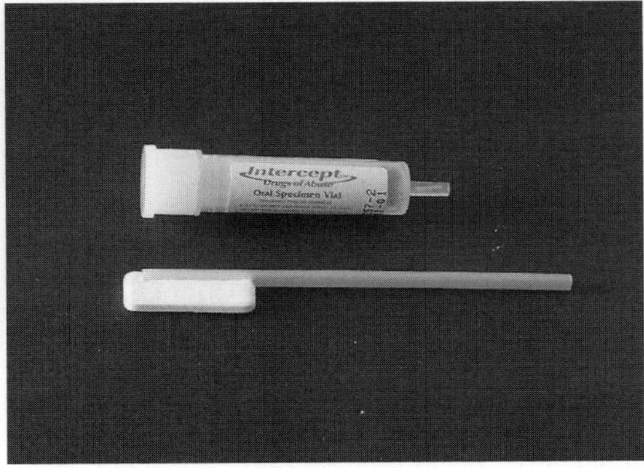

Figure 6.4 The Intercept collection device.

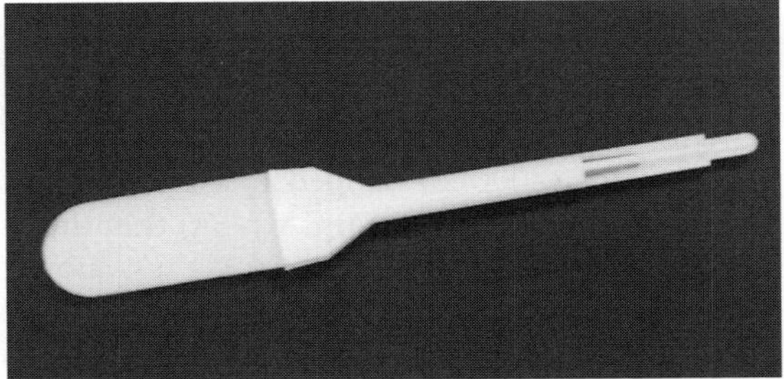

Figure 6.5 The Cozart RapiScan collection device.

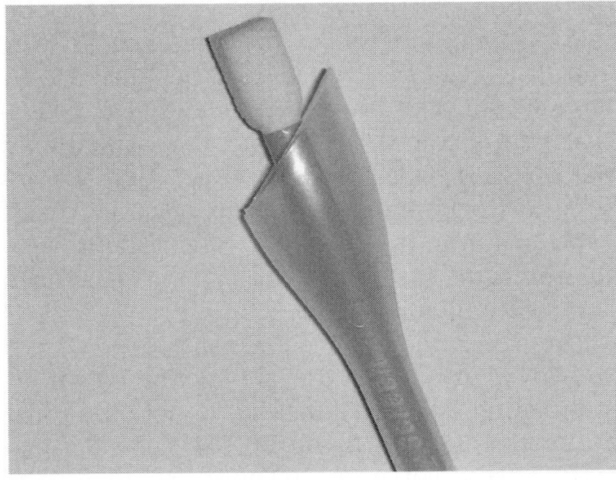

Figure 6.6 The Avitar collection device.

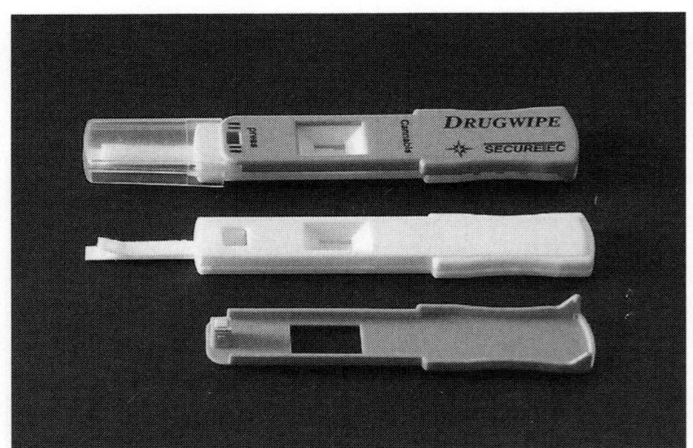

Figure 6.7 The DrugWipe collection device.

Schramm and Smith (1991) and Schramm (1993) developed a small plastic sack (SalivaSac, BioQuant) composed of semipermeable membranes that contains sugars of high relative molecular mass. When it is placed in the mouth, osmotic pressure drives an ultrafiltrate of saliva into the interior of the sack. The drawback is that the sack requires from 10 to 20 minutes (depending on the sack size) to collect sufficient fluid for testing.

Liang *et al.* (2000) developed an aspirator (Life-Point, Rancho Cucamonga, CA, USA) that draws saliva directly from the mouth of the test subject through a tube with a disposable individual sterile mouthpiece. For on-site testing the saliva passes directly into the analyser, which eliminates the need to elute saliva from the collector pad with a buffer and transfer it into an immunoassay cartridge.

For the collection of saliva, generally parotid saliva, small intraoral cups (Schaeffer cup, Curby cup) are available which can be placed over Stensen's duct of the parotid gland. The collection cup is placed in the buccal vestibule with the opening over the duct orifice. Gentle pressure on the cheek over the cup causes air to be expressed from the cup and creates a slight negative pressure that keeps the cup in place until sufficient saliva is collected.

The collection device or method has been shown to influence the pH of the saliva by stimulating saliva flow and hence the drug content of oral fluid according to the Henderson–Hasselbalch equation (O'Neal *et al.* 2000; Kintz and Samyn 2002). Collection devices can also affect the recovery of drugs from oral fluid through retention of the oral fluid in the absorbent, adsorption of the drug on device components and drug recovery from device buffers (O'Neal *et al.* 2000). After the controlled administration of codeine, oral-fluid codeine concentrations were higher in specimens obtained by spitting than in those obtained by absorption devices (O'Neal *et al.* 2000).

Dealing with adulterants

One of the advantages of saliva testing is that the sample is collected under direct observation. Before collection of saliva or oral fluid, the collector should observe the donor for a 10–15-minute period during which the donor does not smoke or consume food or drink. Experience with saliva and breath-alcohol testing is that contaminants, such as ascorbic acid from foods or drink, clear from the oral cavity either by the swallowing of saliva or by dissipation into the general circulation within 10–15 minutes. Also, a simple experiment shows that a person cannot hold saliva, especially saliva that contains liquid or solids, in the mouth for more than 3 minutes without swallowing or dribbling (Jehanli *et al.* 2001). Rinsing of the mouth is not required to collect saliva, and it does not reduce the levels of drugs found in oral fluid.

Sample treatment

Cone (1993) stored collected saliva at −20°C. The OraSure System (OraSure Technologies, Bethlehem, PA, USA) provides for shipping the oral fluid collected with the Intercept pad to a central laboratory for analysis after adding preservative fluid, with no special refrigeration. No sample treatment is required for immunoassay screening of saliva or dilutions of saliva.

If the analyte of interest is unstable in aqueous solutions (e.g. cocaine) or subject to changes by oral fluid bacteria or enzymes (e.g. nitrazepam, flunitrazepam), further efforts at preservation may be required. Freezing the collected oral fluid reduces interference from mucins in pipetting and liquid–liquid extractions for chromatographic confirmation testing. Solid-phase extraction or solid-phase microextraction (SPME) reduces the need for freezing the sample (e.g. Hall *et al.* 1998; Lucas *et al.* 2000).

Analysis of saliva for drugs

Screening tests

Immunoassays to detect drugs in saliva must target or have significant cross-reactivity with the parent drug and lipophilic metabolites. For example, cocaine parent drug and ecgonine methyl ester, heroin and 6-MAM and Δ^9-THC predominate in saliva because of their lipophilicity. When drugs are leached into saliva from buccal depots, as is the case for smoked drugs such as marijuana, smoked cocaine or heroin, parent drug and pyrolysis products predominate in the saliva. Immunoassays developed to detect the hydrophilic metabolites of drugs in urine are not appropriate for saliva screening. In addition, clinical trials and analysis of the sensitivity, specificity and predictive value of different putative cut-offs for saliva screening assays are required before the acceptance of specific immunoassays for saliva drug screening is widely adopted.

On-site testing

A number of on-site test systems for drugs in oral fluid have been developed. These tests are immunochromatographic screening tests. They generally employ lateral diffusion of the oral fluid sample mixed with labelled antibodies in buffer across a linear array of immobilised drugs. When drugs are present in the oral fluid, they bind to the anti-drug antibodies, so the antibodies pass by and do not bind to the corresponding test line that contains the immobilised drug conjugate. Visualisation of the antibody label (colloidal gold, phosphor or other indicator) reveals a lack of response from the array location that corresponds to the drug(s) present.

The first on-site saliva test that utilised an electronic reading device was the Cozart Rapiscan oral fluid drug testing system, developed in 1998, which uses a lateral transfer immunoassay with colloidal gold-labelled anti-drug antibodies (Spiehler 2001). The procedure is typical of those used for on-site oral fluid testing. The saliva specimen is collected from the mouth using a collection pad and placed in a test tube that contains 2 mL run buffer. When placed in the mouth, the collection pad absorbs 1 mL of saliva, which is indicated by development of a blue colour in the indicator section of the handle (see Fig. 6.5). The pad is placed in the tube, where it is diluted with 2 mL of run buffer fluid. The cellulose pad is separated from the plastic handle along a perforated edge. After removing the cap and plastic collector handle, the cotton pad is compressed with a dispenser filter to dispense six drops of the saliva–buffer mixture onto the cassette by directing the tip of the dispense filter tube into the cassette well and gently squeezing the tube.

A fresh disposable cassette and collection kit are used for each test. The cassette or cartridge is inserted into the hand-held instrument for incubation, reading and reporting. The saliva and run fluid rehydrate gold-labelled anti-drug antibodies contained within the cartridge. This mixture travels by capillary action across an array of immobilised drug sites (3–5 minutes for single- and two-panel tests; 12 minutes for a five-panel test). The absence of colour development at an immobilised drug position indicates the presence of drug. The quality-control position contains anti-mouse IgG to ascertain that complete lateral transfer of the specimen has been achieved.

The cassette result (binding of gold-labelled antibody to immobilised drug in the absence of drug in sample) is monitored by the portable, battery-powered reader and reported on the display screen. The results can be printed out on an optional battery-powered printer to provide a permanent record. Results are sent to the printer via the multifunctional port, which also serves to charge the instrument's batteries and to upload new versions of the instrument software, new drug combinations, etc., via an internet interface module.

If the saliva screening test is positive, the remainder of the sample (2.8 mL fluid) may be capped, with tamper-proof tape placed across the cap, and the samples sent to the designated laboratory for confirmation. Alternatively, a urine or blood sample may be collected and sent with the remainder of the positive saliva to the laboratory, depending on the preference of the contracting laboratory (De Giovanni *et al.* 2002).

Other on-site immunochromatographic oral fluid drug tests that use colloidal gold antibody labels are the ORALScreen System (Avitar, Canton, MA, USA; Barrett *et al.* 2001) and Drug-Wipe and DrugRead (Securitec GmbH, Ottobrun bei Munchen, Germany), which employ the Frontline urine dipstick (Boehringer-Manheim GMbH, Manheim, Germany).

A recent on-site immunochromatographic assay uses an up-converting phosphor based on lanthanide particles that absorb infrared light and emit visible light (up-conversion) as the antibody label (Fig. 6.8; Up-Link Rapid Detection system, OraSure Technologies, Inc., Bethlehem, PA, USA). Biological matrices do not up-convert, which eliminates the test background from the autofluorescence. As in the immunochromatographic procedure described above, oral fluid specimens are collected in a device that indicates sample adequacy and retains the oral fluid sample for confirmation testing if required. Specimens are mixed with buffer and introduced to a test cassette. Antibodies labelled with up-converting phosphor microparticles contained on a lateral flow membrane in the cassette are mobilised when the liquid sample flows across the pad. The presence of increasing amounts of drug in the sample decreases the amount of antibody-bound label to the corresponding test line that contains the immobilised drug conjugate. A 10-minute incubation is required. The test simultaneously detects amfetamine, methamfetamine, phencyclidine (PCP) and opiates in oral fluid with 40% or better displacement at 10 μg/L drug (Niedbala *et al.* 2001a). A reader utilising an infrared excitation laser (980 nm) and photomultiplier tube with a filter to determine visible light visualises the location of the bound phosphor-labelled antibody, which indicates whether drugs are present in the oral fluid. Up-converting phosphors that emit visible light at 475, 505, 550 and 720 nm are available. Different phosphors can be used as labels for different anti-drug antibodies, which allows close spacing of the drug conjugate lines on the immunochromatography strip.

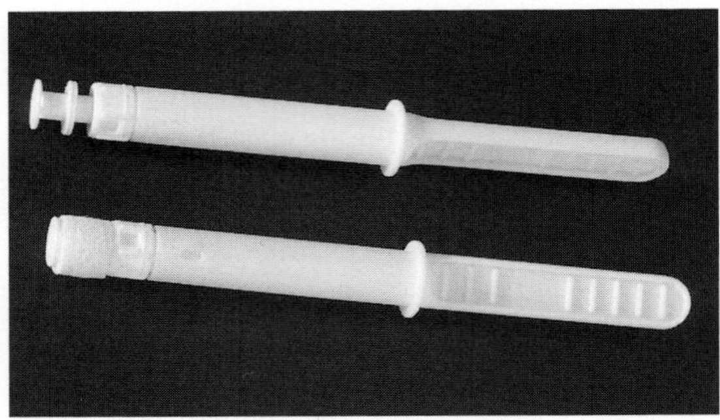

Figure 6.8 The Up-Link collection device.

Confirmation testing

When immunoassays are used as screening tests for drugs in saliva, chromatographic tests should be used for confirmation (Spiehler *et al.* 1988). Like screening tests, confirmation tests for drugs in saliva must be able to detect the parent drug or lipophilic metabolites. They must also be able to detect the levels of drugs that appear in saliva. GC-MS methods have been reported for confirmation of the prescription opiates (Jones *et al.* 2002), opiates and methadone (Moore *et al.* 2001), heroin (Jenkins *et al.* 1995) cocaine (Cone *et al.* 1994; Wang *et al.* 1994), cannabinoids (Kintz *et al.*, 2000c; Fucci *et al.* 2001) and benzodiazepines (Valentine *et al.* 1982). Matin *et al.* (1977) reported a quantitative GC-MS procedure for amfetamine enantiomers in saliva. A tandem immunoaffinity chromatography–HPLC procedure for cannabinoids in oral fluids was published by Kircher and Parlar (1996). GC-MS/MS methods have been published for the confirmation and quantification of cannabinoids in saliva (Hall *et al.* 1998; Niedbala *et al.* 2001a).

Interpretation of saliva drug results

The foremost question in the application of saliva testing to forensic casework is 'What is the relationship of saliva positive results to blood drug concentrations?' Drug concentrations in saliva reflect the free, unbound parent drug and lipophilic metabolites that circulate in the blood.

Since these are the forms of the drug that cross the blood–brain barrier and affect performance and behaviour, saliva is a good specimen for detecting patient compliance with medication, drug involvement in driving behaviour, fitness for duty, or impairment of performance for many drugs. However, efforts to use saliva concentrations to predict blood free-drug concentrations, cerebrospinal fluid (CSF) concentrations or degree of performance impairment in individuals have not reached the accuracy associated with blood measurements. Without knowing the instantaneous saliva pH, saliva drug concentrations may not be extra-polated to give blood drug concentrations. When appropriate cut-off concentrations are employed, saliva drug presence may be associated with recent drug use and, in some cases, with being under the influence of the drug.

Saliva concentrations can be exceptionally high when the route of administration is smoking of the drug, such as with marijuana, cocaine, methamfetamine and heroin, sublingual or buccal adsorption, or snorting of the drug. In cases that involve these routes of administration, 2 to 4 hours must elapse before the contamination of saliva by the remains of the ingested drug are cleared from the mouth and saliva concentrations reflect plasma levels. Marijuana is the exception. Δ^9-THC found in saliva most likely comes from cannabinoids deposited in the oral mucosa as a result of smoking the drug. However, saliva concentrations of Δ^9-THC follow the same time course as the appearance and decline of physiological indices of marijuana's pharmacological effects. The rate of clearance of Δ^9-THC from the oral tissues appears to match the binding and clearance of Δ^9-THC from the central nervous system site of action of cannabinoids.

Pharmacology of drugs in saliva

Saliva alcohol

Ethanol is a low-molecular-weight compound that passes through cell membranes, and does not ionise or bind to plasma proteins. Ethanol distributes to all body fluids in proportion to their water content. The measured saliva : plasma ratio for ethanol, 1.10, is slightly higher than the calculated value, perhaps because of the high blood flow to the salivary glands. Saliva ethanol is in equilibrium with arterial blood rather than the venous blood collected for analysis. Saliva equilibrates rapidly with blood ethanol.

Pharmacology

The passage of ethanol into saliva and the close correlation between saliva and blood alcohol concentrations was reported in the 1930s (Friedemann *et al.* 1938). Jones (1979b, c) reported an ethanol saliva : plasma ratio of 1.077, with a range of 0.84–1.36 in 48 male subjects between 1 and 3 hours after ingestion of 0.72 g/kg ethanol in a fasting condition. Variation was determined by analysis to result equally from inter- and intra-individual components. Individual variation in saliva : plasma ratios showed no systematic variation through the absorption, distribution and elimination phases of ethanol metabolism. Jones (1993) confirmed this value with a measured saliva : plasma ratio of 1.094 in 21 male volunteers. McColl *et al.* (1979) found a highly significant linear correlation between blood ethanol concentrations and those in mixed saliva obtained before and after rinsing and drying the mouth, and parotid saliva. McColl pointed out that this only applies if the saliva ethanol is determined in saliva obtained more than 20 minutes after ingestion of ethanol.

Haeckel and Bucklitsch (1987) reported that ethanol concentrations reached higher peak concentrations in saliva than in peripheral blood. Newman and Abramson (1942) correlated saliva alcohol concentrations with ethanol's effects on performance. Jones (1993) compared saliva, breath and blood concentration–time profiles. Saliva concentrations were higher than blood and breath concentrations. All three correlated equally well with measures of alcohol's effects. Maximum impairment was reached at the same time as peak saliva, blood and breath levels.

Analysis

Ethanol can be analysed in saliva by the same headspace chromatographic (Jones 1978) or enzymatic methods (Jones 1979a) as used for blood (see Chapter 11). Dipstick or reagent strip tests for alcohol have been reported (Tu *et al.* 1992; Pate *et al.* 1993) but were found to be too unreliable for use in determining blood alcohol content (Lutz *et al.* 1993; Pate *et al.* 1993; Wong 2002). Current enzymatic tests have proved more reliable as quantitative tests (Christopher and Zeccardi 1992; Jones 1995; Bendtsen *et al.* 1999; Smolle *et al.* 1999) and several commercial tests for on-site or point-of-collection testing of saliva alcohol are available.

An example of a point-of-collection quantitative test is the QED Saliva Alcohol Test (OraSure, Bethlehem, PA, USA). The saliva or oral fluid is collected by the donor with a cotton swab, which is applied to the test pad (Fig. 6.9). As the saliva moves along the reagent bar by capillary action, any ethanol present is oxidised by alcohol dehydrogenase to give acetaldehyde, with the simultaneous reduction of nicotinamide–adenine dinucleotide (NAD). This results in a cascade of electron donor–acceptor reactions catalysed by diaphorase, and involving FeCN and a tetrazolium salt, that proceeds to production of a purple-coloured endpoint. The length of the resultant purple-coloured bar on the QED device is directly proportional to the concentration of ethanol in the specimen. The alcohol concentration can be read directly from the height of the coloured reaction bar on a printed scale (mg/dL or mg% ethanol), just as in reading a thermometer (Fig. 6.9C). To obtain an accurate reading, the capillary must draw saliva all the way to the top of the device. This is signalled by the development of a purple colour within 5 minutes at the QA spot at the top of the 'thermometer' (Fig. 6.9C).

Since the saliva moves along the reagent bar and reacts directly with the indicator chemicals, any oxidant in the saliva can cause a false positive. The most common oxidant found in saliva is ascorbic acid, commonly added to fruit juices, sodas and soft drinks as a preservative. Ascorbic acid is absorbed in the gums and is still found in the mouth in amounts sufficient to give a false positive with the QED Saliva Alcohol test for up to 10 minutes after drinking some soft drinks and sodas.

The QED Saliva Alcohol test comes in two ranges, 0–150 (which can be read from 0.01 to 0.15 g/dL) and 0–350 (which can be read from 0.02 to 0.35 g/dL). The first, lower, range is for US Department of Transportation (DOT) and driving under the influence (DUI) applications, and the second is for hospital and overdose applications.

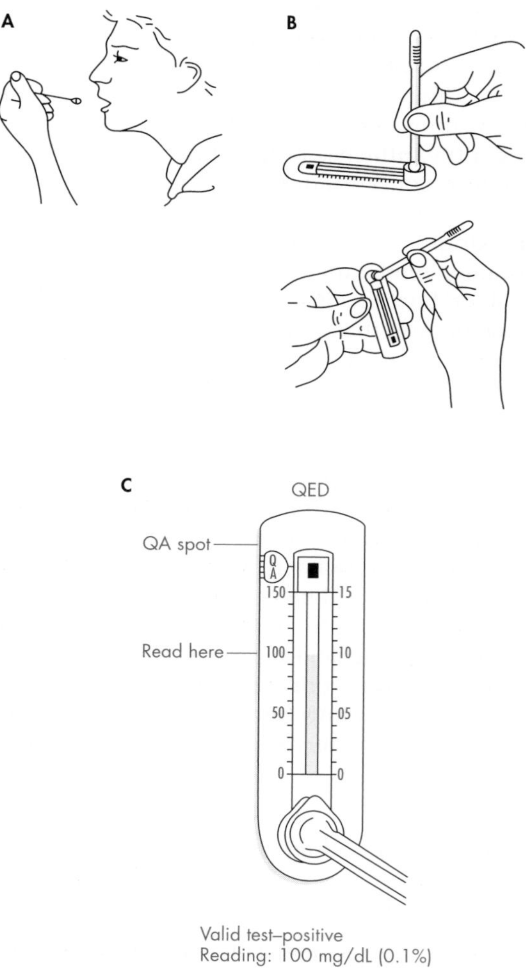

Figure 6.9 The QED Saliva Alcohol Test: (A) collecting saliva; (B) filling the capillary; (C) interpreting the test results.

An example of a headspace enzymatic assay is the On-Site Saliva Alcohol Assay for the qualitative detection of alcohol in urine and saliva (Roche Diagnostics, Nutley, NJ, USA; Ansys Technologies Inc., Lake Forest, CA, USA). The On-Site Saliva Alcohol Assay is similar to the QED Saliva Alcohol Test in that saliva is collected by the donor from his or her own mouth with a cotton swab, and the swab is applied to the specimen well. Since alcohols are volatile, alcohol vapours diffuse from the sample pad to the reaction pad, where they react with alcohol dehydrogenase and diaphorase. The hydrogen released is transferred to the tetrazolium salt and produces a highly coloured formazan dye. The presence of alcohol is indicated by the appearance of a purple plus sign (+) in the result pad. The On-Site Saliva Alcohol Assay does not have a control spot, so an external control must be run in each testing session on an additional test unit. Since the test detects alcohol vapours from the saliva, the saliva sample does not come into contact with the reagents, so there is no possibility of false positives from oxidising agents, such as ascorbic acid, in the saliva. However, the result is qualitative only. The cut-off is 0.02 g%, so a purple plus sign (+) indicates the presence of alcohol at a concentration greater than 0.02 g%.

Interpretation

Saliva ethanol concentrations are an accurate reflection of blood alcohol concentrations, and can subsequently be used to estimate the pharmacokinetics of ethanol in an individual as evidence of impairment and to determine fitness for duty in the workplace.

The DOT has codified saliva ethanol testing for US workplace testing (Department of Transportation 1994). The screening cut-off is 0.02 g% saliva or 0.02 g/210 L of breath. As the saliva alcohol tests are nonspecific chemical screening tests that may react with oxidising agents and with ketones and alcohols other than ethanol, it is necessary to confirm any positive results above 0.02 g% with an independent test based on a different chemical principle. Breath alcohol tests are usually either fuel cells or infrared spectrophotometers with optical filters and computer software safeguards for specificity and sensitivity. Specifically, they must be able to distinguish acetone from ethanol at the 0.02 g% alcohol level. A time limit is placed on confirmation of saliva ethanol results, since ethanol is metabolised rapidly by the liver. Initially, the confirmation breath test had to be performed within 20 minutes. The DOT now requires the confirmation test to be carried out within 30 minutes.

Opiates (heroin, 6-monoacetylmorphine, morphine, codeine and related opiates)

The major metabolite found in oral fluid after heroin use is 6-MAM (saliva : plasma ratio of 6; Cone 1993; Jenkins *et al.* 1994, 1995; Moore *et al.* 2001). The heroin parent drug was found in oral fluid for up to 24 hours after heroin had been smoked and up to 60 minutes after heroin had been injected, with a *S*/*P* ratio after intravenous administration of 2.13, range 0.12–7.2 (Jenkins *et al.* 1995). If heroin is snorted (Cone 1993) or smoked (Jenkins *et al.* 1995), very high levels of heroin (in the mg/L range) may be detected in oral fluid for several hours after use because of deposition of the parent drug in the oral cavity. In addition to heroin and 6-MAM, morphine may be found in saliva after heroin use. An average saliva : plasma ratio of 0.67 (range 0.1–1.82) for morphine in oral fluid after the intravenous administration of heroin was reported by Jenkins *et al.* (1995). Euphoria after heroin use occurs rapidly and diminishes within the first hour, which parallels the time course of heroin in saliva and blood. Miosis caused by heroin peaks approximately 15 minutes after administration by smoking or intravenous injection, and persists for up to 4 hours. Miosis parallels the time course of saliva and blood concentrations of 6-MAM and morphine (Jenkins *et al.* 1994).

Morphine appears in saliva after the administration of morphine sulfate with a saliva : plasma ratio of 0.2 (Cone 1993).

Hydromorphone is found in saliva, with the saliva : plasma ratio in the elimination phase ranging from 0.25 to 2.32 for eight subjects with both inter-individual and intra-individual variation (Ritschel *et al.* 1987). Hydromorphone was detected in saliva by radioimmunoassay for up to 10 hours after intravenous administration of 2–5 mg of hydromorphone.

Pholcodine is found in saliva in the range of 1.5–350 μg/L after oral doses of 20 and 60 mg (Chen *et al.* 1988). The saliva : plasma ratio was 3.6, calculated from the mean areas under the concentration–time curves for plasma and saliva. Pholcodine was detectable in saliva for 20 hours after the last dose on day 11 of chronic dosing.

After administration of codeine, the drug is found in saliva with a saliva : plasma ratio of 3.3 (Cone 1993; Kim *et al.* 2002). O'Neal *et al.* (1999) reported a mean saliva : plasma ratio of 3.7 ± 0.28 when measured 2 to 12 hours after the oral administration of 30 mg of codeine and concluded that saliva codeine concentrations could be used to estimate plasma concentration via the saliva : plasma ratio. Codeine-6-glucuronide was not found in saliva.

O'Neal *et al.* (2000) reported that codeine concentrations in saliva collected by expectoration or draining of unstimulated oral fluid were 1.3–2.0 times higher than codeine concentrations in oral fluid collected by swabbing with absorptive devices (OraSure, Salivette and Finger Collector containing AccuSorb foam). As expected from the Henderson–Hasselbalch equation above, codeine concentrations in unstimulated saliva collected by expectoration were 3.6 times higher than concentrations in specimens collected by expectoration after acidic stimulation by citric acid. Other prescription opiates and opioids reported in oral fluid include hydrocodone, oxycodone (Jones *et al.* 2002), dihydrocodeine (Skopp *et al.* 2001) and fentanyl (Silverstein *et al.* 1993).

Ingestion of 5.2–40 g of poppy seeds produced saliva opiate-positive results at 15 minutes, but not at 1 hour. However, no 6-MAM was found in saliva after ingestion of poppy seeds.

Speckl *et al.* (1999) evaluated a collection device (ClinRep) that consisted of a treated cotton roll which was then centrifuged and the oral fluid collected and filtered before extraction and GC-MS analysis. They reported that the concordance of the analytic results for opiates of the saliva samples with urine was 93% for a cut-off limit of 100 μg/L and 98% for a cut-off limit of 300 μg/L.

Methadone

Lynn *et al.* (1975) and DiGregorio *et al.* (1977a, b) reported that methadone is found in saliva after parenteral administration of methadone. Kang and Abbott (1982) reported a GC-MS method for methadone and 3-ethylidene-1,5-dimethyl-3,3-diphenylpyrrolidine (EDDP) in saliva. The relative metabolic profile for methadone in blood, saliva, urine, sweat and hair is shown in Fig. 6.10.

Wolff *et al.* (1991) found that saliva methadone concentrations could be used to estimate plasma methadone concentrations to monitor consumption of methadone. Since methadone has a pK_a of 8.2, the saliva : plasma ratio is a function of saliva pH. Bermejo *et al.* (2000) reported that the methadone saliva : plasma ratio as a function of saliva pH ranged from 0.6 to 7.2 with an average of 3.7 ($n = 10$) over a measured saliva pH range of 5.0–7.0. In the same specimens, the saliva : plasma ratio of EDDP ranged from 0.2 to 1.8 with an average of 0.89, and was not a function of saliva pH.

Malcolm and Oliver (1997) reported that the saliva : whole blood ratio ranged from 0.45 to 3.4.

Cocaine

Cocaine parent drug is the major analyte found in saliva after cocaine use (DiGregorio *et al.* 1992). In unstimulated saliva, cocaine is ion-trapped in saliva and the saliva : plasma ratio may be 5 or greater (Schramm 1993; Schramm *et al.* 1993). In stimulated saliva, the saliva : plasma ratio ranges from 0.5 to 3.0 (Cone and Menchen, 1988; Cone and Weddington 1989; Jenkins *et al.* 1995; Cone *et al.* 1997). Cocaine appears in saliva immediately after drug administration by intravenous injection (Fenko *et al.* 1990). Benzoylecgonine and ecgonine methyl ester appear in saliva within 15 minutes of cocaine administration and are found in saliva at concentrations similar to those found in blood. Schramm *et al.* (1993) reported a saliva : plasma ratio of approximately 2.5 for benzoylecgonine. Jenkins *et al.* (1995) reported saliva : plasma

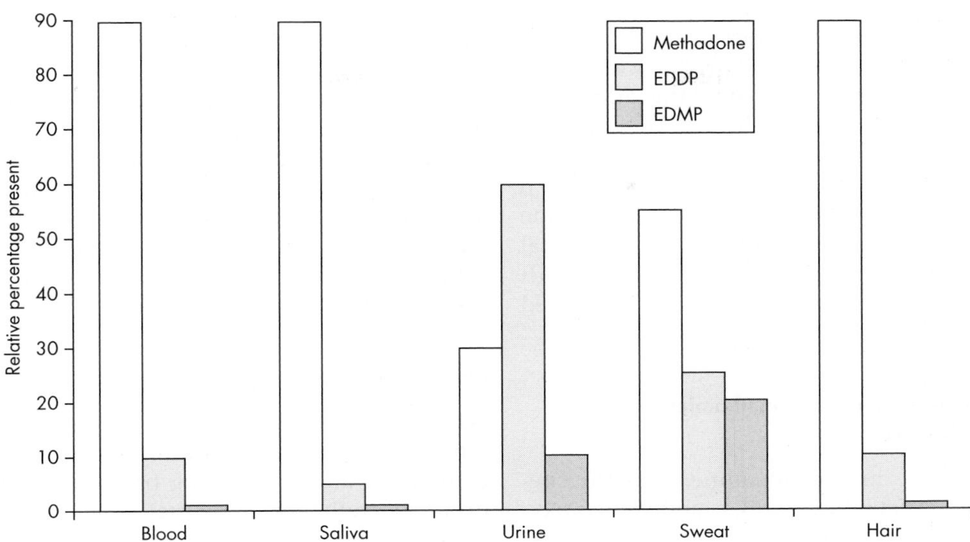

Figure 6.10 Metabolic profile of methadone in blood, saliva, urine, sweat and hair (EDDP, 3-ethylidene-1,5-dimethyl-3,3-diphenylpyrrolidine; EDMP, 2-ethyl-5-methyl-3,3-diphenylpyrroline).

ratios for benzoylecgonine that ranged from 0.02 to 0.66. Norcocaine and *para*-hydroxycocaine may be found in saliva after cocaine administration. Jufer *et al.* (2000) reported a saliva : plasma ratio of 8.7 (range 3.8–13.2) for cocaine, 3.7 (2.3–5.1) for ecgonine methyl ester, 0.4 (0.3–0.5) for benzoylecgonine, 10.3 (5.6–13.6) for norcocaine and 6.1 (2.4–10.8) for *para*-hydroxycocaine. Cocaethylene is found in saliva when ethanol is ingested concurrently with cocaine. In a rat model, Barbieri *et al.* (1994) reported a saliva : plasma ratio of 1.3 for cocaethylene after cocaethylene administration. Jenkins *et al.* (1995) reported that the pyrolysis product of cocaine, AEME, was detected in oral fluid collected after smoking of cocaine, but not in plasma.

Thompson *et al.* (1987) reported that cocaine was found in saliva immediately after intravenous doses of cocaine and that saliva and plasma cocaine concentrations paralleled each other. Saliva cocaine concentrations correlated with the physiological and behavioural effects of the drug. Cocaine saliva : plasma ratios ranged from 0.36 to 9.74. Cone and Weddington (1989) reported detection of cocaine equivalents by immunoassay for 5–10 days after abstinence in heavy cocaine addicts and GC-MS confirmation for 1–2 days. In a more recent study of cocaine and metabolite elimination patterns, Moolchan *et al.* (2000) measured cocaine, benzoylecgonine and ecgonine methyl ester in saliva of admitted cocaine abusers for 12 hours. In the later specimens, metabolites predominated, as is consistent with their longer half-lives in the body. Saliva terminal half-lives were 7.9 h for cocaine, 9.2 h for benzoylecgonine and 10 h for ecgonine methyl ester. Cone *et al.* (1988) reported the correlation of saliva and plasma cocaine concentrations after intravenous cocaine administration with an average half-life of cocaine of 34.7 min in saliva and 34.9 min in plasma. Jenkins *et al.* (1995) reported a detection time for cocaine in saliva of up to 8 hours after intravenous injection and 12 hours after smoking cocaine. Cone *et al.* (1997) reported mean detection times of cocaine in saliva of 3.92 hours after intravenous administration, 5.67 hours after insufflation and 3.17 hours after smoking cocaine.

Jenkins *et al.* (1995) followed cocaine and metabolites in saliva after smoking and intravenous administration of cocaine. They showed that after smoking, cocaine and pyrolysis products of cocaine persisted in saliva for up to 6 hours. Cone *et al.* (1997) compared cocaine appearance in saliva after intravenous, intranasal and smoked administration and found that both the intranasal and smoking routes produced elevated saliva : plasma ratios of cocaine.

Amfetamines (amfetamine, methamfetamine, MDMA, MDA, MDEA)

Amfetamine, methamfetamine, methylenedioxymethamfetamine (3,4-methylenedioxymethamfetamine or 3,4-methylenedioxy-*N*-methylamfetamine; MDMA), 3,4-methylenedioxyamfetamine (MDA) and other amfetamine-class drugs can be found in saliva. Parent drug rather than amfetamine metabolites is found in saliva. The saliva : plasma ratio for amfetamine is 2.76 and for methamfetamine it is 3.98. When amfetamine was administered to subjects as a racemic mixture, both *d*- and *l*-isomers were found in saliva (Wan *et al.* 1978). Saliva has been found to be positive for methamfetamine as long as 50 hours after dosing (Suzuki *et al.* 1989). Cook *et al.* (1993) compared methamfetamine concentrations in saliva and plasma of volunteers who were administered the drug by smoking and intravenous routes.

The excretion profile of MDMA and its metabolites in saliva and in plasma after ingestion of a single 100 mg dose has been reported (Navarro *et al.* 2001). In eight healthy volunteers, salivary concentrations peaked at 1.5 hours after ingestion and the peak values ranged from 1.73 to 6.51 mg/L. These peak values corresponded to an average saliva : plasma ratio of 18.1 (±7.9 SD). The time profile of the S/*P* ratio was also reported, with the peak occurring at 1.5 hours followed by a decline to a plateau between 7.3 and 6.4 at 10 and 24 hours after dosing. MDA was found in saliva at concentrations approximately 4–5% of MDMA concentrations (relative area under the curve; AUC), with highest concentrations between 1.5 and 4 hours after dosing. 4-Hydroxy-3-methoxymethamfetamine (HMMA) was detected in trace amounts in saliva. Samyn *et al.* (2002a) quantified MDMA, MDA and methylenedioxyethylamfetamine (MDEA) concentrations in 50 μL of oral fluid by LC-MS/MS.

Kintz (1997) reported the detection of *N*-methyl-1-(3,4-methylenedioxyphenyl)-2-butanamine (MBDB) in saliva. Peak saliva concentrations were observed at 2 hours, and both MBDB and the demethylated metabolite, BDB, were detected in saliva for 17 hours.

Barbiturates and antiepileptic drugs

Wilson (1993) reviewed the attempts to use saliva for therapeutic drug monitoring of anticonvulsant drugs, including barbiturates. These drugs generally have a neutral or acidic pK_a and many are highly protein bound in blood. Their saliva : plasma ratios are usually less than unity. For example, carbamazepine saliva levels correlate well with dose and blood concentrations. The saliva : plasma ratio for carbamazepine is 0.13–0.33 (Miles *et al.* 1991).

However, the reported phenytoin saliva : plasma ratios vary from 0.01 to 0.25 (average 0.09) for blood total phenytoin and from 1.06 to 2.22 for blood free phenytoin. Phenytoin saliva concentrations do not correlate with blood concentrations or therapeutic effect. They do show compliance or noncompliance, and elevated levels are related to toxicity. Kamali and Thomas (1994) demonstrated, using atropine-induced reductions in saliva flow rate, that the saliva : plasma ratio and saliva phenytoin concentrations were dependant on saliva flow rate, but that this did not account for all of the intra-individual variance in the saliva : plasma ratio for phenytoin.

Phenobarbital saliva : plasma ratios of 0.31–0.63 have been reported (Mucklow *et al.* 1978; Nishihara *et al.* 1979; Wilson 1993). Dilli and Pilai (1980) reported a half-life for pentobarbital in saliva of 17–19 h and for amobarbital of 22–26 hours. Sharp *et al.* (1983) reported saliva secobarbital levels of 210 ± 40 μg/L at 3 hours after oral administration of 50 mg secobarbital. The saliva : plasma ratio was 0.30 ± 0.04. Van der Graaff *et al.* (1986) reported the pharmacokinetics of hexobarbital in plasma and saliva. Wilson (1993) listed the following therapeutic ranges for saliva: carbamazepine 1.4–3.5 mg/L, phenobarbital 5.0–15 mg/L and diphenylhydantoin 1.0–2.0 mg/L. Fabris *et al.* (1989) reported on the influence of pH on saliva phenobarbital content in infants.

Benzodiazepines

Benzodiazepines have an unfavourable saliva : plasma ratio (S/P = 0.01–0.08) because of the acidic pK_a values and a high percentage protein binding in plasma (95–99%); sensitive methods must therefore be used to detect benzodiazepines in saliva (Tjaden *et al.* 1980).

Lucek and Dixon (1980) reported a mean saliva : plasma ratio for chlordiazepoxide of 0.027 ± 0.011. Saliva levels were found to be equal to the concentration of unbound drug in plasma.

Diazepam (pK_a 3.3) and its metabolites are found in saliva at concentrations of 2–5 μg/L with a saliva : plasma ratio of 0.02 (Giles *et al.* 1977, 1981; Dixon and Crews 1978). Giles *et al.* (1980) reported saliva desmethyldiazepam levels in patients who received chronic diazepam therapy. Hallstrom *et al.* (1980) reported a saliva : plasma ratio of 0.016 ± 0.003 for diazepam and 0.029 ± 0.01 for nordiazepam in chronic diazepam users. DeGier *et al.* (1980) reported saliva : plasma ratios of 0.017 ± 0.003 for diazepam, but failed to predict plasma free diazepam levels accurately from saliva diazepam concentrations.

Kangas *et al.* (1979) and Hart *et al.* (1987) reported that saliva concentrations of nitrazepam were considerably lower than the protein-unbound fraction in serum and that monitoring of saliva nitrazepam was of no clinical value. However, Hart *et al.* (1988) reported that while diazepam, nordiazepam and clonazepam are stable in saliva, nitrazepam is unstable in saliva and is rapidly converted into 7-aminonitrazepam on standing in saliva at room temperature.

Samyn *et al.* (2002b) reported the detection of flunitrazepam and 7-aminoflunitrazepam in oral fluid using chemical-ionisation GC-MS. Maximum concentrations were reached 2–4 hours after dosing. Flunitrazepam and its metabolites were not stable in oral fluid specimens, even after treatment with sodium fluoride and refrigeration.

Studies of the effect of benzodiazepines on psychomotor performance and driving performance have compared saliva and plasma concentrations (DeGier *et al.* 1981; Linnoila *et al.* 1983; Jansen *et al.* 1988). Results indicate a good correlation between saliva and plasma concentrations, but poor correlation with psychomotor impairment.

Cannabis (marijuana)

Cannabinoids are excreted in only trace amounts in saliva. Idowu and Caddy (1982) calculated a theoretical saliva : plasma ratio of 0.099–0.129 for Δ^9-tetrahydrocannabinol (Δ^9-THC) and of 0.060–0.099 for 11-OH-Δ^9-THC. The measured saliva : plasma ratio after intravenous injection of labelled cannabidiol is 0.0012 (Ohlsson *et al.* 1986). However, the measured saliva : plasma ratio for THC after smoking marijuana is 10 and is a function of the time since smoking (Cone 1993). Cannabinoids in saliva often result from residuals left in the mouth during ingestion or smoking of marijuana or marijuana products (Niedbala *et al.* 2001b). For this reason, concentrations are highest immediately after smoking and decline rapidly over the first 2–4 hours. In contrast, cannabinoids may not appear in urine or sweat for several hours after smoking (Fig. 6.11). Niedbala *et al.* (2001a) reported an average lag time to urine positive for cannabinoids from 4 hours (GC-MS) to 6 hours (enzyme immunoassay). The advantage of measuring cannabinoids in saliva is that it is an indication of recent use of marijuana.

Just *et al.* (1974) detected Δ^9-THC by two-dimensional thin-layer chromatography and mass spectrometry in saliva extracts for 2 hours after the smoking of a single tobacco cigarette that contained 2.8 mg of Δ^9-THC. Maseda *et al.* (1986) detected Δ^9-THC in saliva using capillary gas chromatography with an electron capture detector for 4 hours after smoking marijuana that contained approximately 10 mg Δ^9-THC. Maseda *et al.* (1986) also reported that saliva Δ^9-THC concentrations at 1 hour were lowered by

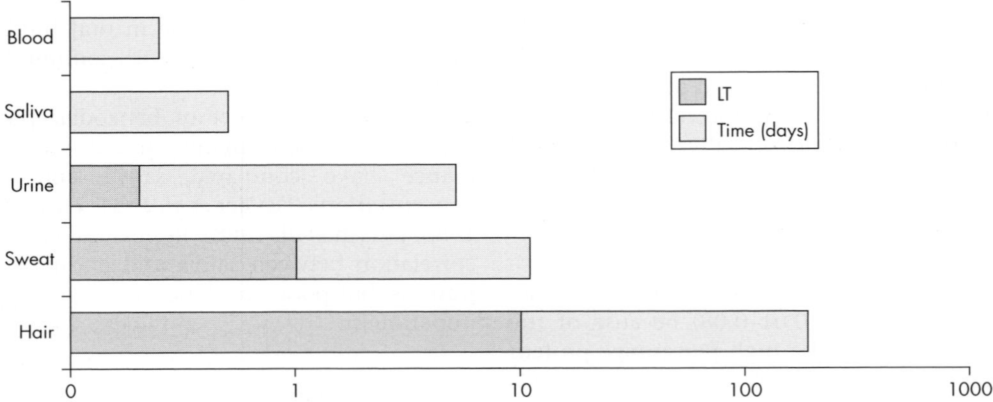

Figure 6.11 The lag time (LT) and window of detection for cannabinoids in blood, saliva, urine, sweat and hair after smoking marijuana.

drinking 200 mL of beer immediately after the marijuana smoking.

No detectable levels of cannabinoids were found in saliva after passive exposure to marijuana smoke.

There were no significant differences in cannabinoid concentration or detection for oral fluid collected simultaneously from the right and left sides of the mouth. Using GC-MS/MS with a 0.5 μg/L Δ^9-THC cut-off concentration, Niedbala *et al.* (2001b) detected Δ^9-THC in oral fluid from 10 subjects who smoked 20–25 mg Δ^9-THC for an average of 34 hours.

Menkes *et al.* (1991) found that saliva levels of THC correlated with rapid heart rate and psychological feelings of a 'high'. Saliva THC concentrations were measured after smoking a cigarette that contained 11 mg THC. Subjective intoxication, measured using a visual analogue scale, and heart rate were correlated significantly with log (saliva THC concentration).

Hall *et al.* (1998) applied solid-phase microextraction (SPME) to the determination of cannabidiol, Δ^8-THC, Δ^9-THC and cannabinol in human saliva by quadrupole ion-trap GC-MS. SPME allows analysis of small saliva samples and eliminates the use of organic solvents. Samyn and Van Haeren (2000) reported on-site testing of drivers with the DrugWipe (Securitec, Munich, Germany) and confirmation by GC-MS after solid-phase extraction and derivatisation. Cannabinoids were confirmed in 10 of 15 subjects (67%), and THC concentrations ranged from 1.4 to 42 μg/L in saliva.

Phencyclidine

PCP has low protein binding in plasma (<10%) and a pK_a of 9.43. From the Henderson–Hasselbalch equation, the saliva : plasma ratio is expected to be greater than unity. After giving oral (1 mg) and intravenous (0.1 or 1 mg) doses of radiolabelled PCP to healthy male volunteers, Cook *et al.* (1982a) reported that the parent drug was found in saliva at concentrations higher than would be expected from the pH differential between plasma and saliva and the binding of the drug in plasma and saliva. The saliva : plasma ratio ranged from 1.5 to 3.0. Saliva was collected by expectoration into glass vials, and saliva pH averaged 6.7 ± 0.17.

PCP is primarily abused by smoking tobacco or marijuana cigarettes that have been dipped into PCP-containing solvents. Inhaled PCP is trapped in the tissues of the mouth. Cook *et al.* (1982b) also reported both PCP and phencyclohexene (PC) were present in plasma after volunteers smoked 100 μg of radiolabelled PCP. The persistence of PCP or PC in saliva after smoking PCP was not reported.

McCarron *et al.* (1984) analysed paired serum and saliva samples from 100 patients suspected of PCP intoxication. Both serum and saliva tests were positive for PCP by radioimmunoassay (RIA) in 70 of the cases, and both were negative in seven cases. In 21 cases with no clinical evidence of PCP intoxication, both serum and saliva RIA were negative in 17 cases, and positive in three cases. Saliva PCP concentrations ranges from 2 to 600 μg/L.

The proposed US workplace cut-off for PCP in saliva is 10 μg/L PCP equivalents by immunoassay and the confirmation cut-off is 10 μg/L PCP (SAMHSA 2000).

Conclusion

Saliva drug concentrations are related to the blood concentration of the unbound, non-ionised parent drug or its lipophilic metabolites for many drugs. For these drugs, saliva concentrations are a function of circulating drug levels in the blood. For many patient populations the ease with which oral fluids are obtained and the avoidance of venepuncture outweighs the inaccuracy of the estimation of drug levels from saliva. This includes clinical uses in infant and paediatric populations, the elderly, and human immunodeficiency virus (HIV)-positive patients. Saliva is useful in pharmacokinetic studies, since multiple specimens can be obtained over time with minimal discomfort to the subject. In forensic practice, saliva drug collection and testing, unlike venepuncture, can be carried out in nonclinical settings, provides information about the presence of drugs, indicates recent ingestion, and may be correlated with psychomotor impairment for some drugs such as marijuana. Finally, in large-scale testing, such as the US workplace drug-testing programmes, collection and testing of oral fluid provides specimens that can be collected under direct observation and that are not easily diluted or adulterated. For this reason, saliva drug testing has been proposed for US federal workplace testing as a specimen for random testing, for testing triggered by reasonable suspicion or cause, and for post-accident testing. Both laboratory-based and on-site saliva drug testing are anticipated in the workplace.

Detection of drugs in sweat

Sweating (perspiration) is primarily a means of temperature regulation. Evaporation of sweat from the skin surface has a cooling effect. In hot conditions or during exercise, muscles heat up due to exertion and more sweat is produced. Sweating can be significantly increased by nervousness and decreased by cold.

The composition of sweat is similar to that of plasma except that sweat does not contain proteins. The exact mechanism of sweat secretion is not well known. Sweat is a filtrate of plasma that contains electrolytes (such as potassium, sodium and chloride) and metabolic waste products such as urea and lactic acid. It also contains odorants such as 2-methylphenol and 4-methylphenol. Production of sweat takes place in sweat glands. As shown in Figure 6.12, in humans there are two kinds of sweat glands: eccrine sweat glands (Fig. 6.12A) and apocrine glands (Fig. 6.12B).

There are approximately 2–3 million sweat glands in the skin of humans. An adult person produces from 100 mL of sweat to as much as 10 L in one day. The eccrine sweat glands are the common type and they are distributed over the entire body, particularly on the palms of the hands, soles of the feet and forehead. They are smaller and are active from birth. Apocrine sweat glands develop during puberty and are mainly present in armpits and the anal-genital area. They produce sweat that contains fatty materials. Apocrine glands typically end in hair follicles rather than pores. The sweat glands are controlled by sympathetic cholinergic nerves which are controlled by the hypothalamus.

Because sweat resembles a filtrate of plasma, water-soluble chemicals such as some drugs and metal ions are found in sweat. The mechanism of the appearance of a drug in sweat is not fully understood. It is believed that the primary mechanism is passive diffusion from blood into sweat glands and transdermal migration of drugs to the skin surface where drugs are dissolved in sweat. Sweat can be collected on sweat wipes or with a sweat patch. There are a few commercially available patches but only one has been approved in the USA as a collecting device (PharmChem

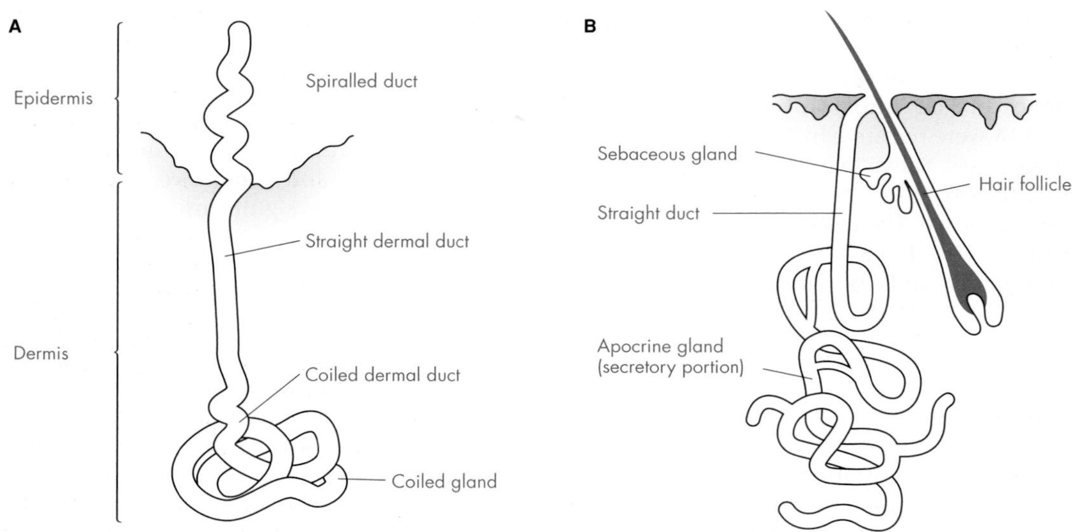

Figure 6.12 Two types of sweat glands: (A) an eccrine sweat gland; (B) an apocrine sweat gland.

Table 6.3 Comparison of urine, sweat and hair testing for cocaine and heroin (National Institute on Drug Abuse, NIDA Notes, Vol. 10, No. 5, 1995)

Issues	Urine	Sweat patch	Hair
Type of measure	Incremental	Cumulative	Cumulative
Invasiveness	High	Low	Low
Detection period	2–3 days	Weeks	Months to years
Risk of false positives[a]	Low	High	High
Risk of false negatives[b]	High	Undetermined	Undetermined
Risk of adulteration	High	Undetermined	Low
Technological development			
Screening assays	Plentiful	Needed	Needed
Confirmation assays	Plentiful	Needed	Needed
Cut-offs	Established	Needed	Needed
Control materials	Plentiful	Needed	Needed
Cost per unit test	Low	Undetermined	High

[a] False positives resulting from environmental contamination of the biological specimen during collection and handling and from passive drug exposure as a result of, for example, contact with skin or exposure to cocaine vapours.
[b] False negatives resulting from the drug detection 'window' of the biological specimen.

Laboratories, Inc., Fort Worth, TX, USA). The main part of a sweat patch is a gauze pad covered by a protective membrane similar to that of an adhesive dressing strip. The membrane has an adhesive perimeter that sticks tightly to the test subject's skin. The sweat patch is usually placed on the subject's upper arm. Sweat patches can be worn for extended periods, they are waterproof and are difficult to tamper with (when removed, the patch cannot be reattached), and they are usually very well tolerated by patients. There are some concerns associated with the use of sweat patches:

- false positives through environmental contamination
- false positives through skin storage
- false positives during application and removal
- no dose–response relationship
- patch wear problems.

It is recommended that the skin be washed with soap and cool water or with a disposable towelette. Then the skin where the patch will be worn is thoroughly cleaned with alcohol wipes prior to patch application. The use of sweat patches detects drug use that occurred just before patch application and while the device remains attached to the skin. Primarily the parent drugs are detected in sweat; however, some drug metabolites can also be found. Drugs of abuse or metabolites detected in sweat include THC, amfetamine, methamfetamine, codeine, morphine, 6-MAM, heroin, PCP, cocaine, benzoylecgonine, ecgonine methyl ester and cocaethylene.

Comparison of urine, sweat and hair testing for cocaine and heroin is presented in Table 6.3.

Currently sweat testing is used in the private sector for monitoring drug use during substance abuse treatment and in the criminal justice system, as well as for return-to-duty and follow-up testing for workplace testing.

References

E. J. Barbieri *et al.*, Rat cocaethylene and benzolylecgonine concentrations in plasma and parotid saliva after the administration of cocaethylene, *J. Anal. Toxicol.*, 1994, **18**, 60–61.

C. Barrett *et al.*, Comparison of point-of-collection screening of drugs of abuse in oral fluid with a laboratory-based urine screen, *Forensic Sci. Int.*, 2001, **122**, 163–166.

B. J. Baum, Principles of saliva secretion, *Ann. New York Acad. Sci.*, 1993, **694**, 17–23.

W. A. Baumgartner and V. A. Hill, Hair analysis for drugs of abuse: decontamination issues, in *Recent Developments in Therapeutic Drug Monitoring and Clinical Toxicology*, I. Sunshine (ed.), New York, Marcel Dekker, 1992, pp. 577–597.

A. M. Baumgartner *et al.*, Radioimmunoassay of hair for determining opiate-abuse histories, *J. Nucl. Med.*, 1979, **20**, 748–752.

W. A. Baumgartner *et al.*, Hair analysis for drugs of abuse, *J. Forensic Sci.*, 1989, **34**, 1433–1453.

P. Bendtsen *et al.*, Monitoring ethanol exposure in a clinical setting by analysis of blood, breath, saliva and urine, *Alcohol Clin. Exp. Res.*, 1999, **23**, 1446–1451.

A. M. Bermejo *et al.*, Saliva/plasma ratio of methadone and EDDP, *J. Anal. Toxicol.*, 2000, **24**, 70–72.

F. Bévalot *et al.*, Analysis of corticosteroids in hair by LC/MS, *J. Chromatogr. B*, 2000, **740**, 227–236.

D. L. Blank and D. A. Kidwell, Decontamination procedures for drugs of abuse in hair: are they sufficient?, *Forensic Sci. Int.*, 1995, **70**, 13–38.

L. W. Cartmell *et al.*, Cocaine metabolites in pre-columbian mummy hair, *J. Okla. State Med. Assoc.*, 1991, **84**, 11–12.

Z. R. Chen *et al.*, Pharmacokinetics of pholcodine in healthy volunteers: single and chronic dosing studies, *Br. J. Clin. Pharmacol.*, 1988, **26**, 445–453.

T. A. Christopher and J. A. Zeccardi, Evaluation of the QED saliva alcohol test: a new, rapid, accurate device for measuring ethanol in saliva, *Ann. Emerg. Med.*, 1992, **21**, 1135–1137.

V. Cirimele *et al.*, Drug concentrations in human hair after bleaching, *J. Anal. Toxicol.*, 1995a, **19**, 331–332.

V. Cirimele *et al.*, Testing human hair for cannabis, *Forensic Sci. Int.*, 1995b, **70**, 175–182.

V. Cirimele *et al.*, Testing human hair for cannabis. III. Rapid screening procedure for the simultaneous identification of THC, cannabinol and cannabidiol, *J. Anal. Toxicol.*, 1996a, **20**, 13–16.

V. Cirimele *et al.*, Detection and quantification of lorazepam in human hair by GC-MS/NCI in a case of traffic accident, *Int. J. Leg. Med.*, 1996b, **108**, 265–267.

V. Cirimele *et al.*, Mise en évidence de l'exposition aux pesticides par analyse des cheveux, *Acta Clin. Belg.*, 1999 (Suppl.), 59–63.

V. Cirimele *et al.*, Identification of 10 corticosteroids in human hair by LC/MS, *Forensic Sci. Int.*, 2000, **107**, 381–388.

E. J. Cone, Saliva testing for drugs of abuse, *Ann. New York Acad. Sci.*, 1993, **694**, 91–127.

E. Cone, Mechanisms of drug incorporation into hair, *Ther. Drug Monit.*, 1996, **18**, 438–443.

E. J. Cone and S. L. Menchen, Stability of cocaine in saliva, *Clin. Chem.*, 1988, 34–1508.

E. J. Cone and W. W. Weddington Jr, Prolonged occurrence of cocaine in human saliva and urine after chronic use, *J. Anal. Toxicol.*, 1989, **13**, 65–68.

E. J. Cone *et al.*, Correlation of saliva cocaine levels with plasma levels and with pharmacologic effects after intravenous cocaine administration in human subjects, *J. Anal. Toxicol.*, 1988, **12**, 200–206.

E. J. Cone *et al.*, Testing human hair for drugs of abuse. II. Identification of unique cocaine metabolites in hair of drug abusers and evaluation of decontamination procedures, *J. Anal. Toxicol.*, 1991, **15**, 250–255.

E. J. Cone *et al.*, Simultaneous measurement of cocaine, cocaethylene, their metabolites and 'crack' pyrolysis products by gas chromatography–mass spectrometry, *Clin. Chem.*, 1994, **40**, 1299– 1305.

E. J. Cone *et al.*, Cocaine disposition in saliva following intravenous, intranasal and smoked administration, *J. Anal. Toxicol.*, 1997, **21**, 465–475.

C. E. Cook *et al.*, Phencyclidine disposition after intravenous and oral doses, *Clin. Pharmacol. Ther.*, 1982a, **31**, 625–634.

C. E. Cook *et al.*, Phencyclidine and phenylcyclohexene disposition after smoking phencyclidine, *Clin. Pharmacol. Ther.*, 1982b, **31**, 635–641.

C. E. Cook *et al.*, Pharmacokinetics of methamfetamine self-administered to human subjects by smoking *S*-(+)methamfetamine hydrochloride, *Drug Metab. Dispos.*, 1993, **21**, 717–723.

C. Dawes and G. N. Jenkins, The effects of different stimuli on the composition of saliva in man, *J. Physiol.*, 1964, **170**, 86–100.

J. J. DeGier *et al.*, Comparison of plasma and saliva levels of diazepam, *Br. J. Clin. Pharmacol.*, 1980, **10**, 151–155.

J. J. DeGier *et al.*, Psychomotor performance and real driving performance of outpatients receiving diazepam, *Psychopharmacology*, 1981, **73**, 340–344.

N. De Giovanni *et al.*, Cozart Rapiscan system: our experience with saliva tests, *J. Chromatogr. B. Anal. Technol. Biomed. Life Sci.*, 2002, **773**, 1–6.

Department of Transportation, 49 CFR Part 40 Procedures for Transportation Workplace Drug and Alcohol Testing Programs. Final Rule, *Federal Register*, 1994, **59**, 7340–7360; 42996–43019.

G. J. DiGregorio *et al.*, Secretion of drugs by the parotid glands of rats and human beings, *J. Dent. Res.*, 1977a, **56**, 502–508.

G. J. DiGregorio *et al.*, Radioimmunoassay of methadone in rat parotid saliva, *Drug Alcohol Depend.*, 1977b, **2**, 295–298.

G. J. DiGregorio *et al.*, Elimination kinetics of cocaine and benzoylecgonine in parotid saliva, serum and urine of adult cocaine abusers, *J. Clin. Pharmacol. Ther.*, 1992, 51–169.

S. Dilli and D. Pilai, Analysis of trace amounts of barbiturates in saliva, *J. Chromatogr.*, 1980, **190**, 113–118.

R. Dixon and T. Crews, Diazepam determination in microsamples of blood plasma and saliva by radioimmunoassay, *J. Anal. Toxicol.*, 1978, **2**, 210–213.

V. Dumestre and P. Kintz, Ephedrine abuse for doping purposes as demonstrated by hair analysis, *J. Anal. Toxicol.*, 2000, **24**, 381–382.

P. Edder *et al.*, Subcritical fluid extraction of opiates in hair of drug addicts, *J. Chromatogr. B*, 1994, **658**, 75–83.

C. Fabris *et al.*, Influence of salivary pH on the correlation between salivary and plasma levels of phenobarbital in the neonatal period, *Minerva Pediatr.*, 1989, **41**, 45–46.

M. Fendrich *et al.*, Validity of drug use reporting in a high-risk community sample: a comparison of cocaine and heroin survey reports with hair tests, *Am. J. Epidemiol.*, 2001, **149**, 955–962.

A. P. Fenko *et al.*, The presence of cocaine and benzoylecgonine in rat parotid saliva plasma and urine after the intravenous administration of cocaine, *Res. Commun. Subst. Abuse*, 1990, **11**, 11–26.

R. Forman, Accumulation of cocaine in maternal and fetal hair. The dose–response curve, *Life Sci.*, 1992, **50**, 1333–1341.

A. Franceschin *et al.*, Detection of morphine in hair with the Abbott TDx, *Clin. Chem.*, 1987, **33**, 2125.

T. E. Friedemann *et al.*, The excretion of ingested ethyl alcohol in saliva, *J Lab. Clin. Med.*, 1938, **23**, 1007–10014.

N. Fucci *et al.*, SPME–GC analysis of THC in saliva samples collected with the "EPITOPE" device, *Forensic Sci. Int.*, 2001, **119**, 318–321.

H. G. Giles *et al.*, Saliva and plasma concentrations of diazepam after a single oral dose, *Br. J. Clin. Pharmacol.*, 1977, **4**, 711–712.

H. G. Giles *et al.*, Diazepam and *N*-desmethyldiazepam in saliva of hospital inpatients, *J. Clin.* Pharm., 1980, **20**, 71–76.

H. G. Giles *et al.*, Disposition of intravenous diazepam in young men and women, *Eur. J. Clin. Pharmacol.*, 1981, **20**, 207–213.

J. P. Goulle *et al.*, Determination of endogenous levels of GHB in human hair. Are there possibilities for the identification of GHB administration through hair analysis in cases of drug-facilitated sexual assault? *J. Anal. Toxicol.*, **27**, 574–580.

R. Haeckel, Factors influencing the saliva/plasma ratio of drugs, *Ann. New York Acad. Sci.*, 1993, **694**, 128–142.

R. Haeckel and I. Bucklitsch, The comparability of ethanol concentrations in peripheral blood and saliva: the phenomenon of variation in saliva to blood concentrations ratios, *J. Clin. Chem. Clin. Biochem.*, 1987, **25**, 199–204.

R. Haeckel and P. Hanecke, Application of saliva for drug monitoring an in vivo model for transmembrane transport, *Eur. J. Clin. Chem. Biochem.*, 1996, **34**, 171–191.

B. J. Hall *et al.*, Determination of cannabinoids in water and human saliva by solid-phase microextraction and quadrupole ion trap gas chromatography/mass spectrometry, *Anal. Chem.*, 1998, **70**, 1788–1796.

C. Hallstrom *et al.*, Diazepam and *N*-desmethyldiazepam concentrations in saliva, plasma and CSF, *Br. J. Clin. Pharmacol.*, 1980, **9**, 333–330.

M. R. Harkey and G. L. Henderson, Hair analysis for drugs of abuse, in *Advances in Analytical Toxicology*, R. C. Baselt (ed.), Chicago, Year Book Medical, 1989, pp. 298–329.

M. R. Harkey *et al.*, Simultaneous quantitation of cocaine and its major metabolites in human hair by gas chromatography chemical ionization mass spectrometry, *J. Anal. Toxicol.*, 1991, **15**, 260–265.

B. J. Hart *et al.*, Complications in correlation studies between serum, free serum and saliva concentrations of nitrazepam, *Methods Find. Exp Clin. Pharmacol.*, 1987, **10**, 21–26.

B. J. Hart *et al.*, The stability of benzodiazepines in saliva, *Methods Find. Exp. Clin. Pharmacol.*, 1988, **10**, 21–26.

G. L. Henderson, Mechanisms of drug incorporation into hair, *Forensic Sci. Int.*, 1993, **63**, 19–29.

G. L. Henderson *et al.*, Cocaine and metabolite concentrations in hair of South American coca chewers, *J. Anal. Toxicol.*, 1992, **16**, 199–201.

G. L. Henderson *et al.*, Incorporation of isotopically labeled cocaine and metabolites into human hair. 1. Dose–response relationships, *J. Anal. Toxicol.*, 1996, **20**, 1–12.

G. L. Henderson *et al.*, Incorporation of isotopically labeled cocaine into human hair: race as a factor, *J. Anal. Toxicol.*, 1998, **22**, 156–165.

K. M. Höld *et al.*, Evaluation of the salivette as sampling device for monitoring β-adrenoceptor blocking drugs in saliva, *J. Chromatogr. B*, 1995, **663**, 103–110.

K. M. Höld *et al.*, Detection of nandrolone, testosterone, and their esters in rat and human hair samples, *J. Anal. Toxicol.*, 1999, **23**, 416–423.

O. R. Idowu and B. Caddy, A review of the use of saliva in the forensic detection of drugs and other chemicals, *J. Forensic. Sci. Soc.*, 1982, **22**, 123–135.

A. A. Jansen *et al.*, Acute effects of bromazepam on signal detection performance, digit symbol substitution test and smooth pursuit eye movements, *Neuropsychobiology*, 1988, **20**, 91–95.

A. N. Jeger *et al.*, Morphin-determination in human hair by instrumental HP–TLC, in *TIAFT Proceedings*, B. Kaempe (ed.), Copenhagen, Mackeenzie, 1991, pp. 250–256.

A. Jehanli *et al.*, Blind trials of an onsite saliva drug test, *J. Forensic Sci.*, 2001, **46**, 206–212.

A. J. Jenkins *et al.*, Pharmacokinetics and pharmacodynamics of smoked heroin, *J. Anal. Toxicol.*, 1994, **18**, 317–30.

A. J. Jenkins *et al.*, Comparison of heroin and cocaine concentration in saliva with concentrations in blood and plasma, *J. Anal. Toxicol.*, 1995, **19**, 359–374.

J. Jones *et al.*, The simultaneous determination of codeine, morphine, hydrocodone, hydromorphone, 6-acetylmorphine and oxycodone in hair and oral fluid, *J. Anal. Toxicol.*, 2002, **26**, 171–175.

A. W. Jones, A rapid head-space method for ethyl alcohol determination in saliva samples, *Anal. Biochem.*, 1978, **86**, 589–596.

A. W. Jones, Assessment of an automated enzymatic method for ethanol determination in microsamples of saliva, *Scand. J. Clin. Lab. Invest.*, 1979a, **39**, 199–203.

A. W. Jones, Distribution of ethanol between saliva and blood in man, *Clin. Exp. Pharmacol. Physiol.*, 1979b, **6**, 53–59.

A. W. Jones, Inter- and intra-individual variations in the saliva/blood alcohol ratio during ethanol metabolism in man, *Clin. Chem.*, 1979c, **25**, 1394–1398.

A. W. Jones, Pharmacokinetics of ethanol in saliva: comparison with blood and breath alcohol profiles, subjective feeling of intoxication and diminished performance, *Clin. Chem.*, 1993, **39**, 1837–1844.

A. W. Jones, Measuring ethanol in saliva with the QED Enzymatic test device: comparison of results with blood and breath alcohol concentrations, *J. Anal. Toxicol.*, 1995, **19**, 169–174.

R. A. Jufer *et al.*, Elimination of cocaine and metabolites in plasma, saliva and urine following repeated oral administration to human volunteers, *J. Anal. Toxicol.*, 2000, **24**, 467–477.

C. Jurado *et al.*, Simultaneous quantification of opiates, cocaine and cannabinoids in hair, *Forensic Sci. Int.*, 1995, **70**, 165–174.

W. W. Just *et al.*, Detection of Δ^9-tetrahydrocannabinol in saliva of men by means of thin layer chromatography and mass spectrometry, *J. Chromatogr.*, 1974, **96**, 189–194.

K. S. Kalasinsky *et al.*, Study on drug distribution in hair by infrared microscopy visualization, *J. Anal. Toxicol.*, 1994, **18**, 337–341.

F. Kamali and S. H. Thomas, Effect of saliva flow rate on saliva phenytoin concentrations: implications for therapeutic monitoring, *Eur. J. Clin. Pharmacol.*, 1994, **46**, 565–567.

G. L. Kang and F. S. Abbott, Analysis of methadone and metabolites in biological fluids with GC/MS, *J. Chromatogr.*, 1982, **231**, 311–319.

L. Kangas *et al.*, Pharmacokinetics of nitrazepam in saliva and serum after a single oral dose, *Acta Pharmacol. Toxicol.*, 1979, **45**, 20–24.

G. Kauert and J. Röhrich, Concentrations of Δ^9-tetrahydrocannabinol, cocaine and 6-acetylmorphine in hair of drug abusers, *Int. J. Leg. Med.*, 1996, **108**, 294–299.

D. A. Kidwell, Analysis of phencyclidine and cocaine in human hair by tandem mass spectrometry, *J. Forensic Sci.*, 1993, **38**, 272–284.

D. A. Kidwell and D. L. Blank, in *Drug Testing in Hair*, P. Kintz (ed.), Boca Raton, CRC Press, 1996, pp. 17–68.

R. Kikura *et al.*, Hair analysis for drug abuse. XV. Disposition of MDMA and its related compounds into rat hair and application to hair analysis for MDMA abuse, *Forensic Sci. Int.*, 1997, **84**, 165–177.

I. Kim *et al.*, Plasma and oral fluid pharmacokinetics and pharmacodynamics after oral codeine administration, *Clin. Chem.*, 2002, **48**, 1486–1496.

P. Kintz, Clinical applications of hair analysis, in *Drug Testing in Hair*, P. Kintz (ed.), Boca Raton, CRC Press, 1996, pp. 267–277.

P. Kintz, Excretion of MBDB and BDB in urine, saliva and sweat following single oral administration, *J. Anal. Toxicol.*, 1997, **21**, 570–575.

P. Kintz, Hair testing and doping control in sport, *Toxicol. Lett.*, 1998, **102**, 109–113.

P. Kintz and N. Samyn, Use of alternative specimens: drugs of abuse in saliva and doping agents in hair, *Ther. Drug Monit.*, 2002, **24**, 239–246.

P. Kintz *et al.*, Nicotine analysis in neonates hair for measuring gestational exposure to tobacco, *J. Forensic Sci.*, 1993, **38**, 119–123.

P. Kintz *et al.*, Testing human hair and urine for anhydroecgonine methylester, a pyrolysis product of cocaine, *J. Anal. Toxicol.*, 1995a, **19**, 479–482.

P. Kintz *et al.*, Simultaneous determination of amphetamine, methamphetamine, MDA and MDMA in human hair by GC-MS, *J. Chromatogr. B*, 1995b, **670**, 162–166.

P. Kintz *et al.*, Testing human hair for cannabis. II. Identification of THC-COOH by GC-MS/NCI as a unique proof, *J. Forensic Sci.*, 1995c, **40**, 619–623.

P. Kintz *et al.*, Hair analysis for nordiazepam by GC-MS/NCI, *J. Chromatogr. B*, 1996, **677**, 241–244.

P. Kintz *et al.*, Codeine testing in sweat and saliva with the DrugWipe, *Int. J. Legal Med.*, 1998, **111**, 82–84.

P. Kintz *et al.*, Testing for anabolic steroids in human hair obtained from two bodybuilders, *Forensic Sci. Int.*, 1999, **101**, 209–216.

P. Kintz *et al.*, Doping control for β-adrenergic compounds through hair analysis, *J. Forensic Sci.*, 2000a, **45**, 170–174.

P. Kintz *et al.*, Pharmacological criteria that can affect the detection of doping agents in hair, *Forensic Sci. Int.*, 2000b, **107**, 325–334.

P. Kintz *et al.*, Detection of cannabis in oral fluid (saliva) and forehead wipes (sweat) from impaired drivers, *J. Anal. Toxicol.*, 2000c, **24**, 557–561.

P. Kintz *et al.*, Testing for GHB in hair by GC/MS/MS after a single exposure. Application to document sexual assault. *J. Forensic Sci.* 2003, **48**, 195–200.

P. Kintz *et al.*, Testing for the undetectable in drug-facilitated sexual assault using hair analyzed by tandem mass spectrometry as evidence. *Ther. Drug. Monit.* 2004, **26**, 211–214.

V. Kircher and H. Parlar, Determination of Δ^9-tetrahydrocannabiniol from human saliva by tandem immunoaffinity chromatography–high-performance liquid chromatography, *J. Chromatogr. B*, 1996, **677**, 245–255.

J. Klein *et al.*, Clinical applications of hair testing for drugs of abuse – the Canadian experience, *Forensic Sci. Int.*, 2000, **107**, 281–288.

E. Klug, Zur Morphinbestimmung in Kopfhaaren, *Z. Rechtsmed.*, 1980, **84**, 189–193.

R. Kronstrand *et al.*, Codeine concentration in hair after oral administration is dependent on melanin content, *Clin. Chem.*, 1999, **45**, 1485–1494.

G. Liang *et al.*, A rapid instrumented fluorescence immunoassay for the detection of tetrahydrocannabinols. *Proceedings of the International Council on Alcohol Drugs and Traffic Safety*, Stockholm, May 22–26, 2000.

M. Linnoila *et al.*, Psychomotor effects of diazepam in anxious patients and healthy volunteers, *J. Clin. Psychopharmacol.*, 1983, **3**, 88–96.

A. C. S. Lucas *et al.*, Solid-phase microextraction in determination of methadone in human saliva by GC/MS, *J. Anal. Toxicol.*, 2000, **24**, 93–96.

R. Lucek and R. Dixon, Chlordiazepoxide concentrations in saliva and plasma measured by RIA, *Res. Commun. Chem. Pathol. Pharmacol.*, 1980, **27**, 397–400.

F. U. Lutz *et al.*, Alco Screen – a reliable method for determining blood alcohol concentration by saliva alcohol concentration? *Blutalkohol*, 1993, **30**, 240–243.

R. K. Lynn *et al.*, The secretion of methadone and its major metabolites in the gastric juice of humans: comparison with blood and salivary concentrations, *Drug Metab. Dispos.*, 1975, **4**, 405–509.

M. Machnik *et al.*, Long-term detection of clenbuterol in human scalp hair by gas chromatography–high resolution mass spectrometry, *J. Chromatogr. B*, 1999, **723**, 147–155.

D. Malamud, Guidelines for saliva nomenclature and collection, *Ann. New York Acad. Sci.*, 1993, **694**, xi–xii.

C. Malcolm and J. S. Oliver, Methadone saliva:blood ratios in the methadone maintenance patients, in *Proceedings of the* 35th *TIAFT Meeting*, Padova, Italy, 1997, pp. 369–375.

P. Mangin, Drug analysis in nonhead hair, in *Drug Testing in Hair*, P. Kintz (ed.), Boca Raton, CRC Press, 1996, pp. 279–287.

C. Maseda *et al.*, Detection of Δ^9-THC in saliva by capillary GC/ECD after marihuana smoking, *Forensic Sci. Int.*, 1986, **32**, 259–266.

S. B. Matin *et al.*, Quantitative determination of enantiomeric compounds: simultaneous measurement of the optical isomers of amfetamine in human plasma and saliva using chemical ionization mass spectrometry, *Biomed. Mass Spectrom.*, 1977, **4**, 118–121.

M. M. McCarron *et al.*, Detection of phencyclidine usage by radioimmunoassay of saliva, *J. Anal. Toxicol.*, 1984, **8**, 197–201.

K. E. McColl *et al.*, Correlation of ethanol concentrations in blood and saliva, *Clin. Sci. (Colch)*, 1979, **56**, 283–286.

D. B. Menkes *et al.*, Salivary THC following cannabis smoking correlates with subjective intoxication and heart rate, *Psychopharmacology*, 1991, **103**, 277–279.

M. V. Miles *et al.*, Intraindividual variability of carbamazepine, phenobarbital and phenytoin concentrations in saliva, *Ther. Drug Monit.*, 1991, **13**, 166–171.

M. R. Moeller, Drug detection in hair by chromatographic procedures, *J. Chromatogr.*, 1992, **580**, 125–134.

M. R. Moeller *et al.*, Identification and quantitation of cocaine and its metabolites, benzoylecgonine and ecgonine methylester in hair of Bolivian coca chewers by GC-MS, *J. Anal. Toxicol.*, 1992a, **16**, 291–296.

M. R. Moeller *et al.*, MDMA in blood, urine and hair: a forensic case, in *Proceedings of the 30th Meeting TIAFT*, T. Nagata (ed.), Fukuoka, Yoyodo Printing Kaisha, 1992b, pp. 347–361.

M. R. Moeller *et al.*, Hair analysis as evidence in forensic cases, *Forensic Sci. Int.*, 1993, **63**, 43–53.

E. T. Moolchan *et al.*, Cocaine and metabolite elimination patterns in chronic cocaine users during cessation: plasma and saliva analysis, *J. Anal. Toxicol.*, 2000, **24**, 458–466.

L. Moore *et al.*, Gas chromatography/mass spectrometry confirmation of Cozart Rapiscan saliva methadone and opiates tests, *J. Anal. Toxicol.*, 2001, **25**, 520–524.

J. C. Mucklow *et al.*, Drug concentration in saliva, *Clin. Pharmacol. Ther.*, 1978, **24**, 563–570.

Y. Nakahara *et al.*, Hair analysis for drug abuse, Part II. Hair analysis for monitoring of methamphetamine abuse by isotope dilution GC-MS, *Forensic Sci. Int.*, 1990, **46**, 243–254.

Y. Nakahara *et al.*, Hair analysis for drugs of abuse. IV. Determination of total morphine and confirmation of 6-acetylmorphine in monkey and human hair by GC-MS, *Arch. Toxicol.*, 1992a, **66**, 669–674.

Y. Nakahara *et al.*, Hair analysis for drug abuse. III. Movement and stability of methoxyphenamine (as a model compound of methamphetamine) along hair shaft with hair growth, *J. Anal. Toxicol.*, 1992b, **16**, 253–257.

M. Navarro *et al.*, Usefulness of saliva for measurement of 3,4-methylenedioxymethamfetamine and its metabolites: correlation with plasma drug concentrations and effect of salivary pH, *Clin. Chem.*, 2001, **47**, 1788–1795.

A. Negrusz *et al.*, Highly sensitive micro-plate enzyme immunoassay screening and NCI-GC-MS confirmation of flunitrazepam and its major metabolite 7-aminoflunitrazepam in hair, *J. Anal. Toxicol.*, 1999, **23**, 429–435.

A. Negrusz *et al.*, Quantitation of clonazepam and its major metabolite 7-aminoclonazepam in hair, *J. Anal. Toxicol.*, 2000, **24**, 614–620.

A. Negrusz *et al.*, Deposition of aminoflunitrazepam and flunitrazepam in hair after a single dose of Rohypnol(r). *J. Forensic Sci.*, 2001, **46**,1143–1151.

A. Negrusz *et al.*, Deposition of 7–aminoclonazepam and clonazepam in hair following a single dose of Klonopin, *J. Anal. Toxicol.*, 2002, **26**, 471–478.

H. W. Newman and M. Abramson, Some factors influencing the intoxicating effect of alcoholic beverage, *J. Stud. Alcohol.*, 1942, **42**, 351–370.

R. S. Niedbala *et al.*, Detection of analytes by immunoassay using up-converting phosphor technology, *Anal. Biochem.*, 2001a, **293**, 22–30.

R. S. Niedbala *et al.*, Detection of marijuana use by oral fluid and urine analysis following single-dose administration of smoked and oral marijuana, *J. Anal. Toxicol.*, 2001b, **25**, 289–303.

L. Nishihara *et al.*, Estimation of plasma unbound phenobarbital concentration by using mixed saliva, *Epilepsia*, 1979, **20**, 37–45.

A. Ohlsson *et al.*, Single-dose kinetics of deuterium-labeled cannabidiol in man after smoking and intravenous administration, *Biomed. Environ. Mass Spectrom.*, 1986, **13**, 77–83.

C. L. O'Neal *et al.*, Correlation of saliva codeine concentrations with plasma codeine concentrations after oral codeine administration, *J. Anal. Toxicol.*, 1999, **23**, 452–459.

C. L. O'Neal *et al.*, The effects of collection method on oral fluid codeine concentrations, *J. Anal. Toxicol.*, 2000, **24**, 536–542.

L. Parton, Quantitation of fetal cocaine exposure by RIA of hair, *Pediatr. Res.*, 1987, **21**, 372A.

L. A. Pate *et al.*, Evaluation of a saliva alcohol test stick as a therapeutic adjunct in an alcoholism treatment program, *J. Stud. Alcohol*, 1993, **54**, 520–521.

H. W. Peel *et al.*, Detection of drugs in saliva of impaired drivers, *J. Forensic Sci.*, 1984, **29**, 185–189.

S. Pichini *et al.*, On-site testing of 3,4-methylenedioxymethamfetamine (Ecstasy) in saliva with DrugWipe and DrugRead: a controlled study in recreational users, *Clin. Chem.*, 2002, **48**, 174–176.

L. Pötsch and H. Leithoff, Fluoreszenzmikroskopische Untersuchungen zum Einbau von Fluorescein in Haare, *Rechtsmedizin*, 1992, **3**, 14–18.

W. A. Ritschel *et al.*, Absolute bioavailability of hydromorphone after peroral and rectal administration in humans: saliva/plasma ratio and clinical effects, *J. Clin. Pharmacol.*, 1987, **27**, 647–653.

L. Rivier, Is there a place for hair analysis in doping control? *Forensic Sci. Int.*, 2000, **107**, 309–323.

M. Rothe *et al.*, Hair concentrations and self-reported abuse history of 20 amphetamine and ecstasy users, *Forensic Sci. Int.*, 1997, **89**, 111–128.

H. Sachs, Forensic applications of hair analysis, in *Drug Testing in Hair*, P. Kintz (ed.), Boca Raton, CRC Press, 1996, pp. 211–222.

H. Sachs and W. Arnold, Results of comparative determination of morphine in human hair using RIA and GC-MS, *J. Clin. Chem. Clin. Biochem.*, 1989, **27**, 873–877.

H. Sachs and P. Kintz, Testing for drugs in hair. Critical review of chromatographic procedures since 1992, *J. Chromatogr. B*, 1998, **713**, 147–161.

H. Sachs and P. Kintz, Consensus of the Society of Hair Testing on hair testing for doping agents, *Forensic Sci. Int.*, 2000, **107**, 3.

H. Sachs and M. Uhl, Opiat-Nachweis in Haar-Extrakten mit Hilfe von GC-MS/MS und Supercritical Fluid Extraction, *Toxichem. Krimtech.*, 1992, **59**, 114–120.

M. Saitoh *et al.*, Rate of hair growth, in *Advances in Biology of Skin*, W. Montagna and R. L. Dobson (eds), Oxford, Pergamon Press, 1969, pp. 183–201.

N. Samyn and Van Haeren, On-site testing of saliva and sweat with DrugWipe and determination of concentrations of drugs of abuse in saliva, plasma and urine of suspected users, *Int. J. Legal Med.*, 2000, **113**, 150–154.

N. Samyn *et al.*, Plasma, oral fluid and sweat wipe ecstasy concentrations in controlled and real life conditions, *Forensic Sci. Int.*, 2002a, **128**, 90–97.

N. Samyn *et al.*, Detection of flunitrazepam and 7-aminoflunitrazepam in oral fluid after controlled administration of Rohypnol®, *J. Anal. Toxicol.*, 2002b, **26**, 211–215.

W. Schramm, Methods for simplified saliva collection for measurement of drugs of abuse, therapeutic drugs and other molecules, *Ann. New York Acad. Sci.*, 1993, **694**, 311–313.

W. Schramm and R. H. Smith, An ultrafiltrate of saliva collected in situ as a biological sample for diagnostic evaluation, *Clin. Chem.*, 1991, **37**, 114–115.

W. Schramm *et al.*, Drugs of abuse in saliva: a review, *J. Anal. Toxicol.*, 1992, **16**, 1–9.

W. Schramm *et al.*, Cocaine and benzoylecgonine in saliva, serum and urine, *Clin. Chem.*, 1993, **39**, 481–87.

M. E. Sharp *et al.*, Monitoring saliva concentrations of methaqualone, codeine, secobarbital, diphenydramine and diazepam after single oral doses, *J. Anal. Toxicol.*, 1983, **7**, 11–14.

J. H. Silverstein *et al.*, An analysis of the duration of fentanyl and its metabolites in urine and saliva, *Anesth. Analg.*, 1993, **76**, 618–621.

G. Skopp *et al.*, Saliva testing after single and chronic administration of dihydrocodeine, *Int. J. Legal Med.*, 2001, **114**, 133–140.

K. H. Smolle *et al.*, QED alcohol test: a simple and quick method to detect ethanol in saliva of patients in emergency departments. Comparison with the conventional determination in blood, *Intensive Care Med.*, 1999, **25**, 492–495.

I. M. Speckl *et al.*, Opiate detection in saliva and urine, a prospective comparison by gas chromatography–mass spectrometry, *J. Toxicol. Clin. Toxicol.*, 1999, **37**, 441–445.

V. R. Spiehler, On-site saliva testing for drugs of abuse, in *Onsite Testing for Drugs of Abuse*, A. Jenkins and B. Goldberger (eds), Totowa, Humana Press, 2001, pp. 95–109.

V. R. Spiehler *et al.*, Certainty and confirmation in toxicology screening, *Clin. Chem.*, 1988, **34**, 1535–1539.

V. R. Spiehler *et al.*, Cut-off concentrations for drugs of abuse in saliva for DUI, DWI or other driving-related crimes, in *Proceedings of the 1999 TIAFT Meeting*, Cracow, Z. Zagadnien Nauk Sadowych, 2000, pp. 160–168.

V. R. Spiehler *et al.*, Validation of Cozart Rapiscan cut-off concentrations for drugs of abuse in saliva, in *Proceedings of the 2000 TIAFT Meeting*, I. Rasanen (ed.), Helsinki, 2001, University of Helsinki, pp. 95–105.

S. Steinmeyer *et al.*, Practical aspects of roadside tests for administrative traffic offences in Germany, *Forensic Sci. Int.*, 2001, **121**, 33–36.

SAMHSA (Substance Abuse and Mental Health Services Administration), Mandatory Guidelines for Federal Workplace Drug Testing Programs 2000, www.health.org/workplace/manguidelines/draft3.htm.

S. Suzuki *et al.*, Analysis of methamfetamine in hair, nail, sweat and saliva by mass fragmentography, *J. Anal. Toxicol.*, 1989, **13**, 176–178.

F. Tagliaro *et al.*, Hair analysis, a novel tool in forensic and biomedical sciences: new chromatographic and electrophoretic/electrokinetic analytical strategies, *J. Chromatogr. B*, 1997, **689**, 261–271.

D. Thieme *et al.*, Analytical strategy for detecting doping agents in hair, *Forensic Sci. Int.*, 2000, **107**, 335–345.

L. K. Thompson *et al.*, Confirmation of cocaine in human saliva after intravenous use, *J. Anal. Toxicol.*, 1987, **11**, 36–38.

U. R. Tjaden *et al.*, Determination of some benzodiazepines and metabolites in serum, urine and saliva by HPLC, *J. Chromatogr.*, 1980, **181**, 227–241.

A. Tracqui *et al.*, HPLC/MS determination of buprenorphine and norbuprenorphine in biological fluids and hair samples, *J. Forensic Sci.*, 1997, **42**, 111–114.

G. C. Tu *et al.*, Characteristics of a new urine, serum and saliva alcohol reagent strip, *Alcohol Clin. Exp. Res.*, 1992, **16**, 222–227.

R. J. Turner, Mechanisms of fluid secretion by salivary glands, *Ann. New York Acad. Sci.*, 1993, **694**, 24–35.

M. Uhl, Determination of drugs in hair using GC-MS/MS, *Forensic Sci. Int.*, 1997, **84**, 281–294.

J. L. Valentine *et al.*, Simultaneous gas chromatographic determination of diazepam and its major metabolites in human plasma, urine and saliva, *Anal. Lett.*, 1982, **15**, 1665–1683.

M. Van der Graaff *et al.*, Pharmacokinetics of orally administered hexobarbital in plasma and saliva of healthy subjects, *Biopharm. Drug Dispos.*, 1986, **7**, 265–272.

S. H. Wan *et al.*, Kinetics, salivary excretion of amfetamine isomers and effect of urinary pH, *Clin. Pharmacol. Ther.*, 1978, **23**, 585–590.

W. L. Wang *et al.*, Simultaneous assay of cocaine, heroin and metabolites in hair, plasma, saliva and urine by GC-MS, *J. Chromatogr. B*, 1994, **660**, 279–290.

J. T. Wilson, Clinical correlates of drugs in saliva, *Ann. New York Acad. Sci.*, 1993, **694**, 48–56.

K. Wolff *et al.*, Methadone in saliva, *Clin. Chem.*, 1991, **37**, 1297–1298.

K. S. Wong, Over-the-counter preliminary alcohol screening devices, *California Assoc. Toxicol. Proc.*, 2002, **30**, 14–16.

G. S. Yacoubian *et al.*, A comparison of saliva testing to urinalysis in an arrestee population, *J. Psychoactive Drugs*, 2001, **33**, 289–294.

M. Yeggles *et al.*, Detection of benzodiazepines and other psychotropic drugs in human hair by GC-MS, *Forensic Sci. Int.*, 1997, **87**, 211–218.

Further reading

Y. H. Caplan and B. A. Goldberger, Alternative specimens for workplace drug testing, *J. Anal. Toxicol.*, 2001, **25**, 396–399.

R. K. Drobitch and C. K. Svensson, Therapeutic drug monitoring in saliva. An update, *Clin. Pharmacokinet.*, 1992, **23**, 365–79.

Drug Policy Alliance, Drug Testing Technologies: Sweat Patch, 2008. http://www.drugpolicy.org/law/drugtesting/sweatpatch_/ (accessed 28.01.08).

Federal Register, Vol. 69, No. 71 (April 13, 2004) Notices.

M. J. Follador *et al.*, Detection of cocaine and cocaethylene in sweat by solid-phase microextraction and gas chromatography/mass spectrometry, *J. Chromatogr. B*, 2004 Nov 5, **811**, 37–40.

R. Haeckel, The application of saliva in laboratory medicine, *J. Clin. Chem. Clin. Biochem.*, 1989, **27**, 221–252.

M. G. Horning *et al.*, Use of saliva in therapeutic drug monitoring, *Clin. Chem.*, 1977, **23**, 157–164.

O. R. Idowu and B. Caddy, A review of the use of saliva in the forensic detection of drugs and other chemicals, *J. Forensic Sci. Soc.*, 1982, **22**, 123–135.

T. Inoue and S. Seta, Analysis of drugs in unconventional samples, *Forensic Sci. Rev.*, 1992, **4**, 90–106.

W. J. Juski and R. L. Milsap, Pharmacokinetic principles of drug distribution in saliva, *Ann. New York Acad. Sci.*, 1993, **694**, 36–47.

S. L. Kacinko *et al.*, Disposition of cocaine and its metabolites in human sweat after controlled cocaine administration. *Clin Chem.*, 2005, **51**, 2085–2094.

D. Kidwell *et al.*, Testing for drugs of abuse in saliva and sweat, *J. Chromatogr. B*, 1998, **713**, 111–135.

H. J. Liberty *et al.*, Detecting cocaine use through sweat testing: multilevel modeling of sweat patch length-of-wear data. *J. Anal. Toxicol.*, 2004, **28**, 667–673.

J. C. Mucklow, The use of saliva in therapeutic drug monitoring, *Ther. Drug Monit.*, 1982, **4**, 229–247.

National Institute on Drug Abuse, NIDA Notes, Vol. 10, No. 5, 1995.

N. Samyn *et al.*, Analysis of drugs of abuse in saliva, *Forensic Sci. Rev.*, 1999, **11**, 1–19.

E. W. Schwilke *et al.*, Opioid disposition in human sweat after controlled oral codeine administration. *Clin. Chem.*, 2006, **52**, 1539–1545.

G. Skopp and L. Potsch, Perspiration versus saliva – basic aspects concerning their use in roadside drug testing, *Int. J. Legal Med.*, 1999, **112**, 213.

7

Postmortem toxicology

G R Jones

Introduction 191
Specimens and other exhibits 191
Analytical toxicology. 198
Interpretation of postmortem toxicology results. 207
Summary 216
References 216
Further reading 217

Introduction

Postmortem toxicology is used to determine whether alcohol, drugs or other poisons may have caused or contributed to the death of a person. It differs fundamentally from clinical toxicology, including therapeutic drug monitoring and emergency toxicology, which is used to assist in the clinical management of a living patient. While drug analysis in clinical toxicology shares some common approaches with postmortem analysis, such as the use of immunoassay, chromatography and mass spectrometry, clinical assays usually need to be modified to give acceptable results with the unique fluids and tissues encountered in postmortem cases. Compared with serum or plasma, and certainly with urine, whole blood contributes a large number of endogenous compounds (e.g. fatty acids, cholesterol and other sterols) that, although present in serum and plasma, are at much lower concentrations in those matrices. However, it is the greater difficulty of interpreting postmortem results that principally differentiates postmortem toxicology from clinical toxicology.

Specimens and other exhibits

Request, receipt and storage

It is the responsibility of the laboratory to advise its clients (e.g. coroner, medical examiner, lawyers, pathologist) what types and amounts of specimens are required for postmortem toxicology testing, and what preservative, if any, should be used. At least one tube of whole blood preserved with 1% sodium fluoride should be provided, to be reserved for testing for ethanol and drugs such as cocaine. Stomach contents and most tissues are usually provided unpreserved. A recommended list of specimens is given in Table 7.1 together with an indication of volumes required for analysis.

The laboratory should provide guidelines on specimen collection and storage as well as a requisition, to be completed by the submitter, which should be sent with the specimens to the laboratory. The requisition serves five primary purposes:

- it identifies the deceased and gives appropriate demographic information and case history (e.g. circumstances of death, relevant medical history, autopsy findings)

Table 7.1 List of recommended postmortem specimens for routine toxicology examination

Specimen	Quantity
Heart blood	25 mL
Peripheral blood	10 mL
Brain	100 g
Liver	100 g
Vitreous humour	All available
Bile	All available
Urine	All available up to 100 mL
Gastric contents	All available (or 100 g and record total present in stomach)

- it identifies the specific specimens and exhibits submitted
- it provides space to identify the testing required
- it identifies the submitter and serves as a chain-of-custody document
- it provides directions and information for packaging and transport of the specimens.

Each specimen must be labelled uniquely to identify the deceased from which the specimen was obtained (i.e. name or case number), and the specimen type. Figure 7.1 gives an example of a requisition for postmortem specimen analysis. The layout, terminology and exact content of such requisitions will vary depending on the particular jurisdiction but the information requested is universally applicable.

The extent of information requested depends on the jurisdiction in which the toxicologist is working. Where most samples are transferred internally within a medical examiner facility, department of forensic medicine or forensic toxicology laboratory, a less-detailed case history or autopsy summary may be required if it can be readily obtained later.

Upon receipt in the laboratory, the specimens submitted must be checked against the information given on the requisition. Where there is more than one specimen of the same type, each container should be labelled uniquely (e.g. A, B, C, . . .), since, with the exceptions of urine, vitreous humour and bile, postmortem specimens are not homogeneous and different containers of the same specimen type (e.g. blood) can sometimes have different drug concentrations. Receipt of the specimens must be recorded, on paper or electronically. That log should include:

- appropriate demographic information
- an adequate description of the specimen and its site of sampling (e.g. femoral blood)
- the approximate volume or mass
- the type of container (e.g. grey-stoppered tube)
- any abnormal appearance of the specimen (e.g. decomposed, heat denatured, bloody urine, and so on).

If preservative has been added to the specimen, as is often the case for blood samples, this should be noted in the log against the appropriate sample.

All laboratories that undertake postmortem toxicology should document the chain of custody. At a minimum, the laboratory should document what was received, from whom, by what means (by hand, courier, mail) and when. Storage of the specimens and exhibits should be secure, and access to specimens and case files should be limited to authorised laboratory personnel. Blood and other tissue specimens should be stored under refrigerated conditions between receipt at the laboratory and analysis. A record should be kept of each occasion the specimen is opened to remove an aliquot. The date when specimens are discarded or returned to the submitter should also be recorded. The length of retention of tissues by the laboratory may be a set period of time (e.g. 3 to 12 months agreed with the client), or the time required to complete any legal proceedings. In the UK there are strict rules on sampling and storage of human tissues and this extends to postmortem samples. Postmortem toxicological analysis is normally requested via the coroner and all samples are officially under his or her jurisdiction. Permission must be obtained from the coroner for disposal of samples.

Specimen types

The specimens available for analysis in postmortem cases may be numerous, or limited to

POSTMORTEM
TOXICOLOGY REQUEST

JUSTICE
Office of the Chief Medical Examiner

47601

SEE REVERSE FOR SPECIMEN AND HANDLING GUIDE

MEDICAL EXAMINER	M.E. LOCATION	NAME OF DECEDENT	SEX
PATHOLOGIST	DATE OF EXTERNAL/AUTOPSY	DATE OF DEATH	AGE
YOUR AUTOPSY NUMBER	EXTERNAL/AUTOPSY LOCATION	PLACE OF DEATH	CME NUMBER

OPERATOR OF VEHICLE/MACHINE? ☐ NO ☐ YES HISTORY OF ALCOHOL ABUSE? ☐ NO ☐ YES HISTORY OF OTHER SUBSTANCE ABUSE? ☐ NO ☐ YES

MEDICATION AVAILABLE/ PRESCRIBED: ______

MEDICAL HISTORY & CIRCUMSTANCES OF DEATH: ______

______

______

IS THERE AN ANATOMIC C.O.D. PRESENT? ☐ NO ☐ YES IS DEATH LIKELY DRUG OR SUBSTANCE RELATED? ☐ NO ☐ YES IS CAUSE PENDING TOXICOLOGY? ☐ NO ☐ YES

ANALYSIS REQUIRED: TOXICOLOGIST MAY EXTEND OR LIMIT ANALYSIS (SEE OVER…)

☐ BLOOD ALCOHOL ☐ OTHER (SPECIFY) ______ NOTE: **MINIMUM** 10 ML BLOOD REQUIRED FOR DRUG SCREEN

☐ CARBON MONOXIDE ☐ NO TESTS REQUESTED (SPECIMENS WILL BE STORED FOR 6 MONTHS)

SPECIMENS SUPPLIED KEY: C COLLECTED NC NOT COLLECTED NA NOT AVAILABLE

C NC NA URINE C NC NA LIVER ☐ ANTEMORTEM SPECIMENS (FOR DELAYED DEATHS):

C NC NA VITREOUS C NC NA STOMACH CONTENTS ______

C NC NA BILE C NC NA BLOOD: SPECIFY COLLECTION SITE: ______

CHAIN OF CUSTODY	INITIALS	DATE
MEDICAL EXAMINER/ PATHOLOGIST		
TRANSPORTED/ DELIVERED BY		
RECEIVED BY		

☐ OTHER SPECIMEN OR PARAPHERNALIA:

______

______

Send with specimen(s) to Toxicology

Figure 7.1 Example of a postmortem toxicology requisition from a Medical Examiner Office. CME, Chief Medical Examiner; C.O.D., cause of death.

blood or a single tissue, depending on the case history and preferences of the submitter. In a relatively recent death, blood, vitreous humour, at least one organ tissue (usually liver) and the gastric contents are commonly collected. However, in the case of severe decomposition, as may occur in a body which has been exposed outdoors for some time, muscle, hair and bone may be the only specimens available.

Although toxicology testing can theoretically be performed on almost any specimen, it is usually limited to those for which there is an appropriate database available to assist with interpretation of the results. This aspect is critical since an important aim of the analysis is to assist in determining the cause of death. An analytical result indicating that there is x µg/mL of drug Y in a sample is not useful unless a conclusion can be drawn as to whether drug Y at level x may or may not have contributed to death. Hence interpretation of results typically requires information on levels of a drug which may arise from therapeutic drug administration and, ideally, levels that may occur via overdose, abuse, poisoning, etc., particularly where these levels have been shown to be fatal.

Proper collection and preservation of postmortem specimens is critical, since there is usually no opportunity to go back for recollection of specimens at a later date as the body will probably have been cremated or buried.

Blood

In living patients the dose of a drug is most closely correlated with its concentration in blood or plasma. Blood has therefore been used as one of the primary specimens in postmortem toxicology. In most cases postmortem blood is relatively fluid and typically has numerous small clots. Sampling can usually be achieved with a syringe and large-gauge needle.

It used to be assumed that postmortem blood was more or less homogeneous in terms of where in the body it is sampled. It is not. Postmortem blood concentrations of many drugs may vary from site to site (see later) due to a process known as postmortem redistribution. As a result, much attention has been focused on the site of collection of postmortem blood samples.

A word of caution may be appropriate about specimen labelling. Samples simply labelled 'blood' may have been collected from almost anywhere in the body. Even samples labelled as 'heart' blood may not have been collected from the heart itself, but drawn blind through the chest wall, and may include pleural or chest fluid, pericardial fluid and even gastric contents if the death was traumatic. On occasion, it might be collected outside the body following a traumatic accident, as pooled blood in a body bag. As the awareness of postmortem redistribution grows, great faith is being placed in the analysis of subclavian and femoral blood compared with cardiac blood. However, the toxicologist should be wary of the anatomic purity of these specimens when large volumes are supplied, and should take this into account when offering an interpretation. Unless the femoral or subclavian veins are ligated, it is very likely that some blood will be drawn from other vessels. For example, a skilled pathologist or technician can sometimes draw as much as 50 mL blood from the femoral vein. However, the femoral vein is relatively small and it is highly likely that much of that volume will be drawn down from the larger iliac vein and inferior vena cava. It is difficult to collect more than 5–10 mL from a ligated femoral vein unless the leg is massaged.

Vitreous humour

Vitreous humour has been used for many years as the preferred specimen for postmortem confirmation of the ingestion of ethanol, since postmortem formation of ethanol (which has been demonstrated in blood and tissues) does not occur to any significant extent in vitreous humour. Even in the presence of elevated concentrations of glucose, fermentation does not occur because the interior of the eye is a sterile medium until the most advanced stages of decomposition. For this reason, vitreous humour is particularly useful for ethanol estimation in decomposing bodies. Vitreous humour has also been used increasingly for the measurement of drugs. For example, digoxin concentrations increase markedly in postmortem cardiac blood, but do not increase significantly in vitreous humour (Vorpahl and Coe 1978). Accordingly, vitreous digoxin concentrations give a better indication of perimortem concentrations than do those in heart blood. It has also been shown that monoacetylmorphine and cocaine may be more stable in vitreous humour than in blood (Lin *et al.* 1997). This presumably results from the relative lack of esterases in the eye as compared with blood. The main disadvantage of vitreous humour is its relatively small volume – about 3 mL in each eye. Another disadvantage is that there is relatively little information in the literature on the concentrations expected after therapeutic doses for most drugs. While the vitreous : blood ratio for some drugs is close to unity, it is considerably less than unity for many drugs. The concentrations of highly lipid-soluble drugs, such as benzodiazepines, are relatively low in vitreous humour compared with whole blood; concentrations of highly protein bound drugs, such as the tricyclic antidepressants, also tend to be much lower (Evenson and Engstrand 1989; Scott and Oliver 2001). The use of vitreous humour is therefore limited by the volume available, and the difficulty of interpretation of the results for many drugs.

Urine

Urine is a useful fluid for toxicology testing, as it comprises more than 99% water and contains relatively few endogenous substances that interfere with chromatography or immunoassay tests. However, there are three disadvantages with urine in postmortem work. Firstly, urine is only available in about 50% of deaths as it is fairly common for the bladder to be voided during the dying process. It is therefore unwise to develop an analytical protocol for postmortem testing that relies solely on the presence of urine for the detection of drugs. Secondly, many drugs are metabolised so extensively that the parent drug is not detected in urine, or is present only at a relatively low concentration. However, if the metabolites are searched for, urine can be a useful fluid, especially for inexpensive methods such as thin-layer chromatography (TLC), in which the metabolite patterns of the tricyclic antidepressants and phenothiazines can be diagnostic. The third disadvantage of urine is that urinary concentrations of most drugs are difficult, if not impossible, to interpret. The correlation between the concentration of drugs in urine and blood is extremely poor. The primary reason for this is that urine is not a circulating fluid but is a waste product collected in the bladder. The concentrations of drugs and metabolites in urine therefore depend on the time of urine formation relative to sampling and drug ingestion. Urine has the advantage of a longer detection window – i.e. drugs can often be detected in urine for a longer period than in blood.

Liver

While many tissues are collected and analysed in postmortem toxicology, liver is the most important. The main reasons are the large amount of tissue available, ease of collection and relative ease of sample preparation compared to other tissues. There is also a relatively large database of liver drug concentrations available in the literature compared to the amount of data for other tissues. Concentrations of many basic drugs are also higher in the liver compared to blood, making detection easier. For example, concentrations of the tricyclic antidepressants are roughly 10–50 times greater in the liver than the blood, partly because of the absorption of drugs from the small intestines by the hepatic portal system. Today, with more sensitive analytical methods, the majority of drugs are detected readily in the blood, and it is not necessary to rely on the liver for their detection. However, liver is an extremely valuable tissue for the analysis of drugs that undergo postmortem redistribution because concentrations in the liver are relatively stable after death. As a result of the increased stability of drug concentrations in liver, analysis of this tissue can be a valuable aid in the interpretation of postmortem toxicology results. Liver concentrations can fall slightly after death through diffusion, although this effect is quantitatively minor. It has also been demonstrated that some local increases in drug concentration can occur because of postmortem diffusion of drugs from the stomach. The only major disadvantage of the liver as a specimen is that it tends to be fatty and can putrefy faster than blood. It is therefore important that analytical methods incorporate some type of clean-up step, and are robust enough to minimise the matrix effect of the tissue.

Stomach contents

Stomach (or gastric) contents are valuable for two primary reasons. After overdosage, drug concentrations in the stomach may be quite high, even after the majority of the drug has passed into the small intestine. Analysis of the stomach contents is uncomplicated by metabolism, so drugs that are metabolised extensively in the body may be detected unchanged. Similarly, drugs that may be difficult to detect in the blood because of extensive distribution in the body might be detected readily in the stomach. In some cases, where death occurred relatively shortly after drug ingestion, it may be possible to see remains of tablets or capsules. If these are sufficiently intact, it may be possible to search them against drug identification databases such as TICTAC (TicTac Communications Ltd.) or, if this is not possible, to analyse a sample of the tablet or capsule to identify the drug. The disadvantage of stomach contents is its composition, which varies from a thin watery fluid to a semisolid, depending on the amount and type of food present. The interpretative value of stomach contents lies in confirming the consumption of an oral overdose. If the total amount of drug detected in the stomach contents is significantly greater than the prescribed dose, the possibility of drug abuse or an overdose should be considered. There are, however, two important caveats. Firstly, stomach contents are rarely homogeneous, and therefore it is difficult to measure accurately the representative concentration of drug in the volume of stomach contents received, unless the contents are homogenised. Most chromatographic assays are based on volumes as small as 1 mL or less, and the potential for sampling errors is consequently great. The second reason why the accurate estimation of a dose in the gastric contents is difficult is that the total stomach contents are often not sent to the laboratory, only a portion being subsampled at autopsy and submitted. Results should therefore be reported as the amount of drug present in the volume or mass of stomach contents received. Specimen collection guidelines should encourage pathologists to submit the complete stomach contents rather than an aliquot.

There are two misconceptions regarding interpretation of drug concentrations in the stomach. Firstly, the concentration (as distinct from the amount) of a substance in the stomach contents is virtually meaningless by itself. Shortly after a therapeutic dose, the concentration of a drug in the stomach may be very high, even if the total amount is not. Secondly, the absence of a large amount of residual drug in the stomach does not necessarily rule out an oral overdose. It may take several hours to die from a drug overdose, during which most or all of the drug could have passed from the stomach to the small intestine, or even have been largely absorbed. On the other hand, consumption of an oral overdose of medicine can result in a formation of a medicine 'mass' or bezoar in the stomach, which may take several hours or even a day or more to dissipate. High concentrations of some drugs can delay gastric emptying. It must therefore be accepted that gastric drug concentrations should never be interpreted on the same basis as those for blood. The detection of a drug or metabolite in the stomach contents does not necessarily mean that the drug was taken orally. Gastric juice is constantly being secreted into the stomach, which in turn is formed from extracellular fluid; this may contain significant amounts of basic drugs and metabolites circulating in the blood. It is also important to bear in mind that gastric juice may have been contaminated with bile from retching or vomiting. In overdose patients administered oral charcoal, large amounts of charcoal in the stomach lead to an underestimation of the total amount of drug present. A review of the record of any antemortem clinical treatment should highlight this possibility.

Other fluids, tissues and organs

Bile has been collected historically, although its usefulness is limited. Previously, bile was valuable because it contains high concentrations of drug conjugates, most notably morphine. Detection of morphine and many other drugs (e.g. benzodiazepines, colchicine and buprenorphine) is, therefore, more likely in the bile than in the blood, in which concentrations may be as much as 1000 times lower. The possibility that drugs in the bile may undergo enterohepatic re-circulation should not be overlooked. With the widespread use of sensitive immunoassays and other techniques, the use of bile as a screening specimen is therefore less valuable than it once was. In addition, bile, like urine, is a waste fluid and, with the possible exception of ethanol, the correlation between blood and bile concentrations of drugs is generally poor.

Brain, kidney and spleen have been used to determine and interpret the concentrations of drugs or other toxins. Brain, and indeed other organ tissues, can be useful in assessing the overall body burden of the drug, although the database of reference values that may assist interpretation is limited. The brain offers the additional advantage that it is a relatively isolated organ and should be unaffected by trauma to the abdomen and chest, although concentrations of many drugs may vary from one region of the brain to another. The measurement of drugs in the brain may therefore be misleading unless the origin of the tissue analysed is identified and there is an adequate database regarding concentrations in that anatomic region.

Drug concentrations in the kidney and spleen have little intrinsic significance, other than as part of the overall assessment of the body burden of a toxin, although the kidney has been found to be useful in determining heavy metal concentrations. Spleen has been used as a secondary specimen for toxins, such as carbon monoxide and cyanide, that bind to haemoglobin.

Injection sites

Forensic folklore indicates that injection sites may be valuable for determining whether someone has been injected with a drug or poison. However, proof of intravenous injection through the analysis of excised tissue around the suspected injection site is unlikely to be convincing, because the drugs will probably be swept away rapidly by the blood circulation. Arguably, a botched injection might leave an extravascular residue. Subcutaneous injection sites offer a better chance of detection, since absorption from them is considerably slower. In either case, it is critical that a control site be excised, for example from the opposite side of the body, in order that it can be analysed alongside the suspected injection sample to compare tissue concentrations. It is easily forgotten that most drugs and other toxins are distributed to virtually every tissue and fluid in the body.

Nasal swabs

Some pathologists collect intranasal samples using cotton-tipped swabs in an attempt to demonstrate nasal administration. However, the same principles apply as for proving a drug was injected at a particular site and interpretation should be undertaken with caution. Using cocaine as an example, if the drug is used one would expect to find small amounts of cocaine, and certainly cocaine metabolites such as benzoylecgonine, in the nasal passage, just through normal secretions. Therefore, without a difficult quantitative assessment, the simple detection of cocaine or its metabolites in nasal swabs does not prove that cocaine was snorted.

Syringes and other items

Detection of some drugs, and particularly non-drug poisons, may be considerably easier in items found at the scene than through analysis of blood alone, and might also assist interpretation of the results. For example, residues of partially dissolved medications found in a drinking glass at a scene of death can be a strong indicator of suicidal intent. Other containers used to mix poisons prior to suicidal consumption (or homicidal administration) can also be useful to the toxicologist. Some pesticides are not detected readily in blood using routine screening procedures but can be detected much more easily in the concentrated residue in a container. Similarly, some potent drugs that are difficult to detect in blood or tissues may be detected in syringes. For example, the interpretation of blood morphine concentrations may be influenced by whether they resulted from use of morphine or diamorphine. Since diamorphine rapidly breaks down in blood, and monoacetylmorphine is only slightly more stable, proof of the use of diamorphine may depend on circumstantial evidence, such as detecting a residue in a syringe. Similarly, finding insulin in a syringe near a person who was not a known diabetic is useful circumstantial evidence of insulin administration. It is otherwise extremely difficult to prove hypoglycaemia in a dead person.

Antemortem specimens

Not infrequently, victims of an accident or overdose may be admitted to hospital, albeit sometimes surviving only briefly, before they die. When that occurs, it is common for blood and sometimes urine and gastric contents to be collected as part of the medical evaluation and treatment. There are at least two reasons why collection and analysis of antemortem specimens can be invaluable, even if death occurs fairly soon after admission to hospital. Firstly, analysis of hospital admission specimens gives a good idea of the circulating blood concentration at the time of admission to the hospital, which by definition is unaffected by postmortem redistribution, and may provide the only reliable indicator of dosage. Secondly, the antemortem specimen may provide the sole opportunity to perform meaningful toxicology if the person survives long enough for alcohol or drugs to be cleared from the body prior to death, or to be diminished to a concentration of limited or no forensic value. Even if blood or plasma collected on admission is not available, clearly timed specimens drawn several hours later may still be useful if allowance is made for clearance and for the presence of drugs administered as part of treatment.

There are some caveats. Blood collected for clinical purposes is usually centrifuged to separate serum or plasma for testing on clinical analysers. However, once separated, the serum or plasma may not be resealed after analysis. This will allow ethanol and other volatile substances such as solvents to evaporate and this possibility should be taken into account if the sample is analysed subsequently for forensic purposes, sometimes several days later. Another problem that can occur with clinical samples is the deterioration of some drugs in unpreserved serum, most notably cocaine. Intuitively, a serum or plasma specimen collected in the casualty or emergency department might be expected to contain higher concentrations of unchanged cocaine than a postmortem blood sample collected later. However, this is often not the case, because postmortem blood is often collected in tubes containing sodium fluoride which inhibits cocaine hydrolysis, whereas clinical samples are typically unpreserved.

Analytical toxicology

Scope of testing

One reason why postmortem toxicology is so challenging is that, in theory, it can require a search for any drug or poison of toxicological significance. However, this approach, while idealistic, is not practicable for any laboratory that receives many hundreds or thousands of cases each year. A more practical approach includes a search for the common drugs of abuse, prescription and non-prescription drugs, followed, as necessary, by specific analyses as indicated by the case history. Any laboratory that claims to perform general 'drug screening' should, at a minimum, have protocols that include gas chromatography (GC) and mass spectrometry (MS) or, as is becoming more common, liquid chromatography–mass spectrometry (LC-MS) and that are not limited to a panel of immunoassay assay screens (e.g. for drugs of abuse). Other substances may be included, depending on the case history. Carbon monoxide should be tested for in garage-related deaths, or circumstances in which malfunctioning fossil-fuel devices are a possibility (e.g. house furnace/boiler, propane-powered devices). Deaths caused by cyanide are often occupationally related (e.g. metal plating, geology, agriculture). In practice, the laboratory investigation is directed by information received from the submitter of the specimens, including basic details of the circumstances of death and the key autopsy findings. No matter how good the laboratory is, some relatively common prescription and non-prescription drugs are not detected readily by commonly used methods. Also, in some geographical regions, particularly those devoted to large-scale agriculture and with relatively limited access to drugs, deaths caused by pesticides and rodenticides may be common, which necessitates a modified approach to drug screening (see Chapter 4). The scope of laboratory testing may vary considerably with case history and is often progressive. Initial negative findings after preliminary testing may prompt further discussions with investigators or pathologists. The death may involve drugs or other poisons that are not detected readily by the screening methods used by the laboratory.

Screening and detection

As noted above, postmortem toxicological analysis usually starts with a drug screen. Certainly, a drug screen can never be a single test, and most commonly is an open-ended panel of tests designed to detect the maximum number of substances of toxicological interest. This approach has often been called a search for the 'general unknown'. Careful distinction must be made between this open-ended approach and a panel or targeted approach, in which the testing protocol only detects specific substances or classes of substances (e.g. drugs of abuse). Such an approach should not be referred to as a drug screen because this misleads the reader of a report into believing that a broader range of substances has been tested for than can possibly be the case. Targeted testing is sometimes justified where the case history strongly indicates that a specific substance is involved, particularly where that substance is not detected by the methods usually employed in the 'general unknown' approach. However, most experienced toxicologists have encountered instances in which the suspected drug was not found, with an entirely different substance detected in a clearly fatal amount. There can be several reasons for this. It may be that the person has consumed some other person's medication. Or it may be that the medications reportedly found at the scene were not those taken. In suicidal deaths, it is not uncommon for the victim or the family to try to hide the evidence of overdose.

In most forensic laboratories a drug screen consists of a panel of immunoassay tests and headspace analysis for alcohol and other volatile substances, combined with one or more broad-based GC or high-performance liquid chromatography (HPLC) procedures, and sometimes TLC and other techniques. The GC screening tests frequently use a nitrogen–phosphorus detector (NPD), since the vast majority of drugs contain nitrogen, and therefore give a response in the detector, whereas non-nitrogenous compounds, such as fatty acids, cholesterol and other lipids, do not. Similarly, most HPLC systems use ultraviolet (UV) or diode array detectors, since the vast majority of drugs absorb light in the region between 210 and 350 nm. However, increasingly, as technology improves and prices decrease, MS is replacing NPDs and electron-capture detectors in GC and in HPLC systems. Virtually all these approaches require some form of specimen preparation and chromatographic techniques such as TLC, GC and HPLC typically require sample extraction.

Specimen preparation and extraction

The first stage of the analytical process involves separation of the drug or compound of interest from the biological matrix in which it is contained. Urine and other nonviscous fluid specimens do not usually require treatment prior to extraction. However, even for relatively fluid blood samples, volumetric measurement with a positive displacement pipette designed for viscous samples, or gravimetric sampling, is preferred. The use of standard glass pipettes is discouraged as being inaccurate with viscous samples. Liquid–liquid extraction or solid-phase extraction (SPE) are both appropriate procedures for extracting drugs from urine and blood. Clotted blood may be homogenised in water or buffer prior to analysis.

The extraction of drugs from solid tissues requires the tissue matrix to be broken down to release drugs into an environment from which they are accessible for solvent extraction. This can be achieved by homogenisation, acid or alkaline hydrolysis, or enzyme digestion. Direct solvent extraction before or after acid or enzymatic digestion has almost superseded the classic protein-precipitation methods. The more sensitive detection methods of GC-MS and LC-MS mean that much smaller amounts of tissue can be processed. Consequently, any emulsion problems that arise are resolved more easily than in the past, when several hundred grams of liver and large volumes of solvent were required. The use of protein-precipitation reagents, such as barium chloride, zinc sulfate and tungstic acid, is discouraged for quantitative work because a significant portion of the analyte may be co-precipitated with the coagulated protein and therefore lost to the analysis.

Homogenisation

Tissues may be homogenised in water or buffer (e.g. Tris buffer). A dilution of one part tissue plus three parts water is common and gives a homogenate sufficiently thin to be pipetted easily, although some laboratories use one part tissue to nine parts water. Use of an efficient homogeniser, such as those that have a 'probe' design that blends, shears and cuts, is preferable. Older-style Waring (food-processor style) blenders or 'stomachers' are less efficient. Tissue homogenates may be analysed without further treatment if they have been prepared with an efficient homogeniser and the assay uses a good internal standard. Care should be taken to prevent exposure of the operator to aerosols that might be formed during the homogenisation process.

A typical procedure is as follows: weigh 5 g liver or other tissue, and cut into small pieces with scissors or a scalpel. Place the tissue in a suitable tube or small beaker and add 15 mL distilled water. Homogenise the tissue to a uniform consistency. For liver and most other tissues, 1–2 mL can subsequently be extracted directly using the protocol in Figure 7.2 for basic drugs. The protocol will extract basic drugs but leave behind lipids and sterols such as cholesterol. The protocol described in Figure 7.3 may be applied for acidic and many neutral drugs. For difficult tissues, e.g. those with a large amount of connective tissue, the enzymatic digestion described below may be useful.

Enzymatic digestion of tissues

Enzymatic digestion involves the use of a robust proteolytic enzyme, such as subtilisin Carlsberg, to digest the tissue to yield an essentially aqueous matrix for extraction, and is suitable for general screening as well as for more specific analysis. It is simple, readily adaptable and provides a protein-free filtrate from which any drugs present may be extracted. It also provides enhanced extraction of many drugs compared with the tungstate, ammonium sulfate, or Stas–Otto methods.

A suitable procedure is as follows: macerate 10 g of liver or other tissue with 40 mL of 1 M tris(hydroxymethyl)methylamine; add 10 mg of subtilisin Carlsberg and incubate in a water-bath at 50–60°C for about 1 h, with agitation. Filter the digest through a small plug of glass wool to remove undissolved connective tissue. Aliquots of this digest may be substituted for the specified biological fluid in most routine screening procedures. The filtered digest has a pH of 8.0 to 9.5.

This method is very useful for the analysis of sectioned injection marks. The superficial fatty skin layer is removed and the remaining muscle layer is analysed as above. If the injection was intramuscular and of recent origin, the drug concentrations should be greater than in a similar tissue sample that does not show an injection mark. If the injection was intravenous, such a distinction cannot be expected. As noted under Injection sites, a sample remote from the suspect injection site should also be analysed as a control for comparison purposes. The enzymatic digestion method's superb ability to 'liquidise' solid tissue can be used for many purposes apart from drug analysis. The recovery of shotgun pellets and small bomb fragments in body tissues is one such application. The preparation of solutions for direct aspiration into atomic absorption instruments for the detection of some metals has also been studied (Lock *et al.* 1981), and its use for the detection of toxic anions and some pesticides also seems feasible.

Drugs that form glucuronide conjugates may be hydrolysed with β-glucuronidase prior to extraction. For example, the determination of morphine in blood is often performed with and without the addition of β-glucuronidase to estimate the unconjugated (free) and 'total' (conjugated plus unconjugated) drug present, and therefore to aid interpretation. Other applications include enhanced detection of benzodiazepines and other drugs in blood and urine.

A typical procedure for the enzymatic hydrolysis of glucuronides is to mix 1 mL blood or urine with internal standard and 1.5 mL buffer and then to add 100 μL of β-glucuronidase obtained from *Helix pomatia*. Mix the solution and allow to incubate at 37°C overnight (ca. 16 h). After incubation, the pH of the solution is adjusted appropriately for solvent extraction or SPE of the drugs of interest.

Acid hydrolysis may be used to cleave glucuronide conjugates. Although more rapid than enzymatic hydrolysis, this method is 'harsher' and should be restricted to acid-stable analytes such as morphine in urine. Acid hydrolysis of blood dramatically increases the amount of potentially interfering substances and may produce a denatured protein mass that reduces analyte recovery.

Liquid–liquid extraction still predominates in most laboratories. The choice of an appropriate solvent is often a matter of experience or tradition. The chosen solvent should ideally extract as much of the target analyte as possible, while minimising the extraction of endogenous substances. Ideally, a solvent should extract the target analyte with a reproducible efficiency of at least 50%, and preferably much higher.

The pH of the specimen influences the extent to which acid and basic drugs are extracted. Addition of a weakly basic buffer, such as sodium borate (pH 9), favours the extraction of weakly basic drugs, as well as most neutral substances. Similarly, the addition of an acidic buffer, such as sodium dihydrogenphosphate, favours the extraction of acidic as well as neutral drugs. The majority of drugs of forensic interest are 'basic' in character, but are often present at relatively low concentrations in blood. It is therefore desirable to have an extraction scheme that incorporates a back-extraction step to eliminate or minimise the extraction of endogenous molecules. An example extraction scheme is shown in Figure 7.2. The sodium hydroxide will force the basic drugs into the lipid-soluble un-ionised form, allowing extraction into the chlorobutane. The chlorobutane is transferred to a fresh tube and the drugs are back-extracted into sulfuric acid. Neutral or acidic substances will remain in the upper chlorobutane layer, which may be pipetted or aspirated to waste. The remaining acid layer is then made basic by addition of sodium hydroxide, and the now un-ionised basic drugs re-extracted with chlorobutane. The upper solvent layer may then be removed and concentrated under nitrogen, prior to analysis by a suitable chromatographic method. This extraction scheme will give extracts that are relatively free of interfering substances. However, it should be noted that morphine and other amphoteric drugs cannot be detected by this method since the phenolic functional group will ionise at high pH, precluding extraction into the solvent. For amphoteric drugs, the basic phase should be less than pH 9.0, and preferably pH 8.0–8.5.

While a similar extraction scheme to that used for basic drugs (but with the additions of acid and base reversed to those of the scheme shown in Fig. 7.2), could be used for strongly acidic drugs, such a method does not efficiently

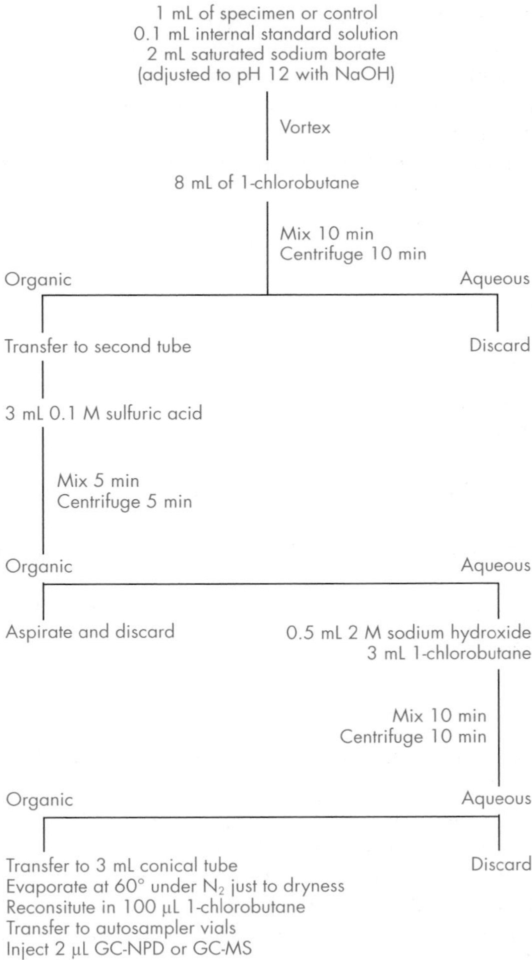

Figure 7.2 Extraction pathway for strong bases.

extract weakly acidic drugs, such as the barbiturates, and neutral drugs, such as meprobamate. Conversely, simple addition of an acidic buffer to whole blood and extraction with a solvent results in the co-extraction of large amounts of endogenous lipid substances. Such extracts may be 'cleaned up' by partitioning between immiscible solvents of different polarities, such as acetonitrile and hexane, as shown in Figure 7.3. The more polar drugs tend to partition into the acetonitrile, whereas the endogenous lipids (fatty acids, sterols) tend to partition into the hexane.

Solid-phase extraction (SPE) has been used for many years in clinical toxicology, although to a lesser extent for postmortem work. SPE usually results in better extraction efficiencies than liquid–liquid methods, especially for more polar analytes. One of the major obstacles to general acceptance in this field has been the difficult nature of postmortem specimens, which are often clotted and laden with solid material that can easily plug the fine material in SPE columns.

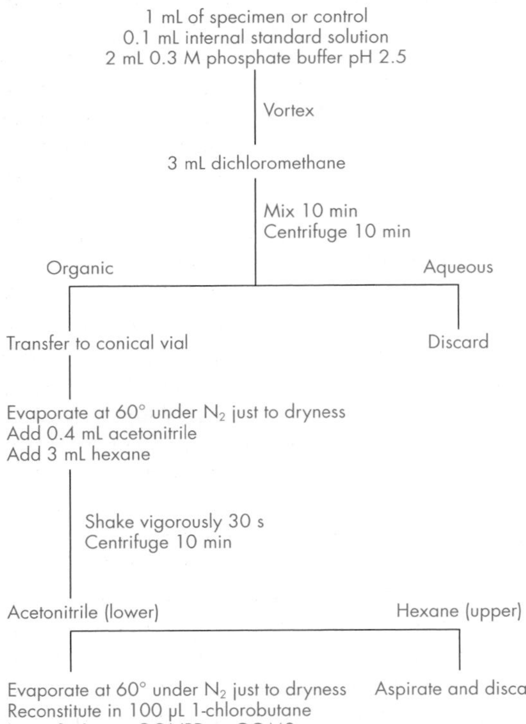
1 mL of specimen or control
0.1 mL internal standard solution
2 mL 0.3 M phosphate buffer pH 2.5
Vortex
3 mL dichloromethane
Mix 10 min
Centrifuge 10 min
Organic
Aqueous
Transfer to conical vial
Discard
Evaporate at 60° under N_2 just to dryness
Add 0.4 mL acetonitrile
Add 3 mL hexane
Shake vigorously 30 s
Centrifuge 10 min
Acetonitrile (lower)
Hexane (upper)
Evaporate at 60° under N_2 just to dryness
Reconstitute in 100 μL 1-chlorobutane
Inject 2 μL onto GC-NPD or GC-MS
Aspirate and discard

Figure 7.3 Extraction pathway for acids and neutrals.

However, improvements in sample preparation techniques and SPE column technology have largely overcome these problems. Use of a good internal standard, appropriate dilution of the sample and centrifugation of residual solid material usually results in a solution that does not plug the column and for which quantitative determination has not been compromised. Despite the inclusion of wash steps, the higher extraction efficiency of SPE columns compared with liquid–liquid extractions can sometimes result in dirtier extracts, although this need not be a problem if specific (e.g. MS) detection methods are used. Manufacturers of SPE columns readily provide sample extraction protocols.

Forensic identification and confirmation

The forensic toxicology profession and the courts have increasingly demanded that the identification of a substance be beyond reasonable scientific doubt. The principle has long been established that forensic identification of an analyte requires the use of two techniques that employ different physical and chemical principles (SOFT/AAFS Guidelines Committee 2006). This approach has the advantage that two completely different scientific techniques are used, which are supportive in arriving at a positive result. It has been argued that forensically acceptable detection and identification of an analyte can be achieved by a single extraction of a postmortem sample followed by GC-MS analysis of that extract. The argument is that GC-MS is a combination of two very different analytical methods – separation of the mixture and determination of retention time being one, and production of the mass spectrum being the other. While this approach is reasonable, it produces a forensically acceptable confirmation only if laboratory contamination and, if possible, contamination of the original specimen can be ruled out. Therefore, at a minimum, the drug should be detected using two different extracts of the same specimen. This is often accomplished incidentally, because separate extracts may be prepared for the initial drug screen and for a subsequent quantitative analysis. Even better is detection and identification of the substance in two different specimens. An example might be detection and identification in a urine specimen, followed by quantification in blood and one or more other tissues. This latter approach increases confidence in the result by ruling out a false-positive finding through contamination from glassware or, indeed, one of the specimens.

Identification of a drug by the use of two similar methods, such as two different immunoassays, is not acceptable, even though such tests may employ different endpoint reactions (e.g. fluorescence polarisation immunoassay (FPIA) and enzyme immunoassay (EIA)). The reason is that the antibodies used may have similar cross-reactivities, even though the designs of the immunoassays as a whole differ. Similarly, identification of a substance on the basis of different retention times (or different relative retention) on two different GC columns is rarely acceptable unless it can be shown clearly that the columns differ markedly in their retention and discrimination characteristics. It should be borne in mind that retention time in GC is dependent on the distribution constant (K) of a substance, that is how it partitions between the stationary phase and the mobile phase, which in the case of GC is a gas. Hence if K is the same for a drug and another substance present in the sample, even if a longer GC column with the same stationary phase is used for the analysis, the two substances will still have the same retention time on the longer column. Thus the emphasis is on selecting a second GC column for which K is different for the drug and the interfering substance.

A caveat to this approach involves simultaneous detection and quantification of ethanol and other specific analytes, such as carbon monoxide. Although two independent methods may be used to identify ethanol, it is still generally accepted that a single GC method is forensically acceptable. Analysis of alcohol using two different columns with non-correlating stationary phases and internal standards provides much greater confidence. The quality of GC methods used in most laboratories, and the fact that few other compounds are likely to be present at such a high concentration, means that erroneous identification of ethanol is unlikely. The few other compounds include methanol, isopropanol and acetone, for which separation from ethanol in the analytical system must be demonstrated. Similar arguments can be made for carbon monoxide, especially when the history clearly indicates that carbon monoxide poisoning is likely. However, in rare circumstances grossly elevated carbon monoxide concentrations may be detected where there is not an obvious source of the poison. In such instances, confirmation by an independent technique is highly desirable (e.g. headspace GC or palladium chloride via a Conway diffusion cell).

Quantification of drugs and other toxins

The vast majority of drugs, metabolites and other toxins are quantified by GC or HPLC, increasingly in combination with MS detection. Simple GC or HPLC detection is usually based on the total peak area produced by the detector (e.g. NPD, flame ionisation detection (FID), UV, diode array detection (DAD)). GC-MS quantification, while it can be based on the total ion signal, is more usually based on the peak area for specific ion fragments – called selected-ion monitoring (SIM). For liquid chromatography coupled to mass spectrometry, MS-MS is more commonly employed to provide sensitivity and specificity. Quantification is still based on peak areas, typically of the product ion of the MS-MS transition monitored. By its nature, SIM GC-MS or LC-MS/MS quantification is considerably more specific and often more sensitive than use of the more traditional GC or LC detectors. This is of particular importance in postmortem work, in which endogenous lipids and putrefactive products can produce significant interference. Other than detection techniques, there are two other major considerations in quantitative postmortem work. The first is the reproducibility and robustness of the extraction procedure. The second is the choice of an appropriate calibration method. Use of an appropriate assay design and sound extraction and calibration methods can minimise the effect of the matrix, especially if the calibrators are prepared in a similar matrix to that being analysed.

Calibration methods

Choice of an appropriate calibration method is critical to obtaining reliable results. Single-point calibrations are generally unacceptable for postmortem toxicology, unless it can be shown that the calibration is stable, reproducible and linear over the desired range, and that appropriate controls are used to validate the calibrations when specimens are being analysed. Multipoint calibrations are preferred, unless the calibration is known to be very stable and linear (e.g. GC-FID headspace ethanol analysis). A minimum of three calibration points is usually recommended, although five or more are preferred, depending on the linearity and precision of the method. An appropriate internal standard is considered almost essential for all GC- or HPLC-based methods to help minimise matrix effects and also to correct for other variables, such as slight differences in transfer volumes when using liquid–liquid extraction or SPE. An internal standard should ideally be similar in chemical structure to the target analyte (e.g. an alkyl analogue). Use of stable isotope analogues (e.g. deuterated) is preferred, where available, because these analogues are virtually identical chemically to their non-deuterated counterparts and hence behave in the same way through sample extraction and analysis. They can only be used where the detection method can differentiate between the deuterated and non-deuterated analogues, meaning that their use is generally linked with MS detection. A good internal standard can provide much greater accuracy and precision than would otherwise be possible with difficult postmortem specimens. Quantitative results are only acceptable if the analyte concentration lies within the validated calibration range (Fig. 7.4). If the concentration lies outside that range, it may be reported as greater than or less than the calibration range, as appropriate, or additional calibrators or controls could be run to validate the calibration in that range. Standard calibration lines should not be extrapolated (Fig. 7.4) and if an accurate result is required when the initial quantification lies outside the scope of the standard curve, the specimen should be diluted and re-analysed.

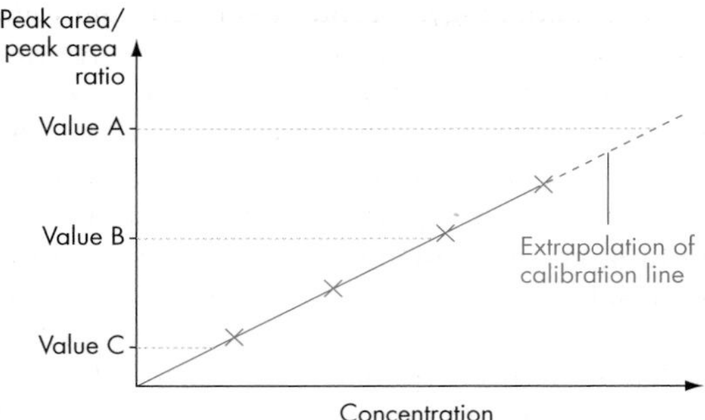

Figure 7.4 Illustration of a calibration line showing values for samples within and outside values for calibrators. Value B lies within the range of the calibrators and can be considered acceptable. Values for A and C are outside the range. Further calibrators should be prepared covering the range for samples A and C. In the case of sample A, it may be possible to dilute the sample and reanalyse using the same set of calibrators if quantification uses peak areas (if peak area ratios are used, then the ratio will not change even if the sample is diluted). Extrapolation of the line to include value A is not correct as the accuracy of the result cannot be guaranteed, although it may be permissible in some circumstances.

Ideally, an assay calibration should be linear and produce a good correlation coefficient (e.g. better than 0.98). Not infrequently the calibration line will be nonlinear and may require a quadratic fit. Some GC or HPLC assays are inherently nonlinear. For example, at very high or low concentrations, ions common to both the analyte and internal standards may cause a deviation from linearity. A large deviation from linearity usually indicates the use of an inappropriate internal standard, poor chromatography, poor analyte recovery during the extraction or that the dynamic range of the detector has been exceeded.

The method of standard addition can be useful in quantitative postmortem analysis. In essence, the specimen being analysed is used as the matrix to prepare calibrators. Preparing standards in solvents is rarely acceptable in toxicological analysis because it does not take into account losses which will occur during extraction processes. Hence the norm is to spike a known mass of the target analyte into a portion of the same matrix as is being analysed. For postmortem toxicology, blood, liver, etc. sampled from a body which may have been recovered some time after death may be in a rather different condition from fresh blood and hence the analyte may behave differently in terms of extraction of the specimen compared with its behaviour in the matrix used for the standards, potentially giving rise to an inaccurate result. Also, interferences may be present in the specimen that are not present in the matrix used for standards, again potentially giving rise to errors. Because the method of standard addition utilises the specimen being analysed, it avoids these difficulties. Multiple calibrators are prepared by adding known amounts of the analyte to tubes that contain the target specimen. An internal standard should be used; if possible, these should be deuterated analogues in MS techniques. The calibration line can be back-extrapolated to the *x*-axis and the concentration determined (see Fig. 7.5). This method can be used with some success for difficult matrices. Ideally, another person in the laboratory should also independently prepare a control (in the same sample matrix).

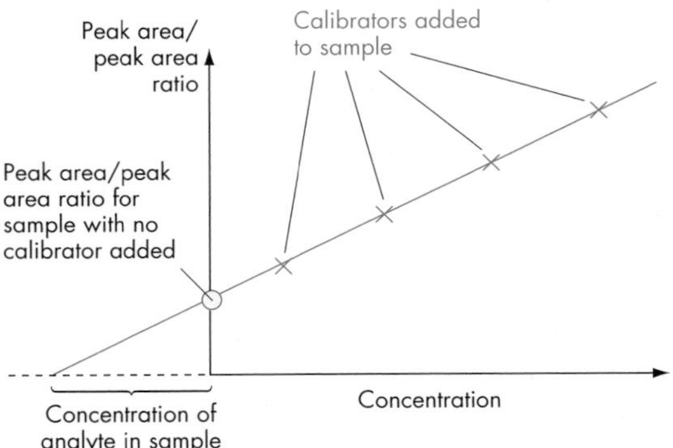

Figure 7.5 Illustration of the graph arising from the standard addition method. The line of best fit, including the value for the sample with no calibrator added, is back-extrapolated to the *x*-axis to determine the concentration of analyte in the sample.

Method validation

It is almost universally accepted that any method used in forensic work must undergo some type of validation (see Chapter 23) to prove that it is fit for purpose, that is that it will provide an accurate answer for the types of samples being analysed and is sufficiently robust to be used by different analysts. However, there is considerable disagreement about the extent of validation required. Perhaps arguably, the extent of validation depends on the specificity and sophistication of the assay, whether the assay is in routine use and the potential consequences of producing an inaccurate result. For example, the legal consequences of a quantitative error in measuring an endogenous analyte, such as adrenaline (epinephrine), are obviously more serious than for, say, strychnine, which ordinarily should not be present in any amount. Similarly, to report an amfetamine analogue as present instead of a decongestant, such as pseudoephedrine, can have serious consequences.

Qualitative methods, such as immunoassay, should be validated for specificity and limit of detection (LOD). It is accepted that most immunoassays cross-react to some extent with analytes other than those targeted, and it is important to know the extent of that cross-reactivity, particularly for structurally related compounds. LOD is important because a class assay (e.g. opiates, amfetamines) may be far less sensitive for some drugs than for others, which allows the possibility of a false negative (the drug not being detected when, in fact, it is present). Where an assay is used to analyse matrices other than those for which it was designed, appropriate validation should be performed. For GC-based and other chromatographic drug screens, it is not usually practical to determine the LOD for every analyte expected to be detected, but the LOD can be determined for representative examples. If the laboratory is asked to determine whether a particular drug is present in a specimen, the laboratory should have some idea what the sensitivity of the assay is, and that it can at least detect potentially toxic concentrations.

A quantitative assay should be validated for accuracy, precision, linearity and LOD. However, it can be argued that some assays are, by their design, self-validating. For example, if a GC-MS-SIM assay uses a good internal standard (ideally a deuterated one), numerous (e.g. six) matrix-matched calibrators, at least one independently prepared matrix-matched control and appropriate acceptance criteria for the calibrators, the calibration as a whole and to the control, the assay could be described as self-validating. If the assay was not accurate, the control result would be out of range. If the assay had poor precision, one or more of the calibrators would not read within an acceptable percentage, when read against the calibration. Specificity can be demonstrated by the appropriate choice of ion ratio qualifiers and lack of chromatographic interference with those ion chromatograms. For some analytes, determination of LOD or limit of quantification (LOQ) is irrelevant if a cut-off is used, or where the analyte concentration is only accepted if within the valid calibration range. Demonstration of that cut-off may be satisfied if it represents the value of the lowest calibrator or control.

Quality control and quality assurance

Quality assurance deals with all aspects of laboratory practice that might influence the accuracy of the final analytical result, and is dealt with elsewhere (see Chapter 23). Quality control (QC) includes the inclusion of material spiked with a known amount of a target analyte. The independently prepared material should be included in an assay to verify that the calibration is accurate within acceptable, defined limits. However, while the routine inclusion of proper QC material should be considered essential, the practice has not been adopted widely in postmortem toxicology testing. Certified reference materials (CRMs) are becoming more widely available, with the National Institute of Standards and LGC Promochem producing drugs of abuse and therapeutic drugs in blood, hair, serum, urine and saliva at certified values. CRM for ethanol has been available for some time. Although time-consuming, spiking analytes into drug-free whole blood with storage at −40°C is an acceptable practice. Ideally, if the control material is prepared in house (in-house reference material), it should be prepared by a person other than the one running the assay, and from different stock material or at the very least from a different weighing of the same powdered stock material. It is not acceptable for an analyst to spike calibrators, and then spike the same solution into separate tubes and call these the controls. Any errors made in the preparation of the standard solution or in spiking calculations would not be uncovered using this approach. It is important that, for quantitative work, acceptance criteria for controls be set and that they be realistic – neither too loose nor unrealistically strict. Failure to meet these criteria should invariably result in corrective action and, as necessary, repeat of the assay. Generally, controls for drugs and other toxins should read within 20% of their nominal value. For some analytes, such as ethanol, criteria such as ± 10% or tighter are more appropriate. If a control is targeted close to the LOQ for the assay, ± 30% may be acceptable for drugs and other toxins. Many laboratories work to some form of set standards. This may be a regional, national or international standards authority. This body will set the criteria for analytical results.

Participation in a suitable proficiency-test programme is another vital component of a good-quality assurance programme and goes a long way to demonstrating competence, as is the accreditation of a laboratory, and inevitably enhances the quality of postmortem toxicology analyses. In such test programmes, the testing laboratory receives material from the programme organiser. It will normally be supplied with information about the sample matrix. Information may or may not be given about the expected analytes. The test laboratory applies the appropriate analyses and then reports their results to the programme organisers. If the result is within accepted limits their performance is deemed acceptable. Testing laboratories can use their success in such performance testing schemes as an assurance of their competence.

Unusual specimen matrices

One of the unique aspects of postmortem toxicology work is that often specimens are received in various states of decomposition or putrefaction. Specimens may be denatured by heat, or mummified. All of these sample types create problems. Samples that are heat denatured are probably the easiest to deal with because the lipid content and concentrations of any putrefactive amines are not much higher than those in relatively fresh postmortem specimens. Heat-denatured samples usually require homogenisation, and for accurate quantitative work may require some type of protease treatment, since a proportion of the analyte may be occluded by coagulated protein. Decomposed and mummified tissues probably create the biggest challenge, because the presence of high concentrations of lipids and putrefactive amines may obscure or interfere with the detection or accurate quantification of target analytes. Even if there is no obvious interference using a specific MS method, there may be a sufficient matrix effect to influence quantitative measurement adversely. Overcoming the effects of specimen decomposition is very difficult and attempts often have limited success. Finding a matrix-matched sample to act as a blank for the preparation of calibrators or controls is difficult, because samples vary tremendously in the nature or extent of decomposition. As noted in the section on calibration methods, the method of standard addition may avoid difficulties in terms of finding a matrix-matched sample. The quantitative determination of analytes in decomposed or other deteriorated samples is invariably less accurate than that in fresher samples. Robust, well-validated methods inevitably produce more reliable results than those that are not.

Other matrices, such as bone, nails and hair, have been analysed successfully for a variety of substances. As with any other matrix, the appropriate use of internal standards (at least for chromatographic assays) and calibrators is important. The more difficult issue may be interpretation of the quantitative results due to lack of suitable databases in these matrices for comparison purposes. It must also be recognised that drugs and toxins typically take time to be incorporated in bone, nails and hair and therefore the results may not provide information about recent intake. More detailed discussion concerning oral fluid and hair are given in Chapter 6.

Limited specimen volume

For a variety of reasons, the volume of postmortem material available for analysis may be very limited. The problem faced by the toxicologist is how to make the best use of that material. With the widespread use of sensitive MS techniques, or even other GC and HPLC detection methods, it should seldom be necessary to base a single assay on more than 1 mL of specimen. However, even with an assay volume as low as or lower than 1 mL, the total amount of specimen may not permit the usual range of tests, or the normal level of sensitivity. Therefore, when such results are reported, it is important to reflect any such shortcomings in the final report, such as a higher LOD, or the inability to perform certain screening tests that otherwise might imply a false negative result.

Interpretation of postmortem toxicology results

When attempting to interpret drug concentrations, forensic toxicologists have traditionally placed a great deal of faith in the assumption that the postmortem concentration of the substance at least approximates that present at the moment of death. Over the years, we have learned that such faith is often misplaced. Even for ethanol, we continue to learn more about its kinetics and disposition during life and changes that occur after death. A thorough understanding of what happens to drugs in the body after death is still lacking, and even for living patients there is a poor correlation between blood concentration and effects. So-called 'therapeutic ranges' have been established for only a relatively small number of drugs, and patient-to-patient variability can be considerable even for these. Some patients exhibit unacceptable side-effects with drug plasma concentrations well within the therapeutic range, whereas plasma concentrations above the therapeutic range are necessary to obtain the desired control with minimal side-effects in others. The problems of interpretation are even greater with postmortem specimens.

Postmortem drug distribution

One of the most important factors to affect the interpretation of postmortem drug concentrations is the phenomenon of 'postmortem redistribution'. The term has been used to describe the movement of drugs within the body after death with the result that the blood concentration of a drug is significantly higher at autopsy than that immediately after death. Postmortem redistribution is a complex phenomenon, and probably involves at least three mechanisms to a greater or lesser degree. The first, and probably the major contributor in most cases, is the release and diffusion of the drug after death from tissues or organs that contain high concentrations (usually the lungs and liver) into nearby cardiac and pulmonary blood vessels. This mechanism has been clearly identified for several drugs, including amitriptyline, for which the concentration in the liver or lungs may be 20–100 times that in the blood. The exact mechanism at a molecular level has not been identified, but it is known that changes in pH and protein structure occur after death, and thereby disrupt the protein binding characteristics of drugs. Therefore, drugs such as the tricyclic antidepressants, which concentrate in the major organs through binding to protein and other molecules, are more likely to undergo redistribution by diffusion along nearby blood vessels. It is worth noting that, although toxicologists have referred to postmortem redistribution from the heart, the bulk of the redistribution occurs from the lungs and liver (Hilberg *et al.* 1994). In contrast to the tricyclic antidepressants, the benzodiazepines undergo very little postmortem redistribution because they are not highly concentrated in the major organs relative to blood. In one case study in which blood was collected from ten separate ligated venous and arterial sites, the marked site dependence in the concentrations of some drugs, but not others, was demonstrated clearly (Jones and Pounder 1987). Figure 7.6 shows the marked site dependence of imipramine and desipramine in the case study, and Figure 7.7 shows the relative lack of site dependence of acetaminophen in the same case.

The second mechanism is simple diffusion after death from a drug depot such as the gastric contents. This is unrelated to release from the major organs because of changes in protein binding. At least two, and possibly three, situations have been identified where this can occur: diffusion or traumatic release from the stomach, agonal aspiration of the stomach contents into the lungs, and continued release from a drug-delivery system. If a drug is present in sufficient concentration in the stomach, diffusion through the stomach wall can occur. Such diffusion can potentially elevate concentrations of drugs in the abdominal blood vessels, such as the abdominal aorta and iliac vein, as well as in tissue such as the liver and kidney (Parker *et al.* 1971). The extent of postmortem diffusion is directly related to both the concentration and total amount of drug in the stomach. Rupture of the stomach in a traumatic accident or suicide can cause artificially elevated drug concentrations by allowing gastric contents to spill into the chest cavity. Under such circumstances even the residue of a single therapeutic dose could produce an erroneous chest blood concentration equivalent to 10 to 100 times that expected after therapeutic doses. In many jurisdictions an autopsy is not performed if the cause of death is obvious, and a less experienced medical examiner might attempt to draw blood from the heart by a blind stick through the chest wall (Logan and Lindholm 1996). Agonal or postmortem movement of the gastric contents into the trachea and lungs can occur after vomiting at the time of death, or as a consequence of handling of the body after death. Marked increases in the concentration of ethanol and drugs can occur through this mechanism, especially into the pulmonary and aortic blood (Pounder and Yonemitsu 1991). In the third situation, markedly increased blood concentrations can occur with at least two different drug delivery devices.

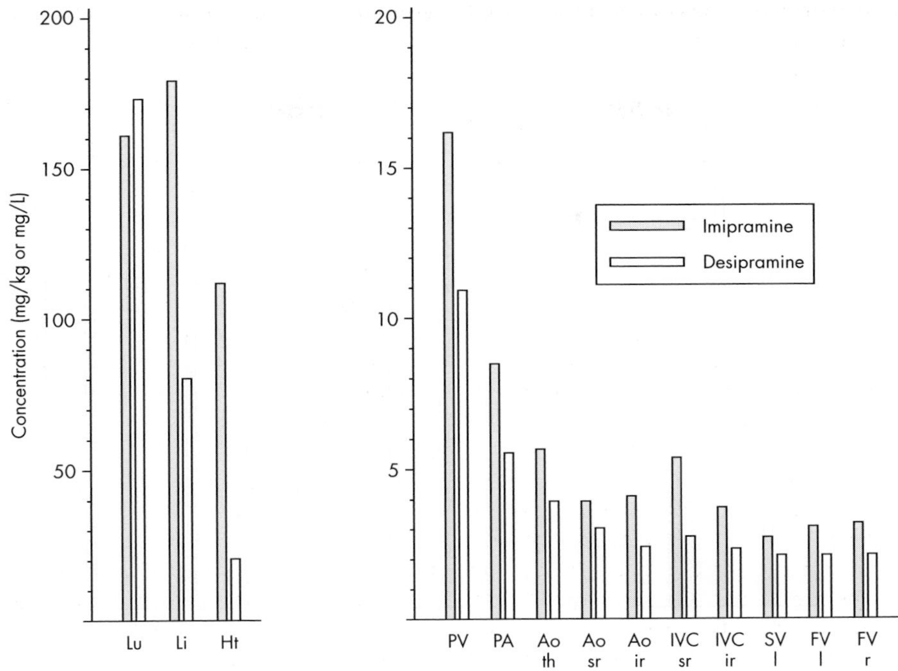

Figure 7.6 Comparison of concentrations of imipramine and the metabolite desipramine in several specimens from the same case. Lu, lung tissue; Li, liver tissue; Ht, heart tissue; PV, pulmonary vein blood; PA, pulmonary artery blood; Ao th, thoracic aorta blood; Ao sr, suprarenal aorta blood; Ao ir, infrarenal aorta blood; IVC sr, suprarenal inferior vena cava blood; IVC ir, infrarenal vena cava blood; SV l, left subclavian vein blood; FV l, left femoral vein blood; FV r, right femoral vein blood. (Based on data from Jones and Pounder 1987.)

Transdermal patches left on a body after death give rise to locally high concentrations of the drug (e.g. fentanyl, nicotine). Transdermal devices rely on passive diffusion across a rate-limiting membrane for drug delivery and, if they are not removed, concentration of the medication in the local area of the patch continues to rise after death, albeit at a slower rate. As there is no blood circulation through the skin after death, the drug is no longer transported away (except by diffusion), which results in a local accumulation of the drug. The concentration gradient between the gel that contains the medication in the patch and the skin is so high that even modest postmortem diffusion can raise postmortem tissue and blood concentrations up to several centimetres away from the patch. The magnitude of such effects depend on the proximity of the patch to the site from which blood was drawn and the postmortem interval. Perhaps more obvious is the situation in which someone dies while receiving analgesics or other medication from an intravenous delivery device (e.g. syringe driver). Intravenous solutions may continue to be pumped into the patient after death, and potentially cause a large local increase in blood concentration (Jenkins *et al.* 1999). While most of these devices are external and readily switched off, some are internal and not obvious until the autopsy is conducted.

The third mechanism is incomplete distribution at the time of death. Even for drugs for which little or no redistribution is thought to occur, marked site-to-site differences in blood drug concentration can occur following an overdose. Since clinical pharmacokinetic studies have shown that a significant arterial–venous difference in concentrations can occur after therapeutic doses, it is reasonable to conclude that even larger differences are likely after

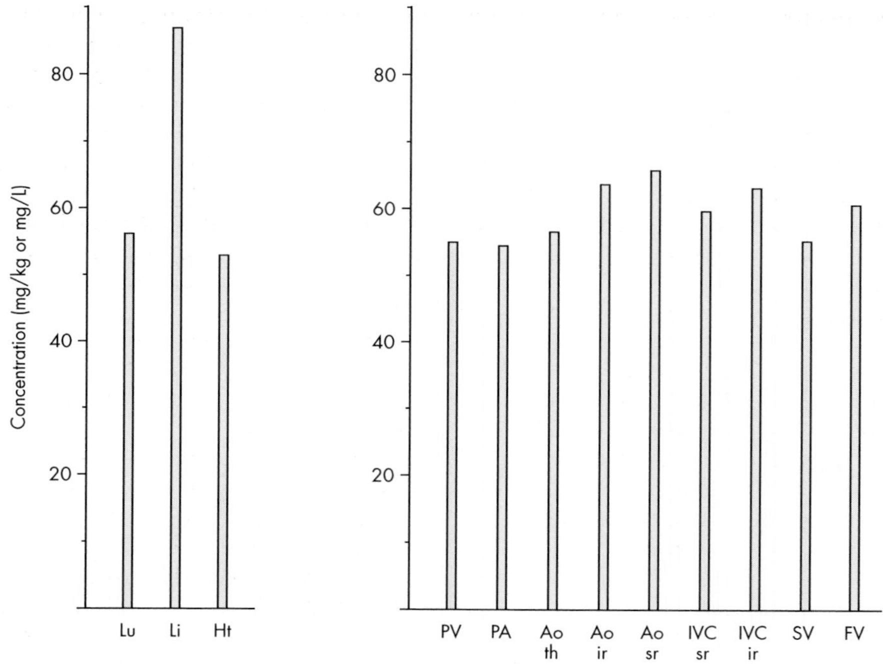

Figure 7.7 Comparison of concentrations of acetaminophen in several specimens from the same case as in Fig. 7.6. Lu, lung tissue; Li, liver tissue; Ht, heart tissue; PV, pulmonary vein blood; PA, pulmonary artery blood; Ao th, thoracic aorta blood; Ao sr, suprarenal aorta blood; Ao ir, infrarenal aorta blood; IVC sr, suprarenal inferior vena cava blood; IVC ir, infrarenal vena cava blood; SV, subclavian vein blood; FV, femoral vein blood. (Based on data from Jones and Pounder 1987.)

massive oral or even intravenous overdoses. In the case of an oral overdose, localised high concentrations are likely in the portal vein, inferior vena cava and right heart and pulmonary vessels. The existence of this phenomenon has been suggested as an explanation for site-to-site differences in unconjugated blood morphine concentrations in diamorphine-related deaths, even though morphine was shown by the same work not to undergo redistribution per se (Logan and Smirnow 1996). It is therefore important to bear in mind that demonstrating site-to-site differences in the blood concentrations of a particular drug does not necessarily prove that the drug undergoes postmortem redistribution. The distinction is an important one. By the nature of postmortem redistribution and postmortem diffusion, increases in blood concentration are time dependent. However, simply to demonstrate that blood samples from two different sites in the body contain different concentrations of a particular drug does not prove that redistribution is likely to occur for that drug in all circumstances.

Ethanol

Although ethanol is a common and relatively well-understood intoxicant, interpretation of postmortem results can be complex. Ethanol can be formed by postmortem fermentation, degraded by bacterial action and redistributed within the body through trauma and other processes.

The postmortem formation of ethanol in the blood, urine and tissues has been well described (Corry 1978). Under appropriate conditions ethanol can be formed in concentrations up to, and exceeding, those set as the statutory limit for driving a motor vehicle in many countries (e.g. 50–100 mg/100 mL blood). What is poorly understood is that concentrations as high as 200–400 mg/100 mL can be formed in exceptional circumstances (Harper and Corry 1988). Conversely, ethanol can also serve as a substrate for many microorganisms such that ethanol concentrations in blood and tissues may initially increase and later decrease. There is no known correlation between the degree of putrefaction of a specimen and the production of postmortem ethanol. Many severely decomposed specimens may contain no ethanol at all, whereas others that appear less severely decomposed may contain concentrations of 80 mg/100 mL or higher.

Other factors can also cause ethanol to be present in postmortem blood as an artefact. It has been demonstrated that when the stomach contains a sufficiently large amount of ethanol, the ethanol may diffuse through the stomach wall and diaphragm and eventually enter into the heart and central blood vessels (Backer *et al.* 1980; Pounder and Smith 1995; Iwasaki *et al.* 1998). Severe trauma, sufficient to rupture the stomach and diaphragm, may allow gastric contents to pass into the chest cavity. In such cases it may be difficult to obtain blood from the usual peripheral vessels. The presence of a small amount of beer or wine, such as might be left after a single drink with lunch, could produce an enormously elevated, but artefactual chest blood ethanol concentration. Another mechanism by which blood alcohol may be elevated is the agonal, or postmortem, movement of gastric contents into the trachea and lungs (Pounder and Yonemitsu 1991). This can lead to elevated blood ethanol concentrations in the major central pulmonary and cardiac vessels and subsequently to erroneous interpretation.

For these reasons, analysis of a second alternative specimen in postmortem cases is recommended. Vitreous humour is the specimen of choice because it remains sterile for a period of days after death and therefore postmortem fermentation does not take place. Only in the case of very severe putrefaction, in which the eye dries out and little fluid is available, is a slight increase in ethanol concentration seen, but the extent of this effect is rarely, if ever, above 20 mg/100 mL (Zumwalt *et al.* 1982). Although an equilibrium between ethanol in the vitreous humour and blood is attained quickly, there may be a lag period during absorption when the vitreous ethanol concentration is slightly lower than that in the blood (Fernandez *et al.* 1989). After equilibrium has been attained, the concentration of ethanol in vitreous humour is about 1.15 times higher than that in blood. This is because ethanol is distributed in the body according to water content and, while vitreous humour contains more than 98% water, whole blood contains on average approximately 85–88% water. Cerebrospinal fluid may be similarly useful, but is more difficult to collect and therefore is less often available for analysis than vitreous humour.

Urine is also a useful fluid for the corroboration of ethanol concentrations in blood. Although concentrations of ethanol in urine average about 1.3 times those in blood, there is considerable variability. Urine is a waste fluid stored in the bladder and, once formed, is largely unaffected by the circulating blood ethanol concentration, unlike ethanol in vitreous humour, which is in equilibrium with the circulating blood. Ethanol can be present in urine and not in blood if sufficient time has elapsed between its consumption and death to allow for clearance from the blood into the bladder. Ethanol can also be detected in urine (sometimes at high concentrations) but not in blood if the donor is a poorly controlled diabetic and if high concentrations of glucose are present. The coexistence of a urinary tract infection (yeast or bacterial) can allow considerable *in vitro* postmortem fermentation to occur in the bladder (Alexander *et al.* 1988). It is virtually impossible to have significant concentrations of ethanol in blood but not in the urine, except as an artefact caused by postmortem fermentation or contamination. The only other exception is where the bladder has been irrigated with warm saline in an attempt to warm a hypothermia victim.

Other postmortem specimens are less useful for ethanol measurement. Bile ethanol concentrations are roughly comparable to those in blood for uncontaminated specimens (Winek *et al.* 1983). However, because of the proximity of the gallbladder to the stomach and liver, bile is of little value where postmortem fermentation or postmortem diffusion are of concern. Similarly, liver and other tissues can undergo postmortem fermentation when bacteria are present. In relatively fresh postmortem tissue, concentrations of ethanol are approximately 50–85% of the corresponding blood concentrations, because of the lower water content of solid tissues. The average liver : blood ratio for alcohol is approximately 0.6 (Jenkins *et al.* 1995).

During metabolism, a small percentage of ethanol is converted to ethyl glucuronide and ethyl sulfate (see Chapter 11). These substances are not known to be formed *post mortem* (Kugelberg and Jones 2007; Høiseth *et. al.*, 2007) and hence finding them in postmortem samples may give an indication of recent ethanol intake before death. Interpretation will depend upon the body fluids, tissues or other specimens in which these substances are found.

Other alcohols and volatiles

The presence of volatiles other than alcohol in postmortem specimens generally, but not always, indicates exposure to, or ingestion of, such compounds. However, some solvents may be formed during life, or by postmortem processes. An example is acetone, which can be present in poorly controlled diabetics at concentrations up to, and sometimes exceeding, 80 mg/100 mL. Acetone is also sometimes present at lower concentrations (e.g. below 10 mg/100 mL) in chronic alcoholics, malnourished individuals and those who suffer from severe stress. Isopropanol can also be present in trace amounts, and is probably formed as a postmortem artefact from acetone (Davis *et al.* 1984). The presence of both isopropanol and acetone can result from solvent ingestion/inhalation (acetone is the major metabolite of isopropanol).

In more northerly climates, methanol is readily available, and accidental or suicidal methanol poisonings are common. Methanol can also be present as an artefact of postmortem change. Methanol is a major ingredient in many embalming fluids, and therefore is present in most embalmed bodies. Some forensic examinations take place in funeral homes, especially in rural areas, and blood or other fluids collected may be contaminated inadvertently with embalming fluid. Less obvious is contamination of motor vehicle accident victims with methanol contained in windshield washer fluid, in which concentrations can be 30% or higher. Blood collected from any site other than from an intact blood vessel has the potential for contamination. It is even possible for the vitreous fluid to be contaminated after the eye has been splashed with windshield fluid.

Drugs and other toxins

Interpretation of the concentrations of drugs in postmortem blood and tissue specimens is complicated because many drugs are unstable *in vivo* and *in vitro*. Interpretation may also be affected by tolerance, inter-individual variation in pharmacological response, drug interactions, the presence or absence of natural disease and the circumstances under which death occurred. For example, cocaine is hydrolysed readily before and after death. It is thought that serum cholinesterase is responsible for the hydrolysis of cocaine to ecgonine methyl ester, while the formation of benzoylecgonine may arise from spontaneous nonenzymatic hydrolysis (Isenschmid *et al.* 1989). Interpretation must therefore depend not only on the concentration of cocaine measured, but also of benzoylecgonine and ecgonine methyl ester. Even when postmortem blood is collected into a tube that contains sodium fluoride (to retard *in vitro* hydrolysis of the cocaine), the degree of hydrolysis that occurs *post mortem* compared with that prior to death is almost impossible to determine. In other words, if relatively high concentrations of cocaine metabolites are detected, it can be difficult to determine whether they resulted from an acute overdose of cocaine or from chronic heavy consumption (bingeing) over a period of several hours or even days. Even if that question could be answered, it is known that cocaine can cause serious and even fatal cardiac arrhythmias at high concentrations, but it is also known that regular cocaine users can snort or inject large doses of cocaine without apparent, serious, short-term toxicity. In contrast, some individuals can develop excited delirium syndrome and die after relatively small doses of cocaine.

Some benzodiazepines (e.g. flunitrazepam, nitrazepam and clonazepam) are known to be unstable *in vitro* and back-calculation of the perimortem concentration is not practical (Robertson and Drummer 1995, 1998). Many other drugs are known to have poor stability in postmortem blood (e.g. chlordiazepoxide, phenelzine, olanzapine, zopiclone). Morphine glucuronide may be converted back into unconjugated morphine in postmortem blood in circumstances in which sufficient bacterial contamination is present to release glucuronidase (Carroll *et al.* 2000).

Blood and/or plasma distribution

One issue that is often overlooked in comparing postmortem data with that from living patients, is that most postmortem laboratories analyse whole blood, whereas clinical laboratories invariably analyse serum or plasma. Many drugs are not evenly distributed between plasma and erythrocytes, and therefore concentrations may be misrepresented by a factor of up to two or more. For example, digitoxin is primarily distributed into plasma, with virtually none in the red cells, with a blood : plasma ratio of 0.5, whereas digoxin has a blood : plasma ratio of close to 1.0 (Lukas and Peterson 1966; Abshagen *et al.* 1971). Similarly, Δ^9-tetrahydrocannabinol (Δ^9-THC) has a blood : plasma ratio approaching 0.5, which indicates that most of the drug is distributed in the plasma, with little in the erythrocytes (Mason and McBay 1985). The significance of this is that most postmortem measurements are conducted on whole blood, whereas many of the pharmacokinetic data are based on plasma measurement. Although the blood : plasma distribution is not likely to have as big an influence on interpretation as postmortem redistribution for some drugs, it is a factor that should not be overlooked, particularly if the analytical results are being compared with those obtained from plasma and/or serum specimens.

Blood and/or tissue distribution

Liver and brain have been used extensively for the postmortem measurement of drugs. Initially, tissues were used because many drugs are present at concentrations of up to 10–50 times that in blood, and because tissues provided a large volume of material for extraction and analysis. This was essential in the days when physical isolation of the poison, crystallisation and pharmacological testing was a goal. As analytical methods improved, analyses for most drugs could be performed on blood, leading to a trend in the analysis of blood alone. However, with the recognition that redistribution and related phenomena could seriously decrease confidence in postmortem blood drug concentrations, analysis of tissues is regaining importance. While concentrations of some drugs can increase by as much as 2- to 10-fold after death in postmortem blood, concentrations in tissues such as liver remain relatively stable. The problem lies with the interpretation of tissue drug concentrations. Unlike in blood, reference ranges for drugs in tissues are not obtainable from clinical studies, and animal data are not directly transferable to humans. Forensic toxicologists have to rely on empirical data from other cases in their own laboratories, or on published material. To be useful, such postmortem data must include cases in which drugs are likely to have been taken in therapeutic doses, not just overdose cases.

The question can be posed, 'How do you convert a tissue concentration into a blood concentration?' You do not. Organs are anatomically distinct entities with different kinetics from blood. Although it is generally true that very high blood concentrations tend to be associated with high tissue concentrations and that a useful relationship can be demonstrated, there is too much variation to attempt mathematical conversion for any single case. Although virtually no studies have examined dose–time–concentration relationship in tissues, and certainly none in humans, some studies have demonstrated marked variation in drug concentrations within an organ, such as the liver and the brain. This further demonstrates why caution must be exercised in attempting to convert tissue concentrations into an equivalent blood concentration. A tissue concentration provides an additional piece of the puzzle. Multiple tissue concentrations provide additional pieces, and help to build a picture of the body burden of the drug in a qualitative sense. This information, together with blood concentrations, information from the autopsy and the circumstances of death, can help formulate informed conclusions about the role of the drugs (if any) in a death.

Pharmacokinetics

Postmortem toxicologists tend to interpret drug concentrations simply in the terms 'What role, if any, did these substances play in the death of this person?' While this question is important, lawyers, judges and the public frequently ask, 'How many tablets did the person take and when did they take them?' The non-scientist readily understands the concept of 'dose' (the number of tablets a person took, compared to the prescribed dose). However, the concept of 'blood concentration' and its relationship (or lack thereof) with time and dose is more difficult to understand. Pharmacokinetics is, in theory, a scientific tool that could bridge the link between the concentration of a drug in the blood and dosage. However, pharmacokinetics can be misapplied in postmortem cases.

Pharmacokinetics is an invaluable tool to help understand the time course of drugs in the body. In the living, it can be used to determine duration of action, inter-individual differences in peak plasma concentrations and clearance, and the likely effectiveness of different pharmaceutical formulations. However, rarely can pharmacokinetics be applied successfully to postmortem toxicology. When clinical pharmacokinetic studies are performed, the dose and time of dose are controlled, and often multiple plasma samples are collected to determine the pharmacokinetic parameters for a drug. For living persons, determination of the dose from a single plasma or blood concentration is fraught with uncertainty. The problem is even more complex for postmortem cases. The most commonequation applied is:

$$\text{Dose (g)} = C\ \text{(g/L)} \times \text{body mass (kg)} \times V_D\ \text{(L/kg)} \qquad (7.1)$$

where C is the concentration of drug in plasma or blood and V_D is the volume of distribution. For postmortem cases, only the body mass of the deceased can be ascertained with certainty and in many cases even this may be inaccurate, for example where decomposition has occurred. The V_D for any given drug typically varies over a range of at least 2-fold in the general population, and frequently more. Theoretically, the concentration of a drug can be determined with reasonable accuracy in the blood sampled. In postmortem cases, there is always uncertainty whether the concentration of drug in the sample was the same, or similar, at the time of death. Furthermore, the use of calculations that involve V_D assumes that absorption of the drug is complete and the drug is in equilibrium throughout the body. In postmortem cases this assumption may be invalid, especially when dealing with acute intoxications or overdoses. As a result, dose calculations may overestimate a dose by as much as 10-fold or more.

Forensic toxicologists have occasionally used analysis of multiple tissue samples from various organs in the body in attempt to overcome the errors inherent in the use of V_D calculations. The approach requires quantitative analysis of tissue from multiple organs and sites to estimate the total body burden of a drug – that is the total amount in the body. At the very least, the major organs such as liver, lungs and brain must be analysed, in addition to skeletal muscle and adipose tissue. Masses measured at autopsy can be used to calculate the total drug in the organs sampled. However, the masses of skeletal muscle and adipose tissue can only be estimated realistically from historical data (Butler 1971; Ciba-Geigy 1971), and may poorly reflect the actual tissue masses in the victim. As previously discussed, the concentration of a drug in the piece of organ or other tissue measured may or may not reflect the average for all of that organ or tissue. Another often overlooked factor is that, after chronic dosing, steady-state levels for some drugs, especially those with a large V_D and long half-life, may be several-fold higher after chronic therapeutic dosing than after a single dose. To summarise, therefore, pharmacokinetic calculations should be attempted with extreme caution, if at all, and any assumptions made should be stated clearly. In most instances, pharmacokinetic calculations using postmortem blood measurements are rarely defensible forensically.

Metabolism and pharmacogenetics

Although the primary pathways of drug metabolism have been understood for at least 20 to 25 years, the extent and mechanisms of drug interactions and pharmacogenetic influences on blood concentrations have only really been elucidated in the past few years. A detailed discussion of pharmacogenetics and drug metabolism is beyond the scope of this chapter; however, some aspects should be highlighted. It is known that 7–8% of the caucasian population are deficient in cytochrome-P450 IID6 (P450IID6), one of the major enzymes responsible for many important oxidative pathways, such as alkyl hydroxylation. That deficiency is determined genetically. As a result, the ability of those affected to metabolise and clear many drugs may be affected seriously. In many instances, even though drug clearance is significantly slower than for those not deficient in P450IID6, it is not as slow as might be predicted because other pathways may compensate. Even if a person is not specifically identified as being deficient in P450IID6, the person or physician may be indirectly aware of it because of an unusual sensitivity to some drugs and the higher prevalence of side-effects. Even in people without deficiencies in drug-metabolising enzymes, drug–drug interactions can result in dangerously elevated concentrations. It has also been recognised that many drugs can inhibit their own metabolism by saturating the primary metabolising enzyme systems. For example, the dose–plasma concentration curve for phenytoin can rise almost exponentially at high therapeutic doses. These variabilities in the relationship between dose and plasma or blood concentration can therefore introduce even more error into any attempt to apply conventional pharmacokinetics to estimate dosage.

There is a great temptation to categorise blood levels in black-and-white terms as being the result of therapeutic doses, or of a suicidal overdose, or perhaps of abuse. Other possibilities are sometimes overlooked when high concentrations of drugs are encountered. One of the simplest ways to determine compliance with prescribed dosage, although not foolproof, is to conduct a medication count. Knowing when the medication was prescribed, how much was dispensed, the dose and the number of days between dispensing and death can often provide a powerful indicator of patient compliance, and whether an overdose is likely or not. Information regarding compliance over a longer period may often be obtained by a review of the pharmacy or medical records. The slowing of drug metabolism with age has been well documented, but this can be overlooked as an explanation for elevated postmortem drug concentrations in the elderly.

Caution against using reference tables

Interpretation of postmortem toxicology results can be very challenging and should only be done with a thorough knowledge of the case history, including autopsy findings, information from the scene and relevant medical history. It is not difficult to interpret a high blood strychnine concentration in a person found dead in a farmhouse together with an open container of strychnine-containing rodent poison and a suicide note. However, how should the toxicologist interpret a moderately high blood concentration of imipramine in an adolescent prescribed the drug for attention-deficit disorder. Could the drug have accumulated? Was the subject suffering from depression? Was he or she complaining of side-effects? Can any medication that remains be accounted for by the time since the prescription was filled and dosage (i.e. a medication count)? Did the autopsy reveal any significant natural disease? Was the behaviour of the subject observed in the immediate period leading to death? Was the death a sudden collapse which was witnessed? Was there a period of emergency hospitalisation leading up to death? If so, what did the medical assessment reveal? Are there any antemortem plasma or blood specimens still available? These are the types of questions that the forensic toxicologist should ask in cases that are anything less than straightforward.

There is a great temptation for forensic toxicologists and others to refer to tables of therapeutic, toxic and fatal concentrations. While these tables may be of some use in clinical toxicology, they are of very limited value for the interpretation of postmortem toxicology results and can be very misleading. Such tables are often drawn extensively from clinical data, seldom take into account tolerance and do not provide for phenomena such as postmortem redistribution. For example, interpretation of morphine and other narcotic concentrations may be very dependent on how long the person has been prescribed the drug and at what dosage. The inappropriate use of tables can result in over- and underestimation of the potential toxicity of a drug depending on the degree of tolerance developed, natural disease and whether other substances are present. The ranges given may not take into account the circumstances of drug use. For example, the therapeutic range for fentanyl when used intravenously as an adjunct to anaesthesia may be greater than 10-fold that after use for analgesia via a transdermal patch. Data compendia may also include cases in which there was a prolonged survival time and the person died from the sequelae of the intoxication (e.g. hypoxia, organ failure), but after medical intervention had prolonged life, resulting in lower blood concentrations. Specific references to case data and further information are lacking in most instances. Experienced postmortem toxicologists rely first on their own case experience, supplemented by compilations of drug monographs, where references to the original published work are available, and the circumstances of the case (Baselt 2002).

Summary

As can be seen from the above, postmortem toxicology is a complex field not only in terms of the types of specimens that may or not be available for analysis but also because of their possible state of decomposition; possible limitations of case history; the potential for any number of substances to be present and the difficulties of screening for all drugs and poisons together with the difficulties of interpretation of results. Despite all these potential difficulties, it can be a fascinating subject area because these difficulties pose interesting analytical and intellectual challenges not found in many occupations.

References

U. Abshagen *et al.*, Distribution of digoxin, digitoxin and ouabain between plasma and erythrocytes in various species, *Naunyn Schmiedebergs Arch. Pharmakol.*, 1971, **270**, 105–116.

W. D. Alexander *et al.*, Urinary ethanol and diabetes mellitus, *Diabet. Med.*, 1988, **5**, 463–464.

C. Backer *et al.*, The comparison of alcohol concentrations in postmortem fluids and tissues, *J. Forensic Sci.*, 1980, **25**, 327–331.

R. C. Baselt, *Disposition of Toxic Drugs and Chemicals in Man*, 6th edn, Foster City, Chemical Toxicology Institute, 2002.

T. C. Butler, The distribution of drugs, in *Fundamentals of Drug Metabolism and Drug Disposition*, B. N. La Du *et al.* (eds), Baltimore, Williams & Wilkins, 1971, pp. 44–62.

F. T. Carroll *et al.*, Morphine 3-D-glucuronide stability in postmortem specimens exposed to bacterial enzymatic hydrolysis, *Am. J. Forensic Med. Pathol.*, 2000, **21**, 323–329.

Ciba-Geigy, *Scientific Tables*, 7th edn, K. Diem and C. Lentner (eds), Basle, Ciba-Geigy Ltd, 1971, pp. 710–711.

J. E. Corry, A review. Possible sources of ethanol ante- and post-mortem: its relationship to the biochemistry and microbiology of decomposition, *J. Appl. Bacteriol.*, 1978, **44**, 1–56.

P. L. Davis *et al.*, Endogenous isopropanol: forensic and biochemical implications, *J. Anal. Toxicol.*, 1984, **8**, 209–212.

M. A. Evenson and D. A. Engstrand, A SepPak HPLC method for tricyclic antidepressant drugs in human vitreous humour, *J. Anal. Toxicol.*, 1989, **13**, 322–325.

P. Fernandez *et al.*, A comparative pharmacokinetic study of ethanol in the blood, vitreous humour and aqueous humour of rabbits, *Forensic Sci. Int.*, 1989, **41**, 61–65.

D. R. Harper and J. E. L. Corry, Collection and storage of specimens for alcohol analysis, in *Medicolegal Aspects of Alcohol Determination in Biological Fluids*, 3rd edn, J. C. Garriott (ed.), Littleton, Year Book Medical Publishers, 1988, pp. 145–169.

T. Hilberg *et al.*, Postmortem release of amitriptyline from the lungs: a mechanism of postmortem drug redistribution, *Forensic Sci. Int.*, 1994, **64**, 47–55.

G. Høiseth *et al.*, *A Study of Ethyl Glucuronide in Postmortem Blood as a Marker of Ante-mortem Ingestion of Alcohol*, Norwegian Institute of Public Health, Division of Forensic Toxicology and Drug Abuse, 2007.

D. S. Isenschmid *et al.*, A comprehensive study of the stability of cocaine and its metabolites, *J. Anal. Toxicol.*, 1989, **13**, 250–256.

Y. Iwasaki *et al.*, On the influence of postmortem alcohol diffusion from the stomach contents to the heart blood, *Forensic Sci. Int.*, 1998, **94**, 111–118.

A. J. Jenkins *et al.*, Distribution of ethanol in postmortem liver, *J. Forensic Sci.*, 1995, **40**, 611–614.

A. J. Jenkins *et al.*, *Unusual Distribution of Morphine in Biological Matrices Following Drug Delivery With an Infusion System*, Boston, American Academy of Forensic Sciences, 1999, p. 272.

G. R. Jones and D. J. Pounder, Site dependence of drug concentrations in postmortem blood – a case study, *J. Anal. Toxicol.*, 1987, **11**, 186–190.

F. C. Kugelberg and A.W. Jones, Interpreting results of post-mortem ethanol specimens: a review of the literature, *Forensic. Sci. Intl.*, 2007, **165**, 10–29.

D. L. Lin *et al.*, Distribution of codeine, morphine, and 6-acetylmorphine in vitreous humour, *J. Anal. Toxicol.*, 1997, **21**, 258–261.

J. Lock *et al.*, Mineral content of reagents used in subtilisin assays, *Med. Sci. Law*, 1981, **21**, 123–124.

B. K. Logan and G. Lindholm, Gastric contamination of postmortem blood samples during blind-stick sample collection, *Am. J. Forensic Med. Pathol.*, 1996, **17**, 109–111.

B. K. Logan and D. Smirnow, Postmortem distribution and redistribution of morphine in man, *J. Forensic Sci.*, 1996, **41**, 221–229.

D. A. Lukas and R. E. Peterson, Double isotope dilution derivative assay of digitoxin in plasma, urine, and stool of patients maintained on the drug, *J. Clin. Invest.*, 1966, **45**, 782–795.

A. P. Mason and A. J. McBay, Cannabis: pharmacology and interpretation of effects, *J. Forensic Sci.*, 1985, **30**, 615–631.

J. M. Parker *et al.*, Post-mortem changes in tissue levels of sodium secobarbital, *Clin. Toxicol.*, 1971, **4**, 265–272.

D. J. Pounder and D. R. Smith, Postmortem diffusion of alcohol from the stomach, *Am. J. Forensic Med. Pathol.*, 1995, **16**, 89–96.

D. J. Pounder and K. Yonemitsu, Postmortem absorption of drugs and ethanol from aspirated vomitus – an experimental model, *Forensic Sci. Int.*, 1991, **51**, 189–195.

M. D. Robertson and O. H. Drummer, Postmortem drug metabolism by bacteria, *J. Forensic Sci.*, 1995, **40**, 382–386.

M. D. Robertson and O. H. Drummer, Stability of nitrobenzodiazepines in postmortem blood, *J. Forensic Sci.*, 1998, **43**, 5–8.

K. S. Scott and J. S. Oliver, The use of vitreous humour as an alternative to whole blood for the analysis of benzodiazepines, *J. Forensic Sci.*, 2001, **46**, 694–697.

SOFT/AAFS Guidelines Committee, *SOFT/AAFS Forensic Toxicology Laboratory Guidelines*, Mesa, Society of Forensic Toxicologists and American Academy of Forensic Sciences Toxicology Section, 2006, pp. 1–24.

T. E. Vorpahl and J. I. Coe, Correlation of ante-mortem and postmortem digoxin levels, *J. Forensic Sci.*, 1978, **23**, 329–334.

C. L. Winek *et al.*, The influence of physical properties and lipid content of bile on the human blood/bile ethanol ratio, *Forensic Sci. Int.*, 1983, **22**, 171–178.

R. E. Zumwalt *et al.*, Evaluation of ethanol concentrations in decomposed bodies, *J. Forensic Sci.*, 1982, **27**, 549–554.

Further reading

W. H. Anderson and R. W. Prouty, Postmortem redistribution of drugs, in *Advances in Analytical Toxicology*, vol. II, R. C. Baselt (ed.), Chicago, Year Book Medical Publishers, 1989, pp. 70–102.

R. C. Baselt, *Drug Effects on Psychomotor Performance*, Foster City, Biomedical Publications, 2001.

R. C. Baselt, *Disposition of Toxic Drugs and Chemicals in Man*, 7th edn, Foster City, Biomedical Publications, 2004.

L. Brunton *et al.*, *Goodman and Gilman's The Pharmacological Basis of Therapeutics*, 11th edn, New York, McGraw-Hill Medical, 2005.

M. J. Ellenhorn, *Ellenhorn's Medical Toxicology: Diagnosis and Treatment of Poisoning*, 2nd edn, Baltimore, Williams & Wilkins, 1997.

S. Karch, *Drug Abuse Handbook*, 2nd edn, Boca Raton, CRC Press, 2006.

B. Levine, *Principles of Forensic Toxicology*, 2nd edn, Washington DC, AACC Press, 2006.

8

Clinical toxicology, therapeutic drug monitoring, *in utero* exposure to drugs of abuse

D R A Uges, M Hallworth, C Moore and A Negrusz

Introduction 219
Clinical toxicology 219
Therapeutic drug monitoring 237
In utero exposure to drugs of abuse . . . 256
References 260
Further reading 260

Introduction

This chapter describes three very important aspects of what can be called 'diagnostic toxicology'. Clinical toxicology discusses all aspects of diagnosis and treatment of various poisonings by examining the patient and evaluating the symptoms, as well as by analysing the specimens collected from the patient for the presence of drug(s). As a result, the proper course of treatment is taken. Therapeutic drug monitoring (TDM) is frequently applied during therapy with drugs which have a narrow therapeutic index in order to avoid or at least minimise the side-effects or more dangerous toxic effects. In addition, because of genetic variations, different people may need different doses of the same drug in order to produce the same pharmacological effect. The phenomenon of *in utero* exposure to drugs and its consequences was fully recognised in early 1990s. As a result, the analysis of specimens collected from both the mother and a newborn is now routinely performed by hospitals and clinics. The main purpose is to reveal the baby's exposure to dangerous drugs during the pregnancy so that the appropriate measures can be taken to assure the child's welfare. In our opinion all three aspects discussed in this chapter are similar and they employ similar analytical techniques starting with less specific but much faster methods in clinical toxicology, methods that are more specific and sensitive but are used for the known drug being monitored in TDM, and finally the most complicated 'looking for unknown' analytical approaches to determine *in utero* exposure.

Clinical toxicology

Hospital toxicology is concerned with individuals admitted to hospital with suspected poisoning and its prime aim is to assist in the treatment of the patient. The range of substances that may be encountered is huge and ideally the hospital laboratory will have the capability to identify and, if required, quantify pharmaceutical agents, illicit drugs, gases, solvents, pesticides, toxic metals and a host of other industrial and environmental poisons in biological fluids. In practice, few laboratories can offer such a comprehensive menu and resources are concentrated on those compounds most often involved in poisoning and for which toxicological investigations are particularly useful to the clinical services. In developed countries, hospital clinical chemistry laboratories are geared to provide these basic services and rely on support from central specialised toxicology laboratories for the rarer cases. Fortunately, in the vast majority of cases the diagnosis can be made on circumstantial and clinical evidence; there is no need for urgent analyses and the analyses can be carried out as a routine exercise. However, when the patient's condition is severe and the diagnosis is not clear, toxicological tests may be crucial and the analytical results must be furnished quickly (usually within 1 to 2 hours of the patient's arrival) if they are to have any bearing on diagnosis and treatment. Ideally, the toxic substance can be both identified and quantified within this time frame. When this is not possible, a qualitative result still has considerable value if the symptoms are consistent with the identified toxin and should be relayed to the clinician without delay.

These time constraints entail an inevitable compromise between speed and analytical accuracy and precision. Consequently, the quantitative methods used may fall short of the standards required, for example, for pharmacokinetic investigations. However, they must be of sufficient quality to allow an appropriate clinical decision to be made. In this area, close liaison between the laboratory personnel and the clinician who manages the patient is essential and can save hours of fruitless effort. An attempt must be made to obtain as much information about the patient as possible. This should include not only the clinical picture, but also any previous medical history of poisoning, details of drugs or other substances to which the patient may have had access and, in cases of accidental poisoning, substances to which the patient may have been exposed. This sort of dialogue between the clinician and an experienced analytical toxicologist can often yield clues as to what the cause of toxicity might be and therefore suggest which tests should be performed as a priority. Close communication must continue if the initial tests prove negative, so that the search has to be widened, or if the clinician requires advice on the interpretation of positive results.

Laboratories that provide analytical toxicology analyses to assist with cases of acute and chronic poisoning often offer additional services in the area of drug abuse. This can range from diagnostic tests to uncover the covert misuse of laxatives and diuretics through to routine screening of urine samples from patients assigned to treatment and rehabilitation programmes. For the latter, the requirement is to establish the drug-taking patterns of new patients and to monitor their subsequent compliance with the prescribed treatment regime. Details of techniques suitable for these services are given in separate sections.

Causes of hospital admissions for poisoning

Social and economic stresses or mental disorders often result in suicide attempts, particularly through drug overdose, which is one of the most common reasons for emergency hospital admissions. Homicidal poisoning is relatively rare, but surviving victims of this practice are often investigated initially in the hospital environment. Individuals who are administered substances without their knowledge to facilitate robbery or sexual abuse may also be admitted to hospital, although in the latter scenario the victims tend to contact the medical services several days after the incident, so the rape drug (gamma-hydroxybutyric acid (GHB), flunitrazepam, alcohol) is no longer detectable. Poisoning in children is mainly accidental, but deliberate poisoning by parents, guardians or siblings does occur. Accidental poisoning usually takes place in the domestic environment, with young children and the elderly particularly at risk. Children may gain access to pharmaceutical products, cleaning agents (bleach, disinfectants), pesticides, alcoholic drinks and cosmetics. The confused elderly may misjudge their intake of medications or be poisoned by inappropriate handling of toxic household products. Both are susceptible to acute or chronic poisoning with carbon monoxide emitted by faulty domestic heating appliances. The workplace is another environment in which accidental poisoning occurs and the analytical results from the hospital laboratory can be important not only in medical diagnosis but also in any subsequent legal investigations that involve insurance claims. On the other hand, the anaesthesiologist wants to know that the poison is not a contraindication for his chosen therapy.

Iatrogenic intoxications occur through inappropriate medical or paramedical treatment. This is an increasing challenge for the toxicologist. Neonates require intravenous dosing and the need to work out doses per kilogram of body mass introduces the risk that the total amount and volume of medicine to be administered may be miscalculated. Other causes of iatrogenic poisoning include drug interactions, use of the wrong route or speed of administration and failure to take note of impaired liver or renal function, which reduces the patient's ability to eliminate the drug. A common example is the accumulation of digoxin in elderly patients with reduced renal function.

Qualitative screening or quantitative analysis?

Laboratories adopt different approaches to hospital toxicology. To a large extent, the range of equipment available and the skills and knowledge of the staff govern the policy adopted. Where resources are scarce, only a limited screen for common drugs and poisons may be carried out, with the main effort directed towards quantitative analyses for toxins indicated by circumstantial evidence and the patient's clinical signs. Specialised toxicology laboratories may pursue a systematic and comprehensive toxicological screen in every case, on the grounds that the clinical and circumstantial indicators are seldom reliable, and then proceed to quantify any substances detected. Whereas the latter approach is more likely to yield useful information, it is expensive and time-consuming. As stated above, close liaison with the clinicians to obtain a comprehensive case history and a full clinical picture can often help to focus the resources on the qualitative and quantitative tests that are most relevant. The guidelines given in Table 8.1 are useful in this context.

Table 8.1 Guidelines to help focus resources on the most relevant qualitative and quantitative tests

Indications for qualitative screening	Indications for quantitative analyses
To distinguish between apparent intoxication and poisoning	When the type and duration of treatment depends on the concentration (e.g. antidotes for paracetamol and thallium)
When information about the patient is lacking (no medical history)	When the prognosis is gauged by the plasma concentration (e.g. paraquat)
When the clinical picture is ambiguous (e.g. seizures)	To distinguish between therapeutic and toxic ingestion of drugs
Where the clinical picture may be caused by a pharmacological group of drugs rather than one particular substance (e.g. laxatives, diuretics)	Mixed intoxications (e.g. methanol and ethanol)
Cases of mixed intoxication (drugs of abuse, alcohol)	Toxicological monitoring (e.g. aluminium, Munchausen's syndrome)
Poisoning with no immediately evident clinical picture (e.g. paracetamol)	Toxicokinetic calculations
Where no reliable or selective quantitative method is available (e.g. herbal preparations)	Research (e.g. efficacy of treatment), education, prevention, etc.
For forensic reasons	
At the special request of the clinician	
For purposes of statistics, research, education, prevention, etc.	

Applications

Confirmation of diagnosis

Most patients who reach hospital in time respond well to measures designed to support the vital processes of respiratory and cardiovascular function and, as mentioned above, toxicological investigations are of only historical value. However, it is still useful to have objective evidence of self-poisoning as this usually instigates psychiatric treatment and follow-up.

Differential diagnosis of coma

When circumstantial evidence is lacking, a diagnosis of poisoning may be difficult to sustain simply on the basis of clinical examination, since coma induced by drugs is not readily differentiated from that caused by disease processes. Apparent poisonings can be caused by hypoglycaemic coma, a cerebrovascular accident, exhaustion (after seizures), brain damage, meningitis, withdrawal symptoms, idiosyncratic reactions (e.g. to theophylline and caffeine), allergic reactions (shock), viral infections or unexpected symptoms of a disease (e.g. Lyme disease). In these situations, toxicological analyses serve either to confirm poisoning as the cause of coma or to rule it out in favour of an organic disorder that requires alternative medical and pathological investigations. A particular, but not uncommon, poisoning is water intoxication, which only can be determined indirectly by sodium serum concentration or osmolarity.

Diagnosis of brain death

A patient with brain death may be a potential donor of organs. In such cases, the patient should have a deep coma of known origin with no indication of a central infection, and have normal metabolic parameters. When the primary cause of coma is drug overdose, it is important to ensure that the drug has been eliminated prior to confirming the diagnosis of brain death. This also applies to drugs that may have been given in therapy. For example, thiopental is often given in the treatment of brain oedema and during neurosurgery. The half-lives of thiopental and its metabolite, pentobarbital, increase if cardiac function is diminished or the patient is hypothermic, and therefore plasma concentrations of both compounds must always be measured. Midazolam and diazepam are also administered frequently in treating cases of brain damage, and the continued presence of active concentrations of these drugs and their metabolites should also be excluded using specific and sensitive procedures, such as high-performance liquid chromatography (HPLC). Even if benzodiazepines or their metabolites cannot be detected, there remains the possibility that some may still be present, for instance hydroxymidazolam glucuronide in active concentrations. This may suggest a provocation test with the specific benzodiazepine antagonist, flumazenil. In all other cases flumazenil is contraindicated in cases of poisoning, as many drugs may induce seizures, which just require a benzodiazepine as antidote. Similarly, the presence of active levels of anticonvulsants (phenobarbital, carbamazepine, phenytoin and valproate), which are also given in the treatment of brain damage, must be excluded. Again, the use of sensitive and specific chromatographic methods is essential.

Influence on active therapy

While supportive therapy remains the cornerstone of the management of acute poisoning, specific antidotes are available for metals (chelation agents), anticholinesterase inhibitors (atropine, pralidoxime, obidoxime), methanol and ethylene glycol (ethyl alcohol, 4-methylpyrazole), paracetamol (*N*-acetylcysteine) and opioids (naloxone). Given a clear diagnosis, a clinician usually administers the antidote without waiting for laboratory confirmation, but subsequent analyses may help to decide whether to continue with the therapy. For example, both parenteral and oral therapy with desferrioxamine in cases of iron poisoning is indicated if patients deteriorate and the serum iron concentration is extremely high. Measurements of cholinesterase activity in serum or red cells are useful in a situation of high-dose infusions of atropine into patients exposed to organophosphorus insecticides or thiocarbamates. Measures designed to reduce the absorption of poisons from the gut, such as the use of emetics, purgatives, gastric lavage and irrigation, are now considered to be of limited value and unwarranted in most cases of poisoning. The efficacy of whole-bowel irrigation is also questionable, although some advocate its use to remove sustained-release or enteric-coated preparations of, for example, iron salts and other potentially lethal poisons that have passed into the small bowel, and in the decontamination of body packers. A single oral dose of activated charcoal has largely replaced other means of reducing absorption, although it is generally useful only when given within 1 hour of ingestion and fails to absorb inorganic ions, alcohols, strong acids or alkalis, or organic solvents.

Techniques to increase the rate of elimination of poisons, such as diuresis, adjusting the urinary pH, haemodialysis and peritoneal dialysis, venous–venous haemofiltration and charcoal haemoperfusion, are now hardly used. Forced diuresis is now frowned upon; it is probably beneficial only in cases of poisoning with thallium and, when coupled with alkalisation of urine, chlorophenoxy herbicides. Alkalisation of urine effectively increases the elimination of salicylates, phenobarbital and chlorophenoxy herbicides. Acidification of the urine has little merit in increasing the elimination of weakly basic substances, such as amfetamines and phencyclidine. Theoretically the elimination of tricyclic antidepressants might be increased by acidification. However, the dangerous effect of this poisoning is the enlarging of the PQ-complex, which toxic cardiac effect requires alkalisation by sodium bicarbonate. Haemodialysis can enhance the elimination of hydrophilic toxins with a small volume of distribution and is useful in treating severe poisoning with salicylates, lithium, methanol, ethylene glycol and chlorophenoxy herbicides. Peritoneal dialysis is by no means as efficient as haemodialysis but is more accessible in remote regions and in developing countries. Haemofiltration also has a role in this context. 'Gut dialysis', or the use of multiple oral doses of activated charcoal, is thought to operate by creating a drug concentration gradient across the gut wall that leads to movement of the drug from the blood in the superficial vessels of the gut mucosa into the lumen. So far, its efficacy has been demonstrated for carbamazepine, dapsone, phenobarbital, quinine and theophylline, and there is evidence for its application in poisoning with calcium antagonists. Most of these procedures carry inherent risks to the patient and, as pointed out above, their applications are limited only to a handful of poisons. Toxicological analyses to identify and quantify the poison should be used to ensure that such interventions are used appropriately and at the same time to prevent overtreatment of patients who would recover without them. Clinical toxicologists have to know the toxic effects of the particular drug. For instance, verapamil, diltiazem, amlodipine and nefidrine are all calcium blockers. However, each has its own required treatment and prognosis.

Medicolegal aspects of hospital toxicology

The primary role of the hospital toxicologist is to assist clinicians in the treatment of poisoned patients, irrespective of any other aspects that surround the case. However, some cases may have a criminal element. These can range from iatrogenic poisoning, in which a patient or relative sues a health authority and its staff for neglect, through to the malicious administration of drugs or poisons by a third party. The latter category includes victims of so-called date-rape, who have been administered drugs such as flunitrazepam, GHB or alcohol to induce confusion and amnesia and facilitate sexual abuse, and nonaccidental poisoning in children. Mothers are the most frequent perpetrators of child poisoning and do so to attract sympathy and attention as a consequence of the child's illness (Munchausen's syndrome by proxy). When these situations arise, the hospital toxicologist is obliged to take special precautions to conserve all residual samples and documentation that may feature subsequently as part of a forensic investigation.

Clinical manifestations and biomedical tests

Specific acute clinical manifestations and vital signs of the patient that can be important in suggesting the cause of poisoning are set out in Table 8.2.

Biochemical tests that gauge the physiological status of the patient are more important in terms of the immediate management of the condition and some of the abnormalities found can also be diagnostic of the type of agent involved (see Table 8.6). These, together with the clinical manifestations and history, provide the basis for the order in which the toxicological tests are carried out.

Other indicative features

Some poisons have characteristic odours that may be discerned on the patient's body, clothes, breath and samples of vomit, as listed in Table 8.3. Colours of the skin and of urine samples can also be useful indicators (Tables 8.4 and 8.5). However, these clues should be interpreted with caution and are not a substitute for proper clinical and toxicological evaluation. The results of biomedical tests are usually available before any toxicological tests have been completed; Table 8.6 highlights their potential diagnostic value.

Assays required on an emergency basis

Table 8.7 lists the toxicological assays (mainly in serum, plasma or blood) that should be performed as soon as possible after admission and highlights those that should preferably be provided by all acute hospital laboratories. Emergency requests for the analysis of rarer poisons may be referred to a specialised centre. Such lists vary according to the pattern of poisoning prevalent in different countries or regions, and Table 8.7 is therefore presented only as a guideline. Notes that indicate the relevance of the assays are also included.

Quality management

It is essential that the whole laboratory process be controlled strictly and subjected to regular internal and external assessments. All administrative and analytical activities should be described in detailed standard operating procedures (SOPs) which should be reviewed and, if necessary, updated at regular intervals. The laboratory should have in place a system of internal quality controls and also participate in external proficiency-testing schemes. Particular attention should be given to the storage of raw analytical data, results and residual samples, and no unauthorised person should have access to patient information. Where possible, the laboratory should seek accreditation by an external authority (see Chapter 23).

Collection and choice of samples

Blood, serum or plasma

Blood is usually easy to obtain and the analytical results can be related to the patient's condition and also be used in pharmacokinetic or toxicokinetic calculations. A 10 mL sample of anticoagulated blood (edetate) and 10 mL of clotted blood should be collected from adults on admission (proportionately smaller volumes from young children). Most quantitative assays are carried out on serum or plasma, but anticoagulated whole blood is essential if the poison is associated mainly with the red cells (e.g. carbon monoxide, cyanide, lead, mercury). Serum from coagulated blood can also be used, although the levels are almost always the same as those in plasma. Serum has the advantage that there is no potential interference from any additive. It is advisable to collect, in addition, a 2 mL blood sample into a fluoride/oxalate tube if ethanol ingestion is suspected. Disinfectant swabs that contain alcohols (ethanol, propan-2-ol) or iodine used to clean the skin prior to venepuncture can contaminate blood samples and should not be used. The vigorous discharge of blood through a syringe needle can cause haemolysis and invalidate a serum iron or potassium assay. Modern sample tubes may have a separation gel layer. Unfortunately these gels can adsorb some drugs (e.g. tricyclic antidepressants) or emitted substances (e.g. toluene).

Table 8.2 Disturbance of clinical features and indications of possible causes

Clinical feature	Disturbances and poisons indicated
General appearance	Restlessness or agitation (amfetamines, cocaine, lysergide (LSD), opiates withdrawal), apathy, drowsiness, coma (hypnotics, organic solvents, lithium)
Neurological disturbances	Electroencephalogram (EEG) (central depressants), motor functions (alcohol, benzodiazepines), speech (alcohol, drugs of abuse), movement disorders (hallucinogens, amfetamines, butyrophenones, carbamazepine, lithium, cocaine, ethylene glycol), reflexes, seizures (most centrally active substances in overdose or withdrawal), ataxia
Vital signs	
Mental status	Psychosis (illicit drugs), disorientation, stupor
Blood pressure	Hypotension (phenothiazines)
	Hypertension (corticosteroids, cocaine, phenylpropanolamines, anticholinergics)
Heart	Pulse, electrocardiogram (ECG) (elevation of QT-time: tricyclic antidepressants, orphenadrine, claritromycine, ofloxazine, erytromycine, haloperidol, pimozide, droperidol)
	Irregularities, torsade de pointes (phenothiazines, procainamide, amiodarone, lidocaine), heart block (calcium blockers, beta-blockers, digitalis, cocaine, tricyclic antidepressants)
Temperature	Hyperthermia (LSD, cocaine, methylenedioxymethylamfetamine (MDMA), serotonin syndrome by selective serotonin reuptake inhibitors (SSRIs), valproate, ritonavir, venlafaxine, dinitro-o-cresol (DNOC), lithium, paroxetine, moclobemide, tramadol)
	Hypothermia (alcohol, benzodiazepines)
Respiration	Depressed (opiates, barbiturates, benzodiazepines)
	Hypoventilation (salicylates)
Muscles	Spasm and cramp (strychnine, crimidine, botulism)
Skin	Dry (parasympatholytics, tricyclic antidepressants)
	Perspiration (parasympathomimetics, cocaine)
	Gooseflesh (strychnine, LSD, opiates withdrawal)
	Needle marks (parenteral injections: drugs of abuse, insulin)
	Colour (red, carboxyhaemoglobin; blue, cyanosis, e.g. with ergotamine; yellow, DNOC)
	Blisters (paraquat, barbiturates)
Eyes	Pinpoint (opiates, cholinesterase inhibitors, quetipine)
	Dilated pupils (atropine, amfetamines, cocaine)
	Reddish (cannabis)
	Reflex, movements, lacrimation, nystagmus (phenytoin, alcohol)
Nose	Nasal septum complications (cocaine)
Kidneys	Rhabomyolysis (ethanol, quinine, heroin, colchicine, chlorophenoxy acids) and secondary causes (causing drugs seizures, agitation, sedation, muscular contraction, hyperthermia, hypokalemia and ischemia)
Chest	Radiography (bronchoconstriction, metals, aspiration)
Abdomen	Diarrhoea (laxatives, organophosphates)
	Obstruction (opiates, sympatholytics such as atropine)
	Radiography (lead, thallium, condoms packed with illicit drugs)
Smell	Sweat, mouth, clothes, vomit (see Table 8.3)

Table 8.3 Odours associated with poisoned patients

Odour	Potential agents or situation
Acetone/nail polish remover	Acetone, propan-2-ol, metabolic acidosis
(Aeroplane) glue	Toluene, aromatic hydrocarbon sniffing
Alcohol	Ethanol (not with vodka), cleaners
Ammonia	Ammonia, uraemia
Bitter almonds, silver polish	Cyanide
Bleach, chlorine	Hypochlorite; chlorine
Disinfectant	Creosote, phenol, tar
Formaldehyde	Formaldehyde, methanol
Foul	Bromides, lithium
Hemp, burnt rope	Marijuana
Garlic	Arsenic, dimethyl sulfoxide (DMSO), malathion, parathion, yellow phosphorus, selenium, zinc phosphide
Mothballs	Camphor, naphthalene, paradichlorobenzene
Smoke	Nicotine, carbon monoxide
Organic solvents	Diethyl ether, chloroform, dichloromethane
Peanuts	Rodenticide
Pears	Chloral hydrate, paraldehyde
Plants with special odours	For example *Taxus*, *Convallaria*
Rotten eggs	Disulfiram, hydrogen sulfide, hepatic failure, mercaptans (additive to natural gas), acetylcysteine
Shoe polish	Nitrobenzene
Turpentine	Turpentine, wax, solvent of parathion, polish

Table 8.4 Typical colours of the skin and poisoning

Colour of skin	Poison or situation
Blue, cyanosis	Hypoxia, methaemoglobinaemia, sulfhaemoglobin
Blue, pigment	Dye (amitriptyline or chloral hydrate tablets), paint
Yellow (jaundice)	Liver damage (alcohol, borate, nitrites, scombroid fish, rifampicin, mushrooms, metals, paracetamol, phosphorus, solvents)
Yellow	Dinitro-*o*-cresol (DNOC)
Reddish	Carbon monoxide
Black, necrosis	Sulfuric acid, burning, intra-arterial injection

Urine

Urine usually contains higher concentration of drugs, poisons and their metabolites than blood and is therefore ideal for qualitative screening. However, in emergency cases, particularly when the patient is unconscious, the delay in obtaining a sample may be unacceptable. Many clinicians are now reluctant to use catheterisation routinely on unconscious patients. A volume of 25–50 mL is sufficient for most purposes.

Table 8.5 Urine colours associated with various poisons

Colour of urine	Poison or drug
Red/pink	Ampicillin, aniline, blackberries, desferrioxamine, ibuprofen, lead, mercury, phenytoin, quinine, rifampicin
Orange	Warfarin, rifampicin, paprika
Brown/rust	Chloroquine, nitrofurantoin

Stomach contents

This sample includes vomit, gastric aspirate or stomach washout. Stomach washout is no longer a routine treatment procedure, but when it is

Table 8.6 Biochemical and haematological abnormalities in poisoning

Abnormality	Indication
Acid–base disturbances	
Metabolic acidosis	Ethylene glycol, salicylate, methanol, cyanide, iron, amfetamines, MDMA
Metabolic alkalosis	Chronic use of diuretics or laxatives
Respiratory acidosis	Opiates
Respiratory alkalosis	Salicylates, amfetamines, theophylline
Increased anion gap	Ethylene glycol
Increased osmolar gap	Alcohols, glycols, valproate
Electrolyte disturbances	
Hypocalcaemia	Ethylene glycol, oxalates, phosphates, diuretics, laxatives
Hyperkalaemia	Digoxin, potassium salts
Hypokalaemia	Theophyllline, insulin, oral antidiabetic drugs, diuretics, chloroquine
Hypernatraemia	Sodium chloride, sodium bicarbonate
Hyponatraemia	MDMA, diuretics, water
Glucose	
Hypoglycaemia	Insulin, oral antidiabetic drugs, ethanol (children), paracetamol (with liver failure)
Liver enzymes	
Raised transaminases	Paracetamol, amfetamines, MDMA, iron, *Amanita phalloides*, strychnine
Haematological	
Anaemia, raised zinc protoporphyrin, basophilic stippling	Lead
Carboxyhaemoglobin	Carbon monoxide
Methaemoglobinaemia	Chlorates, nitrites
Raised prothrombin time	Paracetamol, coumarin anticoagulants

carried out it is important to obtain the first sample of washout rather than a later sample, which will be diluted considerably. If it is obtained soon after the overdose, it may be possible to recognise the presence of undegraded tablets and capsules, or the characteristic odour of certain compounds. Stomach contents can be substituted for urine in toxicological screening, and are useful for identifying poisons derived from plants and fungi, and for other poisons that are difficult to detect in blood or urine. However, as with urine, quantitative analyses serve no purpose, for example, in reflecting the amount of poison absorbed.

Saliva and/or oral fluids

There is growing interest in the use of saliva as an alternative noninvasive test sample and in its potential uses in hospital toxicology, that include caffeine measurements in neonates and 'bedside' tests for drugs of abuse (see Chapter 6).

Other specimens

Meconium, dark green mucilaginous excrements of the newborn, is often used to demonstrate maternal use of drugs (see later). The analytical toxicologist can also be confronted by unusual specimens. For example, a clinician sent unknown pieces of fatty material from a woman's bladder; after analysis it was found to be from a wrongly administered paracetamol suppository.

Toxicological screening

Toxicological screening schemes can be divided into limited, specific or extensive ('general unknown') screening.

Fast limited screening

Immunoassays

Commercially available immunoassays, such as fluorescence polarisation immunoassay (FPIA), enzyme multiplied immunoassay technique (EMIT), radioimmunoassay (RIA) and enzyme-linked immunoabsorbent assay (ELISA; see Chapter 14), give quick qualitative results and, in some cases, a semi-quantitative result in plasma for a variety of substances or groups of compounds. Their limitations in terms of

Table 8.7 Emergency toxicological assays

Assay(s)	Intervention	Comments
Anticholinesterase inhibitors[a]	Atropine, pralidoxime, obidoxime	Measure serum (or preferably red cell) cholinesterase activity
Anti-epileptics (carbamazepine, phenytoin)	Multiple dose-activated charcoal	–
Benzodiazepines	Flumazenil antidote only in severe cases	Consider presence of active metabolites; withdrawal seizures
Beta-blockers	Glucagon, isoprenaline	–
Calcium antagonists	Calcium salt infusions	Verapamil: severe prognosis Nifedipine: acidosis
Carboxyhaemoglobin[a]	Hyperbaric oxygen	No value after administration of oxygen
Chloroquine	High doses of diazepam	Monitor serum K^+
Cocaine	Diazepam, haloperidol	–
Digoxin[a]	Potassium salts, Fab antidote	Monitor serum K^+, measure serum digoxin prior to giving Fab fragments
Ecstasy group (methylenedioxyamfetamine (MDA), MDMA)	Single-dose activated charcoal, diazepam, dantrolene	Check for metabolic acidosis and hyponatraemia, hyperthermia
Ethanol[a]	Haemodialysis	Monitor blood glucose in children
Iron[a]	Desferrioxamine, intravenous + orally	Measure unbound iron; colorimetric assays for serum iron unreliable in presence of desferrioxamine
Isoniazid	Pyridoxine	–
Lithium[a]	Haemodialysis	Measure serum level 6 h after ingestion
Methaemoglobin[a]	Methylene blue	Methaemoglobinaemia caused by nitrites, chlorates, dapsone, aniline
Methanol, ethylene glycol plus other alcohols	Methylpyrazole or ethanol and haemodialysis	Monitor serum ethanol levels to ensure optimum antidote administration
Methotrexate	Folinate, glucarpidase	Measure plasma methotrexate level 36 h after ingestion: <15 μmol/L (see Voraxaze®, Instruction for use)
Opiates	Naloxone	–
Osmolality	–	Increased by alcohol, glycols, severe valproate overdose
Paracetamol[a]	*N*-Acetylcysteine, methionine	Measure serum level at least 4 h after ingestion; prothrombin time and International Normalised Ratio (INR) are useful prognostic indicators
Paraquat (qualitative urine test)[a]	Activated charcoal	Urine test diagnostic; plasma levels useful in predicting outcome
Salicylate[a]	HCO_3^- infusion, haemodialysis	Repeat serum salicylate assays may be needed because of continued absorption of the drug
Strychnine	Diazepam	–
Thallium	Prussian (Berlin) blue orally	Treatment continued until urine thallium levels <0.5 mg/24 h
Theophylline[a]	Multi-dose activated charcoal	Measure serum theophylline in asymptomatic patients 4 h after ingestion
Tricyclic antidepressants	Multi-dose activated charcoal and sodium bicarbonate	QT time

[a] To be provided by all acute hospital laboratories.

specificity and sensitivity must always be considered when interpreting results. Hospital laboratories that provide TDM and screening services for drugs of abuse are ideally placed to invoke these assays as part of a toxicological investigation.

Alcohol dehydrogenase test for ethanol

This quantitative test is based on the oxidation of ethanol to acetaldehyde by alcohol dehydrogenase (ADH) in the presence of nicotinamide–adenine dinucleotide (NAD) and is applicable to serum and plasma. Several commercial ADH kits are available and the test can be performed on routine clinical chemistry analysers. Propan-2-ol and other higher alcohols can also reduce NAD to give positive readings. Methanol and acetone do not react and therefore a gas chromatographic method for alcohols is much preferred.

Toxicological screening by chromatography

Thin-layer chromatography

Thin-layer chromatography (TLC) is usually applied to urine samples or, if these are not available, to stomach contents that have been purified prior to extraction. Any particulate material in the stomach contents should be removed by filtration or centrifugation prior to solvent extraction. Further purification by removal of fats and other dietary material can be carried out using a back-extraction step, as described below.

Many TLC systems have been developed for use in hospital toxicology. These include the commercial Toxilab system, which provides standards for the substances and metabolites most commonly encountered in intoxicated patients. The most generally used mobile phase is chloroform–methanol (9:1 v/v), although some countries now prefer the less toxic dichloromethane to chloroform. In hospital toxicology it is advisable to use at least two separate mobile-phase systems to obtain a more definitive result. Silica-gel plates of 20 cm × 20 cm with or without fluorescent indicator are the most popular, although smaller sizes can also be used.

Gas–liquid chromatography screening for alcohols and other volatile substances

In normal practice it is advisable to measure the more volatile alcohols (methanol, ethanol, acetone and propan-2-ol) separately from the higher alcohols, trichloroethanol and the metabolites of GHB, but for screening it is possible to detect all with two different temperature steps.

Gas chromatographic screening for drugs

Gas–liquid chromatography (GLC) with capillary columns and a nitrogen–phosphorus detector (NPD), or with an electron capture detector (ECD) in series, is a powerful screening system that is sensitive enough to detect many of the compounds of interest in small samples of serum, plasma or whole blood, as well as in urine specimens.

Much greater selectivity and specificity is obtained by coupling the gas chromatograph to a mass spectrometer (see Chapter 21).

HPLC screening using the systematic toxicological identification procedure

The systematic toxicological identification procedure (STIP) system is based on a rapid and simple extraction method followed by isocratic reversed-phase HPLC with diode-array detection. A library of retention times and ultraviolet (UV) spectra is available for about 400 common drugs. A disadvantage of the system is that a large number of drugs elute between 1 and 3 min and this problem is exacerbated with substances devoid of a characteristic UV spectrum (e.g. maximum <210 nm). In such cases a second chromatographic analysis may be required. The technique is also less sensitive than GC screening methods.

In this century liquid chromatography with triple quadrupole mass spectrometric detection (LC-MS/MS) has become increasingly introduced into the clinical laboratory. The quality, robustness, applicability and sensitivity are increasing enormously, but instrument price is decreasing as a result of strong competition between growing numbers of companies.

The great sensitivity of LC-MS/MS makes it possible to precipitate proteins and extract the relevant drugs and their metabolites just by diluting the serum or plasma eight times with an acetonitrile/methanol mixture containing an internal standard. Run times are about 5–7 minutes on average. This method is still lacking a generally available MS library of toxic compounds. Nevertheless, is it quite easy to select a number of relevant drugs on the basis of their masses and collision masses. For instance, if tricyclic antidepressants, selective serotonin reuptake inhibitors (SSRIs), cardiac drugs, anti-convulsants or anti-HIV drugs are suspected, the masses of the relevant drugs in one of these pharmacological groups are selected and within 10 minutes such a series of drugs can be excluded or determined. LC with single MS does not have this possibility owing to lack of sensitivity and selectivity. Although the price of one LC-MS/MS setup equals that of two LC-MS set-ups, one LC-MS/MS has more to offer in TDM and clinical and forensic toxicology than three LC-MS set-ups. Over the next decade an increasing number of laboratories will exchange their HPLC equipment with DAD, ECD and fluorescence detectors for one or two LC-MS/MS instruments.

Tests for specific compounds and groups of compounds

Alcohols, acetone, acetaldehyde and glycols

Ethanol is frequently taken at the same time as other drugs and can intensify the action of depressant drugs. A blood-ethanol determination helps to distinguish this from normal alcoholic intoxication; it is also useful in the clinical assessment of unconscious patients admitted with head injuries and smelling of drink. Children are particularly at risk from hypoglycaemia which may follow the ingestion of alcohol. Methanol is available in a variety of commercial products (antifreeze preparations, windscreen washer additives, duplicating fluids). Acetone is sometimes consumed by alcoholics as a substitute for ethanol; children may take nail cleaner fluid; diabetics may be comatose from high endogenous acetone levels. Acetone is also a metabolite of propan-2-ol. It can be useful to measure acetaldehyde as a toxic metabolite of ethanol, since some patients are unable to metabolise this compound for genetic reasons or because of an interaction with disulfiram, metronidazole, tolbutamide, watercress and other substances. Acetaldehyde is also a major metabolite of paraldehyde. Ethylene glycol is a principal component of automotive antifreeze products. Poisoning by either methanol or ethylene glycol is often associated with severe metabolic acidosis and electrolyte imbalance; therapy with ethanol infusions or other antidotes must be instituted without delay.

Enzymatic assays based on ADH and breath analysers are applicable only to ethanol; a qualitative and quantitative GLC method is required for the other alcohols.

Alcohols in serum by osmolality

If no specific assay for alcohols is available, the osmolal gap should be measured:

$$\begin{bmatrix}\text{measured}\\ \text{mOsmol/kg}\\ \text{in patient's}\\ \text{serum}\end{bmatrix} - \left\{\frac{\text{calculated osmolality}}{0.93}\right\} = \text{osmol gap} \quad (8.1)$$

In practice,

$$\text{osmol gap} = \text{measured mOsmol/kg} - 290 \quad (8.2)$$

$$\text{milligrams of alcohol per litre of serum} = \text{osmol gap} \times \text{relative molecular mass} \quad (8.3)$$

Each measured osmol gap unit = F g/L alcohol in serum; F = 0.026 for methanol, 0.043 for ethanol, 0.05 for ethylene glycol, 0.055 for acetone and 0.059 for propan-2-ol. A negative osmol gap can be caused by a water intoxication (see above) or sodium loss by MDMA.

Screening for abuse of solvents

The term 'glue-sniffing' comes from the abuse of adhesives, which often contain solvents such as toluene, ethyl acetate, acetone or ethyl methyl ketone. These, and similar compounds, also occur in a diverse range of other commercial products that may be abused, such as shoe-cleaners, nail varnish, dry-cleaning fluids, bottled fuel gases (butane and propane), aerosol propellants and fire extinguishers (bromochlorodifluoromethane). The identification, quantification and interpretation of solvents abused are described in detail in Chapter 4.

Antidepressants and antipsychotics

Antidepressants and antipsychotics comprise a diverse group of compounds that includes the tricyclic antidepressants and antipsychotic agents such as phenothiazines, thioxanthenes, butyrophenones, diphenylbutyl piperidines, benzamides and lithium. Other substances, mainly the newer ones, include the SSRIs, monoamine oxide inhibitors (MAOs) and atypical antipsychotics such as clozapine and olanzapine. Tricyclic antidepressants remain an important cause of suicide, and serious poisoning can lead to cardiac disturbances, respiratory depression, metabolic acidosis, convulsions and coma. These are gradually being replaced by the less toxic SSRI compounds such as citalopram, fluoxetine, fluvoxamine, paroxetine and sertraline. These drugs are also used as drugs of abuse. However, the severity of the serotonergic syndrome and the risk of rhabdomyolysis and cardiac conductive failures are often underestimated.

Analysis of antidepressants and antipsychotics by GLC

For detection of the misuse of these drugs, especially the more recent ones and depot preparations, GLC methods have the advantage of producing a lower limit of quantification (LOQ). Alternative systems are described in Chapter 18.

Benzodiazepines, zolpidem and zopiclone

Benzodiazepine tranquillisers are prescribed widely and therefore occur more frequently than any other type of drug in overdose cases. The effects of these drugs in overdose are usually mild, although they may have a synergistic effect when taken with alcohol or other drugs. The anticonvulsive benzodiazepine clonazepam (Rivotril) is also used to detoxify patients with very severe (other) benzodiazepine dependence. Although these drugs do not seem to cause lethal intoxications, reports of deaths from benzodiazepines have been published, most of which refer to elderly people or case of combined overdose of flunitrazepam and opiates. The hypnotic flunitrazepam can also cause a paradoxical effect, which is noticed by hooligans using this benzodiazepine. Over 30 benzodiazepines are available; some of these are both the parent compound and a metabolite of other benzodiazepines. The intrinsic activity varies enormously from one to the other. For example, alprazolam has a therapeutic effect at a serum concentration of 1 μg/L, whereas oxazepam becomes active on average at 1000 μg/L. This phenomenon makes comprehensive screening for the group very difficult. Many of the metabolites (including some glucuronides) are also active. In patients with renal failure the metabolite midazolam glucuronide can still be active even if the parent compound and its hydroxymetabolite are no longer measurable (see also under brain death, p. 222). Several immunoassays are available to screen for the benzodiazepine group in urine. However, in most of these the antibodies do not react with the glucuronides and, therefore, prior enzyme hydrolysis of the urine is required. The hypnotics zolpidem and zopiclone have similar dynamic and toxic activity to the benzodiazepines. Although these are not benzodiazepines, they have a high cross-reactivity with most benzodiazepine immunoassays.

Analysis

All benzodiazepines and their unconjugated metabolites (except the parent drug potassium clorazepate) are extractable from body fluids into an organic solvent and can be quantified in serum or plasma by normal-phase HPLC with UV detection. GC with ECD can also be used (see Chapter 18). All analytes of benzodiazepines, whatever the matrix (blood, urine) or analytical method (immunoassay or chromatography), require a hydrolysis step (see also p. 235, Analytical methods) except when LC-MS/MS is used, as the parent benzodiazepine and all metabolites (including the glucuronides) can be measured as such separately in one run.

Cholinesterase inhibitors (organophosphate and carbamate pesticides)

There are no simple direct chemical tests for these compounds. The toxic effects are usually associated with depression of the cholinesterase activity of the body, and measurement of the plasma or serum cholinesterase can be used as an indication of organophosphorus or carbamate poisoning. Plasma or serum cholinesterase (pseudocholinesterase) is inhibited by a number of compounds and can also be decreased in the presence of liver impairment. Erythrocyte cholinesterase (true cholinesterase) reflects more accurately the cholinesterase status of the central nervous system. However, pseudocholinesterase activity responds more quickly to an inhibitor and returns to normal more rapidly than erythrocyte-cholinesterase activity. Thus, measurement of pseudocholinesterase activity is quite adequate for diagnosing acute exposure to organophosphorus or thiocarbamate compounds, but cases of illness that may be caused by chronic exposure to these compounds should also be investigated by determining the erythrocyte-cholinesterase activity.

Paraquat and diquat

Paraquat (1,1-dimethyl-4,4-bipyridylium chloride) is the most important bipyridyl herbicide. Although deaths are reported from accidental paraquat exposure by inhalation and transdermal absorption, accidental or deliberate intake is nearly always by oral ingestion. Diquat is less toxic than paraquat. Granular preparations usually contain 2.5% of paraquat and 2.5% of diquat; liquid preparations may contain 20% w/v of paraquat only. Measurement of the plasma paraquat concentration is a useful prognostic test and Scherrman *et al.* (1983) have published a nomogram of the relationship between time after ingestion, plasma concentration and probable outcome. The main use of an assay is to prevent overtreatment of patients who are not at risk or who have no chance of survival. Paraquat can be measured in plasma by immunoassay, although the methods are not widely available. HPLC methods have also been described (see Chapter 19).

Chlorophenoxyacetic acid herbicides

Poisoning with chlorophenoxyacetic acids, such as 2,4-dichlorophenoxyacetic acid (2,4-D), 2,4,5-trichlorophenoxyacetic acid (2,4,5-T) and methylchlorophenoxyacetic acid (MCPA), causes metabolic acidosis, myoglobinuria, rhabdomyolysis, elevated liver function tests, hypophosphataemia, miosis and tachycardia. Plasma levels above 100 mg/L are associated with toxic symptoms.

These compounds can be measured spectrophotometrically at a maximum of about 284 nm, or after acid extraction and methylation by gas chromatography with FID or MS detection.

Analgesics: paracetamol, salicylates and other nonsteroidal anti-inflammatory drugs

Acute overdose with most of the nonsteroidal anti-inflammatory drugs (NSAIDs) rarely causes severe toxicity with the exceptions of paracetamol (acetaminophen) and salicylates.

Paracetamol

Paracetamol is widely available as an over-the-counter medicine and is frequently taken in overdose. Paracetamol is metabolised by the liver to *N*-acetyl-*p*-benzoquinoneimine (NAPQI), which is normally inactivated by liver glutathione. After paracetamol overdose, the glutathione stores become depleted to leave toxic amounts of NAPQI to bind to proteins and cause centilobular necrosis. Drugs that induce hepatic P450 enzymes (e.g. phenobarbital) and chronic high ethanol abuse may enhance paracetamol toxicity. Intravenous infusion of *N*-acetylcysteine to replenish the glutathione stores is an effective treatment, especially when given during the early stages of poisoning. During the first 12 h after ingestion of a severe overdose no clinical features other than vomiting may occur. After 12 h, hepatic necrosis causes continued vomiting, which may also induce abdominal pain after 24 h. Signs of jaundice become apparent after 36–72 h and the patient may develop hepatic encephalopathy and hepatic failure. Serum or plasma paracetamol measurements play a crucial role in the early diagnosis; management protocols, and nomograms that relate these to time after ingestion and the likelihood of developing liver damage have been published (Smilstein *et al.* 1991). The sample analysed should ideally not be taken until 4 h after ingestion, since before then the processes of absorption and distribution are incomplete. However, in practice this is not always feasible since the exact time of ingestion may not be known. Measuring a second paracetamol level about 4 h after the first can be useful, especially in cases of staggered overdose, and can give a better indication of prognosis. A half-life of about 4 h indicates a healthy liver and one of about 12 h predicts severe necrosis.

Reliable commercial kits are available for paracetamol measurements in serum or plasma, designed for use on routine clinical analysers and based either on immunoassays (Edinbora *et al.* 1991) or enzymatic reactions (Morris *et al.* 1990). Numerous GC and HPLC methods have also been published.

Salicylates

Salicylic acid is most often derived from acetylsalicylic acid (aspirin) and severe overdose results in respiratory alkalosis and metabolic acidosis. Children below the age of 4 years are particularly susceptible to salicylate poisoning. Continued absorption of aspirin is common after the initial admission to hospital. Sustained-release salicylate preparations may form concretions in the stomach that result in prolonged absorption as they gradually disintegrate. Application of salicylate-containing ointments to abnormal skin can also lead to significant toxicity, as can the use of teething gels in infants. Chronic salicylate poisoning can occur in rheumatic patients who take large doses of aspirin, and salicylism should be considered in any elderly patient with unexpected delirium or dementia. Ingestion of methyl salicylate is rare, but it is potentially more dangerous because of rapid absorption. Treatment of severe salicylate poisoning involves sodium bicarbonate infusions, multiple doses of oral activated charcoal and, in severe cases, haemodialysis. Toxicity is associated with plasma salicylate concentrations of 300 mg/L or greater. Adults with plasma salicylate concentrations less than 450 mg/L and children with plasma salicylate concentrations less than 350 mg/L do not require specific treatment. The slow and continuous absorption of the drug may necessitate repeat plasma salicylate determinations.

Other NSAIDs

Other NSAIDs include the arylacetic acids (e.g. diclofenac), arylpropionic acids (e.g. ibuprofen, ketoprofen, naproxen), heterocyclic acetic acids (e.g. indometacin, ketorolac, sulindac), pyrazolones (phenylbutazone), oxicams (e.g. piroxicam) and mefenamic acid. Most patients who take an overdose of these drugs are asymptomatic, but the chronic use of mixtures of analgesic drugs has been linked to renal damage, including papillary necrosis and chronic interstitial nephritis. Most of these classic NSAIDs were replaced by an increasing number of cyclooxygenase inhibitors (COX-1 and COX-2) but their cardiotoxicity has dramatically decreased their use. These compounds are extractable at acidic pH values and most can be determined by the STIP method or other suitable HPLC methods.

Anti-epileptics (carbamazepine, oxcarbazepine, phenytoin, phenobarbital, primidone, valproate, ethosuximide, clonazepam, clobazam, lamotrigine)

Anti-epileptic drugs are commonly prescribed in combination in epilepsy treatment. Symptoms of acute overdose simulate those of barbiturate poisoning. Laboratories that offer a routine therapeutic drug-monitoring service for these drugs have little difficulty in adapting their normal procedures to the occasional overdose case. Immunoassays for some of the anti-epileptic drugs lack linearity and exhibit different cross-reactivities in the toxic range, and HPLC or GC (see Chapters 19 and 18, respectively) assays are preferred alternatives in toxicological investigations.

Carbon monoxide

Carbon monoxide is one of the most frequent causes of fatal poisoning in developed countries. Common sources of carbon monoxide are vehicle exhaust fumes, smoke from fires and emissions from improperly maintained and ventilated heating systems. More rarely, exposure to dichloromethane vapours from paint strippers, degreasing agents and aerosol propellants can lead to carbon monoxide poisoning because the solvent can be metabolised by mixed-function oxidases to carbon dioxide and carbon monoxide. The affinity of carbon monoxide for haemoglobin is 200–300 times that of oxygen and therefore most of the toxic effects result from diminished oxygen delivery to the tissues. Symptoms progress from headache, nausea, gastrointestinal upset, hyperventilation, hypertension and drowsiness to coma. Chronic poisoning as a result of continuous exposure to small amounts of carbon monoxide leads to nonspecific symptoms, such as headaches, dizziness, fatigue and general malaise, and is often undiagnosed. Elevated carboxyhaemoglobin (COHb) concentrations confirm a diagnosis of carbon monoxide poisoning. When a patient is removed from the contaminated atmosphere the COHb disappears rapidly, particularly if oxygen is administered.

Hospital clinical chemistry laboratories are usually equipped with automated differential spectrophotometers (CO-oximeters) that measure simultaneously the absorption of a blood haemolysate at four or more wavelengths to determine total haemoglobin, the percentage saturation of oxyhaemoglobin and COHb, as well as methaemoglobin and sulfhaemoglobin (Widdop 2002). If such an apparatus is not available, the spectrophotometric method of Rodkey *et al.* (1979) can be used.

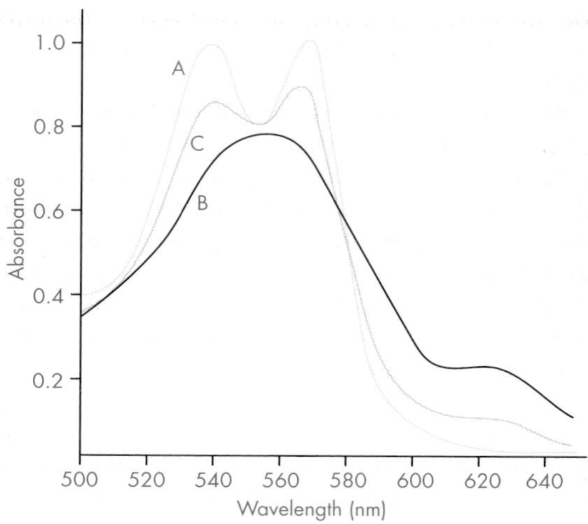

Figure 8.1 Ultraviolet spectra of (A) carboxyhaemoglobin, (B) reduced haemoglobin and (C) a blood sample from a patient poisoned with carbon monoxide.

Quantification of carboxyhaemoglobin in blood by spectrophotometry

Principle When a reducing agent (sodium dithionite) is added to the blood, both the oxygenated form and the methaemoglobin are converted quantitatively to the reduced form, which has the visible spectrum B shown in Fig. 8.1. Carbon monoxide has a much greater affinity for haemoglobin than does oxygen, and the COHb is not reduced by sodium dithionite. Thus, even when treated with sodium dithionite, COHb retains its normal twin-peaked spectrum, marked A in Fig. 8.1. The maximal difference between the spectra of A and B is at 540 nm, while at 579 nm the spectra have the same absorbance (isosbestic point). The percentage saturation of carbon monoxide in a blood sample (A) can be calculated from measurements of the absorbance of the carbon monoxide-free sample (B) and the untreated sample (C), after reduction of each with sodium dithionite.

Standards Gas bottles of pure carbon monoxide can be obtained. Alternatively, commercial reference standards of haemolysed blood in sealed glass ampoules are available (IL, Warrington, UK).

Metals

The detection of poisoning with toxic metals is an important feature of hospital toxicology; in modern laboratories the favoured techniques are atomic absorption spectrophotometry (AAS) and inductively coupled plasma–MS (ICP-MS). Further details of poisoning by metals are described in Chapter 4.

Theophylline and caffeine

Theophylline is prescribed to asthmatic children and adults, but serious toxicity can be caused both by therapeutic excess and by overdose. Clinical features include severe hypotension, cardiac arrhythmias and convulsions. Biochemical disturbances include hyperinsulinaemia, hyperkalaemia, glycosuria and metabolic acidosis. Many theophylline preparations are of the slow-release type, so that the onset of toxic symptoms may be delayed for up to 12 h after overdose. Treatment consists of gastric lavage for patients who reach hospital within 1 h of the overdose and multiple oral doses of activated charcoal, which is thought to be as efficient as charcoal haemoperfusion as an elimination procedure. The plasma theophylline concentration is an important diagnostic test and should be measured urgently. In asymptotic patients levels should be measured 4 h or more after ingestion.

Caffeine is prescribed for neonatal apnoea. It is also an ingredient of many proprietary stimulant preparations and is an important adulterant in drugs of abuse. Some patients have an idiosyncrasy for theophylline or caffeine, developing tachycardia at low serum concentrations. Although the lethal dose is large (about 10 g), severe caffeine intoxication with tachyarrhythmias followed by cardiovascular collapse has caused deaths in children. Caffeine also potentiates the effects of sympathomimetic drugs, which contribute to adverse cardiac disorders.

Commercial immunoassay kits are available to determine theophylline and caffeine in serum or plasma. These drugs can be determined by the STIP chromatography system.

Cardioactive drugs

There are several classes of cardiac drugs. The cardiac glycoside digoxin is the oldest still in use and therapeutic overdose is far more common than deliberate overdose. Serious digoxin overdose has a mortality rate of up to 20% and may be combated by the administration of oral activated charcoal, magnesium sulfate and ovine fragment antidigoxin antibodies. Digoxin is usually measured in serum by immunoassay (see Chapter 14), but the presence of Fab fragments interferes with the assay, as do other cardiac glycosides such as digitoxin. When considering the use of Fab-fragment therapy, a serum digoxin immunoassay carried out prior to administration can be used to calculate the total body burden and the amount of antidote required. Other cardioactive drugs can be measured in serum or plasma by HPLC (Chapter 19) or by GC (Chapter 18).

Drugs of abuse

Drugs of abuse may be taken deliberately or accidentally in overdose, or administered to others by a third party. Laboratory personnel should be aware of potential legal implications that might arise subsequently from any cases that involve drug abuse, and make sure that full documentation is collected and retained. Hospital toxicologists include drugs-of-abuse screening as part of their portfolio of tests provided to aid diagnosis and treatment, and for this purpose urine is the sample of choice. Quantitative assays in serum or plasma are rarely needed urgently and are usually reserved for cases with medicolegal implications. Routine analysis of drugs of abuse in urine also forms part of drug-dependence treatment programmes in which laboratory tests are used to assess the drug-taking pattern of new patients and subsequently to monitor their compliance with treatment. The toxicologist is continuously acquainted with the new trends. For example, oxycodone and buprenophine have become rather popular drugs of abuse.

Analytical methods

Fast immunoassay screening tests are described above and more information can be found in Chapter 5, Chapter 6 and Chapter 14. For routine drug-dependence screening programmes in which large batches of urine samples are analysed daily, the analytical protocol usually comprises rapid automated immunoassay screening using a clinical chemistry analyser followed by the re-examination of positive samples using a more selective chromatographic technique.

Chromatographic analysis of drugs of abuse

Deglucuronidation

Several of these drugs are excreted extensively as glucuronides in the urine. It is therefore recommended that acid or enzymatic hydrolysis of the urine is carried out prior to extraction. Acid hydrolysis is typically performed using 36% hydrochloric acid in a boiling water bath. Enzymatic hydrolysis with β-glucuronidase–sulfatase (from *Helix pomatia* or other species) is a gentler procedure that avoids the destruction of drugs that are acid labile (see p. 200).

Interpretation and advice

An experienced hospital toxicologist is expected not only to provide valid analytical data, but also to assist the clinician in relating the findings to a particular case of poisoning. This may be quite straightforward when the presence of a high concentration of a drug or poison is consistent with the patient's symptoms and the circumstantial evidence. In other cases, factors such as the patient's age, sex, health and previous exposure must be taken into account. For example, addicted patients may have developed a tolerance to extremely high concentrations of opiates, benzodiazepines and ethanol, and exhibit relatively mild toxicity. An elderly invalid with respiratory problems is far more susceptible to an overdose of a central depressant drug than a healthy young adult, and so may have life-threatening symptoms with only moderate plasma concentrations. The route of administration (inhalation, oral ingestion, intravenous injection, etc.) can have a very significant effect on the subsequent toxicity, which must also be taken into account when interpreting plasma concentrations (see Chapter 2). Mixed overdoses of drugs and alcohol are common, and synergistic reactions can confuse the clinical picture. The hospital toxicologist must therefore develop a good background knowledge of drug interactions. However, there are situations in which the analytical results fail to offer an adequate explanation. This can result from mistakes in sample collection, for example when blood samples taken from an arm being used to infuse a therapeutic agent may have very high concentrations of that agent because of contamination. Cleaning the skin with alcohol-based swabs prior to venepuncture can result in apparently huge blood alcohol concentrations. Systems for collecting and referring samples to the laboratory can occasionally break down and the samples received and analysed (with negative results) may be from the wrong patient, or trough and peak levels may be interchanged. Negative results on the correct samples must also be interpreted with caution. The patient may not be poisoned after all and the clinical effects may be caused by an organic disorder. Alternatively, the toxic agent responsible is not detected, which may instigate a wider analytical search or application of a more sensitive assay. A list of therapeutic and toxic concentration ranges for drugs is given in Table 8.8. The hospital toxicologist may also be asked to apply toxicokinetic principles (see Chapter 2) to the quantitative data to answer questions raised by the clinician; examples in which this is relevant are described below.

How much (A) of the poison is still in the body at a serum concentration C?

$$A = C \times V_d \text{ (L/kg body mass)} \times \text{body mass (kg)}$$

where V_d is the volume of distribution.

How long will it take for a measured serum concentration (C_0) to decrease to below the toxic concentration (C_{tox})?

$$C_{tox} = C_0 \times e^{-k_e t}$$

where k_e is the elimination constant, $0.693/t_{1/2}$.

If the elimination is not saturated, the kinetic parameter k_e of the patient can be calculated as follows, using two serum concentrations measured during the elimination phase:

$$\text{Elimination constant } k = \frac{\ln C_1 - \ln C_2}{t_2 - t_1}$$

$$t_{1/2} = \frac{\ln 2}{k} = \frac{0.69}{k}$$

$$\text{Clearance CL} = k \times V_d$$

where V_d is volume of distribution.

What is the efficiency of an extracorporeal elimination treatment?

Severe cases of intoxication sometimes require extracorporeal elimination treatments, such as haemodialysis or haemoperfusion. For the clinician it is important to have an estimate of how many hours the dialysis or haemoperfusion has to be continued and when the next blood should be withdrawn. The efficiency of haemodialysis (or haemoperfusion) can be determined as follows:

- measure the blood flow-rate (mL/min) through the artificial kidney
- as the drug levels are measured in plasma and the drug is cleared from the plasma, the blood flow-rate has to be converted into the plasma flow-rate [blood flow-rate × (1 − haematocrit)].
- measure the drug plasma levels in samples taken before (C_{bef}) and after (C_{aft}) the artificial kidney

- $[(C_{bef} - C_{aft})/C_{bef} \times$ blood flow $\times$ [1 − haematocrit] = clearance (mL/min)
- this extracorporeal clearance has to be added to the physiological clearance of the poisoned patient: $(CL_{own} + CL_{extra} = CL_{total})$
- the half-life time during extracorporeal clearance is: $(\ln 2)/k = 0.69V_d/CL_{total}$.

As an alternative to these formulae, the toxicologist can use a commercially available toxicokinetic or pharmacokinetic software program. The pharmacokinetics software package MW/Pharm (Mediware, University of Groningen, The Netherlands) is very suitable and flexible for both therapeutic drug monitoring (TDM) and toxicological calculations. AutoKinetic by SW Tönnes, Frankfurt, Germany, is a less comprehensive program that uses Microsoft Excel.

Reporting results

Reports (verbal or written) should be submitted to the clinician by an authorised toxicologist who is fully responsible for the results and the advice provided. If the methods used were not validated, this should be indicated to the clinician so that he or she can judge the possible margin of error.

Sources of information

The practice of hospital toxicology requires knowledge and experience of pharmacotherapy, bio-analyses, good laboratory practice, pharmacokinetics, toxicokinetics, pharmacodynamics, basic toxicology, clinical toxicology, forensic toxicology, chemistry, and indications and contraindications of the different treatments. Numerous information sources are available and those listed under Further Reading are among the most useful. It is advisable to consult several sources before giving advice.

Books that deal specifically with poisoning by industrial chemicals, household products and natural toxins are also useful sources of reference.

Therapeutic and toxic concentrations

Table 8.8 lists the therapeutic and toxic serum concentration ranges for a large number of drugs. Therapeutic serum levels are the steady-state concentrations that need to be reached for the drug to exert a significant clinical benefit without unacceptable side-effects. Where concentrations are shown in brackets this refers to extreme, but still acceptable, values. Toxic serum levels are concentrations above which unacceptable, concentration dependent, toxic effects may appear. The toxic levels are expressed as a range, which means that the toxic effects may start somewhere in this range, depending on the patient and his or her clinical history. It should be taken into account that these values are never static and may change with advancing knowledge or with other (therapeutic) uses of the drug. Toxic and, where applicable, normal ranges are also given for substances that have no therapeutic use. It is emphasised that these data are intended merely as guidelines and that there is wide individual susceptibility towards the effects of drugs and poisons. In other words, the physician should treat the patient according to the clinical signs and not the analytical results.

Therapeutic drug monitoring

Introduction

Therapeutic drug monitoring (TDM) may be defined as the use of drug or metabolite monitoring in body fluids as an aid to the management of therapy. Since antiquity, physicians have adjusted the dose of drugs according to the characteristics of the individual being treated and the response obtained. This practice is easiest when the response is readily measurable, either clinically (e.g. antihypertensive drugs, analgesics, hypnotics) or with an appropriate laboratory marker (e.g. anticoagulants, hypoglycaemic agents, lipid-lowering drugs). Dose adjustment is much more difficult (but no less necessary) when drug response cannot be rapidly assessed clinically (e.g. in the prophylaxis of seizures or mania), or when toxic effects cannot be detected until severe or irreversible (e.g. nephrotoxicity or ototoxicity). Provided certain basic conditions are satisfied and appropriate analytical methods are available, the plasma

Table 8.8 Therapeutic and toxic concentrations

Compound	Relative molecular mass	Material[a]	Reference concentration (mg/L) Therapeutic[b]	Toxic[c]
Acebutolol	336.4	S	0.5–1.25	15–20
diacetol	308.4	S	0.65–4.5	–
Acenocoumarol	353.3	S	T, 0.03–0.09; P, 0.1–0.5	T, 0.1–0.15
Acetaldehyde	44.1	B	0–30	100–125
Acetazolamide	222.2	S	(5)10–20	25–30
Acetone	58.1	B	5–20	200–400
Acetylsalicylic acid	180.2	S		
Salicylic acid	138.1	S	50–300	400–500, child 300
Aldrin	364.9	S	0–0.0015	0.0035
Alimemazine	298.4	S	0.05–0.4	0.5
Allobarbital	208.2	S	2–5	10
Allopurinol	136.1	S	P, 1–5	–
oxypurinol	152.1	S	5–15	20
Alprazolam	308.8	S	0.02–0.04	0.075
Alprenolol	249.4	S	0.01–0.2	T, 0.1; P, 1–2
hydroxyalprenolol	266.4	S	0.04–0.065, sum 0.1–0.2	sum T, 0.25–0.3
Aluminium	27.0	S	0–0.02 (0.1)	0.05–0.15
Amantadine	151.3	S	0.3–0.6	1
Amikacin	585.6	S	T, 1–4 (10); P, 15–25 (30)	T, 10; P, 30
4-Aminopyridine	94.1	S	0.025–0.075	0.15–0.2
Amiodarone	645.3	S	1–2.5; T, 0.5–2	3
desethylamiodarone	617.3	S	sum (1–5)	sum 5–8
Amitriptyline	277.4	S	0.05–0.2	–
nortriptyline	263.4	S	sum 0.12–0.25	sum 0.5
Ammonia	17.0	P	0.5–1.7	–
Amobarbital	226.3	S	2–12	>9
Amfetamine	135.2	S	(0.02) 0.05–0.15	0.2
Aniline	93.1	S	–	
Aprindine	322.5	S	0.7–2	2
Arsenic	74.9	B	0.002–0.07	0.1–0.25 (1)
Arsenic	74.9	U	0–0.1	0.2–1
Atenolol	266.3	S	0.2–0.6 (1)	2
Atropine	289.4	S	0.002–0.025	0.03–0.1
Azathioprine	277.3	S	P, 0.05–0.3	–
mercaptopurine	152.2	S	0.04–0.3	1–2
Baclofen	213.7	S	0.2–0.6	1.1–3.5
Barbital	184.2	S	5–30	20
barbiturates				
intermediate acting		S	1–5	10–30
long acting		S	10–40	40–60
short acting		S	1–5	7–10
Benzphetamine	239.4	S	0.025–0.5	0.5
Benztropine	307.4	S	0.08–0.2	0.05
Bismuth	290.0	B	0–0.05	0.1

Boron	10.8	S	0.8–6	20–50
Brallobarbital	287.1	S	4–8	10
Brodifacoum	523.4	S	–	0.02
Bromadiolon	527.4	S	–	0.02
Bromazepam	316.2	S	0.08–0.17	0.25–0.5
bromide	79.9	S	3–30 therapeutic 75–100 (300)	500–1000 (1500)
Bromisoval	223.1	S	10–20	30–40
Buflomedil	307.3	S	0.2–0.5	15–25
Bupivacaine	288.4	S	0.25–0.75; P, 1–4	4–5
Buprenorphine	467.6	S	0.001–0.005	–
Butabarbital (secbutobarbital)	212.2	S	5–15	10
Butalbital	224.3	S	1–10	10–15
Butobarbital	212.2	S	2–15	(14) 32–98
Butriptyline	293.5	S	0.07–0.15	0.4
Cadmium	112.4	B	0–0.0065	0.015–0.05
Caffeine	194.2	S	8–20 (drink 2–5)	30–50
Camazepam	371.8	S	0.1–0.6	2
Carbamazepine	236.3	S	4–12	15
Carbamazepine epoxide		S	0.5–6	15
Carbon monoxide	28.0	B	1–5%	25–35%
Carbon tetrachloride	152.8	S	–	20–50
Carbromal	237.1	S	2–10	15–20
bromide	79.9	S	5–30	300
Carisoprodol	260.3	S	2.5–10	
Chloral hydrate				
trichloroethanol	149.4	S	(2) 5–15	40–70
Chloramphenicol	323.1	S	5–15; T, 5–10; P, 10–20 (25)	25; T, 10
Chlordane	409.8	S	0.001	0.0025
Chlordiazepoxide	299.8	S	0.7–2 (3)	3.5–10
demoxepam	286.7	S	0.5–0.74	1
Chlormezanone	273	S	2.5–9	20
Chloroform	119.4	B	20–50	70–250
Chlorophenoxyacetic acid	221.0	S	–	200
Chloroquine	319.9	S	0.02–0.3	0.5–1
Chlorothiazide	295.7	S	6	–
Chlorpheniramine	274	S	0.017	0.02–0.03
Chlorpromazine	318.9	S	0.05–0.5; child 0.04–0.08	(0.5) 1 (–2); child 0.5
Chlorpropamide	276	S	30–200	200–750
Chlorprothixene	315.9	S	0.03–0.3	0.7 (0.4–0.8)
Chlorthalidone	338.8	S	(blood) 5–10; (plasma) 0.2–1.4	–
Cholinesterase pseudo		S	2000–7000 U/L	1000 U/L
Cimetidine	252.3	S	0.5–1	1.25
Clobazam	300.7	S	0.1–0.4	–
N-desmethylclobazam	286.7	S	2–4	–
Clofibrate	242	S	50–250	–
Clomipramine	314.9	S	0.1–0.25	0.4–0.6
desmethylclomipramine	300.8	S	sum 0.15–0.55	sum 0.6–0.8
Clonazepam	315.7	S	0.03–0.06	0.1–0.12

Table 8.8 (*Continued*)

Compound	Relative molecular mass	Material[a]	Reference concentration (mg/L)	
			Therapeutic[b]	Toxic[c]
Clonidine	229	S	0.0003–0.0015	0.025–0.06
Clopenthixol (zu)	401.0	S	T, 0.002–0.010 (0.015)	0.05–0.1
Clorazepic acid (clorazepate)	314.7	S	–	–
nordazepam	270.7	S	sum 0.25–0.8	sum 2
Cloxacillin	435.9	S	5–30; P, 85	–
Clozapine	326.8	S	0.1–0.6 (0.8); T, 0.1–0.3	0.8–1.3
desmethylclozapine	312.7	S	0.1–0.6	0.7
Cobalt	58.9	B	0.0001–0.0022	–
Cocaine	303.4	S	0.05–0.3	0.25–5
Codeine	299.4	S	T, 0.01–0.05; P, 0.05–0.250	0.3–1
Colchicine	399.4	S	0.0003–0.0024; P, 0.003	0.005
Cyanide	26.0	B	0.001–0.012 (–0.15)	0.5
Cyclizine	266.4	S	0.1–0.25 (0.03–0.3)	0.75
norcyclizine	252.5	S	0.005–0.025	–
Cyclobartital	236.3	S	2–10	10–15
Cyclobenzaprine	275.4	S	0.003–0.036	0.4
Cyclopropane	42.1	P	80–180	–
Ciclosporin	1203	B	T, 0.1–0.4	T, 0.4–0.5
Cytarabine (Ara C)	243.2	S	0.05–0.5	–
Dantrolene	314.3	S	0.4–1.5; T, 0.3–1.4; P, 1–3	–
Dapsone	248.3	S	0.5–5	10–20
Deptropine	333.5	S	–	0.015
Desipramine	266.4	S	0.075–0.25	0.5
Dexfenfluramine	231.3	S	0.03–0.06	0.15–0.25
Dextromethorphan	271.4	S	0.01–0.04	0.1
Dextromoramide	392.5	S	0.075–0.15	0.2
Diazepam	284.7	S	0.125–0.75	1.5
nordazepam	270.7	S	0.2–1.8	–
Diazinon	304.3	S	–	0.05–(0.5)
Diazoxide	230.7	S	10–50	50–100
Dibenzepin	295.4	S	T, 0.025–0.15; P, 0.1–0.5	–
desmethyldibenzepin	281.3	S	sum 0.2–0.4	sum 3
Dichlorophenoxyacetic acid	231.0	S	–	100
Diclofenac	296.2	S	T, 0.05–0.5; P, 0.1–2.5	–
Dicoumarol	336.3	S	8–30 (50)	50–70
Dieldrin	380.9	S	0–0.0015	0.15–0.3
Diflunisal	205.3	S	(9)40–(200)	300–500
Digitoxin	764.9	S	0.01–0.03	0.03
Digoxin	780.9	S	T, 0.0005–0.001	T, (0.0014) 0.0025
Dihydrocodeine	301.4	S	0.03–0.25	0.5–1
Diltiazem	414.5	S	0.05–0.4	0.8
Dimethadione	188.3	S	500–1000	1000
Dinitro-*o*-cresol	198.1	S	1–5	30–60
Diphenhydramine	225.4	S	0.1–1	1

Dipyridamol	504.6	S	1–2; T, 0.1–1	4
Diquat	184.2	S/U	–	0.1–0.4
Disopyramide	339.5	S	2.5–7	8
nordisopyramide	297.5	S	–	sum 8–10
Disulfiram	296.5	S	0.05–0.4	0.5–5
diethyldithiocarbamate	171.3	S	0.3–1.4	–
Domperidon	425.9	S	0.005–0.025 (0.04)	–
Dosulepin (= dothiepin)	295.4	S	0.05–0.15 (0.4)	0.8
desmethyldosulepin	281.5	S	0.01–0.2	0.75
dosulepin *S*-oxide	311.5	S	0.04–0.4	0.65–2
Doxapram	378.5	S	2.7–5.2	–
Doxazosin	451.5	S	0.01–0.15	–
Doxepin	279.4	S	0.02–0.15	0.1
nordoxepin	265.4	S	sum 0.05–0.35	0.5–1
Doxycycline	444.5	S	(1) 5–10	30
Edrofonium	165.2	S	0.15–0.2	–
Enalapril	376.5	S	–	–
desethylenalapril		S	0.01–0.05 (0.1)	–
Encainide	352.5	S	–	–
methoxy-demethylencainide		S	0.06–0.28	–
O-demethylencainide		S	0.1–0.3	0.3
Endrin	380.9	S	0–0.003	0.01–0.03
Ephedrine	165.2	S	0.02–0.2	1
Epirubicin	543.5	S	0.01–0.05	–
Erythromycin	733.9	S	0.5–6; T, 0.5–1; P, 4–12	12–15
Estazolam	294.8	S	0.055–0.2	–
Ethambutol	204.3	S	0.5–6.5	6–10
Ethanol	46.1	B	0–25	1000–2000
Ethchlorvynol	144.6	S	0.5–8	20
Ethinamate	167.2	S	5–10	50–100
Ethosuximide	141.2	S	40–100	(100)150–200
Ethylene glycol	62.1	S	–	200–500
Etidocaine	276.4	S	0.5–1.5	1.6–2
Felodipine	384.3	S	0.001–0.008 (0.012)	0.01–0.015
Fenfluramine	231.3	S	0.05–0.15	0.5–0.7
Fentanyl	336.5	S	0.001–0.002	0.002–0.02
Flecainide	414.4	S	T, 0.45–0.9; P, 0.75–1.25	1.5–3
Fluconazol	306.3	S	5–15 (40)	50–75
Flucytosine	129.1	S	T, 25–50; P, 50–100	100
Flumazenil	303.3	S	0.01–0.05; P, 0.2–0.3	0.5
Flunarizine	404.5	S	0.025–0.2	0.3
Flunitrazepam	313.3	S	0.005–0.015	0.05
Fluoride	19.0	S/U	T0.08–0.15	T, 0.5–2
5-Fluorouracil	130.1	S	0.05–0.3	0.4–0.6
Fluoxetine	309.3	S	0.1–0.45	–
norfluoxetine	295.3	S	0.05–0.35 sum 0.15–0.5 (0.9)	sum 1.5–2.0
Fluphenazine	437.5	S	0.001–0.017	0.05–0.1
Flurazepam	387.9	S	0.0005–0.028	0.15–0.2
desalkylflurazepam	288.7	S	0.04–0.15	sum 0.2–0.5
Fluvoxamine	318.4	S	0.05–0.25	0.65

Table 8.8 *(Continued)*

Compound	Relative molecular mass	Material[a]	Reference concentration (mg/L)	
			Therapeutic[b]	Toxic[c]
Furosemide	330.8	S	2–5 (10)	25–30
Ganciclovir	255.2	S	0.5–5; T, 0.2–1; P, 5–12.5	T, 3–5; P, 20
Gamma-hydroxybutyric acid	104.1	S	0–1; sleep 50–150	100–150
Gentamicin	463	S	T, 0.05–2; P, 4–15	T2
Glibenclamide	494	S	0.03–0.35	0.6
Glutethimide	217.3	S	2–12	12–20
Gold	197.0	S	3–8	10–15
Haloperidol	375.9	S	0.005–0.015 (0.04)	(0.01) 0.05–0.0.5
Halothane	197.4	B	22–84	
Heptabarbital	250.3	S	1–4	8–15
Heptobarbital	218.2	S	50–100	125–150
Hexapropymate	181.2	S	2–5	10–20
Hexobarbital	236.3	S	1–5	8 (10–20)
Hydralazine	160.2	S	(0.05) 0.2–0.9	–
Hydrochlorothiazide	297.7	S	0.07–0.45	–
Hydrocodone	299.4	S	0.002–0.024 (0.05)	0.1
Hydromorphone	285.3	S	0.008–0.032	
Hydroxychloroquine	335.9	S	T, 0.1–0.4; P, 0.5–2.0	0.5–0.8
Hydroxyzine	374.9	S	P, 0.05–0.09	0.1
Ibuprofen	206.3	S	15–30 (5–50)	100
Imipramine	280.4	S	0.045–0.15	0.4–0.5
desipramine	266.4	S	0.075–0.25, sum 0.15–0.3	sum 0.5
Indomethacin	357.8	S	0.5–3	4–6
Iron	35.8	S	0.5–2	6; child 2–8
		B	380–625	–
Isoniazid	137.1	S	T, 0.2–1; P, 3–10	20
Isosorbide dinitrate	236.1	S	0.003–0.018	–
isosorbide mononitrate		S	0.2–0.5	–
Itraconazole	705.6	S	T, >0.25	–
hydroxy-itraconazole		S	sum 1–4	sum 6
Ketamine	237.7	S	0.5–6.5	7
Ketazolam	368.8	S	0.001–0.02	–
nordazepam	270.7	S	0.2–0.6	1–2
Ketoconazole	531.4	S	T, 0.3–0.5; P, 3–10 (20)	–
Labetalol	328.4	S	0.025–0.2	0.5–1
Lamotrigine	256.1	S	2–15	15
Lead	207.2	B	up to 0.3	0.4–0.45
Levomepromazine	328.5	S	0.02–0.15	0.5
Lidocaine (lignocaine)	234.3	S	(1) 1.5–5	7–10
Monoethylglycinexyliclide (MEGX)	206.3	S	0.07–0.175	–
Lisinopril	405.5	S	(0.005) 0.02–0.07	0.5
Lithium	6.9	S	4–10; T, 0.6–1.2 mmol/L	T, 1.5 (2) mmol/L

Loratadine	382.9	S	0.015–0.03	
descarboethoxyloratadine		S	0.007–0.03	
Lorazepam	321.2	S	0.02–0.25	0.3–0.6
Lormetazepam	335.2	S	0.001–0.02	–
Lysergide (LSD)	323.4	S	0.0005–0.005	0.001
Maprotiline	277.4	S	0.075–0.25 (0.1–0.6)	0.3–0.8
desmethylmaprotiline	263.4	S	sum 0.1–0.4	sum 0.75–1
Medazepam	270.8	S	0.01–0.15; P, 0.1–0.5	0.6 (–1)
nordazepam	270.7	S	0.2–0.6	1–2
Mefenamic acid	241.3	S	0.3–20	25
MEGX (liver test)	206.3	S	T, 0.070–0.175	0.05
Meperidine	247.4	S	0.07–0.8	5
Mephenytoin	218.3	S		
desmethylmephenytoin		S	sum 15–40	sum 50
Mepivacaine	246.4	S	2–5.5	6–10
Meprobamate	218.3	S	10–30	30–50
6-Mercaptopurine	152.2	S	0.03–0.08	1–2
Mercury (organic)	200.6	B/U	0–0.01	0.1–0.3
Mercury (inorganic)	200.6	B	0–0.08	0.2
Mesoridazine	386.6	S	0.1–1.1	3–5
Mesuximide	203.2	S	0.04–0.08	–
N-desmethylmesuximide	189.2	S	10–30 (40)	
Methamfetamine	149.2	S	0.01–0.05	0.2–1
Metformin	129.2	S	1–4	5–10
Methadone	309.5	S	0.07–0.1 (0.5)	native 0.2; users 0.75
Methanol	32.0	B	0–1.5	200
Methaqualone	250.3	S	0.4–5	>2
Methotrexate	454.5	S	active 0.005	T, 0.2 (48 h)
Methotrimeprazine	328.5	S	0.02–0.14	–
Methoxsalen	216.2	S	0.1–0.2; T, 0.025–0.1; P, 0.1–0.4	1
Methyldopa	211.2	S	1–5	7–10
Methylenedioxy-methylamfetamine (=XTC. MDMA)	193.0	S	0.1–0.35	0.35–0.5
Methylphenidate	233.3	S	0.005–0.06	(0.5) 0.8
Methyprylon	183.3	S	10–20	12–75 (128)
Metoclopramide	299.8	S	0.04–0.15	0.1–0.2
Metoprolol	267.4	S	0.1–0.6; T, 0.02–0.34	(0.65)–1
Metronidazole	171.2	S	(30)10–30	150 (200)
Mexiletine	179.3	S	0.5–2	2–4
Mianserin	264.4	S	0.015–0.07 (0.14)	0.5–5
desmethylmianserin	250.3	S	sum 0.04–0.125	sum 0.3–0.5
Midazolam	325.8	S	0.08–0.25	1–1.5
Milrinone	211.2	S	0.15–0.25	0.3
Mirtazepine	265.4	S	0.02–0.1 (0.3)	–
desmethylmirtazepine		S	sum 0.05–0.3	sum 1
Moclobemide	268.7	S	T, 0.4–1; P, 1.5–4	5–8
Morphine	285.4	S	0.08–0.12	0.15–0.5

Table 8.8 *(Continued)*

Compound	Relative molecular mass	Material[a]	Reference concentration (mg/L)	
			Therapeutic[b]	Toxic[c]
Nalidixic acid	232.2	S	10–30	40–50
		U	50–200	–
Naloxone	327.4	S	0.01–0.03	–
Naproxen	230.3	S	25–75 (90)	200–400
Netilmicin	475.6	S	T, 0.5–2 (3); P, 7–15 (18)	T4
Nicotine	162.2	S	sum T, 0.001–0.275	
cotinine	176.2	S	sum P, 0.025–0.35	sum 0.3–1
Nifedipine	346.3	S	0.02–0.1 (0.15); T, 0.01–0.02	0.15–0.2
Nickel	58.7	S	0.0015–0.005	–
		U	0.0005–0.006	–
Nitrazepam	281.3	S	0.03–0.12	0.2–0.5
Nitrofurantion	238.2	S	0.5–2 (3)	3–4; child 2
		U	10–400	–
Nomifensine (unbound)	238.3	S	T, 0.02–0.06; P, 0.2–0.6	0.8–0.1
Nordazepam	270.7	S	0.2–0.8 (1.8)	1.5–2
Nortriptyline	263.4	S	0.075–0.25	0.5
Obidoxim	359.2	S	1–10	–
Olanzapine	312.4	S	0.02–0.08 (0.1)	0.2
Opipramol	363.5	S	0.05–0.2 (0.5)	0.5–2 (3)
Orphenadrine	269.4	S	0.05–0.2 (0.6)	0.5–1
tofenacin	255.4	S	sum 0.05–0.2	sum 0.5–2
Oxazepam	286.7	S	(0.15) 0.5–2	2
Oxcarbazepam	252.3	S	as metabolite	–
hydroxycarbazepine		S	12–35	45
Oxprenolol	265.4	S	0.05–0.3 (1.0)	2–3
Oxtetracycline	460.5	S	5–10	30
Oxycodone	315.4	S	(0.005) 0.02–0.05	0.2
Pancuronium (as HBr)	652.8 (732.7)	S	0.1–0.6	0.4
Papaverine	339.4	S	0.2–0.6 (2)	–
Paracetamol (acetaminophen)	151.2	S	10–20 (2.5–25)	T, 75–100; P, 100–150
Paraldehyde	132.2	S	30–200 (300)	200–400
acetaldehyde	44.0	S/B	0–30	100–125
Paramethadione	157.2	S	1.1–5	–
Paraquat	186.3	S/U	–	0.05
Parathion	291.3	S	–	0.01–0.05; workers 0.1–0.2
Paroxetine	329.3	S	(0.01) 0.07–0.15 (0.25)	0.3
Pefloxacin	333.4	S	T, 0.1–6; P, 5–10	25
Penciclovir	253.3	S	T, 0.1–0.3; P, 1.75–2 (orally); P, 10–20 (i.v.)	–
Pentachlorophenol	266.4	S	0–0.1	30
Pentazocine	285.4	S	0.01–0.2 (0.5)	1–2
Pentobarbital	226.3	S	1–10 (25–40)	(5) 8–10

Perazine	339.5	S	0.02–0.35	0.5
Perycíazine	365.5	S	0.005–0.03	0.1
Perphenazine	404.0	S	0.0004–0.03	0.05
Pethidine	247.3	S	0.1–0.8	(1)–2
norpethidine		S	–	0.3–0.5
Phenacetin	179.2	S	5–20	50
Phenazone (antipyrine)	188.2	S	5–25	50–100
Phencyclidine (PCP)	243.4	S	–	0.007–0.24
Phenelzine	136.2	S	0.001–0.002 (0.2)	0.5
Phenmetrazine	177.3	S	0.02–0.25	0.5
Phenobarbital	232.2	S	(10) 20–40	60–80
Phenprocoumon	280.3	S	1–3	5
Phensuximide	189.2	S	4–10; P, 10–20	80
Phenylbutazone	308.4	S	50–100	120–200
Phenylephrine	167.2	S	0.03–0.1 (0.3)	–
Phenylpropanolamine	151.2	S	0.05–0.5	2
Phenytoin [free fraction]	252.3	S	8–20; baby 6–14 [0.2–2]	25; baby 15 [2]
Pimozide	461.6	S	0.001–0.02	–
Pindolol	248.3	S	0.02–0.08 (0.15)	0.7
Pipamperone	375.5	S	0.1–0.4	0.5–0.6
Piperazine	86.1	S	0.02–0.1	0.5
Pipotiazine	475.7	S	0.001–0.06	0.1
Piroxicam	331.3	S	5–10 (20)	–
Platinum (from cisplatin)	195.1	S	0.5–5; P, 10–30	30 T10
Polythiazide	439.9	S	0.002–0.007	–
Prazepam	324.8	S	0.01–0.04	–
nordazepam	270.7	S	0.2–0.8	1–2
Prazocin	383.4	S	0.001–0.075	0.9
Prilocaine	220.3	S	0.5–2 (5)	5
Primidone	218.3	S	T, 5–12	10 (15–20)
phenobarbital	232.2	S	20–40	60–80
Probenecid	285.4	S	40–60; 100–200	–
Procainamide	235.3	S	4–10	10–15
N-acetylprocainamide	277.4	S	2–12; sum T, 5–30	sum 40
Procaine	236.3	S	2.5–10	15–20
Prochlorperazine	373.9	S	0.01–0.05	0.2–0.3
Promazine	284.4	S	0.01–0.4	(1) 2–3
Promethazine	284.4	S	(0.05) 0.1–0.4	1
Propafenone	341.5	S	0.4–1.1 (1.6)	1.1–3
norpropafenone	415.5	S	–	sum 2–3
Propan-2-ol	60.1	B	–	200–400
acetone	58.1	B	–	200–400
Propofol	178	B	narcosis 2–4 (8)	–
Propoxyphen (dextro)	339.5	S	0.1–0.75	1
norpropoxyphen	325.5	S	0.1–0.15	2
Propranolol	259.3	S	T, 0.05–0.15; P, 0.1–0.3	1–2
Propylene glycol	76.1	S	0.05–0.5	1000
Protionamide	180.3	S	T, 0.5; P, 3–8	–
Protriptyline	263.4	S	0.07–0.17 (0.38)	0.5
Pseudoephedrine	165.2	S	0.5–0.8	
Pyrazinamide	123.1	S	30–75	–

Table 8.8 (*Continued*)

Compound	Relative molecular mass	Material[a]	Reference concentration (mg/L)	
			Therapeutic[b]	Toxic[c]
Pyridostigmine	181.3	S	0.05–0.1 (0.2)	–
Quetiapine	383.0	S	(0.025) 0.075–0.5 (0.9)	–
Quinidine	324.5	S	(1) 2–6	(6)–10 (15)
Quinine	324.5	S	1–7 (9.5)	10
Rifampicin	823.0		0.5–1.0	–
desacetylrifampicin		S	sum T, 0.5–1 P, 5–20	20
Risperidone	808.9	S	0.003–0.03	0.08
hydroxyrisperidone	410.5	S	sum 0.02–0.06	0.08
Salbutamol	239.4	S	0.004–0.018	0.03
Salicylic acid	138.1	S	20–300	300–500
Scopolamine	303.4	S	0.0001–0.0003 (0.001)	–
Secobarbital	238.3	S	2–10	>8
Sertraline	306.2	S	0.05–0.25 (0.5)	–
Silver	107.9	B	0–0.005	–
Sotalol	272.4	S	0.5–3 (5)	5–10
Spironolactone	416.6	S	0.1–0.5	–
Strychnine	334.4	S	–	0.075–0.1
Sufentanil	386.6	S	0.0005–0.005 P,0.01–0.02	–
Sultiame	290.4	S	0.5–12.5	12–15
Suramine	1407.2	S	150–250	300
Tacrolimus (FK506)	804	B	T, 0.003–0.01; P, 0.01–0.025	T, 0.015–0.02
Temazepam	300.7	S	0.3–0.9; T, 0.02–0.15	1
Terbinafine	291.4	S	T, 0.01–0.03; P, 0.5–3	–
norterbinafine		S	P, 0.4–0.8	–
Terbutaline	225.3	S	0.001–0.006 (0.01)	0005–0.01
Tetracycline	444.4	S	5–10; T, 1–5	30
Thallium	204.4	B/U	0–0.005	0.1–0.5
Theophylline	180.2	S	8–20; baby 5–10	25–30; baby 15
Thiazinamium	299.5	S	0.05–0.15	0.3
Thiocyanate	58.0	S	1–12 (30)	35–40 (100)
Thiopental	242.3	S	1–5 (25–40)	10 (40–50)
pentobarbital	226.3	S	5–10	10–15
Thioridazine	370.6	S	0.2–1	2 (5)
mesoridazine	386.6	S	0.3 (0.2–1.6)	Large overlap with therapeutic range
sulforidazine	402.6	S	<0.6, sum 0.75–1.5	sum 3
Tin	118.7	S	0.03–0.14	–
Tobramycin	467.5	S	T, 0.5–1.5; P, 5–10 (15)	T, 2; P, 15
Tocainide	193.2	S	4–10	(13–15) 25
Tofenacine	255.4	S	P, 0.025–0.1	0.5–1
Tolbutamide	270.3	S	45–100	400–500
Tolmetin	257.3	S	10–80	–
Tramadol	299.8	B	0.1–0.75	0.8

Trazodone	371.9	S	0.5–2.5; T, 0.3–1.5; P, 1.5–2.5	4
Triameterene	253.3	S	T, 0.01–0.1; P, 0.05–0.2	–
Triazolam	343.2	S	0.002–0.02	–
Trichloroethanol	149.4	S	5–15	40–70
Trichlorophenoxyacetic acid	255.5	S	–	200
Trifluoperazine	407.5	S	(0.001) 0.005–0.05	0.1–0.2
Triflupromazine	352.4	S	0.03–0.1	0.3–0.5
Trihexyphenidyl	301.5	S	0.05–0.2	0.5
Trimethoprim	290.3	S/U	1.5–2.5 (5–10)	15–20
Trimipramine	294.4	S	0.07–0.3	0.5
Valnoctamide	143.2	S	5–25	40
Valproate	144.2	S	50–100 (150)	150–200
Vancomycin	1449.2	S	T, 8–15; P, 20–40	P50
Venlafaxine	313.9	S	0.25–0.5	–
desmethylvenlafaxine	299.8	S	sum 0.2–0.7	sum 1–1.5
Verapamil	454.6	S	0.05–0.35	0.9
norverapamil	440.6	S	sum 0.15–0.6	sum 1
Vigabatrin	129.6	S	T, (1) 5–25	–
Vinblastine	811.0	P	P, 0.25–0.4	–
Vincristine	824.9	P	P, 0.3–0.4	–
Vinylbital	224.3	S	1–4	5
Warfarin	308.3	S	1–3 (7) T, 0.3–3; P, 5–10	10–12
Zidovudine	267.2	S	T, 0.1–0.3; P, 1–1.5	0.5–3
Zolpidem	307.4	S	0.08–0.3	0.5
Zopiclone	388.8	S	0.01–0.05; P, 0.04–0.07	0.15

Concentrations shown in brackets refer to extreme, but still acceptable, values.

[a] B, whole blood (heparinised or edetate); S, serum; U. urine; P, plasma.

[b] Reference concentration (mg/L) during steady state; T, trough level just before drug administration; P, peak level 1 to 2 h after drug administration.

[c] Minimum level or range for which concentration-dependent side-effects or toxic effects have been noticed; –, no values because toxic concentrations not available; T, trough level just before drug administration; P, peak level 1 to 2 h after drug administration.

concentration of a drug or metabolite may serve as an effective and clinically useful surrogate marker of response. However, it must be stressed that TDM is not simply the provision of an analytical result, but a process that begins with a clinical question, and continues by devising a sampling strategy to answer that question, determining one or more drug concentrations using a suitable method and interpreting the result appropriately.

TDM has been routinely practised in clinical laboratories since the mid-1970s, but the scientific foundations of the subject date back to the 1940s, when Marshall first tested the concept that the activity of a drug is dependent on its plasma concentration. In 1960, Buchthal showed a relationship between seizure control and plasma phenytoin concentration in patients being treated for epilepsy, and Baastrup and Schou described the plasma concentration–pharmacological effect relationship for lithium in 1967 (Buchthal *et al.* 1960; Baastrup and Schou 1967). This work coincided with the rise of clinical pharmacology during the 1960s and the demonstration of the fundamental concepts of pharmacokinetics and pharmacodynamics, which underpin the interpretation of drug concentration measurements.

Fundamental concepts

Different patients need different doses of drug to produce the optimum pharmacological effect because individuals vary widely in the way they absorb and dispose of drugs, and in the way they respond to drugs. The steps between prescribing a drug to a patient and obtaining the desired response are summarised in Fig. 8.2, which also indicates the distinction between pharmacokinetics and pharmacodynamics. *Pharmacokinetics* describes the way in which a patient's system handles drugs, and encompasses uptake of drugs into the body, distribution throughout body compartments, metabolism and elimination of drugs (and their metabolites) from the body. These processes are described in more detail in Chapter 2. *Pharmacodynamics* is concerned with the action of pharmacologically active substances with target sites (receptors), and the biochemical and physiological consequences of these actions. For example, the effects of a given tissue concentration of digoxin on cardiac muscle are modified by the potassium concentration, which affects the concentration–response relationship and means that plasma drug concentrations are not the sole determinant of response. In simple terms, pharmacokinetics may be said to be the study of what patients do to drugs, and pharmacodynamics of what drugs do to patients.

If plasma drug concentrations are to be a useful surrogate marker of response, two premises must be fulfilled. The first is that the drug concentration in plasma must accurately reflect the concentration at the site of action (the receptor), which may be located in the plasma compartment itself or may be deep in target tissue. This assumption is true for many drugs, but is far from universal – for example, the blood–brain barrier may mean that plasma concentrations of drugs that act on the brain are unrepresentative of concentrations at the site of action, and adequate concentrations of an antibiotic in the blood may not guarantee effective concentrations at the centre of a poorly perfused abscess (e.g. antituberculosis drugs). The brain/plasma ratio is among other phenomena depending on the PgP-pump, the protein binding and the charge of the substance. There may also be significant time differences between peak concentrations of a drug or its measured active metabolite in plasma and maximum penetration to the receptor, which complicates the interpretation of plasma concentration measurements.

The second premise is that drug concentration at the receptor should provide an accurate index of pharmacological response. This may not be true if other drugs interact with the receptor, if receptor numbers are reduced (e.g. in the phenomenon of tolerance when patients have been on a drug for some time) or if the coupling of receptors to signal transduction pathways is modified.

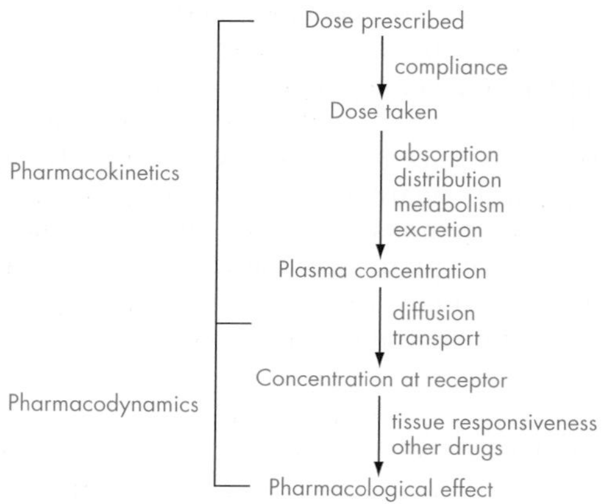

Figure 8.2 Processes involved in drug action.

Criteria to assess the clinical value of drug monitoring

The criteria for TDM to be clinically useful for a particular drug may therefore be developed and summarised as follows:

- Poor correlation between the dose given and the plasma concentration obtained in different patients (wide inter-individual pharmacokinetic variability). Clearly, if the dose given is an effective predictor of plasma concentration in all patients, then measurement of an individual's plasma concentration is superfluous. Compliance testing (determining whether patients actually take the drugs – often now referred to as *concordance* testing) may be a useful adjunct to TDM programmes (see below), but is unlikely to justify such a programme in the absence of other indications for monitoring.

- Good correlation between plasma concentration and pharmacological effect in different patients (low inter-individual pharmacodynamic variability). If plasma concentration measurements do not give accurate information about response, they are at best useless and at worst misleading. So the two premises stated above must be satisfied (plasma drug concentration predicts receptor concentration and receptor drug concentration predicts response). Active metabolites are generally undesirable as they contribute to the effect but make a variable (or zero) contribution to the concentrations, depending on the assay system; for example, a metabolite may have 10% of the biological activity of the parent drug, but show 100% cross-reactivity in an immunoassay. This criterion also normally requires that the action of the drug at the receptor site be essentially reversible. If this is not the case, and the drug binds irreversibly to the receptor, the pharmacodynamic half-life (or duration of effect) may be markedly longer than the pharmacokinetic half-life (or length of time the drug can be detected in the circulation). In this situation, the drug may still be exerting an effect when no drug can be detected in the plasma, and it is difficult to argue that TDM has a useful contribution to make. The exception to this general rule may be some anti-cancer agents, for which an index of the body's total exposure to the drug may predict subsequent response.
- TDM is only clinically relevant for drugs that show significant toxic or undesirable effects at plasma concentrations only slightly above those required for useful effects. If there is a wide margin between effective concentrations and undesirable effects, as is the case for penicillin, effective therapy may be achieved by giving the drug to all patients in large excess, with no need for individualisation of therapy. In contrast, the aminoglycoside antibiotics have relatively narrow margins between effective concentrations and those that produce unacceptable toxicity, so concentration monitoring has an essential role in ensuring maximal effect with minimal toxicity.
- Similarly, TDM is redundant for drugs for which there is a better clinical marker of effect, for example blood pressure, plasma glucose concentration or prothrombin time. Plasma drug concentrations have little to offer in this situation, except in the elucidation of rare cases where a high dose of drug fails to produce the desired effect, when TDM may help differentiate between noncompliance, poor drug absorption, rapid drug metabolism (cytochrome-P450 (CYP) status), receptor dysfunction or the use of the wrong drug for the situation.

Application of these criteria results in a relatively short list of drugs for which concentration monitoring has a proven clinical role. Measurement of other drugs may contribute in isolated cases or particular clinical circumstances, but it cannot be said to be generally useful in dosage.

Indications for drug monitoring

The main reasons for measuring drugs in plasma may be summarised as follows:

- to ensure that sufficient drug is reaching the drug receptor to produce the desired response (which may be delayed in onset, e.g. for antidepressant drugs)
- to ensure that drug (or metabolite) concentrations are not so high as to produce signs or symptoms of toxicity
- as an aid to defining the pharmacokinetic and pharmacodynamic parameters of new drugs or in clinical situations in which these parameters are changing rapidly
- a fourth indication, the detection of noncompliance (poor concordance) with therapy, remains a matter of some controversy. Clearly, if the assessment of compliance is accepted as a valid indication for concentration monitoring, it could be necessary to provide an analytical service for virtually every drug in the pharmacopoeia, at enormous cost. Furthermore, although gross noncompliance with therapy is associated with very low or undetectable concentrations of a drug in the blood, variable compliance can be difficult or impossible to detect, and

the variability between patients that makes dosage individualisation necessary also implies that surprisingly low plasma concentrations for a given dose of drug do not necessarily indicate noncompliance. Noncompliance with therapy can be assessed in other ways, for example by tablet counting, supervision of medication or the use of carefully designed questions that are nonjudgemental (e.g. 'How often do you forget to take your tablets?'). Detection of noncompliance is thus not a primary indication for measuring plasma drug concentrations, although if an analytical service is provided for other reasons, concentration monitoring may have a role for patients with poor symptom control who deny poor compliance despite careful questioning.

Some patients just do not take (all) their medication and save up those not taken for committing suicide later. By controlling the compliance of the patient, the physician can be warned in time. Even if concentration measurements of a drug have been shown to be of proven value, this does not mean that they are required in all situations in all patients who receive the drug. Indeed, indiscriminate use of TDM services has done much to erode the cost-effectiveness of the process, and has frequently harmed rather than helped patient care. As with any laboratory test, a clear clinical question should be formulated before recourse is made to concentration measurements. The question helps to decide what measurements should be made, and how the results can be interpreted. Examples of suitable questions might be 'My patient is not responding to therapy – could this be because of inadequate plasma concentration or is a different drug required?' or 'Could this patient's symptoms be explained by drug toxicity?'. When requesting physicians lose sight of this fundamental principle, and do tests as 'routine', answers without questions are obtained. The dangers of this are well illustrated by the all-too-frequent example of a patient on anticonvulsant therapy for epilepsy who has a 'routine' blood test done in primary care, and the result is found to be significantly above the target or 'therapeutic' range for the drug. The laboratory may then telephone the result as a matter of urgency, and cause an inexperienced physician to react with an inappropriate dose reduction, which precipitates seizures in a patient who was perfectly well controlled on the original dose.

Analytical requirements

Sample

Blood, urine, saliva and hair may be considered as possible samples for TDM analyses. By its very nature hair is a retrospective medium, which can give an indication of drug concentrations in the weeks or months that precede sampling. This is a valuable property in the field of abused drug detection (see Chapter 3), but has little relevance to the individualisation of therapy. Applications of hair analysis to TDM are therefore limited at present, although there have been studies on the long-term monitoring of antipsychotic drugs, such as haloperidol, in psychiatric in-patients. Similarly, the variation of drug concentrations in urine with the degree of urine concentration and state of hydration means that there are no applications in TDM in which urine is preferred to plasma as a sample matrix.

Plasma (or serum) is normally the preferred sample for TDM analyses, but has the disadvantage that it requires an invasive procedure for collection (venepuncture). Some drugs (e.g. many immunosuppressants) are concentrated in the red cells, and whole blood (with an appropriate anticoagulant, e.g. ethylenediaminetetraacetic acid (EDTA)) is more suitable than plasma. When plasma samples are used, care must be taken with anticoagulants and the use of gel separation barriers, both of which can cause interference with some drugs or assay systems. However, in the proven absence of such effects there are no clinically significant differences between serum and plasma, and either may be used. Plasma also contains a considerable amount of protein, and many drugs of interest in the TDM field (e.g. phenytoin) show significant protein binding. This means that the total (free plus protein-bound) concentration of a drug in plasma varies with protein concentration, even though the free (pharmacologically active) concentration remains constant. This variation of measured drug concentration with plasma protein concentration complicates the interpretation of plasma drug levels, and has led to moves to measure only the circulating free (unbound) drug. This can either be achieved *in vitro* by determining the concentration of drug in a plasma ultrafiltrate (obtained by centrifugation of plasma through an appropriate filter or by equilibrium dialysis across a semipermeable membrane) or by sampling an *in vivo* ultrafiltrate. Saliva is sometimes used as the latter, although care must be taken to ensure that the saliva : plasma concentration ratio is constant and unaffected by salivary pH or salivary flow rate. This is not always the case, but where these conditions are satisfied (for drugs that are not ionisable or un-ionised within the salivary pH range, e.g. theophylline, carbamazepine and phenytoin), saliva can provide an effective, noninvasive sample matrix for determination of the pharmacologically active component of a drug in plasma. Saliva sampling can be particularly useful in children or in adults with needle phobia, although there are still problems with collection and potential contamination. Drug concentrations in saliva are normally lower than in plasma or serum, and the matrix itself provides some analytical challenges. For these reasons, salivary monitoring still has not found wide application, although it undoubtedly has a role in some circumstances (see Liu and Delgado (1999) and Chapter 6).

Timing of measurements

The primary requirement for an appropriate specimen if TDM is to be used to assess the adequacy of response is that the specimen be taken when the drug concentration in the body is at a steady state and the effects of any recent dose changes have been allowed to stabilise. The time to reach steady state is determined by the elimination half-life of the drug, and there is a fixed relationship between the number of half-lives that have elapsed since the drug was commenced and the progress towards steady state concentration (see Chapter 2). The plasma concentration after 3.3 half-lives have elapsed is 90% of the predicted steady-state concentration, and 94% of steady-state concentration is reached after four half-lives. For drugs with a long plasma half-life (for example, digoxin and phenytoin), a week or two (or even longer) may be required before steady state is obtained, especially if renal function is poor in the case of digoxin. It is usual to allow at least four elimination half-lives to elapse before monitoring the effect of any dose change, although obviously if toxicity is suspected after a dose change it would be unwise to wait for steady state before checking the plasma concentration. As it takes four half-lives to be at steady state, it takes the same time to eliminate the drug out of the plasma. Amiodarone has an extreme half-life and this can be the reason the clinician cannot wait for the making of an ECG. The amiodarone serum level may be useful for interpretation of its influence on the ECG. Computer programs with the ability to predict steady-state concentrations from measurements made before steady state is attained may also be helpful.

The other issue that relates to the appropriate sample timing is the question of when the sample should be taken in relation to the last dose of the drug. As drugs are normally administered at fixed time intervals, inevitably there is a variation of plasma concentration between one dose and the next. For most purposes, the most reproducible parameter for long-term monitoring is the steady-state trough concentration – a measurement immediately prior to the next oral dose. The importance of precise sample timing depends somewhat on the half-life of the drug – drugs with long half-lives (e.g. phenytoin) show little variation in concentration across the dosage interval, and accurate specimen timing is less important than for short-half-life drugs like theophylline and lithium. For these drugs, toxic symptoms may correlate better with peak plasma concentrations than trough concentrations, and if toxicity is suspected a sample timed at 1–6 h post dose (depending on the release characteristics of the preparation and the speed of absorption) may be more appropriate. Some antibiotics require high peak concentrations and low trough concentrations for optimal effects (e.g. aminoglycosides), while others require the maintenance of high trough concentrations (e.g.

vancomycin). In the case of lithium, a strong case has been made to standardise the sampling time at exactly 12 h post dose. The area under the concentration–time curve (AUC), or the concentration at an intermediate time point, may also be a better predictor of response than either the peak or the trough concentration (e.g. in the case of ciclosporin, where the 2-hour post-dose concentration is now sometimes used). The determination of AUC requires more complex sampling regimes.

Some drugs exhibit a distribution phase immediately after the dose has been given, and for the duration of this phase the plasma concentration is unrepresentative of the pharmacologically relevant receptor concentration. This is particularly the case for digoxin, for which clinically misleading concentrations may be obtained in the first 4 or 5 h following a dose (whether oral or intravenous) while the drug equilibrates between plasma and tissue compartments.

Measurement techniques

A suitable analytical technique is obviously the bedrock of drug analysis, and studies to establish a correlation between plasma drug concentration and response cannot begin until a measurement technique has been developed and validated. The final stage of establishing the clinical value of an assay is prospective randomised controlled trials that compare patients who have been monitored with a control group who have been managed without the aid of concentration monitoring. Unfortunately, there are virtually no drugs for which unequivocal evidence of the clinical benefit of monitoring has been obtained by large-scale trials. Lithium and phenytoin are the best examples.

Much early pharmacokinetic knowledge was obtained from studies using colorimetry, spectrophotometry and spectrofluorimetry (see Chapter 15 for examples of methods), but these methods have now been virtually abandoned for quantitative clinical work because of their lack of specificity. The exception is lithium, which is still frequently measured by atomic absorption or flame emission spectrophotometry, although ion-selective electrodes are displacing spectrometric techniques. Many antibiotics were once measured by bioassay, but this has poor specificity for combinations of drugs and is too slow, imprecise and labour-intensive for present-day applications. Thin-layer chromatography (Chapter 13) is also little used for quantitative measurement of therapeutic concentrations.

The three techniques that are most widely used for routine clinical measurement of drug concentrations are gas chromatography (Chapter 18), high-performance liquid chromatography (Chapter 19) and immunoassays (Chapter 14), with mass spectrometry (Chapter 21) rapidly gaining popularity. In the laboratory for TDM and Toxicology of the first author during 2005–2006, over 120 assays of drugs in serum were converted from HPLC-DAD or immunoassay into validated LC-MS/MS methods. Ion suppression seems to be the optimal analytical technique because of speed, flexibility, sensitivity, reliability and labour saving, and it requires only small sample volume. Selection of the most appropriate method for a given drug or clinical situation is not easy, and the choice depends on the availability of staff, expertise and equipment, the nature of the service to be provided and the range of drugs to be assayed. The widely different chemical natures of the substances to be assayed for TDM purposes means that it is rarely possible to offer a comprehensive service based on a single analytical principle. Also, compromises will usually have to be made between using the best method for each individual analyte and using techniques that allow quantification of a wide range of substances.

The basic requirements of any method are that it should be specific for the substance being assayed (without interference from structurally related compounds or endogenous plasma components), capable of precise quantification, and sufficiently sensitive to detect concentrations normally found in therapy in a sample small enough for clinical work (certainly less than 1 mL plasma and ideally 10–100 μL).

Chromatographic methods

Chromatographic methods are flexible and adaptable to a wide range of compounds. Methods for new compounds can be devised relatively quickly in most cases, compared to immunoassays for which development times can be significant, particularly if a new antiserum must be raised. Chromatographic techniques frequently allow quantification of a range of related compounds in a single run, which has advantages when a number of drugs are prescribed together (e.g. anticonvulsants) or when separate quantification of a drug and its active metabolites is required. The combination of flexibility, specificity and sensitivity makes chromatographic techniques the method of choice for many toxicological applications. However, for TDM purposes they have a number of disadvantages. In comparison to immunoassays they are slower and more labour intensive, frequently demanding a significant level of technical expertise. Sample throughput is usually lower than for automated immunoassays, and sample volume is often higher, which is a particular disadvantage for paediatric applications. Sample preparation is also more laborious, since extraction or formation of a chemical derivative may be required before the chromatographic step.

Both gas chromatography (GC) and high-performance liquid chromatography (HPLC) still have a role, but the previously dominant position of GC in clinical work has steadily been eroded and is probably only relevant in association with mass-spectrometric (MS) detection. HPLC and LC-MS are now the chromatographic methods of choice for most TDM applications

There are different types of mass spectrometry: ion-trap and quadrupole, with hybrids and varying geometries. In recent years, the cost of instruments has fallen dramatically, and LC-MS/MS (LC–tandem MS) is becoming the standard technique for some routine analytes (e.g. the immunosuppressant sirolimus). The flexibility and ease of sample preparation of LC-MS/MS has led to its adoption for a number of drug assays which are not amenable to standard LC for reasons such as poor sensitivity and lack of an available chromophore for UV detection.

Immunoassays

Immunoassays, as conventional separation radioimmunoassays, have been applied to the determination of therapeutic drugs since the late 1960s, and these techniques still have a role when very high sensitivity is required. However, the advent of homogeneous (not requiring a phase separation step) non-isotopic immunoassays in the mid-1970s proved to be the foundation for widespread adoption of commercial immunoassay kits into clinical laboratories. A bewildering variety of techniques are now available, and more details will be found in Chapter 14. These kits have obvious advantages. They are generally technically simple, require little operator skill and are amenable to automation on equipment commonly found in routine clinical laboratories. Sample throughputs can thus be very high, and analysis times very short. Their main disadvantage is lack of specificity, either because of interference from endogenous plasma components (haemoglobin, bilirubin, etc.), which can affect the efficiency of the detection system, or because of cross-reactivity of the primary antibody with metabolites or structurally related compounds. Drugs with a large number of metabolites with similar structures (e.g. benzodiazepines, ciclosporin) pose particular problems in this respect. The development of sophisticated homogeneous non-isotopic systems is now virtually exclusive to large commercial organisations, which limits the practical applicability of immunoassays to compounds for which there is a commercial market for an assay system. It is important to realise that the cross reactivity, selectivity and sensitivity of the available immunoassays may vary, even with the same technique. It was found that FPIA on Abbott's AxSym too often produced false positive results (controlled by GC-MS) whereas FPIA on Abbott's TDx (same samples) did not provide false positive results.

Free-drug concentrations

Free-drug concentrations, as indicated above, may be determined by measuring drug concentrations in a plasma ultrafiltrate obtained by centrifugation of plasma through an ultrafiltration membrane with a molecular weight cut-off of approximately 30 000 a.m.u., by equilibrium dialysis, or by ultracentrifugation. The three separation methods usually give similar results, although systematic differences have been reported and it is advisable to compare the results of two or more techniques when validating a new method. Ultrafiltration is often preferred in the clinical setting as it can be completed more rapidly than the other methods. Where drug binding to protein is temperature dependent, careful control of temperature during the separation step is essential. Monitoring of free-drug concentration undoubtedly provides better clinical information than total concentration monitoring, but the increased methodological complexity and time required have limited its widespread application.

Chirality

The question of stereoselective analyses for therapeutic drugs has attracted increasing attention in recent years. Many pharmacologically active compounds contain a carbon atom linked to four different substituents, and thus have the potential to exist in two different isomeric forms. This property is called *chirality*, and the pairs of mirror-image compounds are termed *stereoisomers* (or *enantiomers*). Frequently, only one stereoisomer possesses a particular pharmacological action, and the other may be inactive or active in a different way. For example, the D-isomer of propoxyphene is a narcotic analgesic, while the L-isomer has no narcotic properties and is used as a cough suppressant. Stereoisomers may also show marked differences in pharmacokinetic properties such as clearance and volume of distribution (Chapter 2), and stereospecific analytical methods able to resolve individual isomers are required if meaningful TDM information is to be obtained. These methods rely on HPLC. Immunoassays are of little use because it is difficult to produce antibodies that react to the different isomers in a way that exactly reflects their biological activity.

Interpretation of results

In the 30 years or so that TDM has been practised in routine clinical laboratories, it has been demonstrated repeatedly that making drug-concentration measurements available to clinicians does not in itself result in improved clinical care. Improved outcome depends on the application of the result to a specific clinical situation with appropriate expertise. This is facilitated by a multidisciplinary approach in which pharmacists, laboratory staff and clinicians work together to share expertise and promote best use of the service. If the laboratory is to provide an effective service, clinicians must be prepared to provide basic data, such as the reason for a particular request, the dose regime, the time of the last dose and the presence of any drugs that may cause pharmacological or analytical interference.

In particular, it is important to understand that the widely quoted (and just as often misused) 'therapeutic ranges' for drugs represent a guide to the approximate concentrations that produce a therapeutic response in the majority of patients, rather than a set of inflexible limits between which patients must be forced. 'Target ranges' has been suggested as a better term, which at least carries the connotation that the ranges are something to aim at rather than implying that all concentrations within the range are therapeutic (and all outside are not). Many patients need plasma drug concentrations above (sometimes substantially above) the upper limit of the therapeutic range for effective therapy, and such concentrations must not provoke a knee-jerk dosage reduction. Specialist clinicians usually appreciate this fact, but nonspecialists frequently do not and the laboratory or pharmacist has an important educational role here. Conversely, plasma drug concentrations below the lower limit of the therapeutic range may produce perfectly satisfactory responses in some patients, for whom arbitrary dose increases to move concentrations into the 'therapeutic range' will merely increase the likelihood of toxicity without added benefit. 'Interpretation' of plasma drug concentrations by comparing them with an arbitrary range and designating them as 'subtherapeutic' or 'toxic' does far more harm than good.

Optimum drug concentrations for a particular patient are highly individual, and depend on many pharmacodynamic factors, as well as on the severity of the underlying disease process. This does not undermine the relevance of TDM, but it does require a degree of interpretative expertise and an understanding of the reason behind a particular request and how the result obtained relates to the clinical question. Whether this expertise resides with the clinician, the pharmacist or the laboratory scientist is less important than the fact that it exists somewhere and can be accessed when needed, although in the nature of the service, laboratory staff are likely to be best placed to monitor interpretation across a range of clinical situations. The cardinal principle, oft repeated but still forgotten, is to treat the patient, not the drug level.

Factors that affect interpretation

As implied above, many factors may affect the interpretation of plasma drug concentrations and it is impossible to go into specific detail within the confines of this chapter. Each of the following may have a bearing on the significance of a particular drug concentration at a particular time.

- pharmacokinetic factors, such as age of the patient, time since the last dose, administration of a loading dose and whether steady state has been achieved
- pharmacodynamic factors, such as receptor density, presence of interfering drugs or drug metabolites and concentration of endogenous substances such as potassium
- clinical factors, such as the severity of the primary condition and the presence of other diseases.

Pharmacodynamic monitoring and pharmacogenetics

We began this section by defining TDM as the use of drug or metabolite measurements in body fluids as an aid to monitoring therapy. In recent years, other methods of controlling drug therapy have been introduced and, though they do not fit the strict definition of TDM, they merit brief mention as they are becoming increasingly important. Pharmacodynamic monitoring is the study of the biological effect of a drug at its target site, and has been applied in the areas of immunosuppressive therapy and cancer chemotherapy. For example, the biological effect of the immunosuppressant ciclosporin can be assessed by measuring the extent of inhibition of calcineurin phosphatase, or the interleukin-2 concentration of peripheral blood lymphocytes. The advantages of such monitoring are that it gives an integrated measure of all biologically active species (parent drug and metabolites), so therapeutic ranges can be defined more closely, and that it is free from the matrix and drug-disposition problems that bedevil TDM for immunosuppressants. The main disadvantage of pharmacodynamic monitoring is that the assays involved are often significantly more complex and time-consuming than the measurement of a single molecular species by chromatography and immunoassay. It is too early to say whether pharmacodynamic monitoring will have a significant role to play in optimising therapy, but it is likely to prove an effective complement to TDM and pharmacogenetic studies.

Pharmacogenetic studies (studies of hereditary influences, including race, on pharmacological responses) have clear and wide-ranging clinical relevance. The enzymes that are responsible for metabolism of drugs and other compounds exhibit wide inter-individual variation in their protein expression or catalytic activity, and result in different drug metabolism phenotypes between individuals. This variation may arise from transient effects on the enzyme, such as inhibition or induction by other drugs, or may be at the gene level and result from specific mutations or deletions. *Pharmacogenetic polymorphism* is defined as the existence in a population of two or more alleles (at the same locus) that result in more than one phenotype with respect to the effect of a drug. The term 'pharmacogenomics' has recently been coined to describe the practice of designing drugs according to individual genotypes to enhance safety and/or efficacy, and undoubtedly represents a massive growth area for 21st-century medicine.

Determination of an individual's ability to metabolise a specific drug, either by administering a test dose of the drug or a compound metabolised by the same enzyme system (phenotyping) or by specific genetic analysis (genotyping) can inform and improve the clinician's ability to tailor drug dosage to the specific requirements of the individual patient. For example, a number of enzymes of the cytochrome P450 superfamily show genetic polymorphisms that account for differences in clinical response. The CYP2D6 isoform metabolises a range of drugs widely used in medicine, including many anti-arrhythmics and antidepressants. Debrisoquine is also a substrate for this isoform, and debrisoquine hydroxylase activity determined by the rate of metabolism of a test dose of debrisoquine has been widely used to determine the CYP2D6 phenotype and the differentiation of poor metaboliser (PM), extensive metaboliser (EM) and ultra-extensive (= ultra-rapid) metaboliser (UEM) phenotypes. However, debrisoquine is no longer available, and dextromethorphan has replaced it as a probe drug for clinical use. Alternatively, genetic analysis can be used to define the CYP2D6 phenotype and identify the alleles associated with the PM phenotype (of which the most common are CYP2D6 *3, *4, *5, *6 and *7). Once determined, the phenotype or genotype can be used to guide the dosage for any of the drugs metabolised by the CYP2D6 isoform. The CYP2D6 enzyme is absent in 5–10% of caucasians, CYP2C19 is absent in 15–30% of Asian people. Some drugs are inhibitors and other enzyme inductors on CYP enzyme 3A4, 2D6, 2C19, 2C9 and/or 1A2.

The combination of classical TDM, pharmacodynamic biomarkers and pharmacogenetics will undoubtedly accelerate the development and facilitate the clinical use of drugs, and will have a major role in delivering therapeutic efficiency and improved patient outcome with less need for plasma concentration monitoring.

In utero exposure to drugs of abuse

Introduction

Various neonatal birth defects are thought to be related to fetal exposure to drugs, alcohol, chemical agents or other xenobiotics. The vast majority of research in the USA has focused on the effects of maternal cocaine use upon the newborn. Cocaine use has been implicated in many cases of placental abruption, maternal hypertension, subarachnoid and intracerebral haemorrhage, premature labour, small head size, reduced birth weight, ruptured uterus and fetal death. Behavioural consequences as neonates reach childhood have also been studied, particularly in cocaine exposed babies. Maternal methamfetamine abuse has similar effects upon the fetus as cocaine, including complications during pregnancy, medical problems in early life and increased rates of premature birth. Neonates exposed to opiates or alcohol often display withdrawal symptoms such as irritability, tremors, hyperactivity and seizures. An early diagnosis of drug exposure is highly desirable in order to provide aid for the long-term development of the child and may help in the prevention of subsequent children from the same mother being exposed to drugs.

To date, urine is the most widely tested biological fluid for the determination of drug exposure during pregnancy. However, it is a difficult sample to collect from newborns, and is only indicative of recent drug exposure (occurring within a few days of birth). As a consequence, the false negative rate is high when urine drug testing is used. Meconium is the first faecal matter passed by a neonate. Many authors have concluded that meconium is a superior sample to neonatal urine for the purposes of determining drug use in pregnancy. However, others disagree with these findings, stating that meconium offers no significant advantage over urinalysis and is in fact a more difficult specimen to process for analysis.

Regardless, meconium testing is now widely accepted as the procedure of choice for the determination of fetal drug exposure. The major advantage of meconium analysis is that it extends the window of detection of drug use to approximately the last 20 weeks of gestation. Meconium is easy to collect and collection is noninvasive to the child. Drugs are stable in meconium for up to two weeks at room temperature and for at least a year when stored frozen. The main disadvantage of meconium is that it is not a homogenous sample because it forms layers depending upon the time of deposition in the intestine. Therefore it must be mixed as thoroughly as possible before analysis to help diffuse the drug throughout the matrix. Also, the testing is more demanding than urinalysis and it is difficult to prepare proficiency or control materials to assess laboratory quality assurance.

Drug use in pregnancy: estimates of abuse

The first nationally representative survey of maternal drug use was conducted under the auspices of the National Institute on Drug Abuse (NIDA). In 1991, NIDA estimated that 5 million women of child bearing age were using illegal drugs, and in 1992 approximately 5% of the 4 million women who gave birth admitted illicit drug use during their pregnancy. The National Pregnancy and Health Survey collected data on 2613 women from 52 rural and urban hospitals (October 1992–August 1993) showing that approximately 5.5% of pregnant women admit to using illegal drugs. Marijuana was the most frequently reported drug, with 2.9% of women admitting use; cocaine users numbered 1.1%. Cigarette and alcohol use was even higher at 20.4% and 18.75%, respectively. The survey also noted ethnic differences in drug use, with the highest use of crack cocaine occurring in African American populations (4.5%) compared to 0.7% Hispanics and 0.4% caucasian women. White women had the highest rates of alcohol use (23%) compared to 15.8% of African Americans and 8.7% of Hispanics. Caucasian women also had the highest rates of cigarette smoking. More recent studies have used meconium to determine maternal drug use, and in 2000, the meconium of 8527 newborns was tested for drugs of abuse. The prevalence of cocaine/opiate exposure in that cohort was 10.7%, although exposure varied by geographical site and was higher in very low-birth-weight babies.

Effects of fetal exposure to drugs

Each year approximately 3–7% of neonates have birth defects and over 60% are of unknown origin. There is increasing speculation that these defects are related to exposure to drugs, alcohol, chemical agents or other xenobiotics *in utero*.

Many drugs are thought to have significant adverse effects upon the neonate, particularly alcohol, but the majority of the illicit drug research has focused upon the effects of cocaine. In the early 1990s a US national survey found that 12 million adults used cocaine and alcohol simultaneously. Cocaine has been reported as a significant contributory factor to many adverse effects encountered in pregnancy. It is known that cocaine may affect the central dopaminergic system, and increased respiratory abnormalities of newborns can be expressed when cocaine is used during pregnancy. An increased number of cardiac problems in neonates born to cocaine-using women has also been reported. Numerous other authors have demonstrated a link between cocaine use and an increase in the number of cases of placental abruption, maternal hypertension, subarachnoid and intracerebral haemorrhage, premature labour, small head size, reduced birth weight, ruptured uterus and fetal death. A significant relationship between drug use during pregnancy and an increased incidence of immune deficiency syndrome in children has also been shown. Several reports on fetal or newborn deaths were published in which maternal cocaine use was a factor. It is now well known that maternal methamfetamine abuse has similar effects upon the fetus as cocaine, including complications during pregnancy, medical complications in early neonatal life and increased rates of premature birth. Heroin-related neonatal effects include opioid withdrawal symptoms such as irritability, tremors, hyperactivity and sometimes even seizures. Opiate abuse also results in the neonatal abstinence syndrome. Mental retardation and dysmorphism have been reported in neonates subjected to high doses of benzodiazepines *in utero*, but in these cases, alcohol may have been a confounding factor.

Formation and composition of meconium

Meconium is the first faecal matter passed by a neonate and is a highly complex specimen. It begins to form between the 12th and 16th weeks of gestation and usually accumulates thereafter until birth. It represents the intestinal contents of the fetus before birth and is a complex matrix, consisting mainly of water but also containing mucopolysaccharides, lipids, proteins, vernix caseosa, bile acids and salts, epithelial cells, cholesterol and sterol precursors, blood group substances, squamous cells, residual amniotic fluid and enzymes. The contents of meconium provide a history of fetal swallowing and bile excretion and it is therefore considered a more accurate history of drug use in the latter half of pregnancy than is neonatal urine. Meconium is usually passed by the neonate 1–5 days after birth, and rarely prior to 34 weeks' gestational age.

Deposition of drugs in the fetus

Drugs and their metabolites have been detected in the urine and plasma of newborn humans and animals. However, it is difficult to determine the metabolic fate of drugs *in utero*. Each of the major metabolic pathways can be promoted by placental and/or fetal enzymes and although the reaction rates appear to increase with gestational age, the presence of a metabolite in the fetus does not necessarily reflect the ability of the fetus to metabolise the drug. It has been suggested that drugs reach the fetus by passive diffusion of small-molecule, lipid-soluble drugs across the placenta. The placenta was thought to be a protective barrier for the fetus, disallowing passive diffusion of drugs; however, the well-documented effects of alcohol and thalidomide do not uphold this theory. The rate of drug transfer through the placenta is affected by the molecular size of the drug, the degree of ionisation of the drug, the hydrophobicity of the drug, blood flow to the placenta and the degree of protein binding to maternal and/or fetal plasma.

The ability of the fetus to swallow amniotic fluid usually begins around the 12th week of gestation. The binding of drugs and metabolites to proteins in the amniotic fluid which is subsequently swallowed by the fetus may account for drug exposure of the fetus.

Drug metabolites may be formed by the fetal liver, and excreted into the bile or urine. From the bile, they are deposited into the meconium; from the urine they are excreted into the amniotic fluid and re-circulated through fetal swallowing. Thus, meconium is a final depository for drugs to which the fetus is exposed. However, some studies concluded that fetal swallowing is not the primary mechanism by which drugs enter the fetus as was previously thought and that in fact there are other routes by which the fetus is drug exposed.

Postmortem analysis of human fetuses exposed to cocaine during pregnancy revealed the presence of cocaine in the meconium of a 17-week old fetus, implying that fetal exposure can be determined even in the case of a very premature fetus. Further, the authors claimed that the amount of cocaine found in the meconium was proportional to the amount of cocaine used by the mother during gestation. Their observations were supported by animal research.

Methods of analysis

Screening meconium for drugs of abuse

Radioimmunoassay (RIA), fluorescence polarisation immunoassay (FPIA) and enzyme multiplied immunoassay technique (EMIT) have all been described as useful analysis methods for screening meconium specimens. Overall, FPIA and RIA have been shown to be more sensitive than EMIT for the detection of cocaine metabolite (benzoylecgonine) in spiked meconium samples. Other comparative research has shown that the CAC Cocaine RIA (DPC Corporation, CA, USA) is the most sensitive assay for meconium screening. Presumably this is because there is significant cross-reactivity with cocaine which is often present in meconium, compared with various other immunoassays which are specific for benzoylecgonine. The original work carried out on meconium used radioimmunoassay for the detection of drugs. In the 1980s, Enrique Ostrea (Department of Pediatrics, Hutzel Hospital, Wayne State University, Detroit, MI, USA) became the first researcher to publish and patent procedures for the screening of drugs of abuse in meconium. In his original method, for each analysis 0.5 g of meconium was collected directly from the diaper. The sample was mixed with distilled water and then concentrated hydrochloric acid, and this homogenate was filtered through glass wool. The filtrate was centrifuged and an aliquot of the supernatant was tested for morphine (heroin metabolite) and benzoylecgonine (cocaine metabolite) using Abuscreen RIA kits. The recovery from drug-free meconium for benzoylecgonine and morphine was 70–105% and 8–97%, respectively. For cannabinoids, methanol was added to meconium. The sample was mixed and allowed to stand at room temperature for 10 minutes then centrifuged. An aliquot of the supernatant was tested for the cannabinoid metabolites by RIA. To date, many other screening procedures have been developed for cocaine, opiates, amfetamines, marijuana, and phencyclidine. The use of ELISA technology has allowed the screening profiles to be expanded since there is no matrix effect normally associated with meconium testing. Direct ELISA screening methods exist for the determination of other drugs such as barbiturates, benzodiazepines, fluoxetine, sertraline, propoxyphene, synthetic opioids, LSD, nicotine and its metabolites (cotinine, *trans*-3′-hydroxycotinine) in meconium.

False positives and false negatives in meconium screening

False negatives It was reported that the method of isolating the drugs from the meconium substantially affects the outcome of the screen. When an essentially clean extract (i.e. drugs are isolated from the matrix using solvent or solid-phase methods) is not used, a high rate of false negative results is observed. The immunoassay technique does not substantially affect the outcome of the analysis, but the sample preparation procedure does.

False positives In a study conducted by Moore *et al.* (1995), 535 meconium samples were chosen which screened positively for at least one of the following drugs: cocaine metabolite, opiates, amfetamines or marijuana metabolite. The screening cut-off levels were 25 ng/g for all drugs except amfetamines (100 ng/g). Of these screen-positive specimens, 285 (53.3%) were subsequently confirmed using GC-MS for one or more of the drugs at cut-off levels of 5 ng/g for all except marijuana metabolite (2 ng/g). Results of the study are presented in Table 8.9.

According to these results, immunoassay screening is falsely positive 46.7% of the time at the cut-off levels used, assuming that the correct drug metabolites are identified in the confirmatory procedure. It is possible that the immunoassay results are not in fact false positives but that there are drug metabolites present in meconium which are contributing to the immunoreactive response. These compounds are subsequently not determined in the confirmatory method, producing false negative results. Probably the most significant advance, to date, in the determination of drugs in meconium was reported by Steele *et al.* in 1993, who determined that for cocaine analysis there was a compound in meconium contributing to immunoreactive response which was not being confirmed by GC-MS. The research group was unable to confirm a significant number of cocaine positive screens using a standard GC-MS assay which identified cocaine, cocaethylene, benzoylecgonine, ecgonine methyl ester and norcocaine. Subsequently, the authors determined that the significant contributor to the immunoassay was *m*-hydroxybenzoylecgonine, a previously unreported metabolite of cocaine in meconium. The authors noted some difficulties with the construction of a standard curve for *m*-hydroxybenzoylecgonine using meconium as the matrix. Following hydrolysis of meconium, the authors also concluded that *m*-hydroxybenzoylecgonine glucuronide has approximately the same immunoreactivity as unconjugated *m*-hydroxybenzoylecgonine.

Table 8.9 Positive screening vs positive confirmation by GC-MS for THC metabolite, cocaine metabolite, opiates and amfetamines

Compound	Positive screen	Positive confirmation	%
THC metabolite	173	97	56.1
Cocaine metabolite	228	135	59.2
Opiates	60	34	56.7
Amfetamines	74	19	25.7

The presence of this metabolite in significant concentrations in meconium demonstrated that the metabolic profile of newborns differs between urine and meconium, and therefore simple application of urine protocol to meconium specimens will cause false negative results. Ethically, it is mandatory to confirm all positives from the preliminary screening by GC-MS and screen-only meconium results should be interpreted with caution.

Confirming meconium for drugs of abuse

There are several published confirmation methods, primarily GC-MS but also HPLC or LC-MS, for the determination of drugs of abuse and their metabolites in meconium. Reported analytes include cocaine, norcocaine, benzoylnorecgonine, cocaethylene, ecgonine methyl ester, *m*-hydroxybenzoylecgonine, and more recently, *p*-hydroxybenzoylecgonine, anhydroecgonine methyl ester and ecgonine ethyl ester, morphine, hydrocodone, hydromorphone, methadone and its principal metabolite, 2-ethylidene-1,5-dimethyl-3,3-diphenylpyrrolidine (EDDP), as well as codeine, methamfetamine and amfetamine, marijuana (11-nor-Δ^9-tetrahydrocannabinol-9-carboxylic acid), phencyclidine, and nicotine and metabolites (cotinine and *trans*-3′-hydroxycotinine). The solid phase extraction or solvent extraction of drugs from meconium is typically followed by instrumental analysis with or without derivatization.

Conclusions

Meconium is considered to be a useful and viable specimen in the determination of drug abuse in pregnancy, since it gives a longer history of drug exposure than neonatal urine. Publications concerning drug testing of meconium are becoming a significant part of medical, toxicological and forensic literature. Screening procedures exist for a number of drugs and confirmatory methods are increasing in number. An early and correct diagnosis of drug exposure is the newborn's best chance of receiving treatment, and the development of good scientific procedures to determine drugs in meconium is of great benefit to society.

References

P. C. Baastrup and M. Schou, Lithium as a prophylactic agent, *Arch. Gen Psychiatry*, 1967, **16**, 162–172.

F. Buchthal *et al.*, Clinical and electroencephalographic correlations with serum levels of diphenylhydantoin, *Arch. Neurol.*, 1960, **2**, 624–631.

L. E. Edinbora *et al.*, Determination of serum acetaminophen in emergency toxicology: evaluation of newer methods; Abbott TDx and second derivative ultraviolet spectrophotometry, *Clin. Toxicol.*, 1991, **29**, 241–255.

H. Liu and M. R. Delgado, Therapeutic drug monitoring using saliva samples. Focus on anticonvulsants, *Clin. Pharmacokinet.*, 1999, **36**, 453–470.

C. M. Moore, D. E. Lewis and J. B. Leikin, False-positive and false-negative rates in meconium drug testing. *Clin. Chem.*, 1995, **41**, 1614–1616.

H. C. Morris *et al.*, Development and validation of an automated enzyme assay for paracetamol (acetaminophen), *Clin. Chim. Acta*, 1990, **187**, 95–104.

F. L. Rodkey *et al.*, Spectrophotometric measurement of carboxyhaemoglobin and methaemoglobin in blood, *Clin. Chem.*, 1979, **25**, 1388–1393.

J. M. Scherrman *et al.*, Acute paraquat poisoning: prognostic and therapeutic significance of blood assay, *Toxicol. Eur. Res.* 1983, **5**, 141–145.

M. J. Smilstein *et al.*, Acetaminophen overdose: a 48-hour intravenous *N*-acetylcysteine treatment protocol, *Ann. Emerg. Med.*, 1991, **20**, 1058–1063.

B. W. Steele *et al.*, *m*-Hydroxybenzoylecgonine: an important contributor to the immunoreactivity in assays for benzoylecgonine in meconium, *J. Anal. Toxicol.*, 1993, **17**, 348–352.

B. Widdop, Analysis of carbon monoxide, *Ann. Clin. Biochem.*, 2002, **39**, 378–391.

Further reading

R. C. Baselt, *Disposition of Toxic Drugs and Chemicals in Man*, 6th edn, Foster City, Chemical Toxicology Institute, 2002.

E. J. Begg *et al.*, The therapeutic monitoring of antimicrobial agents, *Br. J. Clin. Pharmacol.*, 2001; **52**(Suppl 1), 35S–43S.

P. A. M. M. Boermans, *et al.*, Quantification by HPLC-MS/MS of atropine in human serum and clinical presentation of six mild-to-moderate intoxicated atropine-adulterated-cocaine users, *Ther. Drug. Monit.* 2006, **28**, 295–298.

S. Browne *et al.*, Detection of cocaine, norcocaine and cocaethylene in the meconium of premature neonates, *J. Forensic Sci.*, 1994, **39**, 1515–1519.

M. J. Burke and S. H. Preston, Therapeutic drug monitoring of antidepressants: cost implications and relevance to clinical practice, *Clin. Pharmacokinet.*, 1999, **37**, 147–165.

W. Clark and G. McMillin, Application of TDM, pharmacogenomics and biomarkers for neurological disease pharmacotherapy: focus on antiepileptic drugs, *Personalized Med.*, 2006, **3**, 139–149.

R. K. Drobitch and C. K. Svensson, Therapeutic drug monitoring in saliva. An update, *Clin. Pharmacokinet.*, 1992, **23**, 365–379.

M. Eichelbaum, *et al.*, Pharmacogenomics and individualized drug therapy. *Annu. Rev. Med.*, 2006, **57**, 119–137.

R. Eilers, Therapeutic drug monitoring for the treatment of psychiatric disorders. Clinical use and cost-effectiveness, *Clin. Pharmacokinet.*, 1995, **29**, 442–450.

S. I. Johannessen and T. Tomson. Pharmacokinetic variability of newer antiepileptic drugs; when is monitoring needed? *Clin. Pharmacokinet.*, 2006, **45**, 1061–1075.

B. D. Kahan, *et al.*, Therapeutic drug monitoring of immunosuppressant drugs in clinical practice, *Clin. Ther.*, 2002, **24**, 330–350.

J. Leikin and E. Paloucek, *Poisoning & Toxicology Handbook*, 4th edn, New York, Informa Healthcare, 2007.

P. B. Mitchell, Therapeutic drug monitoring of psychotropic medications. *Br. J. Clin. Pharmacol.* 2001, **52**(Suppl 1), 45S–54S.

C. Moore and A. Negrusz, Drugs of abuse in meconium, *Forensic Sci. Rev.*, 1995, **7**, 103–118.

C. Moore *et al.*, Determination of cocaine and its major metabolite, benzoylecgonine, in amniotic fluid, umbilical cord blood, umbilical cord tissue, and neonatal urine: a case study, *J. Anal. Toxicol.*, 1993, **17**, 63.

C. Moore *et al.*, Determination of drugs of abuse in meconium, *J. Chromatogr. B*, 1998, **713**, 137–146.

M. Oellerich *et al.*, Biomarkers: the link between therapeutic drug monitoring and pharmacodynamics. *Ther. Drug. Monit.*, 2006, **28**, 35–38.

S. Pichini *et al.*, Drug monitoring in nonconventional biological fluids and matrices, *Clin. Pharmacokinet.*, 1996, **30**, 211–228.

J. Sanderson, *et al.*, Thiopurine methyltransferase – should it be measured before commencing thiopurine drug therapy? *Ann. Clin. Biochem.*, 2004, **41**, 294–302.

Seyfart, *Poison Index, The Treatment of Acute Intoxication*, 4th edn, Berlin, Pabst Science Publishers, 1997.

B. S. Shastry, Pharmacogenomics and the concept of individualized medicine, *Pharmacogenomics J.*, 2006, **6**, 16–21.

B. E. Smink, *et al.*, Comparison of urine and oral fluid as matrices for screening of thirty-three benzodiazepines and benzodiazepine-like substances using immunoassay and LC-MS-MS, *J. Anal. Toxicol.*, 2006, **30**, 478–485.

S. Soldin, Free drug measurements: when and why? An overview, *Arch. Pathol. Lab. Med.*, 1999, **123**, 822–823.

K. K. Summers *et al.*, Therapeutic drug monitoring of systemic antifungal therapy, *J. Antimicrob. Chemother.*, 1997, **40**, 753–764.

B-L. True, R. H. Dreisbach, *Handbook of Poisoning: Prevention, Diagnosis and Treatment*, Los Altos, Lange Medical Publications, 2001.

T. Uematsu, Therapeutic drug monitoring in hair samples: principles and practice, *Clin. Pharmacokinet.*, 1993, **25**, 83–87.

A. Warner and T. Annesley (ed.), *Guidelines for Therapeutic Drug Monitoring Services*, Washington DC: National Academy for Clinical Biochemistry, 1999 (also published in *Clin. Chem.*, 1998, **44**, 1072–1140).

I. Watson, *et al.*, *Poisoning & Laboratory Medicine*, London, ACB Venture Publications, Association of Clinical Biochemists, 2002.

E. Yukawa, Optimisation of antiepileptic drug therapy: the importance of serum drug concentration monitoring, *Clin. Pharmacokinet.*, 1996, **31**, 120–130.

Table 9.2 *World Anti-Doping Agency Code.* Summary of urinary concentrations above which WADA-accredited laboratories must report findings for specific substances (WADA 2004b)

Substance	Urinary concentration to be reported
Carboxy-THC[a]	>15 μg/L
Cathine	>5 μg/mL
Ephedrine	>10 μg/mL
Epitestosterone	>200 μg/L
Methylephedrine	>10 μg/mL
Morphine	>1 μg/mL
19-Norandrosterone	>2 μg/L males & females
Salbutamol	
as stimulant	>100 μg/L
as anabolic agent	>1000 μg/L
T/E ratio[b]	>4

[a] Carboxy-tetrahydrocannabinol.
[b] Testosterone/epitestosterone ratio.

Table 9.3 Prohibited substances according to the *International Agreement on Breeding and Racing and Wagering* (IFHA 2007)

- Substances capable at any time of acting on one or more of the following mammalian body systems:
  - nervous system
  - cardiovascular system
  - respiratory system
  - digestive system
  - urinary system
  - reproductive system
  - musculoskeletal system
  - blood system
  - immune system except for licensed vaccines
  - endocrine system
- Endocrine secretions and their synthetic counterparts
- Masking agents

According to the IABRW,

> The finding of a prohibited substance means a finding of the substance itself or a metabolite of the substance or an isomer of the substance or an isomer of a metabolite. The finding of any scientific indicator of administration or exposure to a prohibited substance is also equivalent to the finding of the substance.

The basis of such rules is to ban the use of any prohibited substance in racehorses at the time of competition; that is a policy of 'zero tolerance' except for substances controlled by thresholds. The IABRW states that thresholds can only be adopted for:

1. substances endogenous to the horse
2. substances that arise from plants traditionally grazed or harvested as equine feed
3. substances in equine feed that arise from contamination during cultivation, processing or treatment, storage or transportation.

The list of threshold substances taken from the 2007 publication of the IABRW includes arsenic, boldenone, carbon dioxide, dimethyl sulfoxide (DMSO), estranediol (male horse), hydrocortisone, methoxytyramine, salicylic acid, testosterone and theobromine. Substances mentioned above which are detected below the thresholds specified in the agreement are not actionable. For any finding of an endogenous substance above the threshold, the horseracing authority may decide itself or at the trainer's or owner's request to examine the horse further.

In contrast to the policy of 'zero tolerance' of drugs currently adopted by racing authorities, certain drugs are permitted at the time of racing in some other jurisdictions. For example, in North America, concentration thresholds and regulations concerning administration have been set for the widely used nonsteroidal anti-inflammatory drugs (NSAIDs) phenylbutazone and its major metabolite oxyphenylbutazone, flunixin and ketoprofen (Association of Racing Commissioners International (ARCI) Model Rules of Racing (ARCI 2007a)). According to the ARCI, the finding of more than one NSAID in the serum or plasma will be considered a violation. Furosemide is also widely accepted on the North and South American continents with a threshold concentration in serum or plasma set by the RMTC and regulations regarding administration.

The sensitivity of analytical methods used by laboratories to test for drugs in equine body fluids has increased markedly over the past two decades with the introduction of sensitive enzyme-linked immunosorbent assays (ELISAs) and instrumental methods such as gas chromatography–mass spectrometry (GC-MS) and liquid chromatography–tandem mass spectrometry (LC-MS/MS). As a result of this available sensitivity, it is possible that some therapeutic medications may be detected in urine for time periods beyond the point at which the drug continues to exert a pharmacological action. Various approaches have been adopted or proposed to address this issue. In Canada, the racing authorities have adopted a policy of the 'deliberate non-selection of unnecessarily sensitive testing methods for specific substances' (Stevenson 1995). Tobin *et al.* (1999) proposed the development of threshold values for therapeutic substances based upon the determination of the highest no-effect dose for their primary pharmacological effect, such as the use of the heat lamp–abaxial sesamoid block model for local anaesthetics (Harkins *et al.* 1994, 1996). Similarly, Smith (2001) questioned the continued adherence to the policy of zero tolerance for drugs registered for equine veterinary use and suggested the use of pharmacologically determined reporting levels. Smith drew an analogy with other fields – veterinary drug residues in feed, food packaging contaminants and food additives – in which the levels of chemicals of no concern for a biological effect have been determined using pharmacological (toxicological) and pharmacokinetic parameters. For example, maximum residue limits (MRLs) and the acceptable daily intake (ADI) have been determined for many drugs used in veterinary practice for the treatment of livestock.

Reported analytical findings

Human

Data for human sports have been available only since 1987 and are presented for the years 1987, 1990, 1995, 2000 and 2005 in Table 9.4. Figure 9.1 shows the proportion of samples analysed by IOC/WADA-accredited laboratories in the years 1988 to 2005 reported for the three most commonly found prohibited substances: nandrolone, testosterone and salbutamol. Note the marked increase in the reporting of testosterone in recent years following the reduction of the reporting threshold by WADA in 2005.

As shown in Table 9.4, drugs misused in human sport include anabolic steroids, stimulants,

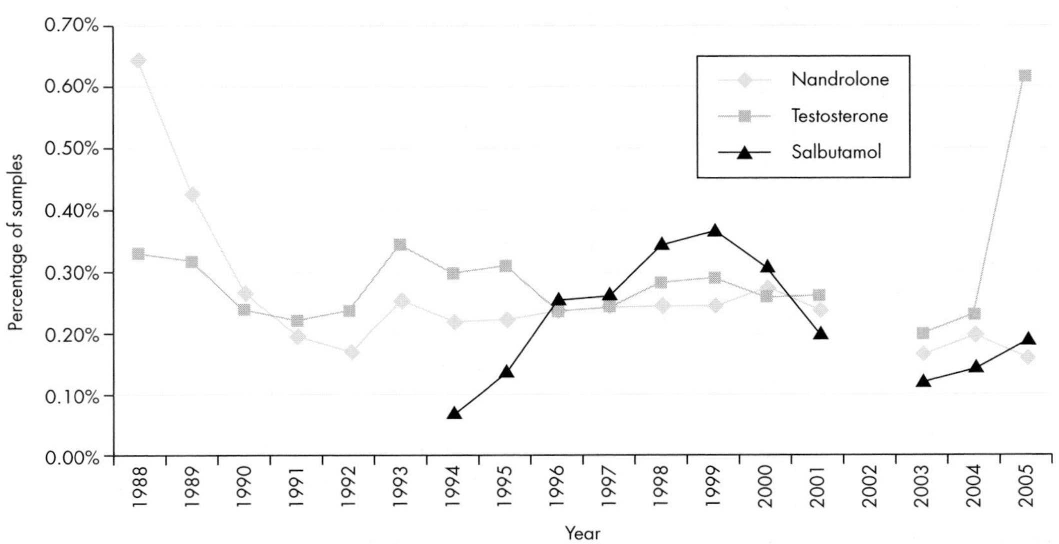

Figure 9.1 The proportion of human sports samples analysed by IOC-accredited laboratories in the years 1988 to 2005 reported for the three prohibited substances most commonly found.

Table 9.4 Prohibited substances most commonly reported by IOC-accredited laboratories, in order of frequency[a]

Number of reports									
Substance	1987	Substance	1990	Substance	1995	Substance	2000	Substance	2005
Nandrolone	262	Nandrolone	192	Testosterone	293	Salbutamol	367	Testosterone	1,132
Pseudoephedrine	100	Testosterone	171	Cannabis	224	Nandrolone	325	Cannabis	503
Testosterone	83	Pseudoephedrine	123	Nandrolone	212	Testosterone	306	Salbutamol	357
Ephedrine	58	Stanozolol	79	Methandienone	132	Cannabis	295	Nandrolone	298
Phenylpropanolamine	57	Phenylpropanolamine	64	Salbutamol	132	Pseudoephedrine	136	Stanozolol	233
Methenolone	42	Ephedrine	43	Pseudoephedrine	102	Ephedrine	129	Amfetamine	194
Stanozolol	37	Codeine	32	Ephedrine	78	Stanozolol	116	Terbutaline	171
Methandienone	27	Methenolone	25	Stanozolol	78	Terbutaline	110	hCG	143
Codeine	26	Amfetamine	24	Methenolone	39	Methandienone	75	Budesonide	116
Amfetamine	24	Methandienone	23	Clenbuterol	31	Lidocaine	64	Ephedrine	93

[a] 1987 was the first year of available data.

glucocorticoids, and peptide and protein hormones such as erythropoietin and human chorionic gonadotropin. Diuretics and masking agents are also commonly found. Of particular interest are the anabolic steroids and glucocorticoids; not only may synthetic analogues be misused, but also testosterone or hydrocortisone. This use of a pseudo-endogenous compound that is either indistinguishable or distinguishable with difficulty from that which is produced naturally by an individual presents interesting analytical problems. Other examples include recombinant growth hormones and recombinant erythropoietins. The biochemical, clinical and analytical aspects of anabolic steroids in sports have been reviewed by Kicman and Gower (2003).

Dietary supplements

In recent years and probably since the passing of the Dietary Supplement and Health Education Act (DSHEA), which requires the US Food and Drug Administration to treat supplements as harmless food products, a large number of food supplements that contain anabolic steroids either deliberately or by contamination have become readily available. This may have given rise to inadvertent violation of the anti-doping rules. An international study by Geyer *et al.* (2004), using GC-MS analysis, showed that of 634 nonhormonal nutritional supplements purchased in 13 countries from 215 different suppliers, 14.8% contained nondeclared androgenic-anabolic steroids (AASs). Of the supplements, 289 were from prohormone-selling companies and 345 were from companies which did not offer prohormone supplements. Prohormones are converted in the body to hormones. Androstenedione and androstenediol are converted in the human system to testosterone. This indicates the problems associated with dietary supplements. Nevertheless, most governing bodies of sport work on the principle of strict liability and it is the responsibility of the competitor in human sport to avoid the administration of a prohibited substance.

Protein hormones

There has been considerable concern in recent years over the use of peptide hormones such as erythropoietin (EPO) and darbepoietin. EPO is a peptide hormone secreted in the kidneys. It has an important role in the regulation of blood cell production. Administration of EPO has been shown to increase erythrocyte production. EPO was originally used to treat patients suffering from kidney disease. These patients often developed anaemia as a result of disruption of EPO production. Athletes recognised the potential for EPO to increase erythrocyte production and hence oxygen uptake.

Human chorionic gonadotropin (hCG) is a glycoprotein hormone produced in the body, particularly during pregnancy. Administration of hCG stimulates testosterone production but does not raise the testosterone/epitestosterone ratio. Initially, this made hCG administration difficult to detect, but methods of detection have now been developed for use in human sports drug testing.

Horseracing

The drugs most commonly detected in horseracing in Europe (France, Germany, Great Britain, Ireland and Italy) over the period 1993 to 1997 were assessed by Smith (2001). The majority of the reported findings (77%) were for substances registered for equine veterinary use. The NSAIDs (including phenylbutazone, flunixin, furosemide and naproxen) accounted for 28% of the reported findings and isoxsuprine for 22%. Isoxsuprine, a vasodilator, is widely used in veterinary practice for the treatment of navicular disease and can be detected in urine for long periods of time after dosing has ceased. Also, as a powder for oral administration through admixture with feed, it can produce serious contamination problems in the stable environment. Procaine and lidocaine accounted for 14% of reported findings and caffeine almost 9%.

For the drugs without market authorisation, anabolic steroids (including testosterone, nandrolone and boldenone) accounted for 36% of the reported findings, xanthines 26% and central nervous system (CNS) stimulant active drugs 12%.

It is interesting to compare these findings with those for reported findings in the USA and Canada over a similar period. If a prohibited substance is reported in a post-race sample from a horse, the IABRW recommends the horse be disqualified. However, as with the Prohibited Substance list, some countries adopt a different policy. In an attempt to harmonise sanctions, the ARCI in North America produced *Uniform Classification Guidelines for Foreign Substances and Recommended Penalties and Model Rules* (ARCI 2007b). Drugs are placed in Classes 1 to 5, with Class 1 agents having a high potential to affect the performance of the horse. Class 1 agents have no place in racing and include opiates, CNS stimulants and psychoactive drugs. Class 2 agents include psychotropics, certain stimulants, depressants, neuromuscular blocking agents and local anaesthetics that could be injected as nerve-blocking agents. These drugs also have the potential to affect racing performance, but it is less than that of Class 1 agents. Class 3 agents include some drugs registered for equine veterinary use and have less potential to affect performance than Class 2 agents. Class 4 includes agents with a recognised therapeutic use and which have less potential to affect performance than Class 3 agents. Examples of drugs from Class 4 include betamethasone, dextromethorphan, diclofenac, flunixin, ibuprofen, phenylbutazone and others. Suspensions from racing and fines are specified for a positive finding for the various drug classes, with Class 1 agents incurring the longest suspensions and highest fines. Also prohibited under the ARCI guidelines is the possession or use of erythropoietin, darbepoietin, oxyglobin and the blood substitute Hemopure.

Carter *et al.* (2001) reported findings for thoroughbred, standardbred and quarterhorses (horses bred for maximum speed over a quarter of a mile) over the period 1995 to 1999 for racing in California, Canada, Florida, Kentucky, Maryland, New York and Ohio. Findings for Class 1 agents, for example, included morphine (15), cocaine, presumably as the major metabolite benzoylecgonine (15), strychnine (3), oxymorphone (2), apomorphine (1), dextromoramide (1) and oxycodone (1). The estimated number of samples tested per annum in Canada and six states within the USA between 1995 and 1999 was 200 000 (Carter *et al.* 2001). For Class 1, 2 and 3 agents, within a four-year period, 39 substances were detected a total of 389 times in an estimated 800 000 samples (incidence of reported findings of 0.049%). For comparison, within Europe, 49 substances were detected a total of 431 times in a four-year period with a total of 97 451 samples – incidence of reported findings 0.44%.

The significant difference in the incidence of reported findings in the two geographical areas can almost certainly be explained by the absence of data for Class 4 and 5 agents in the American study. Many of the substances reported in Europe would fall into these classes within the USA. For example, European racing authorities place significant importance on the detection of anabolic steroids, whereas these are Class 4 agents in the USA and limited testing is applied. Also, NSAIDs and isoxsuprine are Class 4 agents and the level of phenylbutazone and/or oxyphenylbutazone in the reported samples in Europe would be well below the USA threshold (5000 μg/L). The difference in the incidence of reported findings reflects, in part, the difference in philosophical approaches to doping control currently adopted on the two continents: zero tolerance versus permitted medication.

It is interesting to note the influence that the introduction of new or more sensitive tests can have upon reporting statistics. Carter *et al.* (2001) reported 24 findings of Class 1 agents in standardbred racing in the USA over the period 1995 to 1999; 23 of the findings were for the drug metaraminol. These findings were all reported in one state, Louisiana, occurred over a short period of time, and resulted from the introduction of a new test. A similar situation arose with the drug clenbuterol when a more sensitive test was introduced in 1998.

Sampling

Sample collecting procedures must take into consideration both scientific and legal aspects as follows:

- the health of the individual being sampled must be safeguarded
- incorrect labelling, contamination or sample switching must be avoided
- the rights of interested parties, generally the owner and trainer of an animal or the individual or team in human sport, must be safeguarded against error by the analyst.

Human

The *World Anti-Doping Code International Standard for Testing* (WADA 2003b) describes the process for sample collection. The two matrices specified for testing are urine and blood. Urine is the primary matrix used for testing because it is considerably less invasive in terms of sampling compared to blood, offers relatively low health and safety risk compared to blood in terms of sampling and analysis, plus the majority of validated methods have been developed for urine as a testing matrix. Blood may be sampled and used instead of urine provided validated methods of analysis are applied to testing. Blood is used as a test matrix when detecting blood transfusion. The collected sample is split into two: samples A and B.

The IOC and the International Amateur Athletic Federation always provide a second portion for defence use (referred to as the 'B' sample). This is to be opened only after the first sample (referred to as the 'A' sample) has been found to contain a banned drug, and after the competitor has been notified and invited to attend the second analysis, with his or her own expert if the competitor so wishes. The WADA *International Standard for Laboratories* (WADA 2004a) specifies that, 'The 'B' sample confirmation must be performed in the same laboratory as the 'A' sample confirmation. A different analyst must perform the 'B' analytical procedure. The same individual(s) that performed the 'A' analysis may perform instrumental set-up and performance checks and verify results'.

Animal

Article 6 of the IABRW (IFHA 2007) states that a sample collected under a secure chain of custody shall be split into an A sample and a B sample, and this policy is adopted by racing jurisdictions worldwide. If the A sample is reported to contain prohibited substances, the B sample is analysed for those substances, either automatically or at the trainer's request. The analysis is carried out either in the primary laboratory or a nominated secondary laboratory. Within greyhound racing, a split sampling policy generally is not adopted because sometimes only a small volume of urine is available.

Sample matrices

Urine

Urine is the preferred body fluid in all species. Its collection is noninvasive; it is generally available in sufficient quantity; and the drugs or their metabolites tend to be present in relatively high concentrations. The disadvantages are that a drug may be present as its metabolites or in a conjugated form, and the parent drug may be present only in a relatively low concentration. Furthermore, the relationship with the concentration in blood is very imprecise.

Urine is collected almost invariably by voiding naturally. Greyhounds urinate very readily after being released from their transporter; 96% of horses in Britain urinate within 1 hour of racing; humans can generally urinate at will. However, there is the problem of security. Switching of samples is clearly a possibility that must be avoided and particular care is required during the period of waiting before a sample is obtained from a dog or a horse, and because of the desire for privacy on the part of a person. It has been reported that racing cyclists have carried a rubber bladder of (negative) urine under their arm, connected by a rubber tube to the appropriate discharge point. False penises, in a variety of natural colours, are advertised on the internet for purchase. Horse handlers responsible for collecting a urine sample from their horses have been known to substitute a urine sample of their own. One laboratory even received a sample of lager purporting to be horse urine. Incidents such as these emphasise the importance of ensuring that a correct collecting procedure is observed. The WADA guidelines on urine collection (WADA 2004b) specify that urine sample collection shall be witnessed, thereby reducing the chances for supplementation or adulteration. The guidelines specify strict criteria for the entire sampling procedure to minimise the potential for tampering by the athlete or accusations of possible contamination by the sampling personnel.

The odour of urine, and of the residues produced after solvent extraction, generally provide a ready distinction between the species. The presence of appreciable quantities of nicotine, cotinine, caffeine and uric acid in urine provides good evidence of a human source.

Urine samples from greyhounds are caught directly in a bowl held under the animal. For horses, a container held on the end of an extending handle is generally used (e.g. a net held on a metal ring into which is inserted a polythene bag). Metal ladles are unsuitable because the noise produced by the urine that falls into them frequently inhibits the horse from urinating further.

Blood

The principal advantage of a blood sample is that its integrity is easier to safeguard because, usually, it is collected by a doctor or veterinary surgeon experienced in the procedure. In addition, drug concentrations in blood are interpreted more easily than those in urine, and certain drugs that are not excreted in urine in detectable quantities (e.g. reserpine, or human growth hormone) can be detected in blood. In horseracing testing, blood (serum or plasma) is routinely used to determine TCO_2 (total carbon dioxide) level as well as phenylbutazone and/or oxyphenylbutazone and furosemide concentrations. The only disadvantage of blood is the relatively low volume which can be reasonably collected from a human or an animal to perform all necessary tests.

Blood is rarely collected from the greyhound because of the relative ease of urine sampling. In humans, blood is now being collected routinely by some federations (e.g. the International Cycling Union) as a 'health check'. Any competitor whose haematocrit is above 50% is not permitted to compete. This test is intended to limit the use of EPO to stimulate red cell production. However, this test is readily circumvented and depends on too many factors; the use of haemoglobin concentration is preferred. Furthermore, blood samples are also collected for more sophisticated tests to indicate the use of EPO. WADA publish guidelines for sampling blood, with whole blood sampled for detection of blood transfusion and serum for detection of human growth hormone (hGH) and haemoglobin-based oxygen carriers (HBOCs), for example (WADA 2006a). Blood is sampled increasingly in horseracing in much of Europe as a second choice when urine is not obtainable and as the body fluid of choice for pre-race and testing in training samples.

Saliva

The principal disadvantages of saliva are that it is difficult to obtain a useful volume and few drugs are present at a concentration higher than that in plasma. Non-ionised drugs and drugs not protein bound in plasma diffuse passively into saliva. Thus, alkaline saliva (as in the horse) tends to concentrate acidic drugs but, because the percentage of unbound acidic drug in plasma is generally very low, concentrations remain lower than the corresponding total plasma concentrations. For drugs of low lipid solubility, and for high salivary flow rates, equilibrium is not established, which results in concentrations even lower than those predicted on theoretical grounds. The principal value of saliva, therefore, is in the detection of topical contamination that results from fairly recent oral ingestion (see Chapter 6).

Saliva is rarely used in any species for sport drug testing, but it is now increasingly used in workplace drug testing (see Chapter 5).

Hair

The analysis of hair samples to determine the duration and/or frequency of previous drug use is still to be accepted in the sports doping arena and WADA do not specify it as a testing matrix. Analysis of hair still lacks sufficient sensitivity for general application; in addition, the finding of a drug in hair represents prior use of the drug, not what drug is in the circulatory system at the time of test, the guiding principle for most doping controls. Kintz (1998) has reviewed hair testing and doping control in human sport (see also Chapter 6).

Hair analysis has value within horseracing in that it can provide a historical record of drug administrations. This information would be particularly useful for those drugs with no legitimate therapeutic use and long-lasting effects (e.g. anabolic steroids). Reported studies (Whittem *et al.* 1998; Jouvel *et al.* 2000; Popot *et al.* 2001d) have addressed the detection of morphine, diazepam and clenbuterol in horse hair.

Breath

Breath is the preferred sample when testing athletes for alcohol and the WADA guidelines (WADA 2006b) specify procedures for breath alcohol testing.

Analytical approach

Dope is generally administered at or near the therapeutic dose, which results in relatively low concentrations in biological fluids.

Any drug used in human treatment or in veterinary practice may be found. Thus, screening procedures must be both sensitive and of wide coverage, and they differ in detail from other analytical schemes. However, the sports chemist enjoys the advantage of examining relatively constant material, usually in fairly fresh condition. He or she thus has a clearer picture of a normal sample than does the forensic chemist who may be required to examine a wide variety of materials in various states of decomposition. Any sample that fails a screening test is invariably submitted to rigorous confirmatory testing (see below) before an adverse report is issued.

Although the parent drug is the entity normally described in the rules, screening procedures rely upon the detection of either the unchanged drug or its metabolites. The identification of the corresponding metabolites is often useful supplementary evidence to support the identification of the parent drug. Examples may include the detection of 3′- and 4′-hydroxymepivacaine, major metabolites of the local anaesthetic mepivacaine, or nordiazepam after diazepam administration.

Conversely, the absence of any expected metabolites is possible evidence that a sample has been contaminated; this should be refutable by proper chain of custody. Occasionally, the parent drug is not excreted in urine at a detectable concentration, so knowledge of the metabolic pathways in the particular species is essential. An example of this is the identification of 19-norandrosterone and 19-noretiocholanolone in the urine of humans as evidence of the administration of the anabolic steroid nandrolone or a 19-norsteroid precursor. After administration of cocaine, primarily benzoylecgonine and ecgonine methyl ester are detected in urine unless a huge dose of cocaine was given. In that case parent cocaine can also be detected in urine. Some drugs are notable for being excreted in urine almost entirely in conjugated form as, for instance, morphine, apomorphine, fentanyl, nefopam and pentazocine in the horse. When the presence of these drugs is suspected, hydrolysis before extraction is essential because most analytical methods are designed to detect drugs and metabolites in their nonconjugated form. If a hydrolysis procedure is not employed, and the analytical method used is not designed to detect conjugates, the drug may not be detected even though it was administered. LC-MS/MS methods are being designed to detect drugs in their conjugated form, thereby obviating the need for hydrolysis procedures.

Drugs can be used either to improve or to impair athletic performance, though in human sport the latter category of drug is unlikely to be used knowingly. In sports such as greyhound racing and horseracing, however, decreasing an animal's speed can be a profitable exercise, so it is important to monitor sedative drugs in these events. Thus, in horse and dog samples it is essential that all groups be covered.

No single analytical scheme will suffice to cover so many different types of compounds, and various approaches have evolved in racing chemistry and human doping laboratories to address this challenge. Liquid–liquid extractions designed for group separation of drugs followed by thin-layer chromatography (TLC) was used almost universally for many years and is still used widely in North American and some other racing chemistry laboratories. Alternatively, drugs were extracted on styrene–divinylbenzene copolymer XAD-2 resin. The development of solid-phase extraction (SPE) in the cartridge format in the late 1970s and the rapid advances made in the technology associated with the technique have provided an attractive alternative to liquid–liquid extraction in many drug-screening programmes. Immunochemical methods that cover glucocorticosteroids were first introduced into equine drug-screening programmes in the 1970s. However, in the late 1980s, ELISAs were developed specifically for equine drug-testing programmes and are now widely used to support TLC and instrumental screening programmes.

Human sports drug-testing laboratories have not employed TLC typically and do not use ELISA extensively, but used XAD-2 and now, more commonly, C_8 and C_{18} SPE. Liquid–liquid extraction is still commonly employed in laboratories for some drug classes. Instrumental methods (GC using nitrogen–phosphorus detection (GC-NPD), high-performance liquid chromatography using ultraviolet detection (HPLC-UV), GC-MS and LC-MS(/MS)) are the predominant analytical methods in most animal and human sports drug-testing laboratories. Even if not routinely used for screening, some sort of TLC technology is sporadically used by many laboratories to isolate or purify a compound of interest followed by the analysis of so called scrape from the TLC plate by GC-MS, LC-MS, etc.

Solvent extraction and thin-layer chromatography

In general, the choice of solvent is dictated by the wide range of drugs to be covered, or the need to extract a specific drug as in confirmatory analysis procedures.

The classic extraction–TLC methods used primarily by North American laboratories for drug testing in animal sports provide coverage for a wide range of basic, acidic and neutral drugs. Individual aliquots of urine, in some cases following pre-treatment, are extracted at various pH values and with a range of organic solvents. The extracts are applied to TLC plates run in a variety of solvent systems, and the TLC plates are sprayed with a range of reagents, often in sequence.

Ion pair (IP) extraction can be used to optimise the extraction of weak acids, weak bases and zwitterionic compounds. The ion pairing buffer (phosphate buffer with bromothymol blue) is added to the urine and the pH adjusted to 7.4. Drugs are extracted with dichloromethane : 2-propanol (3 : 1) and aliquots of the extract are applied to two TLC plates. The developed plates are examined under UV light and subjected to a range of visualisation reagents.

Steroids are extracted from urine using ethyl acetate after adding saturated sodium borate solution and washing the extract in 15% sodium sulfate in sodium hydroxide solution. The extract is run in a TLC system of chloroform : ethyl acetate : methanol (50 : 45 : 5 v/v); the plate is dried and then re-run in Davidow reagent. The steroids are visualised by spraying with a mixture of sulfuric acid : ethanol (50 : 50 v/v) and heating (high heat) with a hot-air blower or hot plate to develop dark oxidation spots.

Solid-phase extraction

In many racing chemistry laboratories throughout the world, SPE has replaced liquid–liquid extraction for the isolation of drugs from both urine and plasma. Based upon the studies of Shackleton and Whitney (1980), the early applications of SPE to racing chemistry were in the use of C_{18} bonded-phase cartridges to the isolation of anabolic steroids and their metabolites from equine urine (Dumasia *et al.* 1986). With the development of a range of more polar phases and, more importantly, ionic phases, the technique evolved to provide a simple, rapid, robust and efficient approach to the fractionation of drugs from biological fluids. Retention through a cation-exchange mechanism isolated the basic drugs, whereas an anion-exchange mechanism isolated acidic drugs. Foster *et al.* (1990) have reported an automated SPE procedure for drugs in horse urine. Following initial extraction using Tox-Elut cartridges (cartridges that contain a specially modified form of diatomaceous earth), basic and acid–neutral drugs were separated using a cation-exchange cartridge. Further purification of the acid–neutral fraction was achieved using silica SPE cartridges.

However, mixed-mode cartridges with retention mechanisms based upon both hydrophobic interactions and ion-exchange processes have found wide application in racing chemistry and many other disciplines associated with drug analyses. Dumasia and Houghton (1991) reported the application of the mixed mode cartridge for the extraction of beta-agonists, beta-antagonists and their metabolites in horse urine prior to their analysis by GC-MS. Westwood and Dumasia (1994) automated this approach for the general screening of basic drugs and their metabolites from horse urine.

Wynne *et al.* (2001b) reported a multi-eluate approach to the SPE extraction of biological fluids to detect drug residues. The method employs the mixed-mode cartridge (C_8–cation exchange) to separate the basic and acidic–neutral fractions. The acidic–neutral fraction was fractionated on a second mixed-mode cartridge (C_{18}–anion exchange; Figure 9.2).

Mixed-mode phases are also available in new poly(styrene–divinylbenzene) sorbents, produced by combining two classes of polymeric sorbents, copolymeric and functionalised polymers. The treatment of the functionalised polymer with sulfonic acid provides cation-exchange characteristics. These cartridges have been shown to be effective in the extraction of a number of basic drugs from equine urine (Stanley *et al.* 2001).

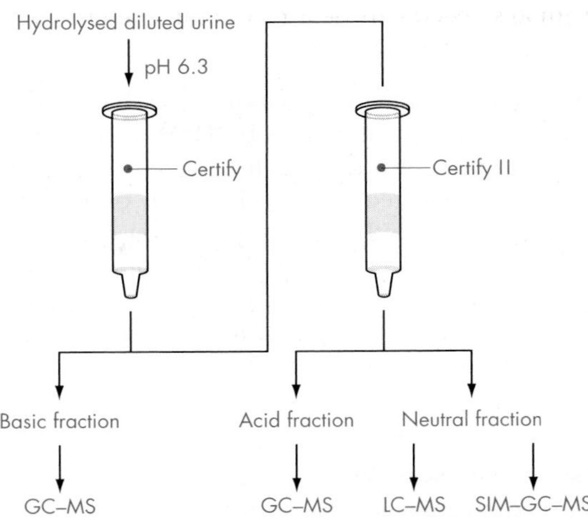

Figure 9.2 Multi-eluate approach to SPE of biological fluids to detect drug residues.

One of the major problems encountered in the SPE of horse urine, particularly if automated procedures are used, is cartridge blockage. This is primarily because of the viscous nature of horse urine and, to a lesser extent, suspended material. This problem has been addressed (Wynne *et al.* 2001a, 2001c) using non-conditioned SPE (NC-SPE). The sorbents used in this technique are highly cross-linked with a unique combination of hydrophilic and lipophilic moieties and thus do not require conditioning. They have good flow characteristics and can be applied to the extraction of a wide range of drugs. Wynne *et al.* (2001c) suggested the application of NC-SPE for the pre-extraction of horse urine before application of the recovered extract to mixed-mode cartridges. The application of SPE to veterinary drug abuse has been reviewed by Wynne (2000).

Automation

One of the advantages of SPE is its ease of automation, and many laboratories have introduced commercial SPE robotics for the unattended extraction of samples. Teale *et al.* (2000) have also reported the development of an automated on-line SPE GC-MS screening procedure for basic drugs in horse urine. The approach uses commercial SPE robotics linked via a programmable temperature vaporising (PTV) injector to a commercial bench-top GC-MS system.

Gas chromatography and gas chromatography–mass spectrometry

Gas chromatography has been the workhorse analytical technique of most doping testing laboratories for many years. Originally GC was combined with flame ionisation detection (FID), nitrogen-phosphorus detection (NPD) and, for some drugs, electron capture detection (ECD). The advent of relatively inexpensive benchtop GC-MS instruments has made GC-MS the analytical technique of choice where analytes are amenable to chromatographic separation by GC. GC offers the capability of separating a large number of substances in a single analytical run making it ideal for screening purposes. Operation of mass spectrometry in selected-ion monitoring (SIM) mode gives enhanced sensitivity, while operation in scan mode enables the mass spectrum of a drug identified in a sample to be assessed for match against the mass spectrum of an authenticated standard of the drug. It may also be possible to identify, presumptively, unexpected and/or interfering substances using mass spectral libraries or, in some instances, comparison with literature spectra.

As noted previously, caution must be exercised when analysing by GC drugs that are excreted in urine as conjugates and an appropriate method of hydrolysis must be incorporated into the analytical procedure.

Various derivatisation procedures are employed to make polar and/or thermally labile analytes more amenable to analysis by GC. Anabolic steroids, which are difficult to chromatograph without chemical conversion, are normally silylated and analysed as trimethylsilyl derivatives. Derivatisation has also been found to be useful for the analysis of drugs that do not produce characteristic ions without chemical conversion.

Liquid chromatography–mass spectrometry

With the development of atmospheric-pressure ionisation techniques, LC-MS has found increasing application in doping control in animal and human sports for both the qualitative and quantitative analysis of drugs. Screening methods have been developed in animal sports testing for corticosteroids (Tang *et al.* 2001) and diuretics (Eenoo *et al.* 2001). Methods developed for individual drugs include hydrocortisone (Samuels *et al.* 1994), triamcinoloneacetonide (Koupai-Abyazani *et al.* 1994b), levodopa and its metabolites (Koupai-Abyazani *et al.* 1994a), clidinium bromide (Ryan *et al.* 1996) and glycopyrrolate (Teale and Houghton 1994). The technique has also been applied to the analysis of intact steroid conjugates isolated from horse urine with particular reference to the quantification of testosterone sulfate (Dumasia *et al.* 1996).

Product-ion scan MS/MS has facilitated the development of screening procedures for large numbers of compounds in a single analysis. Leung *et al.* (2007) reported the high-throughput screening of 75 basic drugs in equine plasma by LC-ESI-MS/MS, with sub-parts per billion levels of detection. LC-ESI-MS/MS has also been used for the analysis of eight major anabolic steroids with three ion transitions used for confirmation (Guan *et al.* 2005). The limit of quantification was 25 pg/mL for boldenone; 50 pg/mL for normethandrolone, nandrolone and methandienone, and 100 pg/mL for testosterone, tetrahydrogestrinone, trenbolone and stanozolol.

In human sports drug testing, LC-MS and LC-MS/MS are being used increasingly in several areas. Barron *et al.* (1996) developed a direct method to determine anabolic steroids in human urine by on-line SPE LC-MS. Thevis *et al.* (2001) used LC-MS/MS for the rapid screening of samples for beta-blockers. Diuretics have been screened by LC-MS techniques (Ventura *et al.* 1991) and by LC-MS/MS (Thieme *et al.* 2001). The sulfate conjugate of 19-norandrosterone has been analysed by LC-MS/MS in negative electrospray ionisation mode (Strahm *et al.*, 2007) with a lower limit of quantification of 200 pg/mL, emphasising the applicability of LC-MS for the analysis of drug conjugates. The role of LC-MS(/MS) in doping control has been reviewed by Thevis and Schanzer (2007).

Isotope ratio mass spectrometry

Combustion isotope ratio MS (CIRMS) (see Figure 3.31) is now used routinely by some WADA accredited laboratories. After injection, the sample flows through the column and the compounds of interest are separated on the column. Eluted compounds are then combusted oxidatively in a combustion reactor. Nitrogen oxides are removed by reduction to nitrogen and water is then removed by passing the eluent through a water separator. The sample is then introduced into the ion source of the MS by an open split interface. CIRMS provides an additional tool to help distinguish a person whose testosterone to epitestosterone ratio may be naturally beyond the normal range from an individual who has administered testosterone. The synthetic testosterone has a different proportion of ^{13}C to the more abundant ^{12}C than the normal endogenous steroid (de la Torre *et al.* 2001). The extracted steroids are separated by GC and then converted into CO_2 and the relative amounts of ^{12}C to ^{13}C as CO_2 determined for each eluting steroid in turn. Typically, the testosterone metabolites androsterone and etiocholanolone or androstanediols are monitored (Aguilera *et al.* 2000), or the metabolites 5α-androstanediol and 5β-androstanediol (Shackleton *et al.* 1997b; Aguilera *et al.* 2001), often comparing the results with pregnanediol or pregnanetriol as endogenous internal standards (Shackleton *et al.* 1997a; Aguilera *et al.* 1999). Aguilera *et al.* (1997) have also used GC-CIRMS to detect exogenous hydrocortisone administration to the horse.

Confirmatory methods

In human sports drug testing, MS is essential for the definitive identification of a prohibited substance, with the exception of peptide hormones and glycoproteins, such as human chorionic gonadotropin (hCG) for which a validated immunoassay is required for detection and quantification. For confirmation of these substances, a second different immunoassay is required. Specific techniques and methodologies for other peptide hormones and glycoproteins such as human growth hormone (hGH) and EPO are currently being considered.

Industry guidelines for horseracing laboratories state that for regulatory identification, MS or a similarly definitive technique, if applicable to the analyte in question, must be included.

Criteria for identification

WADA generally expects a capillary gas chromatographic retention time (or relative retention time) match between the sample and a reference standard, analysed using the same procedure in the same assay, of 1% or better and three diagnostic ions in the mass spectra to match to within 20% or better of the relative abundance of each ion.

Although mass spectral library data may be useful in the early phase of substance identification, especially in generic screening procedures, they are not considered sufficiently reliable for the final identification. Similarly, published data are used more to assure reliability than directly for substance identification.

Horseracing laboratories are required to have established and documented chromatographic and mass spectrometric criteria that the analyte of interest in the test sample must have in common with the reference material for identification purposes. To assist in this process, the racing industry, primarily through the efforts of the Association of Official Racing Chemists, has produced the guidelines *Accreditation Requirements and Operating Criteria for Horseracing Laboratories*, published by the International Laboratory Accreditation Co-operation (ILAC) (ILAC 1997). ILAC require that validation of methods by testing laboratories conform to ISO 17025 (ILAC 2002).

WADA requires laboratories to be accredited to ISO 17025 (see Chapter 23) to be eligible for WADA accreditation, whereas animal-racing authorities only recommend laboratories to be accredited to ISO/IEC 17025 (ISO/IEC 2005).

ISO 17025 (ISO/IEC 2005) requires traceability of measurements and in the sports fields this is considered to be met, when identifying a prohibited substance, by the direct comparison with a reference material analysed in parallel or in series with the test sample. A reference standard is generally accepted as a chemical with a well-established structure. The material may be characterised structurally within the laboratory using appropriate techniques or validated against a certified reference material or by comparison with uncontroversial published data. A reference material may also be an isolate from a urine or blood sample after an authenticated administration, provided that the analytical data from it is sufficient to justify fully its identity as a metabolite from the substance administered. Chemical reference standards are often not available and hence there is the need to use authenticated administrations for comparison purposes. Many of the most common substances are now available with certificates of analysis, and thereby fully meet the generic traceability requirements of ISO 17025.

The required documentation for the analytical certificate is clearly set out in ISO 17025, but merely requires a statement as to the substance found. However, in some jurisdictions, analytical data must also be provided with the certificate, but this is rarely clearly specified and often gives grounds for claims by lawyers that data are being concealed; there is clearly a need for harmonisation of the requirements. Further information on quality control and assessment is contained in Chapter 23.

Threshold analysis

Thresholds may be set either in the rules for laboratory reporting or as a penalty threshold (e.g. furosemide, flunixin, phenylbutazone and ketoprofen in serum in the equine, carboxy-tetrahydrocannabinol, cannabis metabolite in human urine). In either case, the laboratory needs a protocol to determine whether the specified threshold has been exceeded. Fully validated assays are used in these cases, with suitable quality-control samples run concurrently with the sample being assessed to assure the assay validity.

Anabolic steroids

In human sport, anabolic steroids are used as body-building drugs, sometimes in very large quantities, in events such as weightlifting and shot-putting. In horseracing, their use seems to be more general. They are said to improve a horse's appetite and to produce behavioural changes of a masculinising type in geldings and mares, though they may also be used in stallions. There are broadly two chemical types based upon the androstane and estrane ring systems: those with a 17α-alkyl group, which are active orally but possess hepatotoxicity, and 19-nor derivatives administered by injection. Although steroidal oestrogens and some stilbenes reputedly possess anabolic activity and are employed in beef production, they do not appear to be used as doping agents.

Studies (Houghton 1977; Houghton and Dumasia 1979, 1980; Dumasia and Houghton 1981, 1984; Dumasia *et al.* 1983) have shown the metabolism of the veterinary anabolic agents nandrolone, testosterone, boldenone and trenbolone in the horse to be complex, with both phase I and phase II processes playing important roles. Nandrolone has been shown to be endogenous to the male horse (Houghton *et al.* 1984) and this, and testosterone, are controlled by threshold values (see Table 9.2). Metabolism of 17α-alkyl anabolic agents has also been studied in the horse (Schoene *et al.* 1994; McKinney *et al.* 2001). These studies have thus been essential to identify key analytes for the development of screening and confirmatory analysis methods.

Radioimmunoassay and subsequently ELISA procedures have been developed for these veterinary anabolic agents (Jondorf 1977; Jondorf and Moss 1977) and commercial assays are currently available. Also, the identification of the major metabolites for these steroids has enabled the development of multi-residue GC-MS screening procedures (Dumasia *et al.* 1986; Houghton *et al.* 1986). The metabolism differs markedly from that in humans, with the reduction of the 4-ene-3-one group and epimerisation at C17 being major phase I pathways. Phase II processes also differ markedly, with sulfate conjugation playing an important role in horses, but a minor role in humans. Thus the developed methods for screening and confirmatory analysis by mass spectrometric methods require steps for cleavage of both glucuronic acid and sulfate conjugates.

The metabolism of anabolic steroids in humans has been documented, especially by Schanzer and co-workers (e.g. Schanzer and Donike 1993; Schanzer 1996). Synthetic anabolic steroids used in humans may be detected readily by the use of GC-MS analysis. Detection of the administration of pseudo-endogenous compounds (i.e. compounds that are virtually identical to those of endogenous origin, such as testosterone), present a more complex problem although the use of CIRMS (see above) has greatly assisted obtaining evidence to prove administration. There are several methods to indicate that testosterone has been administered to a male human. Natural testosterone production is controlled by a feedback mechanism that involves the pituitary gland, and administration of testosterone suppresses the natural production of pituitary hormones, such as luteinising hormone (LH) and follicle-stimulating hormone (FSH). GC-MS analysis may be used to measure the testosterone concentration in urine, and immunoprocedures to determine LH and hence the urinary ratio of total (free plus conjugated) testosterone to LH. Testosterone is measured in nmol/L, and LH in International Units of Human Menopausal Gonadotropin 2nd International Reference Preparation per litre (HMG-IR2/L). A ratio in excess of 200 is abnormal (Brooks *et al.* 1979).

In female humans, whose pituitary hormones may be suppressed by the use of oral contraceptives, the testosterone to LH ratio is of little evidential value. Instead, a method suitable for both males and females is to measure the ratio of total testosterone to epitestosterone using GC-MS. In this method, the bis(trimethylsilyl) derivative is formed and the intensity of the molecular ions at m/z 432, under electron-impact conditions for both of the steroid derivatives, is used to determine the ratio (Donike and Zimmermann 1980). The internationally accepted limit for the ratio is 6, although WADA currently requires reports to be issued whenever a ratio of 4 is reached. A method to detect the administration of dihydrotestosterone, the more active metabolite of testosterone, has also been proposed (Kicman *et al.* 1995) based on the perturbation of the endogenous hormone profile following administration. Isotope ratio MS is also now used to assist detection of the administration of testosterone and related compounds.

Sampling carried out only at the time of competition has enabled the misuser to switch from using a preferred synthetic anabolic steroid to testosterone or to a synthetic anabolic steroid that is eliminated rapidly in sufficient time to escape detection. Thus sampling out-of-competition and with minimum notice as well as at competitions is now accepted as the optimal approach to detecting, and thereby limiting, the use of anabolic steroids in humans.

Mass spectral and chromatographic data for many anabolic steroids and their metabolites have been published by Ayotte *et al.* (1996). Kicman and Gower (2003) have reviewed the use of anabolic steroids in sports, including analytical perspectives.

Diuretics

Diuretics, and especially furosemide, are widely used in horse racing to prevent so-called exercise-induced pulmonary haemorrhage (EIPH). They are also used in weightlifting and other competitions classified by weight. The diuretic furosemide is permitted in horse racing in most of the USA but with strict conditions pertaining to administration. The dilution of the urine which results from diuretic use can render detection of some other drugs more difficult.

Diuretics have a wide variety of chemical structures but can be detected in urine by HPLC or by TLC using silica gel G plates and ethyl acetate as the mobile phase. A method applicable to human urine using extractive alkylation and GC-MS is given in Lisi *et al.* (1991, 1992), or LC-MS/MS (Thieme *et al.* 2001) may be used.

Protein hormones

Currently, in human sports drug testing, methods are accepted for the analysis of hCG and for EPO only. Tests for hCG are based on immunoprocedures (Cowan *et al.* 1991; Laidler *et al.* 1994). A method to identify the different isoform pattern of recombinant EPO from that of endogenous material using isoelectric focusing (Figure 9.3) has been developed recently (Lasne and Ceaurriz 2000; Lasne 2001), whereas a method based on the perturbation of a number of blood parameters (haematocrit, reticulocyte haematocrit, percentage macrocytes, serum EPO and soluble transferrin receptor; Parisotto *et al.* 2001) was used at the Sydney Olympics in 2000. New forms of EPOs are now reaching the marketplace. Catlin *et al.* (2002) have published the detection of the administration of darbepoietin, a novel erythrocyte-stimulating protein (with a half-life about three times that of endogenous human EPO), using the isoelectric focusing method of Lasne and Ceaurriz (2000). Interestingly, this method has been used to confirm the presence of recombinant EPO in the canine as well as detecting human urine substituted for canine urine (Bartlett *et al.* 2006).

A test to prove growth hormone (GH) administration was first adopted at the Athens Olympics in 2004. Since recombinant GH does not contain the 20 kDa isoform, the absence of this isoform is the basis of this test (Wu *et al.* 1999). An alternative approach is based on using a discriminant function with the GH-sensitive substance insulin-like growth factor 1 (IGF-1)

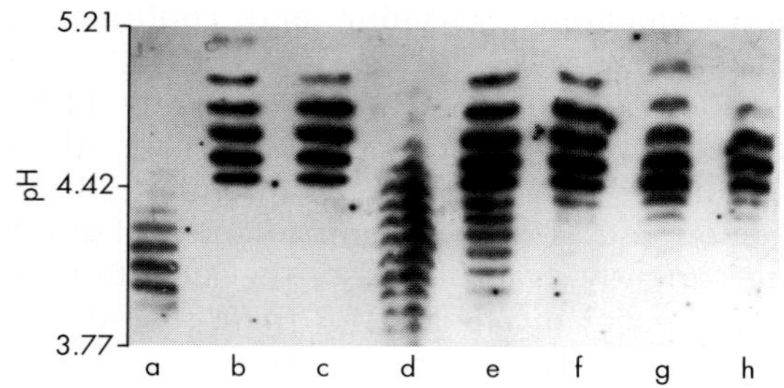

Figure 9.3 Autoradiograph of isoelectric patterns of exogenous and endogenous erythropoietin (EPO). Images were obtained by chemiluminescent immunodetection of blotted EPO after isoelectric focusing. Lanes: a, Purified commercial human urinary natural EPO (Sigma); b, recombinant EPO-β (Neorecormon, France); c, recombinant EPO-α (Eprex, France); d, urine from a control subject; e, f, urine from two patients treated with Neorecormon EPO for post-haemorrhagic anaemia; g,h, urine from two cyclists from Tour de France 1998 (samples concentrated by ultrafiltration). Note the 'mixed' appearance of the pattern in lane e. The cathode is at the top; pH values are indicated on the left. (Reprinted with permission from Macmillan Publishers Ltd from F. Lasne and J. D. Ceaurriz, Recombinant erythropoietin in urine, *Nature*, **405** (6787), page 635, © 8 June 2000.)

produced by the liver and procollagen type III (P-III-P) (Sonksen 2001; Powrie *et al.* 2007). This latter approach has the benefit of a longer detection time than the isoform method.

Rumour concerning the abuse of GH in horseracing has been circulating for a number of years, but interest in developing methods for its control intensified in 1998 with the approval, in Australia, of recombinant equine GH for veterinary use. IGF-1 has been confirmed as a universal marker to detect abuse of the three commercially available recombinant GH variants (equine, porcine and bovine GH) which were shown to be active in the horse (De Kock *et al.* 2001b). However, as IGF-1 is endogenous to the horse, the current international rules of racing would require its control through a threshold value.

In a collaborative study, IGF-1 levels in normal serum samples of horses in South Africa, Australia and the UK were determined by an immunoradiometric assay (IRMA) and were shown to have a distribution close to normal (De Kock *et al.* 2001c). Also, significant increases in IGF-1 levels in serum have been demonstrated after GH administration (De Kock *et al.* 2001b; Faustino-Kemp *et al.* 2001; Noble and Sillence 2001; Popot *et al.* 2001a, 2001b).

LC-MS methods for IGF-1 determination have been developed (Bobin *et al.* 2001; De Kock *et al.* 2001a) to support screening on the basis of immunochemical methods. In addition, LC-MS has been shown to provide a viable approach for the quantification of IGF-1 (Popot *et al.* 2001c; Guan *et al.* 2007).

Misuse of recombinant human erythropoietin (rhEPO) in horses, supposedly to improve performance, has received wide publicity. However, the horse is a natural blood doper in that, under exercise, contraction of the spleen can increase haematocrit by 33%. Thus misuse of rhEPO presents a serious threat to the welfare of the horse, as its administration coupled with splenic contraction could result in a marked increase in blood viscosity. This increase in an animal undergoing severe exercise could have serious health implications. Some physiological implications of rhEPO administration to horses were reviewed by McKeever (1996).

ELISA tests to detect rhEPO administration to horses and greyhounds have been evaluated and shown to be effective in serum (Tay *et al.* 1996). The double Western blotting technique developed by Lasne and Ceaurriz (2000) for EPO analysis in urine has also been evaluated in the horse (Y. Bonnaire, LAB, France, personal communication) and shown to be effective. As the natural equine EPO does not cross-react with the antibody used in the test, the test provides a better distinction between positive and negative samples when applied to equine urine as opposed to human urine.

References

R. Aguilera *et al.*, Detection of exogenous hydrocortisone in horse urine by gas chromatography combustion carbon isotope ratio mass spectrometry, *J. Chromatogr. B*, 1997, **702**, 85–91.

R. Aguilera *et al.*, Screening urine for exogenous testosterone by isotope ratio mass spectrometric analysis of one pregnanediol and two androstanediols, *J. Chromatogr. B*, 1999, **727**, 95–105.

R. Aguilera *et al.*, A rapid screening assay for measuring urinary androsterone and etiocholanolone delta C-13 (parts per thousand) values by gas chromatography/combustion/isotope ratio mass spectrometry, *Rapid Commun. Mass Spectrom.*, 2000, **14**, 2294–2299.

R. Aguilera *et al.*, Performance characteristics of a carbon isotope ratio method for detecting doping with testosterone based on urine diols: controls and athletes with elevated testosterone/epitestosterone ratios, *Clin. Chem.*, 2001, **47**, 292–300.

ARCI 2007a *The Association of Racing Commissioners International Model Rules of Racing*, 2007 (http://oa-rtip.org/industry/download-rules.html) (accessed 15.04.08).

ARCI, 2007b *Uniform Classification Guidelines for Foreign Substances and Recommended Penalties and Model Rules*, Lexington, ARCI, 2007.

C. Ayotte *et al.*, Testing for natural and synthetic anabolic agents in human urine, *J. Chromatogr. B*, 1996, **687**, 3–25.

D. Barron *et al.*, Direct determination of anabolic steroids in human urine by on-line solid-phase extraction liquid chromatography mass spectrometry, *J. Mass Spectrom.*, 1996, **31**, 309–319.

C. Bartlett *et al.*, Detection of the administration of human erythropoietin (HuEPO) to canines, *Anal. Toxicol.*, 2006, **30**, 663–669.

S. Bobin *et al.*, Approach to the determination of insulin-like-growth-factor-I (IGF-I) concentration in plasma by high-performance liquid chromatography–ion trap mass spectrometry: use of a deconvolution algorithm for the quantification of multiprotonated molecules in electrospray ionization, *Analyst*, 2001, **126**, 1996–2001.

R. V. Brooks *et al.*, Detection of anabolic steroid administration to athletes, *J. Steroid Biochem.*, 1979, **11**, 913–917.

W. G. Carter, Medication violations and penalties for RCI Class 1, 2 and 3 foreign substances: a preliminary report, in *Proceedings of the 13th International Conference of Racing Analysts and Veterinarians*, R. B. Williams *et al.* (eds), Newmarket, R & W Publications (Newmarket) Ltd, 2001, pp. 303–309.

D. H. Catlin *et al.*, Comparison of the isoelectric focusing patterns of darbepoetin alfa, recombinant human erythropoietin, and endogenous erythropoietin from human urine, *Clin. Chem.*, 2002, **48**, 2057–2059.

D. A. Cowan *et al.*, Effect of administration of human chorionic-gonadotropin on criteria used to assess testosterone administration in athletes, *J. Endocrinol.*, 1991, **131**, 147–154.

S. S. De Kock *et al.*, Growth hormone abuse in the horse: preliminary assessment of a mass spectrometric procedure for IGF-1 identification and quantitation, *Rapid Commun. Mass Spectrom.*, 2001a, **15**, 1191–1197.

S. S. De Kock *et al.*, Administration of bovine, porcine and equine growth hormone to the horse: effect on insulin-like growth factor-1 and selected IGF binding proteins, *J. Endocrinol.*, 2001b, **171**, 163–171.

S. S. De Kock, *et al.*, Growth hormone abuse in the horse: establishment of an insulin-like growth factor base, in *Proceedings of the 13th International Conference of Racing Analysts and Veterinarians*, R. B. Williams *et al.* (eds), Newmarket, R & W Publications (Newmarket) Ltd, 2001c, pp. 94–97.

X. de la Torre *et al.*, C-13/C-12 isotope ratio MS analysis of testosterone, in chemicals and pharmaceutical preparations, *J. Pharm. Biomed. Anal.*, 2001, **24**, 645–650.

M. Donike and J. Zimmermann, Preparation of trimethylsilyl, triethylsilyl and *tert*-butyldimethylsilyl enol ethers from ketosteroids for investigations by gas chromatography and mass spectrometry, *J. Chromatogr.*, 1980, **202**, 483–486.

M. C. Dumasia and E. Houghton, Studies related to the metabolism of anabolic steroids in the horse – the identification of some 16-oxygenated metabolites of testosterone and a study of the Phase II metabolism, *Xenobiotica*, 1981, **11**, 323–331.

M. C. Dumasia and E. Houghton, Studies related to the metabolism of anabolic-steroids in the horse – the Phase I and Phase II biotransformation of 19-nortestosterone in the equine castrate, *Xenobiotica*, 1984, **14**, 647–655.

M. C. Dumasia and E. Houghton, Screening and confirmatory analysis of β-agonists, β-antagonists and their metabolites in horse urine by capillary gas chromatography–mass spectrometry, *J. Chromatogr.*, 1991, **54**, 503–513.

M. C. Dumasia *et al.*, Studies related to the metabolism of anabolic steroids in the horse – the metabolism of 1-dehydrotestosterone and the use of fast atom bombardment mass spectrometry in the identification of steroid conjugates, *Biomed. Mass Spectrom.*, 1983, **10**, 434–440.

M. C. Dumasia *et al.*, Development of a gas chromatographic–mass spectrometric method using multiple analytes for the confirmatory analysis of anabolic steroids in horse urine. 1 Detection of testosterone phenylpropionate administrations to equine male castrates, *J. Chromatogr.*, 1986, **377**, 23–33.

M. C. Dumasia, *et al.*, LC/MS analysis of intact steroid conjugates: a preliminary study on the quantification of testosterone sulfate in equine urine, in *Proceedings of the 11th International Conference of Racing Analysts and Veterinarians*, D. E. Auer and E Houghton (eds), Newmarket, R & W Publications (Newmarket) Ltd, 1996, pp. 188–194.

P. van Eenoo *et al.*, Screening for diuretics in urine by LC/MS, in *Proceedings of the 13th International Conference of Racing Analysts and Veterinarians*, R. B. Williams *et al.* (eds), Newmarket, R & W Publications (Newmarket) Ltd, 2001, pp. 214–221.

J. Faustino-Kemp *et al.*, The use of IGF-I as a marker for detecting administration of growth hormone, in *Proceedings of the 13th International Conference of Racing Analysts and Veterinarians*, R. B. Williams *et al.* (eds), Newmarket, R & W Publications (Newmarket) Ltd, 2001, pp. 321–323.

S. J. Foster *et al.*, An automated solid phase extraction procedure for some diuretics and similar drugs in horse urine with HPLC detection, in *Proceedings of the 8th International Conference of Racing Analysts and Veterinarians*, J. P. Rogers and T. Toms (eds), Johannesburg, The Jockey Club of Southern Africa, 1990, pp. 3–10.

H. Geyer *et al.*, Analysis of non-hormonal nutritional supplements for anabolic-androgenic steroids – results of an international study, *Int. J. Sports Med.*, 2004, **25**, 124–129.

F. Y. Guan *et al.*, Detection, quantification and confirmation of anabolic steroids in equine plasma by liquid chromatography and tandem mass spectrometry, *J. Chromatogr. B*, 2005, **829**, 56–68.

F. Y. Guan *et al.*, LC-MS/MS method for confirmation of recombinant human erythropoietin and darbepoetin alpha in equine plasma, *Anal. Chem.*, 2007, **79**, 4627–4635.

J. D. Harkins *et al.*, Determination of the local anaesthetic efficiency of procaine, cocaine, bupivacaine and benzocaine, in *Proceedings of the 10th International Conference of Racing Analysts and Veterinarians*, P. Kallings *et al.* (eds), Newmarket, R & W Publications (Newmarket) Ltd, 1994, pp. 303–306.

J. D. Harkins *et al.*, Determination of highest no-effect dose (HNED) for local anaesthetic responses to procaine, cocaine, bupivacaine and benzocaine, *Equine Vet. J.*, 1996, **28**, 30–37.

E. Houghton, Studies related to the metabolism of anabolic steroids in the horse: 19-nortestosterone, *Xenobiotica*, 1977, **7**, 683–693.

E. Houghton and M. C. Dumasia, Studies related to the metabolism of anabolic steroids in the horse: testosterone, *Xenobiotica*, 1979, **9**, 269–279.

E. Houghton and M. C. Dumasia, Studies related to the metabolism of anabolic steroids in the horse: the identification of some 16-oxygenated metabolites of 19-nortestosterone, *Xenobiotica*, 1980, **10**, 381–390.

E. Houghton *et al.*, The identification of C-18 neutral steroids in normal stallion urine, *Biomed. Mass Spectrom.*, 1984, **11**, 96–99.

E. Houghton *et al.*, Development of a gas chromatographic–mass spectrometric method using multiple analytes for the confirmatory analysis of anabolic steroid residues in horse urine. 2. Detection of administration of 19-nortestosterone phenylpropionate to equine male castrates and fillies, *J. Chromatogr.*, 1986, **383**, 1–8.

IFHA, *International Agreement on Breeding and Racing and Wagering*, Boulogne, International Federation of Horseracing Authorities, 2007 (http://www.horseracingintfed.com/resources/200; accessed 04.02.2008). (See also http://www.horseracingintfed.com/racingDisplay.asp?section=6; accessed 04.02.2008.)

ILAC, *Accreditation Requirements and Operating Criteria for Horseracing Laboratories*, ILAC G-7, Rhodes, International Laboratory Accreditation Cooperation 1997 (see http://www.ilac.org (accessed 25.01.08).

ILAC, *The Scope of Accreditation and Consideration of Methods and Criteria for the Assessment of the Scope in Testing*, ILAC, G18, International Laboratory Accreditation Cooperation 2002 (see http://www.ilac.org) (accessed 25.01.08).

ISO/IEC 17025, *General Requirements for the Competence of Calibration and Testing Laboratories*, Geneva, ISO, 2005.

W. R. Jondorf, 19-Nortestosterone, a model for the use of anabolic steroid conjugates in raising antibodies for radioimmunoassays, *Xenobiotica*, 1977, **7**, 671–681.

W. R. Jondorf and M. S. Moss, On the detectability of anabolic steroids in horse urine, *Br. J. Pharmacol.*, 1977, **60**, 297–298.

C. Jouvel *et al.*, Detection of diazepam in horse hair samples by mass spectrometric methods, *Analyst*, 2000, **125**, 1765–1769.

A. T. Kicman *et al.*, Proposed confirmatory procedure for detecting 5-α-dihydrotestosterone doping in male athletes, *Clin. Chem.*, 1995, **41**, 1617–1627.

A. T. Kicman and D. B. Gower, Anabolic steroids in sport: biochemical, clinical and analytical perspectives, *Ann. Clin. Biochem.*, 2003, **40**, 321–356.

P. Kintz, Hair testing and doping control in sport, *Toxicol. Lett.*, 1998, **102–103**, 109–113.

M. R. Koupai-Abyazani *et al.*, Identification of levodopa and its metabolites in equine biological fluids by liquid chromatography–atmospheric pressure ionisation mass spectrometry, in *Proceedings of the 10th International Conference of Racing Analysts and Veterinarians*, P. Kallings *et al.* (eds), Newmarket, R & W Publications (Newmarket) Ltd, 1994a, pp. 123–126.

M. R. Koupai-Abyazani *et al.*, Determination of triamcinolone acetonide in equine serum and urine by liquid chromatography–atmospheric pressure ionisation mass spectrometry, in *Proceedings of the 10th International Conference of Racing Analysts and Veterinarians*, P. Kallings *et al.* (eds), Newmarket, R & W Publications (Newmarket) Ltd, 1994b, pp. 209–213.

P. Laidler *et al.*, New decision limits and quality-control material for detecting human chorionic gonadotropin misuse in sports, *Clin. Chem.*, 1994, **40**, 1306–1311.

F. Lasne, Double-blotting: a solution to the problem of non-specific binding of secondary antibodies in immunoblotting procedures, *J. Immunol. Methods*, 2001, **253**, 125–131.

F. Lasne and J. D. Ceaurriz, Recombinant erythropoietin in urine, *Nature*, 2000, **405**, 635.

G. Leung *et al.*, High throughput screening of sub-ppb levels of basic drugs in equine plasma by liquid chromatography–tandem mass spectrometry. *J. Chromatogr. A*, 2007, **1156**, 271–279.

A. M. Lisi *et al.*, Screening for diuretics in human urine by gas chromatography–mass spectrometry with derivatization by direct extractive alkylation, *J. Chromatogr. B*, 1991, **563**, 257–270.

A. M. Lisi *et al.*, Diuretic screening in human urine by gas chromatography–mass spectrometry – use of a macroreticular acrylic copolymer for the efficient removal of the coextracted phase-transfer reagent after derivatization by direct extractive alkylation, *J. Chromatogr. B*, 1992, **581**, 57–63.

K. H. McKeever, Erythropoietin: a new form of blood doping in horses, in *Proceedings of the 11th International Conference of Racing Analysts and Veterinarians*, D. E. Auer and E Houghton (eds), Newmarket, R & W Publications (Newmarket) Ltd, 1996, pp. 79–84.

A. R. McKinney *et al.*, Metabolism of methandrostenolone in the horse: a gas chromatographic–mass spectrometric investigation of phase I and phase II metabolism, *J. Chromatogr. B*, 2001, **765**, 71–79.

G. K. Noble and M. N. Sillence, The potential of mediator hormones as markers of growth hormone abuse in racehorses, in *Proceedings of the 13th International Conference of Racing Analysts and Veterinarians*, R. B. Williams *et al.* (eds), Newmarket, R & W Publications (Newmarket) Ltd, 2001, pp. 88–90.

R. Parisotto *et al.*, Detection of recombinant human erythropoietin abuse in athletes utilizing markers of altered erythropoiesis, *Haematologica*, 2001, **86**, 128–137.

M. A. Popot *et al.*, Detection of equine recombinant growth hormone administration in the horse, in *Proceedings of the 13th International Conference of Racing Analysts and Veterinarians*, R. B. Williams *et al.* (eds), Newmarket, R & W Publications (Newmarket) Ltd, 2001a, pp. 98–104.

M. A. Popot *et al.*, IGF-I plasma concentrations in non-treated horses and horses administered with methionyl equine somatotropin, *Res. Vet. Sci.*, 2001b, **71**, 167–173.

M. A. Popot *et al.*, High performance liquid chromatography–ion trap mass spectrometry for the determination of insulin-like growth factor-I in horse plasma, *Chromatographia*, 2001c, **54**, 737–741.

M. A. Popot *et al.*, Determination of clenbuterol in horse hair by gas chromatography–tandem mass spectrometry, *Chromatographia*, 2001d, **53**(Suppl.), S375–S379.

J. K. Powrie *et al.*, Detection of growth hormone abuse in sport, *Growth Horm. IGF Res.*, 2007, **17**, 220–226.

M. Ryan *et al.*, Detection and confirmation of clidinium bromide in equine urine using LC/MS/MS and GC/MS techniques, in *Proceedings of the 11th International Conference of Racing Analysts and Veterinarians*, D. E. Auer and E Houghton (eds), Newmarket, R & W Publications (Newmarket) Ltd, 1996, pp. 488–493.

T. Samuels *et al.*, Applications of bench-top LC/MS to drug analysis in the horse: I. Development of a quantitative method for urinary hydrocortisone, in *Proceedings of the 10th International Conference of Racing Analysts and Veterinarians*, P. Kallings *et al.* (eds), Newmarket, R & W Publications (Newmarket) Ltd, 1994, pp. 115–118.

W. Schanzer, Metabolism of anabolic androgenic steroids, *Clin. Chem.*, 1996, **42**, 1001–1020.

W. Schanzer and M. Donike, Metabolism of anabolic steroids in man – synthesis and use of reference substances for identification of anabolic steroid metabolites, *Anal. Chim. Acta*, 1993, **275**, 23–48.

C. Schoene *et al.*, Preliminary study of the metabolism of 17-alpha-methyltestosterone in horses utilizing gas chromatography–mass spectrometric techniques, *Analyst*, 1994, **119**, 2537–2542.

C. H. L. Shackleton and J. O. Whitney, Use of Sep-pak cartridges for urinary steroid extraction: evaluation of the method for use prior to gas chromatographic analysis, *Clin. Chim. Acta*, 1980, **107**, 231–243.

C. H. L. Shackleton *et al.*, Confirming testosterone administration by isotope ratio mass spectrometric analysis of urinary androstanediols, *Steroids*, 1997a, **62**, 379–387.

C. H. L. Shackleton *et al.*, Androstanediol and 5-androstenediol profiling for detecting exogenously administered dihydrotestosterone, epitestosterone, and dehydroepiandrosterone: potential use in gas chromatography isotope ratio mass spectrometry, *Steroids*, 1997b, **62**, 665–673.

R. L. Smith, The zero tolerance approach to doping control in horseracing: a fading illusion, in *Proceedings of the 13th International Conference of Racing Analysts and Veterinarians*, R. B. Williams *et al.* (eds), Newmarket, R & W Publications (Newmarket) Ltd, 2001, pp. 9–14.

P. H. Sonksen, Insulin, growth hormone and sport, *J. Endocrinol.*, 2001, **170**, 13–25.

S. D. Stanley *et al.*, Unique functionalised polymeric columns for solid phase extraction, in *Proceedings of the 13th International Conference of Racing Analysts and Veterinarians*, R. B. Williams *et al.* (eds), Newmarket, R & W Publications (Newmarket) Ltd, 2001, pp. 241–244.

A. J. Stevenson, The Canadian approach: limitations on analytical methodology, in *Testing for Therapeutic Medications, Environmental and Dietary Substances in Racing Horses*, T. Tobin *et al.* (eds), Lexington, The Maxwell H. Gluck Research Center, 1995, pp. 99–104.

E. Strahm *et al.*, Direct detection and quantification of 19-norandrosterone sulfate in human urine by liquid chromatography–linear ion trap mass spectrometry, *J. Chromatogr. B*, 2007, **852**, 491–496.

P. W. Tang *et al.*, Analysis of corticosteroids in equine urine by liquid chromatography–mass spectrometry, *J. Chromatogr. B*, 2001, **754**, 229–244.

S. Tay *et al.*, Evaluation of ELISA tests for erythropoietin (EPO) detection, in *Proceedings of the 11th International Conference of Racing Analysts and Veterinarians*, D. E. Auer and E Houghton (eds), Newmarket, R & W Publications (Newmarket) Ltd, 1996, pp. 410–414.

P. Teale and E. Houghton, Application of bench-top LC/MS to drug analysis in the horse: II. Analysis of glycopyrrolate, in *Proceedings of the 10th International Conference of Racing Analysts and Veterinarians*, P. Kallings *et al.* (eds), Newmarket, R & W Publications (Newmarket) Ltd, 1994, pp. 119–122.

P. Teale *et al.*, Gas chromatography/mass spectrometry screening of post race equine urine samples for basic drugs using automated on-line extraction, in *Proceedings of the 12th International Conference of Racing Analysts and Veterinarians*, B. Laviolette and M. R. Koupai-Abyazani (eds), Newmarket, R & W Publications (Newmarket) Ltd, 2000, pp. 44–46.

M. Thevis *et al.*, High speed determination of beta-receptor blocking agents in human urine by liquid chromatography/tandem mass spectrometry, *Biomed. Chromatogr.*, 2001, **15**, 393–402.

M. Thevis and W. Schanzer, Current role of LC-MS(/MS) in doping control, *Anal. Bioanal. Chem.*, 2007, **388**, 1351–1358.

D. Thieme *et al.*, Screening, confirmation and quantitation of diuretics in urine for doping control analysis by high-performance liquid chromatography–atmospheric pressure ionisation tandem mass spectrometry, *J. Chromatogr. B*, 2001, **757**, 49–57.

T. Tobin *et al.*, Testing for therapeutic medications: analytical/pharmacological relationships and 'limitations' on the sensitivity of testing for certain agents, *J. Vet. Pharmacol. Ther.*, 1999, **22**, 220–233.

R. Ventura *et al.*, Approach to the analysis of diuretics and masking agents by high-performance liquid chromatography–mass spectrometry in doping control, *J. Chromatogr. B*, 1991, **562**, 723–736.

WADA 2003a, *The World Anti-Doping Code*, World Anti-Doping Agency, 2003, Montreal, Canada (http://www.wada-ama.org).

WADA 2003b, *The World Anti-Doping Code International Standard for Testing v.3.0*, 2003, World Anti-Doping Agency (http://www.wada-ama.org).

WADA 2004a, *World Anti-Doping Code International Standard for Laboratories v.4.0*, World Anti-Doping Agency, Aug. 2004 (http://www.wada-ama.org).

WADA 2004b, *World Anti-Doping Program Guidelines for Urine Sample Collection v.4*, World Anti-Doping Agency, June 2004 (http://www.wada-ama.org).

WADA 2005, *World Anti-Doping Code International Standard for Therapeutic Use Exemptions* (In force 1 January 2005), World Anti-Doping Agency, Nov. 2004 (http://www.wada-ama.org).

WADA 2006a, *World Anti-Doping Program Guidelines for Blood Sample Collection v.5*, World Anti-Doping Agency, Jan. 2006 (http://www.wada-ama.org).

WADA 2006b, *World Anti-Doping Progam Guidelines for Breath Alcohol Collection, v.1.0*, World Anti-Doping Agency, July 2006 (http://www.wada-ama.org).

WADA 2008, *The World Anti-Doping Code, The 2008 Prohibited List*, International Standard, World Anti-Doping Agency, Sept. 2007 (http://www.wada-ama.org).

S. A. Westwood and M. C. Dumasia, A note on mixed-mode solid phase extraction of basic drugs and their metabolites from horse urine, in *Sample Preparation for Biomedical and Environmental Analysis*, D. Stevenson and I. D. Wilson (eds), New York, Plenum Press, 1994, pp.163–166.

T. Whittem *et al.*, Detection of morphine in mane hair of horses, *Aust. Vet. J.*, 1998, **76**, 426–427.

Z. Wu *et al.*, Detection of doping with human growth hormone, *Lancet*, 1999, **353**, 895.

P. M. Wynne, The application of SPE to veterinary drug abuse, in *Solid Phase Extraction*, M. J. K. Simpson (Ed.), New York, Marcel Dekker, 2000, pp. 273–306.

P. M. Wynne *et al.*, An improved method for the automated extraction of anabolic steroids from equine urine, in *Proceedings of the 13th International Conference of Racing Analysts and Veterinarians*, R. B. Williams *et al.* (eds), Newmarket, R & W Publications (Newmarket) Ltd, 2001a, pp. 245–251.

P. M. Wynne *et al.*, A multi-eluate approach to solid phase extraction of biological fluids for detection of drug residues, in *Proceedings of the 13th International Conference of Racing Analysts and Veterinarians*, R. B. Williams *et al.* (eds), Newmarket, R & W Publications (Newmarket) Ltd, 2001b, pp. 232–240.

P. M. Wynne *et al.*, Reduced blocking rates through application of a new NC–SPE sorbent to the extraction of equine urine, in *Proceedings of the 13th International Conference of Racing Analysts and Veterinarians*, R. B. Williams *et al.* (eds), Newmarket, R & W Publications (Newmarket) Ltd, 2001c, pp. 445–452.

10

Drug-facilitated sexual assault

A Negrusz and R E Gaensslen

Introduction and basic terms 287
The extent of the problem 288
History and legislation 289
Drugs used to facilitate sexual assault 290
Specimens and analytical methods 296
Summary 297
References 297
Further reading 298

Introduction and basic terms

This chapter gives a general overview of drug-facilitated sexual assault (DFSA), including the drugs associated with DFSA and approaches for sampling and analysis to investigate allegations of these offences.

Sexual assault perpetrated on mainly women, but also on men, while they are incapacitated by so-called 'date-rape' drugs recently became the focus of many investigations conducted by law enforcement agencies in many countries including the USA. During the past decade a marked increase in reports of this crime as well as in the number of scientific publications on the subject has been observed. The list of sedative drugs associated with sexual assault is long and among others includes flunitrazepam with other benzodiazepines such as diazepam, temazepam, clonazepam, oxazepam, as well as gamma-hydroxybutyrate (GHB), ketamine and scopolamine. In a typical scenario, a potential sexual offender surreptitiously spikes the drink of an unsuspecting person with a sedative drug for the purpose of 'drugging' and subsequently sexually assaulting the victim while the victim is under the influence of this substance. Victims usually report loss of memory during and after these incidents. They wake up in unfamiliar places, inappropriately dressed and often with the sense but not the actual recollection of having had sex. Most recent studies conducted in the USA and UK and described later in this chapter clearly show that other drugs and alcohol play an important role in facilitating sexual assault.

Sexual assault usually refers to a broad range of sexual offences from inappropriate touching or contact to actual penetration of intimate parts of a victim's body without consent. The term includes a completed rape, i.e. vaginal, anal and/or oral penetration in the case of a female victim (and oral and/or anal penetration in the case of a male victim) by penis, fingers or objects. In the USA sexual assault may be defined in different terms in the laws of different states (e.g. sexual battery, criminal sexual assault, rape, etc.). Rape is usually nonconsensual sexual intercourse, and in some states it refers only to penile-vaginal penetration. In the UK, rape is nonconsensual peno-vaginal or peno-anal penetration and fellatio and cunnilingus are indecent assault. Rape is often accomplished by a perpetrator using force or threat of force, but force or threat of force is not a required element. It has been established that approximately 80% of all rapes are 'acquaintance rapes' committed by a person known to the victim. Only 20% are 'stranger rapes' when the victim has no prior relationship with the offender. The determining factor is consent. Absence of consent makes the sexual contact a sexual assault.

Drug-facilitated sexual assault (DFSA) means a completed rape perpetrated upon a victim, usually a woman, who is mentally and physically incapacitated by drugs given to her surreptitiously by another person or persons, or as a result of voluntary consumption of alcohol and/or drugs and involuntary ingestion of another drug administered surreptitiously. DFSA may also include situations where the victim is sexually assaulted after voluntary use of drugs and/or alcohol. There is some evidence too that some 'date-rape' drugs may be used recreationally, and that sexual assaults can occur while a person is under their influence. These cases are also drug-facilitated sexual assaults, even though the drug may not have been surreptitiously administered to the victim by the perpetrator. It does not matter whether the victim was given the drugs unknowingly or was using the drugs recreationally. The crucial aspect is that any sexual act is nonconsensual.

The extent of the problem

The number of reported sexual assaults in the USA, for example, according to the FBI Uniform Crime Report, is presented in Table 10.1. Both the number and the rate of reported rapes declined throughout most of the 1990s, reaching a low in 1999. It is also well known that the number of *reported* rapes is significantly lower than the actual number. In 1999, for example, the Bureau of Justice Statistics estimated that there were over 141 000 cases of sexual assault, 58% more than the number actually reported to the police.

Until the late 1990s, there were no reliable data or estimates of the fraction of sexual assaults – actual or reported – that involved drugs typically associated with sexual assault. The only published data in the USA directly relevant to the prevalence issue are based on analysis of approximately 1200 urine specimens from a random collection of cases submitted to the investigators by forensic science/toxicology laboratories nationwide, specifically in order to screen for and identify alcohol and 'date-rape' drugs and other drugs (ElSohly and Salamone 1999). Approximately 60% of all samples tested were positive for one or more drugs, although not necessarily those typically associated with DFSA. GHB was detected in about 4% of samples. About 8.2% of the specimens had confirmed benzodiazepines, but flunitrazepam was seen in only a few cases.

A similar study was carried out in the UK (Scott-Ham and Burton 2005). Whole blood and/or urine from 1014 cases of alleged DFSA were analysed for alcohol, common drugs of abuse and drugs associated with DFSA. Where the presence of a sedative or disinhibiting drug was detected, the researchers used information provided by the police and, where necessary, follow-up discussion with complainants to try to distinguish between voluntary use and involuntary ingestion of the drug. Voluntary use was considered to be voluntary therapeutic use or

Table 10.1 Number of reported sexual assaults (SA) – FBI Uniform Crime Report

Year	Number of SA	Rate/100 000
1990	102 560	41.2
1991	106 590	42.3
1992[a]	109 060	42.8
1993	106 010	41.1
1994	102 220	39.3
1995	97 460	37.1
1996	96 252	36.3
1997	96 153	35.9
1998	96 144	34.5
1999[b]	89 411	32.8
2000	90 178	32.0
2001	90 863	31.8
2002	95 136	33.0
2003	93 433	32.1

[a] The highest.
[b] The lowest.

abuse of a drug. Involuntary ingestion was where the complainant alleged that the drug was 'given to them by another person without their knowledge'. All samples were screened for drugs of abuse (amfetamine, methamfetamine and ecstasy; barbiturates; benzodiazepines; cannabis; cocaine; methadone and opiates) by enzyme immunoassay (EIA) followed by confirmatory analysis by gas chromatography–mass spectrometry (GC-MS) and/or high-performance liquid chromatography (HPLC). All samples were subjected to GC-MS analysis for the detection of drugs associated with DFSA and their metabolites, with a colorimetric test used to screen for trichlorinated compounds. Alcohol only was detected in 31% of cases; illicit drugs only in 19% of cases; and illicit drugs and alcohol in 15% of cases. For the purposes of the study, illicit drugs were considered to be cannabis, cocaine, ecstasy, amfetamine, heroin and ketamine (where self-reporting indicated abuse of ketamine rather than involuntary ingestion). A sedative drug was detected in 18% of cases but most of these were considered to be voluntary use as opposed to involuntary ingestion. Only 2% of the total cases examined were considered as involuntary ingestion, i.e. where the drug was not self-administered, although it was noted that 'in a minority of the cases only, it was not always possible to obtain sufficient information to decide whether or not the complainant has taken the drug voluntarily' and also that the information recorded by police officers investigating a case was often minimal. It was also concluded that 'the low number of identified deliberate spiking cases (2%) may not necessarily reflect the true number of DFSA cases that have occurred'. Reasons given for this were that samples may not have been provided sufficiently quickly or that a urine sample was not provided, both situations potentially leading to non-detection of a sedative drug even though it may have been administered. There were an additional nine cases where a sedative drug was alleged to have been forcibly administered. Of the 21 cases considered as involuntary ingestion, sedative drugs identified included benzodiazepines (diazepam, temazepam, lorazepam, nitrazepam and lormetazepam), zopiclone, GHB, antihistamines (diphenhydramine), and sedative antidepressants (mirtazepine). Ecstasy was implicated in three cases of alleged DFSA in the study. Flunitrazepam was not detected in any of the samples analysed, although it is often considered one of the major drugs associated with DFSA.

A systematic study to estimate the prevalence of drug-facilitated sexual assault was carried out at the University of Illinois at Chicago. Four clinics in different US jurisdictions were provided with sexual assault kits and asked to enrol sexual assault complainants. Subjects provided two urine specimens and a hair specimen and completed a questionnaire describing the assault as well as any drugs they were using. The three specimens were then analysed to evaluate the self-reporting of illegal drugs and the number of drugs found in the subjects. Following this analysis, the results were combined with the subject's account of the assault and evaluated as to whether DFSA was a possibility. Approximately 140 subjects were enrolled and the drugs analysed for were found in 61.8% of the subjects, with 4.9% positive for the classic 'date-rape' drugs. For the evaluation of the validity of self-reporting of drug use, three drugs were included: marijuana, cocaine and amfetamines. The investigators hypothesised that sexual assault complainants would be more truthful in their reporting than other populations studied. However, in this study, subjects positive for these drugs reported their usage approximately 40% of the time only. Approximately 4.2% of the subjects were evaluated as having been victims of DFSA through surreptitious drugging. Flunitrazepam was found in specimens collected from four victims participating in the study. When voluntary drug use by the subject is included, 35.4% of subjects were estimated to have been possible victims of DFSA. The true value of DFSA in this study is most likely to be between these two estimates.

History and legislation

Increased numbers of incidents of drug-facilitated sexual assault in the USA in the early 1990s, especially the illegal use of flunitrazepam to facilitate sexual assault, have prompted federal legislation known as the 'Drug-Induced Rape Prevention & Punishment Act of 1996' [21 U.S.C. Sec. 841(b)(7)]. The legislation provides criminal penalties of up to 20 years imprisonment for any person who distributes a controlled substance, such as Rohypnol (flunitrazepam), to a person with the intent to commit a crime of violence, including rape. On 18 February 2000, President Bill Clinton signed another very important piece of legislation, the 'Hillory J. Farias and Samantha Reid Date-Rape Drug Prohibition Act of 2000' (Public Law 106–172) placing GHB on Schedule I of the Controlled Substances Act schedules, and requiring that the Secretary of Health and Human Services submit to Congress annual reports which estimate the number of incidents of the abuse of 'date-rape' drugs. This legislation was prompted and named after two teenage girls, Samantha and Hillory, who died after GHB was surreptitiously added to their soft drinks.

In 1998, during the Annual Meeting of the American Academy of Forensic Sciences in San Francisco (California), an international committee on drug-facilitated rape was formed. Two years later, the Committee became one of the regular committees of the Society of Forensic Toxicologists. More recently, during the 2002 Annual Meeting of the Society of Forensic Toxicologists in Dearborn (Michigan), three subcommittees were formed. One of the subcommittees is to work on recommendations for, and approaches to, toxicological investigations of drug-facilitated sexual assault. As a first step, the subcommittee identified all potential drugs and substances detected or suspected in biological specimens collected from victims. The compounds are presented in Table 10.2.

Drugs used to facilitate sexual assault

Flunitrazepam

The best-known but by no means the only drug associated with sexual assault is flunitrazepam manufactured by Roche under the name Rohypnol®. Flunitrazepam (5-(2-fluorophenyl)-1,3-dihydro-1-methyl-7-nitro-2*H*-1,4-benzodi azepin-2-one)) belongs to the 7-nitro group of benzodiazepines. Its hypnotic effect predominates over the sedative, anxiolytic and muscle-relaxing effects of other compounds from the same pharmacological group (Figure 10.1). Flunitrazepam is available in oral tablets and in injectable form in about 80 countries around the world. It has a much stronger affinity for the gamma-aminobutyric acid (GABA) receptor than diazepam (Valium®). In fact, it is 10 times as potent as diazepam. Flunitrazepam is readily (80–90%) absorbed through the gastrointestinal tract and metabolised almost completely by the liver. Its metabolism includes reduction to 7-aminoflunitrazepam and then to the *N*-glucuronide, demethylation to the *N*-demethyl metabolite, hydrolysis to the 3-OH metabolite and then to the *O*-glucuronide. Approximately 90% of its metabolites are excreted through the urine and 10% in the faeces. Deaths involving flunitrazepam in conjunction with other central nervous system (CNS) depressants, such as ethanol, but also due to overdose of flunitrazepam alone, have been reported.

The first seizure of Rohypnol in the USA took place in 1989, and reports of the misuse of the drug have increased since then. Flunitrazepam is often used to enhance the effects of heroin, alcohol or marijuana. Rohypnol tablets are smuggled into the USA (mainly from Mexico) and sold with street names such as Roofies, Rophies, Roopies, Rib, Rope, Pappas, Peanuts, Pastas, Forget pills, Ro-shays, Roaches and Roche 2. In the early 1990s flunitrazepam was identified as the drug of choice in DFSA. As of 1996, the prescription, sale and importation of flunitrazepam into the USA has been banned. Rohypnol is available in the UK as a prescription drug. Roche have reformulated tablets so that they give a blue colour when dissolved in water, thereby alerting drinkers to the fact that their drinks have been spiked.

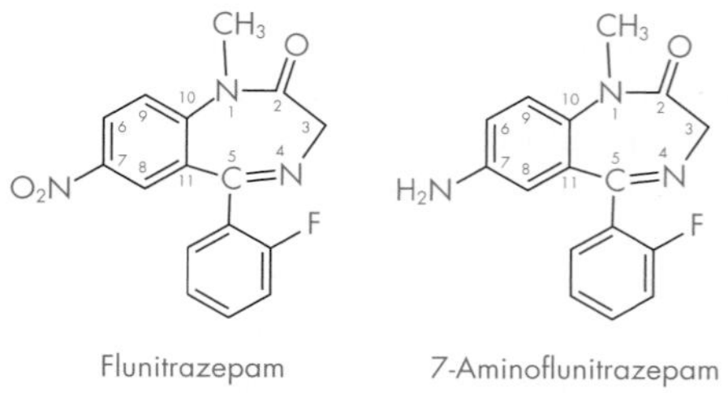

Flunitrazepam   7-Aminoflunitrazepam

Figure 10.1 Chemical structure of flunitrazepam and its major metabolite 7-aminoflunitrazepam.

Table 10.2 Recommended maximum detection limits for common DFSA drugs and metabolites in urine samples (courtesy of Dr Marc LeBeau)

Target analytes	Parent drug	Trade names / 'street names'	Recommended maximum detection limit
Ethanol			
Ethanol	Ethanol	Alcohol, ethyl alcohol, 'booze'	10 mg/dL
GHB and analogues			
Gamma-hydroxybutyrate	Gamma-hydroxybutyrate	Xyrem, 'GHB', Easy Lay', 'G', 'Georgia Home Boy', 'Grievous Bodily Harm', 'Liquid Ecstasy', 'Liquid E', 'Liquid G', 'Liquid X', 'Salty Water', 'Scoop', 'Soap'	10 μg/mL
	1,4-Butanediol	'1,4-BD', 'Enliven', 'Inner G', 'Revitalize Plus', 'Serenity', 'SomatoPro', 'Sucol B', 'Thunder Nectar', 'Weight Belt Cleaner', 'White Magic'	
	Gamma-butyrolactone	'GBL', 'Blue Nitro', 'G3', 'Gamma G', 'G.H. Revitalizer', 'Insom-X', 'Invigorate', 'Remforce', 'Renewtrient', 'Verve'	
Benzodiazepines			
Many benzodiazepines are biotransformed into glucuronide-conjugated metabolites. To improve detection limits and times, it is recommended that laboratories use instrumental techniques that will detect the glucuronide metabolites or hydrolyse urine specimens to free the conjugate before extraction.			
Alprazolam; α-hydroxy-alprazolam	Alprazolam	Xanax, Niravam	10 ng/mL
Chlordiazepoxide	Chlordiazepoxide	Librium, Libritabs	10 ng/mL
Clonazepam; 7-aminoclonazepam	Clonazepam	Clonapin, Klonopin, Rivotril	5 ng/mL
Diazepam	Diazepam	Valium, Diastat, Dizac	10 ng/mL
Flunitrazepam; 7-aminoflunitazepam	Flunitrazepam	Rohypnol	5 ng/mL
Lorazepam	Lorazepam	Ativan	10 ng/mL
Nordiazepam	Diazepam, Chlordiazepoxide		10 ng/mL
Oxazepam	Oxazepam, Diazepam, Chlordiazepoxide, Nordiazepam, Temazepam	Serax	10 ng/mL
Temazepam	Temazepam, Diazepam	Normison, Restoril	10 ng/mL
Triazolam; 4-hydroxy-triazolam	Triazolam	Halcion	5 ng/mL
Marijuana			
11-Carboxy-THC	Tetrahydrocannabinnol (THC)	Marinol, Dronabinol, 'Marijuana', *Cannabis sativa*	10 ng/mL

Continued

Table 10.2 *(Continued)*

Target analytes	Parent drug	Trade names / 'street names'	Recommended maximum detection limit
Barbiturates			
Amobarbital	Amobarbital	Amytal	25 ng/mL
Butalbital	Butalbital	Esgic, Fioricet , Fiorpap, Fiorinal	
Pentobarbital	Pentobarbital, Thiopental	Nembutal	
Phenobarbital	Phenobarbital, Primidone		
Secobarbital	Secobarbital	Seconal, Tuinal	20 ng/mL
Over-the-counter medications			
Brompheniramine; desmethylbrompheniramine	Brompheniramine	Alatapp, Bromaline, Bromanate, Bromfed, Bromphen, Dimetane, Dimetapp, Myphetane, Polytine, Puretane	10 ng/mL
Chlorpheniramine Desmethylchlorpheniramine	Chlorpheniramine	Aller Chlor, Chlor-Trimeton, Coricidin, Deconamine, Efidac, Kronofed, Teldrin	
Dextromethorphan	Dextromethorphan	Benylin, Romilar, Delsym	
Diphenhydramine	Diphenhydramine	Banophen, Belix, Benadryl, Dermarest, Excedrin PM, Hydramine, Sleepinal, Sleep-Eze 3, Tylenol PM, Unisom Sleep Gels	
Doxylamine; desmethyldoxylamine	Doxylamine	Unisom, Bendectin	
Antidepressants			
Amitriptyline; nortriptyline	Amitriptyline	Elavil, Endep	10 ng/mL
Citalopram; desmethylcitalopram	Citalopram	Celexa, Cipramil	
Desipramine	Desipramine, Imipramine	Norpramin, Pertofrane	
Doxepin; desmethyldoxepin	Doxepin	Sinequan, Adapin, Zonalon, Prudoxin	
Fluoxetine; norfluoxetine	Fluoxetine	Prozac, Sarafem	
Imipramine	Imipramine	Tofranil	
Paroxetine		Asimia, Paxil	
Sertraline; norsertraline	Sertraline	Zoloft	
Narcotic and non-narcotic analgesics			
Codeine	Codeine		10 ng/mL
Fentanyl	Fentanyl	Actiq, Duragesic, Sublimaze, Innovar	
Hydrocodone	Hydrocodone	Anexsia, Hycodan, Lorcet, Lortab, Norco, Panacet, Vicodin, Zydone	
Hydromorphone	Hydromorphone	Dilaudid, Palladone	
Meperidine Normeperidine	Meperidine	Demerol, Mepergan	

Methadone; EDDP[a]	Methadone	Dolophine	
Morphine	Morphine	Avinza, Astramorph, Duramorph, Kadian, MSIR, MS Contin, Oramorph, Roxanol	
Oxycodone	Oxycodone	Oxycontin, Oxyir, Roxicodone, Percodan, Percocet, Percolone, Roxicet, Tylox	
Propoxyphene; norpropoxyphene	Propoxyphene	Darvocet, Darvon, Wygesic	
Miscellaneous drugs			
Carisoprodol	Carisoprodol	Soma	50 ng/mL
Clonidine	Clonidine	Catapres, Combipres, Clorpres, Duraclon	1 ng/mL
Cyclobenzaprine	Cyclobenzaprine	Flexeril	10 ng/mL
Ketamine	Ketamine	Ketalar	1 ng/mL
Norketamine			
Methylenedioxy-amfetamine	Methylenedioxy-amfetamine		10 ng/mL
Methylenedioxy-methamfetamine	Methylenedioxy-methamfetamine		
Meprobamate	Meprobamate, Carisoprodol	Equagesic, Equanil, Micrainin, Miltown	50 ng/mL
Phencyclidine	Phencyclidine		10 ng/mL
Scopolamine	Scopolamine	Isopto Hyoscine, Scopace, Transderm Scop	
Valproic acid	Valproic acid	Depacon, Depakene, Valproate	50 ng/mL
Zolpidem	Zolpidem	Ambien	10 ng/mL
Stimulants			
While the drugs listed below do not possess the pharmacological effects typically associated with DFSA drugs, owing to their popularity it is recommended that screens for these drugs and metabolites be conducted at the detection limits listed or better.			
Amfetamine	Amfetamine, methamfetamine	Adderall	50 ng/mL
Cocaine; benzoylecgonine	Cocaine		50 ng/mL
Methamfetamine	Methamfetamine	Desoxyn	50 ng/mL

[a]EDDP, 2-ethylidene-1,5-dimethyl-3,3-diphenylpyrrolidine.

Gamma-hydroxybutyrate

Other drugs that have been implicated in sexual assault include gamma-hydroxybutyrate (GHB) (synonym: gamma-hydroxybutyric acid) and related compounds which are converted to GHB such as gamma-butyrolactone (GBL) and 1,4-butanediol (1,4-BD) shown in Figure 10.2. Figure 10.3 shows the metabolic transformation of GBL and 1,4-BD to GHB by alcohol dehydrogenase, aldehyde dehydrogenase and lactonase. GHB is sold on the streets under names such as Salty Water, Scoop, Soap, Liquid X, Natural Sleep-500 and Liquid Ecstasy. It is used in date rape because it is effective rapidly, is relatively easy to manufacture and obtain, and is alleged to have aphrodisiac properties. Possession, sale and clandestine manufacturing of GHB are illegal in many countries including the USA, UK and Japan. Since July 2002, GHB has been approved in the USA for treatment of narcolepsy.

GHB is rapidly metabolised and eliminated from the body. The detection window for blood is about 6 hours and for urine is about 8 hours. GHB is endogenously produced in the human body and in some foods and this needs to be taken into account when carrying out an analysis for GHB (see Specimens and Analytical Methods on p. 296).

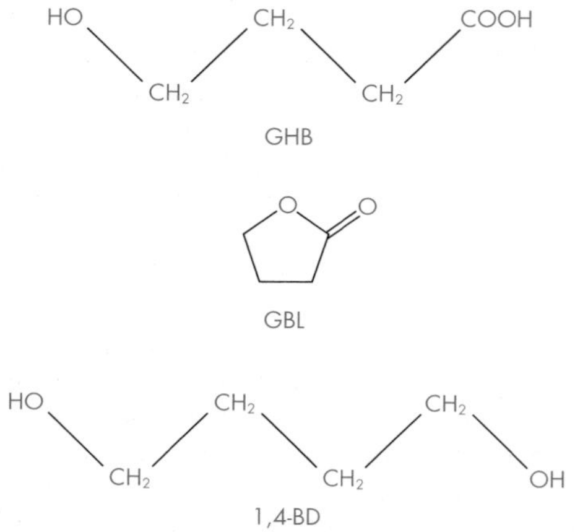

Figure 10.2 Chemical structure of gamma-hydroxybutyrate (GHB), gamma-butyrolactone (GBL) and 1,4-butanediol (1,4-BD).

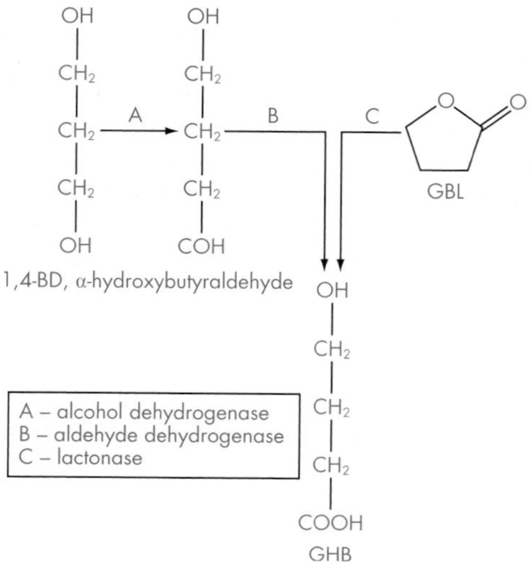

Figure 10.3 Metabolic transformation of GBL and 1,4-BD to GHB.

Ketamine

The general anaesthetic ketamine (Ketalar®, Ketaject™, Vetalar™) is used in human and veterinary medicine for induction of anaesthesia for short surgical procedures and routine veterinary examination. It was introduced to the market in the 1960s as a unique anaesthetic agent. It is structurally related to phencyclidine (PCP), but has only 25% of the psychotomimetic activity of PCP. The pharmacology of ketamine is complex. Like PCP, ketamine has activity at multiple sites in the brain. It primarily acts as a glutamate antagonist by noncompetitively binding to the PCP receptor located in the ion channel of the *N*-methyl-D-aspartate (NMDA) receptor complex. It sterically blocks the cation channel gated by the NMDA receptor, impeding the flow of Na^+ and Ca^{2+} ions into the neuron and resulting in disruption of glutamate-mediated transmission at these sites throughout the brain. The (*S*)-isomer is more potent in displacing the NMDA ligand from its receptor than is (*R*)-ketamine. In addition, ketamine facilitates monoamine transmission by inhibiting the reuptake of dopamine, noradrenaline (norepinephrine) and serotonin, resulting in an accumulation of these neurotransmitters in synapses. It also acts on the opiate system as an agonist at the μ-opiate receptor. When abused, ketamine can produce psychotic symptoms and cognitive impairment that may persist for up to 3 days. Clinically, ketamine has been used to induce schizophrenia as a model of psychosis. Like PCP, ketamine induces short-lived psychotic symptoms in non-schizophrenic volunteers.

Ketamine is rapidly metabolised, with the principal metabolites being an active metabolite, norketamine, and an inactive metabolite, 6-hydroxynorketamine. Ketamine is demethylated to norketamine by the liver microsomal cytochrome P450 system, specifically the isoforms CYP3A4, CYP2B6 and CYP2C9 (Figure 10.4). In the USA, ketamine is regulated as a Schedule III controlled substance.

Recently, there has been a resurgence of interest in ketamine due to its appearing as a 'club drug' at rave parties and at bars. On the streets it is known as 'K', 'Special K' and 'Cat Valium' and by many other names. The primary

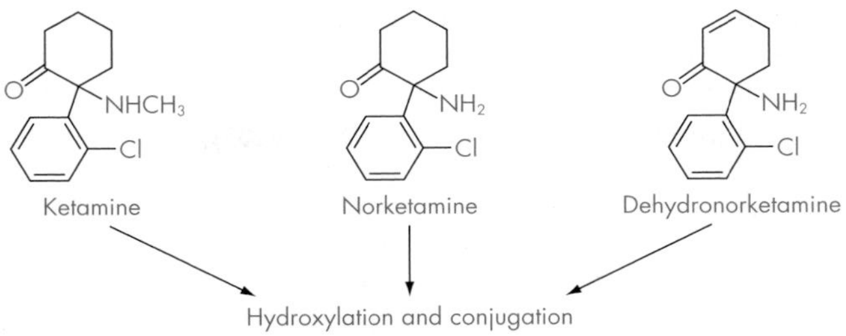

Figure 10.4 Metabolism of ketamine.

source for ketamine is diversion from veterinary clinics where it is available as a parenteral solution. Ketamine is used in a liquid form, its pharmaceutical preparation, or as a powder formed by allowing the solvent of the injectable to evaporate. It is taken voluntarily by intramuscular injection or by the intranasal or oral routes. Ketamine can be ingested involuntarily when it is unknowingly added to a drink to induce a stupor for drug-facilitated sexual assault, i.e. as a 'date-rape' drug.

Clonazepam

Clonazepam (5-(2-chlorophenyl)-1,3-dihydro-7-nitro-2*H*-1,4-benzodiazepin-2-one) is an anticonvulsant benzodiazepine and it displays many of the effects common to all benzodiazepines. It is available in tablets containing 0.5 mg, 1 mg and 2 mg under the trade names Klonopin™, Clonex™, Iktorivil™ and Rivotril™. It is a CNS depressant that results in loss of voluntary muscle control and loss of inhibition, and reduces anxiety. Like some other benzodiazepines, it causes anterograde amnesia. Clonazepam is metabolised in the liver to 7-aminoclonazepam by reduction of the 7-nitro group (Figure 10.5). This is followed by hydroxylation at the 3-carbon and subsequent glucuronidation. Almost all of the parent drug is metabolised – less than 0.5% of clonazepam is excreted unchanged in the urine. The elimination half-life from plasma has been described as being between 19 and 60 hours. The apparent volume of distribution ranges between 1.5 and 6.2 L/kg. After a 2 mg dose of clonazepam, the peak concentration of both parent compound and 7-aminoclonazepam in blood occurs 2 hours after ingestion. The onset of action of clonazepam is between 30 and 60 minutes, and duration of action may last up to 12 hours. Clonazepam is a highly potent benzodiazepine with a relatively low affinity for the benzodiazepine receptor. It must cross the blood–brain barrier to get to its site of action. The ability of a drug to cross this barrier depends on protein binding, lipid solubility and ionisation constant. Clonazepam is largely non-ionised at physiological pH and relatively water insoluble, so it readily crosses biological membranes and therefore rapidly passes from the blood to the brain. It has also been shown to decrease seizure activity and is approved by the Food and Drug Administration only for use in the treatment of seizures. Clonazepam is a DEA Schedule IV drug, available by prescription in the USA.

Owing to the physiological effects after clonazepam ingestion, it has the potential to be abused in drug-facilitated sexual assault situations. Clonazepam causes decreased inhibition, reduced anxiety, and a loss of voluntary muscle control. In addition, it causes anterograde amnesia, impairing the victim's memory of events occurring shortly after ingestion of the

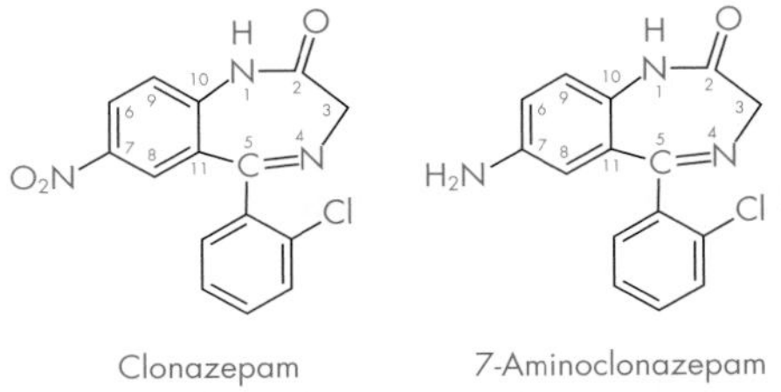

Figure 10.5 Chemical structure of clonazepam and its major metabolite 7-aminoclonazepam.

drug. These qualities may make clonazepam attractive to potential sexual offenders. Another fact that makes clonazepam particularly dangerous as a date-rape drug is that it is sometimes sold under the same street name 'Roofies' as flunitrazepam.

Alcohol and other drugs

Other sedative drugs associated with DFSA include scopolamine, barbiturates, muscle relaxants such as carisoprodol, cyclobenzaprine and meprobamate, diphenhydramine and other benzodiazepines. As shown from the studies of Scott-Ham and Burton (2005) and the University of Illinois at Chicago, alcohol and/or other drugs are also important in cases where DFSA is alleged and, in fact, may play a greater role than the sedative drugs typically associated with this crime. One of the major conclusions arising from Scott-Ham and Burton's work is that 'There are a variety of drugs that can be used for this type of crime [DFSA] and investigators should not concentrate only on the possible use of GHB and Rohypnol' and also that 'Alcohol consumption and use of illicit drugs should be considered as significant "risk factors" in such cases'.

Drugs used in DFSA have depressant effects on their users. Symptoms reported by victims of alleged drug-facilitated rape include confusion, decreased heart rate, dizziness, drowsiness, impaired judgement, impaired memory, lack of muscle control, loss of consciousness, nausea, reduced blood pressure and reduced inhibition. All these effects can be synergistically enhanced if the drug is taken with alcohol. In addition, drugs used in DFSA induce amnesia, presumably one of the main reasons for their selection as 'date-rape' drugs.

Specimens and analytical methods

One of the most important issues that needs to be considered in a DFSA investigation is the sensitivity of both screening and confirmatory techniques, since some of the compounds, e.g. benzodiazepines, are typically used in a single low dose. There is the added complication that victims of DFSA often do not report the incident until sometime after the event owing to amnesia and doubt about what may have happened, and possibly other psychological reasons. Sufficient time may have elapsed for most, if not all, of the drug to have been metabolised and eliminated from the more usual matrices sampled for toxicological testing (e.g. blood and urine).

Preliminary screening techniques for drugs in urine include enzyme multiplied immunoassay (EMIT), fluorescence polarisation immunoassay (FPIA), and Abuscreen OnTrak and OnLine imunoassays (Roche Diagnostics). Enzymatic hydrolysis followed by the extraction of benzodiazepines, including flunitrazepam and 7-aminoflunitrazepam, is frequently performed in order to increase the sensitivity of the assay. Confirmatory methodologies include gas chromatography–mass spectrometry with electron ionisation (EI-GC-MS) and both positive (PCI-GC-MS) and negative (NCI-GC-MS) chemical ionisation detection. In developing background information for the construction and optimisation of analytical methods for the drugs and their metabolites, one important component is a controlled, clinical dosing study with the drugs. In such a study, healthy volunteers are given single doses of a drug under careful medical supervision, then monitored for drug and metabolite concentrations in urine and hair for several days afterwards. In recent years, substantial analytical progress has been achieved in the USA and in France, allowing the detection for extended periods of selected benzodiazepines and GHB in urine and hair after a single low dose. As noted above, this is important because DFSA victims often do not report the incident immediately after the assault. Thus, it would not be unusual for a urine or blood analysis to provide a negative result when the drug had in fact been ingested, because of the likelihood of a single low dose, urine volume and the length of time since the drug was taken. Many drugs are deposited in hair and hence it may be possible to detect traces of drug in hair some time after an alleged DFSA.

As noted above, GHB is produced endogenously in the body. However, because of this endogenous production, it has been proposed that exogenous sources of GHB should only be considered when levels in blood and urine exceed 5 and 10 μg/mL, respectively. GBL is hydrolysed to GHB, particularly at high pH (Del Signore *et al.* 2005) and hence, if an analysis is carried out to differentiate between GBL and GHB, attention must be paid to minimising hydrolysis. It has also been reported that there can be site-dependent production of GHB in the early postmortem period (Moriya and Hashimoto, 2005) such that higher levels of endogenous GHB may occur in postmortem samples. This aspect should be taken into account when analysing for GHB in post-mortem samples. Shima *et al.* (2005) noted that the alpha-hydroxybutyric acid (AHB) and beta-hydroxybutyric acid (BHB), isomers of GHB, are also produced endogenously in the body and that levels of BHB in urine are considerably higher than levels of GHB. As the mass spectra of the various isomers are similar, there needs to be good chromatographic separation of the various isomers when using GC-MS or LC-MS to avoid inaccurate identification and quantification. Saudan *et al.* (2005) applied for the first time a method using continuous flow gas chromatography–combustion–isotope ratio mass spectrometry (GC-C-IRMS), described in Chapter 3, to discriminate between endogenous and exogenous (synthetic) GHB in blood. Significant differences in the carbon isotope ratio ($^{13}C/^{12}C$) were found between endogenous and synthetic GHB. The method can presumably be applied to other biological specimens including urine.

Summary

Much has been made of the drug-facilitated sexual assault problem in the popular media and, to some extent, in the scientific literature. There is no doubt that the involvement of flunitrazepam and some other benzodiazepines, ketamine, GHB and some other drugs with similar pharmacological effects in sexual assaults is a relatively new problem. The true extent of the problem is not yet known.

The need for methods to detect these drugs in the body fluids and/or hair of complainants has drawn forensic toxicologists into the analysis of sexual assault evidence. This development has prompted considerable research on the development of better, more sensitive methods of detection for the drugs and their metabolites. Controlled clinical studies on the time course of drug and metabolite elimination of some of the substances have also been done where feasible.

Considerable progress has been made over the past 20 or so years in the standardisation of sexual assault evidence collection protocols and devices. These efforts have been coordinated in many places by groups with representation from police, prosecutors, clinicians, victim services advocates and forensic laboratories. Until now, however, there has never been any need to consider or discuss the routine collection of urine and/or hair for forensic toxicological analysis. To the extent that the 'date-rape' drug phenomenon turns out to be a major problem, there will have to be significant changes in the initial response to complainants, in evidence collection kits, in the kind of forensic analysis done, and in follow-up procedures. This has already been recognised by the Metropolitan Police in the UK who have issued 'Early evidence kits' and protocols for investigation of DFSA. The kits permit collection of urine and mouth swabs (to detect signs of oral sex) and the protocols stress the need for timely sample collection. Improvements in drug detection methodology and knowledge of drug elimination will help in designing those changes in order that they prove most useful in assisting victims, and identifying and convicting perpetrators of drug facilitated sexual assault.

References

A. G. Del Signore *et al.*, ^{1}H NMR analysis of GHB and GBL: Further findings on the interconversion and a preliminary report on the analysis of GHB in serum and urine. *J. Forensic Sci.*, 2005, **50**, 81–86.

The Drug-Induced Rape Prevention and Punishment Act of 1996 (Act), 21 U.S.C. Sec. 841(b)(7) (http://www.usdoj.gov/ag/readingroom/drugcrime.htm).

M. A. ElSohly and S. J. Salamone, Prevalence of drugs used in cases of alleged sexual assault. *J. Anal. Toxicol.*, 1999, **23**, 141–146.

F. Moriya and Y. Hashimoto, Site-dependent production of γ-hydroxybutyric acid in the early postmortem period. *Forensic Sci. Int.*, 2005, **148**, 139–142.

Public Law 106–172, February 18, 2000: the Hillory J. Farias and Samantha Reid Date-Rape Drug Prohibition Act of 2000 (http://lcweb2.loc.gov/law/usa/us060172.pdf).

C. Saudan, *et al.*, Detection of exogenous GHB in blood by gas chromatography-combustion-isotope ratio mass spectrometry: implications in postmortem toxicology. *J. Anal. Toxicol.,* 2005, **29**, 777–781.

M. Scott-Ham and F. C. Burton, Toxicological findings in cases of alleged drug-facilitated sexual assault in the United Kingdom over a 3-year period. *J. Clin. Forensic Med.*, 2005, **12**, 175–186.

N. Shima *et al.*, Urinary endogenous concentrations of GHB and its isomers in healthy humans and diabetics. *Forensic Sci. Int.*, 2005, **149**, 171–179.

Further reading

M. P. Juhascik *et al.*, An estimate of the proportion of drug-facilitated sexual assault in four US locations, *J. Forensic Sci.*, 2007, **52**, 1396–1400.

M. Juhascik *et al.*, Development of an analytical approach to the specimens collected from victims of sexual assault, *J. Anal. Toxicol.*, 2004, **28**, 400–406.

M. A. LeBeau and A. Mozayani (eds), *Drug-Facilitated Sexual Assault: A Forensic Handbook*, San Diego, Academic Press, 2001.

11

Alcohol, drugs and driving

B K Logan, R G Gullberg, A Negrusz and S Jickells

Introduction 299
Alcohol and driving 308
Drugs and driving 317
References 321

Introduction

Forensic aspects of alcohol, drugs and driving

Driving under the influence (DUI) of alcohol (DUIA) or drugs (DUID) is responsible for thousands of accidents each year (National Highway Traffic Safety Administration 1993; Wennig and Verstraete 2000). In many countries, laws have been introduced to control drink-driving together with procedures to detect and prosecute impairment, and to treat and rehabilitate offenders. Alcohol is clearly still the largest contributor to impaired driving, but the additional impact of drug impairment on driving has also become a focus in recent years. Forensic toxicologists play an important role in many aspects of DUI, particularly in measuring the pharmacological relationship between drug or alcohol use and impairment. They have a primary role in analysing samples from drivers suspected of being impaired, interpreting results and presenting information in court. The consequences to the offender (arrest, detention, trial, legal expenses, fines, loss of licence, imprisonment) are serious, and defendants deserve assurances that laboratories carrying out measurements employ appropriate analytical safeguards and standards, and that individuals who interpret results have the necessary education and qualifications.

A typical scenario for procedures relating to DUI is as follows:

1. Police see a vehicle being driven erratically or are called to the scene of an accident.
2. Police question the driver and look for signs of impairment (see sections below).
3. Police assess impairment using tests such as the horizontal gaze nystagmus test and walk and turn test (see Fig. 11.2).
4. Police carry out roadside screening tests for breath alcohol (BrAc) and/or drugs.
5. If tests indicate the driver is over the legislative limit for BrAc and/or if drugs are present, the driver is taken to a police station or other authorised test facility and an evidential breath alcohol test carried out and/or a sample of blood taken for laboratory testing.
6. The blood sample is analysed for blood alcohol by headspace gas chromatography (Fig. 11.3) (if evidential BrAc testing has not been carried out) and for the presence of drugs if impairment through drugs is suspected.
7. The driver may be prosecuted depending on the test results and circumstances of the case.

Effects of alcohol on driving

Ethanol is the most commonly encountered alcohol in terms of DUI. Consumption of ethanol is legal in many jurisdictions where it is generally considered socially acceptable if consumed in moderation.

Other alcohols are occasionally encountered in terms of DUI. Methanol is a highly toxic substance. It is not generally consumed knowingly but may be consumed by accident, particularly by persons desperate to consume alcohol who are unaware of the toxicity of methanol. Other alcohols such as isopropanol (propan-2-ol) and ethylene glycol can cause impairment but, as for methanol, consumption of these substances is uncommon.

Alcohol is readily absorbed through the stomach and, in particular, through the small intestine, with virtually 100% of an oral dose is absorbed in healthy persons. It transfers readily to the bloodstream owing to its high water solubility and is then distributed rapidly throughout the body, portioning into all tissues, particularly those with a high water content. Alcohol is metabolised (Fig. 11.1A) in the liver, although some is eliminated unchanged. Although the major pathway for metabolism is oxidation via

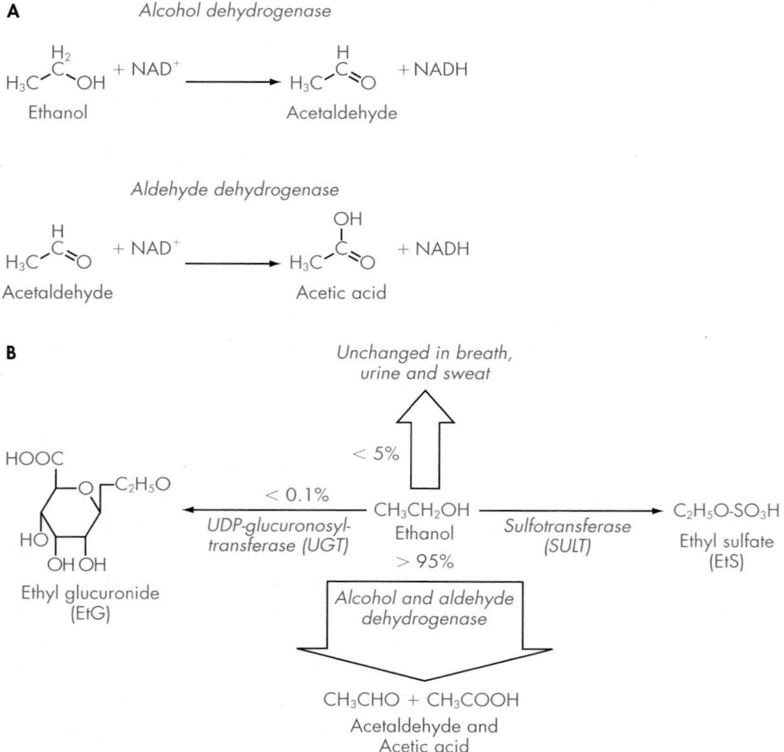

Figure 11.1 Metabolism of ethanol. (A) Showing the major metabolic pathway. (B) Showing the minor conjugation reactions with sulfate and glucuronic acid.

acetaldehyde to acetic acid, a small percentage of ethanol is conjugated to give ethyl glucuronide and ethyl sulfate (Fig. 11.1B).

Being volatile, alcohol can diffuse into free air and hence can pass from the pulmonary system into the lungs where it is expelled in breath. This excretion of alcohol in breath makes breath alcohol testing possible. Food present in the stomach can slow the absorption of ethanol.

Ethanol (hereafter referred to as alcohol) is a central nervous system (CNS) depressant. The precise mechanism by which alcohol affects cognition and psychomotor control is not understood completely, but the fact that it does so is very well documented, and is well understood by most members of the public. To understand the effects of alcohol on driving, the complexity of the driving task itself must be appreciated. Driving is a complex process that requires the simultaneous integration of psychomotor tasks, hand–eye coordination, muscle control and cognitive tasks. Moreover, since driving is a divided-attention task, the driver does not have the luxury of focusing exclusively on any one of these components, but rather must attend to all appropriately, monitor a number of sensory inputs, and prioritise each task depending on changing circumstances. Drug or alcohol use can affect the execution of individual tasks, and their effects are therefore more pronounced on more complex tasks, of which driving is a textbook example.

Alcohol causes a slowing of nerve conduction, which results in slower reaction times, difficulty in processing and integrating information, and consequently diminished performance in divided-attention tests. Individuals are overtly affected differently at different blood alcohol concentrations (BACs). This results from a variety of factors, which include prior exposure to alcohol, degree of both acute and chronic alcohol tolerance, innate physical condition and any associated limitations. Sometimes the effects of alcohol are not obvious to a casual or lay observer and must be assessed by tasks that challenge those abilities most subject to alcohol effects (see p. 306, discussion of identifying impairment). An individual can be affected by alcohol to the extent that it can interfere with driving before some of these overt signs of intoxication (e.g. staggering and slurred speech) appear. The BAC at which all individuals are affected in their driving by alcohol consumption is a continuing topic of discussion among forensic toxicologists, although most toxicologists agree that any individual with a BAC above 1.5 g/L would display overt signs of being affected on close inspection, even by a lay witness.

Effects of drugs on driving

CNS depressants

Like alcohol, many drugs produce CNS depression, either as a desired effect or as a side-effect of the drug. Hence much of the above discussion of alcohol applies to these types of drugs. Table 11.1 presents some common drugs with CNS depressant activity that have been implicated in impaired driving cases. Driving has been shown to be affected in driving simulators, in on-road driving studies and from epidemiological and anecdotal reports for many drugs, including cannabis, cocaine, methamfetamine, 3,4-methylenedioxymethamfetamine (MDMA), carisoprodol, phencylidine (PCP), ketamine, opioids, benzodiazepines and gamma-hydroxybutyric acid (GHB), as recently reviewed in two special issues of *Forensic Science Reviews* (vol. 14, 2002, and vol. 15, 2003). Combining alcohol with prescription or recreational drugs causes an additive or synergistic effect. It is not only illegal drugs which are implicated in DUID cases. One of the most commonly encountered examples in DUID casework is that of chronic pain patients. A patient who suffers from back pain might be prescribed one or two centrally acting muscle relaxants such as carisoprodol or cyclobenzaprine, a barbiturate such as butalbital, an opioid analgesic such as propoxyphene, hydrocodone or oxycodone, a sleeping aid such as zolpidem,

Table 11.1 CNS depressant drugs frequently associated with driving impairment

Antidepressants	Sedatives/hypnotics	Analgesics	Antipsychotics	Anticonvulsants	Muscle relaxants	Antihistamines
Alprazolam[a]	Flunitrazepam[c]	Tramadol[a]	Chlorpromazine[a]	Phenobarbital[b]	Carisoprodol[b]	Diphenhydramine[b]
Amitriptyline[a]	Lorazepam[c]	Codeine[a]	Mesoridazine[a]	Phenytoin[b]	Diazepam[a]	Chlorphenamine[b] (chlorpheniramine)
Amoxapine[a]	Zopiclone[a]	Morphine[a]	Thioridazine[a]	Carbamazepine[b]	Cyclobenzaprine[b]	Brompheniramine[b]
Butalbital[b]	Zolpidem[a]	Oxycodone[a]	Tiotixene[a]	Clonazepam[c]		
Butobarbital[b]	Zaleplon[a]	Hydrocodone[a]	Loxapine[a]			
Clomipramine[a]						
Gamma-hydroxybutyric acid[c]	Hydromorphone[a]	Amoxapine[a]				
Clonazepam[c]	Toluene	Dextropropoxyphene[a]				
Desipramine[a]	Xylene	Pentazocine[a]				
Diazepam[a]	Ethyl chloride	Fentanyl[a]				
Dosulepin[a] (dothiepin)	Cloral hydrate	Methadone[a]				
Doxepin[a]	Amylobarbital[b]	Pethidine[a]				
Imipramine[a]	Clomipramine[a]					
Meprobamate[b]						
Nortriptyline[a]						
Oxazepam[c]						
Trazodone[a]						
Triazolam[c]						
Trimipramine[b]						

[a] Basic drugs.
[b] Weakly acidic or neutral drugs.
[c] Weakly basic drugs.

and often an antidepressant drug to treat the depression that typically accompanies chronic pain. The resultant combined effect makes a reduction in driving performance very likely. Whether impairment is a result of legitimate prescription use or not is immaterial from a public safety standpoint, and a driver impaired by use of prescription drugs must be subject to the same penalties as a recreational drug user.

Cannabis

Cannabis (marijuana) is a very popular recreational drug. Obtained from the plant *Cannabis sativa*, the leaves and flowering parts contain a variety of cannabinoids that posses psychoactive effects, the predominant one being Δ^9-tetrahydrocannabinol (Δ^9-THC). Cannabinoids have significant behavioural and physiological effects, which contribute to changes in a person's ability to drive safely. The drug is popular for its relaxation-promoting and euphoric properties, accompanied by sedation and, in the right dose and setting, by hallucinations. Accompanying effects include altered time and distance perception, a reduced ability to concentrate, impaired learning and recall, increased appetite and mood changes. Associated physiological effects include increased pulse and blood pressure, and bloodshot eyes. Loss of the ability of the eyes to focus on objects has also been reported.

The predominant effects with respect to driving are sedation and the effects on concentration, divided attention, perception, and temporal and spatial orientation. The sedative effects can be similar to those of CNS depressants, and the associated driving behaviours are similar also.

Although a number of papers have been published in the scientific literature regarding cannabis use and driving impairment, it is difficult to draw hard and fast conclusions about the exact effect of cannabis on driving: the dose needed to bring about impairment and the length of time the drug may affect impairment. This is due to differences in aspects such as time of observation of behaviour after administration, dose administered, duration of effect between individuals, lack of appropriate control groups, and cannabis use combined with alcohol or other drugs. The general picture is that there is a higher percentage of cannabinoid-positive blood or urine samples (indicating use) in drivers involved in accidents or arrested for impaired driving than in the general population.

A limited number of studies have been performed in which subjects have been administered cannabis and then tasked with driving in electronic driving simulators, or actually operating vehicles on open or closed driving courses. These studies have been reviewed by Huestis (2002), and reveal evidence of minor to moderate, but significant, reduction in driving performance at the doses given. However, some drivers actually improved in performance after the cannabis dose. This effect of improved driving performance has also been seen in some alcohol-intake studies where a slight improvement was seen at low blood alcohol levels. In The Netherlands, on-road driving studies gave findings consistent with earlier studies (Robbe and O'Hanlon 1993, 1999), i.e. that cannabis use did impair driving ability. No correlation was found between the blood THC concentrations and the degree of effect. It was also shown that, when cannabis was taken in combination with alcohol, the effects on driving were increased.

In summary, cannabis is a psychoactive drug with effects on mood, concentration and judgement in addition to its sedating properties, all of which contribute in a dose-related fashion to impairment of vehicle operation. Compared to many other drugs, the level of impairment after mild-to-moderate single-dose recreational use is low, equivalent to a BAC in the range 0.3–0.7 g/L. Combining alcohol and cannabis produces a greater impairment than either alone, and cannabis use should be considered when determining what may have produced impairment in subjects with low BACs. The blood THC and metabolite concentrations are not well correlated with effect, although some authors have explored the possibility of relating these concentrations to time since last use (Huestis *et al.* 1992).

CNS stimulants

In contrast to the sedation-inducing drugs discussed above, stimulants generally increase neuronal activity which, in moderation, may not be entirely detrimental. Caffeine can revive the drowsy driver, and patients with attention deficit disorder (ADD) or narcolepsy can benefit from appropriate doses of methylphenidate or amfetamine. However, stimulant drugs can upset the delicate neural homeostasis in a healthy individual. Stimulants, principally cocaine and the amfetamines, are used recreationally for their excitatory, euphorigenic properties. In this context they produce intense overwhelming and distracting effects. After acute administration, users report feeling elated, powerful, having superior intellect and insight, and intense sexual arousal and stimulation. Time may appear to pass more quickly, speech becomes faster and less coherent, and users can become impatient and agitated, sometimes to the point of violence. These perceptual changes are accompanied by increases in pulse and blood pressure, pupillary dilation, sweating and psychomotor restlessness, manifested as pacing, fidgeting and scratching. Simple reaction time may be improved under the influence of stimulants, but this is only one component of driving; in fact, complex reaction time, which demands impulse control, intelligent decision-making and appropriate response, may be affected adversely. The intensity of these effects depends on the dose, the route of administration, and to some extent the user's experience with, and tolerance to, the effects of the drug. Inevitably, these effects, when combined, are detrimental to complex task performance and make drivers less attentive, while the psychomotor excitation demands greater focus on muscle control and vehicle operation. These opposing effects result in poorer driving. As with any other drugs, the effects are likely to become more apparent when demands are high, such as driving in bad weather, in heavy traffic, in an unfamiliar environment or in a defective vehicle.

In addition to these acute effects, humans display both acute and chronic tolerance to the effects of stimulants. With cocaine and the amfetamines, the initial excitatory, euphoric phase can be followed by a withdrawal phase, the intensity of which depends on the duration and intensity of drug use. During the withdrawal phase, subjects are typically fatigued, lack energy, and can be irritable, depressed and restless. Sometimes delusions and pseudohallucinations can occur, and the subject can become psychotic. Often this is called the 'crash' phase, during which the subjects sleep a fitful restless sleep, sometimes for days in the case of methamfetamine withdrawal. Drivers have been reported as being lethargic, sleepy, with very poor lane discipline (weaving), and frequently drive at high speed, drive off the road or drive into oncoming traffic.

Blood cocaine and amfetamine drug concentrations must be interpreted with caution, since a single blood drug measurement does not predict what phase of intoxication the subjects may be experiencing, and consequently what pattern of effects are likely to predominate. Nonetheless, blood drug concentrations can show whether drug use is consistent with recreational doses in the case of cocaine, and may help distinguish between legitimate dosing of amfetamines (e.g. in the treatment of narcolepsy, ADD or eating disorders) and recreational use. The doses of stimulant drugs required to produce the sought-after euphoric effects are accompanied inevitably by deterioration in driving performance.

Hallucinogens

Drugs with hallucinogenic properties have an obvious deleterious effect on driving. Inability to distinguish illusion from reality results in poor decision-making and consequently poorer driving. Drugs such as psilocibe mushrooms, mescaline, lysergide (LSD), ketamine and PCP can produce fully formed hallucinations, seeing objects, shapes or individuals that are not present, synaesthesias or blending of sensory information such as 'seeing' sounds, or 'hearing' colours. Ketamine and its psychomotor effects on driving have been evaluated (Mozayani 2002). Many other drugs can produce milder hallucinations, including, as noted earlier, cannabis and stimulants.

Methylenedioxy-substituted amfetamines, such as MDMA, methylenedioxyamfetamine (MDA) or methylenedioxyethamfetamine (MDEA) can also produce hallucinations, particularly tactile ones that enhance sensitivity to touch. However, the predominant impairing effects of that class of compounds appear more related to their excitatory and stimulant properties (Logan and Couper 2001).

The legal environment

In order to establish legislative limits for DUI, information on drug or alcohol intake and the effects on impairment must be available. Alcohol, the most widely abused drug, is the best understood in terms of use-related impairment. Numerous studies have been carried out measuring alcohol consumption, levels in the body and associated psychomotor performance (Moskowitz and Robinson 1988; Moskowitz and Fiorentino 2000). These studies indicate that alcohol consumption does result in impairment. Most jurisdictions have adopted limits on the level of alcohol which is considered acceptable/unacceptable for an individual to have in their system while operating a motor vehicle. The limits differ greatly between jurisdictions. Norway and Sweden have adopted a 'zero tolerance' policy, that is persons should not drive after consumption of alcohol. However, to allow for analytical inaccuracy in measuring levels of alcohol and to account for ingestion of ethanol from alcohol-containing food and medicines, they have set a standard of 0.2 g/L, i.e. 0.2 g alcohol per litre of blood (a concentration roughly equivalent to that achieved by the consumption of one alcoholic drink in a 67.5 kg male over 1 hour), as the blood alcohol concentration above which all individuals are assumed to be impaired. In the rest of Europe, Australia and North America, the legislated BAC limits generally vary between 0.5 and 1.0 g/L; 0.5 g/L is permitted in Australia and much of Europe (Belgium, Denmark, Finland, France, Germany, Greece, Italy, The Netherlands), and 0.8 g/L in the United Kingdom and in most of North America (but with 1.0 g/L permitted in some states in the USA). The limit in Japan is 0.3 g/L. Some jurisdictions set alternative lower limits for younger (presumably less experienced) drivers, or drivers of commercial vehicles (i.e. buses and large trucks). Most jurisdictions also have an alternative offence of driving while affected by the consumption of alcohol 'to the slightest degree', or some such similar language, to allow prosecution of individuals intoxicated by BACs below the statutory threshold. Some jurisdictions also have BAC levels above which more serious charges may be brought.

As noted above, alcohol is known to diffuse from the blood into the lungs and can be eliminated via breath. The relationship between levels in blood and breath has been established, thereby permitting the introduction of breath alcohol testing; legislative limits for breath alcohol have been introduced in many jurisdictions.

Legislating against driving under the influence of drugs presents a greater difficulty since there is less information available about how drugs impair driving, or how impairment can be associated with a quantitative measure of the drug in a person's system. It is relatively simple to carry out studies on alcohol intake and impairment because alcohol is legal in most countries and hence can be administered for studies without raising undue ethical considerations. This is not the case with many drugs, particularly those such as cocaine, opiates and amfetamines which are generally regarded as prohibited substances in most countries. Deliberately administering these substances to test impairment raises considerable ethical issues, particularly at concentrations simulating recreational use. Even for the studies which have been carried out, there seems to be no simple correlation between blood concentrations of the drug and effects on impairment. Thus, unlike for alcohol, in many jurisdictions there are no readily accepted values for drug concentrations in body fluids at or above which it is assumed a person's driving will be impaired. Consequently, many jurisdictions have introduced impairment tests for individuals suspected of drug impaired driving. These are typically tests of co-ordination skills but may also include observation of physical parameters such as pupil size. Although such tests may indicate impairment, for prosecution purposes the link to impairment through drug intake must be made. This is demonstrated generally through a chemical test of blood or urine, and more recently of oral fluid. The relative merits of these sample types is discussed later. Where the law is set so that no actual concentration limit is set for the offence, a toxicologist is generally relied upon to provide the necessary link between the use of that drug, the significance of any of the quantitative results and the drug's potential effects on psychomotor skills, particularly those related to driving. Some jurisdictions have adopted quantitative '*per se*' limits for drugs in blood or urine above which the person's driving is assumed impaired. These laws are generally based on the principle that the use of some drugs is illegal, or that they are used principally for recreational purposes and not necessarily on whether there is a demonstrated link between the limit set and impairment. The pharmacological merits and limitations of this approach are made evident in a later section.

Identifying the drug- or alcohol-impaired driver

Before the drug- or alcohol-impaired driver can be subjected to chemical tests, he or she must be caught. Studies carried out in the USA by the National Highway Traffic Safety Administration have identified several characteristics which may indicate that a person is driving under the influence of alcohol (or drugs) (see Table 11.2). The final column in the table indicates the probability of the driver being impaired.

Once a driver is stopped by the police, the officer looks for other evidence of intoxication, such as:

- smell – e.g. the smell of alcohol or burning cannabis
- bloodshot eyes
- unusual behaviour or responses by the driver to an officer's questions (including slow or slurred speech and physical responses), inappropriate answers to simple questions
- flat, dull, or excited demeanour
- unusually large or small pupils, unusual eye movements
- impairment of fine motor skills (e.g. difficulties with removing documents from wallet, dropping documents).

The presence of alcohol containers or drug paraphernalia which could be readily accessed by the driver (e.g. on the passenger seat), while not evidence of drug or alcohol use *per se*, should not be overlooked.

Generally, after noting the presence of some of these indicators or clues, the officer asks the subject to get out of the vehicle. This provides an opportunity to observe some gross motor skills. Table 11.3 documents clinical signs and symptoms and associated blood alcohol levels taken from a study by Dubowski (1994). The police may ask the subject to carry out some tasks which are designed to test psychomotor and cognitive abilities, and divided-attention skills. If drug influence is suspected, documenting the physiological parameters influenced by the use of these drugs (pulse, blood pressure, muscle tone, eye movement, pupil size and reaction to light, etc.) can assist in identifying the class or classes of drugs that might account for the observed impairment.

It is quite straightforward to identify a subject under the influence of a CNS depressant, since these signs are well documented for alcohol. Often noted are problems with fine or coarse motor control, staggering gait (ataxia), loss of balance, impairment in divided-attention tests, slurred speech and glassy and/or bloodshot eyes. Readily observable horizontal gaze nystagmus (HGN) is a consistent and common feature of CNS depressant intoxication (see Fig. 11.2). Subjects often have a sleepy or dazed appearance, have difficulty understanding questions or responding appropriately and may be disoriented to time and place. Driving behaviours commonly noted are a direct consequence of the CNS depressant effects on coordination and attention, such as weaving within or between lanes, failure to notice and obey traffic signals, failure to obey posted speed limits, wide turns, no use of turn signals and driving at night without lights.

Tests of impairment

Historically, a variety of roadside impairment tests have been used to assist with the assessment of whether a driver is impaired. Picking up coins, counting backwards, serial addition or subtraction, alphabet recitation, standing on one leg, etc., have all had their proponents, but

Table 11.2 Visual detection of DUI motorists (National Highway Traffic Safety Administration 1993)

Behaviour[a]	Probability of being impaired (p)
Problems maintaining proper lane position: weaving[b], weaving across lane lines[b]; straddling a lane line; swerving; turning with a wide radius; drifting; almost striking a vehicle or other object	0.50–0.70
Speed and braking problems: stopping problems (too far, too short or too jerky; accelerating or decelerating for no apparent reason; varying speed, slow speed (15 km/h (10 mph) or more under limit)	0.45–0.70
Vigilance problems: driving in opposing lanes or wrong way on one-way system; slow response to traffic signals; slow or failure to respond to officer's signals; stopping in lane for no apparent reason; driving without headlights at night[c]; failure to signal or signal inconsistent with action[c]	0.55–0.65
Judgement problems: following too closely; improper or unsafe lane change; illegal or improper turn (too fast, jerky, sharp, etc.); driving on other than the designated roadway; stopping inappropriately in response to an officer; inappropriate or unusual behaviour (throwing, arguing, etc.); appearing to be impaired	0.35–0.90
Post stop clues: difficulty with motor vehicle controls; difficulty exiting the vehicle; fumbling with driver's licence or registration documents; repeating questions or comments; swaying, unsteady or balance problems; leaning on the vehicle or other object; slurred speech; slow to respond to the officer and/or the officer must repeat; provides incorrect information, changes answers; odour of alcoholic beverage from the driver	>0.85

[a] Any two cues, $p \geq 0.50$.
[b] Weaving plus any other cue, $p \geq 0.65$.
[c] $p > 0.50$ when combined with any other cue: driving without headlights at night; failure to signal or signal inconsistent with action.

many are not suitable for use because of their dependence on the subject's fluency in a particular language, or their normal ability to count or perform simple mathematics. By far the most popular test battery now employed in North America involves three tests: the walk-and-turn test (WATT), the one-leg-stand test (OLST), and an assessment of horizontal gaze nystagmus (HGN). In the UK, field impairment tests include the WATT, OLST plus the finger-and-nose test, pupillary examination, and the modified Romberg balance test. Other countries use these or similar tests to assess impairment. Some of these tests are illustrated in Figure 11.2.

None of these field sobriety/field impairment tests have been validated specifically for different patterns of drug use. The value of these types of test is to demonstrate an inability on the part of the subject to integrate simple psychomotor and cognitive skills and, therefore, to show evidence of impairment. In some jurisdictions, the results of the various tests have been associated with the influence of specific classes of drugs. For example, dilated pupils are linked with use of stimulants, hallucinogens and cannabis, whereas constricted pupils are associated with use of narcotic analgesics (e.g. heroin, morphine).

Once it is established that the subject appears impaired, the next step should be a test for drugs or alcohol at the roadside. This can help confirm or otherwise whether the subject has alcohol or other drugs in their system and, in the case of alcohol, whether the level is approaching or above the legal limit. Depending on the roadside test result, the subject may be released or may be detained for further sampling and/or testing. Further testing may be required for prosecution

Table 11.3 Effects of alcohol on psychomotor and cognitive skills (Dubowski 1994)

Blood alcohol concentration (g/L)	Stage of alcoholic influence	Clinical signs and symptoms
0.1–0.5	Subclinical	No apparent influence; behaviour nearly normal by ordinary observation; slight changes detectable by special tests
0.3–1.2	Euphoria	Mild euphoria, sociability, talkativeness; increased self confidence, decreased inhibitions; diminution of attention, judgement and control; beginning of motor sensory impairment; slowed information processing; loss of efficiency in finer performances tests
0.9–2.5	Excitement	Emotional instability, loss of critical judgement; impairment of perception, memory and comprehension; decreased sensitory response, increased reaction time; reduced visual acuity, peripheral vision and glare recovery; sensory motor incoordination, impaired balance, drowsiness
1.8–3.0	Confusion	Disorientation, mental confusion and dizziness; exaggerated emotional states (fear, rage, sorrow, etc.); disturbances of vision (diplopia, etc.), and of perception, colour, form, motion, dimensions; increased pain threshold; increased muscular incoordination, staggering gait; slurred speech, apathy, lethargy
2.5–4.0	Stupor	General inertia approaching loss of motor function; markedly decreased response to stimuli; marked muscular incoordination; inability to stand or walk; vomiting, incontinence of urine or faeces; impaired consciousness and respiration, possible death
3.5–5.0	Coma	Complete unconsciousness, coma, anaesthesia; depressed or abolished reflexes; subnormal temperature; incontinence of urine and faeces; impairment of circulation and respiration; possible death; death from respiratory arrest
4.5+	Death	

purposes as the types of field tests used are often insufficiently robust for legislative purposes.

The best-known and most robust field test for alcohol is the roadside breath-alcohol test. A variety of devices are available. Most are based on electrochemical detection, although devices incorporating chemical reactions which produce a colour change in the presence of alcohol are available.

Enzymatic tests with a colour endpoint have also been developed for the field measurement of saliva alcohol. Such tests may have some potential value as screening tests in instances where the subject cannot provide breath, such as if injured and immobile.

For drug testing, a variety of commercial products are available for use in the field, most of which are based on an immobilised immunoassay test strip. These are usually designed for use with sweat, saliva or urine. There is considerable debate about these tests (operator dependency; limited range of drugs tested for) and they are not typically accepted for evidential purposes. However, they provide some form of screening to enable police to decide whether a driver does have drugs in their system and hence whether they should be taken in for further testing.

Alcohol and driving

Alcohol measurement

When testing for impairment through alcohol, the most common matrices for testing are blood and/or breath. Less usually, testing is carried out

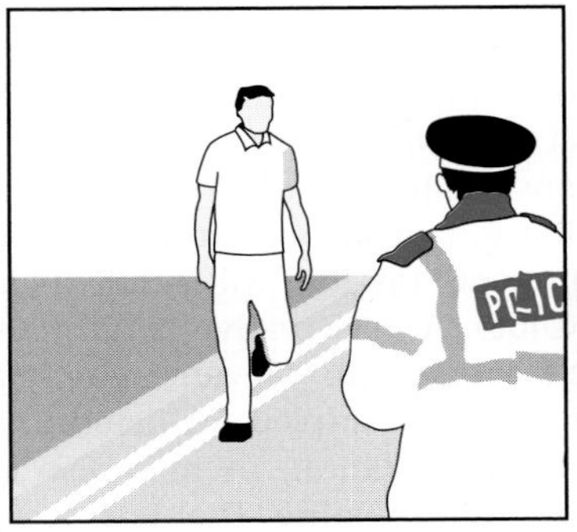

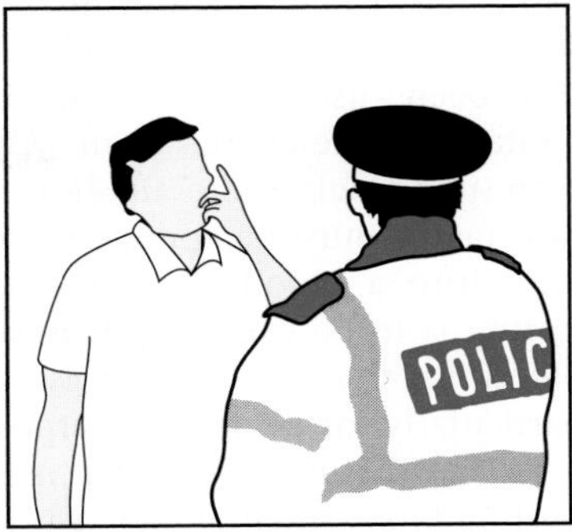

Stand on one leg test

For this test the driver must raise the right foot six to eight inches off the ground and keep their hands by their sides.
They must then count 'one thousand and one, one thousand and two' and so on until the officer tells them to stop.
The officer checks whether the subject sways, hops, puts their foot down or raises their arms.

Walk and turn test

The driver must walk along a real or imaginary line putting one foot directly in front of the other, heel to toe. They must take nine steps in this manner, counting out loud. When the ninth step has been taken they must leave the front foot on the line and turn around using a series of small steps with the other foot. After turning they must take another nine heel to toe steps along the line.

Finger and nose test

The driver stands with feet together, hands out in front palms side up and closed with the index finger extended. The officer then asks the driver to tilt their head back and he then calls out a sequence of left and right commands and the driver must touch their nose with the corresponding index finger and then lower their head.

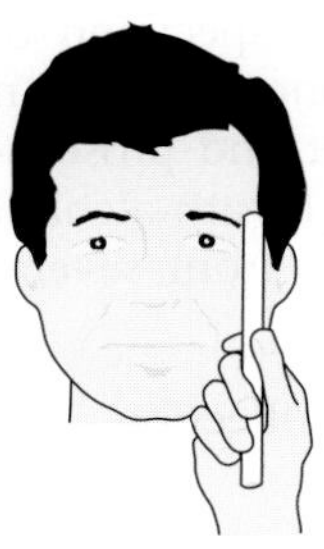

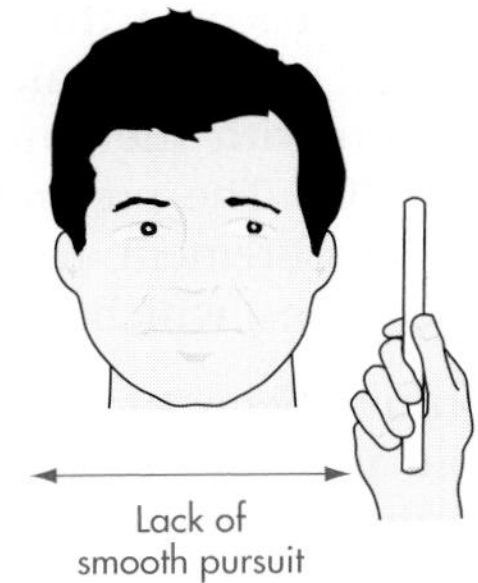

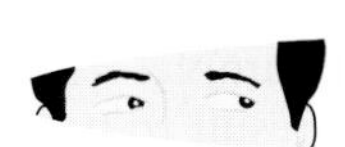

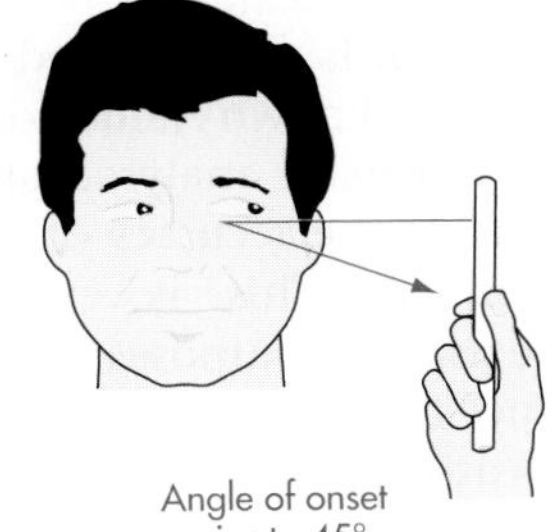

Horizontal Gaze Nystagmus test

An object is held in front of the driver's eyes. This is then moved to one side and then the other while the driver is asked to hold their head still and follow the movement of the object with their eyes. The officer observes the motion of the driver's eyes. If the driver is not impaired through drugs or alcohol their eyes should follow the object with a steady gaze. If they are impaired, the motion of the eyes will be jerky and the driver may have difficulty keeping their head still with a tendency to move the whole head in order to track the object.

Figure 11.2 Examples of tests used to assess impairment through alcohol and drugs (http://www.police.homeoffice.gov.uk/news-and-publications/publication/operational-policing).

on urine or saliva, but these matrices are not so well recognised when prosecuting for driving under the influence of alcohol.

Blood

Historically, blood-alcohol testing was the first method employed to determine a subject's alcohol consumption or intoxication (Jones 1996). Early methods involved distillation of alcohol from the blood, followed by oxidation and titration. These methods have been replaced almost entirely with enzymatic and gas chromatographic methods.

Enzymatic methods have the advantage that they can be automated readily, and can allow an alcohol test to be added to a panel of other blood chemistry tests, particularly in a hospital setting.

Clinical alcohol tests are carried out on plasma or serum. It is important to know which matrix has been used for testing because plasma contains more water than whole blood and correspondingly more alcohol. Hence a conversion factor must be applied to convert a plasma level into a blood alcohol level. If enzymatic testing is to be carried out, measurement using blood as the test matrix is to be preferred, particularly for evidential purposes.

By far the most popular method for determining blood alcohol is by gas chromatography (GC). This technique has the advantages of being semi-automatable, extremely reproducible and compatible with multiple sample types. Both packed column and capillary column procedures are acceptable for forensic blood-alcohol analysis, although most modern GCs operate with capillary columns. Headspace GC methods are normally applied (see Fig. 11.3) because ethanol is volatile and hence a complex sample clean-up procedure to extract the ethanol is not required. Some form of standard with a known value for ethanol concentration is normally analysed alongside test samples to enable the accuracy of the analytical result to be verified. This is exceedingly important for legislative purposes, particularly in view of the fact that a successful prosecution may result in a driver losing their means of making a living, or in the case of charges of dangerous driving may result in lengthy imprisonment. Certified standards can be purchased which are used in the determination of blood alcohol concentrations. These standards are analysed alongside test samples. If the result for the certified reference material is within the permitted tolerance, then results for samples can be accepted as accurate.

The disadvantage of using blood for testing is that a police surgeon, forensic medical examiner or other clinically qualified person is normally required to take a blood sample. Very few, if any, police departments have their own medical examiner and hence the norm is for the examiner to be called to the station to take a sample. It may take some time before they arrive, during which time metabolism and excretion of alcohol will be occurring. Many persons have an aversion to needles and this can also give rise to sampling problems. Caution must also be exercised with blood samples to minimise possibilities of microbial contamination (as this may give rise to extraneous production of alcohol) and to prevent volatilisation of alcohol from improperly sealed containers (as this will result in an incorrect test value). A preservative is normally added to blood samples to prevent microbial growth. When blood is sampled for determination of alcohol concentration, there is also an associated delay in obtaining the test result because the sample is sent to a specialist laboratory for analysis. This delay in knowing the test result can be stressful for the driver suspected of DUI and delays the police in taking action to prosecute impairment. For the above reasons, many police forces prefer breath testing.

Breath

Breath has become the biological specimen of choice for measuring alcohol concentration in association with the enforcement and prosecution of DUI. The preference for breath-alcohol (BrAc) measurement has resulted from several considerations, which include:

- noninvasive nature of sample collection
- rapid analysis and result
- minimal operator training
- sampling and analysis allowed in non-laboratory environment
- acceptable metrological properties of current instrumentation that demonstrate fitness-for-purpose
- minimal cost
- legislative mandates and parliamentary or high court and/or supreme court endorsement.

These factors have combined to establish breath-alcohol analysis as the most common forensic analysis employed in drink-driving enforcement.

As breath-alcohol analysis is typically performed in a police station or other non-laboratory environment by a trained user (but who is not a chemist or forensic scientist) it must be performed with the minimum possible input or influence on variability in the test result from the subject or operator.

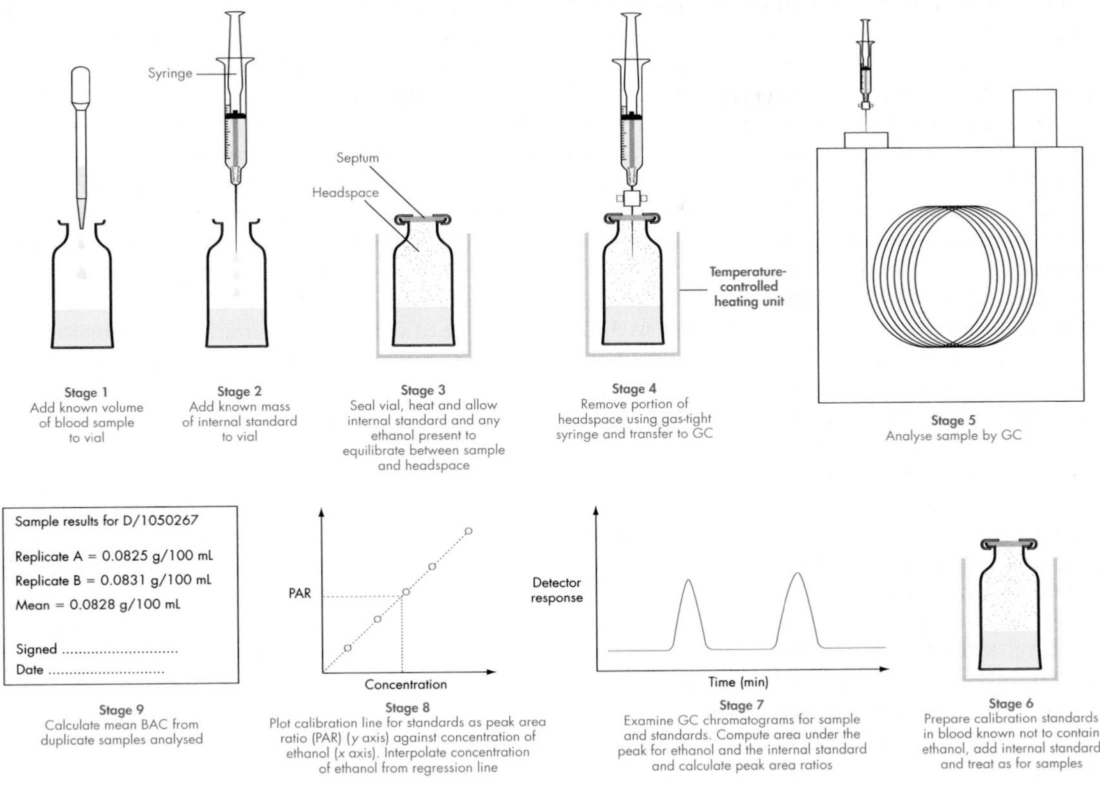

Figure 11.3 An illustration of headspace GC analysis to determine blood alcohol concentration.

At a very minimum, a sound forensic breath-test protocol which is to be used for prosecution purposes should include:

1. Trained and qualified breath-test instrument operators
2. Validated instrumentation which is re-calibrated on a routine basis
3. At least 15 minutes pre-exhalation observation
4. Internal instrument standards verifying calibration
5. Duplicate breath samples with appropriate agreement (i.e. ± 10% of the mean)
6. External control standards (wet bath or gas)
7. Blank tests between all analyses
8. Printout of all results
9. Error detection systems throughout the test procedure

If the subject has recently consumed alcohol and there has not been time for this to dissipate from the mouth, an erroneously high BrAc value will be obtained. This presence of residual alcohol is often referred to as mouth alcohol. A period of at least 15 minutes should be allowed to elapse between the last drink the subject is known to have consumed and the breath alcohol test to ensure any mouth alcohol has dissipated. In addition, all instruments should be evaluated periodically according to an established quality-assurance procedure to ensure optimal analytical performance, including accuracy, precision, linearity and critical-system evaluations (e.g.

acetone detection, radiofrequency interference detection, mouth alcohol detection, etc.).

Breath-alcohol instrumentation

The first instruments for breath-alcohol testing employed chemical reactions involving a colour change. Concerns were raised about the specificity and accuracy of these and they have largely been replaced by devices employing the optical absorption of infrared (IR) energy according to Beer's law (see Chapter 15) making this a quantitative determination. Such instruments include the Camic Datamaster (Camic Ltd, UK) and the Lion Intoxilyzer (Lion Laboratories, UK). Specificity needs to be taken into account when using IR because other volatile organic substances which may be present in breath will also absorb in the IR and may produce a false reading. Examples of such substances include volatiles produced by ketosis and volatile solvents such as toluene and paint thinners which may be present via solvent abuse, the workplace or home decorating and repairing. Most evidential breath-alcohol instruments employing IR incorporate multiple wavelengths to increase specificity for ethanol (Fig. 11.4). During the 1980s, fuel-cell technology, which operates on the principle of electrochemistry, also emerged as a useful analytical method in forensic breath-alcohol measurement. Although fuel cells have been employed typically in screening devices, their technology has improved dramatically in recent years. Instruments employing both IR and fuel-cell methodologies to quantify ethanol in breath for evidential purposes include the Alcotest 7110 (Draeger Safety) and the Intoximeter (Intoximeters Inc., USA). The advantage of the combined IR and fuel-cell instruments is that two different methodologies are used for measurement, thereby maximising the chance of detecting the presence of volatile substances other than alcohol and minimising the possibility of a false result.

Urine and saliva

Urine

Urine has been used in some jurisdictions as a specimen for forensic alcohol testing. It is amenable to analysis by both the enzymatic and chromatographic methods described above. However, its major limitations are collection and interpretation. If observed, urine collection raises privacy issues; if not observed, it raises issues of chain of custody, and the potential for substitution or dilution. With respect to interpretation, urinary alcohol concentration is an indirect measurement of BAC. Urine is formed in the kidneys as an ultrafiltrate of blood. There-

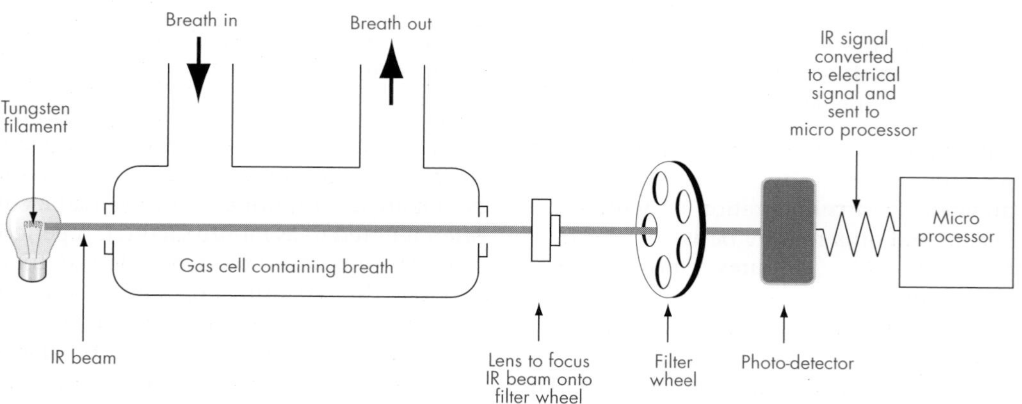

Figure 11.4 Schematic of an IR breath testing instrument. The instrument contains a series of filters whose function is to indicate whether other substances are present which might interfere with quantification of BrAc concentration. The instrument uses the ratios of the C—H vibrational stretching modes of ethanol at 2873.56 cm^{-1} and 2949.85 cm^{-1} to check whether interfering substances are present.

fore, a factor must be applied to account for the higher water content. Of more importance, however, is that, since urine is formed over time, the urine alcohol concentration is an average corresponding to the blood concentration over the time during which the urine was formed and collected in the bladder. Since this can cover an appreciable amount of time (up to several hours), even a urine sample corrected for water content may not reflect the true BAC at the time of urine collection. To correct for this, for forensic purposes urine is generally collected for analysis about an hour after an initial void. The subject is directed to empty his or her bladder, after which he or she is allowed a period of time (approximately an hour) during which new urine corresponding to their current BAC is formed and collected for testing. Such complications and the associated problems of interpretation mean that urine alcohol determination is not a preferred forensic approach, although it is acceptable in many jurisdictions. Problems with interpretation are generally overcome by adopting a statutory '*per se*' urine alcohol offence – i.e. if the measured value exceeds the set restriction, the driver is considered to be 'impaired' or 'under the influence' and an offence is deemed to have been committed.

Oral fluid

Saliva, or oral fluid (as it is more correctly known), is a plasma ultrafiltrate produced through the parotid and other glands in the oral cavity. Many drugs, including alcohol, that are present in the blood therefore also appear in the saliva. Oral fluid can, however, be subject to contamination from recent oral intake of drugs and alcohol, or simply from retaining these in the mouth and expelling them without ingestion. Contamination can last for some time, depending on the drug's lipophilicity and water solubility. Alcohol, for example, is generally dissipated from the mouth by absorption and exhalation within 15 min. A 15–20 min waiting period is therefore standard in an evidential breath-testing environment, prior to the subject being offered an evidential breath test, and a similar waiting period is essential for a test of salivary alcohol. A number of vendors sell salivary alcohol test strips, based on the principle of enzymatic oxidation. These are used most appropriately as screening devices, since their quantitative accuracy is highly operator-dependent. They are, however, often sold directly to the public for self-testing, and it is possible that people may make inappropriate decisions about driving based on an inaccurate test, and may ignore the legal prohibition against driving while affected, irrespective of BAC.

There is, however, a good correlation between circulating blood alcohol and saliva alcohol and, if for some reason a blood or breath sample cannot be provided, a properly collected and preserved oral fluid sample can be subjected to a gas chromatographic analysis with the appropriate forensic safeguards. For these purposes, oral fluid should be collected in a tube with minimal headspace to prevent loss and an enzyme inhibitor to inhibit post-collection alcohol production.

Interpretation and presentation of alcohol results

The measurement process is not complete until the test results have been interpreted appropriately and presented clearly to those responsible for making a decision based on them. Too often, most effort is directed towards ensuring the highest integrity of the measurement process with less consideration given to the clear communication of the results and their possible limitations.

Appropriate interpretation of blood-, urine-, oral fluid- or breath-alcohol results begins with a thorough understanding of the purpose of the measurement and the process that produced them. The results of a roadside screening test, for example, are interpreted differently from an evidential test result. The roadside breath test is generally undertaken to establish alcohol use and provide probable cause for an arrest, to be followed by a more highly controlled evidential test. In many jurisdictions, the roadside screening test is not considered acceptable for prosecution purposes and only the result of an evidential test will be accepted by the courts.

As with any forensic evidence, alcohol results must be presented to the court along with a brief explanation of the measurement process. This allows the court to put the measurement results in their appropriate context and assign the relevant weight. Pre-trial meetings with the legal representatives are always useful to discuss the testimony and any unique issues in the case. It is very important that scientists present themselves as objective and impartial expert witnesses, and they should be an advocate for the evidence, acknowledging its strengths and weaknesses but giving an unbiased and objective opinion about the most likely interpretation.

The expert witness should be prepared to present the basic principles of the analytical method and describe the instrument in terms that can be understood by a lay person. The legal basis for the approval of the instrumentation and method (e.g. administrative rules, statutory law or case law) must also be presented to establish the legal foundation for admissibility. When new technology is first introduced into a jurisdiction, a legal judgment is typically made to establish whether the technology has gained general acceptance within the relevant scientific community. In the US this is referred to as a Frye (Frye vs. United States 1923) or Daubert (Daubert vs. Merrell Dow Pharmaceuticals 1993) standard. To present the technical features of modern instruments in simple terms can be a challenge for the forensic scientist. For example, in a breath-test case the use of some very basic visual aids to illustrate the principles of IR absorption and the basic components of the instrument can be very helpful.

Alcohol results should be presented and interpreted according to the legislative definitions and framework to which a particular country or state adheres. For instance, in the UK, the blood-alcohol limit is quoted as 80 mg/100 mL and the breath-alcohol limit 35 μg/100 mL. In the USA, corresponding values are 0.08 g/100 mL and 0.08 g/210 L, respectively. It is also worth bearing in mind that conversion factors used, for example, to translate breath-alcohol levels into blood-alcohol levels and vice versa may also differ slightly from country to country.

The expert witness must be prepared to acknowledge the uncertainty inherent in measurement results. All measurements possess uncertainty that arises from both systematic and random sources (see Chapter 23). Estimates of uncertainty become particularly important when the results are near the critical prohibited levels. Obviously the more replicate determinations that can be carried out on a sample the better, because the mean value is likely to be closer to the true value (assuming the procedures are accurate) compared with the situation where a single replicate is analysed. However, it is not practical to analyse large numbers of replicates for reasons of time and cost, and also because there may be a limited volume of sample available for analysis. Hence the norm is for duplicate subsamples to be analysed or, in the case of breath alcohol determinations, for the alcohol concentration in two separate exhalations of breath to be determined. The mean of the values is then reported. However, as noted above, there will be an uncertainty associated with the result reported. Ideally, the results presented to the court are accompanied by an estimate of their uncertainty. This provides relevant information that allows the court to weigh the evidence in view of the required fitness-for-purpose and also to make a decision regarding the offence as defined in the statute; for example, whether the level of alcohol in the breath of the defendant was higher or lower than the legislative limit. Even when the estimate of uncertainty does not accompany the results presented in court, the forensic scientist should be prepared to determine and present these estimates. Although several methods exist to determine and present measurement uncertainty (Ellison *et al.* 2000), one useful and intuitive method is to provide a confidence interval for the individual's mean breath-alcohol concentration (Gullberg 2003). A similar approach can be taken for BAC results.

Retrograde extrapolation or back-calculation of alcohol concentration

Many jurisdictions express an offence under DUI as having, or exceeding, a specified alcohol concentration 'at the time of driving'. Some time is likely to have elapsed between the time that a person is stopped for suspicion of DUI and the time at which either evidential breath alcohol testing is carried out or samples are taken for laboratory testing to determine blood alcohol.

During this time, the level of alcohol in a person's system will change owing to distribution, metabolism and excretion processes. Thus the level at the time of evidential testing or sampling will not be the same as it was at the time the driver was questioned initially. There is then a need to provide some retrograde estimate of a subject's blood- or breath-alcohol concentration at the time the DUI offence occurred. Several terms are applied to this estimate, including retrograde extrapolation, back-calculation, estimating back, back-extrapolation or relating back. All refer to the process of applying basic principles of pharmacokinetics to arrive at an estimate of a person's blood or breath alcohol result at a prior time based on a measured concentration at a later time. An example might serve to illustrate its application (see Fig. 11.5).

Back-calculation estimations generally assume two extremes of likely alcohol elimination rates based on published data for alcohol elimination in impaired drivers (Jones and Andersson 1996) which are used to estimate the upper and lower likely limits of the alcohol concentration at a particular time prior to testing or sampling together with a 'most likely' elimination value.

Back-calculation estimations, as illustrated by Figure 11.5, rely on the following assumptions:

- the subject's BrAc concentration (BrAC) or BAC is on the linear elimination portion of the concentration–time curve at the time of arrest
- the elimination rate remains linear and constant throughout the time from arrest to breath-alcohol analysis
- the subject's true elimination rate for the time in question is captured between the extreme limits employed in the calculation (i.e. $0.009 < \beta < 0.029$)
- the measurements of the subject's BrAC or BAC provide acceptably accurate and precise estimates of the subject's true BrAC or BAC, respectively.

The acceptability of this type of calculation is often challenged legally, but it is admissible for forensic purposes as long as the expert provides the extrapolated estimates and the assumptions used in the calculation and the uncertainties involved.

Figure 11.6 is a graphical representation of the data shown in Figure 11.5. The broad range for the extrapolated results is seen clearly.

Widmark's equation

A question that is often asked as part of a DUI investigation is 'How much alcohol is the suspect likely to have consumed to have produced the blood or breath alcohol determined by testing?' or alternatively, 'Is the subject's recollection of how much alcohol they drank conversant with the blood or breath alcohol value determined?'

During the early part of the 20th century, E. M. P. Widmark, a Swedish physician, did much of the foundational research regarding alcohol pharmacokinetics in the human body (Widmark 1981). In addition, he developed an algebraic equation that allowed any one of seven variables to be estimated given the other six. According to Widmark's equation (11.1), the amount of alcohol consumed (N) is a function of these several variables:

$$N = f(W, r, C_t, \beta, t, z) \tag{11.1}$$

where N is the amount of alcohol consumed, W is the body mass, r is the volume of distribution (a constant), C_t is the BAC, β is the alcohol elimination rate, t is the time since the first drink and z is the volume of alcohol per drink.

These variables are related according to equation (11.2):

$$N = \frac{Wr(C_t + \beta t)}{0.8z} \tag{11.2}$$

where N is the number of drinks consumed, W is the body mass in ounces (or kg), r is the volume of distribution (a constant relating the distribution of water in the body in L/kg), C_t is the BAC in kg/L, β is the alcohol elimination rate in kg/L/h, t is the time since the first drink in hours, z is the volume of alcohol per drink in fluid ounces (or L) and 0.8 is the density of ethanol (i.e. 0.8 ounces per fluid ounce or 0.79 g/mL). It should be noted that the units used to measure body mass and mass of alcohol in the drink (i.e. $0.8 \times$ volume of alcohol in the drink) must be the same. A different value is used for the

An individual is stopped and arrested for DUI at 20:00 (8:00 p.m.). For some reason (distance, accommodating passengers, waiting for a tow truck, etc.) the officer is not able to obtain a breath sample from the subject until 22.30 (10:30 p.m). At that time the subject provides duplicate samples according the jurisdiction's protocol and obtains results of 0.068 and 0.073 g/210 L. The jurisdiction has a prohibited BrAC of 0.08 g/210 L while operating a motor vehicle. The forensic scientist is asked to perform a retrograde extrapolation in this case and proceeds as follows.

A careful review of the officer's case report should be conducted. The scientist must make some assumption about the time when the subject finished his or her last drink. We will assume for this example that the subject indicated this to be at 18:30 (6:30 p.m), 1.5 h before the arrest. Based on this time of 1.5 h, we can reasonably conclude that the subject's peak BrAC had been achieved by the time of the offence and the subject was on the linear descending portion of the BrAC versus time curve at the time of arrest. We also note that there is an interval of 2.5 h between the time of arrest and the time of the breath analyses. This is sufficient time to ensure that a difference in mean BrAC can be measured given the typical variability observed in forensic BrAC measurements. The retrograde extrapolation calculation should be made based on the mean breath alcohol result, 0.0705 g/210 L in this case.

We next assume two extremes of likely alcohol elimination rates based on published data for alcohol elimination in impaired drivers (Jones and Andersson 1996) and determine the upper and lower likely limits of the extrapolated estimate according to the equation

$$B_1 = B_2 + \beta t$$

where B_1 (g/210 L) is the estimate of prior alcohol concentration based on B_2 (g/210 L), the alcohol concentration measured during the test (at 22:30 (10.30 pm)), β is the elimination rate (g/L/h or, for this example, g/210 L/h) and t is the time elapsed between arrest and testing. The lower and upper limits for β are 0.009 and 0.029 g/210 L/h, respectively.

Substituting the test value in the equation and the upper and lower elimination rates:

$$\text{for } \beta = 0.009 \text{ g/210 L/h: } B_1 = 0.0705 + (0.009)(2.5) = 0.0930 \text{ g/210 L}$$
$$\text{for } \beta = 0.029 \text{ g/210 L/h: } B_1 = 0.0705 + (0.029)(2.5) = 0.143 \text{ g/210 L}$$

This approach gives the upper and lower limits of the likely extrapolated result, with a 95% confidence interval, based on the normal alcohol elimination rates in the drinking-and-driving population. In this example both estimates exceeded the statutory *per se* limit of 0.08 g/210 L and hence it is concluded that the driver's BrAC would have exceeded the statutory limit at the time of the arrest.

For jurisdictions expressing BrAC limits in other units, e.g. µg/100 mL, calculations are made in the same way but substituting the appropriate values for β in µg/100 mL.

Figure 11.5 An example of retrograde extrapolation (back-calculation).

volume of distribution for males and females. Women generally have a higher proportion of fat relative to water compared to men and hence on a mass basis men have a higher percentage of water per unit mass. As alcohol is water soluble and therefore partitions preferentially into the aqueous phase, the volume of distribution is greater in men than women. The generally accepted value of r for men is 0.68 L/kg and for women is 0.55 L/kg.

The examples shown in Figure 11.7 illustrate typical uses of the Widmark equation in DUI cases. Table 11.4 illustrates typical ranges of values for the alcohol content of different beverages, which can help to define 'a drink' in terms of its percentage alcohol content by volume.

Figure 11.8 illustrates a typical Widmark alcohol concentration–time curve for an individual who consumed alcohol on an empty stomach. The rapid rise to the peak concentration, typical of empty-stomach consumption, is observed along with the classic linear elimination portion of the curve. Widmark's equation was applied to this individual by computing the

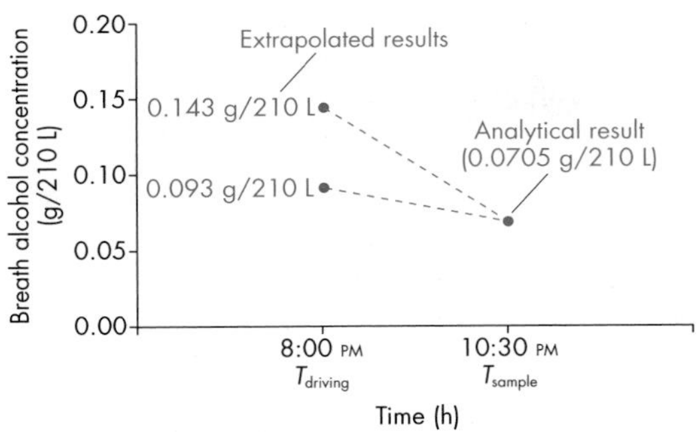

Figure 11.6 Retrograde extrapolation example.

Table 11.4 Typical ranges for the alcohol content of different beverages

Beverage	Alcohol content (vol%)
Mild ale, bitter, cider	2.5–4
Light ale, lager, stout, strong ale	4.5–8
Wine	10–14
Martini, sherry, port	18–22
Gin, rum, whisky (70° proof)	40 and above

estimated BrAC (see below) as a function of time. A linear estimation curve is observed below that of the subject's actual BrAC curve. For this individual, Widmark's method (using the assumed r and β parameters) underestimated the actual BrAC. Experimental plots such as this are useful to assess the validity of the Widmark estimation methods but cannot normally be applied in DUI cases because BAC or BrAC values are typically taken at a single point in time and hence the full pharmacokinetic dataset required is not available.

Using breath alcohol results in Widmark's equation

Most forensic cases that utilise Widmark's equation employ breath alcohol rather than blood alcohol results. Thus when using BrAC results, they must be converted into an estimated BAC before introducing the value into the equation. This introduces another factor that has uncertainty: the BAC/BrAC conversion factor. Typically, the breath and corresponding blood alcohol values are assumed to be the same (using a conversion factor of $K_{BAC/BrAC} = 2100$). This is reasonable in forensic cases, since substituting their BrAC typically benefits the defendant by providing an underestimate of their true BAC. These principles should be kept in mind when working with Widmark's equation.

Ethyl glucuronide and ethyl sulfate

A small proportion of ethanol is metabolised to give ethyl glucuronide (EtG) and ethyl sulfate (EtS). These metabolites are proving to be useful biomarkers of alcohol consumption and have been used to show recent alcohol consumption in drink-driving incidents. It is known that ethanol can be produced in the body by fermentation after death. Hence the finding of ethanol from analysis of blood or urine sampled *post mortem* from a driver who has died in motor vehicle accident cannot be taken as evidence of alcohol consumption prior to death. Studies indicate that EtG is not produced *post mortem* (Schloegl *et al.* 2006; Høiseth *et al.* 2007). Hence if these substances are found in *post mortem* blood or urine this is indicative of alcohol consumption *ante mortem*.

Drugs and driving

Choice of specimen for drug testing in impaired driving cases

As noted above, oral fluid may be used in some jurisdictions as a matrix in roadside tests to detect whether a driver has drugs in their system. These tests are generally based on immunoassay-type kits and in many jurisdictions are not considered acceptable for evidential purposes. In some jurisdictions, testing using oral fluid is not accepted, even for screening purposes, and roadside tests rely on impairment tests as described above. Thus the norm would be for a driver suspected of driving under the influence of drugs to be screened using a roadside test or assessed using an impairment test and, if the test

Example 1

A male weighing 180 lb is apprehended for drink driving. A test indicates his BAC is 0.15 g/100 mL. He claims to have drunk 3 beers (12 fl oz per beer, 4% alcohol by volume) 5 hours before the test. Is this consistent with his BAC? Using equation (11.2) we substitute the appropriate information: r = 0.68 L/kg, BAC (C_t) = 0.15 g/100 mL ≡ 0.0015 kg/L, β = 0.15 g/L/h ≡ 0.00015 kg/L/h and t = 5 h, to estimate the number of drinks (N) consumed:

$$N = \frac{(180\ \text{lb})\ (16\ \text{oz/lb})\ (0.68\ \text{L/kg})\ (0.0015\ \text{kg/L} + [(0.00015\ \text{kg/L/h})\ (5\ \text{h})])}{0.8\ (0.48\ \text{fl oz/drink})}$$

Not that it was necessary to convert the weight of the person to oz for the calculation, the C_t value to kg/L and the β value to kg/L/h. Solving for N we find

$$N = \frac{1958.4\ (0.00225)}{0.384} = 11.5\ \text{drinks}$$

Example 2

The next most-common use of Widmark's equation is to estimate the BAC (C_t) given the number of drinks consumed. We now assume the following: a female weighing 57 kg, r = 0.55 L/kg, β = 0.17 g/L/h, t = 4 h had consumed seven 30 mL glasses of 80 degree proof vodka. Employing equation (11.2), we introduce the information given and solve for C_t as follows:

$$7 = \frac{(57\ \text{kg})\ (0.55\ \text{L/kg})\ [C_t + 0.00017\ \text{kg/L/h})\ (4\ \text{h})]}{0.8\ (0.024\ \text{L/drink})}$$

Because we are interested in finding C_t, we rearrange this equation as follows:

$$C_t = \frac{(7)(0.8)(0.024)}{(57)(0.55)} - (0.00017)(4)$$

$$C_t = 0.0036\ \text{kg/L or } 0.360\ \text{g/100 mL}$$

Figure 11.7 Use of the Widmark equation.

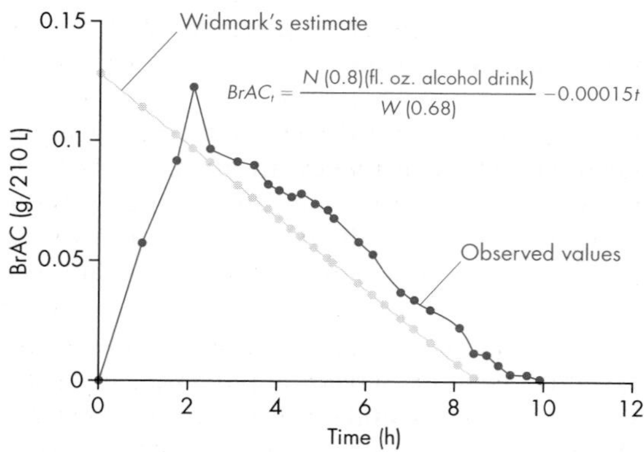

Figure 11.8 Comparison of actual BrAC with the Widmark estimate.

indicated drug(s) to be present, the suspect would be taken in so that samples could be taken for evidential testing. Specimens of choice for evidential testing are urine and blood.

As seen in Chapter 2, drugs and metabolites are typically excreted in urine. Depending on the drug, it or its metabolites may be detected well after the effect of the drug has disappeared. Thus, while urine can be considered an excellent specimen for answering the question, 'Did the donor of the specimen at some time prior to provision of the specimen use or ingest this drug?', it is of little use in determining, in isolation, whether the subject was impaired or intoxicated at the time the sample was collected. Instead, the investigator must rely on objective evidence of impairment (slurred speech, staggering, inappropriate conduct or response, poor coordination, glassy stare, agitation, restlessness, etc.) to provide the necessary connection between the observed bad driving and the urine drug test result. The toxicologist can then use his or her specialised knowledge to assess whether the observed effects could be consistent with the known properties of the drugs detected. It should also be borne in mind when using urine as a test matrix that, after administration of a drug, it may take some time before the drug is metabolised and excreted. Therefore, if a drug was ingested not long before the driver was stopped and tested, and urine was taken as the test specimen the test result may be negative, even though the drug is present in the body and exerting an effect in the subject.

In spite of these limitations, urine has become a popular specimen for drug testing in impaired driving cases because of the ease with which it may be collected (although there are privacy and associated chain-of-custody issues to be addressed), and its ease of screening in the laboratory by immunoassay on automated instruments.

Blood is a preferred specimen for collection and analysis in an impaired driving investigation, since blood drug concentrations can usually be related to some degree to published concentrations associated with known doses or patterns of recreational use. The blood concentration inevitably, however, is also a function of both the dose and the time since last dose, and whether the use is acute or chronic. Typically, this information is unavailable or unreliable. Relationships between blood concentration and any specific degree of impairment or effect on driving have been established for very few drugs. Apart from alcohol, the exception to this may be other members of the depressant drug class, which have been studied to a greater degree. As a result, the interpretation of blood drug concentrations still needs to be treated with caution, and the full range of possible ingestion patterns, and likely effects, should be considered. In the laboratory, blood drug analysis is more challenging, and many clinical laboratories are not properly equipped for this. Blood is more difficult to collect, and requires a qualified person to collect the sample who may not be available at the roadside or at the time the suspect is apprehended.

Oral fluid is being explored as a possible alternative to blood, because of its ease of collection at the roadside. Oral fluid may also prove useful in countries with laws that prevent the collection of blood. Recent studies, however, have shown that the relationship between blood and oral fluid drug concentrations is not always predictable and, again, it suffers from the same lack of ability to correlate a concentration to a specific degree of effect. At present, oral fluid drug testing to demonstrate effect is not widely accepted in the field. Hair drug testing is well established, but has little application in impaired driving toxicology because the time frame in which it can demonstrate drug use (weeks to months) is usually not relevant to the time of driving.

Laboratory approaches to drug testing in DUID cases

After a subject has been arrested for suspected driving while impaired through drugs, the sample that is taken and sent to the testing laboratory should be subject to a broad screen for common drugs relevant to the patterns of recreational drug use in the jurisdiction, as well as for common CNS-acting prescription and over-the-counter drugs.

Most laboratories begin with an immunoassay screen. These assays are often class-specific rather than drug-specific, and their value is more to rule out the presence of certain drug classes than to provide a comprehensive test. Toxicologists should also be sensitive to the fact that immunoassays will not detect all types of drugs present, may produce different intensities of response to members of the same drug class and may fail to identify completely important members of a class of drugs. Immunoassay tests should, wherever possible, be supplemented by chromatographic tests to include as many of the locally relevant drugs as possible. Without this, the possibility of failing to identify a drug or metabolite that has caused impairment is significant.

Immunoassay drug screening

Many different types of immunoassay screening tests are available commercially. The techniques in most widespread use include enzyme multiplied immunoassay technique (EMIT), enzyme-linked immunosorbent assay (ELISA), kinetic interaction of microparticles in solution (KIMS) and fluorescence polarisation immunoassay (FPIA). Radioimmunoassay is also a suitable technique but is tending to be replaced in many laboratories for health and safety and environmental reasons. When applied properly, any of these techniques is suitable for drug screening in DUID cases. Although the specificity of immunoassay tests have improved markedly, there is always the possibility of a false positive result, i.e. of the test showing a positive result even though no drug or metabolite is present in the test specimen. Hence immunoassays must be treated as a screening technique only, and should not be considered proof of the identification of a compound without a complementary confirmatory analysis. Additionally, since the sensitivity of the immunoassay panel is limited, and cross-reactivities within a class of drug vary widely, it may be necessary to conduct GC-MS analysis when a drug is indicated specifically (e.g. via symptoms seen in roadside sobriety tests; drug paraphernalia in the driver's vehicle; odour of drugs noticed in the suspect's vehicle when first stopped), even if the immunoassay result is negative.

Drug confirmation

The 'gold standard' for confirmatory identification of drugs in biological samples is GC-MS, although LC-MS(/MS) methods are being developed which can be considered equally acceptable. A clean-up procedure is generally applied to the sample to separate the drug(s) and metabolites from the sample matrix and to concentrate the drugs so that they can be more readily detected and quantified. A commonly applied approach is to exploit the fact that many drugs are basic or acidic. Sample clean-up techniques are manipulated to separate basic drugs from weakly acidic or neutral drugs before each fraction is analysed by GC-MS and/or LC-MS/MS. As different laboratories employ different analytical strategies, details of these will not be given. Detailed strategies can be found in *Clarke's Analysis of Drugs and Poisons* (Moffat *et al.* 2004).

Determining an appropriate protocol for the laboratory

While attention should be paid to the opinion of the arresting officer about what drugs are suspected in any given case, the toxicologist should apply a good broad-spectrum drug screen to be able to exclude the possibility of other drugs with similar effects. For example, an individual withdrawing from intravenous amfetamine use may appear drowsy and have constricted pupils, poor psychomotor performance and injection marks. These symptoms may appear to be caused by a narcotic analgesic, and consequently a test only for opiates would not disclose the true agent responsible.

The class of CNS depressants is probably the most challenging analytically, since it includes some chemically very diverse drugs, from solvents and inhalants to long- and short-acting benzodiazepines, antidepressants, antihistamines and novel recreational drugs such as gamma-hydroxybutyric acid and butane-1,4-diol. Practically speaking, an escalation approach is the most economical and effective, beginning with the commonly encountered drugs and expanding and adding assays for drugs that could account for the symptoms observed.

It is critical that laboratories performing this work observe accepted standards for forensic analysis, including: maintaining security and chain of custody, maintaining written protocols for commonly performed procedures, validating method accuracy through use of appropriate standards and controls, verifying the identity of any drugs reported, using MS wherever possible, implementing the scientific review of data, participating in proficiency testing programmes and ensuring that staff have appropriately documented qualifications and training.

References

Daubert vs. Merrell Dow Pharmaceuticals, 509 U.S. 579 (1993).

K. M. Dubowski, Quality assurance in breath-alcohol, *J. Forensic Sci.*, 1994, **35**, 1414–1423.

S. L. R. Ellison *et al.*, *Quantifying Uncertainty in Analytical Measurement*, 2nd edn, EURACHEM/CITAC, 2000.

Frye vs. United States 54 App DC 46 293F 1013 (1923).

R. G. Gullberg, Breath alcohol measurement variability associated with different instrumentation and protocols, *Forensic Sci. Int.*, 2003, **131**, 30–35.

G. Høiseth *et al.*, A study of ethyl glucuronide in post-mortem blood as a marker of ante-mortem ingestion of alcohol. *Forensic Sci. Int.*, 2007, **165**(1), 41–45.

M. Huestis, Cannabis (marijuana) – effects on human performance and behavior, *Forensic Sci. Rev.*, 2002, **14**, 15–60.

M. A. Huestis *et al.*, Blood cannabinoids II. Models for the prediction of time of marijuana exposure from plasma concentrations of delta-9-tetrahydrocannabinol (THC), and 11-nor-9-carboxy-deltahydrocannabinol (THCCOOH), *J. Anal. Toxicol.*, 1992, **16**, 283–286.

A. W. Jones, Measuring alcohol in blood and breath for forensic purposes – a historical review, *Forensic Sci. Rev.*, 1996, **8**, 1–32.

A. W. Jones and L. Andersson, Influence of age, gender, and blood-alcohol concentration on the disappearance rate of alcohol from blood in drinking drivers, *J. Forensic Sci.*, 1996, **41**, 922–926.

B. K. Logan and F. J. Couper, Methylenedioxymethamfetamine (MDMA, ecstasy) and driving impairment, *J. Forensic Sci.*, 2001, **46**, 1426–1433.

A. C. Moffat, M. D. Osselton and B. Widdop (eds), *Clarke's Analysis of Drugs and Poisons*, 3rd edn, London, Pharmaceutical Press, 2004.

H. Moskowitz and D. Fiorentino, *A Review of the Literature on the Effects of Low Doses of Alcohol on Driving-Related Skills*, DOT/HS 809 028, Washington DC, National Highway Traffic Safety Administration, 2000.

H. Moskowitz and C. D. Robinson, *Effects of Low Doses of Alcohol on Driving-Related Skills: A Review of the Evidence*, DOT-HS-807-280, Washington DC, US Department of Transportation, National Highway Traffic Safety Administration, 1988.

A. Mozayani, Ketamine – effects on human performance and behavior, *Forensic Sci. Rev.*, 2002, **14**, 123–132.

National Highway Traffic Safety Administration, Highway Safety Programs; Model specifications for devices to measure breath alcohol, Federal Register, 1993, **58**, 48705–48710.

H. W. J. Robbe and J. F. O'Hanlon, *Marijuana and Actual Driving Performance*, DOT HS 808 078, Washington DC, US Department of Transport, 1993.

H. W. J. Robbe and J. F. O'Hanlon, *Marijuana, Alcohol and Actual Driving Performance*, DOT HS 808 939, Washington DC, US Department of Transport, 1999.

H. Schloegl *et al.*, Stability of ethyl glucuronide in urine, post-mortem tissue and blood samples, *Int. J. Legal Med.*, 2006, **120**, 83–88.

R. Wennig and A. Verstraete, Drugs and driving, in *Forensic Science, Handbook of Analytical Separations*, M. J. Bogusz (ed.), Amsterdam, Elsevier Science, 2000, pp. 453–457.

E. M. P. Widmark, *Principles and Applications of Medicolegal Alcohol Determination*, Davis CA, Biomedical Publications, 1981, pp. 107–108.

12

Forensic chemistry and solid dosage form identification

J Ramsey

Introduction 323
Dosage forms 324
Examination of unknown products 331
References 333

Introduction

History

Tablets and capsules are a surprisingly modern development. Thomas Brockedon was granted a patent in 1843 'for manufacturing pills and medicinal lozenges by causing materials, when in a state of granulation, dust or powder, to be made into form and solidified by pressure in dies'. In 1884, Burroughs Wellcome & Co. applied for the term 'tabloid' to be made a registered trademark. It is said that Henry Wellcome (1853–1936) derived this word from 'tablet' and 'alkaloid' and used it to mean highly effective drugs in a compressed, concentrated form. The *British Pharmacopoeia* (*BP*) of 1885 included a monograph for Glyceryl Trinitrate Tablets. No others appeared until 1945 when the Seventh addendum to the *BP* of 1932 still only contained 35 tablets. Tablets and later dosage forms, such as gelatin or starch capsules, and sugar-coated tablets (dragées), proved to be particularly well suited to mass production.

Tablets and capsules are now commonplace and a large number of consumer products are available in this form, not only medicines, but also products such as sweeteners (sugar substitutes), confectionery (mints), detergents and even toys (indoor fireworks, jumping beans).

Legitimate medicines supplied as tablets and capsules, such as the barbiturates (Tuinal, Seconal), methaqualone (Mandrax, Quaalude) and amfetamines (Drinamyl) were commonly misused in the 1960s. Legitimate capsules were also emptied and used to conceal heroin in the 1970s. Illicit drugs were rarely seen as tablets or capsules until the early 1990s, when the drugs now commonly known as ecstasy flooded the club–dance scene, first in Europe and later the USA. Currently, many millions of illicitly made tablets that contain methylenedioxymethamfetamine (MDMA) or its homologues and analogues are consumed each week. This 'normalisation' of tablets as an illicit dosage form has resulted in an expansion of illicitly produced tablets that contain other drugs, principally amfetamine and methamfetamine, in other countries, particularly in Southeast Asia (Thailand, Myanmar (Burma)).

The need for tablet and capsule identification arises for many reasons in both healthcare and law-enforcement practice. Treatment of the poisoned patient may be assisted by identification of the product responsible, even though most patients are treated symptomatically. The agent responsible for the poisoning, if a tablet or capsule, may often be identified more rapidly than the diagnosis may be made by the analysis of body fluids. However, the tablets found alongside the patient are not necessarily the same as those that were taken. Pharmacy practice generates many identification enquiries, such as the rogue tablet found in a tablet bottle or the customer who wants 'some more of these', but does not know what they are. In Europe, 'parallel imports' are common, because it is cheaper to import some medicines from other countries. The imported drugs, even if manufactured by the same company, usually have a different physical appearance from the familiar native product. Patients, when prescribed a generic form of a medicine, might receive an unfamiliar product of foreign origin and request confirmation that an error has not been made. A constantly changing melange of products in circulation also results from takeovers and mergers within the pharmaceutical industry (when the physical appearance of products is changed to meet new corporate identity standards). Consequently, patients, pharmacists and law officers are continually faced with unfamiliar products.

Changes in legislation may also generate new reasons to perform identifications; for example, when anabolic androgenic steroids came under the Misuse of Drugs Act in the UK in 1996 both the Police and Her Majesty's Customs and Excise (now Her Majesty's Revenue and Customs) were suddenly required to be able to recognise them.

The misuse of pharmaceutical products, such as the benzodiazepines (particularly temazepam and diazepam), and an illicit drugs scene in which users like to experiment, results in solid dosage forms being much more prevalent. Drug-assisted sexual assault may also involve drugs supplied as tablets and capsules (e.g. flunitrazepam). The trading across national boundaries via the internet of so-called 'lifestyle drugs' used to treat obesity (e.g. phentermine, orlistat), impotence (sildenafil, vardenafil, tadalafil), baldness (finasteride) or smoking cessation (bupropion) also results in enquiries to identify unfamiliar products.

The current 'harm minimisation' strategy to counteract drug misuse, which involves informing users, potential users and parents honestly about the risks of drug misuse, has alerted parents and those responsible for the welfare of youngsters (e.g. teachers) to the possibility that those in their charge might be in possession of illicit (illegal) drugs. In turn, this has meant that many more enquiries are made to healthcare professionals regarding the identification of suspect materials. Many enquiries are made to community (retail) pharmacists regarding 'tablets' found in the possession or proximity (bedrooms, school playgrounds) of young people.

Some confectionery may coincidentally resemble medicines and some may even be deliberately designed to resemble drugs (such as sugar cigarettes). Small white tablets marked with a P, an O or an L purported to be the material from the holes in the centre of Polo Mints caused much concern when they were found out of context, such as in a school playground (Young 1997; Ramsey 2001).

Dosage forms

Pills

'Pills' proper are an outdated dosage form seldom encountered in modern pharmacy practice. Technically, pills are a small rounded mass, usually handmade, and are intended to be swallowed whole. However, the word is in common usage as a generic term for all solid dose forms, e.g. ecstasy pills, slimming pills or contraceptive tablets ('the pill'). Some branded products still use the word, but this usually refers to small sugar-coated tablets (Beechams Pills, Ex-Lax Pills).

Tablets

Tablets are compressed dosage forms that contain both active ingredients and inactive materials called excipients, which include diluents, adhesives, binders, fillers, lubricants, disintegrants and colours. Tablets need to be strong enough to withstand transport and handling, yet still disintegrate and release the active ingredients when consumed. The behaviour of the tablet depends on the production methods, the various excipients and their effect on the active ingredient. The physical form of the active ingredient (particle size) and the particular salt are also important.

The identification of a tablet is usually based on the physical appearance or the analytical determination of the active drug and seldom depends upon the nature of the excipients. However, examination of the gastric contents, after gastric lavage (now less favoured) or at post-mortem, with a polarising microscope for the presence of starch granules may indicate the recent consumption of tablets or capsules.

Illicit tablets

Seizures of millions of illicit tablets, mostly 'ecstasy', have been made in many countries, (e.g. UK, France, Germany, Belgium, The Netherlands, USA, China, Poland). These tablets are usually marked with a distinctive logo that often belongs to large commercial organisations (automobile manufacturers, mobile phone makers, fashion designers), or are cartoon characters or simple text or currency symbols.

The investigation of the illicit production of the synthetic phenethylamines (MDMA, amfetamine) may require the examination of the clandestine 'laboratories' that produce the active ingredient as well as tablet-making facilities. Information may be gleaned on the synthetic route to the active substance and batch characteristics by analysis of the impurity profile of the finished tablet (van Deursen *et al.* 2006).

Moulded tablets

Small numbers of tablets may be made by moulding, a similar process to that once used in pharmacies. The active ingredient, a diluent and some form of binder (gum or adhesive) are pressed into a mould and allowed to set. Perforated metal sheet or even pegboard may be used as the mould. This dose form was common for lysergic acid diethylamide (lysergide, LSD) in the UK in the 1970s. Small 'microdots' (2.4 mm in diameter and 1.3 mm thick, weighing 5 mg: Fig. 12.1) were produced in large numbers using sheets of perforated metal.

The product shown in Figure 12.2 is from a London club's 'amnesty bin'. The tablet is made from plaster-of-Paris to resemble an ecstasy tablet, but it contains no active ingredients.

Compressed tablets

Legitimate products

Modern commercial compressed tablets are made with highly automated machines that use multiple sets of dies and punches in clean-room conditions. Strict quality-assurance procedures ensure that the product is manufactured to close tolerances, so there is little variation in physical appearance (size, weight, colour), content of active ingredient and bioavailability.

Illicit tablets

Small numbers of tablets may be made using drilled metal plates and hammer-driven punches or by screw-driven hand presses. Most illicit tablets are made by similar machines to those used by the legitimate manufacturers, but in

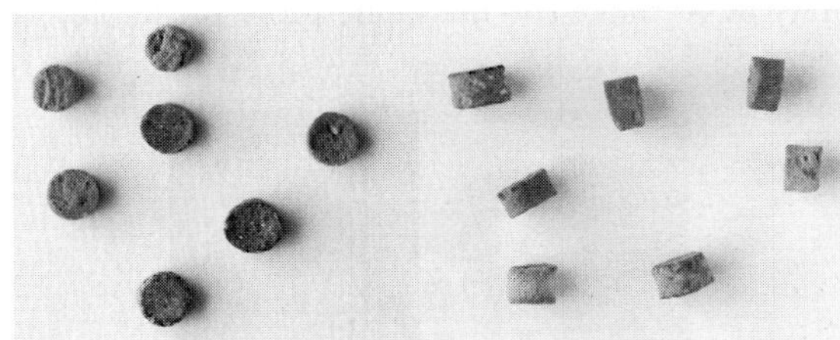

Figure 12.1 LSD tablets ('microdots') made using perforated metal sheet. (Courtesy of TICTAC Communications Ltd.)

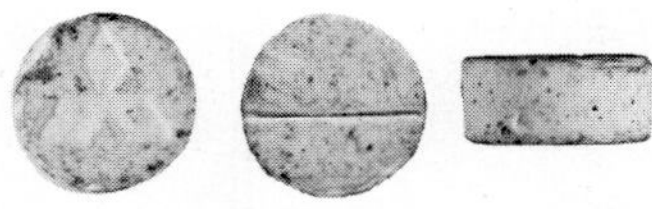

Figure 12.2 Fake ecstasy tablet made from plaster-of-Paris, taken from a London club's 'amnesty bin'. (Courtesy of TICTAC Communications Ltd.)

very different conditions (Fig. 12.3). The equipment needed to satisfy the demand for ecstasy tablets (estimated at one million each week in the UK) has to be highly automated. The machines may be in poor condition and the dies and punches may be damaged and leave characteristic visible imperfections on the tablets they produce, which may provide valuable intelligence. The so-called 'ballistic' examination of tablets for these imperfections (using techniques like those for the examination of firearms and ammunition) by forensic laboratories was once common, but is no longer carried out routinely in the UK.

The variability of dimensions and dose of illicitly produced tablets is often much greater than that found in legitimate tablets, despite the use of similar machinery. Tablets pressed in the same die must all have the same diameter, but can vary greatly in thickness depending on the fill weight and the degree of compression. This may affect both the dose and the disintegration time and hence the bioavailability of the active compound.

Coated tablets

Tablet cores may be coated with layers of sucrose, a thin film of resin or a soluble wax. This may be to make the medicine more palatable, to protect the active ingredient from exposure to air, light or moisture, to delay the absorption until it reaches the small intestine or to extend the duration of action. Products may also be coated to give them a more attractive appearance. Sugar-coated tablets vary more in dimensions (both size and weight) than uncoated or film-coated products. Markings printed on sugar-coated tablets may often rub off quite easily. The sugar coating also tends to 'round off' the edges of the core, so that sharp edges become rounded. Sugar-coated tablets may closely resemble confectionery in both appearance and taste, at least initially, and may be consumed inadvertently by children who believe them to be sweets (candy).

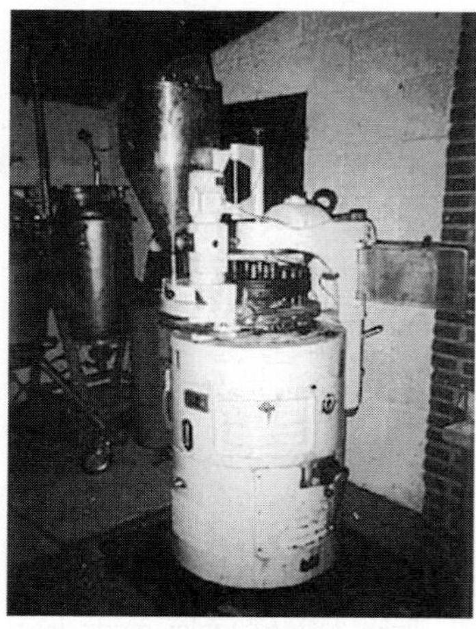

Figure 12.3 Commercial tablet machine used to produce illicit tablets. (Courtesy of TICTAC Communications Ltd.)

Counterfeits

There are many examples of counterfeit or substandard pharmaceutical products that are fraudulently labelled with respect to their source or content. Their use has resulted in failure of treatment or even poisoning (Reidenberg and Conner 2001). Less surprisingly, products of uncertain origin appear on the drug-abuse scene. Diazepam tablets that appear to be professionally made and of foreign origin are commonly in circulation in the UK (Fig. 12.4), but neither the manufacturer nor the importer is known.

Anabolic agents in ampoules and tablets, purportedly from reputable manufacturers, have been detected that do not contain the active ingredient stated on the packaging. For example, the counterfeit product shown in Figure 12.5 was found to contain testosterone, and not boldenone as stated on the packaging, where the word steroid was incorrectly spelled.

Illicit tablets of similar appearance, probably made in the same machine, may also contain different active ingredients. Examples of the tablet shown in Figure 12.6 have

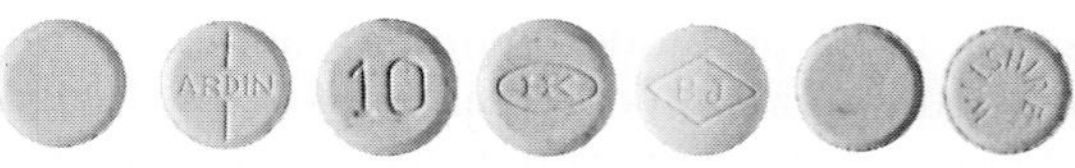

Figure 12.4 Diazepam tablets that appear to be professionally made but are of unknown origin. (Courtesy of TICTAC Communications Ltd.)

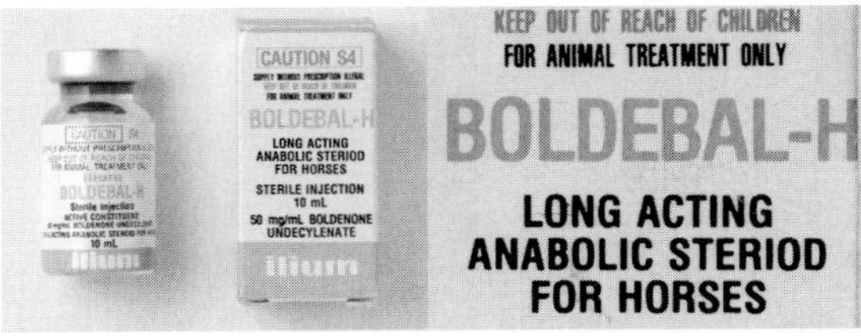

Figure 12.5 Counterfeit anabolic steroid (Boldebal-H) packaging with spelling mistake. (Courtesy of TICTAC Communications Ltd.)

been found to contain methyltestosterone, methandrostenalone or clenbuterol.

Individual legitimate pharmaceutical tablets may also be modified by hand to look like other products and so increase their value. The half-scored tablet in Figure 12.7 had a Y-shaped marking (similar to the Mercedes motor manufacturer's logo) carved on to make it resemble an ecstasy tablet.

Capsules

Capsules are popular consumer dosage forms because their slender shape makes them easy to swallow, and they effectively mask any unpleasant taste or odour of their contents. Most capsules consist of two parts, a cap and body, and are made from gelatin. These shells are made using precision-machined moulds, to which the liquid gelatin adheres, forming both the cap and body sections. High-speed machinery removes the gelatin shell layers from the moulds and then joins, prints and packages them. The two parts may be the same or different colours, or may be transparent.

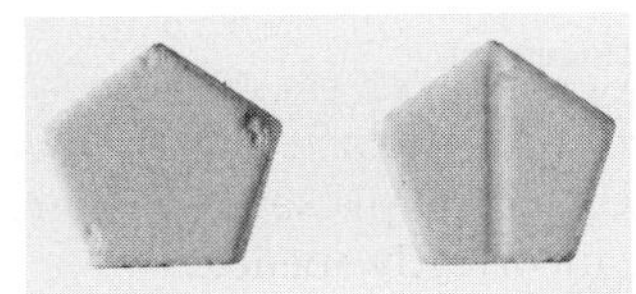

Figure 12.6 Illicit tablet seen with different active ingredients (either methyltestosterone, methandrostenalone or clenbuterol). (Courtesy of TICTAC Communications Ltd.)

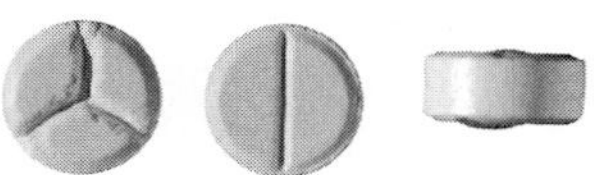

Figure 12.7 Legitimate tablet modified to look like an ecstasy tablet. (Courtesy of TICTAC Communications Ltd.)

Capsule filling

Small numbers of capsule shells may be filled by hand or by highly automated filling machines able to fill many thousands of capsules per hour. The contents may be powder, controlled-release granules, herbal material or, less commonly, liquid.

Capsule printing

Capsules are usually marked, although the printing may rub off, particularly on oil-filled soft gelatin products. The printing may not be on the cap or body consistently (Fig. 12.8). This is particularly noticeable when the cap and body are different colours.

Special capsules

Special capsules made from cellulosic (hydroxypropylmethylcellulose) raw materials and printed with natural printing inks satisfy vegetarian and cultural (e.g. Kosher or Halal) needs. Wider diameter capsules are designed for double-blind clinical trials to allow containment and blinding of large-diameter or uniquely shaped tablets.

Very small gelatin capsules are used for oral dosage to rodents in preclinical studies and are specially designed for performing preclinical trials, such as pharmacokinetic, pharmacodynamic and safety studies.

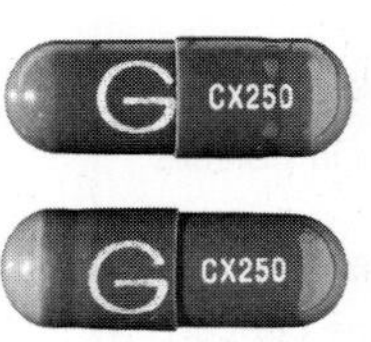

Figure 12.8 Examples of capsule showing marking reversed on cap and body. (Courtesy of TICTAC Communications Ltd.)

Liquid-filled capsules

Soft gelatin capsules are commonly used to contain liquid or semi-liquid preparations (Fig 12.9). Some have abuse potential. Encapsulated liquid preparations of temazepam had to be modified and subsequently discontinued because the contents were being withdrawn with a syringe and needle and injected intravenously, intramuscularly or even intra-arterially, which caused severe lesions (Dodd *et al.* 1994).

Special two-piece hard gelatin capsules may be sealed for secure containment of liquids and semi-solids. The overlapping portion is moistened during the filling process and the cap and body effectively weld together as they dry. Two-piece capsules (Fig. 12.10) may be secured with a sealing band of shellac to prevent leakage of, or tampering with, the contents.

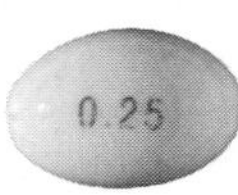

Figure 12.9 Soft gelatin capsule containing liquid. (Courtesy of TICTAC Communications Ltd.)

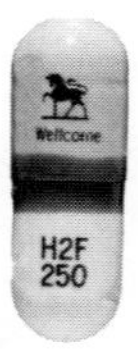

Figure 12.10 Cap and body capsule with sealing band. (Courtesy of TICTAC Communications Ltd.)

Transdermal devices

Potent drugs, with suitable solubility characteristics, that require extended dosing may be given in preparations designed to deliver the drug through the intact skin (transdermally; Table 12.1). The dosage forms may be creams, sprays or patches that resemble adhesive wound dressings (Elastoplast, Band aid). Patches are usually either transparent or in colours to match skin tones. Some are marked with names or codes, while others are completely unmarked.

The misuse of transdermal patches that contain fentanyl has been reported; fentanyl may be extracted from these patches and used as a source of the drug for injection or they may even be dried and smoked (Marquardt and Tharratt 1994; Purucker and Swann 2000).

Table 12.1 Preparations designed to deliver the drug through the intact skin

Drugs delivered in transdermal devices	Function
Estradiol	Hormone replacement
Testosterone	Hormone replacement
Norethisterone (norethindrone)	Hormone replacement
Nicotine	Tobacco withdrawal
Glyceryl trinitrate (nitroglycerin)	Antianginal
Fentanyl	Analgesic
Hyoscine (scopolamine)	Motion sickness
Rotigotine	Treatment of Parkinson's disease
Diclofenac	Anti-inflammatory
Buprenorphine	Analgesic
Oxybutynin	Anticholinergic
Other compounds in patches	
Citronella oil	Insect repellent
Tropical orchid aroma	Appetite control
Capsicum (cayenne pepper)	Counter irritant
Arnica montana (leopard's bane)	Counter irritant
Methyl salicylate	Analgesic
Ferrite magnet	Pain relief?

Novel preparations

There are many novel dosage forms, some of which are used when the fast- or slow-controlled release of an active ingredient is required.

Melts

The product Maxalt melt 10 mg contains the antimigraine drug rizatriptan. Although approximately 13 mm in diameter, it weighs only 64 mg and is intended to be taken without water (Fig. 12.11).

Slow-release products may have cores that do not disintegrate in the gut and may be found intact at postmortem examination in stomach contents. These cores are also found in other circumstances, such as in homes for the elderly and psychiatric institutions, with the outer coating removed (presumably after having been spat out).

The Adalat tablet (Fig. 12.12) has such a core (Fig. 12.13); it is a complex device with a laser-drilled hole that is clearly visible in a yellow layer. The core is revealed when the coating, which is pink, is removed; this is a common identification enquiry.

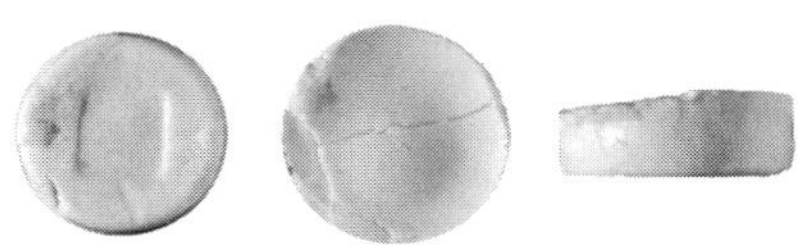

Figure 12.11 Maxalt melt, anti-migraine treatment designed to be taken without water. (Courtesy of TICTAC Communications Ltd.)

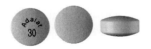

Figure 12.12 Adalat tablet (coated). (Courtesy of TICTAC Communications Ltd.)

Figure 12.13 Adalat tablet of Figure 12.12 with coating removed. (Courtesy of TICTAC Communications Ltd.)

Veterinary products

Relatively few veterinary medicines for use in large animals are supplied as tablets or capsules because it is usually easier for a veterinary practitioner to administer an injection to an animal. However, treats and worming preparations and medicines for domestic animals are commonly sold as tablets. Animal treats may have markings reminiscent of those on ecstasy tablets.

Some products may be very large: Coppinox 27 copper supplement capsules for cattle are 24 mm long and weigh over 25 g.

Impregnated paper

LSD is commonly supplied impregnated into small absorbent paper 'stamps', which usually carry a distinctive marking. Large sheets are perforated so they may be torn into individual doses on quarter-inch or 7 mm squares. They are impregnated by dipping the sheet into a solution of the drug in a solvent (or by spraying the sheet with a solution), often vodka or ethanol. More rarely the solution of the drug may be applied to the individual paper squares on the sheet with a dropper. The pattern may be complete for each square or may extend across multiple squares or the whole sheet (Fig. 12.14). The patterns are classified by law enforcement agencies by a *Prototype number*. LSD has also been impregnated in gelatin squares (window panes) or on sugar lumps and supplied as moulded tablets.

Other very potent illicit drugs (e.g. 4-bromo-2,5-dimethoxyamfetamine (DOB); 2,5-dimethoxy-4-chloroamfetamine (DOC); 2,5-dimethoxy-4-iodoamfetamine (DOI)) may also be seen, though rarely, impregnated into paper.

Confectionery

Some confectionery is commonly mistaken for illicit drugs. Sweets, mainly mints, may look like medicines or illicit drugs, particularly when out of the original packaging (Fig. 12.15).

Sugar-coated chocolate drops (Smarties, M&Ms) may also be confused with sugar-coated tablets, particularly when they bear markings for

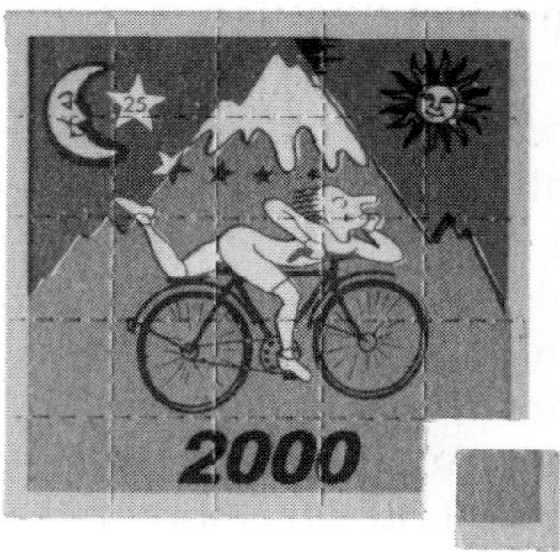

Figure 12.14 LSD-impregnated paper sheet with a pattern that covers multiple doses (the small square is a single dose). (Courtesy of TICTAC Communications Ltd.)

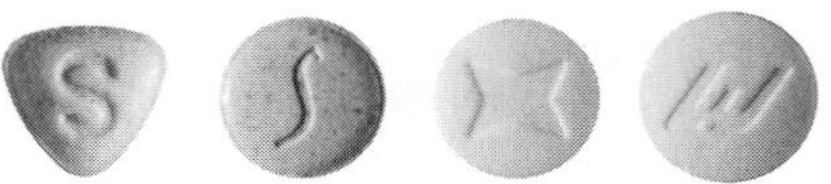

Figure 12.15 Confectionery that resembles ecstasy tablets. (Courtesy of TICTAC Communications Ltd.)

special promotions (Fig. 12.16). The TICTAC database (see later) contains over 120 different Smarties.

Sweeteners (sugar substitutes) in tablet form regularly result in identification enquiries when they are found in or near food or out of context in schools or public places (Fig. 12.17).

Purposes of identification

Community

Community pharmacy practice sometimes requires the identification of tablets and capsules.

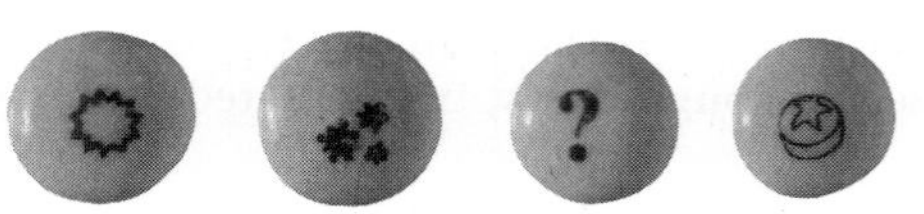

Figure 12.16 Sugar-coated chocolate drops. (Courtesy of TICTAC Communications Ltd.)

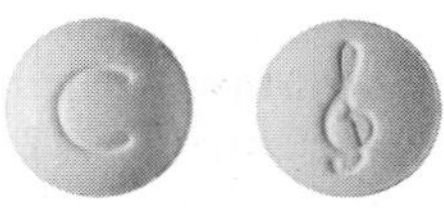

Figure 12.17 Sweeteners that are mistaken for drugs. (Courtesy of TICTAC Communications Ltd.)

Customers may become anxious when dispensed unfamiliar generic products, particularly when they are dispensed mixed batches. Parallel imported products may also cause anxiety and confusion. Patients on large amounts of medication may become confused and may report the presence of 'rogue' tablets.

Anxious parents may also rely on community pharmacists for advice on suspect 'drugs' found around the home. While abused drugs are more likely to be in tablet form than ever before, many such enquiries result from the discovery of confectionery and sweeteners in unlikely circumstances.

Hospital

The treatment of acute poisoning rarely depends upon the identification of a tablet or capsule. However, confirmation of the identity of medicines brought in with the patient may be of value. Those who treat drug abusers also frequently require identifications. Many abused drugs are in tablet form and most drug abusers use multiple-drug types. Enquiries to identify the benzodiazepines (particularly temazepam and diazepam) and opiate/opioid analgesics (codeine and dihydrocodeine in the UK, dihydrocodeinone in the USA) are particularly common.

Pharmaceuticals

The pharmaceutical manufacturers need to be able to recognise their own products as a public service and also, from time to time, check proposed markings for new products to ensure they are not currently in use. They also need to investigate allegations that batches of their products contain 'rogue' tablets.

General

The practice of workplace drug testing requires medical review officers (MROs) to investigate whether the medication declared by the testee is consistent with the results of the subsequent laboratory analysis of a urine sample. The medication is frequently declared in insufficiently precise terms that require clarification (e.g. declared as 'Anadin', or described as 'pink headache tablets'). Suspicious tablets may also be found in the workplace (e.g. gymnasia, food production plants, off-shore oil rigs).

Forensic

Identifications are carried out in the law-enforcement sector for many reasons by many different agencies. HM Revenue and Customs need to be able to recognise suspected contraband in luggage, particularly now that controls on anabolic agents are in force. Prisons need to be able to screen drugs in the possession of remand prisoners and to investigate contraband and enforce the status of drug-free wings. Police benefit from ready access to identification resources to make decisions about items discovered during searches and to prevent unnecessary submissions for laboratory analysis.

The international proliferation of ecstasy (MDMA and similar compounds) has created the requirement to investigate the illicit production of these tablets. This is an international trade in which the same or similar tablets are found all over the world. They are commonly marked with logos from all manner of consumer products and companies, particularly those that produce trendy products of appeal to the youth market. The TICTAC database (see below) currently has over 1200 logos, most from illicit products.

Another aspect is the identification of solid dosage forms from the scene of a fatality at which death by an overdose of drugs is suspected.

Examination of unknown products

Unnecessary submissions and expensive laboratory time may be saved if solid dosage forms can be recognised from their physical appearance. They may be identified with a high degree of confidence if they have sufficiently characteristic features, if the appearance can be accurately described and if an appropriate database is available.

The method of identification used depends upon why the identification is required, the speed with which a result is needed, the nature of the unknown and the resources available. When a rapid identification is required for clinical purposes, and if the unknown is likely to be a legitimate pharmaceutical, it is usually sufficient just to locate it in a commercial database, particularly if it carries a distinctive marking. The treatment of the patient is likely to be symptomatic and is unlikely to depend solely on the identification of the product. If the identification is for forensic purposes and the product is likely to be illicit or has no distinctive features, a chemical analysis is required. However, a preliminary search of a database can save much time and expense and can guide the subsequent analysis.

Solid dosage form identification databases

History

The legitimate pharmaceutical products available vary greatly from country to country. National pharmacopoeias define medicines available in each country, but generally do not provide much data on physical appearance. The physical appearance of branded medicines usually differs when marketed in different countries and manufacturers are seldom familiar with their own products from other countries. Several identification systems have been developed in the UK over the years. There are no international databases of the physical appearance of legitimate solid dosage forms. Paradoxically, there is more uniformity in illicit tablets found in different countries; the same designs and logos on ecstasy tablets are seen all around the world.

TICTAC (The Identification CD-ROM for Tablets and Capsules)

TICTAC (http://www.tictac.org) is a UK commercial database supplied every 13 weeks on CD-ROM, with interim updates provided via the internet. It is used by both healthcare and law-enforcement professionals. TICTAC includes data on over 22 000 solid dosage forms from the UK and Eire, and contains both legitimate and illicit drugs. It includes over 65 000 pictures of the products, chemical structures of the active ingredients and reactivity with immunoassay reagents. An index of street slang for drugs and drug-related activities is also included (Oliver 1992; Ramsey and Woolley 2001).

IDENTIDEX

IDENTIDEX is a commercial text-only database of largely American products. It is supplied as part of the Micromedex suite of medical information programs on CD-ROM (IDENTIDEX System 2001).

Logo Index

The Logo Index is a database produced by the Drug Enforcement Administration in the USA. It was published sporadically as a book and also on floppy disk. It contained text only information on mainly US products and included data on both legitimate and illicit products (Franzosa 1995).

Drug Identification Bible

The *Drug Identification Bible* has an alphabetical index of markings (imprints) on almost 14 000 American tablets and capsules; it also has almost 900 pictures of controlled prescription drugs. It is published annually (Marnell 2001).

The Compendium of Pharmaceutical Specialities

The *Compendium of Pharmaceutical Specialities* (CPS) is a Canadian compendium with pictures of most pharmaceuticals (Canadian Pharmacists Association 2001). It is available in hard copy and on CD-ROM.

Confirmation of identity

Confirmation of identity may be required if the product is not identified uniquely or if the consequences of an error demand that identification be confirmed. The analysis can be quite challenging for some products, such as multivitamins and minerals, herbal products, homeopathic remedies and steroids.

Colour tests have been promoted for use by purchasers of ecstasy tablets at dance venues, either by organisations that offer a service or by the users themselves (Spruit 2001; Winstock *et al.* 2001). The Marquis reagent and more recently the Mecke or modified Mecke reagent and Mandelins reagent are available to the public for this purpose on the internet (Winstock *et al.* 2001).

Confirmation of identity may be required for a variety of reasons:

- identification of illicit products
- unequivocal identification for forensic purposes
- detection of adulteration
- detection of the substitution of capsule contents
- identification of products not in commercial databases
- investigation of counterfeit or substandard products.

It may often be achieved by suspending a whole tablet or a scraping from a tablet or a portion of a capsule contents in a solvent, such as ethanol or methanol, and analysing it by spectroscopic methods (UV, IR, MS) or chromatographic methods (TLC). Analysis can present significant analytical challenges and may require structural elucidation using proton NMR spectroscopy.

The analysis of non-active ingredients (excipients in legitimate medicines or diluents in illicit drugs) may be of value in investigating counterfeit medicines or the origin of illicit drugs. Near-IR spectroscopy, particularly when linked with microscopy, is a valuable technique for this purpose (see Chapter 16). Polarised-light visible microscopy may be used to identify excipients such as the starches (e.g. maize, potato) used as disintegrants.

The confirmation of identity of herbal products is difficult and may require microscopic examination for plant fragments by a specialist and chromatographic analysis (often TLC) for indicator compounds. The genetic characteristics of traditional Chinese herbal drugs are under investigation at the Royal Botanic Gardens at Kew (London, UK) and may be of value for the confirmation of their identity in the future.

References

Canadian Pharmacists Association, *CPS Compendium of Pharmaceuticals and Specialities*, 36th edn, Ottowa, Canadian Pharmacists Association, 2001.

T. J. Dodd *et al.*, Limb ischaemia after intra-arterial injection of temazepam gel: histology of nine cases, *J. Clin. Pathol.*, 1994, **47**, 512–514.

E. S. Franzosa and C. W. Harper, *The Logo Index for Tablets and Capsules*, 3rd edn, Washington DC, US Department of Justice, Laboratory Support Section, Office of Forensic Sciences, 1995.

IDENTIDEX System, Colorado, Micromedex Healthcare Series, 2001 (http://www.micromedex.com/products/identidex/).

T. Marnell, *Drug Identification Bible*, Grand Junction, Amera-Chem, Inc., 2001.

K. A. Marquardt and R. S. Tharratt, Inhalation abuse of fentanyl patch, *J. Toxicol. Clin. Toxicol.*, 1994, **32**, 75–78.

J. Oliver (ed.), Knowledge based systems in forensic toxicology – Computer aided tablet and capsule identification, in *Forensic Toxicology*, Proceedings of 26th International Meeting of TIAFT, Glasgow, Edinburgh, Scottish Academic Press, 1992.

M. Purucker and W. Swann, Potential for duragesic patch abuse, *Ann. Emerg. Med.*, 2000, **35**, 314.

J. D. Ramsey, Confusing product, *Pharm. J.*, 2001, **264**, 295.

J. D. Ramsey and J. M. Woolley, *TICTAC 6.4*, London, TICTAC Communications Ltd, 2001 (http://www.tictac.org).

M. M. Reidenberg and B. A. Conner, Counterfeit and substandard drugs, *Clin. Pharmacol. Ther.*, 2001, **69**, 189–193.

I. P. Spruit, Monitoring synthetic drug markets, trends, and public health, *Subst. Use Misuse*, 2001, **36**, 23–47.

M. M. van Deursen *et al.*, Organic purity profiling of 3,4-methylenedioxymethamphetamine (MDMA) tablets seized in the Netherlands., *Science & Justice*, 2006, **3**, 135–152

A. R. Winstock *et al.*, Ecstasy pill testing: harm minimization gone too far? *Addiction*, 2001, **96**, 1139–1148.

R. Young, Drug alert over mint with no hole, *The Times*, 1997, January 6, p. 3.

13

Colour tests and thin-layer chromatography

W Jeffery and C F Poole

Introduction 335
Colour tests 335
Thin layer chromatography 343
References 372
Further reading 372

Introduction

This chapter covers colour tests and thin layer chromatography (TLC). Although these approaches have different mechanisms in terms of the underlying scientific principles, they both serve a similar function in toxicology: that of providing a relatively rapid and inexpensive indication of the presence or absence of a substance and an indication of the identity of a substance. The emphasis for colour tests is on 'indication'. Such tests do not provide confirmation of identity. This is also the case for TLC unless it used in association with some form of detection which provides confirmation of identity. TLC coupled with mass spectrometry (MS) is available and will provide this certainty, but such systems are not in widespread use in most toxicology laboratories. If the identity of a substance is required, more sophisticated techniques need to be employed such as gas chromatography (GC) or high-performance liquid chromatography (HPLC) in combination with MS. As we will see from the final section in this chapter, preparative TLC can be used as a separation technique prior to analysis by, for example, MS, nuclear magnetic resonance (NMR) or Fourier transform–infrared (FTIR) methods. TLC can be used quantitatively but, in comparison with techniques such as GC or HPLC with their associated sensitive detectors, does not offer comparable sensitivity when substances are present at very low concentrations. However, sensitivity using TLC may be perfectly adequate for analysis of drugs and poisons in stomach contents, urine, etc., in cases of poisoning and overdose, and to identify drugs and poisons in powders, tablets, solutions, etc.

Colour tests

Colour tests (sometimes referred to as chemical spot tests) provide toxicologists and drug analysts with one of the first tools for the presumptive identification of drugs and poisons. These colour tests are most usefully applied to pharmaceuticals and scene residues and, to a lesser extent, to biological fluids such as stomach contents, urine, etc. They are used to place the unknown into a specific class of compounds or to eliminate categories or classes of compounds. These colour tests remain popular for many reasons. They are simple to perform and no extensive training is required. As such, they appeal in situations where laboratory facilities may be very limited, for example in parts of the developing world. They can be performed in the field by police officers or technicians, require minimal reagents, are inexpensive, and give immediate results that can be viewed by the naked eye. In many instances, colour tests can also be used as TLC location reagents, applied by spraying or dipping (see p. 357). Some of the tests can also be carried out by the micro technique described by Clarke and Williams (1955).

Colour tests are particularly important in clinical toxicology (Chapter 8), especially where a patient is being treated in accident and emergency, and clinical symptoms may indicate some form of poisoning. In these circumstances, the clinician needs to know as quickly as possible what substance or substances are involved in order to initiate treatment. Under these circumstances, colour tests can provide an indication of compound class far more rapidly than immunoassays and chromatographic techniques such as GC and HPLC. Examples of colour tests that are particularly important in this respect include Trinder's test for salicylates; the Fujiwara test for halogenated hydrocarbons (e.g. dry cleaning reagents) (see Fig. 13.1); furfuraldehyde test for carbamate pesticides; test for cholinesterase inhibitors (organophosphate pesticides); sodium dithionite test for paraquat and diquat pesticides; and various tests for paracetamol including the ferric chloride test, Folin–Ciocalteu, Liebermann's and Nessler's tests.

Colour tests are widely used by police authorities and customs to detect drugs of abuse. Important tests include the Marquis test (for opiates and amfetamines), Mandelin's test for amfetamines, Scott's test for cocaine and the Duqenois–Levine test for cannabis. Colour tests have also been developed for gamma-hydroxybutyric acid (GHB) and its precursor gamma-butyrolactone (GBL).

Colour tests range from those that rely on reactions with certain functional groups (e.g. Folin–Ciocalteu for phenols), those that are almost specific for a given group (e.g. FPN reagent for phenothiazines), through to those that give diagnostic colours with a wide range of compounds (e.g. the Marquis test, see Fig. 13.1 where virtually the whole colour spectrum can be encountered, depending on the drug present).

Some tests give similar colour response for markedly different classes of drugs. The Marquis test exemplifies this with drugs as chemically disparate as butriptyline, diamorphine, guiafenesin and procyclidine all giving a violet colour. It follows that colour tests are only an indication of the presence of a compound or class of compounds and that all tests must be confirmed by more specific methods. This is especially important where test results may ultimately result in custodial sentences.

Basic tests for drug substances and products

The World Health Organization (WHO) has published *Basic Tests for Drugs* (WHO 1998), which includes pharmaceutical substances, medicinal plant materials and dosage forms. The United Nations (UN) has published *Rapid Methods for Drugs of Abuse* (UN 1994). The basic tests described, which are designed to verify the identity of drug substances and medicinal products and to detect gross contamination, use a limited number of readily available reagents and equipment. Overall, the combined books offer compound-specific tests for approximately 500–600 products and are based on a combination of organoleptic checks and simple physicochemical tests, such as colour reactions and melting-point determinations.

Semi-quantitative TLC methods have also been developed as basic tests using a limited number of solvent systems and detection systems. References to these tests are given in WHO (1998).

It should be remembered that basic tests are not, in any circumstances, intended to replace pharmacopoeial requirements, but should be used as a rapid and inexpensive means to verify identity and strength of drugs and medicinal products, and possibly to detect poor-quality counterfeit and other substandard products. In the event that suspect products are detected, these should be tested for compliance against pharmacopoeial requirements.

Given the very large number of colour tests which are available, it is beyond the scope of this textbook to list every test and the reader is referred to *Clarke's Analysis of Drugs and Poisons* (Moffat *et al.* 2004) and to the UN *Rapid*

Fujiwara test (general reagent for halogenated hydrocarbons)

Reagent
Freshly prepared 20% (w/v) *sodium hydroxide solution.*

Method
Mix together 2 mL of the reagent and 1 mL of pyridine. Add the sample (1 mL of urine) and heat in a water-bath at 100°C for 2 min with shaking.

Indications
A red–pink colour in the pyridine layer indicates the presence of compounds that possess at least two halogen atoms bound to one carbon atom. These include chloramphenicol, chlorbutanol, chloroform, dichloralphenazone, trichloroethane, trichloroethanol, trichloroacetic acid and trichloroethylene. Chloral hydrate and dichlorophenazone do themselves react, but are excreted in urine as trichloroacetic acid. No colour is given by dicophane (DDT) or carbon tetrachloride, although massive exposure to the latter solvent may lead to a positive urine test because of the presence of chloroform as a contaminant. 2,2,2-Trichloroethanol gives a yellow colour. The LOD is 1 mg/L.

As can be seen, this is a simple and rapid test making it exceedingly useful in clinical evaluation of suspected poisoning. In these circumstances the more sophisticated chromatographic techniques such as GC and HPLC are not appropriate because it simply takes too long to carry out the required analysis. Colour tests can provide a rapid indication of the substance present allowing clinical treatment to be applied as quickly as possible.

Marquis test
The Marquis test is a useful broad-spectrum test used mostly for opium alkaloids and amfetamines.

Reagent
Carefully mix 100 mL of concentrated *sulfuric acid* with 1 mL of 40% (v/v) *formaldehyde solution* (stable for several weeks if protected from light).

Method
Add a drop of the reagent to the sample on a white tile.

Indications
Various colours that represent the whole of the visible spectrum are given by a large number of compounds. Structures that tend to maintain the response to the reagent at the violet end of the spectrum are, in decreasing order of efficacy: ring sulfur (with or without aromatic ring); ring oxygen (with aromatic ring); extra-ring oxygen or sulfur (with aromatic ring); aromatic compounds that consist entirely of C, H, N. Thus, there is a tendency for the response to the Marquis reagent to move gradually towards longer wavelength (i.e. through green to orange and red) as the ratio of C, H, N to the other groups in the molecule rises (see the table below). In practice, it is often difficult to differentiate colours as specifically as shown below, particularly within a particular colour range. For example, there are five colours listed under 'red' but differentiation between e.g. black-red and brown-red may not be as easy as indicated. This is particularly the case where the Marquis test is used to identify street drugs. Drugs supplied at street level are typically 'cut' or 'adulterated' with a wide variety of substances to maximise the profit for dealers. Adulterants can include sugars, other drugs such as caffeine, paracetamol and topical anaesthetics (e.g. lidocaine, procaine), talc, etc. For drugs sold in tablet form such as MDMA, adulterants will include substances used to produce tablets. These substances can interfere in the colour reaction. The presence of strong acid can char organic substances, again interfering with the colour produced.

The LOD values for the Marquis test are: 1 μg for codeine sulfate, mescaline sulfate, methadone-HCl; 5 μg for lysergide tartrate, methamfetamine-HCl and morphine; 10 μg for amfetamine-HCl and diamorphine HCl.

The advantage of the Marquis test (and similar colour tests) is that it is simple to carry out, inexpensive, requires virtually no specialised equipment, can be applied in a wide variety of situations, does not require extensive operator training and gives a rapid result. Contrast this with the more sophisticated chromatographic techniques which, although they provide a far more confirmatory answer are not simple to carry out, require specialist equipment, need to be carried out in specialist facilities with highly trained operators, are costly and take longer to give a result.

Colours with the Marquis test

Colour	Compound
Red	Alprenolol, benzylmorphine (→ violet), buphenine, dimethothiazine, etenzamide, etilefrine, fenclofenac (slow), fenpiprane, fluphenazine, flurbiprofen, hexoprenaline, labetalol (→ brown–red), maprotiline, mephenesin carbamate, mequitazine (slow), mesoridazine (→ violet), methoxyphenamine, metopimazine, mexiletine, nadolol, pentazocine (→ green), pericyazine, phenazopyridine, phenoperidine, phenylephrine, piperacetazine, prenylamine, thebaine (→ orange), thiethylperazine (→ green), thioproperazine, tiotixene, tolpropamine, tranylcypromine (→ brown), vinblastine
Orange–red	Alverine, amfetamine-HCl, bethanidine, diphemanil, flupentixol, methamfetamine-HCl
Violet–red	Thioridazine (→ blue–green)
Black–red	Doxepin-HCl
Brown–red	Alphaprodine, doxepin, trihexyphenidyl
Pink	Alimemazine, fenoprofen, fluopromazine, metoprolol, promazine, promethazine, trifluoperazine
Orange	Adrenaline (→ violet), aletamine, amfetamine (→ red→ brown), anileridine (slow), benactyzine (→ green→ blue), benzethonium, benzilonium (→ green→ blue), benzfetamine, bunamidine (→ red), carbetapentane (slow), carfenazine (→ red–violet), chlorphentermine, clidinium (→ blue), cyclandelate (slow), cycrimine (→ red), dehydroemetine, dimethyltryptamine, dipyridamole, ethacridine (→ red), ethoheptazine, ethylnoradrenaline (→ brown), famprofazone, fenbufen (→ brown), fencamfamin, fenethylline, fentanyl, harmine, indapamide (→ violet), indometacin, isothipendyl, ketobemidone, lachesine (→ green→ blue), lymecycline, mepenzolate (transient), mephentermine (→ brown), mescaline, methamfetamine, metanephrine (→ violet–brown), methacycline, methanthelinium, methindizate (→ green), methylphenidate, methylpiperidyl benzilate (→ green→ blue), 5-methyltryptamine (→ brown), α-methyltryptamine (→ brown), *N*-methyltryptamine, nefopam (→ brown), nomifensine (slow), normetanephrine (→ violet–brown), oxeladin, oxytetracycline, pentapiperide, pethidine, phenethylamine, phenformin (→ brown), phentermine, piminodine, pipenzolate (→ green→ blue), piperidolate, pizotifen (→ red), poldine methylsulfate (→ green→ blue), primaquine, profadol (→ red–brown), prolintane (→ brown), propantheline, prothipendyl, psilocybine, rolitetracycline, spiramycin, tetracycline, trimethoprim, trimethoxyamfetamine, tryptamine, veratrine, xylometazoline
Red–orange	Chlorprothixene
Pink–orange	Diuron
Yellow–orange	Orphenadrine, pipradrol
Brown–orange	Amitriptyline
Yellow	Acriflavine (→ red), amiloride, azacyclonol, benzquinamide, benzatropine, bromazine, broxaldine, broxyquinoline, caramiphen, chlordiazepoxide, chlorphenoxamine (→ green), chlortetracycline (→ green), chlortalidone, cinchophen, clefamide, clemastine (green rim), colchicine, conessine (→ orange), cyclizine, demeclocycline (→ green), deptropine, diethyltryptamine (→ brown), 2,5-dimethoxy-4-methylamfetamine, diphenhydramine, diphenidol, diphenylpyraline, doxycycline, ethoxzolamide, ethylmorphine (→ violet→ black), furaltadone, halquinol, hydrocodone (→ brown→ violet), hydromorphone (→ red→ violet), hydroxyephedrine, isoetarine (→ orange), lidoflazine, lorazepam, mepacrine, methyldopa (→ violet), methyldopate (→ violet), norcodeine (→ violet), orciprenaline, oxycodone (→ brown→ violet), oxyphenbutazone, phanquone, phenbutrazate (slow), phentolamine, phenyramidol, pindolol (→ brown), pramoxine (→ green), proflavine (→ orange), salbutamol, salinazid, sodiumcromoglicate, solanine (→ violet), terbutaline, tetrabenazine, thebacon (→ violet), tofenacin, triamterene, trimetazidine (fades), vancomycin, viprynium embonate, zomepirac (100°C, → orange)

Orange–yellow	Methylphenidate-HCl, stanozolol
Yellow–pink	Methadone-HCl
Green	Berberine, carbaryl, chelidonine, harman, norharman, oleandomycin, propranolol, protriptyline, pseudomorphine, sulindac (slow)
Yellow–green	Acepromazine (→ red), verapamil (→ grey)
Blue–green	Tolnaftate
Brown–green	Harmaline
Grey–green	Cyproheptadine, deserpidine, naphazoline, oxypertine, phenindamine, protokylol, rescinnamine, reserpine (→ brown)
Blue	Clofibrate, embutramide, nicergoline (→ grey)
Grey–blue	Mebhydrolin, 1-naphthylacetic acid
Violet	Alimemazine, apomorphine (→ black), azatadine, benorilate, bisacodyl, buprenorphine, butriptyline, captodiame, chloropyrilene, chlorpromazine, clofazimine, codeine, diamorphine, diethylthiambutene, dihydrocodeine, dimethindene (→ blue), dimethoxanate, doxorubicin, doxylamine, etoxazene, guaifenesin, guanoxan, hexocyclium metilsulfate, mepyramine, 6-monoacetylmorphine, morphine, nalorphine, normorphine, oxprenolol, oxycodone-HCl, oxyphenisatine, pecazine, penthienate, pentazocine, perazine, perphenazine, phenoxybenzamine, phenyltoloxamine, pholcodine, pimozide, pipoxolan (→ grey), prochlorperazine, procyclidine, profenamine, promazine, promethazine, proquamezine, solanidine, thenium, thiopropazate, tricyclamol, viloxazine
Red–violet	Acetophenazine, benzoctamine, bephenium hydroxynaphthoate, cefaloridine, chlophedianol (→ brown), dihydromorphine, ethomoxane, isoxsuprine, lobeline, methdilazine, propiomazine, tramazoline, trifluomeprazine, trifluoperazine, triflupromazine, trimeperidine
Blue–violet	Methocarbamol, levomepromazine, morantel, neopine, noscapine (fades), pyrantel
Brown–violet	Butaperazine, dopamine, methylenedioxyamfetamine, tridihexethyl
Grey–violet	Diprenorphine, oxymorphone, pyrrobutamine, thenalidine, trihexyphenidyl
Black–violet	Dextropropoxyphene (→ green), methapyrilene, thenyldiamine
Brown	Bibenzonium, carbidopa, cyclazocine (→ green), diclofenac (slow), dimoxyline, dosulepin, doxepin, ergometrine, ergotamine, erythromycin, hordenine (→ green), ibuprofen (100°, → orange), isoprenaline (→ violet), lysergamide, methadone, naloxone (→ violet), naproxen, narceine (→ green), noradrenaline, pethidine-HCl, phentermine, phenazocine, rimiterol (→ black), serotonin (slow), syrosingopine, tyramine (→ green)
Red–brown	Biperiden, debrisoquine, methyl benzoquate, oxetacaine, phenprobamate, trimetozine, tripelennamine
Orange–brown	Benethamine (→ brown), clomocycline, nortriptyline
Yellow–brown	Moxisylyte, ritodrine, triacetyloleandomycin, tylosin
Green–brown	Alcuronium, bufotenine, psilocin
Violet–brown	Clomifene, diethazine, levomethadyl acetate (→ grey–green), methoxamine (→ green)
Grey–brown	Dihydroergotamine, methylergometrine, octafonium
Grey	Butorphanol, diaveridine (→ violet–brown), ibogaine (→ orange) lysergide, methoserpidine, methysergide, pholedrine (→ green)
Blue–grey	Acetorphine (→ yellow–brown), etorphine (→ yellow–brown)
Black	Methylenedioxyamfetamine
Blue–black	Methylenedioxyamfetamine
Green–black	Lysergide

Figure 13.1 Examples of colour tests: the Fujiwara test for halogenated hydrocarbons and the Marquis test for opiates and amfetamines.

Methods for Drugs of Abuse and WHO *Basic Tests for Drugs* for details of the various tests available. The important aspects to remember with regard to colour tests are their place in the analytical scheme (rapid, diagnostic tests) and the limitations of these tests.

Interpretation of colour tests

Colour descriptions

Colours exhibited by these tests cannot be described with any accuracy. They may vary in intensity or tincture with the concentration of compounds in the test samples and the presence of extraneous material. In addition, their assessment is always a subjective one, even in people with normal colour vision. For example, the Marquis test is stated to give a black or blue-black colour with MDMA and a green-black with lysergide (Fig. 13.1). Even in the pure form these colours may not be readily distinguishable; add this to the fact that most drugs of abuse are more routinely encountered diluted with a variety of other substances, and one can begin to appreciate the difficulties that can arise in the real world with colour tests. Some of the complexes formed are unstable, so that the colour changes or fades with time.

Effects of ionic form

Salts may give different colours from those of the corresponding acid or base. In general, free acids or bases that have been isolated from the test material by an extraction process give better colours than their salts. The colour of a salt may be modified by the nature of the other ions present. For example, all hydrochloride salts give a red colour in Mandelin's test and a blue colour with Koppanyi–Zwikker reagent (prior to adding pyrrolidine). Basic salts of weak acids may produce different colours because of a change in pH. Where a compound has been extracted from biological material, these factors should not create any difficulty since it will be present in the form of the base. However, when applying the tests to pharmaceutical preparations, where the compounds are usually present as salts, this can cause problems. To overcome this, the material can be extracted in much the same way as for biological samples to derive the free base. Bromide and iodide salts can be converted into the nitrate before testing.

Use of the colour tests lists

The system typically adopted in colour tests uses ten basic colours: the spectral colours (red, orange, yellow, green, blue and violet), together with pink, brown, grey and black. Where there is a variation in hue, this is indicated by combining two colours (e.g. red–brown) (see Fig. 13.1). The second-named colour is considered to be the dominant one. For example, red–brown is listed under brown, whereas brown–red is listed under red. When interpreting results, it is often necessary to search lists given for tests under two main colours (e.g. for red–brown the lists under both red and brown should be consulted). This takes account of the subjective nature of colour assessment. An arrow between two colours (e.g. red→brown) indicates that the colour changes during the course of the test. Occasionally, the colour displayed by a test solution in reflected light may be different from that in transmitted light, in which case the solution is described as dichroic. A combined colour may be obtained when more than one drug is present or the drug itself is coloured, which limits the value of the tests for biological samples.

Practical points

Performing colour tests

Tests are usually carried out either in clear glass test-tubes or on white glazed porcelain tiles (spotting tiles), which give a uniform background against which colours can be assessed. For drugs, most colour tests are designed to work on about 1 mg, either as the solid form or as a dried extract of this amount.

A sample known not to contain the compound of interest should be tested at the same time as the test sample. This enables a comparison of the colours produced by the sample and by the reagent blank. Ideally, the blank sample should have the same matrix as the test sample (e.g. for urine tests use analyte-free urine), since this takes account of the effects of extraneous materials. Otherwise, water is usually adequate.

Before making a final decision on the result of a test, the reaction of the unknown should be compared with that of a reference substance tested under exactly the same conditions. The reference substance should, ideally, be spiked a blank sample of the same type as the sample; for example, if the sample to be tested is a urine sample then the reference sample should be added to a sample of urine known not to contain the compound of interest.

Validation of a colour test

It is essential to validate all tests and test reagents for sensitivity and specificity; O'Neal *et al.* (2000) have outlined a suitable method for a chemical spot test.

Application of colour tests to sample extracts

Several solvent extraction schemes have been devised to fractionate compounds on the basis of their acidic, neutral or basic characteristics (see Moffat *et al.* 2004). The tests listed in Table 13.1 can be applied to evaporated extracts.

Table 13.2 summarises tests that can be applied to detect some of the most important drug groups and other poisons.

Colour reagents and thin-layer chromatography

Many common colour-test reagents are used routinely as locating reagents in TLC (e.g. acidified iodoplatinate solution, Dragendorff's reagent, Marquis reagent, Van Urk's reagent) (see below). These reagents may be applied by spraying or dipping. In high-performance TLC (HPTLC) it is more common to use an automated dipping device for applying locating reagents. It is worth noting that the preparation of the spray or dip equivalent of a colour reagent may differ slightly from that of the colour reagent preparation itself because spray reagents may need to be of a somewhat different viscosity to enable application to TLC plates.

It is also the case that the reaction and resultant colour that marks the presence of a certain substance obtained from spraying a reagent on TLC plates may differ from that obtained from a direct colour test and, in some cases, will not yield any results. This is because of pH effects, that is, whether the TLC plate has been dipped in 0.1 M sodium hydroxide and the substance tested is acidic in character (i.e. the free acid of a

Table 13.1 Tests that can be applied to evaporated extracts

Fraction	Test
Strong acid	Aromaticity
	Ferric chloride
	Folin–Ciocalteu reagent
	Liebermann's reagent
	Millon's reagent
	Nessler's reagent
Weak acid	Aromaticity
	Coniferyl alcohol
	Diazotisation
	Ferric chloride
	Folin–Ciocalteu reagent
	Koppanyi–Zwikker reagent
	Liebermann's reagent
	Mercurous nitrate
	Millon's reagent
	Nessler's reagent
Neutral	Aromaticity
	Furfuraldehyde
	Koppanyi–Zwikker reagent
	Liebermann's reagent
	Mercurous nitrate
	Nessler's reagent
Basic	Amalic acid test
	p-Dimethylaminobenzaldehyde
	Ferric chloride
	Formaldehyde–sulfuric acid
	Forrest reagent
	FPN reagent
	Liebermann's reagent
	Mandelin's reagent
	Marquis reagent
	Nessler's reagent
	Sulfuric acid

Table 13.2 Indication of which tests can applied to detect some of the most important drug groups and other poisons

Substance/functional group	Useful tests/reagents
Alcohols	Potassium dichromate
Alkaloids and nitrogenous bases	Dragendorff's reagent
Amides (aliphatic)	Nessler's reagent
Aldehydes (aliphatic)	Schiff's reagent
Amfetamines	Marquis test, Mecke test, Froehde's reagent and Mandelin's test
	Sodium nitroprusside–acetone
Antidepressants	Marquis test
Barbiturates	Dille–Koppanyi reagent
	Koppanyi–Zwikker reagent
	Mercurous nitrate
	Vanillin reagent
	Zwikker reagent
Benzodiazepines	Formaldehyde–sulfuric acid
Cannabis	Duquenois reagent
Carbamates (non-aromatic)	Furfuraldehyde
Cocaine	Cobalt thiocyanate
	p-Dimethylaminobenzaldehyde
	Mandelin's test
	Scott's test
Chlorinated phenols	Nitric acid (fuming)
Chlorinated hydrocarbon insecticides	Nitric–sulfuric acid
Cyanide	Ferrous sulfate (B)
	Sodium picrate
Cyanide groups	Sodium picrate
Dithiocarbamates	Sodium nitroprusside
Ergot alkaloids	*p*-Dimethylaminobenzaldehyde
Halogenated hydrocarbons	Fujiwara test
Imides	Koppanyi–Zwikker test
Ketones	Sodium nitroprusside
Methadone	Cobalt thiocyanate
	Mandelin's test
	Marquis test
	Tetrabromophenolphthalein ethyl ester
Mono-substituted pyridine ring	Cyanogen bromide
Nitrates and nitrites	Ferrous sulfate
Opiates	Marquis, Mecke, Froehde's, Mandelin's tests
Oxidising agents	Diphenylamine
Paraquat/diquat	Sodium dithionate
Phencyclidine	Cobalt thiocyanate
	p-Dimethylaminobenzaldehyde
	Tetrabromophenolphthalein ethyl ester
Phenols	*p*-Dimethylaminobenzaldehyde
	Ferric chloride
	Folin–Ciocalteu reagent
	Millon's reagent

Phenothiazines	Ferric chloride
	Formaldehyde–sulfuric acid
	Forrest reagent
	FPN reagent
Phenylpyrazolines	Nitrous acid
Primary aromatic amines	Coniferyl alcohol
	Diazotisation
Primary and secondary amines	Dragendorff's reagent
	Simon's test
Propoxyphene	Cobalt thiocyanate
	Froehde's reagent
	Liebermann's test
	Tetrabromophenolphthalein ethyl ester
Quaternary ammonium compounds	Tetrabromophenolphthalein ethyl ester
Quaternary amines	Dragendorff's reagent
Quinines	Cobalt thiocyanate
	Thalleioquin
Quinones	Methanolic potassium hydroxide
Reducing agents	Benedict's reagent
Salicylates	Ferric chloride
	Trinder's reagent
Steroids	Antimony pentachloride
	Naphthol sulfuric acid
	Sulfuric acid
Sulfonamides	Copper sulfate
	Koppanyi–Zwikker reagent
	Mercurous nitrate
	Nitrous acid
Sulfur-containing	Palladium chloride
	Sodium nitroprusside
Tertiary amines	Dragendorff's reagent
	Tetrabromophenolphthalein ethyl ester

salt post-extraction). However, this aspect of colour reagents and their use in TLC as sprays can often give clues as to the drug's or substance's chemistry.

Thin layer chromatography

TLC is a widely used technique for the separation and identification of drugs. It is equally applicable to drugs in their pure state, to those extracted from pharmaceutical formulations, to illicitly manufactured materials, and to biological samples.

In its simplest form, TLC can be regarded as the separation of substances on a planar surface coated with a stationary phase. The mobile phase moves across the planar surface from one edge to the other and substances separate out according to their distribution between the stationary phase and mobile phase (see Fig. 13.2). As we will see in the discussion that follows, this is a simple view of TLC and many adaptations and refinements have been made to this basic procedure to enable rather sophisticated separations.

TLC as we know it today was established in the 1950s (see Fig. 13.3) with the introduction of standardised procedures that led to improved

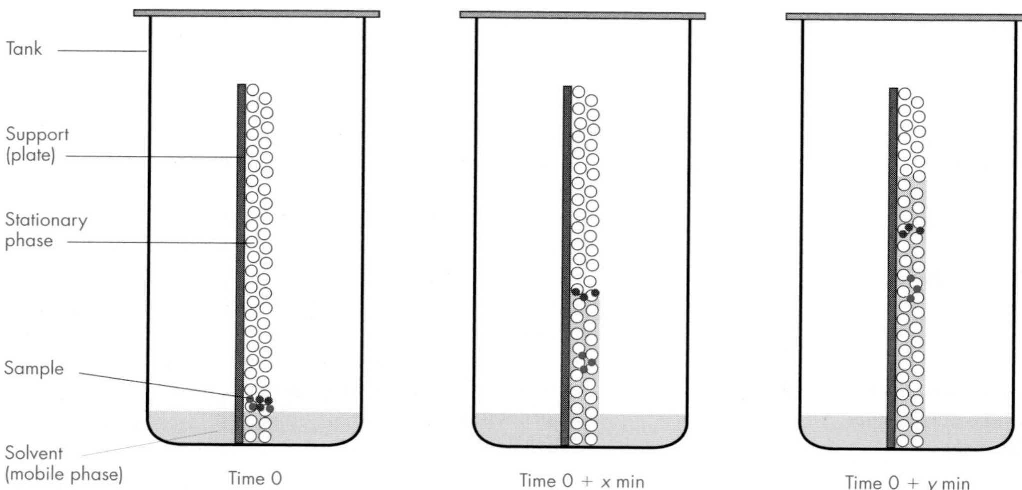

Figure 13.2 Illustration of a TLC separation. The sample mixture is spotted at one end of the support plate and placed in the mobile phase. The mobile phase moves across/through the stationary phase carrying the components of the sample with it. The components of the sample partition between the mobile phase and stationary phase. Assuming the correct conditions are chosen, this results in a separation of substances on the plate.

separation performance and reproducibility, and paved the way for its commercialisation and an increase in the number of published applications. The 1970s saw the introduction of fine-particle layers and associated instrumentation required for their correct use. In this form, TLC became known as high-performance TLC, instrumental TLC or modern TLC to distinguish it from its parent, now generally referred to as conventional TLC. High-performance TLC has not displaced conventional TLC from laboratory studies and the two approaches coexist today because of their complementary features (Table 13.3). Conventional TLC provides a quick, inexpensive and portable method for qualitative analysis. It requires minimal and readily available instrumentation and uses easily learned experimental techniques. HPTLC is characterised by the use of kinetically optimised layers for faster and more efficient separations; it takes advantage of a wider range of sorbent chemistries to optimise selectivity and requires the use of instrumentation for convenient (automated) sample application, development and detection. HPTLC provides accurate and precise quantitative results based on in-situ measurements and a record of the separation in the form of a chromatogram, such as the example in Fig. 13.6 on p. 348. While all modern laboratories are capable of drug analysis by conventional TLC, only those laboratories equipped with the necessary instrumentation for HPTLC have this option. Preparative TLC is used when one or more components of a sample are required in bulk for further studies, such as for identification by NMR, MS, FTIR, etc. Layers on preparative TLC plates are thicker than on conventional plates to allow higher sample loading. Particle size may also be larger.

In the basic TLC experiment, the sample is applied to the layer (stationary phase) as a spot or band near to the bottom edge of the layer. The separation is carried out in a closed chamber either by either contacting the bottom edge of the layer with the mobile phase, which advances through the layer by capillary forces as in Fig. 13.2, or by forcing the mobile phase to move through the layer at a controlled velocity by means of an external pressure source or centrifugal force. A separation of the sample results from the different rates of migration of the sample components in the direction travelled by the mobile phase, dependent upon their distribution between the stationary and

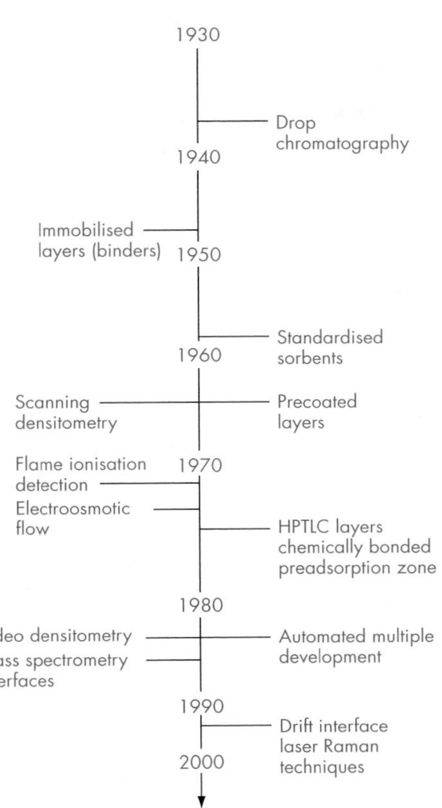

Figure 13.3 Time line depicting the evolution of modern TLC.

mobile phases. After development and evaporation of the mobile phase, the sample components are separated in space, their position and quantity being determined by visual evaluation or in-situ scanning densitometry aided by the formation of easily detected derivatives by post-chromatographic chemical reactions, as required.

The distance the sample has moved along the plate is then noted and is compared with the distance moved by the mobile phase. This is referred to as the retardation factor, or R_F value, and is the fundamental parameter used to characterise the position of a sample zone in a TLC chromatogram. For linear development it represents the ratio of the distance migrated by the sample compared to the distance travelled by the solvent front:

$$R_F = \frac{Z_X}{Z_f - Z_0} \tag{13.1}$$

where Z_X is the distance travelled by the sample from its origin, $(Z_f - Z_0)$ is the distance travelled by the mobile phase from the sample origin, Z_f is the distance travelled by the mobile phase measured from the mobile phase level at the start of the separation, and Z_0 is the distance from the sample origin to the mobile phase level at the start of the separation. The boundary conditions for R_F values are $1 > R_F > 0$. The R_F value is generally calculated to two decimal places. Some authors prefer to tabulate values as whole numbers, as hR_F values equivalent to $100R_F$, in which case values are between 0 and 100.

Standards of substances anticipated to be present are normally analysed alongside samples in order to compare their spatial location relative to samples and their response to the detection method used. R_F values for standards are compared with those for samples.

Separations by column liquid chromatography (HPLC) and TLC occur by essentially the same physical process. The two techniques are frequently considered as competitors, when it would be more realistic to consider them as complementary. The attributes of TLC that provide for its co-existence as a complementary technique to HPLC are summarised in Table 13.4. TLC methods are most effective for the low-cost analysis of a large number of samples (e.g. drug screening in biological fluids and tissues, determination of the botanical origin and potency of traditional herbal medicines, stability testing and content uniformity testing), for the rapid analysis of samples that require minimum sample clean up, or where TLC allows a reduction in the number of sample preparation steps (e.g. analysis of samples containing components that remain sorbed to the stationary phase or contain suspended microparticles). TLC also provides advantages for the analysis of substances with poor detection characteristics that require post-chromatographic chemical treatment for detection. In other cases, HPLC methods are generally preferred, particularly if the sample matrix is very complex and/or

Table 13.3 Characteristic properties of silica gel precoated TLC layers

Parameter	High-performance TLC	TLC
Plate dimensions (cm^2)	10 × 10	20 × 20
Layer thickness (mm)	0.1 or 0.2	0.1–0.25
Starting spot diameter (mm)	1–2	3–6
Diameter of separated spots (mm)	2–6	6–15
Solvent front migration distance (cm)	3–6	10–15
Time for development (capillary flow) (min)	3–20	20–200
Detection limits[a]		
Absorption (ng)	0.1–0.5	1–5
Fluorescence (pg)	5–10	50–100
Nominal particle size range (μm)	3–7	5–20
Apparent particle size (μm)[b]	5–7	8–10
Minimum plate height (μm)	22–25	35–45
Optimum velocity (mm/s)	0.3–0.5	0.2–0.5
Porosity		
Total	0.65–0.70	0.65–0.75
Interparticle	0.35–0.45	0.35–0.45
Intraparticle	0.28	0.28

[a] For drugs with favourable detection properties.

[b] Determined by chromatographic measurements. Precoated TLC layers are prepared from silica gel with a narrower particle size range than typical bulk materials available for self-made layers.

sample components have very similar distribution coefficients, for separations by size-exclusion and ion-exchange chromatography, and for trace analysis using selective detectors unavailable for TLC.

Stationary phases

Conventional TLC plates can be prepared in the laboratory by standardised methods, but reproducible layer preparation is easier to achieve in a manufacturing setting. Few laboratories prepare their own plates today, finding it more efficient to purchase TLC plates from commercial suppliers.

Precoated plates for high performance, conventional and preparative TLC are available in a range of sizes and different layer thickness, supported on glass, aluminium or plastic backing sheets. To impart the desired mechanical stability and abrasion resistance to the layer, a binder such as poly(vinyl alcohol), poly(vinyl pyrrolidone), gypsum or starch in amounts from 0.1% to 10% (w/w) is incorporated into the layer. An ultraviolet (UV) indicator, such as manganese-activated zinc silicate of a similar particle size to the sorbent, may be added to the layer for visualisation of separated samples by fluorescence quenching. TLC plates with a narrow preadsorbent zone located along one edge of the layer are available to aid manual sample application.

Silica gel is the most important stationary phase for TLC, with other inorganic oxide adsorbents, such as alumina, kieselguhr (a silica gel of low surface area) and Florisil (a synthetic magnesium silicate), of minor importance. Most silica gel sorbents have an average pore size of 6 nm and are designed for the separation of small molecules (relative molecular mass <700). The chromatographic properties of the inorganic oxide adsorbents depend on their surface chemistry and specific surface area. For silica gel, silanol groups (—Si—OH) are the dominant adsorption sites (Fig. 13.4). The complementary

Table 13.4 Attributes of TLC providing the link to contemporary applications in drug analysis

Attribute	Application
Separation of samples in parallel	Low-cost analysis and high-throughput screening of samples requiring minimal sample preparation
Disposable stationary phase	Analysis of crude samples (minimising sample preparation requirements) Analysis of a single or small number of samples when their composition and/or matrix properties are unknown Analysis of samples containing components that remain sorbed to the separation medium or contain suspended microparticles
Static detection	Samples that require post-chromatographic treatment for detection Samples that require sequential detection techniques (free of time constraints) for identification or confirmation
Storage device	Separations can be archived Separations can be evaluated in different locations or at different times Convenient fraction collection for coupled column–layer chromatography
Sample integrity	Total sample occupies the chromatogram, not just that portion of the sample that elutes from the column

sample properties that govern retention are the number and type of functional groups and their spatial location (see Fig. 13.5).

The influence of functional group properties on selectivity is illustrated in Fig. 13.6 for the separation of ethynyl steroids. The steroids with phenolic groups are the most strongly retained, followed by hydroxyl groups, and then ketone and ester groups. Subtle separation differences through steric hindrance at a functional group and differences in ring conformations are also seen, which allow the separation of steroids with very similar chemical properties.

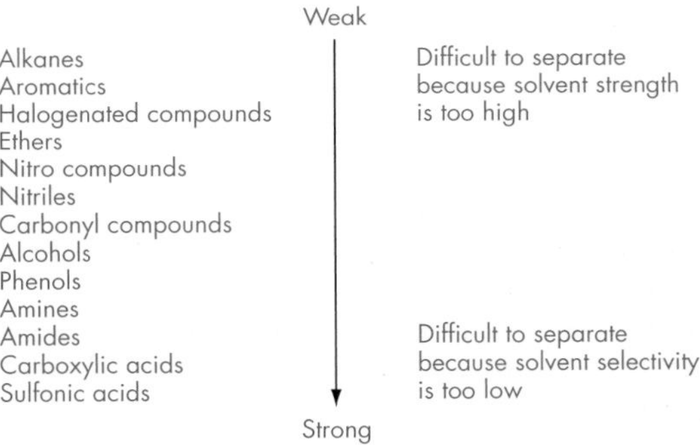

Figure 13.5 General adsorption scale for separations by silica gel TLC.

Separations on silica gel are considered as 'normal' phase separations (see pp. 514 and 515), where the stationary phase is polar relative to the mobile phase. TLC separations can be carried out in reversed-phase mode. In this mode, the mobile phase is more polar than the stationary phase. Chemically bonded stationary phase layers are prepared from silica gel by reaction with various organosilane reagents to form siloxane bonds. The degree of chemical bonding can be varied to form stationary phases with a high coverage of bonded phase and few residual silanol groups on the silica surface to phases with a lower bonded phase coverage and more (higher concentration or proportion of) residual silanol groups (Table 13.5). Reversed-phase alkylsiloxane-bonded layers with a high level of surface bonding cannot be used with mobile

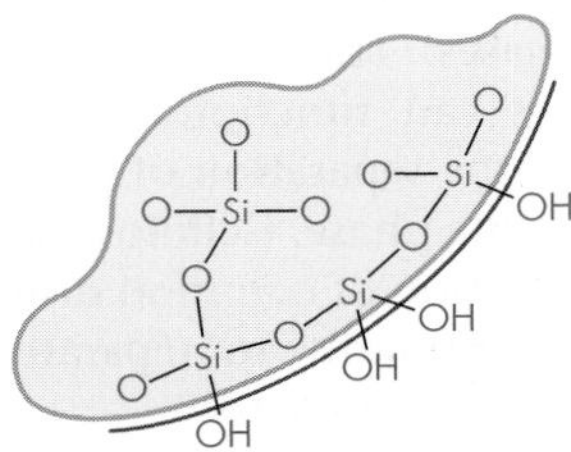

Figure 13.4 Structure of silica gel.

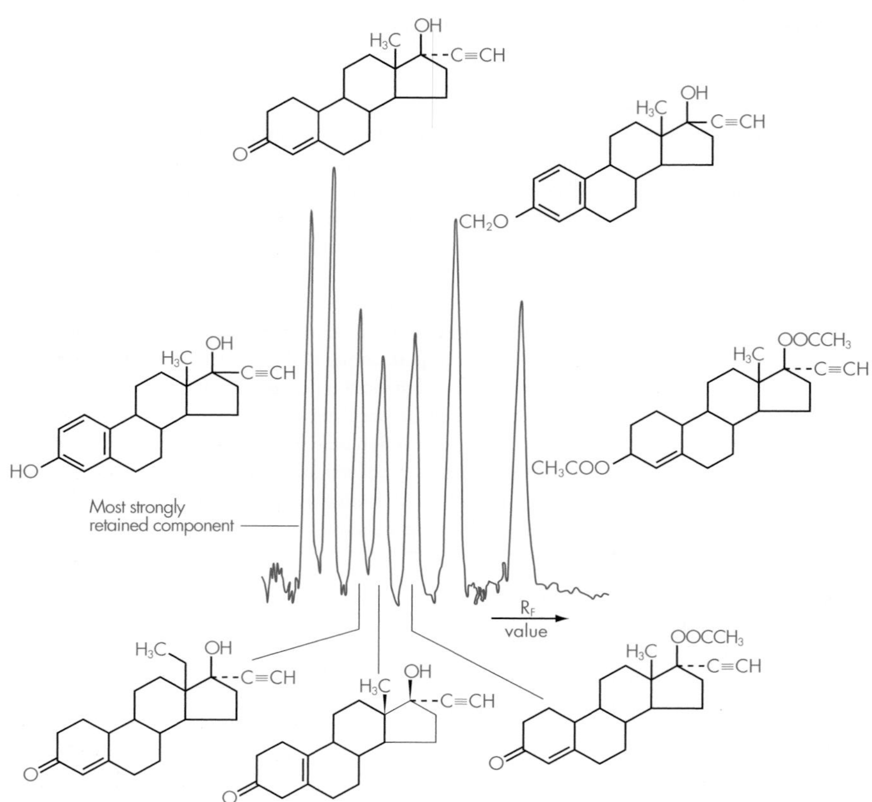

Figure 13.6 Separation of ethynyl steroids (birth-control pill components) by high-performance TLC. Two 15 min developments with the mobile phase hexane–chloroform–carbon tetrachloride–ethanol (7:18:22:1) on a silica gel 60 high-performance TLC plate. Chromatogram was recorded by scanning densitometry at 220 nm.

phases that contain a significant amount of water (>30% v/v) because of the inadequate mobile-phase velocity generated by capillary forces. Water compatibility for alkylsiloxane-bonded layers is achieved by increasing the particle size of the silica support material, using a reproducible although lower degree of silanisation, and by using modified binders. These layers are referred to as water wettable and are used for all types of reversed-phase separations, while layers with a high degree of silanisation are used predominantly with non-aqueous mobile phases. Alkylsiloxane bonded phases are used primarily (but not exclusively) for the separation of water-soluble polar drugs and weak acids and bases after ion suppression (buffered mobile phase) or ion-pair formation. Water compatibility is not a problem for chemically bonded phases where the bonded group is polar in nature e.g. aminopropylsiloxane or spacer-bonded propanediol (Table 13.5). These phases can be used for both normal- and reversed-phase separations. For separations that cannot be achieved on silica gel, the polar chemically bonded phases are the most widely used stationary phases. The 3-aminopropylsiloxane-bonded layers can function as a weak anion exchanger for the separation of polyanions with a buffered mobile phase. Cellulose layers provide only weak retention of common drug substances and are used primarily to separate very polar compounds in biochemistry.

TLC has found limited use for the separation of enantiomers. The most widely used approach

Table 13.5 Retention properties of silica based chemically bonded layers

Type of modification	Functional group	Application[a]
Alkylsiloxane	$Si—CH_3$	For reversed-phase separations generally, but not exclusively
	$Si—C_2H_5$	Separation of water-soluble polar organic compounds (RPC)
	$Si—C_8H_{17}$	Weak acids and bases after ion suppression (RPC)
	$Si—C_{18}H_{37}$	Strong acids and bases by ion-pair mechanism (RPC)
Phenylsiloxane	$Si—C_6H_5$	Of limited use for drug analysis
Cyanopropylsiloxane	$Si—(CH_2)_3CN$	Useful for both RPC and NPC In NPC it exhibits properties similar to a low-capacity silica gel In RPC it exhibits properties similar to short-chain alkylsiloxane-bonded layers (it has no selectivity for dipole-type interactions)
Aminopropylsiloxane	$Si—(CH_2)_3NH_2$	Used mainly in NPC and IEC; limited retention in RPC Selectively retains compounds by hydrogen-bond interactions in NPC; separation order generally different to that in silica gel Functions as a weak anion exchanger in acidic mobile phases (IEC)
Spacer bonded propanediol	$Si—(CH_2)_3OCH_2CH(OH)CH_2OH$	Used in NPC and RPC, but more useful for NPC because of low retention in RPC Polar drugs selectively retained by hydrogen bond and dipole-type interactions in NPC; more hydrogen-bond acidic and less hydrogen-bond basic than aminopropylsiloxane-bonded layers in NPC; more retentive than aminopropylsiloxane-bonded layers in RPC Similar retention to short-chain alkylsiloxane-bonded layers, but different selectivity for hydrogen-bonding drugs

[a] NPC, normal-phase chromatography; RPC, reversed-phase chromatography, IEC, ion-exchange chromatography.

employs ligand-exchange chromatography on reversed-phase layers impregnated with a solution of copper acetate and (2*S*,4*R*,2*RS*)-*N*-(2-hydroxydodecyl)-4-hydroxyproline. Separations result from stability differences in diastereomeric complexes formed between the drug, copper and the proline selector. Suitable drugs for this application require an amino acid or α-hydroxycarboxylic acid group for complex formation. A more versatile approach to the separation of enantiomeric drug substances by reversed-phase TLC is the use of chiral selectors, such as cyclodextrins or bovine serum albumin, as mobile-phase additives.

Technique

The technique of TLC involves a number of separate steps, namely:

- preparing the layer
- applying the sample
- developing the plate
- detecting the separated zones
- identifying the separated substances.

These steps are described below.

Layer pretreatments

Prior to chromatography it is common practice to prepare the stationary phase layer for use by any or all of the following steps: washing, conditioning and equilibration. TLC plates may also be cut to preferred sizes using scissors for plastic- or aluminium-backed plates and diamond or carbide glass-cutting tools for glass-backed plates. Newly consigned precoated layers are invariably contaminated, or quickly become so, because of residual contaminants from the manufacturing process, contact with packaging materials and adsorption of materials from the atmosphere. To remove contaminants, single or double immersion in a polar solvent, such as methanol or propan-2-ol, for about 5 min is generally superior to predevelopment with the mobile phase. For trace analysis, sequential immersion and predevelopment may be required to obtain the best results.

For inorganic oxide adsorbents the absolute R_F value and the reproducibility of R_F values depend on the activity of the stationary phase. The latter is controlled by the adsorption of reagents, most notably water, through the gas phase. Physically adsorbed water can be removed from silica gel layers by heating at about 120°C for 30 min. Afterwards, the plates should be stored in a grease-free desiccator over blue silica gel. Heat activation is not normally required for chemically bonded layers. Equilibration of activated layers by exposure to the atmosphere is extremely rapid and layer activation is at times an unnecessary step. In modern air-conditioned laboratories, layers achieve a consistent level of activity that should provide sufficient reproducibility for most separations. Inorganic oxide layers can be adjusted to a defined activity by exposure to a defined gas phase in an enclosed chamber. Since manipulation in the atmosphere almost certainly readjusts this activity, it is best performed after application of the sample zones in a developing chamber that allows both layer conditioning and development in the same chamber (e.g. a twin-trough chamber), or in a separate conditioning chamber immediately before development. Atmospheres of different constant relative humidity can be obtained by using solutions of concentrated sulfuric acid or saturated solutions of various salts (*CRC Handbook of Chemistry and Physics*, 2007). Acid or base deactivation can be carried out in a similar manner by exposure to, for example, ammonia or hydrochloric acid fumes.

Sample application

Drugs are applied to TLC plates as spots or bands with a homogeneous distribution of material within the starting zone. For high-performance layers, starting spot diameters of about 1.0–2.0 mm are desirable, corresponding to a sample volume of 100–200 nL if applied by a dosimeter (micropipette). For conventional TLC plates, sample volumes 5- to 10-fold greater are acceptable. Attention should be paid to the solvent used for sample dissolution and application. Desirable properties of the sample solution are summarised in Table 13.6.

If scanning densitometry is used for detection, manual sample application with hand-held devices is inadequate. For densitometry, the starting position of each spot must be known accurately, which is achieved easily with mechanical devices that operate to a precise grid mechanism. Also, the sample must be applied to the layer without disturbing the surface, something that is nearly impossible to achieve using manual application.

Sample application devices for TLC encompass a wide range of sophistication and automation. The most popular devices for quantitative TLC use the spray-on technique. A controlled nitrogen-atomiser sprays the sample from a syringe or capillary, to form narrow, homogeneous bands on the plate surface. The plate is moved back and forth under the atomiser on a

Table 13.6 Solution requirements for sample application

Property	Requirements
Sample solvent	Good solvent for the sample to promote quantitative transfer from the sample application device to the layer Low viscosity and sufficiently volatile to be easily evaporated from the layer (dilute viscous samples if possible with a volatile solvent of low viscosity) Wet the sorbent layer to provide adequate penetration of the layer by the sample (a potential problem for alkylsiloxane-bonded layers and aqueous sample solutions) Weak chromatographic solvent to minimise predevelopment during sample application (ideally, if used as a chromatographic solvent the least-retained sample component should have $R_F < 0.1$)
Aqueous solutions	Dilute if possible with a water-miscible solvent that forms a lower boiling-point azeotrope Apply in small increments or, if spray-on techniques are used, with a slow application rate Use layers with a preadsorption zone and refocus the sample prior to development
Suspensions	Filter before attempting sample application Otherwise use layers with a preadsorption zone and an extraction solvent that mobilises the components of interest for refocusing

translational stage to apply bands of any length between zero (spots) and the maximum transit length of the spray head. Bands are typically 0.5 or 1.0 cm in length, with the longer bands used primarily for preparative-scale separations. The rate of sample deposition can be adjusted to accommodate sample solutions of different volatility and viscosity. An advantage of spray-on devices is that different volumes of a single standard solution can be applied for calibration purposes and the standard addition method of quantification is carried out easily by over-spraying the sample already applied to the layer with a solution of the standard. Fully automated sample applicators can be programmed to select samples from a rack of vials and deposit fixed volumes of the sample, at a controlled rate, to selected positions on the plate. The applicator automatically rinses itself between sample applications and can spot or band a whole plate with different samples and standards without operator intervention.

Glass microcapillaries for conventional TLC and fixed-volume dosimeters (which consist of a 100 or 200 nL platinum–iridium capillary sealed into a glass-support capillary) for HPTLC are also commonly used for sample application and require less sophisticated instrumentation. The capillary tip is brought into contact with the plate surface using a mechanical device to discharge its volume. A click-stop grid mechanism is used to provide an even spacing of the samples on the layer and a frame of reference for sample location during scanning densitometry.

Layers with a preadsorbent zone (a narrow zone prepared from a silica gel of low surface area with weak retention) simplify some aspects of sample application. This allows relatively large sample volumes or dirty samples to be applied to the preadsorption zone and their reconcentration to a narrow band at the interface between the preadsorbent and separation zones by a short development prior to chromatography. However, since the distribution of the sample may not be even within the band, the quantitative accuracy of densitometric measurements may be impaired using this approach.

Although manual sample application is not advised for quantification, it is acceptable for qualitative purposes. A variety of glass microcapillaries are available for sample application. In some of these, the microcapillary is calibrated and the use of a thin wire inside the capillary enables positive displacement of the sample to enable quantitative application.

Development

The principal development techniques in TLC are linear, circular and anticircular, with the velocity of the mobile phase controlled by capillary forces or forced-flow conditions. Circular TLC typically employs centrifugal force in the separation. The sample is applied as a band at the centre of a circular plate. The plate is then spun in a centrifugal manner, with the mobile phase in contact with the centre of the plate. The centrifugal force causes the mobile phase to move radially across the plate to the outer edge, with separation of the components of the sample taking place in the process. The separation process can either be interrupted and the separate bands developed or the bands can be allowed to develop right to the edge of the plate and then be collected for further examination. Anticircular TLC operates in a reverse manner, with the sample and mobile phase applied at the outer edge of a circle.

In any of these modes, continuous or multiple development can be used to extend the application range. Radial development is used rarely for drug analysis. Forced-flow development requires sophisticated equipment not commonly found in analytical laboratories, and is not described here.

For linear (or normal) development, samples are applied along one edge of the plate and the separation developed for a fixed distance in the direction of the opposite edge. Viewed in the direction of development, the chromatogram consists of a series of compact symmetrical spots of increasing diameter or, if samples are applied as bands, in rectangular zones of increasing width (Fig. 13.7).

In continuous development, the mobile phase is allowed to traverse the layer under the influence of capillary forces until it reaches some predetermined position on the plate, at which point it is evaporated continuously. Evaporation of the mobile phase usually occurs at the plate atmospheric boundary using either natural or forced evaporation. Continuous development is used primarily to separate simple mixtures with a short development length and a weaker (more selective solvent) than employed for normal development.

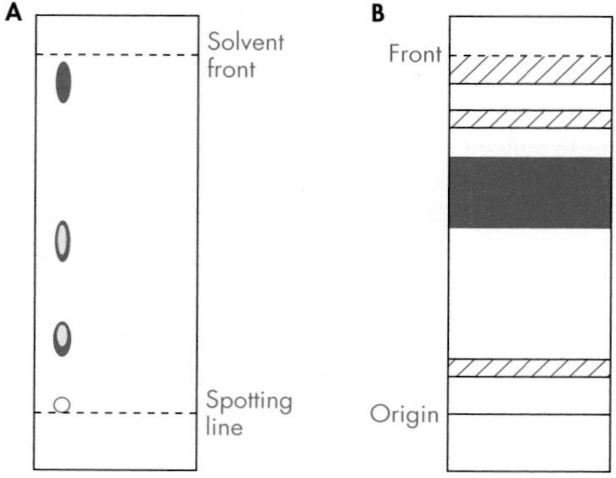

Figure 13.7 Development of TLC plate with (A) sample applied to the plate as a spot and (B) sample applied to the plate as a band.

In unidimensional multiple development, the TLC plate is developed for some selected distance, then either the layer or the mobile phase is withdrawn from the developing chamber, and adsorbed solvent is evaporated from the layer before repeating the development process. The principal methods of unidimensional multiple development are summarised in Table 13.7. Multiple development provides a very versatile strategy for separating complex mixtures, since the primary experimental variables of development distance and composition of the mobile phase can be changed at any development step, and the number of steps can be varied to obtain the desired separation. Multiple development provides a higher resolution of complex mixtures than does normal or continuous development; it can easily handle samples of a wide polarity range (stepwise gradient development); and, because the separated zones are usually more compact, it leads to lower detection limits. Equipment for automated multiple development is commercially available.

For drug mixtures that span a wide retention range, some form of gradient development is required to separate all the components in either a single chromatogram or in separate chromatograms for successive developments. Continuous solvent-composition gradients, as commonly employed in HPLC, are used rarely in TLC. These require experimental conditions that

Table 13.7 Multiple development techniques

Method	Features
Multiple chromatography	Fixed development length Same mobile phase for each development The number of developments can be varied Drugs that are difficult to separate should be repeatedly developed with solvents that produce low R_F values corresponding to the most selective mobile phase for the separation The maximum zone centre separation for two drugs of similar migration properties occurs when the zones have migrated 0.63 of the solvent front migration distance
Incremental multiple development	Variable development length: (a) first development is the shortest; (b) each subsequent development is increased by a fixed distance; (c) last development length corresponds to the maximum useful development distance Same mobile phase for each development The number of developments can be varied Provides better separations than multiple chromatography
Increasing solvent-strength gradients	Uses incremental multiple development Fractionates sample into manageable subsets Optimises separation of each subset Complete separation of all components is not achieved at any segment in the development sequence
Decreasing solvent-strength gradients	Uses incremental multiple development First development employs the strongest solvent with a weaker solvent for each subsequent step Final separation recorded as a single chromatogram

are less convenient than those for mobile-phase step gradients. In addition, step gradients can be constructed easily to mimic a continuous linear gradient, with the added advantage that the zone refocusing effect can be employed to minimise zone broadening. Gradients of increasing solvent strength are used to fractionate complex mixtures by separating just a few components in each step. Individual drugs are usually identified and quantified at the intermediate steps at which the drugs of interest are separated. In this way, the zone capacity can be made much larger than predicted for a complete separation recorded as a single chromatogram. However, this approach is tedious when many components are of interest and it is difficult to automate. Alternatively, if incremental multiple development is used, the sample can be separated for the shortest distance in the strongest mobile phase, with each subsequent, longer development using mobile phases of decreasing solvent strength. This strategy is most useful when the final separation is to be recorded as a single chromatogram, but it is limited in zone capacity because all the components must be located between the sample origin and the final solvent front. The two approaches for exploiting solvent-strength gradients are thus complementary and selection is made based on the properties of the sample. The decreasing solvent-strength gradient approach is the operating basis of automated multiple-development (AMD) chambers.

In two-dimensional TLC the sample is spotted at the corner of the layer and developed along one edge of the plate. The solvent is then evaporated, and the plate is rotated through 90° and redeveloped in the orthogonal direction. If the same solvent is used for both developments, the sample is redistributed along a line from the corner at which the plate was spotted to the corner diagonally opposite (see Fig. 13.8). In this case, only a small increase in resolution can be anticipated. For a more efficient separation system, the resolved sample should be distributed over the entire plate surface. This can be achieved only if the selectivity of the separation mechanism is complementary in the orthogonal directions. Using two solvent systems with complementary selectivity is the simplest approach for this, but it is often only partially successful. In many cases the two solvent systems differ only in their intensity for a given set of properties and are not truly orthogonal. Chemically bonded layers can be used in the reversed-phase and normal-phase modes, and these enable the use of additives and buffers as a further way to adjust selectivity. The acceptance of two-dimensional TLC for quantitative analysis will depend, though, on providing a convenient method for in-situ detection and data analysis. It seems unlikely that two-dimensional development will be more widely used in TLC, except for qualitative analysis, until the problems of detection are solved.

Development chambers

The development process in TLC can be carried out in a variety of vessels that differ significantly in design and sophistication. For convenience these are often categorised under the headings of normal (N-chamber) and sandwich (S-chamber), and further subdivided according to whether the internal atmosphere is saturated (N_S or S_S) or unsaturated (N_U or S_U). Sandwich chambers have a depth of gas phase in front of the layer of less than 3 mm, with other chamber designs indicated as normal chambers. Saturation of the vapour phase is achieved by using solvent-saturated pads or filter papers as a chamber lining.

The twin-trough chamber is the most popular of the simplest TLC developing chambers. It consists of a standard rectangular developing tank with a raised, wedge-shaped bottom. The wedged bottom divides the tank into two compartments, so that it is possible either to develop two plates simultaneously or to use one compartment to condition the layer prior to development (Fig. 13.9).

The horizontal developing chamber (Fig. 13.10) can be used in either the normal or sandwich

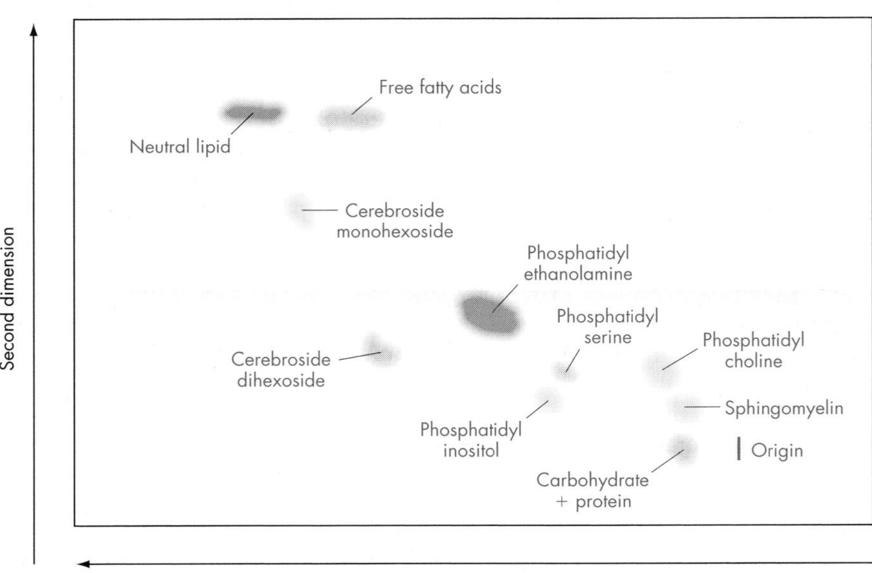

Figure 13.8 Two-dimensional TLC as illustrated by the separation of lipid compounds. (Adapted from Parsons and Patton 1967.)

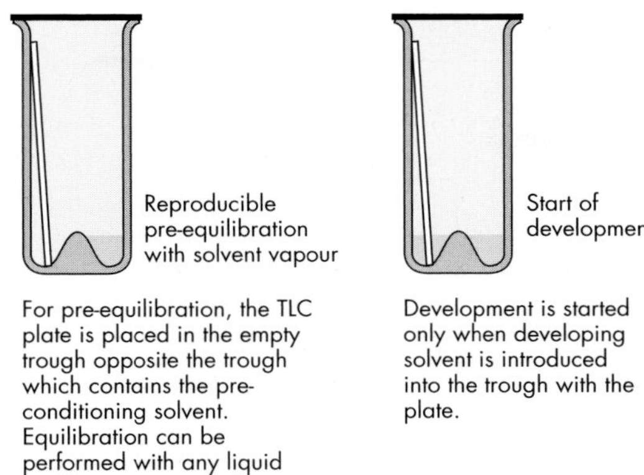

Reproducible pre-equilibration with solvent vapour
Start of development
For pre-equilibration, the TLC plate is placed in the empty trough opposite the trough which contains the pre-conditioning solvent. Equilibration can be performed with any liquid and for any period of time.
Development is started only when developing solvent is introduced into the trough with the plate.

Figure 13.9 Diagram showing pre-equilibration of plate and development in twin trough tank.

configuration for either conventional edge-to-edge or simultaneous edge-to-centre development. Starting the development simultaneously from opposite edges allows the number of samples separated to be doubled in the same time. The sandwich configuration of the horizontal developing chamber is not suitable for mobile phases that contain volatile acids, bases or large amounts of volatile polar solvents, such as methanol or acetonitrile, because of the restricted access of the saturated vapour phase to the dry portion of the separation layer.

The automated developing chamber increases laboratory productivity and improves the reproducibility of separations by providing precise control of layer conditioning, mobile-phase composition, solvent-front migration distance and drying conditions. This chamber can be used in the normal or sandwich configuration with all the operational features preselected on a microprocessor-based control unit and monitored by sensor technology.

The AMD chamber (Fig. 13.11) provides the necessary conditions and control for automated separations by incremental multiple development with a decreasing solvent-strength gradient. The operating parameters of layer conditioning, solvent-front migration distance, mobile-phase composition and drying time for each development, and the total number of developments for the separation, are entered into the computer-based control unit. The complete separation sequence is carried out without further intervention. Each development is typically 3–5 mm longer than the previous one and, depending on the complexity of the desired mobile phase gradient, a total of 10–30 developments is used, which requires 1.5–4.5 h for completion.

Detection

About 1–10 μg of substances derivatised to form a coloured product can be detected by visual inspection of a TLC plate. The quantitative reproducibility is rarely better than 10–30%. This may be adequate for qualitative methods, but for reliable quantification, in-situ spectrophotometric methods are preferred as they are more accurate and far less tedious and time consuming than excising zones from the layer

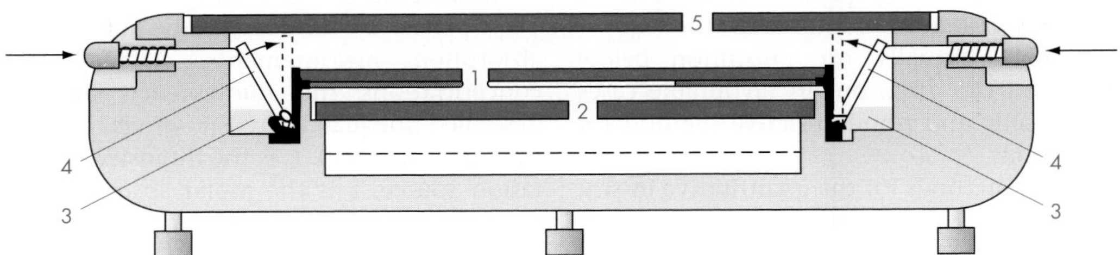

Figure 13.10 Illustration of a horizontal developing chamber: **1**, TLC plate; **2**, removable counter plate to convert the chamber from normal to sandwich configuration; **3**, mobile-phase reservoirs; **4**, glass slide to direct mobile phase flow; **5**, glass cover plate. Raising the glass slide (4) to contact the edge of the layer (1) causes the mobile phase to flow through the layer from the solvent reservoir (3). If both glass slides are raised simultaneously, development occurs from both sides to the middle, which allows the simultaneous development of samples applied along the two edges of the layer.

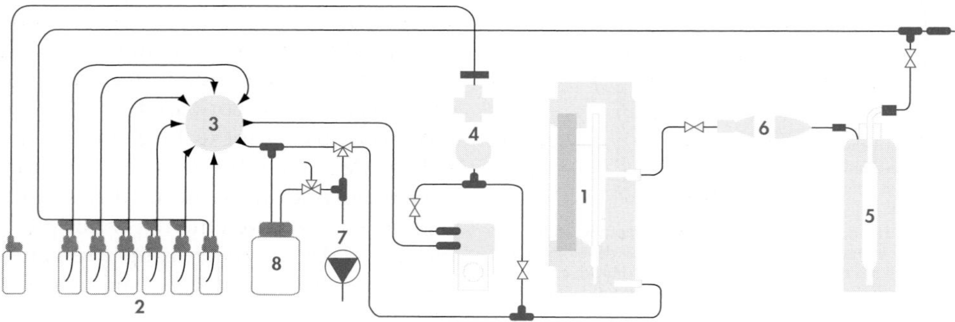

Figure 13.11 Illustration of the automated multiple-development chamber: **1**, developing chamber; **2**, solvent reservoirs; **3**, solvent-selection valve; **4**, solvent mixer; **5**, wash bottle for preparation of the gas phase for layer conditioning; **6**, gas-phase reservoir; **7**, vacuum pump; **8**, solvent waste reservoir. All operations of this chamber are managed by a programmable control unit and initiated as time sequences. A sequence starts with a conditioning step in which the vapour phase stored in reservoir (5) is pumped into the developing chamber (1). During conditioning the mobile-phase composition is mixed by withdrawing the desired solvents from their storage bottles (2) and transferring the desired volumes to the mixer. At the selected time the mobile phase is pumped into the developing chamber and ascends the layer to the desired height, determined by an optical position monitor. The solvent is then drained from the chamber to waste (8) and the vacuum pump (7) engaged to remove solvent vapours from the chamber. The next segment of the sequence is then commenced according to the program entered into the control unit, until all the segments are complete and the separation is finished.

for determination by conventional solution spectrophotometry.

A fluorescence-quenching technique can be used for detection. This involves visualisation of UV-absorbing compounds on TLC plates that incorporate a fluorescent indicator. The zones of UV-absorbing substance appear dark against the brightly fluorescing background of a lighter colour when the plate is exposed to UV light of short wavelength. The method is not universal, since it requires overlap between the absorption bands of the indicator (λ_{max} ~ 280 nm with virtually no absorption below 240 nm) and the drug, but in favourable cases it is a valuable and nondestructive method for zone location.

All optical methods for the quantitative in-situ evaluation of TLC chromatograms are based upon measuring the difference in optical response between a sample-free region of the layer and regions of the layer in which separated substances are present. Reflectance measurements can be made at any wavelength from the UV to the near infrared (185 to 2500 nm). The relationship between signal and sample amount in the absorption mode is nonlinear, and does not conform to any simple equation. The principal method of quantification in TLC is by calibration using a series of standards that span the concentration range of the drug to be determined. The calibration curve is usually based on a second-order polynomial fit for the calibration standards, with individual samples quantified by interpolation only.

The determination of drugs that fluoresce on TLC plates is fundamentally different from absorption measurements. At low sample concentrations the fluorescence signal F is described adequately by $F = \varphi I_0 \varepsilon b C$, where φ is the quantum yield, I_0 is the intensity of the excitation source, ε is the molar absorption coefficient, b is the thickness of the TLC layer and C is the sample amount. With the exception of the sample amount, all terms in this expression are constant, or fixed by the experiment, and therefore the fluorescence emission is linearly dependent on the sample amount (over two or three orders of magnitude).

Derivatisation reactions

There is a long history of the use of derivatisation reactions in TLC to visualise colourless compounds. Many of these reactions are of a qualitative nature, which was not a problem when TLC was used rarely for quantification. Some of these reactions have been adapted to the demands of quantitative scanning densitometry, as either pre- or post-chromatographic treatments, and new reagents and methods have been added specifically for quantitative measurements in TLC.

In post-chromatographic reactions the reagents can be applied to the layer through the gas phase or by evenly coating the layer with a solution of the reagents. Gas-phase methods are fast and convenient but are restricted by the number of useful reagents. Examples include iodine, ammonia and hydrogen chloride, which are applied by inserting the layer into a tank that contains a saturated atmosphere of the reactive vapour. Spraying or dipping are used to apply reagents in solution to the layer. Spray techniques that use simple atomisers have long been used in TLC, but application of reagent by this method is quite difficult to perform well. The homogeneity of the reagent distribution over the layer depends on many factors, such as the droplet size, distance between the spray device and layer, direction of spraying and discharge rate of the reagent. If ventilation of the workspace is inadequate, spray techniques can be a potential health hazard. For quantitative analysis, immersion of the layer into a solution of the reagents in a controlled manner, referred to as dipping, is the preferred technique, since it does not rely on manual dexterity and produces superior results in scanning densitometry. Some spray reagents do not make good dipping solutions because they contain solvents that are too aggressive or viscous for convenient application (aqueous concentrated acids and bases, for example). Dipping solutions are usually less concentrated than spray reagents and water is often replaced by an alcohol for adequate permeation of reversed-phase layers. In general, it is necessary to reformulate spray solutions in order to produce suitable solutions for dipping and, possibly, to change the reaction conditions. Automated low-volume dipping chambers provide a uniform speed and dwell time for the immersion process; this typically requires only a few seconds and is long enough to impregnate the layer with solution but not long enough to wash sample components off the layer.

Post-chromatographic derivatisation reactions can be classified as reversible or destructive depending on the type of interaction between the reagents and separated drugs, and as selective or universal based on the specificity of the reaction. The most common reversible methods employ iodine vapour, water, fluorescein, or pH indicators as visualising reagents. In the iodine vapour method, the dried plate is enclosed in a chamber that contains a few crystals of iodine; components on the chromatogram are stained more rapidly than the background and appear as yellow–brown spots on a light yellow background. Removal of the plate from the visualisation chamber and allowing the iodine to evaporate can reverse the reaction.

Spraying a TLC plate with water reveals hydrophobic compounds as white spots on a translucent background when the water-moistened plate is held against the light.

Solutions of pH indicators (e.g. bromocresol green, bromophenol blue) are widely used to detect acidic and basic drugs.

Irreversible methods are more common for quantification and comprise hundreds of reagents based on selective chemistries, although this number has reduced to relatively few standard visualisation operations in routine use. Some typical examples used in drug identification are summarised in Table 13.8. Reagents that are specific to functional groups or selective for compound classes can be applied to determine low levels of substances in complex matrices such as biological fluids and plant extracts.

The fluorescence response for drugs and their derivatives on TLC layers is sometimes less than that expected from solution measurements; it is observed at different excitation and emission wavelengths from those used in solution; and it may decrease with time. Adsorption onto the sorbent layer provides additional nonradiative pathways for the dissipation of the excitation energy, which is most probably lost as heat to the surroundings and reduces the observed fluorescence signal. The extent of fluorescence

Table 13.8 Some common visualisation reagents for drug identification in TLC

Name	Reagent	Application
Bratton–Marshall	2% *N*-(1-Naphthyl)ethylenediamine dihydrochloride in ethanol (95%)	Aromatic and primary amines, sulfonamides, benzodiazepines
Tillman	Dissolve 0.1 g of sodium salt of 2,6-dichlorophenol indophenol in 100 mL of ethanol	Organic acids
Dragendorff	(a) 17% (w/v) bismuth nitrate in 20% aqueous acetic acid (b) 40% (w/v) potassium iodide in water Mix 4 parts of (a) with 1 part of (b) and 14 parts of water	Alkaloids, miscellaneous, drugs
Fast Black K	0.5% (w/v) aqueous solution of Fast Black K salt	Aliphatic primary and secondary amines, amphetamines and phenols and heterocyclics
Fluorescamine	(a) 25 mg of fluorescamine in 100 mL acetone	Primary amines, sulfonamides
FPN	(a) 0.05 M ferric chloride solution (b) 5% (w/v) perchloric acid Mix 1 part (a) with 50 parts (b)	Phenothiazines, dibenzazepines
Platinic chloride	(a) 5% (w/v) aqueous platinic chloride solution (b) 10% (w/v) aqueous potassium iodide Mix 5 mL of (a) with 45 mL of (b) and dilute to 100 mL with water	Quaternary ammonium compounds, alkaloids
Acidified platinic chloride (acidified iodoplatinate)	As for platinic chloride but add 5 mL conc. HCl to the final solution	As above
Mandelin	Dissolve 1.2 g ammonium metavanadate in 95 mL of water and carefully add 5 mL of concentrated sulfuric acid	Acid drugs
Marquis	Add 0.2–1.0 mL of 37% formaldehyde solution carefully to 10 mL of concentrated sulfuric acid	Alkaloids, beta-blockers, amfetamines, phenothiazines
Ninhydrin	0.5 g ninhydrin plus 10 mL HCl diluted to 100 mL with acetone	Primary and secondary amines
Potassium permanganate, acidified	1 g potassium permanganate in 100 mL 0.25 M sulfuric acid	Drugs with unsaturated aliphatic bonds
Van Urk	Dissolve 1 g *p*-dimethylaminobenzaldehyde in 100 mL ethanol and add 10 mL concentrated HCl	Indoles, amines, sulfonamides, pesticides

quenching often depends on the sorbent used for the separation and is generally more severe for silica gel than for chemically bonded sorbents. In most cases, impregnating the stationary-phase layer with a viscous liquid, such as liquid paraffin or Triton X-100, before evaluating the separation enhances the emission signal (in favourable cases 10- to 200-fold). The general mechanism of fluorescence enhancement is assumed to be dissolution of the sorbed solute with enhancement in response being due to the fraction of solute that is transferred to the liquid phase, where fluorescence quenching is less severe. Viscous solvents are employed to minimise zone broadening from diffusion in the liquid phase during the measurement process.

Slit-scanning densitometers

Commercial instruments for scanning densitometry usually allow measurements in the reflectance mode by absorbance or fluorescence. Most instruments employ grating monochromators for wavelength selection and spectrum recording in the absorbance mode. For fluorescence measurements, a filter which transmits the emission wavelength envelope but attenuates the excitation wavelength is placed between the detector and the plate. The separations are scanned at selectable speeds up to about 10 cm/s by mounting the plate on a movable stage controlled by stepping motors. A fixed sample beam is shaped into a rectangular area on the plate surface, through which the plate is transported in the direction of development. Each scan, therefore, represents a lane of length defined by the solvent-front migration distance and width by the slit dimensions of the source.

The data from scanning densitometry can be plotted as a densitogram, i.e. a plot of absorbance (y-axis) versus distance (x-axis) (Fig. 13.6). It resembles the chromatograms obtained by GC and HPLC separations, but in these separations the x-axis is time. Standards are typically run alongside samples. The area under the curve is computed for the samples, plotted to give a calibration line and then sample values interpolated from the calibration line. TLC with scanning densitometry permits the use of internal standards, provided an internal standard is selected that can be visualised in the same way as the samples (e.g. if it is derivatised in the same way or if it fluoresces). If an internal standard is used, the absorbance ratio of the peak area of the standard substance/peak area of the internal standard is plotted on the y-axis of the calibration. Scanning densitometers can also record a spectrum of the substance corresponding to each spot. This can help determine spot purity by comparing the sample spectrum with that of a standard analysed alongside and/or help in identifying the substance.

Distorted chromatograms can be corrected by track optimisation, in which the sample zones are integrated as if the slit had moved along an optimum track from peak maximum to peak maximum. In modern TLC the relative standard deviation from all errors, instrumental and chromatographic, can be maintained below 2–3%, which makes it a very reliable quantitative tool.

Image analysers

For image analysers, scanning takes place electronically using a combination of a computer with video digitiser, light source, monochromators and appropriate optics to illuminate the plate and focus the image onto a charged-coupled-device (CCD) video camera. The captured images are initialised, stored and transformed by the computer into chromatographic data. Background subtraction and thresholding are common data-transformation processes. Image analysers provide fast data acquisition, simple instrument design and convenient software tools that search and compare sample images. Technological limitations currently prevent image analysers from competing with mechanical scanners in terms of sensitivity, resolution and available wavelength-measuring range. They have proved popular for less-demanding tasks, for the development of field-portable instruments and as a replacement for photographic documentation of TLC separations.

Other instrumental detection methods

Radioisotope-labelled drugs and their metabolites can be detected selectively with good sensitivity by imaging detectors that use windowless gas-flow proportional counters as detectors. The proportional counter is filled with a mixture of argon and methane gas, which is ionised locally by collision with beta or gamma rays produced by radioactive decay in the sample zones that contain radioisotopes. The local bursts of ionised gas molecules are sensed by a position-sensitive detector and stored in computer memory. These signals are accumulated for quantitative measurements.

Flame ionisation has been used to detect samples of low volatility that lack a chromophore for optical detection. The separation is performed on specially prepared, thin, quartz rods with a surface coating of sorbent attached by sintering. The rods are developed in the normal way, usually held in a support frame that also serves as the scan stage after the rods have been removed from the developing chamber and dried. The rods are moved at a controlled speed through a hydrogen flame and the signal is processed in a similar manner to that with the flame ionisation detector used in gas chromatography. The linear working range of the detector is about 3–30 μg for most substances. There are few reported applications in drug analysis.

General interfaces are available for the in-situ measurement of mass, infrared and Raman spectra of separated zones on TLC plates. Individual results in terms of sensitivity and spectral quality are impressive, but none of these methods is used routinely in drug analysis laboratories. This is a possible area for development.

Identifying the separated substances

The R_F value is affected too adversely by measurement difficulties and by variations in experimental and environmental conditions to be a useful identification parameter on its own. When standard substances are available, it is common practice to run standards and samples in the same system for improved confidence in identification based on R_F values. If scanning densitometry is used, an acceptable agreement in R_F values is generally supported by the automated matching of specific absorbance ratios or full spectra for the samples and standards.

In drug-screening programmes, in which simultaneous separation of standards and samples is impractical, the certainty of drug identification is improved by simultaneous separation of a series of related standard substances that allow the experimental R_F values to be corrected to standardised R_F values from automated library searches:

$$hR_F(X)^c = hR_F(A)^c + [\Delta^c/\Delta][hR_F(X) - hR_F(A)] \tag{13.2}$$

where

$$\Delta^c = hR_F(B)^c - hR_F(A)^c$$
$$\Delta = hR_F(B) - hR_F(A)$$

and $hR_F(X)$ is the R_F value for substance X, $hR_F(A)$ and $hR_F(B)$ are the R_F values for the standard substances that bracket $hR_F(X)$, and ^{c} indicates the corrected value for X and the accepted values for A and B.

Alternatively, a calibration curve of experimental R_F values against the accepted R_F values for the standards can be prepared and used to transpose experimental R_F values to corrected R_F values. Typically, four evenly spaced standard substances with the sample origin ($hR_F = 0$) and solvent front ($hR_F = 100$) are included as additional reference points.

Database searches

Database searches are used in systematic toxicological analysis to identify suspect substances in biological fluids and post-mortem tissue samples. Extracted samples are separated in one or more standard TLC systems. The corrected R_F values, often combined with the results of sequential post-chromatographic colour reactions, are then entered into the search program. The input data are automatically compared against a database of reference drugs, common metabolites, natural contaminants, etc., for identification. A number of chemometric procedures can be used for data analysis, but the most common approach is based on the mean list method.

It is assumed that the errors in individual measurements are random and can be described by a standard deviation. The precision of the separation system can then be described as the mean of the standard deviation of all substances separated in the system, called the system mean standard deviation. This allows a confidence interval or window to be assigned to the system as some multiple (typically three) of the system mean standard deviation. Each R_F value in the system database that appears in the window could be confused with the original substance. The number of substances identified as above is called the list length. Repeating the process for all R_F values in that system and averaging the individual list lengths provides the mean list length for that system. The mean list length indicates, on average, the number of substances in the database that qualify as candidates for the identification of a single drug. The shorter the mean list length, the greater the information potential of the system. Combining the results from additional retention parameters in complementary standard separation systems, colour reactions, spectroscopic data, etc., minimises the mean list length to the point that only a small number of candidate compounds for the unknown are indicated. More specific tests can then be used to identify the unknown from among the small number of indicated possibilities. For systematic drug identification in forensic toxicology, commonly two or more complementary TLC systems combined with the results from several in-situ sequential colour reactions are used. For drugs of toxicological interest, a mean list length from 2 to 10 is possible.

Systematic drug identification

One of the most difficult tasks the forensic toxicologist can face is to investigate a suspicious death when there is no information to guide them as to what substances may be present in samples submitted for analysis. The toxicologist is trying to find an answer to the question 'Is there any drug or poison present that may have contributed to death?' This is the proverbial 'needle-in-a-haystack' situation. A systematic approach must then be taken.

Systematic toxicological analysis takes advantage of the separation of an unknown substance in standard TLC systems (or other chromatographic systems) to establish the probable identity of the substance by reference to a database of candidate compounds using a statistical comparison approach, such as the mean list method. Suitable chromatographic techniques for systematic toxicological analysis must meet the following criteria:

1. The drugs must exhibit acceptable chromatographic properties in the separation system.
2. The R_F values for the drugs must be distributed evenly over the full R_F range.
3. The R_F values are standardised in such a way that good interlaboratory reproducibility is obtained.
4. When more than one separation system is used, there must be a low correlation of R_F values in the selected systems.

TLC systems that meet these requirements are described below.

Since pH-dependent extractions are customarily used in drug extraction and work-up procedures, different TLC systems are used to separate acidic and basic drugs, with neutral drugs likely to occur in both fractions. The Committee for Systematic Toxicological Analysis of The International Association of Forensic Toxicologists (TIAFT) recommended 11 separation systems for drug identification (Table 13.9). Four systems (1 to 4a) are to separate neutral and acidic drugs and seven systems (4b to 10) are to separate neutral and basic drugs. Reference data are available for about 1600 toxicologically relevant substances. For general drug screens, the use of two separation systems with a low correlation is recommended: systems 2 and 4(a) for neutral and acidic drugs and systems 5 and 8 for neutral and basic drugs (systems 7 and 8 are nearly as good). Combining colour reactions with the TLC data improves the certainty of identification significantly. Four colour reactions are carried out on the same plate in sequence. After each step the colour is noted and encoded by means of a colour chart (1, yellow; 2, orange; 3, brown; 4, red; 5, purple; 6, black; 7, blue; 8, green; 0, no spot observed). The sequence consists of formaldehyde vapour and Mandelin's reagent, water, fluorescence under 366 nm irradiation and modified Dragendorff's reagent. Other sequential colour reactions can be encoded and utilised in the same way. The Merck Tox Screening System (MTSS) contains the TIAFT TLC database and several other useful tools for searches using other chromatographic and spectroscopic databases and user-created databases. Hard-copy lists of R_F values are also available (de Zeeuw, 1992)

Romano *et al.* (1994) presented data for 443 drugs in four TLC systems using high-performance silica gel TLC plates (Table 13.10). These systems use slight modifications of the mobile-phase compositions recommended by TIAFT. The UniTox system uses three TLC systems (Table 13.11). System 1 is designed to separate neutral and acidic drugs and systems 2 and 3 to separate basic, amphoteric and quaternary drugs. Two of the separation systems are based on reversed-phase separations designed to complement the more familiar silica gel separations. The database contains over 375 drugs of

Table 13.9 TLC systems recommended by TIAFT for systematic toxicological analysis (drug database, de Zeeuw *et al.* 1992)

TLC system						
No.	Mobile phase	Chamber type	Stationary phase	Reference compounds[a]	hR_F[c]	Error window[b]
(1)	Chloroform–acetone (4:1)	Saturated	Silica gel	Paracetamol	15	7
				Clonazepam	35	
				Secobarbital	55	
				Methylphenobarbital	70	
(2)	Ethyl acetate	Saturated	Silica gel	Sulfathiazole	20	8
				Phenacetin	38	
				Salicylamide	55	
				Secobarbital	68	
(3)	Chloroform–methanol (9:1)	Saturated	Silica gel	Hydrochlorothiazide	11	8
				Sulfafurazole	33	
				Phenacetin	52	
				Prazepam	72	
(4a)	Ethyl acetate–methanol–25% ammonia (17:2:1)	Saturated	Silica gel	Sulfadimidine	13	11
				Hydrochlorothiazide	34	
				Temazepam	63	
				Prazepam	81	
(4b)	Ethyl acetate–methanol–25% ammonia (17:2:1)	Saturated	Silica gel	Morphine	20	10
				Codeine	35	
				Hydroxyzine	53	
				Trimipramine	80	
(5)	Methanol	Unsaturated	Silica gel	Codeine	20	8
				Trimipramine	36	
				Hydroxyzine	56	
				Diazepam	82	
(6)	Methanol–*n*-butanol (3:2) containing 0.1 mol/L sodium bromide	Unsaturated	Silica gel	Codeine	22	9
				Diphenhydramine	48	
				Quinine	65	
				Diazepam	85	

(7)	Methanol–25% ammonia (100:1.5)	Saturated	Silica gel impregnated with 0.1 mol/L KOH in methanol and dried	Atropine	18	9
				Codeine	33	
				Chlorprothixene	56	
				Diazepam	75	
(8)	Cyclohexane–toluene–diethylamine (15:3:2)	Saturated	Silica gel impregnated with 0.1 mol/L KOH in methanol and dried	Codeine	6	8
				Desipramine	20	
				Prazepam	36	
				Trimipramine	62	
(9)	Chloroform–methanol (9:1)	Saturated	Silica gel impregnated with 0.1 mol/L KOH in methanol and dried	Desipramine	11	11
				Physostigmine	36	
				Trimipramine	54	
				Lidocaine	71	
(10)	Acetone	Saturated	Silica gel impregnated with 0.1 mol/L KOH in methanol and dried	Amitriptyline	15	9
				Procaine	30	
				Papaverine	47	
				Cinnarizine	65	

[a] Concentration of reference standards, 2 mg/mL of each substance.

[b] Error window defined as three times the mean standard deviation.

general toxicological interest, including a large number of amfetamines.

The Toxi-Lab system is a TLC kit for toxicological drug screening; it contains equipment for extraction, development, detection and identification. Separations are performed on unsupported, particle-embedded glass-fibre sheets with holes punched in them to receive samples and standards as extraction or reference disks. A combination of silica gel and reversed-phase separations together with sequential colour reactions is used for identification and confirmation purposes. The database is designed for computer searches with results entered in a standard format.

Pesticides are a further class of toxic substances of interest to systematic toxicological analysis because of their general availability, toxicity and potential confusion with drugs. Erdmann *et al.* (1990) developed a database for 170 commonly used pesticides separated in three standardised TLC systems (Table 13.12). The systems in Table 13.12 supplement those in Table 13.9, in which many common pesticides migrate with the solvent front. Systems 1 and 2 are recommended for general screening and system 3 for the identification of special compounds not distinguished in the first two systems.

General applications

Thousands of general and validated methods are available for the determination of drugs as pharmaceutical products and in biological fluids. Since the zone capacity of TLC systems is small, there are no general methods for drugs as a class, but there are a large number of methods for individual drugs defined by therapeutic or chemical categories. These still represent substantial diversity driven by the need to optimise selectivity for each group of substances taken for analysis. This information can provide a useful starting point for system selection, but is no general substitute for systematic method development. For these reasons universal methods for general drug analysis do not exist and earlier attempts at systematised approaches for different drug categories have failed to keep pace with the growth in number of drugs in those categories. In addition, systems recommended for the separation of individual drug categories rarely prove optimal for the separation of individual drugs and their impurities or metabolites.

Method development

What does the analyst do when the conventional systems fail to separate substances of interest? In such cases there is a need to develop a suitable method for separation. A trial-and-error approach is possible, but it is more sensible to take a systematic approach.

For TLC, the development technique to be used when analysing a sample is selected based on the number of detectable components in the mixture and their polarity range (Table 13.13). It may not be necessary to separate each and every component from one another. Depending on the aim of the separation it may only be necessary to separate the components of major interest from each other and from the less important components. The less important components may not need to be separated individually.

A single development with capillary-controlled flow may be too difficult or impossible for mixtures that contain more than eight to ten components of interest. In addition, if the range of polarities is too wide, multiple development techniques using mobile phase gradients are likely to be required to enable separation of all components.

Method development is easier if standards for the relevant compounds are available. Standards simplify zone tracking (i.e. where a component has 'run' on a plate) and enable detection characteristics and the possibility of spectroscopic resolution of incompletely separated zones to be established. Standards are also required for calibration if quantification is required and to construct spectral libraries for identification purposes. The expected concentration range of relevant compounds may indicate that derivatisation will be required in order to detect substances at the levels at which they are present in samples and to increase zone separation of neighbouring compounds if one compound is a minor component with similar migration properties to a major component.

Table 13.10 The separation systems recommended by Romano *et al.* (1994) for systematic toxicological analysis by TLC (drug database: Romano *et al.* 1994)

TLC system					
No.	Mobile phase	Chamber type	Stationary phase	Reference compounds	hR_F^c [a]
(1)	Ethyl acetate–methanol–30% ammonia (17:2:3)	Saturated	Silica gel	Morphine	25
				Strychnine	44
				Aminopyrine	70
				Cocaine	85
(2)	Cyclohexane–toluene–diethylamine (13:5:2)	Saturated	Silica gel	Clobazam	15
				Aminopyrine	29
				Mebeverine	47
				Amitriptyline	60
(3)	Ethyl acetate–chloroform (1:1)	Saturated	Silica gel	Caffeine	9
				Ketamine	24
				Flunitrazepam	44
				Prazepam	61
(4)	Acetone	Saturated	Silica gel impregnated with 0.1 mol/L KOH in methanol and dried	Imipramine	20
				Pericyazine	37
				Aminopyrine	62
				Lidocaine	78

[a] Error window estimated as 7–9% R_F^c.

Table 13.11 The UniTox system for systematic toxicological analysis by TLC (drug database, Ojanpera 1995; additional compounds (amfetamines) in Ojanpera *et al.* 1991)

TLC system						
No.	Mobile phase	Chamber type	Stationary phase	Reference compounds	hR_F[c]	Error window
(1)	Methanol–water (13:7)	Unsaturated	Octadecylsiloxane-bonded silica gel	Diazepam	16	4
				Secobarbital	35	
				Phenobarbital	54	
				Paracetamol	74	
(2)	Toluene–acetone–94% ethanol–25% ammonia (45:45:7:3)	Saturated	Silica gel	Codeine	16	5
				Promazine	36	
				Clomipramine	49	
				Cocaine	66	
(3)	Methanol–water–concentrated hydrochloric acid (50:50:1)	Unsaturated	Octadecylsiloxane-bonded silica gel	Hydroxyzine	20	4
				Lidocaine	46	
				Codeine	66	
				Morphine	81	

Table 13.12 Standardised TLC systems for the screening of pesticides (pesticide database, Erdmann *et al.* 1990)

TLC system					
No.	Mobile phase	Chamber type	Stationary phase	Reference compounds	hR_F[c]
(1)	Hexane–acetone (4:1)	Saturated	Silica gel	Triazophos	21
				Parathion-methyl	30
				Pirimiphos-methyl	49
				Quintozene	84
(2)	Toluene–acetone (19:1)	Saturated	Silica gel	Carbofuran	20
				Azinophos-methyl	42
				Methidathion	56
				Parathion-ethyl	85
(3)	Chloroform–acetone (1:1)	Saturated	Silica gel	Nicotine	11
				Ioxynil	39
				PCP	60
				Methabenzthiazuron	85

Space considerations prohibit further discussion and presentation of the many hundreds of systems for TLC and associated visualisation reagents used in toxicological analysis. The reader is referred to Moffat *et al.* (2004) for further details on solvent systems, visualisation reagents and R_F values for a wide range of drugs and poisons.

Table 13.13 Zone capacity calculated or predicted for different conditions in TLC

Development method	Dimensions	Zone capacity
Predictions from theory		
Capillary-controlled flow	1	<25
Forced flow	1	<80 (up to 150 depending on pressure limit)
Capillary-controlled flow	2	<400
Forced flow	2	Several thousand
Based on experimental observations		
Capillary-controlled flow	1	12–14
Forced flow	1	30–40
Capillary-controlled flow (AMD)	1	30–40
Capillary-controlled flow	2	About 100

A general guide to the selection of stationary phases for TLC separations is summarised in Fig. 13.12. Silica gel is generally the first choice to separate drugs of low molecular weight that are soluble in moderately polar organic solvents. Reversed-phase chromatography on chemically bonded layers is generally used to separate drugs that are difficult to separate on silica gel because of inadequate retention, inadequate selectivity or zone asymmetry. Ionic compounds and easily ionised compounds are frequently separated by reversed-phase chromatography using buffered mobile phases (weak acids and bases) or ion-pair reagents (strong acids and bases). Only a limited number of stationary phases are available for ion-exchange chromatography, which is not a widely used separation mechanism in TLC.

Since the solvent used for the separation is evaporated prior to detection, a wider range of UV-absorbing solvents are commonly used in TLC than is the case for HPLC. Solvents must be of high purity, since nonvolatile impurities and stabilisers remain sorbed to the stationary phase and can cause problems in the detection step. Multicomponent mobile phases can produce a mobile-phase gradient in the direction of development through demixing. If demixing is complete, zones with sharp boundaries are formed, which separate the chromatogram into sections of different solvent composition and therefore selectivity. Demixing effects are less apparent when saturated developing chambers are used. These considerations hinder optimisation strategies based on the composition of the mobile phases as popularised in HPLC.

The selection of a mobile phase to separate simple mixtures need not be difficult and can be arrived at quickly by guided trial and error methods. A solvent of the correct strength for a unidimensional development should be selected which migrates the sample components into the R_F range 0.2–0.8, or thereabouts and, if of the correct selectivity, distributes the sample compo-

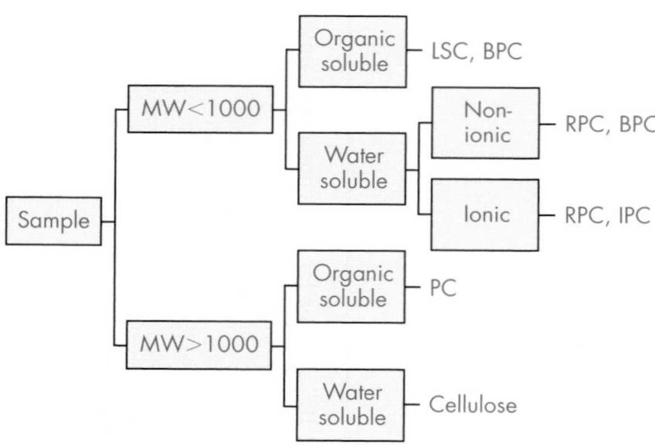

Figure 13.12 Mode selection guide for TLC. LSC, liquid–solid chromatography on an inorganic oxide layer; BPC, liquid–solid chromatography on a chemically bonded layer; RPC, reversed-phase chromatography with a chemically bonded layer and an aqueous organic mobile phase; IPC, ion-pair chromatography with reversed-phase separation conditions; PC, precipitation chromatography used to separate polymers based on solubility differences in a mobile-phase solvent gradient.

nents evenly throughout this range. Solvent systems can be screened in parallel using several development chambers, as prescribed in the PRISMA model (see Fig. 13.13) (Nyiredy *et al.* 1985a,b, 1988; Dallenbach-Tölke *et al.* 1986).

To select suitable mobile phases, the first experiments are carried out on TLC plates in unsaturated chambers with ten solvents, chosen from the different selectivity groups, indicated by bold type in Table 13.14. After these screening experiments with single solvents, the solvent strength is either reduced or increased so that the substance zones are distributed in the R_F range 0.2–0.8. If the substances migrate into the upper third of the plate, the solvent strength is reduced by dilution with hexane (the strength-adjusting solvent). If the substances remain in the lower third of the plate with the single solvents, the solvent strength is increased by the addition of a strong solvent, such as water or acetic acid. A similar procedure is followed in the reversed-phase mode, except that solvent selection is limited to water-miscible solvents and water is used as the strength-adjusting solvent. From these trial experiments, those solvents that show the best separation are selected for further optimisation in the second part of the model.

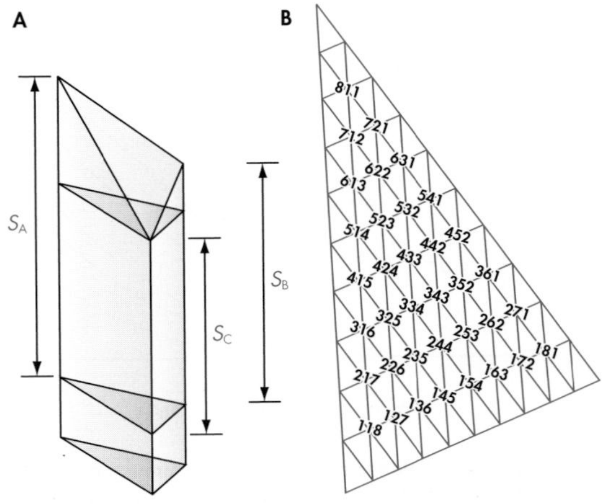

Figure 13.13 The PRISMA mobile-phase optimisation model, showing the construction of the prism and the arrangement of selectivity points on the top face or horizontal plane cut through the prism.

Table 13.14 Solvent-strength parameters and selectivity groups for solvents used for separations on silica gel

Selectivity group	Solvent
I	*n*-Butyl ether, diisopropyl ether, methyl *t*-butyl ether, **diethyl ether**
II	*n*-Butanol, **propan-2-ol**, propan-1-ol, **ethanol**, methanol
III	**Tetrahydrofuran**, pyridine, methoxyethanol, dimethylformamide
IV	**Acetic acid**, formamide
V	**Dichloromethane**, 1,1-dichloroethane
VI	**Ethyl acetate**, methyl ethyl ketone, **dioxane**, acetone, acetonitrile
VII	**Toluene**, benzene, nitrobenzene
VIII	**Chloroform**, dodecafluoroheptanol, water

Between two and five solvents can be selected to construct the PRISMA model for solvent optimisation. Modifiers required to maintain an acceptable zone shape, such as acids and ion-pair reagents, can be added in a low and constant concentration, so that their influence on solvent strength can be neglected. The PRISMA model (Fig. 13.13) is a three-dimensional geometrical design that correlates solvent strength with selectivity of the mobile phase. The model consists of three parts: the base or platform (represents the modifier), the regular part of the prism with congruent base and top surfaces, and the irregular truncated top prism (frustum). The lengths of the edges of the prism (S_A, S_B, S_C) correspond to the solvent strengths of the neat solvents (A, B, C). Since the selected solvents usually have different solvent strengths, the lengths of the edges of the prism are generally unequal and the top plane of the prism is not parallel and congruous with its base. If the prism is cut parallel to its base at the height of the lowest edge (determined by the solvent strength of the weakest solvent, solvent C in Figure 13.13, the lower part gives a regular prism, and the top and any planes, which represent weaker solvents diluted with a strength-adjusting solvent, are parallel equilateral triangles. The upper frustum of the model is used for mobile-phase optimisation of polar drugs in normal phase TLC, while the regular part is used to separate moderately polar drugs in normal-phase TLC and all separations by reversed-phase TLC.

For polar compounds, optimisation is always started on the top irregular triangle of the model, either within the triangle, when three solvents are selected, or along one side, for binary mobile phases. Any solvent composition on the face of the triangle can be represented by a three-co-ordinate selectivity point (P_S), each co-ordinate corresponding to the volume fraction of the solvent at that position on the triangle (see Fig. 13.13B). Optimisation is commenced by selecting solvent combinations that correspond to the centre point P_S = 333 and three other points close to the apexes of the triangle P_S = 811, 181 and 118. If the separation obtained is insufficient, other selectivity points are tested around the solvent combination that gave the best separation. On changing the selectivity points on the top triangle, the solvent strength changes as well, especially when the solvent strengths of the solvents used to construct the prism are significantly different. The solvent strength should be adjusted with the strength-adjusting solvent as required to maintain the separation in the optimum R_F range. Failure to obtain the beginning of a separation requires that a new prism be constructed, using a different solvent for at least one of the edges.

For reversed-phase TLC, the solvation-parameter model provides a convenient computer-aided approach to method development. Suitable water-miscible solvents with a range of selectivity include methanol, propan-2-ol, 2,2,2-trifluoroethanol, acetonitrile (or dioxane), acetone (or tetrahydrofuran) and dimethylformamide (or pyridine). For optimisation of systems (stationary phases and binary mobile phases), preliminary results in the form of system maps (a continuous plot of the system constants against mobile-phase composition) are required. System maps are a permanent record of the system properties used in all calculations and are available for most common layers and indicated solvents for selectivity optimisation. For each computer-simulated separation a retention map is calculated from the system map and displays the computed R_F values as a continuous function of the binary mobile-phase composition. A typical retention map for the computer-predicted separation of analgesics on an octadecylsiloxane-bonded layer with 2,2,2-trifluoroethanol–water mixtures as the mobile phase is shown in Figure 13.14. Solvent compositions that result in an acceptable zone separation are identified easily by visual inspection. Computer simulation of retention maps allows those systems (defined as a combination of stationary and mobile phase) likely to provide an acceptable separation to be identified before experimental work commences. The agreement between model predicted and experimental R_F values is generally good, typically better than 0.05 R_F units. A mixture-design approach is used to extend this method to ternary solvent mixtures.

For drug mixtures of a wide polarity range, stepwise changes in solvent composition are required to achieve a satisfactory TLC separation. Models to calculate migration distances using incremental multiple development with increasing and decreasing solvent-strength gradients have been described, but are complicated and not widely used. Optimised gradients for automated multiple development are usually

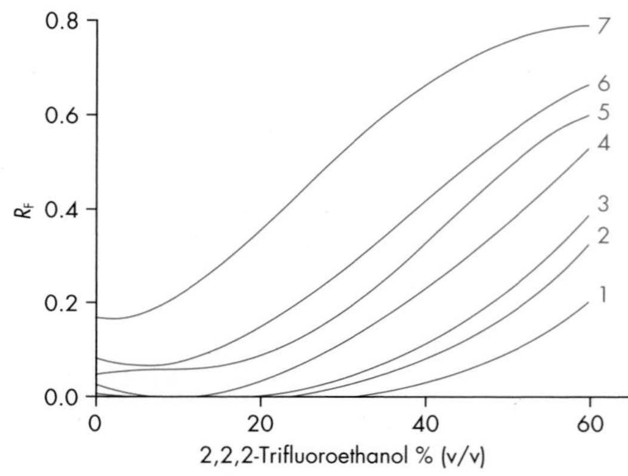

Figure 13.14 Retention map for the simulation of the separation of analgesics by reversed-phase TLC on an octadecylsiloxane-bonded layer with 2,2,2-trifluoroethanol–water as the mobile phase. **1**, Chlorphenamine (chlorpheniramine); **2**, ibuprofen; **3**, naproxen; **4**, phenacetin; **5**, aspirin; **6**, caffeine; **7**, paracetamol (acetaminophen).

arrived at by more pragmatic means. Methods based on a universal gradient commence with methanol, end with hexane, and use either dichloromethane or methyl *t*-butyl ether as the intermediate solvent for separations on silica gel. By scaling and superimposing the chromatogram of the separation above the theoretical gradient profile, those regions of the chromatogram that affect the separation are easily identified. The solvent composition for the initial and final development steps is adjusted to eliminate those portions of the gradient that do not contribute to the separation. The gradient shape is modified to enhance resolution in those regions of the chromatogram that are separated poorly or to minimise regions devoid of sample zones. For moderately complex mixtures this approach is often satisfactory. If, after the above adjustments, the separation is inadequate it is necessary to identify a more selective solvent for problem regions in the gradient. The PRISMA model can be used at this point to identify more selective solvents to incorporate into the gradient as a replacement for the initial, terminal or base solvent.

Preparative thin-layer chromatography

Preparative TLC is used mainly to purify drugs or to isolate drug metabolites and impurities in amounts of about 1–100 mg for subsequent use as reference materials, structural elucidation, biological activity evaluation and other purposes. Scale-up from analytical TLC is achieved by increasing the thickness of the layer (loading capacity increases with the square root of the layer thickness) and by increasing the plate length used for sample application. Precoated TLC plates for preparative chromatography vary in size from 20 cm × 20 cm to 20 cm × 40 cm and are coated with 0.5–10 mm thick layers, with the most popular thickness being 1.0–2.0 mm. As the average particle size (~25 μm) and size distribution (5–40 μm) are larger for preparative layers, and as sample overload conditions are used commonly in preparative chromatography, invariably inferior separations in a longer time (~1–2 h) are obtained compared with analytical separations. Resolution can be increased significantly by using wedge-shaped, gradient-thickness layers. These layers have a uniform increase in thickness from 0.3 mm at the bottom to 1.7 mm at the top. Sample bands are focused during migration by the negative mobile-phase velocity gradient created by the layer geometry.

Sample application is a critical step in preparative TLC, and if performed improperly can destroy all or part of the separation. The sample, usually as a 5–10% (w/v) solution in a volatile solvent, is applied as a band along one edge of the layer to give a maximum sample load of about 5 mg/cm for each millimetre of layer thickness. Sample loads are usually lower for difficult separations and for cellulose and chemically bonded layers. Any of the automated band applicators for analytical TLC are suitable for sample application in preparative TLC. Manual sample application by syringe or glass pipette must be performed carefully to avoid damaging the layer and producing irregularly shaped migrating zones. A short predevelopment, of about 1 cm with a strong solvent, is often useful to refocus manually applied bands. Preparative layers with a preadsorbent zone are useful for manual sample application, since the focusing mechanism can be used to correct for poor sample-application technique. In all cases, it is important that the sample solvent is evaporated fully from the layer prior to the start of the separation to avoid the formation of distorted separation zones. It is usual to leave a blank margin of 2–3 cm at each vertical edge of the plate to avoid uneven development as the solvent tends to move differentially at the edges of the plate.

Most of the changes in preparative TLC over the past decade have occurred in the method of development. Conventionally, ascending development in large-volume tanks that hold a number of preparative layers in a rack is commonly used. In laboratories that perform preparative TLC on a regular basis, higher resolution and shorter development times are achieved by using forced-flow development or rotation planar chromatography (accelerated development using centrifugal force). These methods allow conventional development and elution with on-line detection and automated fraction collection to be used.

After development, physical methods of zone detection are used to identify the sample bands of interest. Layers that contain a UV indicator for fluorescence quenching or the adsorption of iodine vapours are useful for this purpose because they are nondestructive. If a reactive spray reagent is used for visualisation, it should be sprayed on a small strip of the chromatogram only, so as not to contaminate the remainder of the material. Some form of masking arrangement can be employed to protect the area of the plate where the spray reagent is not to be applied. Once the bands of interest are located (by examining the area of the plate which has been sprayed), the corresponding zones in the non-sprayed area are scraped off the plate carefully with a spatula or similar tool. A number of devices based on the vacuum-suction principle for removing the marked zones from the plate are also available. Soxhlet extraction, liquid extraction or solvent elution with a polar solvent is used to recover drugs from the sorbent. For solvent extraction, water is often added to dampen the silica gel prior to extraction with a water-immiscible organic solvent. Chloroform and ethanol (methanol is less suitable because of its higher silica solubility) are widely used for solvent elution. Colloidal silica can be removed by membrane filtration prior to vacuum stripping of the solvent.

References

E. G. C. Clarke and M. Williams, *J. Pharm. Pharmac.*, 1955, **7**, 255–262.

CRC Handbook of Chemistry & Physics, 88th edn, D. R. Lide (ed.), Boca Raton, CRC Press, 2007.

Dallenbach-Tölke, K. Nyiredy, Sz., Meier, B. and Sticher, O., Optimization of overpressured layer chromatography of polar, naturally occurring compounds by the 'PRISMA' model, *J. Chromatogr.* 1986, **365**, 63–72.

R. A. de Zeeuw *et al.* (eds), *Thin-Layer Chromatographic R_F Values of Toxicologically Relevant Substances on Standardized Systems*, Weinheim, VCH, 1992.

F. Erdmann *et al.*, A TLC screening programme for 170 commonly used pesticides using the corrected R_F value (R_F^c value), *Int. J. Legal. Med.*, 1990, **104**, 25–31.

A. C. Moffat, M. D. Osselton and B. Widdop (eds), *Clarke's Analysis of Drugs and Poisons*, 3rd edn, London, Pharmaceutical Press, 2004.

Sz. Nyiredy *et al.*, The 'PRISMA' optimization system in planar chromatography, *J. Planar Chromatogr.*, 1988, **1**, 336–342.

Sz. Nyiredy *et al.*, 'PRISMA': Ein Modell zur Optimierung der mobilen Phase für die Dünnschichtchromatographie, vorgestellt anhand verschiedener Naturstofftrennungen, *Planta Med.*, 1985a; **51**, 241–246.

Sz. Nyiredy *et al.*, 'PRISMA': A geometrical design for solvent optimization in HPLC, *HRC & CC* 1985b, **8**, 186–188.

I. Ojanpera, Thin-layer chromatography in forensic toxicology, in *Practical Thin-Layer Chromatography. A Multidisciplinary Approach*, B. Fried and J. Sherma (eds), Boca Raton, CRC Press, 1995, pp. 193–230.

I. Ojanpera *et al.*, Screening for amphetamines with a combination of normal and reversed phase thin-layer chromatography and visualization with Fast Black K salt, *J. Planar Chromatogr.*, 1991, **4**, 373–378.

C. L. O'Neal *et al.*, Validation of twelve chemical spot tests for the detection of drugs of abuse, *Forensic Sci. Int.*, 2000, **109**, 189–201.

J. Parsons and S. Patton, Two-dimensional thin-layer chromatography of polar lipids from milk and mammary tissue, *J. Lipid Res.*, 1967, **8**, 696–698.

G. Romano *et al.*, Qualitative organic analysis. Part 3. Identification of drugs and their metabolites by PCA of standardised TLC data, *J. Planar Chromatogr.*, 1994, **7**, 233–241.

UN, *Rapid Methods of Drugs of Abuse. A manual for use by national law enforcement and narcotic laboratory personnel.* A United Nations Publication, St/Nar/13/Rev.1, 1994.

WHO, *Basic Tests for Drugs*, Geneva, World Health Organization, 1998.

Further reading

Colour tests

F. Bamford, *Poisons, Their Isolation and Identification*, 3rd edn, London, Churchill, 1951.

K. W. Bentley, *The Chemistry of Morphine Alkaloids*, Oxford, Clarendon Press, 1954.

E. G. C. Clarke, The isolation and identification of alkaloids, in *Methods of Forensic Science*, Vol. 1, F. Lundquist (ed.), London, Wiley, 1962, pp. 1–241.

P. W. Enders, A simple color test on quaternary ammonium compounds, in *Reports on Forensic Toxicology*,

H. and R. Brandenberger (eds), Mannedorf, Branson Research, 1985, pp. 195–198.

F. Fiegl, *Spot Tests in Organic Analysis*, 7th edn, Amsterdam, Elsevier, 1966.

F. Fiegl and V. Anger, *Spot Tests in Inorganic Analysis*, 6th edn, New York, Elsevier, 1972.

R. F. Flanagan *et al.*, *Basic Analytical Toxicology*, Geneva, World Heath Organization, 1995.

T. A. Gonzales *et al.*, Colour reactions for the identification of non-volatile organic poisons, in *Legal Medicine, Pathology and Toxicology*, 2nd edn, New York, Appleton–Century–Crofts, 1954, pp. 1191–1255.

S. H. Johns *et al.*, Spot tests: a colour chart reference for forensic chemists, *J. Forensic Sci.*, 1979, **24**, 631–649.

C. A. Johnson and A. D. Thornton-Jones (eds), *Drug Identification*, London, Pharmaceutical Press, 1966.

F. Musshoff *et al.*, Hallucinogenic mushrooms on the German market – simple instructions for examination and identification, *Forensic Sci. Int.*, 2000, **113**, 389–395.

E. G. Saker and E. T. Solomons, A rapid inexpensive presumptive test for phencyclidine and certain other cross-reacting substances, *J. Anal. Toxicol.*, 1979, **3**, 220–221.

B. C. Sangalli, A new look at qualitative toxicology. Spot tests in the emergency department, *Vet. Hum. Toxicol.*, 1989, **31**, 445–448.

E. Stair and M. Whaley, Rapid screening and spot tests for the presence of common poisons, *Vet. Hum. Toxicol.*, 1990, **32**, 564–566.

I. Sunshine (ed.), *Methodology for Analytical Toxicology*, Cleveland, CRC Press, 1975.

US Department of Justice, *NILECJ Standard for Chemical Spot Tests for Preliminary Identification of Drugs of Abuse*, Washington DC, US Department of Justice, July, 1978.

US Department of Justice, *NILECJ Standard for Chemical Spot Tests for Preliminary Identification of Drugs of Abuse*, Washington DC, US Department of Justice, July, 1981.

Thin-layer chromatography

R. A. de Zeeuw *et al.*, Potential and pitfalls of chromatographic techniques and detection modes in substance identification for systematic toxicological analysis. *J. Chromatogr. A*, 1994, **674**, 3–13.

B. Fried and J. Sherma (eds), *Practical Thin-Layer Chromatography. A Multidisciplinary Approach*, Boca Raton, CRC Press, 1995.

F. Geiss, *Fundamentals of Thin-layer Chromatography*, Heidelberg, Huethig, 1987.

H. Jork *et al.*, *Thin-Layer Chromatography Reagents and Detection Methods*, Weinheim, VCH, Vol. 1 1990; Vol. 2 1992.

O. H. Klungel *et al.*, The potential of the X-rite reflection spectrometer in systematic toxicological analysis by thin-layer chromatography, *J. Planar Chromatogr.*, 1993, **6**, 112–116.

Sz. Nyiredy, *Planar Chromatography. A Retrospective for the Third Millennium*, Budapest, Springer Medical, 2001.

C. F. Poole, *The Essence of Chromatography*, Amsterdam, Elsevier, 2003.

C. F. Poole, Planar chromatography at the turn of the century, *J. Chromatogr. A*, 1999, **856**, 399–427.

C. F. Poole and N. C. Dias, Practitioner's guide to method development in thin-layer chromatography, *J. Chromatogr. A*, 2000, **892**, 123–142.

E. Reich and A. Schibli, *High Performance Thin-Layer Chromatography for the Analysis of Medicinal Plants*, New York, Thieme, 2006.

J. Sherma and B. Fried (eds), *Handbook of Thin-Layer Chromatography*, 3rd edn, Routledge, USA, 2003.

H. Wagner *et al.*, *Plant Drug Analysis*, Berlin, Springer-Verlag, 1984.

I. D. Wilson *et al.*, *Encyclopaedia of Separation Science*, Vols 1–10, London, Academic Press, 2000.

14

Immunoassays

C Hand and D Baldwin

Introduction 375
Basic principles of immunoassay 377
Heterogeneous immunoassays 382
Homogeneous immunoassays 386
Automation of immunoassay 388
Analysis of alternative samples to urine 388
Quality control, calibration, standardisation and curve fitting 389
References 391

Introduction

Immunoassays have a firm place among routine methods for the analysis of drugs in biological fluids and other matrices. The technique may be used by the smallest or largest of laboratories, with methods that range from single-use point-of-care tests for the analysis of a single sample to fully automated systems capable of analysing thousands of samples per day. Regardless of format, all immunoassays are based on the interaction of a target molecule (antigen) with a corresponding antibody.

When applied to drug testing, competitive immunoassay techniques are normally used. These use an antibody specific for the drug or drug class being assayed, and a labelled form of the same drug or a labelled form of the antibody to generate a measurable signal. Immunoassays are also often referred to in terms of the method used to detect whether the drug under study is present. Radioimmunoassay (RIA) and enzyme-linked immunosorbent assay (ELISA) are examples. RIA is popular because of its high sensitivity, its ability to analyse large numbers of samples rapidly and also because preliminary extraction stages are not required. The drug immunoassay involves setting up a competition for binding to the antibody between antigen (drug) in the sample and a fixed amount of antigen added as part of the test system (Fig. 14.1). Labelling of this added antigen or antibody with a suitable marker and measuring the signal generated by a suitable analytical measurement enables results to be compared with a calibration curve made from a set of standards with known amounts of added drug. Alternatively, the result from a sample or set of samples can be compared with a single-point 'cut-off' calibrator to give a simple positive or negative qualitative result. The technique is capable of high sensitivity, with μg/L quantities easily detectable and ng/L possible with specialist assays.

The basic technique consists of placing a fixed quantity of an antibody in a tube together with a fixed quantity of the labelled drug, and the test sample that contains the drug to be assayed. The specific binding sites on the antibody bind both the labelled drug molecules and the unlabelled drug molecules present in the test sample. The proportion of labelled drug molecules bound is inversely proportional to the number of unlabelled drug molecules.

Immunoassays are divided into two types depending on whether, after the antibody binding reaction has taken place, there is a need to separate the bound and free fractions of the assay before measuring the signal: in RIAs, the radioactivity is measured. However, there is no difference between the signals produced by bound and free labelled drug so that it is necessary to separate the two before measurement. These assays are referred to as heterogeneous immunoassays. Since the amount of radiolabelled drug that remains in the solution, or is bound to the antibody, depends on the concentration of unlabelled drug, measurement of the radiolabelled drug in either the bound or the free form gives an estimate of the original concentration of unlabelled drug. Heterogeneous immunoassays (see below) using non-isotopic labels have widely replaced RIA, but in this case it is the bound fraction that is measured because a large excess of enzyme is present in the free fraction. With RIA, a calibration curve is constructed in which the percentage of labelled drug bound to the antibody is plotted against the concentration of drug (Fig. 14.2).

For assays in which the drug is labelled with an enzyme or a fluorescent substance, the measurement is of an optically detected change, such as ultraviolet absorption, fluorescence or luminescence. In certain types of optical immunoassays, there is a difference between the signals generated by the free and the bound labelled drug. Thus, no separation step is necessary and these are referred to as homogeneous immunoassays. The difference between the signals may arise because the signal can be suppressed on binding, produced on binding, or altered on binding.

Immunoassays for drugs can therefore be separated into two main groups:

- homogeneous immunoassays do not require antibody-bound antigen and free (unbound) antigen to be separated before measurement of the signal
- heterogeneous immunoassays require the separation of antibody-bound and free antigen before measurement of the signal.

Both types of assay have wide application in the drug-testing field, each with its advantages and disadvantages. Detailed descriptions of different types of assay within each group are given below.

Immunoassays offer a flexible approach to the analysis of various biological fluids for the presence or absence of drugs. They provide a rapid and convenient method to screen large numbers of samples in a variety of matrices and they

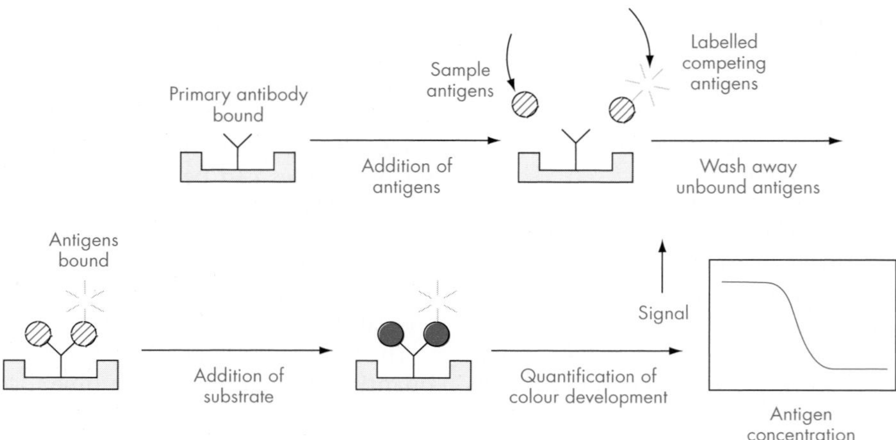

Figure 14.1 Enzyme-linked immunosorbent assay (ELISA) illustrating the principles of immunoassay. The sample is applied to the antibody which is typically coated in the wells of a 96-well plate. Labelled antigen is then added and the solution is incubated for a set period during which time the antigen (drug) and labelled antigen compete in binding to the antibody. Non-bound antigen and other non-bound substances are then washed away. The amount of bound, labelled antigen is then measured.

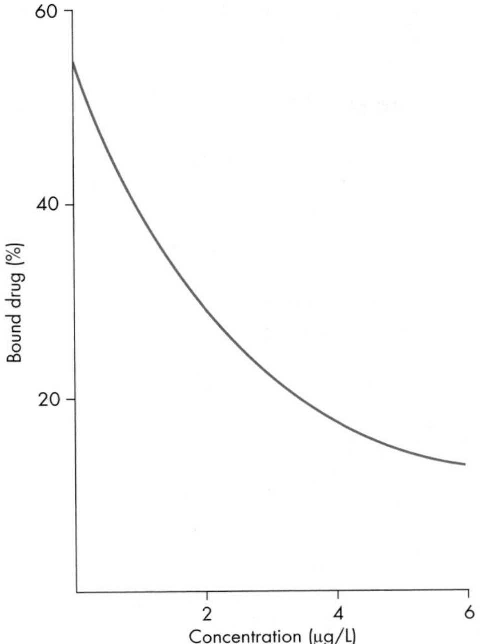

Figure 14.2 Calibration curve for an immunoassay.

allow the differentiation of negative specimens and thus avoid the need for further, more complicated and expensive processing or investigation. Where specific assays are available they can be used to quantify accurately and precisely the concentration of drug in a sample as required for therapeutic drug monitoring (TDM) in a plasma, serum or blood sample.

Immunoassay has become the method of choice for TDM and the principles and considerations described here for immunoassay are applicable to toxicology and drug screening. The main differences between these applications is the degree of quantification required (TDM requires fully quantified results), and the selection of antibodies with the required cross-reactivity profiles. For example, TDM assays may require highly specific antibodies that are reactive only with a single chemical entity, whereas immunoassays used in toxicology or drug-abuse screening may be designed to be broadly cross-reactive with a whole drug group.

Labels used in immunoassay include radioisotopes, enzymes, chemiluminescent molecules, particles (such as colloidal gold or latex beads) and fluorescent molecules. Immunoassay formats vary from systems designed for rapid point-of care testing of a single sample through to fully automated systems that can process thousands of samples per day.

The first RIA method, published by Yalow and Berson (1959), was for the analysis of insulin. This heralded the beginning of a field of analysis that is now used routinely across the disciplines of clinical chemistry, endocrinology, pharmacology and toxicology. Antibodies raised against morphine by Spector and Parker (1970) were used in the development of an immunoassay using a radioactive tracer (RIA) and many variants have followed since. From an end-user's viewpoint, the vast majority of immunoassays used today are in the form of commercially available, easy to use, automated, semi-automated or simple point-of-care tests. However, the immunochemistry used to produce these test kits involves many intricate interactions of biochemicals with the sample under test. This chapter describes the principles of immunoassay as they specifically relate to testing for the presence of drugs and discusses the major types of immunoassay in common use.

Basic principles of immunoassay

Antibody production

All immunoassays require the use of antibodies. It is this element of the system and the way in which it is produced that is the key to the performance of the assay.

Antibodies are proteins – immunoglobulins (Ig) – produced by beta-lymphocytes in response to an immunogen. There are many different immunoglobulins (IgG, IgA, IgM, IgE and IgD), but mostly IgG is used in immunoassay design. The IgG molecule can be represented simply by the letter 'Y' with two antigen binding fragments, 'Fab' (antibody binding fragment) at the top (the arms of the Y) and the 'Fc' (crystalline fragment) at the base (the stem of the Y) (Fig. 14.1) Drug molecules are too small to provoke an immune response, so drug immunogens are created by conjugation of a drug or drug derivative to a larger carrier protein to give an immunogen through a process called haptenisation. Host animals for antibody production are usually rabbits, sheep or goats for polyclonal antisera, or mice for the production of monoclonal antibodies.

Suitable carrier proteins include bovine serum albumin (BSA), immunoglobulins or keyhole limpet haemocyanin (KLH). The aim of the haptenisation process is to conjugate multiple derivatised drug molecules (the hapten) to the carrier protein. This conjugation is usually via a —COOH or —NH_2 moiety on the drug or via a similar group introduced by derivatisation.

The position on the drug molecule used for haptenisation to the protein determines the specificity of the resultant antibodies. Knowledge of the metabolism of the drug and information on structurally related compounds are important when beginning the antibody synthesis. For example, Figure 14.3 shows the molecular structure of morphine, in which the carbon atoms at positions 3, 6, 2 and the N-group are all readily amenable to derivatisation and thus enable conjugation to a carrier protein. The position through which the drug molecule is conjugated to the protein is 'hidden' from the immune system and so changes to the target molecule at the conjugation position do not usually affect the binding of the antibody.

The example of morphine is a good illustration of how this can be used to the advantage of the immunoassay developer or the analyst using the assay. If an immunogen were produced via the 3-position it would no longer be a specific determinant against which the antibodies are raised. Hence the resultant antibody is likely to display cross-reactivity with the major metabolite of both morphine and diacetylmorphine (heroin), namely morphine-3-glucuronide. It would also recognise codeine (3-*O*-methylmorphine). The production of morphine antibodies using 3-position haptenisation is used commonly to produce broad cross-reacting 'anti-opiate' antibodies. The cross-reactivity to different opiates varies from one antiserum or antibody to another. It is important that each antiserum or antibody be characterised fully by the assay developer.

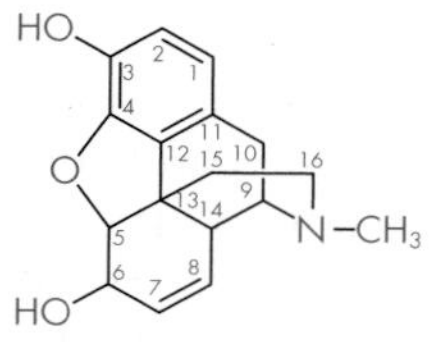

HO
O
HO
N–CH_3
1 2 3 4 5 6 7 8 9 10 11 12 13 14 15 16

Figure 14.3 Structure of morphine.

Production of morphine antibodies via the 6-position gives better specificity to morphine relative to codeine and morphine-3-glucuronide, and is expected to produce antibodies that display good cross-reactivity to 6-monoacetylmorphine and the active metabolite morphine-6-glucuronide. Both of these cross-reactions may be desirable, depending on the purpose to which the antibody is being put.

To produce a more specific assay for morphine, derivatisation and conjugation via the nitrogen group can be utilised. This leaves the 3- and 6-positions as the antigenic determinants and therefore produces antibodies that are more likely to be specific for morphine without cross-reactivity to codeine or dihydrocodeine, for example. An N-linked antiserum will, however, give potential for cross-reactivity with molecules such as normorphine, which have an alteration at the N-position.

Another consideration during antibody production is the use of a 'bridge' molecule. This is employed as a chemical spacer between the hapten and carrier protein to allow better access to the drug for potential antibodies. It is important to remember that the immune response in the host animal may also produce antibodies to the whole immunogen – not just the drug molecule – which includes the bridge molecule. Interference from 'bridge antibodies' can be avoided or minimised by using a different chemical spacer from that used in immunogen synthesis when conjugating the drug-signal reagent.

The measure of the strength of the binding between an antigen and an antibody is described by the affinity constant. This binding is non-covalent and reversible and reaches equilibrium. High-affinity antibodies bind faster than low-affinity antibodies and perform better in immunochemical methods.

Monoclonal antibodies versus polyclonal antisera

Polyclonal antisera contain a complex mixture of antibodies raised during the immunisation process. By comparison, a monoclonal antibody is a single entity that results from the isolation of a single antibody-producing cell. In drug immunoassays, the higher-affinity antibodies produced by polyclonal antisera can sometimes be preferable to the lower-affinity antibodies produced by a monoclonal system.

Polyclonal antisera

Immunisation of a rabbit or a sheep usually proceeds with 20 to 100 μg of the protein-conjugated hapten, which can be mixed with an adjuvant to stimulate the immune system. This produces an immune response that consists mainly of IgM followed by IgG. This response is further stimulated by additional immunisations of a similar or lower dose at regular intervals – typically every 3–4 weeks for 20 weeks or longer. Test bleed samples of approximately 1–2 mL are taken at 10–14 days post injection, at which point the immune response (and therefore antibody titre in the serum) is at its highest.

After analysis of the test bleeds, a larger antiserum sample can be drawn. This can be as much as several hundred millilitres when using larger host animals (e.g. sheep). Antisera yield can vary from hundreds to many thousands of tests per millilitre depending on the success of the immunisation programme and the type of assay in which they are employed. It is not the absolute volume of serum that is important, but rather the amount and quality of antibodies contained therein.

Using standard separation methods, such as ammonium sulfate precipitation, Protein A separation and/or ion-exchange chromatography, antisera can be purified for further use. Affinity chromatography can be beneficial in certain circumstances and involves passing the antiserum over a column that contains an immobilised form of the drug of interest. In this way it is possible to fractionate a complex polyclonal antiserum. In some cases purification is not necessary and the antiserum (i.e. the serum itself) can be used with simple dilution.

Monoclonal antibodies

Monoclonal antibodies offer the advantage of a continuous supply of antibodies with the same characteristics, so once a good antibody is selected it can be used indefinitely.

After immunisation and successful test bleeds, monoclonal antibodies are made by the fusion of mouse lymphocytes (or lymphocytes from other species) from the spleen with myeloma cells. The resultant hybridoma cells are separated by limiting dilution to give single cells that secrete single monoclonal antibodies. This technique was first described in 1975 and is now in routine use (Kohler and Milstein 1975).

Monoclonal antibodies generally have lower affinity than polyclonal equivalents, which can lead to less-sensitive assays. Monoclonal antibodies are not more specific than polyclonal antisera, but once a specific antibody is selected, the cell line can be stored and the antibody produced indefinitely. Note that in drug testing, it is possible for an antibody to be too specific, as it may be desirable to have broad cross-reactivity to a drug family (such as benzodiazepines) or to a single drug and its metabolites (such as buprenorphine).

Monoclonal antibodies offer the advantages of purity and homology, which is useful for circumstances in which the antibody is being labelled or conjugated as part of the immunoassay set-up – for example when being labelled with an enzyme or coated with colloidal gold.

Other molecular biology and recombinant techniques, such as phage display (Chiswell and McCafferty 1992), in which the genetic code is harnessed to produce antibodies, give an exciting additional source of this important immunoassay component.

Antibody dilution curves

Once an immunisation is underway, the quality of the antiserum is assessed by means of an antiserum dilution curve. This demonstrates the binding of the antibody to the target drug and is an indication of the antibody's affinity for the antigen. Using a heterogeneous enzyme immunoassay (EIA) as an example, a test bleed of rabbit anti-cotinine was coated onto a microplate at different dilutions in bicarbonate buffer (pH 9) using incubation overnight at room temperature. The resultant binding to different titres of horseradish peroxidase-labelled cotinine is shown in Figure 14.4. Dilutions of the enzyme–drug conjugate for this type of experiment can be made in simple phosphate buffer (pH 7.4) with a small amount of protein (e.g. BSA at 0.05% w/v) to prevent nonspecific binding (NSB) of materials to the assay tube. The hook (or apparent peak) seen in Fig. 14.4 at high antiserum concentrations is caused by a combination of steric hindrance and saturation of coating antibody to the microplate.

Once the concentration of antibody (titre) that produces the desired response is selected, it is necessary to check that the antibody also responds as required with the target drug (i.e. that the target drug successfully competes with the labelled drug for binding to the antibody). The improved performance with subsequent test bleeds for samples taken from a rabbit immunised with a buprenorphine–protein immunogen

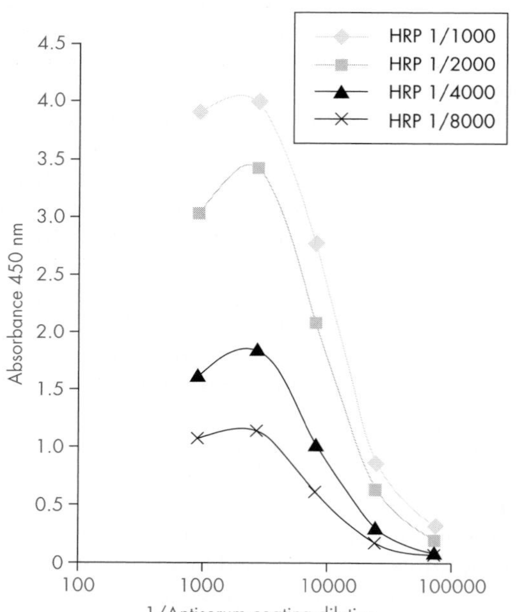

Figure 14.4 Titration curve for rabbit anti-cotinine antiserum with cotinine (HRP, horseradish peroxidase).

is shown in Figure 14.5. It is possible to gain useful information by combining both the experiments described above and analysing both a positive and negative sample at each antibody dilution. In this way, binding and displacement can be seen at each antibody titre.

Careful titring of the labelled drug derivative and antibody dilution can improve the assay characteristics, and the assay can be optimised further by the addition of other proteins, surfactants and stabilisers to the assay buffer.

An immunisation programme usually involves the injection of between three and six animals with the same antigen. If suitable antibodies are not produced after several immunisations, it may be necessary to start the programme again with different animals and possibly a different immunogen.

Analytical specificity

The analytical specificity or cross-reactivity of an immunoassay provides an indication of how the assay responds to other drugs relative to the drug used as a calibrator or standard. The cross-reactivity profile of the immunoassay is important when assessing whether it is suitable for a particular task. For example, determination of cocaine use by the analysis of a urine specimen requires the immunoassay to exhibit good cross-reactivity to the urinary metabolite benzoylecgonine. By contrast, the assay needs to demonstrate good cross-reactivity to cocaine if the samples to be analysed are saliva or hair extracts, since high concentrations of the parent drug relative to metabolites are found in these specimens.

With classic competitive immunoassays (such as RIA and EIA), cross-reactivity is often calculated relative to the amount of drug that displaces 50% of the antibody-bound signal reagent. In the drug-testing field it is common to add a known amount of drug to the assay and record what response is given. Percentage cross-reactivity is then calculated as:

$$\text{Cross reactivity (\%)} = \frac{\text{Apparent concentration of target drug}}{\text{Concentration of added drug}} \times 100 \tag{14.1}$$

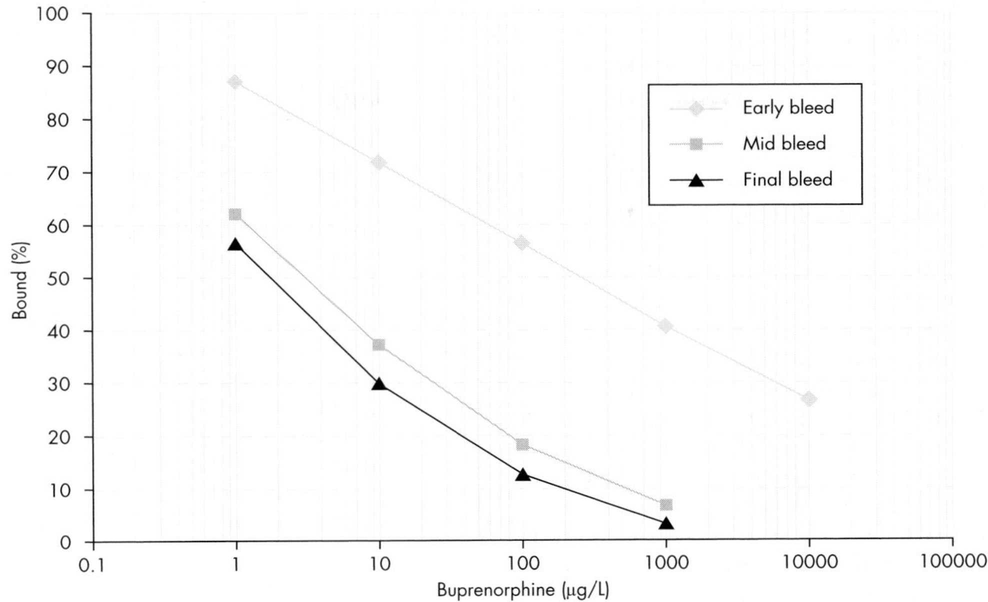

Figure 14.5 Comparison of early, mid and final test bleeds for anti-buprenorphine antisera.

For example, if in an opiate assay (calibrated with morphine standards) to which a solution of 1000 ng/mL of codeine is added as a test sample, the result from the assay read against the morphine calibration curve is 100 ng/mL, the cross-reactivity of codeine in the assay relative to morphine is 10%, i.e.

$$\text{Cross reactivity (\%)} = \frac{100\ \mu\text{g/L apparent morphine}}{1000\ \mu\text{g/L added codeine}} \times 100 = 10\,\% \tag{14.2}$$

However, for many drug immunoassays it is not sufficient to test cross-reactants at a single concentration. Several concentrations must be prepared in the sample matrix under test and the effect on the assay examined, effectively making a calibration or standard curve for each potential cross-reactant.

The graph in Figure 14.6 illustrates curves for five compounds, with compound A used as the calibrator. The important feature of many drug immunoassays is that some drugs show parallel cross-reactivity to the calibrator substance (e.g. B and E in Fig. 14.6), while others exhibit non-parallel cross-reactivity. In the example shown, compound D would have been thought to have low cross-reactivity if it had been tested at high concentrations only (1000 and 2000 µg/L). At a concentration of 10 µg/L, it is closer to 100% cross-reactive, while at low levels (1 µg/L) compound D exhibits 400% cross-reactivity relative to compound A.

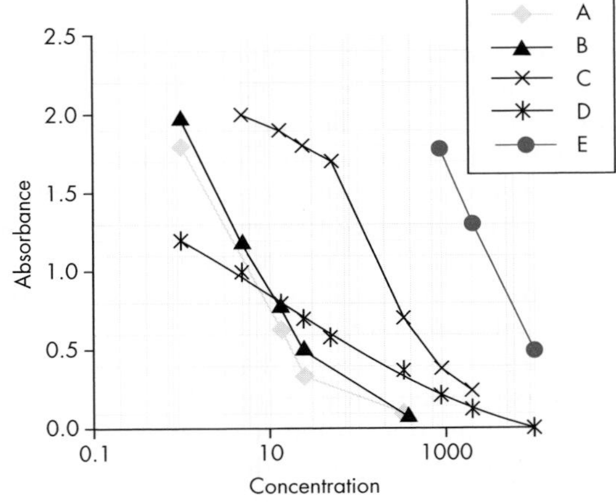

Figure 14.6 Different cross-reactivity reactions using one compound (compound A) as a reference. Concentration is µg/L.

Nonparallel cross-reactivity can be seen within a drug group for both parent drug(s) and metabolite(s). Isomeric forms can also exhibit different cross-reactivity profiles and it is common to see different reactivity between (+)-amfetamine and (−)-amfetamine.

Drugs tested for cross-reactivity indicate to the analyst which compounds might be appropriate for subsequent confirmatory analysis after a positive immunoassay result. Drugs that show little or no cross-reactivity *in vitro* can give strong immunoassay positives from people who take the drug *in vivo*. For example, benzfetamine is converted into methamfetamine and amfetamine, but the parent drug would not show cross-reactivity in many methamfetamine or amfetamine immunoassays.

The important factor with regard to antibodies from an analyst's perspective is to know the characteristics of the antibody used in the immunoassay. Knowledge of the type of immunoassay used is important when considering the next stage of the analytical process, for example gas chromatography–mass spectrometry (GC-MS). If an immunoassay is used to demonstrate the use of a drug by measuring its metabolites in urine, the confirmation method should be configured appropriately. This can be achieved by the introduction of hydrolysis steps so that, for example, glucuronide metabolites, which are detected by the immunoassay screen, can then be analysed as the parent drug compound by GC-MS. Other metabolites may exist to which the immunoassay may be directed, as with the buprenorphine metabolite norbuprenorphine, and consideration must be given to the most appropriate substance to target by GC-MS. It is normal practice to set a lower cut-off for confirmatory analysis than that used for the initial screening method.

The above assay design features have important consequences when using immunoassay for samples other than urine (e.g. saliva, hair and blood). For example, if the drug in the sample is largely present in parent form in saliva or hair, the antibody and immunoassay must be directed to the parent molecule rather than to the metabolites.

Heterogeneous immunoassays

Heterogeneous immunoassays require the separation of bound and free antigen before measurement of the signal because of a lack of difference in the signal generated from the antibody-bound drug or free-label. The separation step of heterogeneous assays gives two distinct advantages over homogeneous assays. Firstly, potential endogenous interference from the sample produced by whole blood or highly discoloured urine is removed at the wash stage prior to signal development. This has the benefit that preliminary sample-extraction steps are not required. Secondly, the reaction has lower limits of detection compared to homogeneous assays. This difference is illustrated by the ability to use whole blood directly in a heterogeneous test kit, whereas extraction of the blood sample is generally required before analysis in a homogeneous method (Perrigo and Joynt 1995) and in the detection of potent drugs such as LSD (Cassells *et al.* 1996; Kerrigan and Brooks 1999). Other applications for heterogeneous assays include screening of hair and saliva, in which drug concentrations are significantly lower than in urine.

Enzyme immunoassays

The terms enzyme immunoassay (EIA) and enzyme-linked immunosorbent assay (ELISA) are often used interchangeably to outline non-isotopic assays and, more loosely, to describe heterogeneous and homogeneous assays.

Within the context of heterogeneous methods, EIA and ELISA have widely replaced RIA as the assay system because of the advantages already outlined. EIA methods are based upon antibody capture using labelled antigen systems, while ELISA methods are based on labelled antibodies. Both types of immunoassays are competitive systems.

Antibody-capture systems

Figure 14.7 is a schematic representation of an EIA based on a microplate antibody capture. The system uses anti-drug antibodies coated onto a microplate well by passive absorption. A microplate is a tray of 96 wells (each having a volume of approximately 400 μL) that are generally arranged as 12 × 8-well strips. The coating can be achieved by simply adding a solution of the antiserum or purified antibody in a bicarbonate buffer at pH 9 using high-precision pipettes. A suitable incubation period (e.g. overnight at room temperature) allows the antibodies to bind to the plastic microplate well. Following this incubation, the solution is washed from the solid phase and dried to leave an antibody-coated well. In some cases, a secondary coating of a non-relevant protein is performed to increase stability of the solid-phase antibody and to prevent nonspecific binding of assay components to the plastic well of the microplate. This process forms part of the reagent manufacturing process of commercial kits provided as a dry microplate with the antibody pre-coated.

In running the assay, a sample (10–50 μL) is added to the microplate followed by a buffered solution (typically 100 μL) that contains a fixed amount of drug labelled with an enzyme such as horseradish peroxidase or alkaline phosphatase. The plate is then left for sufficient time to allow the horseradish peroxidase-labelled drug and any drug present in the sample to compete for

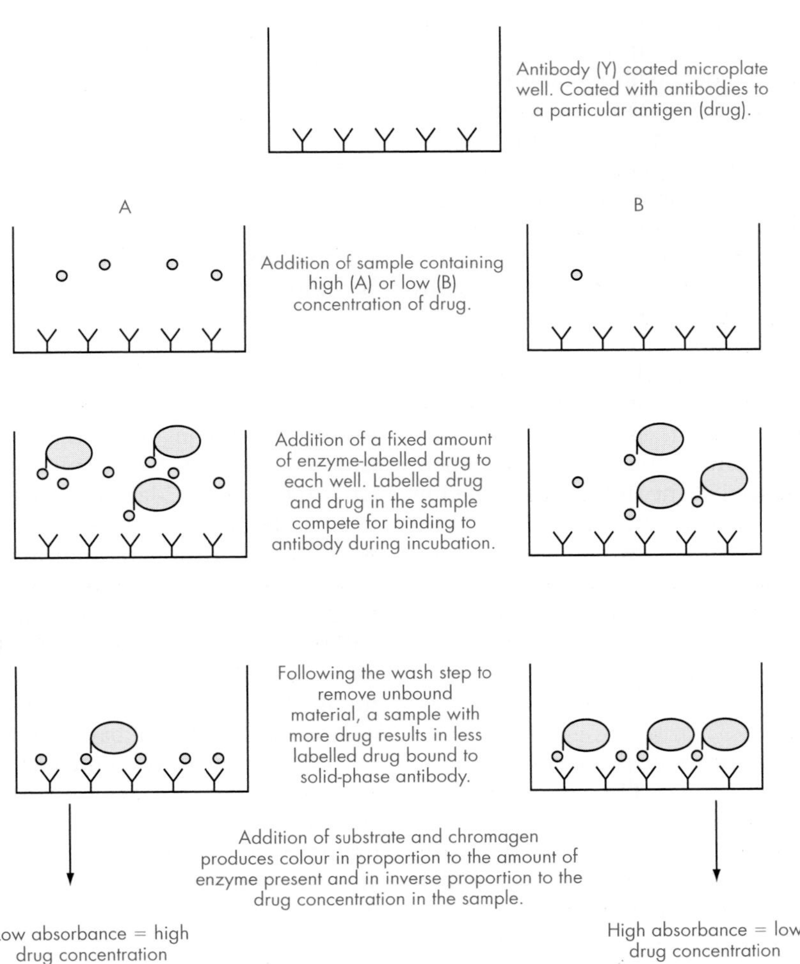
Antibody (Y) coated microplate well. Coated with antibodies to a particular antigen (drug).
A
B
Addition of sample containing high (A) or low (B) concentration of drug.
Addition of a fixed amount of enzyme-labelled drug to each well. Labelled drug and drug in the sample compete for binding to antibody during incubation.
Following the wash step to remove unbound material, a sample with more drug results in less labelled drug bound to solid-phase antibody.
Addition of substrate and chromagen produces colour in proportion to the amount of enzyme present and in inverse proportion to the drug concentration in the sample.
Low absorbance = high drug concentration
High absorbance = low drug concentration

Figure 14.7 A heterogeneous EIA.

binding to the solid-phase antibody. This is referred to as the incubation period. In the absence of drug, the maximum binding of the enzyme label occurs. Increased amounts of drug in the sample result in decreased amounts of antibody-bound enzyme label. After the incubation period, the microplate is washed with a suitable buffer (the separation step) to remove all traces of unbound enzyme label. Antibody-bound enzyme conjugate (and antibody-bound drug) is left immobilised to the wall of the antibody-coated microplate.

After the wash step, a substrate reagent is added to the microplate well and left to develop colour. The substrate of choice for horseradish peroxidase is dilute hydrogen peroxide with tetramethylbenzidine (TMB) as chromagen, which is available as a liquid-stable, ready-to-use product. TMB provides a blue coloured signal that can be measured at 630 nm using a standard laboratory microplate reader. In routine use, the colour development is stopped, after it has developed over a 20–30 min incubation period, by the addition of 1 M dilute sulfuric acid. This causes a shift in absorbance that is read at 450 nm. The whole assay process described here can be fully automated or performed with the simplest of laboratory equipment.

The amount of enzyme-labelled drug bound to the solid-phase antibody, and therefore available for colour development, is inversely proportional to the amount of drug in the specimen. The colour produced at the final stage of the EIA is therefore inversely proportional to the amount of drug in the specimen, which gives a calibration curve similar to that found with RIA (Fig. 14.2).

Enzyme-linked immunosorbent assay, antibody-labelled systems

Competitive ELISA procedures are similar to the antibody-coated microplate EIA described above. The difference is that the anti-drug antibody is enzyme labelled rather than the drug. A drug derivative is coated onto the plastic well, which serves as a way to separate bound and free fractions.

The drug is conjugated to a protein using a process similar to that used to prepare an immunogen. This must be a different protein from the one used as the carrier protein to make the antibody in order to prevent binding of anti-protein antibodies made during the immunisation process. The protein–drug conjugate can be coated to the microplate well in the same manner used for coating antibodies in EIA (see above). During the assay, using similar procedures to those described for EIA, competition occurs between the drug in the sample and the immobilised drug for binding to an enzyme-labelled anti-drug antibody. Following incubation, a wash step is used to separate bound and free fractions, and leave labelled antibody immobilised to the solid-phase drug derivative on the microplate well wall. The amount of labelled antibody that is bound, and responsible for the signal generation, is inversely proportional to concentration of drug in the sample.

Radioimmunoassay

RIA was the forerunner of heterogeneous immunoassays. Difficulties associated with the handling and storage of radioactivity, disposal of radioactive waste and the half-life of the radioactive labels have resulted in RIA being replaced largely by non-isotopic EIA methods.

Two main types of RIA have been used for drug testing based on the isotope employed. An isotopic drug label is termed a tracer. Use of tritium (^{3}H)- or ^{14}C-labelled drug allows an identical molecular structure of tracer to the drug being tested, although counting the beta emissions involves an organic-based scintillation fluid and a sophisticated beta scintillation counter. Use of the gamma-emitting ^{125}I as tracer allows faster and more efficient counting and a number of research (Hand *et al.* 1986) and commercial RIAs were based on this isotope.

The immunoassay principle for RIA is the same as that for EIA described above. Antibody-coated tubes have been used to good effect with iodinated tracers. Simple decanting easily separates the bound and free fractions, and allows quantification of the bound fraction using a gamma counter. Other ways to separate bound and free fractions include the use of a second antibody precipitation step. This requires a centrifuge to form a pellet of bound material that can be counted after the free fraction has been decanted or aspirated. Magnetic beads and other particles coated with a second antibody have also been used to aid this separation of the bound and free fractions. Dextran-coated charcoal has been used to absorb free tracer from solution, and thereby allow the antibody-bound fraction in the supernatant to be counted (Bartlett *et al.* 1980).

Chemiluminescence immunoassays

Chemiluminescence offers the potential for increased sensitivity by an order of magnitude greater than RIA. However, such increased sensitivity would result in detection limits far greater than those of current confirmation techniques and so chemiluminescence assays have not gained popularity in either urine screening or toxicology.

The signal generated in a chemiluminescent immunoassay is caused by compounds that emit light during a chemical reaction. The flash of light can be extended by the addition of enhancers to the system. Enhanced luminescence, as seen with luminol in the presence of horseradish peroxidase and substituted phenols, causes a prolonged 'glow' of light that is easier to measure (Whitehead *et al.* 1983). Substrates that provide chemiluminescent end-points for other enzyme labels are available, such as adamantyl dioxetane phosphate, as used with alkaline phosphatase in the DPC Immulite system (Hand 1994).

Fluorescent labels

Fluorescent end-points for heterogeneous immunoassays are based on a fluorescent label or fluorophore. The principle of fluorescence relies on the 'Stokes' shift' or movement of wavelength from that used to excite the fluorophore to the detection wavelength at which light is emitted from the fluorophore. The labels can be used in an immunoassay in the same way as a radioactive label or by using an enzyme label to generate a fluorescent molecule.

An example of this type of signal system utilises an alkaline phosphatase enzyme label and 4-methylumbelliferyl phosphate substrate. The substrate is converted into the fluorescent 4-methylumbelliferone, which can be detected by a suitable fluorimeter. When using the assay procedure described for the heterogeneous EIA above, the fluorescence obtained is inversely proportional to the amount of drug in the sample.

The use of fluorescent labels in toxicology testing has not gained wide popularity because of the interference from endogenous sample components.

Lateral flow methods

There is a growing trend in the immunoassay sector to develop point-of-care tests. The Syva Emit system (see Homogeneous Immunoassays, p. 386) on small analysers such as the ETS, has allowed drug testing outside the laboratory for many years (Centofanti 1994). The use of inexpensive, easy-to-use single disposable cartridges or slides for a variety of drugs has accelerated this trend.

Single-use cartridges are basically variants of a competitive ELISA assay run on a solid-phase strip rather than inside a well or tube. These tests use particles as the means of signal generation and are mostly used with antibodies that have been labelled with colloidal gold or coloured latex spheres. This technique was established for urine drug testing and can also be applied to serum, whole blood (using a suitable filter pad to separate red cells) and saliva (employing a suitable collection method).

Figure 14.8 illustrates the 'lateral flow' or 'immuno-chromatographic assay' process for a single analyte. As with ELISA, an antigen–protein derivative is fixed to a solid-phase. In this case it is bound to a nitrocellulose membrane as a line or series of dots at a defined position (Fig. 14.8A). Labelled antibody (typically labelled with colloidal gold or coloured latex) is located in a pad that overlaps with the nitrocellulose membrane.

When the pad is wetted with sample, the labelled antibody rehydrates and flows from the

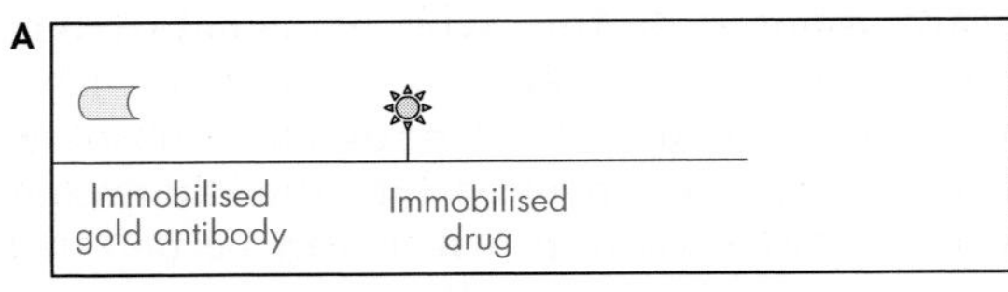

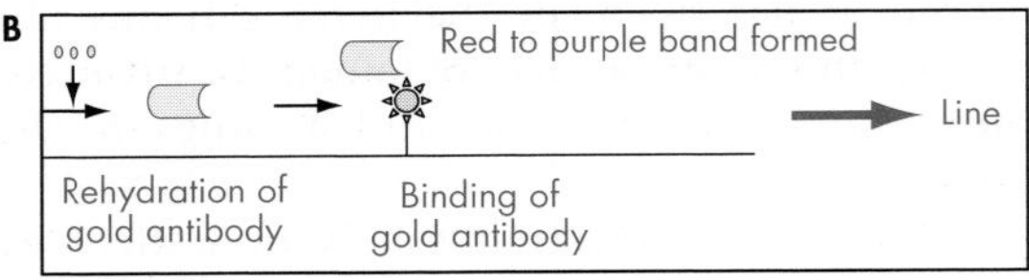

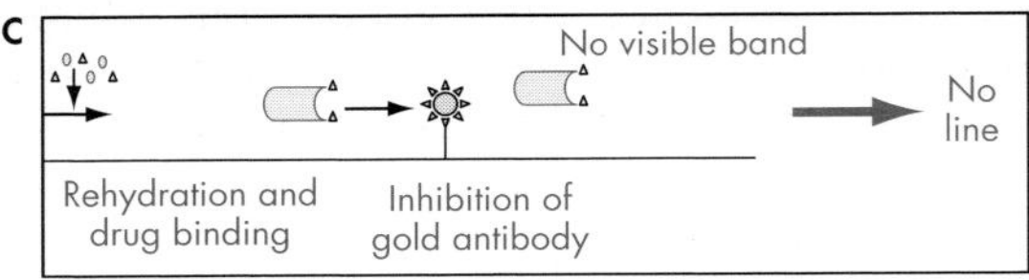

Figure 14.8 A competitive lateral flow immunoassay.

pad onto the membrane by capillary action. As the sample and rehydrated gold-labelled antibody flow along the membrane, any drug in the sample binds to the labelled antibody and inhibits it from binding to the immobilised drug on the membrane (Fig. 14.8C). If no drug is present in the sample, the rehydrated antibody binds to the immobilised drug and a visible line is formed (Fig. 14.8B). Separation of bound and free drug continues, as part of the assay process, with the movement of liquid across the membrane, leaving either bound material (a visible line) or free material (no visible line) to travel to an absorbent end-pad. As with ELISA, the amount of colour developed (or line formed at the site of the immobilised drug) is inversely proportional to the amount of drug present in the sample.

The addition of a control line on the membrane provides an indication that sufficient fluid has passed through the length of the test strip and thus an indication that the test has been performed correctly. Control lines typically use anti-IgG antibodies to capture excess drug-specific labelled antibody.

The addition of a number of drug-derivative lines in different positions on the nitrocellulose membrane together with suitable matching labelled antibodies allows the analysis of multiple drugs at the same time from a single sample.

The majority of these tests are interpreted visually, and the reagents are titrated and optimised such that there is no colour or line present when the 'cut off' concentration of analyte is present. Recent developments have overcome the problems of visual interpretation associated with lateral flow tests. This has been achieved by developing a small portable reader based on digital imaging. The benefits are that the line can be determined more accurately, the result can be quantified if required and the subjectivity of visual interpretation is removed (Spiehler *et al.* 2000).

Homogeneous immunoassays

Homogeneous immunoassays do not require the separation of bound and free fractions, and as a result have been automated successfully in a number of different systems.

The most widely used and most cost-effective immunoassay used to screen large numbers of urine samples when there is no need for high sensitivity is the homogeneous EIA marketed by Syva (Dade-Behring) for many years as EMIT (enzyme multiplied immunoassay technique). This method, for use for the analysis of morphine, was first published in 1972 (Rubenstein *et al.* 1972).

The EMIT technique is based on the enzyme activity of a drug-labelled enzyme, glucose-6-phosphate dehydrogenase (PDH), modulated by antibodies raised against the drug. Enzyme activity (in the presence of glucose-6-phosphate) results in the conversion of nicotinamide–adenine dinucleotide (NAD) to the reduced form NADH, and the subsequent increase in absorbance at 340 nm is monitored spectrophotometrically.

Addition of the anti-drug antibody results in binding to the drug-labelled enzyme, which effectively reduces the enzyme activity (Fig. 14.9). Any drug in the sample competes with the drug-labelled enzyme in binding to the antibody, which allows unbound enzyme to become active and thereby increases absorbance

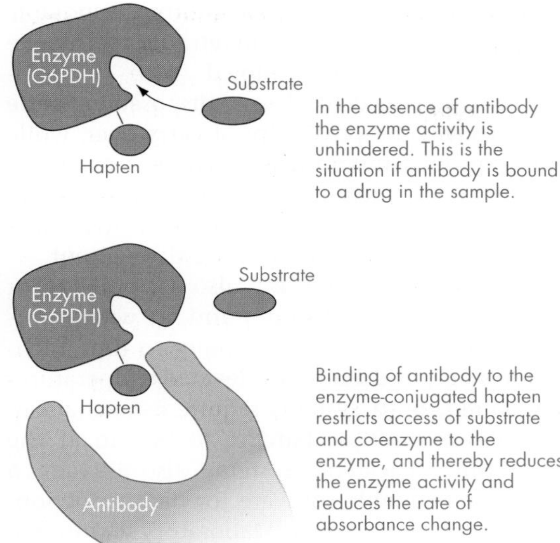
Enzyme (G6PDH)
Substrate
Hapten
In the absence of antibody the enzyme activity is unhindered. This is the situation if antibody is bound to a drug in the sample.
Enzyme (G6PDH)
Substrate
Hapten
Antibody
Binding of antibody to the enzyme-conjugated hapten restricts access of substrate and co-enzyme to the enzyme, and thereby reduces the enzyme activity and reduces the rate of absorbance change.

Figure 14.9 A homogeneous enzyme multiplied immunoassay technique (EMIT).

at 340 nm. Increasing amounts of drug in the sample produce increased enzyme activity and hence an increase in the rate of change of absorbance at 340 nm.

The use of bacterial PDH, which uses NAD as coenzyme, avoids interference from endogenous PDH, which uses nicotinamide–adenine dinucleotide phosphate (NADP). Earlier examples of the technique used lysozyme (Rubenstein *et al.* 1972) or malate dehydrogenase (Ullman and Maggio 1980; Kabakoff and Greenwood 1981).

CEDIA, cloned enzyme donor immunoassay

A more recent variant on the homogeneous enzyme immunoassay is the CEDIA system. This system, like EMIT, uses the binding of an antibody to influence the activity of an enzyme. Competition for binding by drug present in the sample results in an increase in enzyme activity.

The CEDIA principle (Henderson *et al.* 1986) relies on the spontaneous complementation of two genetically engineered fragments of β-galactosidase from *Escherichia coli*. The polypeptide chain of the enzyme is presented as two inactive fragments, the large fragment, termed enzyme acceptor (EA), and a small fragment, enzyme donor (ED), which contains the 5% of enzyme missing from the EA portion. By conjugating hapten to the ED fragment, the addition of antibodies that bind the hapten can prevent the formation of an intact, and therefore active, enzyme. Any drug present in the sample competes for antibody-binding sites, such that an increase in drug concentrations yields less binding of antibody to the ED fragment and therefore results in more enzyme activity which can be monitored spectrophotometrically.

Fluorescence polarisation immunoassay

Fluorescence polarisation immunoassay (FPIA) is another example of a homogenous immunoassay, and uses fluorescein-labelled antigen as the tracer molecule (Dandliker *et al.* 1973). It has been widely used as the basis of assay systems to analyse drugs in urine (Colbert *et al.* 1985).

The fluorescein-labelled antigen rotates rapidly when not bound by an antibody. When bound by the antibody, the rotation is slowed dramatically compared to the unbound molecule. To generate the assay signal, a fluorimeter shines light, at the excitation wavelength for fluorescein, through a vertical polarising filter. Rapidly rotating unbound fluorescein molecules emit light in a different plane from the incident light, whereas the relatively stationary antibody-bound fluorescein returns light in a similar plane, which is detected via the polarising filter.

Drug added via the sample competes for binding to the antibody with the fluorescein-labelled hapten, thereby reducing the amount of fluorescein bound to the antibody, which results in less emitted fluorescence being detected via the polarised filter. The background fluorescence found with many biological samples means it is usual to take a blank reading of the sample and reagents before the addition of the fluorescent tracer to the mixture. This method is the basis of the Abbott ADx system.

Microparticle methods

Agglutination of microparticles has been used as a signal system in homogeneous assay-based methods. Agglutination reactions for drugs use particles, generally latex, that have drug conjugated onto them. Addition of antibody (which has two binding sites) to the drug-coated particles causes bridging between antibodies and the particles to produce agglutinates. The drug present in a sample, added to the mixture of antibody and drug-conjugated particles, competes for antibody-binding sites and therefore prevents agglutination. In this type of assay the degree of agglutination is inversely proportional to the amount of drug in the sample.

The basis of the Roche Abuscreen Online system termed KIMS (kinetic interaction of microparticles in solution) involves monitoring the rate of agglutination via spectrophotometric means.

Automation of immunoassay

The ability of an immunoassay to screen large numbers of samples has lead to the development of a number of different automated solutions. These can be tailored to meet the requirements of laboratories using either semi-automated systems through to full automation with walk-away capability. Automation of a heterogeneous assay sequence up to the separation step is referred to as the 'front-end', while those steps post separation are termed 'back-end'. Full automation of all stages requires a system able to carry out the separation stage. Front-end automation involves an accurate pipetting mechanism for samples and reagents. This is achieved by employing a robotic sample processor that facilitates the automatic transfer of samples (with bar code recognition) from primary tubes to reaction wells (or tubes). This transfer can be done in batch mode (i.e. all samples are pipetted from one destination to another) or by random access (i.e. the selective transfer of sample to one or more different reaction wells) and can be read directly from an imported work-list.

Sampling can be done using either disposable pipette tips or a fixed polytetrafluoroethylene (PTFE)-coated probe coupled with a high-precision syringe drive. Use of disposable pipette tips removes the possibility of carry-over, while fixed probe instruments require extensive washing to reduce carry. As this increases the processing times, multiple probe instruments have been developed to increase throughput.

Back-end automation can also use pipettes for the reagents (e.g. substrate) and, as with front-end systems, can have the ability to time incubation stages and maintain elevated temperatures if required. Both systems require a mechanism that allows multiple batches to be run at the same time. Back-end systems also include a reader and suitable software for data reduction, and can be interfaced with laboratory mainframe computers.

Full automation is essentially a combination of front- and back-end systems that incorporates a suitable mechanism to complete the separation phase. For microplates this involves a simple 'on-board' washer that automatically dispenses and aspirates wash fluid. Similar systems have been developed for tube washing, although the size constraint means these are stand-alone modules. The process of automation of heterogeneous enzyme immunoassays is well developed and is widely used in blood-bank laboratories in which many thousands of tests can be processed per day. Automation of homogeneous assays is less complex as they do not require a separation step. The most widely used systems, such as the EMIT, CEDIA and OnLine methods, are readily automated on modern clinical chemistry analysers. These analysers are able to pipette accurately, control temperature and measure rates of absorbance. The throughput of the instrument can range from a hundred up to a thousand tests per hour.

Analysis of alternative samples to urine

Immunoassays for drugs have been widely employed in the analysis of urine samples. Other sample matrices, such as whole blood, serum, hair extracts, saliva and sweat, can be used successfully. Heterogeneous assays are ideally suited to these alternative matrices. Their inherent sensitivity provides the lower limits of detection required for forensic use and the wash step endows the ability to deal with difficult matrix effects. Correct selection of antibody allows the assay system to be targeted towards specific drugs or metabolites.

Immunoassays are generally designed for a particular use and sample type. With testing for drugs of abuse the assay is often designed for urine specimens, whereas therapeutic drug assays are generally designed for plasma or serum. Situations can arise in which the drug of interest is in a different matrix from that for which the kit has been validated, so the onus is on the user to test and validate this new application. Urine and serum immunoassay kits are widely available and assays for other matrices, which include blood, cerebrospinal fluid, fingernails, hair, meconium, saliva, stomach contents and sweat, have been developed successfully.

Many assays can be adapted to work with different matrices, although it is advisable to consult the kit manufacturer prior to making kit adaptations. After discussion and advice from the developer or manufacturer of an assay, the next step is to obtain similar samples to the test case; it is essential to try and match these as closely as possible, with special reference to the type of preservative used. Some samples (e.g. bottled beer) are readily available and it should be possible to obtain the exact brand under test, so that the alcohol and other ingredients are matched identically. In cases such as aged, putrefied whole blood, it can prove more difficult to obtain and select a sample matrix.

Once a suitable sample matrix has been obtained, known amounts of the drug of interest are added to the sample matrix. The concentrations are usually chosen to fall within the range of the kit. The high sensitivity of immunoassays means it is often possible to introduce a dilution factor without compromising the limit of detection in the sample. For example, if the limit of detection of the confirmatory method is 100 μg/L, use of an EIA with a cut-off of 10 μg/L allows the use of a 1:10 dilution factor. Such a dilution reduces potential interference without compromising overall sensitivity.

Heterogeneous immunoassays are more robust and tolerant of different types of sample matrices than homogeneous assays because of the separation stage of the assay.

A common finding, often described as a 'matrix effect', is that the newly created calibration curve is not usable through adverse interference. This can arise from an inherent interference from the sample itself with the signal system or from interference with the antibody–antigen reaction. Homogeneous immunoassays are more prone to interference since the sample is present during the signal-generation stage. Reducing the sample load by dilution in a suitable buffer or using a smaller test volume should reduce the effect. Unfortunately, the trade-off is that the limit of detection and curve shape might be sacrificed. Liquid- or solid-phase extraction of the sample can be used when direct application of the sample fails.

Quality control, calibration, standardisation and curve fitting

It is common practice to perform laboratory-based immunoassays as a batch or a single run that contains calibration and control material together with unknown samples. From the calibrators (or standards), a calibration curve can be derived and a concentration for the unknown sample can be determined. Inclusion of samples with known drug concentration (controls) at regular intervals allows an assessment of reproducibility within the batch. Duplication and control of reproducibility forms the basis of 'within run' precision assessment.

Inclusion of the same quality-control material in consecutive runs gives an indication of run-to-run reproducibility. This can be supplemented with the inclusion of previously analysed patient or test samples. Together with monitoring curve parameters, these components allow an opinion to be formed as to the acceptability of the batch-to-batch precision when compared with predefined parameters.

Drug immunoassays can be run in a number of ways, depending on user requirements. Urine drug screening may only require a simple qualitative (positive or negative) result. Fully quantitative results are required for diagnostic purposes or TDM. In forensic applications, an assay run in a semi-quantitative mode (with a small number of calibrators) provides an estimated concentration. This estimated concentration is useful when progressing to a confirmation stage (e.g. GC-MS).

For quantitative assays, the curve fit between data points is important and a number of curve-fitting options are available. Some manufacturers supply 'closed' curve-fitting programs that determine the fit, and calibrator ranges are fixed on all instruments of that particular make. Open systems allow the user to select a suitable fit and transformation for the particular application. Care should be taken with this selection, as it is possible to mismatch the curve fit and immunoassay. Common problems include automated systems that attempt to fit a straight line to a curve or poorly fit the points of a curve. There is no substitute for the operator checking the raw data from an assay.

For toxicological analysis, it is often appropriate to use a point-to-point curve fit (while accepting that the curve when far from a point is less accurate). Other examples of curve fits include spline and four-parameter fits. The overriding consideration is to ensure, by validating the method, that the chosen fit connects the data points in the most suitable way. A simple example of how the same assay can produce different results because of data handling is shown in Figure 14.10. Both curves are plotted using the same results, but in Series 1 extra calibrator points are plotted. The curves plotted for Series 2 work perfectly satisfactorily as a 'semi-quantitative' assay, but give inaccurate numerical results at points where the point-to-point curve fit is not suitable to provide a quantitative answer (illustrated best in Fig. 14.10 at the 100 μg/L region). The introduction of extra calibrators provides a more robust curve more suited to quantification of drug concentration. The addition of extra calibrators also ensures that a single calibrator point does not unduly bias the curve. In Figure 14.10, using Series 2 any small error or change to the 200 μg/L calibrator alters the curve significantly, but with Series 1 the curve is held by the 100 μg/L calibrator point.

Sample adulteration

Specimen donors (i.e. patients, employees, detainees) may not want the immunoassay drug screen to perform correctly and may take steps to adulterate their specimen. This is largely a problem associated with screening of urine for drugs of abuse; hair, blood and saliva are less likely to be adulterated. Steps to counter this problem include observing the collection of the sample, together with physical and chemical tests to confirm that the sample is voided freshly and from the individual being tested. Tests include measurement of sample temperature at the point of collection, on-site or laboratory tests of pH, relative density and urinary creatinine concentration. More specific tests can be performed for particular adulterants.

The effect of sample adulteration differs depending on the assay type. Some assays produce false-negative results, whereas others produce artificially elevated results.

The key to the successful application of immunoassay as part of a testing regimen is knowledge of the characteristics of the assay in use and knowledge of the limitations as well as the benefits of each of the many variants of the method.

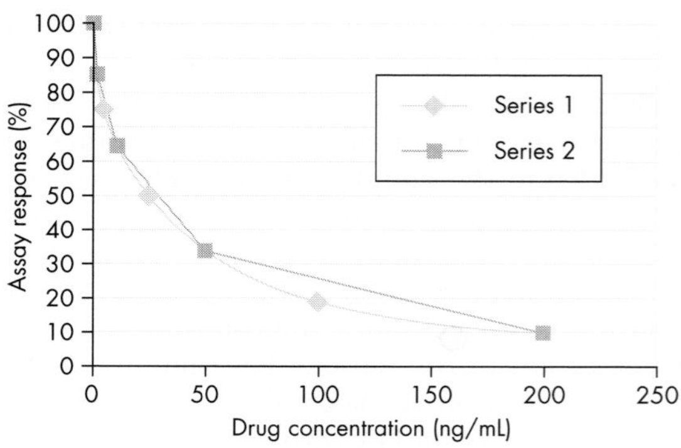

Figure 14.10 Example to illustrate how different curve-fitting programs can influence the results of an immunoassay.

Spectral selectivity, and in some cases detection sensitivity, can be enhanced significantly by the various chemical and instrumental techniques outlined above. Such methods should, of course, be validated by applying the conventional analytical criteria of accuracy (against a reference method), linearity, precision and independence from interfering substances.

The scope of UV and visible (UV-visible) spectrophotometry can be further extended when combined with a chromatographic separation step, such as high-performance liquid chromatography (HPLC). The LC eluent is directed post-column to a UV-visible spectrophotometer to enable the detection of substances absorbing in the UV-visible region. Traditionally, absorption was measured at a single wavelength, but the development of rapid-scanning detectors based on linear photodiode arrays permits spectra to be acquired during the elution of peaks. Computer-aided manipulation of these spectra has led to new strategies for the examination of chromatographic peak purity, based on classic techniques in spectroscopy. Figure 15.2A shows the relatively limited information available from measurement at a single wavelength compared with the additional information available from photodiode array detection (DAD) (Fig. 15.2B) (Lindholm *et al.* 2003).

Spectral libraries of UV-visible spectra are available commercially and these, combined with computers enable the development of archive-retrieval methods for spectral characterisation.

Nomenclature

In the UV and visible spectrum, the energy of photons associated with electronic transitions

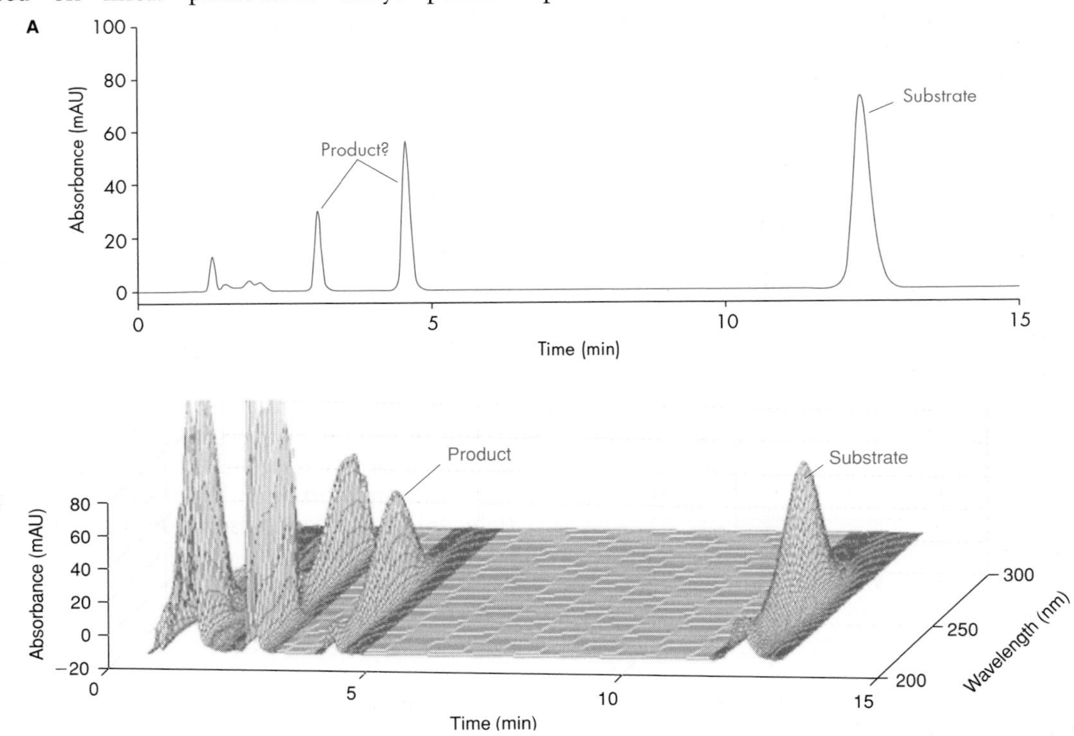

Figure 15.2 HPLC analysis of a sample taken from the genetically modified bacterial fermentation of the steroid progesterone to produce 9α-hydroxyprogesterone. (A) HPLC chromatogram from absorbance measured at 245 nm. (B) HPLC chromatogram from absorbance measured with diode-array detector (DAD) between 220 and 400 nm. Monitoring absorbance only at 245 nm did not permit the peak due to the product to be identified. The 3D plot from HPLC-DAD allowed the peak for 9α-hydroxyprogesterone to be clearly identified. (Reprinted from J. Lindholm *et al.*, Use of liquid chromatography–diode-array detection and mass spectrometry for rapid product identification in biotechnological synthesis of a hydroxyprogesterone, *J. Chromatogr. A*, 2003, **992**, 85–100 with permission from Elsevier.)

lies in the range 147–630 kJ/mol. This energy (ΔE) can be expressed in terms of the principal parameters that define electromagnetic radiation, namely frequency μ (Hz), wavelength λ (nm) and wavenumber $\bar{\nu}$ (cm^{-1}):

$$\Delta E = h\mu = \frac{hc}{\lambda} = hc\bar{\nu} \qquad (15.1)$$

where h is Planck's constant, and c is the velocity of radiation *in vacuo*.

The positions of peaks are sometimes described in terms of wavenumber, which has the advantage of being a linear function of energy, but this term is much more frequently used in infrared spectrophotometry. The practical unit most often used in UV and visible spectrophotometry is wavelength (λ), usually expressed in nanometres (nm). The older units of wavelength, millimicron (mμ) and ångström (Å) are not recommended terms. The position of maximum absorption of a peak is designated λ_{max}.

The wavelength span is conventionally divided into two ranges: the UV extends from 200 nm to about 400 nm; the visible range extends from about 400 nm to 800 nm. Outside these limits, the 'far UV' or 'vacuum UV' extends from 10 nm to 200 nm, and the 'near infrared' from 0.8 μm to about 3 μm (see Fig. 15.3).

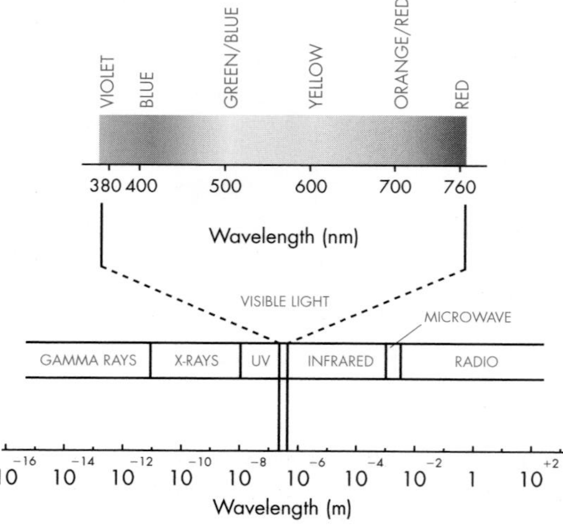

Figure 15.3 Radiation spectrum highlighting the visible region of the spectrum.

A molecular grouping specifically responsible for absorption is termed a chromophore, and is usually a conjugated system with extensive delocalisation of electron density, for example the benzene ring. Any saturated group, with little or no intrinsic absorption of its own, that modifies the absorption spectrum when attached directly to a chromophore is described as an auxochrome, examples being —OR, —NR_2, —SR. Auxochromes are considered to exert their effect through partial conjugation of their polarisable lone-pair electrons with those of the adjacent chromophore. However, if the lone pair of electrons is involved in bonding, as for example in the case of a protonated quaternary ammonium group, the auxochromic effect vanishes. This property can be used for molecular characterisation, as discussed below.

When developing analytical methods, it is important that an analyst can recognise whether or not a molecule will absorb in the UV-visible region from a consideration of the chemical structure of the substance.

Laws of absorption spectrophotometry

The extent of absorption of radiation by an absorbing system at a given monochromatic wavelength is described by the two classic laws of absorptiometry, which relate the intensity of radiation incident on the absorbing system (I_0) to the transmitted intensity (I) (Fig. 15.4). Lambert's (or Bouguer's) law concerns instrumental factors, and states that at a given concentration (c) of a homogeneous absorbing system, the transmitted intensity (I) decreases exponentially with increase in absorption pathlength (l).

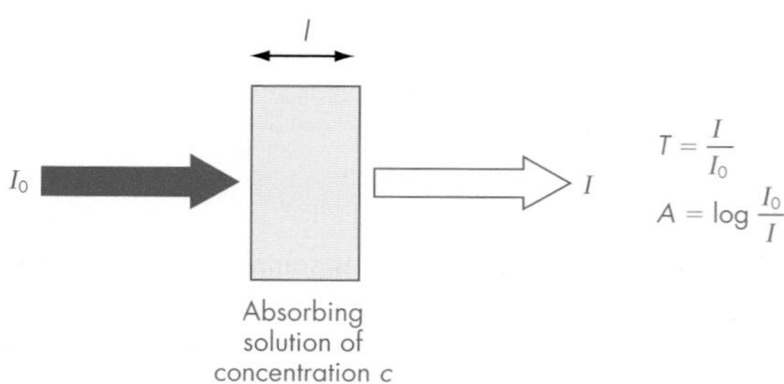

Figure 15.4 Attenuation of a beam of radiation by an absorbing solution.

The complementary Beer's law deals with concentration and states that for a layer of defined pathlength (l), the transmitted intensity (I) decreases exponentially with the increase in concentration (c) of a homogeneous absorbing system. Combination of these observations gives the familiar Beer–Lambert law:

$$\log \frac{I_0}{I} = \varepsilon c l \tag{15.2}$$

where ε is the molar absorption coefficient of the system.

The logarithmic term is linearly related to concentration and pathlength, and is referred to as absorbance (A). The older terms extinction (E) and optical density (OD) are not recommended, although they are often found in the literature. Transmittance ($T = I/I_0$) and percentage transmittance [$\%T = 100(I/I_0)$] are not linear functions of concentration and pathlength but can be related readily to absorbance:

$$A = \log \frac{I_0}{I} = \log \frac{1}{T} = 2 - \log(\%T) \tag{15.3}$$

The molar absorption coefficient (ε) is defined as 'the absorbance of a 1-molar solution in a cell of 1 cm pathlength' with units of M^{-1} cm^{-1} (L mol^{-1} cm^{-1}).

The term *specific absorbance* is also used, denoted by $A^{1\%}_{1\,cm}$ or A (1%, 1 cm) or A^1_1. This is defined as 'the absorbance of a 1% w/v solution in a cell of 1 cm pathlength' (g (100 mL)$^{-1}$ or g/100 mL). It was formerly known as the 'specific extinction coefficient', symbol $E^{1\%}_{1cm}$ or E (1%, 1 cm).

$$\frac{A^1_1}{10} = \frac{\varepsilon}{M_r} \tag{15.4}$$

where M_r is the relative molecular mass.

Absorbance is often expressed in logarithmic form in cases where spectra are to be compared. The logarithmic form of the Beer–Lambert law expresses the effects of molar absorption coefficient (ε), concentration (c) and pathlength (l) as additive terms

$$\log A = \log \varepsilon + \log c + \log l \tag{15.5}$$

Validity of the Beer–Lambert law

The validity of the Beer–Lambert law is affected by a number of factors. If the radiation is nonmonochromatic, that is its spectral bandwidth is greater than about 10% of the drug absorption bandwidth at half-height, the observed absorbance will be lower than the 'true' limiting value for monochromatic radiation. Thus, sharp bands are more susceptible than broad bands to absorbance error on this account. Moreover, if the absorbing species is nonhomogeneous, or if it undergoes association, dissociation, photodegradation, solvation, complexation or adsorption, or if it emits fluorescence, then positive or negative deviations from the Beer–Lambert law may be observed. Stray-light effects and the type of solvent used may also lead to noncompliance with the Beer–Lambert law.

Stray-light effects

Stray light is radiation at wavelengths different from those desired. It may arise from light scattering or other defects within the instrument, or it may be caused by external radiation. In the absence of stray light, the observed absorbance tends to a constant value as the concentration of a sample is increased because all light is absorbed and no light reaches the detector. However, if stray light is present and reaches the detector, this will give rise to a negative deviation from the Beer–Lambert law. Stray-light errors are more likely to be observed near the wavelength limits of an instrument, at which the radiation intensity of the source and the efficiency of the optical system are reduced, especially below 220 nm and at the crossover point between the UV and the visible lamps (about 320–400 nm). Errors may become serious if the solvent absorbs strongly or if a strongly absorbing sample is measured by difference spectrophotometry.

Solvent effects

The solvent often exerts a profound influence on the quality and shape of the spectrum. For example, many aromatic chromophores display vibrational fine structure in nonpolar solvents, whereas in more polar solvents this fine structure is absent because of solute–solvent interaction effects (see also Fig. 15.1). A classic case is phenol and related compounds, which have different spectra in cyclohexane and in aqueous solution. In aqueous solutions, the pH exerts a profound effect on ionisable chromophores because of the differing extent of conjugation in the ionised and the non-ionised chromophore. This change of spectrum with pH and associated change in the ionic state of a molecule and conjugation is illustrated in Figs 15.11 and 15.12 (p. 409) for phenobarbital and other barbituric acids. Note the shift in absorption to higher wavelengths as the conjugation is increased (increase in alternating double and single bonds in the molecule).

The quality of spectral measurement is affected directly by the type and purity of the solvent used. Each solvent has a cut-off wavelength (which corresponds to about 10% transmittance) and this varies with solvent purity (Table 15.1). A solvent should not be used below its cut-off wavelength, even though reference-cell compensation is employed, because of the greater risk of stray-light effects. The UV spectra of some solvents are illustrated in Fig. 15.5. The UV cut-off of solvents must be borne in mind when selecting solvents for HPLC mobile phases, particularly for analytes that absorb only in the low UV. A solvent should be selected with a lower UV cut-off than the absorption wavelength of the analyte.

Table 15.1 Cut-off points equivalent to 10% transmittance for spectroscopic solvents

Solvent	Wavelength (nm)
Water (distilled) or dilute inorganic acid	190
Acetonitrile (HPLC, far-UV grade)	200
Acetonitrile	210
Butyl alcohol	210
Cyclohexane	210
Ethanol (96% v/v)	210
Heptane	210
Hexane	210
Propan-2-ol	210
Methanol	210
Ether	220
Sodium hydroxide (0.2 M)	225
Tetrahydrofuran	215
Ethylene dichloride	230
Methylene chloride	235
Chloroform (stabilised with ethanol)	245
Carbon tetrachloride	265
N,N-Dimethylformamide	270
Benzene	280
Pyridine	305
Acetone	330

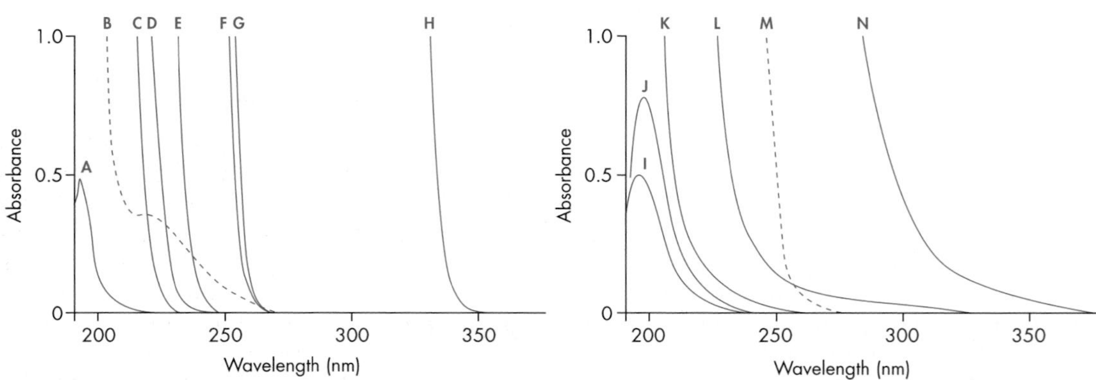

Figure 15.5 UV absorption of solvents (HPLC-grade unless otherwise stated): (A) acetonitrile (far-UV grade); (B) methyl *t*-butyl ether; (C) acetonitrile; (D) 1–chlorobutane; (E) methylene chloride; (F) acetic acid (AR grade); (G) ethyl acetate; (H) acetone; (I) hexane; (J) isooctane; (K) methanol; (L) tetrahydrofuran; (M) chloroform; (N) diethylamine (AR grade).

Some cautionary comments may be appropriate at this point. It is better to use single- or double-distilled water and to avoid deionised water, which can be contaminated with absorptive fragments of ion-exchange resin or contain bacterial metabolites; these can contribute significantly to nonspecific absorption at low wavelengths. Ethanol is normally used as the 96% v/v strength, since dehydrated alcohol is usually contaminated with traces of benzene added to form the azeotropic mixture for distillation. Acetonitrile can vary noticeably in quality, depending on the supplier. The grade supplied for use in HPLC is usually to be recommended. Acetone, sometimes used to clean cells, is highly absorptive and not always easily removed, despite its volatility and aqueous solubility. Chloroform and carbon tetrachloride absorb strongly at about 250 nm and should therefore only be used for measurements at wavelengths above about 280 nm. Given the safety considerations of chlorinated solvents, use of these is best avoided if possible. Ether, although transparent down to 220 nm, presents particular problems because of its volatility (unstable standard solutions) and inflammability. Although absorptivity is considered to be relatively insensitive to temperature changes, organic solvents in general suffer from high temperature-coefficients of expansion, so that for ultimate precision a cell provided with a thermostat may be required.

Instrumentation

General considerations

The basic components of analytical instruments for absorption and fluorescence spectroscopy are alike in function and general performance requirements. Most spectroscopic instruments are made up of five components:

- stable source of radiant energy
- wavelength selector that permits the isolation of a restricted wavelength region
- sample container
- radiation detector, which converts radiant energy to a measurable signal (usually electrical)
- signal processor and readout.

Colorimeters

Colorimeters usually employ a single tungsten radiation source in combination with broad-band (~30 nm) optical filters of nominal wavelength, or narrow-bandwidth interference filters with a defined wavelength for use in the visible range. The range of linearity of the colorimeter may be constrained by the relatively broad spectral bandwidths employed, and therefore should be checked carefully for each type of assay.

Single-beam spectrophotometers

These differ from the colorimeter in using a prism or a high-quality diffraction grating monochromator, together with an additional intense source of UV radiation, usually a deuterium (or hydrogen) lamp. The function of the monochromator is to separate the source radiation such that light of a narrow wavelength band only is transmitted to the sample. They are capable of high precision, particularly in the optimum absorbance range (0.3–0.6 absorbance units). The reference and sample cells must be moved manually in and out of the radiation beam at each wavelength, so it is not practicable to scan a spectrum using such a device.

Double-beam spectrophotometers

Double-beam spectrophotometers (Fig 15.6) use similar high-quality optical components to those in the single-beam instrument. However, the radiation from the monochromator is split into two identical beams by a rotating mirror. One beam passes through the sample and the other through the reference cell, before being recombined to focus on the detector. Each signal is processed appropriately by the detector electronics to measure the absorbance 10 to 20 times per second. The advantage of the double-beam set-up is that the absorbance of the cell and solvent is automatically compensated for so that the resultant spectrum is that of the sample only. A scan motor drives the monochromator to give a constant wavelength change per second, which is synchronised with a recorder or digital plotter to present the spectrum. For broad bands, scan speeds up to 2 nm/s can be employed. However, some computer-controlled spectrophotometers with fast data-processing capabilities can scan at rates approaching 20 nm/s, and still maintain spectral fidelity even for sharp peaks.

Diode-array spectrophotometers

Diode-array spectrophotometers (referred to as diode-array detectors, DAD, or photodiode-array, PDA, detectors) employ multichannel detectors (Fig 15.7). The most commonly encountered detector of this type is the linear photodiode array. The reversed-optics mode is employed, so that radiation is passed through the sample or reference cell, then dispersed by a diffraction grating polychromator and detected by a device that comprises several hundred diodes. Each photodiode registers the integrated intensity of radiation incident on it, which is determined by the spectral dispersion : photodiode ratio. If, for example, a 200 nm bandwidth of radiation is dispersed across 256 photodiodes, the nominal resolution per photodiode is 0.78 nm.

A spectrum in a specified range is acquired within 20 ms. The analogue signals from each photodiode are digitised and transferred to a computer, where they are corrected for dark-current response and transformed to absorbance. A number of digital techniques are available to increase sensitivity, extending the use of rapid-scanning detectors to multicomponent analysis, reaction kinetics, tablet dissolution tests, process control and detection in HPLC (Fell *et al.* 1982). (See also Chapter 19 for a discussion of the use of the DAD in HPLC.)

Coupled techniques

Where large numbers of samples must be analysed quickly, the use of automated instruments becomes viable. One path is to use the automated sample handling in the flow injection analysis (FIA) technique.

FIA is an example of a continuous flow system: the sample becomes part of a flowing stream in which the unit operations of the analysis take

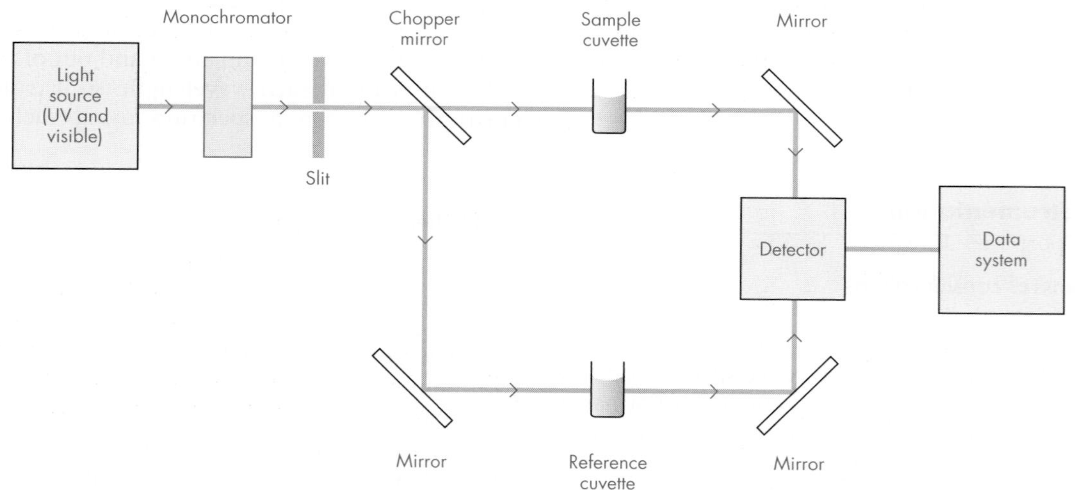

Figure 15.6 Double-beam spectrophotometer. The source radiation (UV from a deuterium lamp or visible from a tungsten lamp) is transmitted to the sample cuvette and reference cuvette via a series of mirrors, passing through a monochromator (diffraction gating). Note that the same radiation source is transmitted through the sample and the reference cuvette. The chopper mirror is a half-mirror which is constantly rotated. This allows the light to pass to the sample when the mirror is not in the light path and to be transmitted to the reference when the mirror rotates back into the light path.

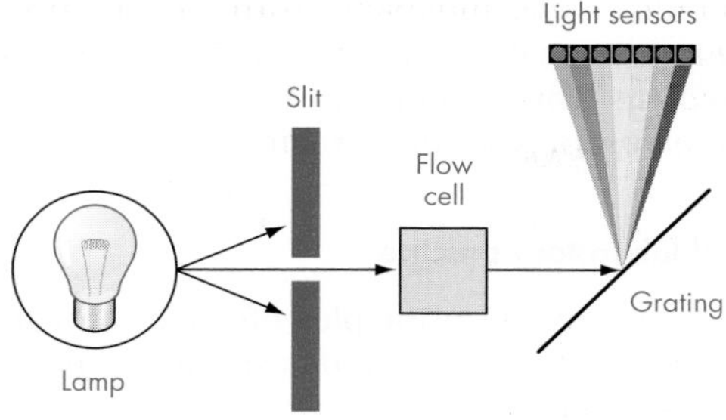

Figure 15.7 Schematic of a diode-array detector. Compare with Figure 15.6 for the double-beam spectrophotometer for the reverse geometry whereby, in the DAD, the radiation is dispersed by the diffraction grating *after* passing through the sample and is then detected by the array of photodiodes.

place as the sample is carried from the injection point to a flow-through measuring device (such as a photometer) and finally to waste. The intensity of the radiation that reaches the detector is recorded continuously; when an absorbing species is passing through, a sharp peak is generated, with the height of the peak proportional to the analyte concentration. Sample sizes injected are mostly in the range 10–30 μL.

Instruments are available with the ability to carry out manipulations such as in-line heating, in-line distillation, in-line UV-digestion or in-line extraction, so that UV and/or visible spectroscopy can be used for a wide variety of compounds.

For complex sample matrices, the limited specificity of spectroscopic methods can be an important drawback and a restriction for analysis. This restriction can be overcome by coupling liquid chromatography with a suitable detector, thereby enabling separation and detection of a wide variety of substances including macromolecules and ionic species in complex mixtures. Detection systems used depend upon the nature of the component of interest, but the most widely used detectors in liquid chromatography are based upon UV or visible radiation. Photometers often make use of the 254 nm and 280 nm lines from a mercury source, because many organic functional groups absorb in this region. However, to achieve adequate specificity, often diode arrays are used, which are able to display an entire spectrum as an analyte exits the column (liquid chromatography with diode-array detector (LC-DAD)). Compared to single-wavelength detection, which provides no information about peak purity, the diode array's full spectral comparison provides results with a far greater confidence level (see Fig. 15.2).

Generally, the LC-DAD technique is applied for toxicological screening. Substances are identified on the basis of both retention time and UV spectrum (Bogusz and Wu 1991; Lambert *et al.* 1995; Tracqui *et al.* 1995; Elliott and Hale 1998). The diode array can also be connected to a mass spectrometer (LC-DAD-MS), where MS increases the sensitivity and gives an extra confirmation of the component's identity.

Instrument performance checks

While instruments with conventional optics may require frequent calibration because they have many moving parts, diode-array spectrophotometers with no moving parts are extremely reproducible and stable, in both the short and the long term.

Following the recommendations of the *European Pharmacopeia* (Council of Europe 2008) for UV and visible spectrophotometry, the wavelength and the absorbance must be calibrated.

Wavelength

The wavelength scale must be verified using the absorption maxima of holmium perchlorate solution, the lines of a hydrogen or deuterium discharge lamp, or the lines of a mercury vapour lamp. The permitted tolerance is ±1 nm for the UV range and ±3 nm for the visible range.

Absorbance

The absorbance should be checked using suitable filters or a solution of potassium dichromate of 60 mg/L in 0.005 M sulfuric acid at the wavelengths indicated in Table 15.2.

Table 15.2 Wavelengths at which absorbance should be checked

Wavelength (nm)	Specific absorbance (A_1^1)	Maximum tolerance
235	124.5	122.9–126.2
257	144.5	142.8–146.2
313	48.6	47.0–50.3
350	107.3	105.6–109.0

Stray light

The level of stray light should be assessed, since it increases with instrument age. It may be detected at a given wavelength with suitable filters or a 1.2% w/v potassium chloride solution. The *European Pharmacopeia* (Council of Europe 2008) requires that the absorbance be greater than 2 at a wavelength of 198 nm when compared with water as compensation liquid.

Resolution

In some assays it is necessary to specify the minimum desirable resolution, since changes in the spectral bandwidth (or monochromator slit-width) can seriously affect the observed absorbance of sharp peaks. The *European Pharmacopoeia* (Council of Europe 2008) requires that the spectral bandwidth employed should be such that further reduction does not lead to an increase in measured absorbance. This is particularly important for drugs that have aromatic or strongly conjugated systems (e.g. diphenhydramine, phenoxymethylpenicillin, and amphotericin A and B). In such cases, a spectral bandwidth of more than 1 nm leads to a reduction in observed absorbance at the peak maximum (and conversely an increase in absorbance at a peak minimum), since the recorded absorbance is the mean of that over the whole bandwidth at that wavelength. Although increasing the slit width gives a better signal-to-noise ratio, a slit width of 2 nm is adequate for most bands, with 1 nm or 0.5 nm being used for very sharp peaks.

For qualitative analysis the resolution can be measured by recording the spectrum of a 0.02% solution of toluene in hexane. The minimum ratio of the absorbance at the maximum at 269 nm to that at the minimum at 266 nm is stated in the monographs of the *European Pharmacopoeia* (Council of Europe 2008).

Good laboratory practice

According to the principles of good laboratory practice (GLP), the apparatus should be periodically inspected, cleaned, maintained and calibrated according to the laboratory's Standard Operating Procedures. Records of procedures should be maintained. Calibration should, where appropriate, be traceable to national or international standards of measurements. Instrument manufacturers are now integrating GLP into their instruments. Examples of this include a logbook database in which lamp changes and defects are registered. Also, a key-lock function is now a common part of a quality system to avoid effects from unwanted keystrokes.

Sample preparation and presentation

The most frequent mode of sample presentation is as a dilute solution, although gases and solid surfaces can also be examined. Combinations of UV and visible spectrophotometry or spectrofluorimetry with HPLC are particularly advantageous for sensitive and selective detection of chromophores and/or fluorophores.

Cells

In the visible region, a matched pair of glass cells can be used, but they are inappropriate for the UV region because of the poor transmission properties of glass in this range (Fig. 15.8). Fused-silica or quartz cells have high transmittance from 190 to 1000 nm, and are therefore the cells of choice. The pathlength employed is usually 1.00 cm. Cells of longer pathlength are used for poorly absorptive drugs and/or where the concentration is low. Flow cells designed to minimise turbulent flow through the cell are used to monitor changes in absorbance during a reaction, for tablet dissolution studies, or for

HPLC. Care should be taken that the cell walls do not block the radiation beam, otherwise variable errors are introduced. Most removable cells have two clear faces through which the incident and transmitted radiation pass and two non-clear faces. The cell should be handled via the non-clear faces, thereby avoiding contamination of the clear faces. The cell should be aligned in the instrument so that the radiation passes through the clear faces. Cells provided with a thermostat are used for studies on enzymatic and other processes in which temperature is a key parameter.

The meticulous handling and care of cells is a necessary condition for precise and accurate measurement. Cells should be cleaned carefully, filled with an appropriate solvent and matched for absorbance to less than 1%. Each pair of cells should be marked on the base in soft pencil to identify the set and its normal orientation. The tolerance on the pathlength of the cells used is ±0.005 cm (Council of Europe 2008).

When filled with the same solvent, the cells intended to contain the solution to be examined and the compensation liquid must have the same transmittance. If this is not the case, an appropriate correction must be applied. It is convenient to designate the more strongly absorbing cell as the 'sample' cell, the other cell being coded as 'reference'. In this way the cell constant (i.e. the difference in absorbance at the measurement wavelength when filled with solvent) will be positive and can thus be subtracted from each absorbance reading. Moreover, the possibility of 'oscillating error' introduced by randomly changing the cell orientation during a series of measurements is eliminated. The 'cell constant' should be checked regularly at the measurement wavelength when filled with an appropriate solvent, or by scanning the baseline over the wavelength range.

Cells should be cleaned scrupulously after use. If they have contained aqueous solutions, they can be cleaned readily by repeated rinsing with distilled water or by soaking overnight in a very dilute solution of detergent. Special detergents should be used to clean cells contaminated with biological material. Cells that have been used with organic solvents require special care, with a sequence of solvents ending in spectroscopic ether being convenient to obtain dry, clean cells. In all cases, the manufacturer's instructions should be followed, when available. Sharp glass or metal objects should not be introduced into a cell, lest the internal surface be scratched. The outside optical surfaces should be polished

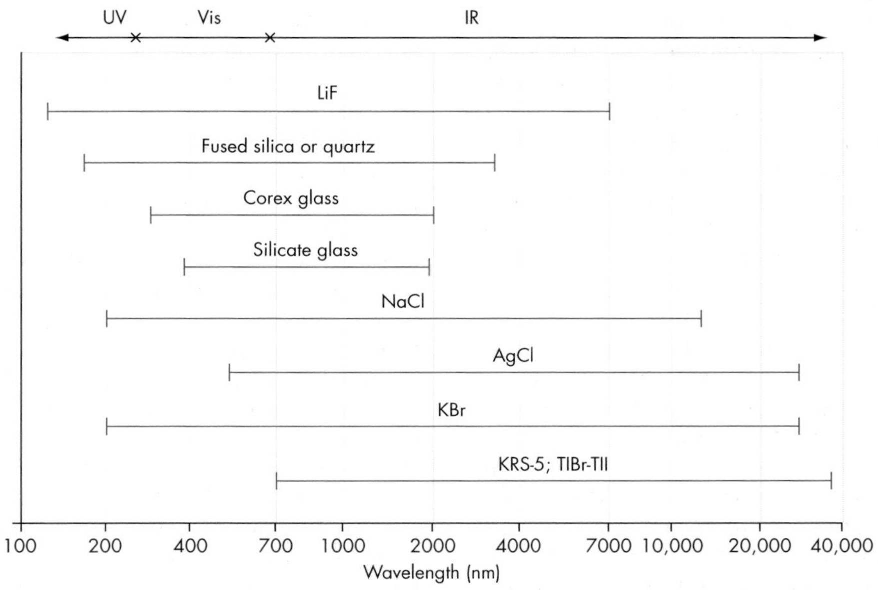

Figure 15.8 Transmittance range for various optical materials (from Skoog *et al.* 1996, p. 529).

before use with a soft cloth or photographic lens tissue. Cells should be stored in pairs, dry and in a protective container.

The types of cells used for HPLC–UV-visible and capillary electrophoresis (CE)–UV-visible are small and delicate and need to be in a precise orientation with the radiation beam to function efficiently. These cells are typically not removed from the instrument unless absolutely necessary. If maintenance is required, the instrument handbook should be consulted and extreme care should be taken in handling the cells.

Solvents

Solvents used in spectrophotometry must meet certain requirements to ensure successful and accurate results. The solvent chosen must dissolve the sample, yet be compatible with cuvette materials.

The solvent chosen must also be relatively transparent in the spectral region of interest. To avoid poor resolution and difficulties in spectrum interpretation, a solvent should not be used for measurements near or below its UV cut-off (i.e. the wavelength at which absorbance for the solvent alone approaches one absorbance unit). The cut-offs of common solvents are listed in Table 15.1.

Once a solvent is selected on the basis of physical and spectral characteristic, its purity must be considered. The absorbance curve of a solvent, as supplied, should be smooth (i.e. have no extraneous impurity peaks in the spectral region of interest). Solvents especially purified and certified for spectrophotometric use are available from suppliers.

Good laboratory practice

According to GLP, chemicals, reagents and solutions should be labelled to indicate identity (with concentration if appropriate), expiry date and specific storage instructions. Information concerning source, preparation date and stability should be available. The expiry date may be extended on the basis of documented evaluation or analysis.

Records, including test-item and reference-item characterisation, date of receipt, expiry date, and quantities received and used in studies should be maintained. Handling, sampling and storage procedures should be identified in order that the homogeneity and stability are assured, and that contamination and mix-up are precluded. Storage containers should carry information on identity, expiry date and specific storage instructions. The stability of test and reference items under storage and test conditions should be known for all studies.

Data processing and presentation of results

Single component systems

Where only one component in the sample absorbs significantly, the wavelength is chosen to coincide with the centre of a broad maximum in the spectrum to minimise wavelength-setting errors. For example, for 1,2,4,5-tetrazine in aqueous solution, a wavelength of 535 nm would be appropriate (see Fig. 15.1). If the spectrum has no suitable maximum, a flat absorption minimum can be used, provided that the consequent loss of sensitivity is acceptable. Wavelengths near the extremities of the UV and visible ranges must be avoided, because of the effects of stray-light errors.

Accurate measurements of a drug in solution may be difficult because of nonspecific absorption, i.e. absorption by other components in the sample. In these circumstances, the geometric correction devised by Morton and Stubbs (1946) is sometimes applied. This assumes that the nonspecific absorption varies linearly with wavelength over the range measured. Taking a solution of pure drug, two equi-absorptive points are selected, one at a lower wavelength (λ_1) and the other at a higher wavelength (λ_3) than that of the peak maximum (λ_2). Any irrelevant absorption in the sample increases the observed absorbance of one equi-absorptive point (usually λ_1) more than the other (λ_3). A simple geometrical calculation involving absorbances at λ_1 and λ_3 enables the absorbance at λ_2 to be corrected for the nonspecific absorption (Donbrow 1967). The assumption of linearity of the irrelevant absorption can be tested by subtracting the theoretical curve for the calculated quantity of pure material and inspecting the residual difference spectrum.

The classic example of a pharmacopoeial assay based on the Morton–Stubbs correction is that for vitamin A alcohol and the ester (*British Pharmacopoeia* 2002, p. 1783). Other techniques proposed for the correction of nonspecific absorption include difference spectrophotometry, second-derivative spectrophotometry, the use of orthogonal polynomials, and chemical or physical transformation of the drug to give absorption at a longer wavelength.

Multicomponent systems

The absorption spectra of two or more drugs of interest often overlap. Hence if two or more components with overlapping absorption spectra are in the sample matrix, problems can arise. Subject to certain conditions, the Vierordt method of simultaneous equations can be employed to obtain the individual concentrations (Glenn 1960). If each of n drugs obeys the Beer–Lambert law over the concentration range of interest, and if the law of additivity of absorbances applies, then the total absorbance, A_T^λ, observed at any wavelength λ is given by the sum:

$$A_T^\lambda = \sum_{i=1}^{n} A_i^\lambda = \sum_{i=1}^{n} k_i^\lambda c_i \ell \qquad (15.6)$$

where the subscript i denotes each component in the system. The term k_i^λ represents the specific absorbance ($A_{1\,\text{cm}}^{1\%}$) or the molar absorptivity ε ($\text{L mol}^{-1}\,\text{cm}^{-1}$), as determined by the units selected for concentration c_i.

For a two-component system, two wavelengths λ_1 and λ_2 are selected (as discussed below) and two corresponding simultaneous equations are set up:

$$A_T^{\lambda_1}/\ell = k_1^{\lambda_1} c_1 + k_2^{\lambda_1} c_2 \qquad (15.7)$$

$$A_T^{\lambda_2}/\ell = k_1^{\lambda_2} c_1 + k_2^{\lambda_2} c_2 \qquad (15.8)$$

Equations (15.7) and (15.8) readily yield the concentration of each component, c_1 and c_2, by conventional algebra.

The selection of appropriate wavelengths and the use of accurate absorptivity values are clearly crucial. Generally, λ_1 is the λ_{max} for component 1, while λ_2 is the λ_{max} for component 2, provided that at these wavelengths the absorptivity of the overlapping component is small. If the spectra of both components are very similar, the errors of the method increase appreciably as the difference between the absorptivity ratios tends to zero.

Although this method should apply to the analysis of three or more components, in practice it is often difficult to select wavelengths that fulfil all the requisite conditions.

The limit test for amphotericin A (a tetraene, λ_{max} 300 nm) in the antifungal antibiotic amphotericin (consisting primarily of amphotericin B, a heptaene, λ_{max} 380 nm) is an example of such a two-component analysis (*British Pharmacopoeia* 2007).

Difference spectrophotometry

Difference spectrophotometry is a method of compensating for the presence of extraneous materials in a sample that would otherwise interfere with the spectrum of the drug being determined. It involves the measurement of the absorbance difference, at a defined wavelength, between two samples in one of which a physical or chemical property of the drug has been changed. It is assumed that the spectrum of the drug can be changed without affecting the spectrum of the interfering material. Alternatively, the absorbance difference may be measured between the sample and an equivalent solution without the drug. Difference spectrophotometry is sometimes described as 'differential spectrophotometry', but this term is not recommended because of its possible confusion with derivative spectrophotometry.

Many suitable methods for physical and chemical modification of the drug absorbance have been reported. For example, the bathochromic effect (also discussed later) is used in the difference spectrophotometric assay of barbiturates. The absorbance of the sample at about pH 10 (A_{10}), to which the mono-anionic species contributes (A_B) (see p. 409, Fig. 15.11), is used to compensate for the absorption of interfering endogenous materials (A_M) that have been carried through the extraction procedure. The sample absorbance at pH 13 (A_{13}) (see Fig. 15.11), to which the di-anionic species (A_D) contributes, is measured at about 260 nm with reference to the sample absorbance at pH 10 (A_{10}), so that:

$$A_{13} = A_D + A_M \tag{15.9}$$

$$A_{10} = A_B + A_M \tag{15.10}$$

Thus:

$$\Delta A = A_{13} - A_{10} = A_D - A_B \tag{15.11}$$

If

$$\Delta\varepsilon = (\varepsilon_D - \varepsilon_B) \tag{15.12}$$

then

$$\Delta A = \Delta\varepsilon \ell c \tag{15.13}$$

Thus, the difference absorbance can be related readily to concentration by prior calibration of the constant $\Delta\varepsilon$, or the concentration may be found by simple proportion:

$$\Delta A_{test}/\Delta A_{standard} = c_{test}/c_{standard} \tag{15.14}$$

It should, however, be established that ΔA is a linear function of concentration (c) over the range required. It is convenient to select for the analytical wavelength a value that corresponds to a maximum in the difference spectrum, obtained by scanning the sample and reference solution over an appropriate wavelength range.

Difference spectrophotometry can be used for quality control in cases where the interfering material is well defined, because an appropriate dilution of a suitable reference solution can be used in the reference cell. The difference absorbance is, however, susceptible to systematic error when there is uncertainty in the concentration of interfering materials in the samples to be assayed. This error increases in proportion to the ratio of the molar absorptivity of the interference to that of the drug.

A further technique to correct for absorptive interferences by difference measurement is based on *dual-wavelength spectrophotometry* (not to be confused with dual-beam spectrophotometry). In dual-wavelength spectrophotometry, two monochromatic beams at different wavelengths are passed through the same sample. One wavelength (λ_1) is generally characteristic of the drug, while the other (λ_2) is selected carefully so that the absorbance is equivalent to the level of absorptive interference (A_m^{λ}) anticipated at the analytical wavelength (λ_1). Thus, the second radiation beam is analogous to the reference cell employed in conventional difference spectrophotometry, and the difference in absorbance at the two wavelengths (ΔA) represents the absorption of drug (A_m^{λ}) corrected for interference:

$$A^{\lambda^2} = A_n^{\lambda_1} + A_m^{\lambda_2} \tag{15.15}$$

and since

$$A^{\lambda_2} = A_m^{\lambda_1} \tag{15.16}$$

then

$$\Delta A = A^{\lambda_1} - A^{\lambda_2} = A_n^{\lambda_1} \tag{15.17}$$

A classic application of this method is the correction of Rayleigh scatter in samples of biological origin.

Derivative spectrophotometry

In derivative spectrophotometry, the absorbance (A) of a sample is differentiated with respect to wavelength (λ) to generate the first, second or higher-order derivatives:

$A = f(\lambda)$,	zero order
$dA/d\lambda = f'(\lambda)$,	first derivative
$d^2A/d\lambda^2 = f''(\lambda)$,	second derivative

and so on.

Derivative spectra often yield a characteristic profile, in which subtle changes of gradient and curvature in the normal (zero-order) spectrum are observed as distinctive bipolar features

(Fig. 15.9). The first derivative of an absorption spectrum represents the gradient at all points of the spectrum and can be used to locate 'hidden' peaks, since $dA/d\lambda = 0$ at peak maxima (Fig. 15.9). However, second- and higher even-order derivatives are potentially more useful in analysis.

The even-order derivatives are bipolar functions of alternating sign at the centroid (i.e. negative for 2nd, positive for 4th, etc.), whose position coincides with that of the original peak maximum (Fig. 15.9). To this extent, even-derivative spectra bear a similarity to the original spectrum, although the presence of satellite peaks that flank the centroid adds a degree of complexity to the derivative profile. A key feature is that the derivative centroid peak width of a Gaussian peak decreases to 53%, 41% and 34% of the original peak width, in the second, fourth and sixth orders, respectively. This feature can increase the resolution of overlapping peaks. However, the increasingly complex satellite patterns detract from resolution enhancement in higher derivative spectra.

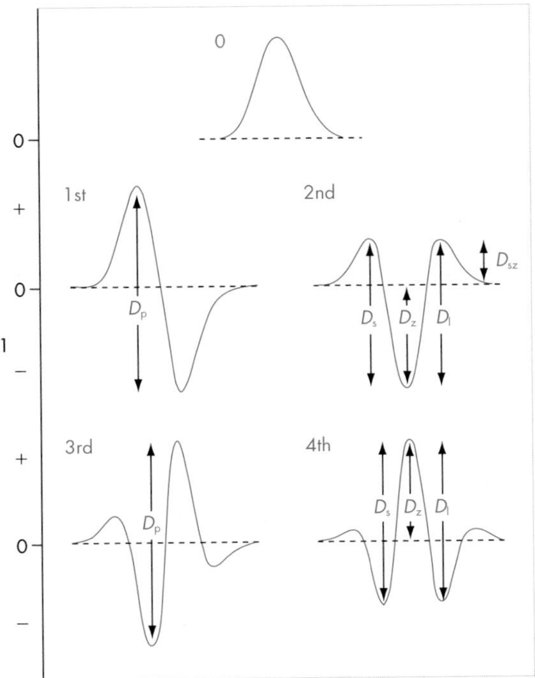

Figure 15.9 First to fourth derivatives of a Gaussian peak, and some graphical measures of derivative amplitude (D): D_p, peak-to-peak; D_s, peak-to-satellite at short wavelength; D_z, peak-to-derivative zero; D_l, peak-to-satellite at long wavelength; D_{sz}, satellite peak-to-derivative zero.

Although transformation of a spectrum to its second- or higher-order derivative often yields a more highly characteristic profile than the zero-order spectrum, the intrinsic information content of the data is not increased; indeed, some data, such as constant 'offset' factors, are lost. The advantage of the derivative method is that it tends to emphasise subtle spectral features by presenting them in a new and visually more accessible way. The method is generally applicable in analytical chemistry and can be used equally for resolution enhancement of electrochemical, chromatographic or thermal analysis data. It is widely used in near infrared spectroscopy (see Chapter 16).

Derivative spectrophotometry has found application in clinical, forensic and biomedical analysis (Gill *et al.* 1982). In forensic toxicology, the suppression of the absorption from interfering substances by second-derivative spectrophotometry is well demonstrated in studies on amfetamine in a homogenised liver extract (Fig. 15.10). The characteristic absorption spectrum of amfetamine (Fig. 15.10C) is masked by interfering substances in a homogenised liver extract suspected to contain amfetamine (Fig. 15.10A). The second-derivative spectrum of the liver extract reveals a very similar spectrum to the second-derivative spectrum for amfetamine (Figs. 15.10B and D, respectively), clearly illustrating the use of this data treatment technique.

Interpretation of spectra and qualitative analysis

Spectrophotometric measurements with UV or visible radiation are useful for detecting components that contain unsaturated groups or atoms such as sulfur or halogens. A drug, its impurity or a metabolite can also be transformed selectively so that the spectrum is shifted to the visible region and away from interference caused by another drug, formulation components, or

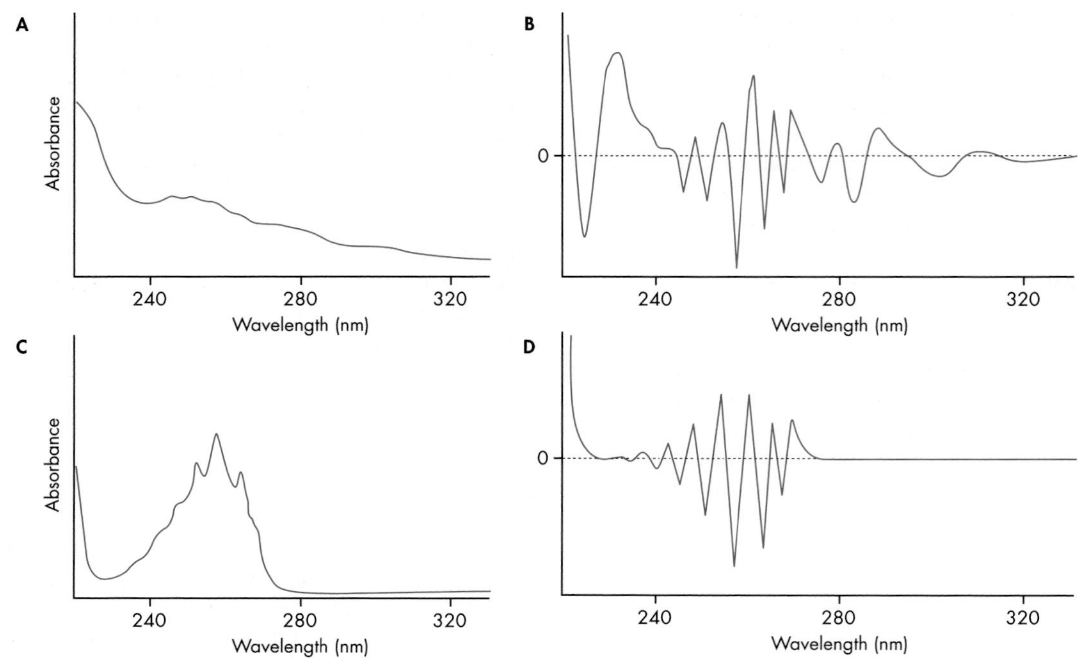

Figure 15.10 Detection of amfetamine in homogenised liver extract. Standard zero-order (A) and second-derivative (B) spectra of the liver extract, compared with the standard zero-order (C) and second-derivative (D) spectra of amfetamine. Solutions were in 0.1 M sulfuric acid. (From Gill *et al.* 1982.)

biological substances, and thereby confer a further degree of specificity.

However, specific identification of a compound can rarely be made on the basis of UV spectral evidence alone. Often, the spectrum serves as confirmatory evidence of identity, in support of other analytical data such as nuclear magnetic resonance (NMR), MS, IR. The general approach usually followed in qualitative applications is first to establish by independent means (e.g. chromatography) that the material consists substantially of one absorbing component. Spectra are then recorded in aqueous acidic, basic and ethanolic or methanolic solution. The wavelengths of the principal peaks and the corresponding absorptivity values are noted for each solvent system. The data are then compared with data for UV absorption maxima for standard substances tabulated in wavelength order. A number of compounds with absorbing properties similar to the test substance are identified (using a wavelength window of ± 2 nm) as potential candidates for the unknown substance. One must be aware that, in general, the UV-vis spectrum of a metabolite of a component closely matches the spectrum of the component itself.

Further evidence of substance identity can be deduced from the absorptivity ratios of peaks within a spectrum; moreover as has already been discussed, the change in these ratios together with the shift in peak positions as the pH is changed can be diagnostic. If a drug molecule ionises reversibly (i.e. without degradation), the family of curves for a constant concentration in acidic and basic solvents displays one or more isosbestic points at characteristic wavelengths, at which the absorbance is constant at all values of pH.

Spectral shifts are among the most useful diagnostic features in drug molecules that possess ionisable groups. A marked *bathochromic shift* (or 'red' shift) to longer wavelengths in alkaline solution is observed not only for most of the phenolic drugs, such as the phenolic oestrogens, but also in the case of hydroxypyridines, ketones, benzodiazepines, pyridones and nitro-compounds. The bathochromic shift is often large (<10 nm) and accompanied by an increase in molar absorptivity (*hyperchromic effect*) and loss of any fine structure.

This effect has been exploited, for both qualitative and quantitative purposes, for the analysis of barbiturates. In acidic or neutral solution, barbiturates show little absorption above 230 nm (Fig. 15.11A), but in 0.05 M borax buffer (pH 9.2), ionisation yields an intense conjugated chromophore (Figs 15.11B and 15.12) with a well-defined maximum near 240 nm (A_1^1 = 400–450). In sodium hydroxide solution (pH 13), a second stage of ionisation occurs (except in *N*-substituted derivatives) to further extend the conjugation and give a peak maximum near 255 nm (Figs 15.11C and 15.12). However, solutions in alkali are unstable through ring-opening, so that measurements must be made rapidly.

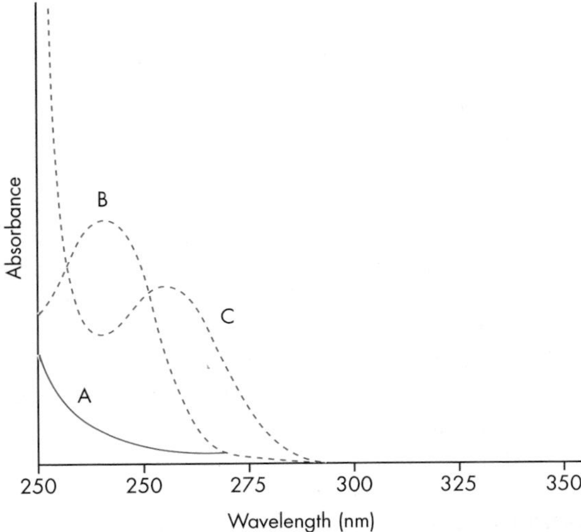

Figure 15.11 Effect of pH on the UV spectrum of phenobarbital. Curve A: nonionised barbiturate in 0.1 M hydrochloric acid. Curve B: mono-anion in 0.05 M borax buffer (pH 9.2). Curve C: di-anion in 0.5 M sodium hydroxide (pH 13).

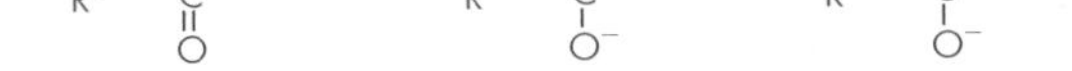

Figure 15.12 Dissociation of C5–substituted barbituric acids: (A) undissociated free acid; (B) mono-anion; (C) di-anion.

The *hypochromic* or 'blue' shift to shorter wavelengths is shown by aromatic amines in acid solution and is highly characteristic for many drugs. On acidification, the protonated quaternary ammonium group no longer participates in the chromophore, so that the spectrum is shifted to shorter wavelengths, sometimes by as much as 30 nm, with a sharp fall in absorptivity (*hypochromic effect*).

In addition to their use in characterising a chromophore, pH-induced shifts can also be exploited to shift a spectrum along the wavelength scale to obtain an interference-free window in which to measure an ionisable species in a mixture.

Solvent effects

A solvent for UV and visible spectroscopy must be transparent throughout the region of interest and should dissolve a sufficient quantity of the sample to give well-defined peaks. Moreover, consideration must be given to possible interactions with the absorbing species. For example, polar solvents, such as water, alcohols, esters and ketones, tend to suppress vibrational fine structure and should thus be avoided when spectral detail is desired. Nonpolar solvents, such as cyclohexane, often provide spectra that more closely approach that of a gas (see also Fig. 15.1). In addition, the polarity of the solvent often influences the position of absorption maxima. Consequently, a common solvent must be employed when comparing spectra for the purpose of identification.

When using an HPLC-UV system, any effects on the spectral characteristics of a substance brought about by various mobile phases must be considered when comparing spectra generated in this manner with those recorded from acidic, neutral and alkaline solutions. Moreover, potential effects brought about during gradient elution HPLC, in which the composition of the mobile phases is constantly changing, should be borne in mind. With acetonitrile, methanol, ethanol, propan-2-ol and other water-miscible solvents, no essential changes in the spectra may occur and direct comparison with other databases is feasible. However, changes in pH can have a significant effect on the UV spectra of compounds involved in an acid–base equilibrium (e.g. carboxylic acids, phenols, thiophenols) and compounds with basic nitrogen atoms. Direct comparison of spectra with other compendia of data, including those listed in the Collections of data on p. 419, is only valid when the mobile phases have the same pH.

Quantitative analysis

Fundamental basis

The basic principle of most spectrophotometric measurements involves comparing, under well-defined conditions, the absorption of radiation by the substance in an unknown amount with the same absorption of radiation by a known amount of the material being determined. In general, to obtain the maximum sensitivity it is best to work with radiation of a wavelength that is approximately equal to that for which the solution exhibits a maximum selective absorption.

Assuming that the linear range for compliance with the Beer–Lambert law has been established and that the drug concentration has been adjusted within the optimum range for the type of instrument concerned, two approaches to quantification may be employed:

- reference standards
- specific absorbance.

Reference standards

If an acceptable reference standard of the drug is available, and if the calibration graph passes through zero, measurement of replicates of the standard (at a comparable concentration) and of the test solutions are performed in bracketing sequence (i.e. each group of samples is preceded and followed by the standard), under identical conditions of solvent and temperature and using the same pair of matched cells. Each result should be corrected for the cell constant. The concentration of the test sample is then found by reference to the results from the standards. Where UV-visible is coupled to liquid chromatography, it is more usual to run a series of calibration standards where the concentration of the standards covers a known but varying range. The calibration standards are analysed first, then the test samples. Where large sample batches are analysed, it is good practice to analyse one of the standards after every 10 samples. A calibration line is plotted and the values for the samples are interpolated from the calibration line.

Specific absorbance

The specific absorbance can be used to calculate the sample concentration, using the absorbance measured in the specified solvent. A check on the accuracy of the absorbance scale is clearly essential. Wavelength accuracy is not so important.

The practical usefulness of reference-specific absorbance values (A_1^1) clearly depends on a number of factors. These include the state of purity of the substance, the solvent conditions originally used to establish the reference data, the precise conditions employed in the reference instrument and the extent to which they correspond with those of a particular test laboratory. It is therefore wise to ascertain the status of any absorptivity data in the literature. If a sample of the drug concerned is available in pure form, it is good practice to establish periodically a 'local' value of the absorptivity and to use this in calculating sample concentrations.

Linearity issues

The validity of the Beer–Lambert law should be established for each drug under the measurement conditions to be used over an appropriate concentration range. For single-beam instruments, the absorbance range for precise measurements is between about 0.3 and 0.6 absorbance units, the optimum being at 0.43 absorbance units. For double-beam spectrophotometers, the optimum range lies between 0.6 and 1.2 absorbance units. Five or more standard solutions, with absorbances that span the working range, should be measured in duplicate in a matched pair of cells against the solvent as reference; the residual absorbance difference between the cells when filled with solvent (the cell constant) should be subtracted from each individual measurement and checked regularly.

The linearity of an analytical method is determined by mathematical treatment of the absorbance data of the standard solutions across the claimed range of the method. The treatment is normally a calculation of a regression line $y = ax + b$, with y being the absorbance and x the concentration, by the method of least squares. The linearity is usually expressed by means of a correlation coefficient r, where:

$$r = \frac{\sum_i (c_i - \bar{c})(A_i - \bar{A})}{\sqrt{\left(\sum_i (c_i - \bar{c})^2\right)\left(\sum_i (A_i - \bar{A})^2\right)}} \qquad (15.18)$$

for all n points with i from unity to n.

When $r = 1$, there is a perfect correlation. Usually, r values better than 0.995 can be obtained.

The intercept should not differ significantly from zero. If a significant non-zero intercept is obtained, it should be demonstrated that there is no effect on the accuracy of the method.

Linearity should be evaluated graphically in addition to or alternatively to a mathematical evaluation. The evaluation is made by visual inspection of a plot of absorbance A as a function of analyte concentration c. If any systematic positive or negative deviation is found, additional points should be inserted and the linear working range established.

International Conference on Harmonisation Validation Criteria

The main objective of validation of an analytical procedure is to demonstrate that the procedure is suitable for its intended purpose. The objective of an analytical procedure should be understood clearly, since this will govern the validation characteristics that need to be evaluated. Typical validation characteristics that should be considered according to the International Conference on Harmonisation of Technical Requirements for Registration of Pharmaceuticals for Human Use (ICH) are:

- accuracy
- precision (repeatability and intermediate precision)
- specificity
- detection limit
- quantification limit
- linearity and range.

All these characteristics are also listed and explained in the USP 30 (USP 2007). For the quantitative determination of impurities, all these criteria should be evaluated, while for limit tests the specificity and detection limit are most relevant. For assays, all characteristics except detection limit and quantification limit are normally evaluated.

For linearity, the ICH recommends a minimum of five concentrations to be measured.

Fluorescence spectrophotometry

General considerations and theoretical background

As noted in the introduction to this chapter, many of the comments applied to spectrophotometry measured in the UV-visible region also apply to fluorescence spectrophotometry. However, there are some fundamental differences which apply to fluorescence spectrophotometry; not least the molecular basis of fluorescence itself. The consequences of this are that there are some differences in instrumentation, sample treatment and data interpretation that merit a discussion of fluorescence spectrophotometry in addition to UV-visible.

Molecular fluorescence is an emission process in which molecules are excited by the absorption of electromagnetic radiation. The excited species then relax to the ground state, giving up their excess energy as photons.

There are several ways an excited molecule can give up its excess energy and relax to its ground state. Two of the most important of these mechanisms are nonradiative relaxation and fluorescent relaxation.

Nonradiative relaxation can occur through collisions between excited molecules and molecules of the solvent, by giving excess energy to solvent molecules. When relaxation takes place by fluorescence, bands of radiation are produced as the excited molecules relax to several energy states, which are very close in energy level and thus in wavelength (Fig. 15.13). Fluorescence occurs only from the lowest vibrational level of an excited electronic state.

Molecular fluorescence bands are made up largely of lines that are longer in wavelength (lower in energy) than the band of absorbed radiation responsible for their excitation. This shift to longer wavelength is sometimes called the Stokes' shift. For that reason, the absorption or excitation spectrum and the fluorescence spectrum for a compound often appear as approximate mirror images of one another. The most useful region for the fluorescence technique is 200–800 nm.

Fluorescence spectrophotometry is usually the method of choice for quantitative analytical purposes if applicable. It has assumed a major role in analysis, particularly the determination of trace contaminants in our environment, industries and bodies, because for applicable compounds fluorescence spectrometry gives high sensitivity and high specificity. The selectivity of fluorescence methods is greater than that of absorption methods, as fewer substances fluoresce than absorb radiation in the UV or

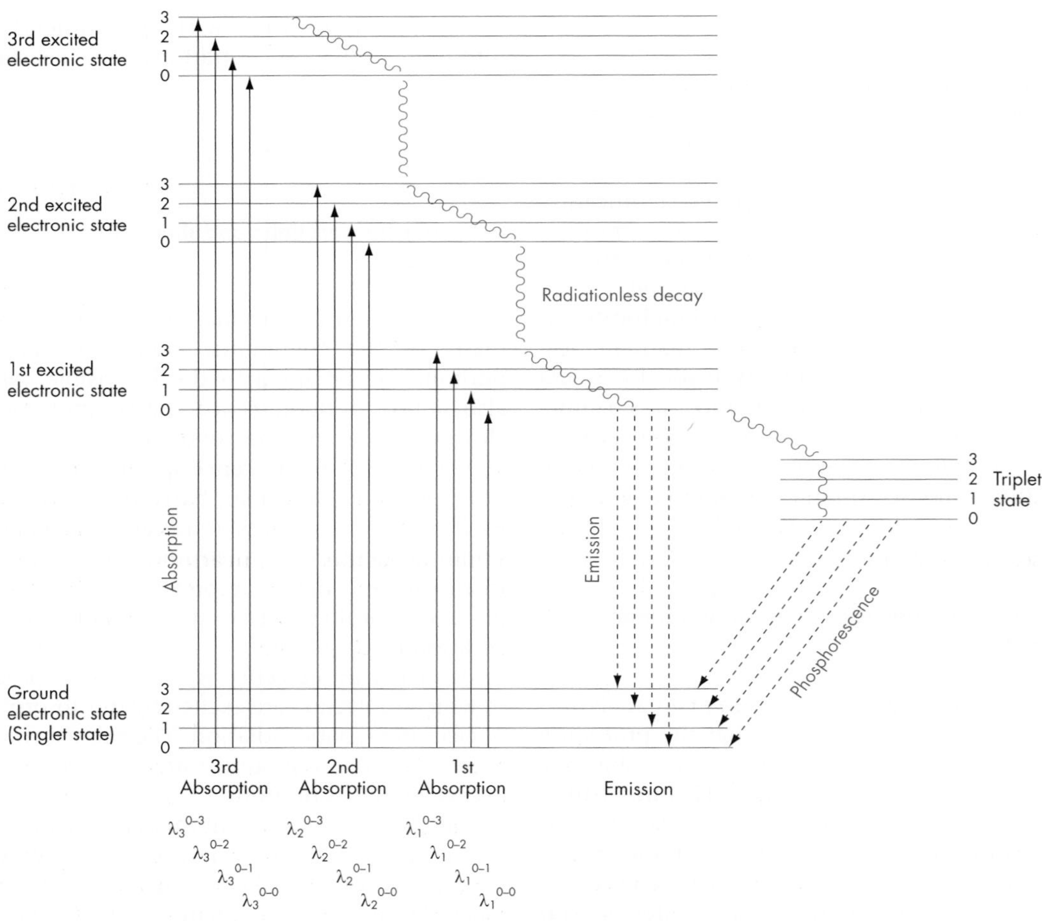

Figure 15.13 Normal absorption (excitation), radiationless decay, and fluorescence of an isolated chromophore.

visible region. Furthermore, fluorescence is more selective because both the emission and the absorption spectra can be obtained. Fluorescence is usually also more sensitive than absorption methods, as it is always easier to measure a small signal against a very small zero background than to measure a small difference between large signals. However, the phenomenon of fluorescence itself is subject to more rigorous constraints on molecular structure than is absorption, such that only a relatively limited number of substances exhibit fluorescence. It is possible to introduce a fluorophore by chemical reaction (derivatisation) and this is widely employed in spectrophotometry to take advantage of the sensitivity and specificity of fluorescence.

Nomenclature

A term used in fluorescence is quantum efficiency, described by the quantum yield (i.e. the ratio of the number of molecules that fluoresce to the total number of excited molecules). Highly fluorescent molecules can have quantum efficiencies that approach unity. Some drugs possess rather high quantum efficiencies for fluorescence, such as quinine and lysergide (LSD).

All absorbing molecules have the potential to fluoresce. They do so if fluorescent emission occurs at a greater rate than relaxation by nonradiative ways. The kind of relaxation process is highly dependent on the molecular structure. Compounds that contain aromatic rings give the most intense and most useful fluorescence emission. Substitution on an aromatic ring causes shifts in the excitation wavelength spectrum and in fluorescence efficiency. Substituents such as $—NH_2$, $—OH$, $—OCH_3$ and $—NHCH_3$ groups often enhance fluorescence, while $—Cl$, $—Br$, $—I$, $—NO_2$ or $—COOH$ are electron-withdrawing groups that can lead to a complete reduction of fluorescence (e.g. aniline fluoresces while nitrobenzene does not). The molecular grouping responsible for fluorescence is sometimes described as a fluorophore.

Fluorescence is particularly favoured in rigid molecules, as molecular rigidity reduces deactivation by nonradiative processes (fewer internal vibrations). This is also why certain organic chelating agents are more fluorescent when complexed with a metal ion.

Laws of fluorescence spectrophotometry

The power of fluorescent radiation I_f is proportional to the radiant power of the excitation beam absorbed by the system:

$$I_f = K'(I_0 - I) \qquad (15.19)$$

The constant K' depends upon the quantum efficiency of the fluorescence. To relate I_f to the molar concentration c of the fluorescing molecule, Beer's law can be used:

$$I/I_0 = 10^{-\varepsilon \ell c} \qquad (15.20)$$

By substituting Equation (15.20) into (15.19) we obtain:

$$I_f = K' I_0(1 - 10^{-\varepsilon \ell c}) \qquad (15.21)$$

After expansion of the exponential term, and provided $\varepsilon lc < 0.05$, we can write:

$$I_f = 2,3\ K' \varepsilon \ell c I_0 \qquad (15.22)$$

or at constant I_0:

$$I_f = Kc \qquad (15.23)$$

Thus, a plot of the fluorescence power of a solution versus the concentration of the emitting species should be linear at low concentrations. Limiting factors for linearity are not only the concentration of the solute, but also factors such as the blank fluorescence, quenching and absorption of exciting radiation by the solvent.

Quenching and other special effects

When the fluorescence of a species is attenuated as a result of its reaction with an analyte, the signal decreases. This effect is called quenching and can be used for quantification purposes, primarily for the determination of anions. Quenching can also be an unwanted effect in the case of dissolved oxygen (see p. 416).

Also, if the analyte is too concentrated, self-quenching may occur when fluorescing molecules collide and lose their excitation energy by radiationless transfer. The fluorescence versus concentration curve may have a maximum and then actually show a decrease in fluorescent power with increasing concentration. It is imperative in quantitative determinations to be aware of this problem, since a given fluorescent power can correspond to two values of concentration.

Instrumentation

General considerations

As noted for UV-visible, the basic components of analytical instruments for absorption and fluorescence spectroscopy are alike in function and general performance requirements. However, some special conditions apply to instruments for measuring fluorescence. Such instruments are generally referred to as fluorimeters.

Single-beam fluorimeters

A single-beam fluorimeter consists of a radiation source (usually a mercury or xenon lamp), a primary filter (excitation), a sample cell, a secondary filter (emission) and a fluorescence detection system. In most such fluorimeters the detector is placed on an axis at 90° from that of the exciting beam. This right-angle geometry permits the exciting radiation to pass through the test specimen and not contaminate the output signal received by the fluorescence detector. However, the detector unavoidably receives some of the exciting radiation as a result of the inherent scattering properties of the solutions themselves, or if dust or other solids are present. Filters are used to eliminate this residual scatter. The primary filter selects the short-wavelength radiation able to excite the test specimen, while the secondary filter is normally a sharp cut-off filter that allows the longer wavelength fluorescence to be transmitted, but blocks the scattered excitation (see Fig. 15.14). Most fluorimeters use photomultiplier tubes as detectors. The photocurrent is amplified and read out on a meter or recorder.

Scanning spectrofluorimeters

When at least one monochromator (grating or prism) is used instead of a filter, the instrument is called a spectrofluorimeter. The use of gratings instead of filters makes the instrument superior in wavelength selectivity, flexibility and convenience. More complex spectrofluorimeters employ two diffraction gratings (or prisms) to select the fixed excitation wavelength (λ_{ex}) and the fixed wavelength (λ_f), together with a high-intensity xenon source, scanning motors and electronic compensation for variations in source intensity as the wavelength is varied.

Coupled techniques

As with UV-visible detectors which are coupled to HPLC, for components of interest that fluoresce, the chromatographic system can be equipped with a fluorimetric detector (LC-FL). In

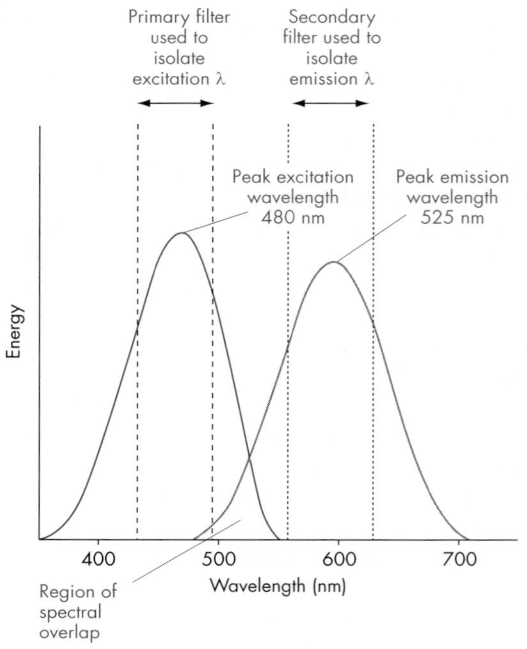

Figure 15.14 Illustration of filters used to isolate wavelengths for excitation and emission.

the case of weakly fluorescent or nonfluorescent drugs, a number of well-characterised derivatisation reactions are available. These include dansyl chloride (5-dimethylaminonaphthalene-1-sulfonyl chloride) for primary and secondary amines (Fig. 15.15) and phenolic hydroxyl groups, and fluorescamine 4-phenylspiro-[furan-2(3*H*), 1′-isobenzofuran]-3,3′-dione, fluorogenic 2,1,3-benzoxadiazoles and *o*-phthalaldehyde for primary amines. Derivatisation reactions of this type have extended the scope of fluorescence detection in HPLC significantly.

A fluorescence detector can be coupled with capillary electrophoresis (CE-FL) or ion chromatography to determine charged components in complex mixtures.

Instrument performance checks

In fluorescence the calibration of excitation and emission monochromator wavelengths should be checked regularly by the use of sharp lines from the instrument's own radiation source (e.g. xenon lines at 450.1, 462.4, 467.1 and 473.4 nm) or the use of sharp fluorescence peaks in solutions or glasses of trivalent lanthanide ions (terbium, europium). Other fluorescence standards in common use are ovulene and other polycyclic aromatic hydrocarbons with fine vibrational structures such as naphthalene and anthracene. In practice, it is necessary only to calibrate one monochromator, since the other can then be calibrated by the Rayleigh scattered

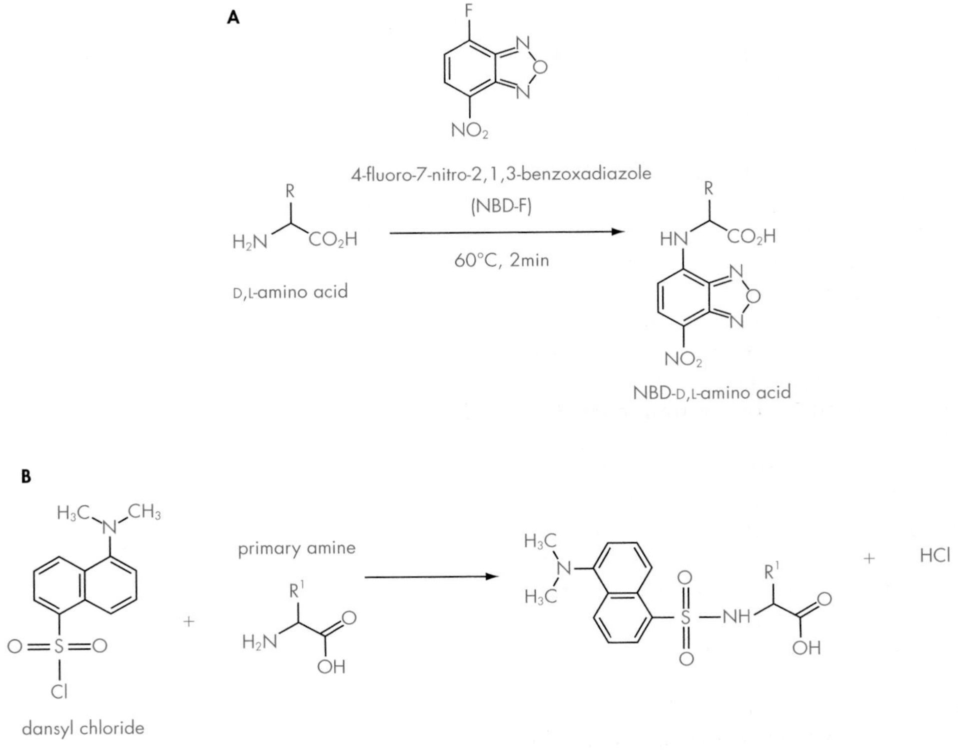

Figure 15.15 Example of derivatisation to produce a fluorescent derivatives. (A) Derivatization of an amino acid using NBD-F. (B) Derivatisation of a primary amine using dansyl chloride.

radiation using a sample of colloidal silica in the sample position. The use of an auxiliary light source, such as a mercury light pen, is the least satisfactory method for wavelength calibration.

Sample preparation and presentation

The most frequent mode of sample presentation is as a dilute solution, although gases and solid surfaces can also be examined. Combinations of spectrofluorimetry with HPLC are particularly advantageous for sensitive and selective detection of fluorophores. A fluorescence detector can be combined in series with a UV-visible detector to provide additional information from analysis of complex mixtures (e.g. to differentiate fluorescent and nonfluorescent substances).

Cells

Specimen cells used in fluorescence measurements may be round tubes or rectangular cells similar to those used in absorption spectrophotometry, except that they are polished on all four vertical sides. A convenient test specimen size is 2 to 3 mL, but some instruments can be fitted with small cells holding 100–300 μL or with a capillary holder that requires an even smaller specimen volume.

Temperature regulation is often important in fluorescence spectrophotometry. For some substances, fluorescence efficiency may be reduced by as much as 1–2% per degree of temperature rise. In such cases, if maximum precision is desired, temperature-controlled sample cells are useful. For routine analysis, it may be sufficient to make measurements rapidly enough so that the specimen does not heat up appreciably from exposure to the intense light source (USP 2007).

Solvents

Change of solvent may markedly affect the intensity and spectral distribution of fluorescence. It is inadvisable, therefore, to alter the solvent specified in established methods without careful preliminary investigation. Many compounds are fluorescent in organic solvents but virtually nonfluorescent in water. Thus, a number of solvents should be tried before it is decided whether or not a compound is fluorescent. In many organic solvents, the intensity of fluorescence is increased by elimination of dissolved oxygen, which has a strong quenching effect. Oxygen may be removed by bubbling an inert gas, such as nitrogen or helium, through the test specimen.

Data processing and presentation of results

Analytical fluorimetry

The fluorescence properties of a compound are characterised by two spectra. An excitation spectrum is obtained by monitoring the fluorescence at a convenient fixed wavelength λ_f, while scanning the excitation monochromator at a fixed speed up to a wavelength no higher than λ_f. The excitation spectrum should, in principle, be comparable with the absorption spectrum. The fluorescence spectrum is obtained by illuminating the sample at a convenient fixed excitation wavelength λ_{ex} and scanning the emission monochromator at a fixed speed over a wavelength range no lower than λ_{ex}.

Some spectrofluorimeters are able to scan the excitation and emission monochromators synchronously to yield fluorescence spectra which are generally simpler and considerably sharper than the conventional fluorescence spectrum. With computer-aided spectrofluorimetry, the acquisition and digital storage of fluorescence spectra are possible. These can then be manipulated in various ways to give the derivative spectrum (see equivalent section for UV-visible above) in which fine structure is accentuated, the difference spectrum, or multiwavelength spectral deconvolution, to calculate the concentration of known overlapping components (Winfield *et al.* 1984).

In another digital technique, a series of fluorescence spectra are acquired while sequentially stepping the excitation wavelength. When these spectra are combined to give a matrix of (I_f, λ_f, λ_{ex}), a three-dimensional isometric projection is presented. This type of graphic presentation is described as an 'emission–excitation matrix' or 'fluorogram' (Fig. 15.16). The data can also be plotted as the equivalent two-dimensional plot of isointensity contours in the (λ_f–λ_{ex}) plane (Fig. 15.17). Three-dimensional graphics are increasingly used for the qualitative comparison of fluorescent molecules, as in the example of promethazine and its principal degradation product, promethazine sulfoxide (Figs 15.16 and 15.17).

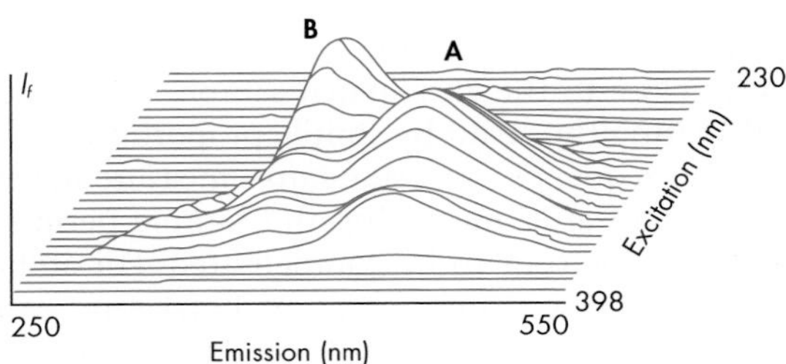

Figure 15.16 Isometric projection of emission–excitation matrix of fluorescence intensity (I_f) for promethazine hydrochloride (A) and promethazine sulfoxide (B) in buffer at pH 3.0. (From Fell *et al.* 1981.)

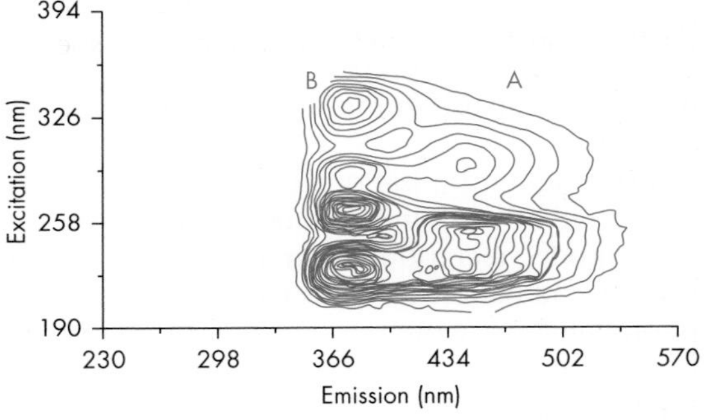

Figure 15.17 Contour plot of emission–excitation matrix of promethazine hydrochloride (A) and promethazine sulfoxide (B) in buffer at pH 3.0. (From Clark *et al.* 1985.)

Interpretation of spectra and qualitative analysis

For compounds with appropriate fluorescence properties, spectrofluorimetry gives high sensitivity and high specificity. High sensitivity results from the difference in wavelengths between the exciting and fluorescence radiation. This results in a signal contrasted with an essentially zero background; it is always easier to measure a small signal directly than a small difference between two large signals, as is done in absorption spectrophotometry. High specificity results from dependence on two spectra, the excitation and emission spectra, and the possibility of measuring the lifetimes of the fluorescent state. Although in biological samples the fluorescence intensity of interfering substances may be relatively high, the sensitivity and selectivity of the method are generally such that fluorescent drugs and their metabolites can be analysed more readily than by conventional spectrophotometry. Two compounds that are excited at the same wavelength but emit at different wavelengths are readily differentiated without the use of chemical separation techniques. Likewise, two compounds may fluoresce at the same wavelength but require different excitation wavelengths, thus enabling differentiation. Also, a fluorescent compound in the presence of one or more nonfluorescent compounds is readily analysed fluorimetrically, even when the compounds have overlapping absorption spectra. Nonfluorescent or weakly fluorescent compounds can often be derivatised with strong fluorophores, which enables them to be determined quantitatively.

Many fluorescent species contain ionisable groups with fluorescent properties sensitive to pH. In some cases only one of the ionised species may be fluorescent. Examples are the barbiturates, which only fluoresce at an elevated pH in the di-anionic form. Phenol fluoresces at pH 7, but at pH 12, when it is converted into its anion, there is no fluorescence. Therefore, the relationship of fluorescence intensity with pH should always be examined as part of the method development.

Fluorescence intensity and wavelength often vary with the solvent. In most molecules, fluorescence decreases with a decrease in solvent viscosity as the probability of intermolecular energy transfer tends to be enhanced. The same effect occurs with an increase in temperature.

Quantitative analysis

Fundamental basis

Excitation spectra are usually used to confirm the identity of components and to select an optimum excitation wavelength for quantitative analysis. The emission spectrum is then used for analytical applications.

Spectrofluorimetry differs from absorption spectrophotometry in not yielding an absolute scale of values, as it depends on the number of excited molecules and their method of relaxation. For this reason it is essential to employ a reference standard for quantitative measurements.

The linear relationship between the power of fluorescence and the concentration of the fluorescing solute forms the basis for quantification, the linearity constant for which may be established by calibration with standards. A plot of fluorescence readings against the concentration of the reference solutions furnishes the calibration curve.

Linearity and baseline issues

In dilute solution, the fluorescence intensity (I_f) for defined values of λ_{ex} and λ_f is related linearly to molar concentration (c), according to the approximate relationship:

$$I_f = Kc \text{ at } \lambda_{ex}, \lambda_f \quad (15.24)$$

under constant instrumental conditions.

Sensitivity can be increased by working at high excitation powers to give larger signal-to-noise ratios. Since the source intensity can change from time to time, fluorescence signals are not measured as absolute parameters. They are expressed rather in terms of relative fluorescence. All measurements are made relative to reference standards of known concentration. All readings must be corrected for background fluorescence.

A necessary condition is that the total absorbance ($=\varepsilon lc$) of the system should not exceed 0.05 absorbance units; otherwise progressively greater negative deviations from linearity are observed. At high drug concentrations, fluorescence intensity reaches a plateau. Beyond this, fluorescence intensity actually decreases with increasing concentration, because of inner-filter effects (self-quenching), in which ground-state molecules absorb the fluorescence emitted by excited molecules.

It is essential to establish the range of linearity of the calibration curve of I_f versus c, using at least five standard solutions, for which the condition that absorbance at the wavelength of maximum excitation is <0.05 absorbance units holds. Samples are usually analysed by single-point bracketing, taking a standard conveniently close to the anticipated sample value and calculating the result by simple proportion.

The sequence of standard measurements before and after measuring the sample permits any baseline drift to be compensated. For additional assay security, two-point bracketing can be employed, in which two standard solutions, one higher and the other lower than the concentration observed for the sample, are used in bracketing sequence. Two-point bracketing becomes too onerous when large sample numbers are to be analysed, as may be the case in HPLC-FL. In this situation, standards are analysed first, followed by samples, with a standard analysed after approximately every 10 samples. This compensates for any baseline drift whilst maintaining a reasonable time for analysis.

Instrumental limitations caused by instability of the radiative source can be overcome by the ratio mode operation. A small fraction of the exciting radiation is directed to a reference photodetector, which is chosen primarily for wide wavelength response. The output signal is used as a monitor and, as the excitation radiation increases or decreases in power because of fluctuations in the source, there is a corresponding increase or decrease in relative fluorescence.

References

M. Bogusz and M. Wu, Standardized HPLC/DAD system, based on retention indices and spectral library, applicable for systematic toxicological screening, *J. Anal. Toxicol.*, 1991, **15**, 188–197.

British Pharmacopoeia, Vol. I, London, The Stationery Office, 2002.

British Pharmacopoeia, London, The Stationery Office, 2007.

Council of Europe, *European Pharmacopoeia*, 6th edn, Strasbourg, Council of Europe, 2008.

B. F. Clark *et al.* Pharmaceutical applications of variable-angle synchronous scanning fluorescence spectroscopy, *Anal. Chim. Acta*, 1985, **170**, 35–44.

M. Donbrow, *Instrumental Methods in Analytical Chemistry*, Vol. II, *Optical Methods*, London, Pitman, 1967.

S. P. Elliott and K. A. Hale, Applications of an HPLC–DAD drug-screening system based on retention indices and UV spectra, *J. Anal. Toxicol.*, 1998, **22**, 279–289.

A. F. Fell *et al.*, Analysis for paraquat by second- and fourth-derivative spectroscopy, *Clin. Chem.*, 1981, **27**, 286–292.

A. F. Fell *et al.*, Computer-aided multichannel detection in high-performance liquid chromatography, *Chromatographia*, 1982, **16**, 69–78.

R. Gill *et al.*, The application of derivative UV-visible spectroscopy in forensic science, *J. Forensic Sci. Soc.*, 1982, **22**, 165–171.

A. L. Glenn, The importance of extinction ratios in the spectrophotometric analysis of mixtures of two known absorbing substances, *J. Pharm. Pharmacol.*, 1960, **12**, 595–608.

W. E. Lambert *et al.*, Systematic toxicological analysis of basic drugs by gradient elution of an alumina-based HPLC packing material under alkaline conditions, *J. Anal. Toxicol.*, 1995, **19**, 73–78.

J. Lindholm *et al.* Use of liquid chromatography–diode-array detection and mass spectrometry for rapid product identification in biotechnological synthesis of a hydroxyprogesterone, *J. Chromatogr. A*, 2003, **992**, 85–100.

R. A. Morton and A. L. Stubbs, Photoelectric spectrometry applied to the analysis of mixtures and vitamin A oils, *Analyst*, 1946, **71**, 348–356.

D. A. Skoog *et al.*, *Fundamentals of Analytical Chemistry*, 7th edn, Philadelphia, Saunders College Publishing, 1996.

A. Tracqui *et al.*, Systematic toxicological analysis using HPLC/DAD, *J. Forensic Sci.*, 1995, **40**, 254–262.

USP, *USP 30/NF 25*, Rockville, United States Pharmacopeial Convention, 2007.

S. A. Winfield *et al.*, The fluorimetric determination of salicylic acid using computer-based multicomponent analysis, *J. Pharm. Biomed. Anal.*, 1984, **2**, 561–566.

Collections of data

Absorbances at 220 nm and absorption maxima for over 200 compounds:

M. Bogusz and M. Wu, Standardized HPLC/DAD system, based on retention indices and spectral library, applicable for systematic toxicological screening, *J. Anal. Toxicol.*, 1991, **15**, 188–197.

Absorption maxima for 311 pharmaceuticals, toxicants and drugs of abuse:

A. Tracqui *et al.*, Systematic toxicological analysis using HPLC/DAD, *J. Forensic Sci.*, 1995, **40**, 254–262.

Ultraviolet spectral data for 119 drugs:

E. M. Koves and J. Wells, Evaluation of a photodiode array–HPLC-based system for the detection and quantitation of basic drugs in postmortem blood, *J. Forensic Sci.*, 1992, **37**, 42–60.

Ultraviolet absorption maxima for over 1000 compounds:

T. Mills III and J. C. Roberson, *Instrumental Data for Drug Analysis*, Vol. 4, Amsterdam, Elsevier, 1987.

High-performance liquid chromatographic database of retention indices and UV spectra:

M. Bogusz and M. Erkens, Reversed-phase high-performance liquid chromatographic database of retention indices and UV spectra of toxicologically relevant substances and its interlaboratory use, *J. Chromatogr A*, 1994, **674**, 97–126.

Database with molecular ultraviolet spectra:

C. Burgess and A. Knowles, *Techniques in Visible and Ultraviolet Spectrometry*, Vol. I, 2nd edn, London, Chapman and Hall, 1981.

Ultraviolet spectra (2682) run between 195 nm and 380 nm under isocratic high-performance chromatography conditions:

F. Pragst *et al.*, *UV Spectra of Toxic Compounds*, 4th edn, Happenheiml, Verlag Dr Dieter Helm, 2002.

Isocratic reversed-phase high-performance chromatography system with diode-array detection. A library of retention times and UV-spectra is available for about 400 common drugs (see Chapter 1):

Systematic Toxicological Identification Procedure (STIP) http://home.worldonline.nl/[[sim]]sint1166.

Further reading

C. Burgess and A. Knowles (eds), *Standards in Absorption Spectrometry*, London, Chapman and Hall, 1984.

A. G. Davidson, Ultraviolet–visible spectrophotometry, in *Practical Pharmaceutical Chemistry*, 4th edn, A. H. Beckett and J. B. Stenlake (eds), London, Athlone Press, 1988.

LabCompliance, GLP for analytical laboratories: http://www.labcompliance.com.

S. Gorog, *Ultraviolet–Visible Spectrophotometry in Pharmaceutical Analysis*, Boca Raton, CRC Press, 1995.

ICH: International Conference on Harmonisation of Technical Requirements for Registration of Pharmaceuticals for Human Use: http://www.ich.org.

R. D. Maier and M. Bogusz, Identification power of a standardized HPLC–DAD system for systematic toxicological analysis, *J. Anal. Toxicol.*, 1995, **19**, 79–83.

J. N. Miller (ed.), *Standards in Fluorescence Spectrometry*, London, Chapman and Hall, 1981.

NIST: National Institute of Standards and Technology., NIST Chemistry WebBook: http://webbook.nist.gov.

M. Pesez and J. Bartos, *Colorimetric and Fluorimetric Analysis of Organic Compounds and Drugs, Clinical and Biochemical Series*, Vol. 1, New York, Marcel Dekker, 1974.

Scientific Institute of Public Health, *Belgian GLP Compliance Monitoring Programme Manual*, Brussels, Scientific Institute of Public Health – Louis Pasteur, 1999.

D. A. Skoog *et al.*, *Fundamentals of Analytical Chemistry*, 7th edn, Philadelphia, Saunders College Publishing, 1996.

E. L. Wehry (ed.), *Modern Fluorescence Spectroscopy*, Vols 3 and 4, New York, Plenum Press, 1981.

H. H. Willard *et al.*, *Instrumental Methods of Analysis*, 7th edn, Belmont, Wadsworth, 1988.

16

Infrared spectroscopy

A Drake (with 'Near infrared' by *R D Jee*)

Introduction 421
Instrumentation 425
Data processing. 428
Instrument calibration. 429
Sample preparation 431
Sample presentation 432
Interpretation of spectra 441
Qualitative analysis 442
Quantitative analysis 447
Collections of data 447
Near infrared 448
References 453
Further reading 454

Introduction

Infrared (IR) spectroscopy is the study of the scattering, reflection, absorption or transmission of IR radiation in the spectral range 800 to 1 000 000 nm (0.8 to 1000 μm). In older literature (pre-1970), IR radiation was referred to in terms of wavelengths as microns (μm: micrometres). Nowadays, the wavenumber ($\overline{\nu}$) unit is used almost exclusively. The relationship between wavenumber in cm^{-1} and wavelength (λ) in μm is given by:

$$\overline{\nu} = \frac{10^4}{\lambda} \quad (16.1)$$

The IR spectrum can be divided into three sub-regions:

- 12 500 to 4000 cm^{-1} (0.8 to 2.5 μm; near IR)
- 4000 to 400 cm^{-1} (2.5 to 25 μm; mid IR)
- 400 to 10 cm^{-1} (25 to 1000 μm; far IR).

The mid IR region (often referred to simply as infrared) is the main focus of this chapter because it is the wavelength region used most widely in the analysis of drugs and other substances. A short discussion of near IR is given towards the end of the chapter, highlighting the particular advantages that IR analysis in this region can offer.

The energy associated with electromagnetic radiation is given by Planck's equation:

$$E = \frac{hC}{\lambda} \quad (16.2)$$

where E is the energy, h is Planck's constant, C is the velocity of light and λ is the wavelength of light.

IR radiation can excite molecular vibrations (and associated molecular rotations). At room temperature, a molecule is generally in its ground electronic state where it sits in its ground vibrational state. Provided the incoming IR radiation has the appropriate energy (wavelength, wavenumber), resonant absorption occurs to excite the molecule to a particular higher vibrational state. Vibrational transitions give rise to an absorption spectrum characteristic of the compound. Several factors characterise this absorption spectrum: the number of absorption features and their associated wavenumbers, the strength (intensity) of the absorption features, and the sharpness of these features.

Energy and wavenumber of infrared absorption by molecular vibration

Molecules can undergo two types of vibrations, namely stretching vibrations that involve changes in bond length and bending vibrations that involve changes in bond angles. The vibrational modes associated with the methylene group —CH_2— are illustrated in Figure 16.1.

Theoretically, a 'nonlinear' molecule has ($3N-6$) such modes of vibration, where N is the number of atoms in the molecule. These are called fundamental modes and require IR energy in the range 4000–400 cm^{-1} (mid IR) to become excited. Not all vibrations in a molecule are assignable in an IR spectrum; generally, only the most prominent are readily assigned to a given vibrational mode. These characteristic vibrations are a good way to detect the existence of functional groups in a chemical compound. The precise wavenumber at which a particular vibration absorbs light is associated with bond strength and the atomic masses of the atoms in the bond. The wavenumbers required for the excitation of typical vibrations are given in Table 16.1.

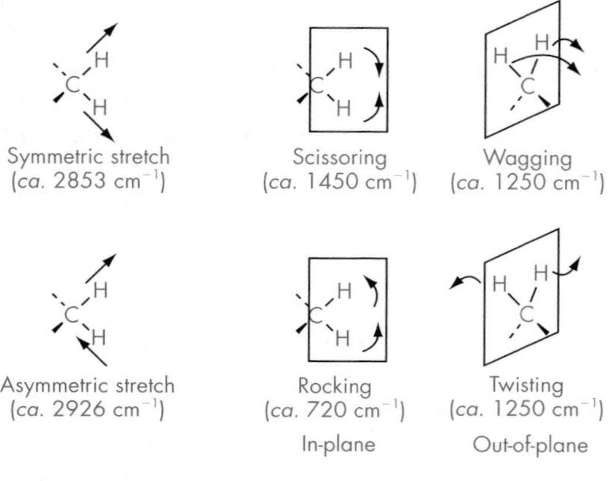

Figure 16.1 Molecular vibrations of the methylene CH_2 group. (Courtesy of D. L. Pavia *et al.*, 1979.)

In addition, there are overtones (the excitation of a vibration to a double or higher frequency) and combinations that are the sum or difference of two or more fundamental bands. No fundamental vibrations require energy greater than 4000 cm^{-1} to become excited. All vibrations in the near IR are therefore overtones or combination bands. The reader is referred to spectroscopic texts for a more detailed explanation of the origin of IR bands (e.g. Williams and Fleming 1995, and others listed in the Further Reading).

Changes in the wavenumber of a band can be related to changes in either the structural environment or the physical state of the molecule. However, many bands in the complex region from 1800 to 400 cm^{-1}, which is usually referred to as the 'fingerprint region', remain of

Table 16.1 Important vibrations and IR frequencies

Wavenumber (cm^{-1})	Vibration
3600–2500	O—H stretch, broad, strong (prominent)
3400	N—H stretch, broad, medium (prominent)
3000	C—H aromatic stretch
2900	C—H aliphatic stretch, strong
1800–1650	C=O stretch strong (prominent) Ester R—O—C=O, ca. 1740 cm^{-1} Ketone C=O, ca. 1715 cm^{-1} Carboxylic acid HO—C=O, ca. 1705 cm^{-1} Amide H_2N—C=O, ca. 1650 cm^{-1}
1300–1000	C—O stretch, strong
1800–400	Forest of vibrations – fingerprint region

unconfirmed origin. Many of the bands are characteristic of the molecule as a whole and cannot be assigned directly to particular bonds. Nevertheless, inspection of IR spectra can form the basis of qualitative analytical work in IR spectroscopy to confirm the identity of a sample. A complete molecular structure cannot be deduced directly from an IR spectrum. Rather, functional groups are identified and total molecular identity is confirmed by comparison with IR spectra in a compendium or by comparison with a reference substance of known provenance run under the same conditions.

Strength of molecular vibration absorption

Traditionally, an IR spectrum is reported as a plot of percentage transmittance ($T\%$) against wavenumber $\bar{\nu}$. The IR transmission spectrum of a polystyrene film used to calibrate the wavenumber scale is given in Figure 16.2.

The absorption of light in Fig. 16.2 is registered as the reduced transmission of light, i.e. a proportion of the incident radiation is absorbed by the sample. The non-absorbed radiation (transmitted) is detected by the detector. The simple ratio of the transmitted intensity to the incident intensity is known as the transmittance. The percentage transmittance is 100 times the transmittance (see Fig. 16.3).

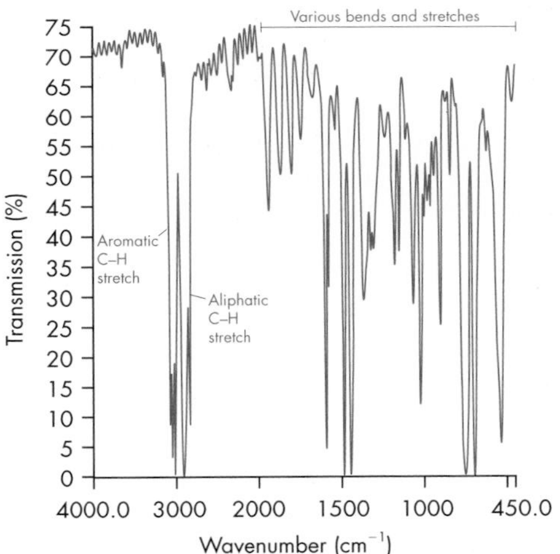

Figure 16.2 Transmission spectrum of a polystyrene film.

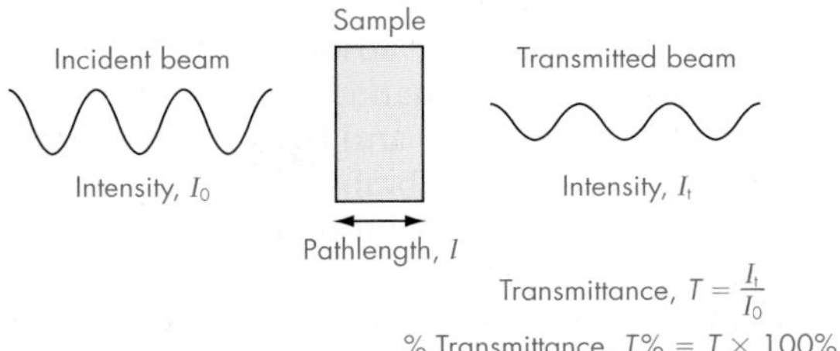

Figure 16.3 Transmission of light by a sample.

The absorption of light is quantified through Beer's law as:

$$A = \log \frac{I_0}{I_t} = \varepsilon c l \tag{16.3}$$

where A is the absorbance, c is the molar concentration, l is the pathlength of the sample and ε is the molar absorption coefficient, also referred to as the molar extinction coefficient. Note that the terms I_0 and I_t are used to differentiate between incident radiation (I_0) and the transmitted radiation (I_t). Absorbance is the log of the inverse of transmittance:

$$A = \log \frac{I_0}{I_t} = \log \frac{1}{T} \tag{16.4}$$

The various vibrational modes have different tendencies to absorb, giving different molar extinction coefficients, and therefore they have different intensities in the spectrum. The carbonyl (C═O) stretch in the 1750 to 1650 cm^{-1} range has a particularly strong transition electric dipole moment, and therefore ε is large for a vibration (approximately 100) and the carbonyl absorption is a very prominent feature. The C═O stretch is said to be 'allowed' spectroscopically. The C—H stretching mode generates a lower transition electric dipole moment and the ε value is smaller at ~10. However, there are usually many C—H bonds in a molecule and the additive absorption of these makes the C—H vibration a prominent feature.

The stretches of symmetrical bonds, such as H—H (hydrogen gas), —C—C— (ethane), O—O (oxygen) and N—N (nitrogen), do not have a transition dipole moment and therefore $\varepsilon \rightarrow 0$ and these stretches are not observed and are said to be 'forbidden'. Similar vibrations in complex molecules do absorb, but extremely weakly. On the other hand, gases such as NO, NO_2, CO, CO_2, SO_2, CH_4 and H_2O (water vapour) do have IR-active vibrations that can be measured to monitor environmental levels. The low value of ε and low concentrations of these gases mean that cells used in the analysis of gases by IR are very long (up to 1 m or more). Water vapour and CO_2 present in the normal atmosphere produce absorption effects in an IR spectrometer in the absence or presence of a sample. High-precision work when determining IR spectra benefits from flushing the sample environment with dry air or nitrogen. The water vibrations centred at 3782 cm^{-1} and 1587 cm^{-1} show a fine structure associated with the rotations of the water molecule.

The actual movement of charge during a vibration is, in practice, very small and a value of ε of approximately 200 is a practical upper limit. In tables of IR data, the intensity of a vibrational band is designated as vs (very strong), s (strong), m (medium) or w (weak) to reflect the variation in absorption coefficient (intensity of spectral feature). The measurement of IR intensity was unreliable for older designs of instrument, which made quantitative work in the IR unreliable. This is less true for modern instruments.

The spectroscopic character of overtones and combinations is less well defined. Accordingly, ε in the near IR is low and absorption is detected only for concentrated solutions with an absorption that may be too strong for spectral regions in which ε is larger. The molar absorption coefficient, ε, is largely responsible for determining the sensitivity of an analysis.

Width of an infrared absorption band

In ultraviolet (UV) and visible electronic absorption spectroscopy, absorption is limited to the excitation of a single electron in a chromophore, albeit to one of several excited states. An electronic spectrum is rarely composed of more than three prominent spectral features. However, the energy required to excite an electron is enough also to excite associated vibrational and rotational states, and the absorption profile is broad. The UV–visible spectrum is characterised by only a few broad features. A typical half-height width of a UV–visible absorption is between 2000 and 5000 cm^{-1}.

The IR spectrometer sees the excitation of bond vibrations and associated rotational motions. In contrast to UV-visible, the IR spectrum comprises many relatively sharp features that provide an excellent fingerprint for identification. A typical half-height width of an IR absorption band is 10–20 cm^{-1}. The UV and IR spectra for hydrocortisone are shown in Figure 16.4, illustrating the broad spectral features of the UV spectrum relative to the information-rich IR spectrum with its far sharper features. Note that the region above 2000 cm^{-1} is not shown in Fig. 16.4B.

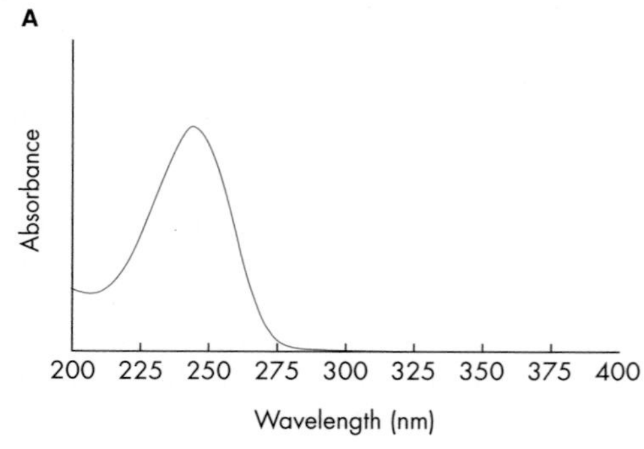

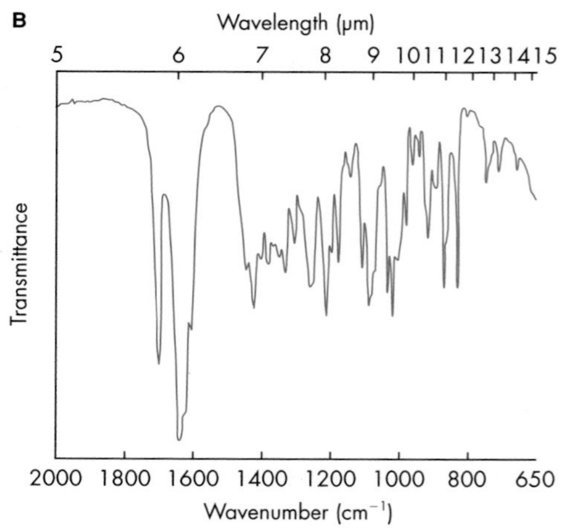

Figure 16.4 (A) UV spectrum and (B) IR spectrum of hydrocortisone.

Instrumentation

Dispersive spectrometers

Conventional spectrometers start with an appropriate light source focused onto the entrance slit of a monochromator that splits the light up into its wavelength components. The monochromator exit slit selects a particular emerging wavelength. The monochromatic light passes through a sample where it may or may not be absorbed before being detected by a light detector (photomultiplier or photodiode). This type of spectrometer is known as a dispersive instrument. To measure transmittance or absorbance, both the incident intensity and the transmitted intensity need to be measured at every wavelength.

Single-beam dispersive spectrometers

With a single-beam instrument, the I_0 spectrum is measured first with air (or appropriate solvent) as a reference in the light beam. In a separate measurement the I_t spectrum of the sample is recorded. Computers allow data to be stored and processed automatically. To ensure accuracy and precision, all components in the instrument (light source, detector and electronics) need to be very stable to ensure that I_0 does not drift.

Nowadays, single-beam dispersive IR spectrometers are likely to be found only in monitoring processes (e.g. environmental pollution).

Double-beam spectrometer

Double-beam spectrometers are designed to compensate for instrument drifts and to eliminate the need to determine I_0 and I_t in separate measurements. The layout of a typical double-beam spectrometer is illustrated in Fig. 16.5. Dispersive instruments in the IR have the sample located next to the light source before the monochromator, unlike their UV-visible counterparts.

In a double-beam instrument, IR light from the source, typically an electrically conducting element such as a Globar (an electrically-heated silicon carbide rod) maintained at about 1000 K, equally illuminates two mirrors M_1 and M_2. The light from mirror M_1 acts as the reference beam; the light from M_2 is the sample beam. Mirrors M_3 and M_4 send the light beams to mirrors on a mechanical chopper. The mechanical chopper is a rotating disc carrying mirrors that alternately reflect the reference and sample beams into the monochromator. After passage through the monochromator, monochromatic light from the sample and reference beams is detected alternately by the single detector as the wavelength drive changes the wavelength that passes to the detector. In the reference-beam chopper period the detector registers I_0 and in the sample-beam chopper period I_t is measured. The alternating signals are amplified and their ratio is calculated to give $I_t/I_0 = T$ or $\log(I_0/I_t) = A$. The preferred detector, certainly by the 1980s, was deuterated triglycine sulfate (TGS). This is a pyroelectric detector with an electrical resistance very sensitive to heat (IR intensity).

All measurements can be made simply with air in the reference beam. Placing a cell with solvent in the reference beam enables compensation for unwanted absorption (e.g. from solvents in which the sample is dissolved). The measurement cell pathlengths in the reference and sample beams must be identical. A computer interfaced with the spectrometer enables post-measurement

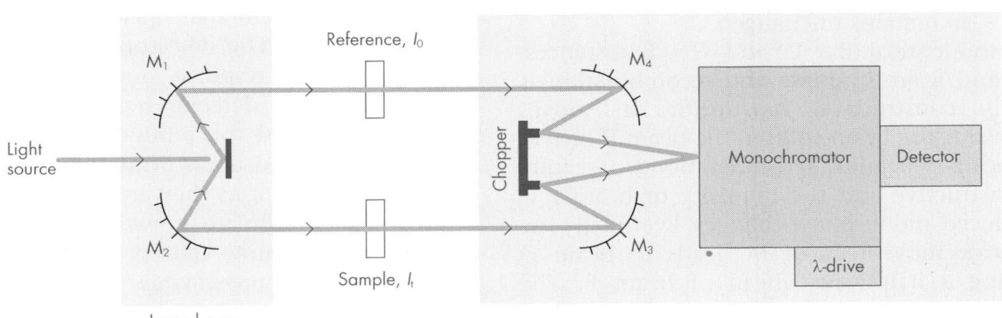

Figure 16.5 Double-beam dispersive IR spectrometer.

subtraction of the reference spectrum from the sample spectrum.

The amount of polychromatic IR light that hits the detector from the natural, black-body, room-temperature radiation of the cell compartment walls can be 10-fold or more than the desired monochromatic IR radiation from the reference or the sample. This background radiation is stray light that severely affects the accuracy of the I_0/I_t value. Locating the sample before the monochromator ensures that the 'chopped' signal selected by the detector system is related almost exclusively to light derived from either the sample or reference beams. Artificial reduction of absorbance values is thereby greatly reduced. However, locating a sample close to an IR source can cause deleterious heating effects.

Interferometric spectrophotometers

By far the most commonly encountered IR spectrometer in analytical laboratories is the Fourier transform (FTIR) spectrophotometer. FTIR spectrometers have the sample next to the detector after wavelength selection. This reduces heat effects from having a sample in proximity to an IR source. Locking into the mirror oscillation frequency coupled with the signal filtering associated with the Fourier transform and the improvements in optics and detectors makes this preferred sample position viable.

The FTIR spectrometer incorporates an interferometer in place of a monochromator. The way a FTIR spectrometer operates is shown schematically in Fig. 16.6:

- If the mirror M_1 is set to oscillate along the optic axis, the distance travelled by beam (B + D) varies, while the distance travelled by (C + E) remains unchanged.
- With identical (B + D) and (C + E) distances, D and E are in-phase and recombination is fully constructive. As mirror M_1 moves towards the beam splitter, the beam D arrives 'ahead' of beam E; recombination is not fully constructive and the intensity of beam F is reduced and its phase changes. Eventually the mirror movement of M_1 leads to beam D being a half wave ahead of beam E. The recombination is now fully destructive and the intensity of beam F becomes zero. At this point, the movement of M_1 is reversed past the oscillation mid-point to eventually make D retarded compared to E, to give zero intensity at half-wave retardation before returning to the mid-point of the oscillation.
- As the mirror moves back and forth through a single mirror oscillation period, the intensity of a single wavelength of IR light varies considerably. In practice, all wavelengths are passing through the system simultaneously. Therefore, the total IR light intensity registered as falling on the detector during a single mirror oscillation period is very complicated and takes the form illustrated in Fig. 16.7.
- The signal illustrated in Fig. 16.7 is now subjected to a mathematical procedure called Fourier transformation. This extracts the light intensity versus wavelength (wavenumber) information.
- With no reference or sample in the beam, this measurement is the background or I_0 spectrum, which is stored in the computer to be used as the I_0 for all subsequent transmittance (I_t/I_0) or absorbance [$\log(I_0/I_t)$] measurements during the working session.
- A measurement is now made with the sample in place. A similar interferogram is created. This is also subjected to Fourier transformation to produce a sample light-intensity throughput spectrum.
- Subsequent data manipulation in the computer produces the transmission or absorption spectrum of the sample.

Technical details

- The IR source is a Globar or similar proprietary 'hot' element that operates at approximately 1300 K. The detector for FTIR needs to have a fast response and low inherent noise. The TGS detector remains the most widely employed for routine use. Pyroelectric devices based upon lithium tantalite are becoming popular as they are less expensive, have greater ordinate linearity and present better temperature stability (TGS linearity falls off above approximately 32°C). For high-precision work with lower noise, liquid-nitrogen-cooled semiconductor detectors are

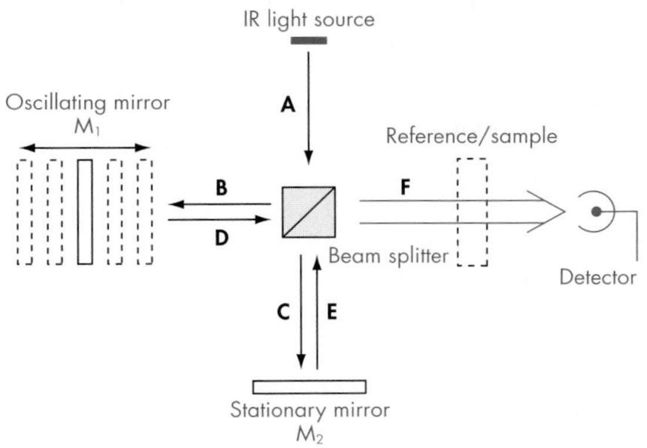

Figure 16.6 Layout of an IR interferometer (FTIR spectrometer).

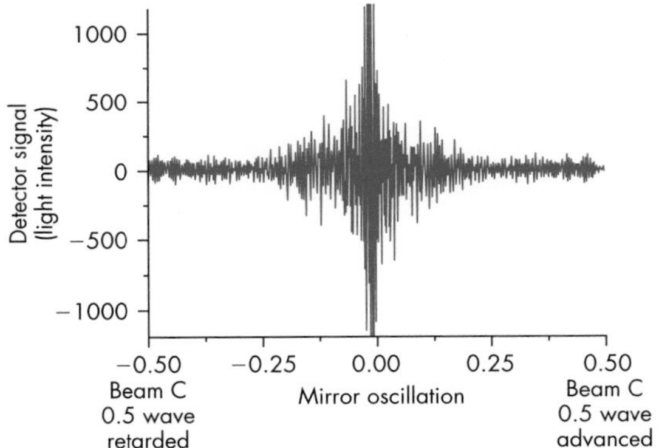

Figure 16.7 Interferogram produced by a single-mirror oscillation.

available based on indium–antimonide (In–Sb), indium–gallium–arsenide (In–Ga–As) or mercury–cadmium–telluride (Hg–Cd–Te).

- FTIR spectrometers have advantages over dispersive instruments. The interferometer offers greater light collection and throughput. More light means less noise and greater sensitivity. The multiplex advantage concerns the very nature of the interferometric measurement. All wavelengths are observed for a single scan at the same time. In a dispersive instrument, only one wavelength is detected at any one time. In the interferometer, more time is spent effectively measuring each wavelength, even though the total scan time may be the same. More time to measure each wavelength means lower noise and greater sensitivity.
- Two options are available to the FT technique: either a spectrum can be scanned much faster than a dispersive instrument, or the same time as for the dispersive instrument can be spent measuring a spectrum to present lower noise results. In practice, a single mirror oscillation in the interferometer produces a spectrum scan in a fraction of a second. A dispersive instrument scan can take up to 10 minutes. Taking 10 minutes over an FTIR measurement allows the averaging of very many scans. The signal-to-noise (S/N) ratio in an IR spectrometer is proportional to $\sqrt{}$ (number of scans). Accumulating and averaging 1, 4, 16, 64, 256 or 1024 scans produces a signal-to-noise improvement of 1-, 2-, 4-, 8-, 16- or 32-fold, respectively.
- The level of stray light associated with FTIR spectroscopy is low, typically less than 0.02%, because the technique is devoid of imperfect gratings and the signals selected are associated only with the oscillating mirror movement. Absorbance values remain linear up to two absorbance units, which in turn leads to more accurate quantitative measurements, even with strongly absorbing bands.
- Resolution is generally excellent over the whole spectrum, with an effective measurement spectral bandwidth of 1 cm^{-1} being achieved readily.

The increased sensitivity and scanning speed of FTIR spectrometers and associated sensitive cooled semiconductor detectors enables IR microscopes and gas chromatographs to be coupled to FTIR spectrometers, thereby expanding the types of samples that can be analysed by FTIR. The ability to couple a microscope opens up possibilities for examining minute quantities of a contaminant, for example in tablets or other pharmaceutical preparations; mapping the homogeneity/inhomogeneity of tablets; and identifying individual layers in laminate polymers.

Data processing

All modern IR spectrometers are computer controlled, with measured data stored digitally. Computer control simplifies the process of running instruments and allows the easy implementation of standard operating procedures (SOPs).

Computers readily allow changes between spectral units. In the early days, the IR spectrum of a compound was reported as percentage transmittance as a function of wavelength in microns (μm). By the 1970s, percentage transmittance as a function of wavenumbers became the preferred form. The computer allows the ready conversion between transmittance and absorbance and between microns and wavenumbers. Presentation in terms of absorbance/wavenumber is likely to become increasingly familiar.

Computers readily allow accumulation of spectra. The spectrum of a weak sample can be scanned repeatedly to give an averaged spectrum with appreciably reduced noise and an improvement in sensitivity. For example, there is little difference between the spectra of carbon disulfide and of benzocaine in carbon disulfide (Fig. 16.8), but with spectrum manipulation, a good spectrum of benzocaine is readily obtained (Fig. 16.9). The amount of benzocaine in the cell was approximately 4 μg but only about one quarter of this was in the IR beam. Each spectrum was recorded in less than 30 seconds.

Digitised spectra can be corrected easily for solvent absorption or the presence of impurities. Various mathematical procedures can be applied, which include baseline corrections and levelling, smoothing, the determination of peak bandwidths, and the calculation of absorption band areas. Derivative spectra can be produced to help distinguish the contributions of overlapping components in an absorption band.

The identification and interpretation of spectra are assisted greatly by computer analysis. Spectra can be readily overlaid for comparison. The spectrum of a sample can be compared with a library of spectra (database) and a list of the compounds of best fit can be either displayed on a screen or printed out. The presence of certain functional groups can also be confirmed.

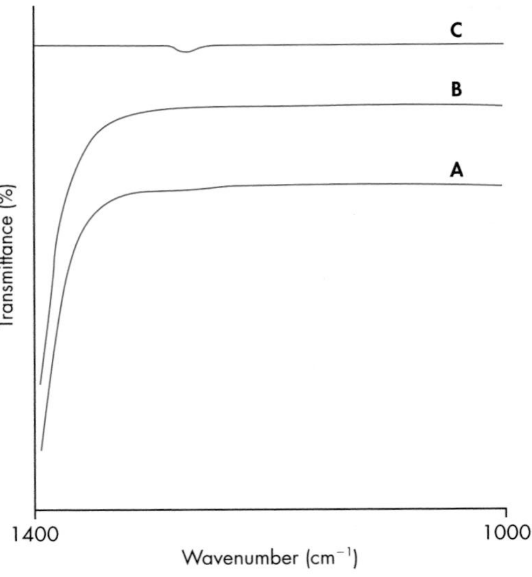

Figure 16.8 IR spectrum of benzocaine in carbon disulfide (A), carbon disulfide (B), and the difference spectrum (A − B) (C). (Courtesy of Perkin-Elmer Ltd.)

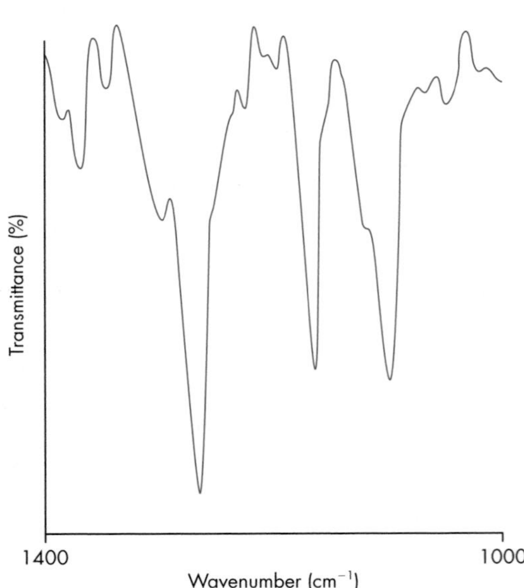

Figure 16.9 The difference spectrum of benzocaine shown in Fig. 16.8 (curve C) smoothed, corrected for baseline contribution and with percentage transmittance scale expanded 200 times. (Courtesy of Perkin-Elmer Ltd.)

Instrument calibration

Calibration of a spectrometer is critical. If the instrument is not calibrated correctly the data obtained will be inaccurate.

Six factors need to be considered when calibrating an IR spectrometer:

- wavelength (wavenumber) scale
- absorbance scale
- stray light
- spectral resolution
- data resolution
- time scale of measurement (time constant).

Wavelength (wavenumber) scale

The wavelength (wavenumber) scale is a critical parameter in infrared, particularly where computer matching of spectra is employed for identification purposes. As noted in discussions later in this chapter, computer matching relies on comparison of the major absorbance bands in the IR spectrum. The data system calculates the wavenumbers corresponding to the main absorbance bands for the sample and then, in effect, compares these with the wavenumbers for the main absorbance bands in the reference library spectra. If the wavenumbers are not accurate for the sample spectrum, the data system will not produce a correct library match.

A card carrying an accredited transparent film of polystyrene (0.035 mm in thickness) is used to calibrate the wavelength (wavenumber) scale. The spectrum should have the form illustrated in Figs 16.2 and 16.10. Peak locations and tolerances recommended in the *British Pharmacopoeia* (British Pharmacopoeia Commission 2007) are given in the inset in Fig. 16.10.

Absorbance scale

Unfortunately, there are no internationally recognised standards for IR spectra. The absorbance scale is set in the factory with the aid of complicated optics. Filters are available in the 4000–2000 cm^{-1} range. The high background blackbody radiation that falls on the detector from sources other than the sample means the ideal absorbance for good signal-to-noise ratio is approximately 0.4.

Stray light

Stray light can be tested by introducing a neat solvent or very high-concentration sample into the sample beam so that at the wavelength (wavenumber) of interest the expected absorbance is in excess of $A = 5$. All the relevant light at this wavelength (wavenumber) has been effectively absorbed.

Spectral resolution (spectral bandwidth)

In dispersive instruments, the spectral bandwidth (SBW) is set by the entrance and exit slits of the monochromator. In the FTIR spectrometer, the 'depth' of the Fourier transformation sets SBW with typical values of 1 cm^{-1}, 2 cm^{-1} and 4 cm^{-1} available in the spectrometer control software. The narrower the SBW the more faithfully are sharp absorption bands registered; however, the noisier the spectrum (less light), the more time (accumulations) is required to keep the noise level down.

The *British Pharmacopoeia* (British Pharmacopoeia Commission 2007) recommends the following to ensure good spectral resolution:

> For monochromator instruments, record the spectrum of a polystyrene film 35 μm in thickness. The difference x [Fig. 16.10] between the percentage transmittance at the transmission maximum A at 2870 cm^{-1} and that at the transmission minimum B at 2849.5 cm^{-1} should be greater than 18. The difference y between the percentage transmittance at the transmission maximum C at 1589 cm^{-1} and that at the transmission minimum D at 1583 cm^{-1} should be greater than 10.
>
> For Fourier-transform instruments, use suitable instrument resolution with the appropriate apodisation prescribed by the manufacturer. The resolution is checked by suitable means, for example by recording the spectrum of a polystyrene film approximately 35 μm in thickness. The difference between the absorbances at the absorption minimum at 2870 cm^{-1} and the absorption maximum at 2849.5 cm^{-1} is greater

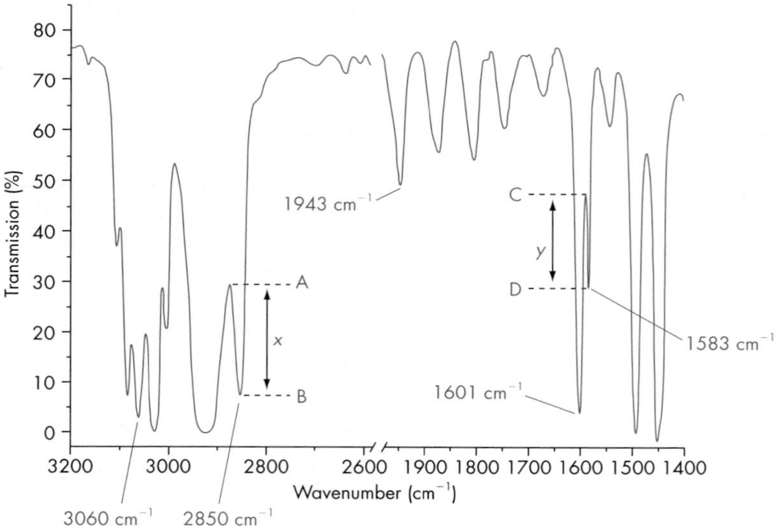

Transmission minima (cm^{-1})	Acceptable tolerance (cm^{-1})	
	Monochromator instruments	Fourier transform instruments
3060.0	±1.5	±1.0
2849.5	±2.0	±1.0
1942.9	±1.5	±1.0
1601.2	±1.0	±1.0
1583.0	±1.0	±1.0
1154.5	±1.0	±1.0
1028.3	±1.0	±1.0

(British Pharmacaopoeia 2007.)

Figure 16.10 Zoomed-in regions of the IR spectrum of a 40 μm thick polystyrene film indicating the location of critical parameters. A whole spectrum is illustrated in Fig. 16.2.

than 0.33. The difference between the absorbances at the absorption minimum at 1589 cm^{-1} and the absorption maximum at 1583 cm^{-1} is greater than 0.08.

This recommendation is very specific for a 35 μm thick film of polystyrene.

Data resolution

In a computer, spectra are stored as lists of wavenumber and transmittance (absorbance) data pairs. These *X*,*Y* data pairs are plotted on demand. A sufficient number of data points are required to give an undistorted picture. Too many points may be unnecessary and require excessive memory allocations. Figure 16.11 illustrates the effects of spectral and data resolution on the spectral integrity of the IR spectrum of a 0.04 mm thick polystyrene film.

The terms spectral resolution and data resolution are often confused. Some instruments, in modifying the Fourier transform mathematics to reduce the SBW, also produce a change in the data resolution of the spectra computed. The 1154 cm^{-1} band of polystyrene is reproduced in Fig. 16.11 measured with different SBW and data resolution. Viewing the spectra presented in Fig. 16.11 indicates that data resolution can be a more important issue than spectral resolution. In

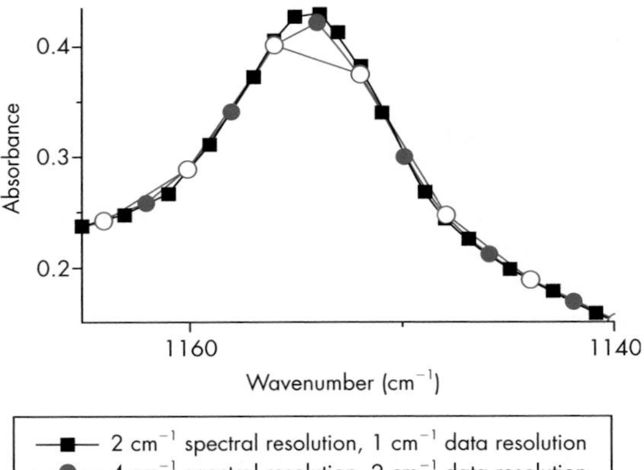

Figure 16.11 Zoomed-in region of the IR spectrum of a 0.04 mm thick polystyrene film illustrating the effect of spectral bandwidth and data resolution.

general, for typical drug molecules, a SBW of 4 cm^{-1} is probably sufficient to describe faithfully the natural bandwidth of a vibrational absorption band. However, a data resolution of 1 cm^{-1} is preferred to ensure that the measured data are a faithful representation of the capability of the spectrometer. Increasing SBW, reducing data resolution, or both, can reduce noise.

Time scale of measurement (time constant, averaged scans)

In analogue dispersive instruments, the scan speed refers to the rate of rotation of the monochromator diffraction grating, which in turn controls the rate-of-change of the wavelength (wavenumber) that comes from the monochromator exit slit. The instrument has an inherent controllable response time (time constant). Scanning too rapidly means that measured peaks are distorted and flattened (reduced intensity): the instrument is being run too fast for the electronics to cope with the changing signal from the detector. A scan should be fast enough to avoid time wastage, yet slow enough to leave the spectrum undistorted. The longer the response time (i.e. the larger the time constant), the lower the noise and the longer the time required to measure spectra. The choice of time response versus scan speed is sample dependent and needs to be selected according to experience.

In a FTIR spectrometer, the scan speed is set by the oscillation rate of the moving mirror and the computer Fourier transformation speed. A typical spectrum can be accumulated in a second or so. The instrument operator has no control of this. The time to measure an FTIR spectrum is set by the number of scans accumulated and averaged, and the speed of the computer (see Technical Details under Interferometric Spectrophotometers on p. 426).

Sample preparation

A major advantage of IR spectroscopy is the ability to measure relatively heterogeneous materials and poorly characterised samples, particularly in condensed phases (e.g. creams, powders, crystalline materials). By their nature, these samples are often not chemically pure and IR spectroscopy can identify or confirm the existence of major constituents. IR spectroscopy is often used to demonstrate that a sample is concordant with expectation.

Nevertheless, it is essential to have pure samples to act as standards for IR spectroscopy. A major difficulty can be that of purifying and handling a few micrograms of material without substantial losses, although these problems have largely been overcome by using fractional crystallisation or chromatography as a prelude to IR spectroscopy. On-line FTIR spectroscopy is possible, but is largely a research tool. Nowadays, the identification of samples in minute amounts is achieved by other techniques, such as nuclear magnetic resonance (NMR) spectrometry and mass spectrometry (MS) (see Chapter 21). This is particularly the case with hyphenated techniques, which involve the use of spectrometric methods on-line with a chromatographic process. Nevertheless, IR spectroscopy has an important role to play in identifying functional groups. FTIR is also widely used in the analysis of drugs of abuse and can be particularly useful in differentiating salt from free-base forms of a drug.

Sample presentation

IR spectra can be measured in the gas, liquid or solid phase. However, most compounds of interest are solids at room temperature. In principle, an IR spectrum can be obtained from as little as 1 μg of a compound. From a practical point of view, quantities of the order of 200–1000 μg are much easier to handle. Very small quantities require greater sensitivity to be achieved with microcells, placing as much material as possible in the IR beam. Microcells require beam-condensing optics to focus as much light as possible through the microcell assembly.

Glass and silica contain SiO—H and Si—O bonds that can vibrate and strongly absorb IR radiation. Therefore, cell windows need to be fabricated from ionic materials with bonds that do not have vibrations. Crystal lattice vibrations cause absorption in the far IR. Barium fluoride (and calcium fluoride) are excellent for aqueous media, although window absorption prevents measurements below 1000 cm^{-1}. Silver chloride windows are water resistant and will allow transmission down to 400 cm^{-1}, but are friable. The most popular IR window material is sodium chloride, which is transparent down to 600 cm^{-1}. However, NaCl is a water soluble material and caution needs to be exercised in solvent choice when preparing thin films from solution on this material.

Gases

In normal laboratory experiments, IR spectroscopy is used only rarely for analysis in the gas phase. Gases are likely to be at a very low concentration and special long-path, airtight gas cells are required. These cells normally have sodium chloride windows, and mirrors may be used to reflect the light through the gas cell several times to achieve a very long pathlength. The detection of environmental gases is a typical application of gas-phase IR spectroscopy. Gas-phase analysis is carried out when FTIR is used as a detector coupled to GC. Even for GC-FTIR, a long pathlength cell referred to as a 'light pipe' is used in the detector to help increase the sensitivity of detection.

Liquids and solutions

Liquids have a very high molarity. Thus chloroform, with a relative molecular mass of 119.4 and density 1.48 g/mL, can be said to be 12.4 M. According to Beer's law, to detect the C—H stretch ($\varepsilon \approx 10$) with absorption $A = 0.4$, the pathlength required, given by $l = A/(\varepsilon c)$, is approximately 3×10^{-3} cm – i.e. very short!

Neat nonvolatile liquids can be measured simply by placing a drop between two IR transparent plates and pressing the plates together to ensure a narrow (<0.1 mm) measurement pathlength (Fig. 16.12). Volatile liquids may need proper sealed liquid cells to prevent volatilisation.

When samples in solution are to be analysed, liquid cells can be used. These typically consist of two parallel transparent windows (0.1–0.01 mm apart) separated by a precise gasket made of Teflon or lead and fitted with inlet and outlet ports. Cells with variable pathlengths are also available, in which one window is retained on a screw that can be finely adjusted to give a precise pathlength in the 0.1–0.01 mm range. These cells are particularly useful for varying pathlength to accommodate for solvent absorption and variations in concentration ranges. If the absorbance is too strong, the pathlength of the cell can be reduced.

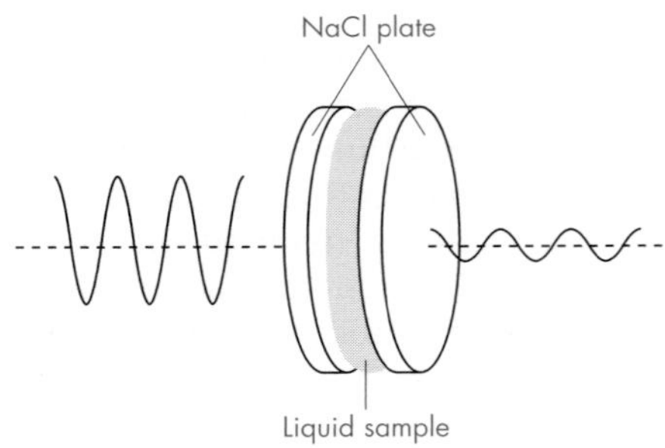

Figure 16.12 Liquid sample or Nujol mull sandwiched between two NaCl plates.

The number of solvents suitable for IR spectroscopy is limited because most solvents suitable for the dissolution of organic solutes will also absorb in the IR and hence will have their own IR spectrum. The spectrum of the solution is then a combination of the solute and the solvent. The measurement of the IR absorption of a solute is only possible in a spectral range for which the solvent is relatively transparent. Carbon tetrachloride and carbon disulfide, which lack hydrogen and contain a minimal number of bond types, are often suggested as the most useful solvents because they have relatively few absorption bands in the IR region. However, they have relatively poor solubilisation characteristics, particularly for polar solutes. In practice, solvent choice is based upon solubility and IR transparency at the wavenumber of interest. Deuterated solvents can help open regions for analysis. Chloroform can be replaced by deuterochloroform and water with deuterated water. Acetonitrile, toluene and dioxane are also good solvents to consider. Solvent absorption can be accounted for in a computer by comparison of the solution and solvent spectra. Spectral subtraction can be carried out, but caution should be observed when doing this.

To overcome the inherent absorption of solvents and the relatively low extinction coefficient of a vibrational transition, pathlengths should be narrow and concentrations of solutes high. The concentration of the test compound is usually about 5–10%, but concentrations up to 20% (w/v) can be employed. With these high concentrations, hydroxyl and amino compounds often exhibit bands caused by intermolecular hydrogen bonding. Interactions between the compound and the solvent can occur, which may result in changes in the intensity and wavenumber of bands in different solvents and the breakdown of Beer's law.

IR solvents are often volatile and require very short pathlengths. This combination can lead to solvent evaporation, which produces large concentration changes. In the older style IR spectrometers, the heat of IR radiation could cause evaporation – this is less of a problem with FT systems with the sample placed after the interferometer. An example is presented here of the determination of the amount of dimeticone in a cream formulation.

Dimeticone can be extracted from creams with 4% (w/w) liquid paraffin in toluene and quantified by reference to standard solutions based upon the Si—O stretching vibration at 1260 cm^{-1} in a 0.1 mm sodium chloride liquid cell (Fig. 16.13).

Solids

Solids are by far the most common sample types analysed by IR. They are generally examined either as thin films or as dispersions in either liquids or solids. The ideal sample for IR transmission measurements is clear, visually transparent and homogeneous. This can be difficult to achieve with solids. Heterogeneous samples that are optically poor with large sample particles can introduce light scattering and the Christensen effect. Light scattering becomes significant when the particle size is more than 1/20th the wavelength of the incident light. Light scattering produces a spectrum offset that is curved, with high light scattering at shorter wavelengths/higher wavenumbers and lower light scattering at longer wavelengths/lower wavenumbers. The Christensen effect, which results from severe refractive index changes at the sample surface, leads to distorted band shapes. Peaks take on an S-shape with an apparent reduced (or even negative) absorption at the longer wavenumber edge. As a result, asymmetric bands may be observed that vary in position and intensity from true values. For transmission measurements, the sample must, ideally, have the appearance of a 'perfect glass'. To reduce the light scattering and the Christensen effect, all components of the sample must have a very small particle size (≤ 1 μm) and must be dry; samples should be ground until particle sizes are less than 1 μm.

The polymorphic form of a solid sample can affect the IR spectrum. This is an important issue in the pharmaceutical industry, as the rate of dissolution of a solid drug can depend upon its crystal morphology. Polymorphic forms and the factors that influence their formation can be investigated simply by means of a diamond anvil

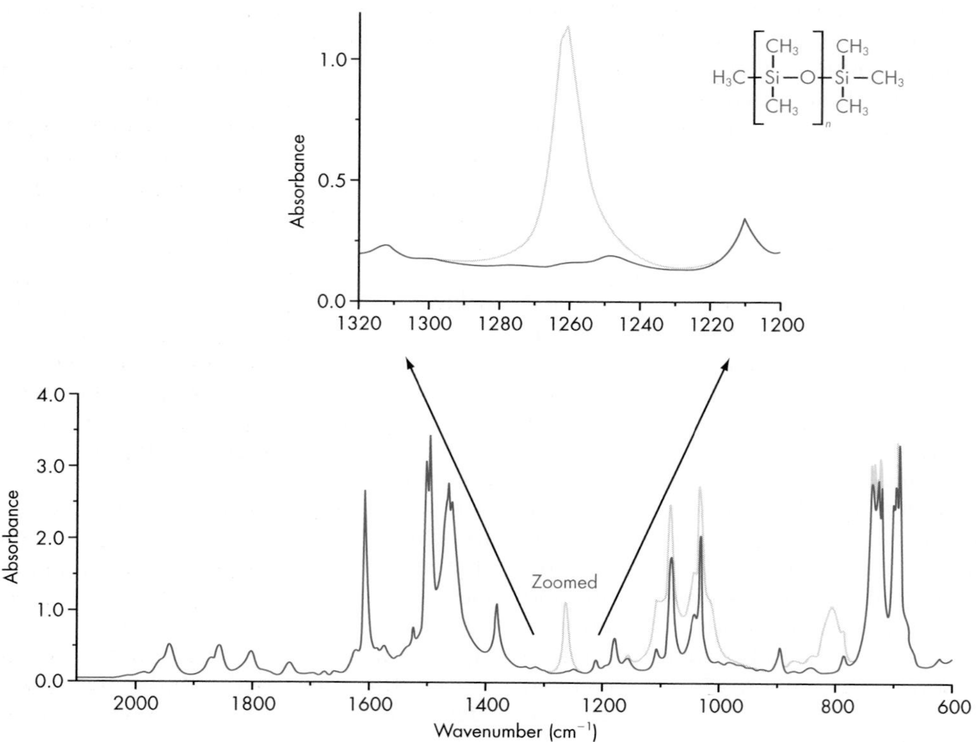

Figure 16.13 The IR spectrum of dimeticone dissolved in 4% (w/w) liquid paraffin in toluene. Heavy line: 4% (w/w) liquid paraffin in toluene. Light line: 1.5% (w/v) dimeticone dissolved in 4% (w/w) liquid paraffin in toluene.

in which the sample is crushed between two diamond windows (see Fig. 16.14). This means of sampling does not change the polymorphism of the sample, unlike some sample presentation techniques such as alkali halide discs.

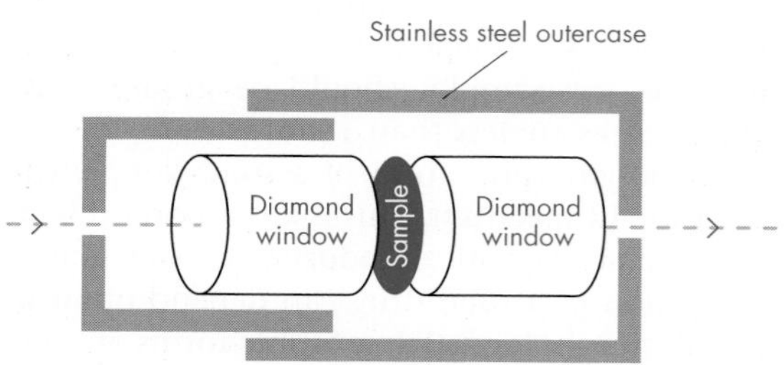

Figure 16.14 Diamond anvil.

Mulls

Solid compounds are dispersed in a liquid, such as liquid paraffin (Nujol). The finely powdered compound (about 1–10 mg) is mixed with one drop of the liquid and ground in an agate mortar. The test sample must have the constituency of a smooth thin cream. The mull is spread onto an alkali halide plate, usually NaCl or KBr, and another plate is placed on top, taking care to exclude air bubbles. The plates are pressed together strongly. A disadvantage of this method is that the spectrum of the mulling agent is superimposed upon that of the sample. Consequently, liquid paraffin cannot be used if the C—H stretching vibrations are to be examined, and a halogenated liquid, such as 'Fluorolube' (a fluorinated hydrocarbon) or hexachlorobutadiene, must be employed.

Although widely used in the past, mulls have been superseded by techniques such as attenuated total reflectance and diffuse reflectance (see p. 437) which offer simpler sampling techniques and avoid the need for spectral subtraction.

Alkali halide discs

The technique of dispersing the compound in an alkali halide has been used widely in the identification of drugs. Originally, KBr was used and the technique is still often referred to as the 'KBr technique'. However, potassium chloride (KCl) is superior to KBr because it is less hygroscopic. Storage of the alkali halide in an 80°C oven helps to ensure anhydrous conditions.

The finely powdered, dry, test compound (about 1 mg) is mixed with the alkali halide (about 250 mg) and ground either mechanically in an agate ball mill or by hand in an agate mortar. A texture approaching that of talcum powder is a good consistency. The mixture is then pressed under a load of approximately 10 tons of force in a purpose-designed press to produce an optically good, thin disc (Fig. 16.15). A vacuum helps to retain dry conditions and smooth disc formation. The load is applied for 10 minutes.

If only small quantities of the compound are available (about 200 μg), a thin cardboard mask with a slot in the centre can be used. The mask is placed in the die and the slot is filled with the mixture before pressing. A mask is often employed routinely because it provides a support for the alkali halide and so enables the disc to be handled more easily. Microdiscs of diameter down to 0.5 mm can be prepared using metal (lead or stainless steel) discs of 13 mm diameter with a hole of the appropriate size in the centre. The hole is filled with KBr (about 1 mg) that contains from 0.05% to 0.2% of the sample, which is then pressed in the usual way. The metal discs should be washed before use in both polar and nonpolar solvents and finally in good-quality acetone to remove traces of oil and grease, which may produce artefacts in the C—H region of the spectrum. The method may fail if excessive pressure is used, as this causes deformation of the lead disc.

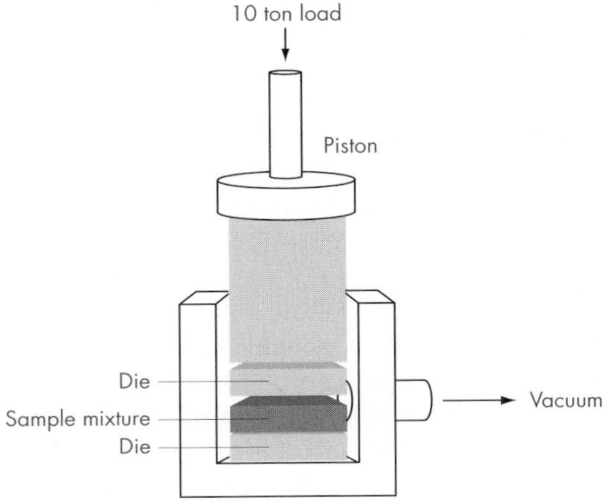

Figure 16.15 KBr disc press.

Another useful technique consists of dissolving the compound in a small volume of chloroform and drawing it into a Hamilton-type syringe held in a repeater holder. A small cluster of fine KBr particles is picked up on the end of the needle by a trace of chloroform expressed from the needle. The solvent is evaporated gently and the rest of the solution is fed into the KBr from the syringe as it evaporates. A disc is then made from the powder. It is important that the end of the needle be cut at right angles to the shaft and ground flat; those supplied for use with liquid chromatographs are suitable. For compounds which are bases, one must decide whether to evaporate solvents without the addition of hydrochloric acid, and accept the consequent loss of certain amines by volatilisation, or to add hydrochloric acid and accept the reduced solubility of the amine hydrochlorides in chloroform. Considerable losses of the sample by evaporation may occur for other types of compound (e.g. phenols), particularly when dilute solutions are used.

KBr is hygroscopic which means it is sometimes difficult to remove the last trace of water, and so silver chloride may be used instead. An indentation about 0.8 mm deep and slightly wider is made in the centre of a small piece of silver chloride sheet, and a solution (about 0.1 μL) that contains as little as 500 ng of substance is placed in the indentation and gently warmed to evaporate the solvent. The sheet is then placed in a die, which produces a cone of silver chloride with the sample embedded in it. A similar cone of plain silver chloride is mounted in the reference beam. Excellent spectra can be obtained with this technique.

The alkali halide discs can be stored in a dry environment and give good spectra several years after preparation. A well-prepared disc should have over 80% transmittance in regions where the sample does not absorb, although it will not necessarily be visually clear. It is not always easy to obtain a good disc when a very small amount of a recovered drug is available. In these circumstances, attenuation of the reference beam can 'sharpen' the spectrum. Another technique is to heat the alkali halide disc to about 80°C for 30 to 60 minutes with an IR lamp to evaporate any absorbed water. However, the high temperature accentuates the disadvantages of the alkali halide disc technique. In addition, the following artefacts have been observed:

- formation of anhydrides from carboxylic acids
- ketals and cyanohydrins reverting to the parent ketone
- loss of water from secondary alcohols.

Several disadvantages are inherent in the alkali halide disc technique. The alkali halides that are generally used are hygroscopic, and it is very difficult to exclude all traces of water. This often results in an O—H band in the spectrum. A number of compounds that contain O—H groups either form hydrogen bonds with the alkali halide or are adsorbed on its surface, so the method is unsuitable if the O—H band is to be examined. In such cases, polytetrafluoroethylene (PTFE) powder can sometimes be used in place of the alkali halide. Polymorphism occurs in many compounds and the grinding and pressing can alter the crystal form and consequently the spectrum. Splitting of bands also frequently occurs. Another disadvantage is the possibility that chemical changes will occur during the preparation of the disc. For example, double decomposition can occur:

$$\text{Base}\cdot\text{HCl} + \text{KBr} \rightarrow \text{Base}\cdot\text{HBr} + \text{KCl}$$

Hydrochlorides should, preferably, be examined in KCl. Bromide may be oxidised to bromine by some compounds, particularly strong oxidising agents, which may result in a disc becoming either discoloured or having yellow–brown spots. If the sample is a potential oxidising agent, other techniques of sample preparation should also be used to check the reliability of the spectra obtained from the alkali disc.

Organic compounds that contain nitrogen in a functional group should not be used with plates that are made of thallium bromide and thallium iodide as they appear to react with the plates.

Despite these disadvantages, the technique is still very useful for solid drugs. The advantages are that, besides being easy to use, the absorption of the alkali halide is very low and the quantity of compound required is small. The discs can easily be stored for reference purposes or the compound can be recovered if required.

Thin films

This method is of use if it is necessary to obtain spectra free from the dispersing media. The film can be prepared either by melting the solid and pouring it onto a suitable plate or by evaporation of a solution on an IR transparent plate (e.g. an NaCl disc).

Measurement of strongly absorbing or strongly light scattering samples

IR light incident on solid, powders or other materials such as creams is transmitted only poorly, if at all, because of the long pathlengths and light scattering. Neat liquids and solutions need very narrow pathlengths to overcome solvent absorption. However, scattered light or reflected light can be monitored in these cases and these techniques can be used to examine intact pharmaceutical preparations.

Light scattering

IR light falling on a powder can be reflected in two ways. The light can be reflected truly in the sense of mirror reflection (angle of incidence equals the angle of reflectance); this is known as specular reflectance. Alternatively, the IR light can be scattered, in the Rayleigh scattering sense, over all angles with a scattering intensity related to particle size; this is often referred to as diffuse reflectance. Specular reflectance is related to the refractive index of the sample, and intensity versus wavenumber data are difficult to interpret. Diffuse reflectance, on the other hand, is more simply related to light intensity; if the light is absorbed at the surface, it cannot be scattered back. A typical apparatus, often given the acronym DRIFT (diffuse reflectance IR Fourier transform spectroscopy), accessory is illustrated in Fig. 16.16. The sample is placed on a sample tray located beneath two ellipsoidal mirrors M_3 and M_4. Heterogeneous powders and fibres often benefit from being ground and 'diluted' with KBr. Pure KBr can be used as the reference material in a separate measurement for the reference spectrum. A good sample can be produced by rubbing a solid sample with English Abrasives paper P220C silicon carbide to produce a sample of approximately 150 μg over a 35 mm^2 area.

Diffuse reflectance is a measure of intensity versus wavenumber data, normally in a single-beam configuration. To ensure that measurements are at least approximately proportional to

A Drift attachment

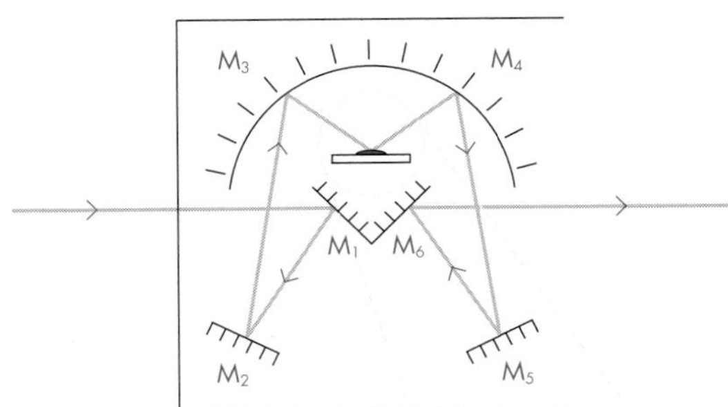

B Zoomed view of sample tray

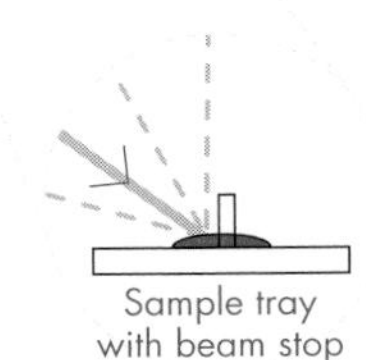

Figure 16.16 DRIFT attachment: IR radiation from the interferometer strikes mirror M_1 and is directed onto the sample tray by mirrors M_2 and M_3. In (A) the pure reflection path is highlighted. In practice, a beam stop (B) blocks the specular reflectance and only the diffuse reflected (scattered) beam is collected by mirrors M_3 and M_4 and directed towards the detector by mirrors M_5 and M_6.

concentration, a Kubelka–Munk transformation can be applied (Kubelka and Munk 1931).

$$\text{Kubela–Munk spectrum} = \left[\frac{\left(1 - \dfrac{\text{Sample spectrum}}{\text{Reference spectrum}}\right)^2}{2\left(\dfrac{\text{Sample spectrum}}{\text{Reference spectrum}}\right)}\right] \quad (16.5)$$

Alternatively, data can be presented as [−log(reflectance spectrum)] versus wavenumber.

The advantage of DRIFT analysis is the ease of sample preparation, particularly for powders which are simply mixed with KBr and presented to the FTIR, thereby reducing sampling time compared with KBr disc preparation.

Attenuated total reflectance

Light that arrives at an appropriate angle to the boundary between two media (or materials) with appropriate refractive indices n_1 and n_2 can be reflected back into the first medium (Fig. 16.17A). This is known as internal reflectance. For this to happen, the light beam must have at least sampled the second medium, if only to a depth of approximately 10 μm. The light in this fine slice of the second medium is referred to as an evanescent wave. If the second medium has absorption properties, this is sensed by the evanescent wave and the reflected beam has a reduced (attenuated) intensity, the attenuated total reflectance (ATR). The detected beam now provides intensity versus wavenumber characteristics that are effectively the absorption spectrum of the second medium.

Several proprietary attachments on the market are based upon a single rhomboid prism, of which an example is illustrated in Figure 16.17B. Suitable optical materials for medium 1 are zinc selenide (ZnSe), germanium and diamond. A sample well is created on the side of the rhomboid optical block. A typical ZnSe block is 50 mm × 1 or 2 mm, which gives 15–45 reflections, depending on rhomb angles. In this case, 5 to 10 μm sections of medium 2 are sampled 7–22 times, which results in an effective optical pathlength of the order 35–220 μm. The pathlength is reproducible and samples are easy to change in comparison with the equivalent simple transmission spacer cell, although the

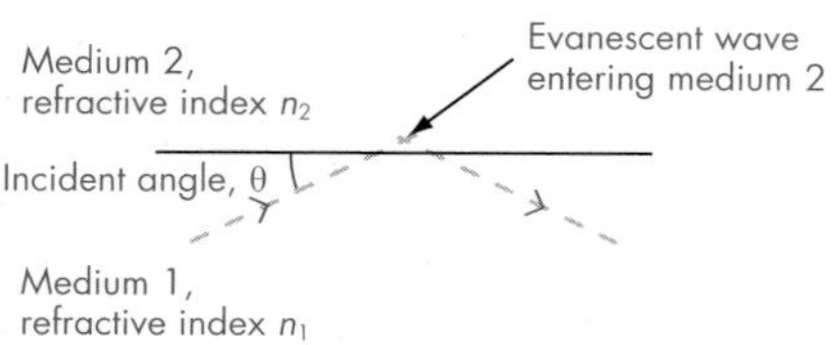

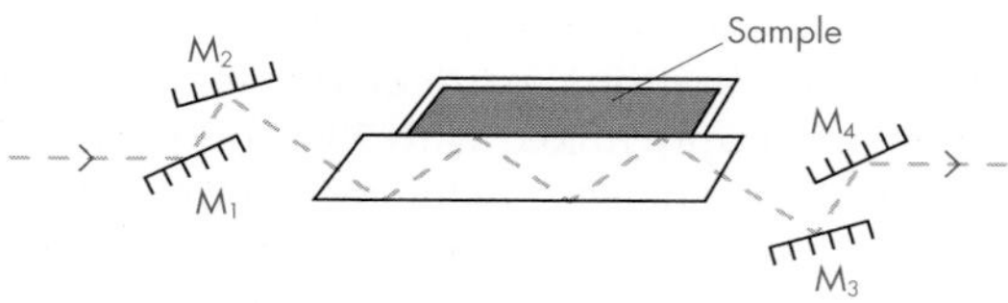

Figure 16.17 (A) Evanescent wave senses medium 2. (B) The attenuated total reflectance attachment, with light directed by mirrors M_1 and M_2, enters the rhomboid prism at 90°. Here the sample is measured twice (two internal reflections) before the light exits the prism at 90° and is directed to the detector by mirrors M_3 and M_4. In practice, there can be as many as 45 reflections.

latter may be preferred for simple solutions. Any material that forms a good optical contact with the prism can, in principle, be measured (solutions, oils, waxes, creams, pastes, powders and films).

More sophisticated devices exist, such as the DuraSamplIR attachment (Fig. 16.18) supplied by SensIR Technologies, Warrington, UK. The IR radiation from the interferometer is directed into a ZnSe prism by mirror M_1. Subsequent internal refection directs the IR radiation through a diamond prism, where the evanescent wave is reflected back through the ZnSe prism and then onto the detector via mirror M_2. In principle, a powder sample, with no sample preparation, is placed on the diamond prism surface, where it is compacted by a plunger. Powders, films, solutions, etc., can all be measured with equal ease and no sample pretreatment. This device produces excellent results in minimal time and baselines are flat as the technique is not dependent on light scattering.

The initial cost of ATR accessories may seem high compared to purchase of KBr to make discs, but the outlay is recouped quickly owing to cost savings in the time taken to analyse samples.

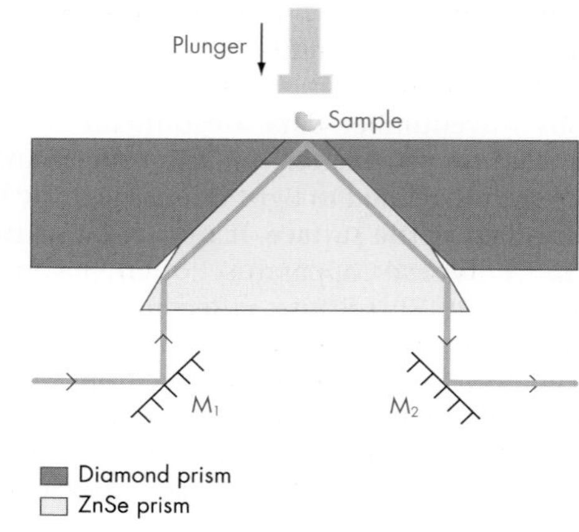

Figure 16.18 The DuraSamplIR attachment.

Non-pure samples

Numerous situations arise in the analysis of drugs and in forensic toxicology where the analyst wishes to use IR to identify an unknown substance or to confirm that a sample contains a particular substance. Examples include identifying components in suspect drugs of abuse seized alongside a dead body; confirming that a particular poison is present in a sample of stomach contents, and so on. Drugs of abuse as used at 'street' level are rarely pure. Hence analysis by IR will yield a spectrum of all components present that absorb in the IR region. Identifying a single component in this mixed spectrum is usually difficult if not impossible, particularly where the component of interest is present at low concentrations. When the starting material is a residue from the evaporation of a solvent extract of urine, blood, tissue or is a mixture of unknown substances, the most suitable method of purification is some form of chromatography.

Thin-layer chromatography

Suitable systems for thin-layer chromatography (TLC) are described in Chapter 13. After separation, solutes are present on the TLC plate as spots or bands intimately associated with the stationary phase. TLC separations can be carried out by normal-phase TLC or by reversed-phase operation (see Chapter 13). Normal-phase TLC typically employs silica gel as the stationary phase. Reversed-phase TLC uses organic stationary phases, typically long-chain hydrocarbons, covalently bonded to silica gel. Reversed-phase TLC should be avoided if IR is to be used for identification because it is difficult to remove the spot without also removing the organic stationary phase, giving rise to a mixed IR spectrum. Furthermore, location reagents must be chosen with care, and a destructive reagent, such as the Marquis reagent for alkaloids (which contains concentrated sulfuric acid), should not be used. Nondestructive reagents such as iodoplatinate solution can be used because the coloured complex is decomposable to yield the original compound. However, even this procedure may introduce extraneous peaks into the spectrum and, ideally, location reagents are best avoided. If the compound cannot be detected under UV light, it could be applied to the thin-layer plate twice and only a portion of the chromatogram sprayed, which thus allows location of substances but also permits the unsprayed portion to be eluted.

The use of aqueous acid or alkali to elute the compound from the thin-layer plate, followed by solvent extraction of the aqueous solution, is more efficient than direct solvent extraction of the adsorbent. In one method of direct extraction, the adsorbent is scraped from around the spot, the glass adjacent to the spot is carefully cleaned and the adsorbent is eluted *in situ* directly onto a wall of potassium bromide (KBr) built around the tip of the spot. The KBr is then pressed into a disc. This technique is only suitable for well-resolved spots. Elution of the spot sideways reduces contamination from compounds that are not resolved as well. The recovery of material from chromatograms varies from nil to over 70%. Compounds that contain hydroxyl and carboxyl groups, which can readily form hydrogen bonds with the solid support, tend to be recovered in low yield. Considerable interference in the 1100 cm^{-1} region is found with some adsorbents and compounds.

In a variation of this method, the thin-layer adsorbent is placed in the bottom of a glass vessel together with a triangular 'wick' of compressed KBr. Solvent is added and it rises up the wick and evaporates from the upper region. The compound is conveyed up the wick by the solvent and accumulates at the tip of the triangle, which is then cut off, dried, and used to prepare a disc. About 10 μg of compound is required to produce a satisfactory spectrum. The advantage of this technique is that the lower part of the KBr wick acts as a filter and removes finely divided adsorbent, which can give rise to spurious peaks.

In a further method, the thin-layer adsorbent is scraped onto a small amount of KBr powder in the hub of an 18-gauge metal hypodermic needle. A 1 mL glass syringe is filled with pure solvent and connected to the needle, and the compound is eluted dropwise onto a mound (10 mg) of dry KBr powder. Each drop of solvent is allowed to evaporate completely before the elution of the next drop. The powder and solute are then mixed and pressed into a disc.

Eluted material almost always includes unwanted extraneous matter co-extracted from the thin-layer chromatogram. Thus it is advisable to use the eluent from a 'blank' area as a reference solution. Contamination from plasticisers, solvents and dirty glassware can also be a serious problem when a spectrum has to be obtained from a few micrograms of a compound. Even momentary contact of dry adsorbent with plastic tubing can remove appreciable quantities of plasticisers. Hence the following precautions should be taken:

- use the minimum amount of the purest adsorbent available
- elute with less than 1 mL of a solvent that contains $<$0.0001% (1 ppm) of nonvolatile residue
- keep sample handling to a minimum
- clean all glassware with an efficient detergent in an ultrasonic bath
- avoid contact of materials and samples with plastics.

Gas chromatography

Gas chromatography (see Chapter 18) can provide a very convenient method of obtaining pure samples for IR spectroscopy. However, the sample can still be contaminated with impurities eluted from the stationary phase. The effluent from the chromatograph is a hot vapour and the problem is to obtain small quantities in a form suitable to present to the spectrometer. The spectrum of the vapour can be recorded directly or the compound can be trapped and then its spectrum recorded. Unfortunately, there is no entirely satisfactory method for the direct coupling of a gas chromatograph to a standard dispersive IR spectrometer. The outlet of the gas chromatograph can be split and one part connected to a heated cell (or light pipe) placed in the beam of an IR spectrometer. The gas flow is then stopped, trapping the sample in the cell, and the spectrum is recorded in the vapour phase. This technique can provide acceptable spectra of volatile compounds such as butyl acetate, which has a strong carbonyl band, but spectra of less-volatile compounds such as caffeine and phenylbutazone are more difficult to obtain. The temperatures of the connecting pipe and cell are clearly of great importance to keep the compounds as vapours. The coupling of a gas chromatograph to a Fourier transform instrument is much more satisfactory because the speed of scanning is sufficiently rapid to enable the spectrum of a compound to be recorded as it is eluted. Nevertheless, the temperatures of the cell and pipework are still of critical importance. GC-FTIR is now a well established analytical technique with instruments available from several major instrument manufacturers. Sensitivity is not as good as that given by detectors such as flame ionisation detectors (FID) or MS and this has restricted the workplace use of what is otherwise a very powerful analytical instrument.

It is possible to trap analytes separated by GC and then analyse off-line by IR. The method used to trap a compound post GC depends on whether it is a solid or a liquid at room temperature and, if the latter, on its volatility. Ways in which small samples can be obtained from a gas chromatograph in a form suitable to present to the spectrometer are described below. The main difficulty, common to all these methods of collecting fractions, is to determine the optimum temperature of the outlet tube from the chromatograph and the temperature of the collecting device. This problem can only be solved by trial and error.

It should be borne in mind that many GC detectors are destructive (e.g. FID, alkali flame ionisation detectors (AFID)) and this must be taken into account in determining at what point in the system the sample can be collected.

Cooled tubes

Most techniques to collect the effluent employ cooled tubes of glass or metal, but it is difficult to obtain good recoveries of a few micrograms of compounds of different volatilities by any one technique. Drugs such as the barbiturates and phenothiazines can be recovered in 50–70% yields in glass or metal capillary tubes held at room temperature, whereas more volatile drugs, such as the amfetamines, need to be cooled in liquid nitrogen or solid carbon dioxide (Curry *et al.* 1968; De Leenheer 1972).

Alkali halide tubes

A straight tube that contains a plug of powdered alkali halide is connected to the outlet of the chromatograph. The effluent condenses on the halide, which can then be pressed into a disc. This technique is most useful for compounds that are solid at room temperature.

High-performance liquid chromatography

High-performance liquid chromatography (Chapter 19) provides a very convenient method of purification, particularly if gas chromatography is either inapplicable or if derivatisation of the compound is necessary to enable chromatographic separation. Unlike gas chromatographs, liquid chromatographs are usually operated at or only slightly above ambient temperature, and detectors such as UV-visible and diode-array detection are nondestructive. Thus, the appropriate fraction of eluate can be collected by holding a test-tube or vial under the exit port as the substance of interest elutes. This can either be done via knowledge of the time at which the substance elutes or by monitoring the detector response and collecting the sample as the peak inflection starts.

The method used to retrieve the sample from the eluate to present to the IR spectrometer depends upon whether the compound is a solid or a liquid and, if the latter, on its volatility and the quantity present. All the common solvents absorb in the IR region. However, with the data-processing facilities of modern IR spectrometers, this is not a great disadvantage. The spectrum of the solvent can be recorded and then subtracted from the combined spectra of the compound and solvent to give a difference spectrum. If the concentration of the sample is low, the difference spectrum can be enhanced either by repetitive scanning and signal averaging or by expansion of the ordinate scale. In many cases, however, the amount of material is too small to enable the compound to be collected and transferred to standard cells.

Alternatively, the compound can be recovered by evaporation of the solvent. However, evaporation also concentrates any nonvolatile impurities in the solvent, so the use of pure solvents is essential. Another possible source of contamination is the packing material used in liquid chromatography columns. Many of these materials are based on silica gel and appreciable amounts of silica may be dissolved by certain solvents. Collecting from reversed-phase HPLC can be more difficult owing to the presence of water from the mobile phase, particularly where this will cause problems with spectral interpretation. Evaporation of water requires heating of the sample, which may lead to solute degradation or loss by volatilisation.

Microsublimation

This simple technique can be highly effective in purifying certain compounds (Fig. 16.19). Drugs may be sublimed from an evaporated solvent extract in the tube onto the cold finger of the apparatus, and the sublimate transferred by grinding the KBr powder gently with the cold finger.

Interpretation of spectra

A nonlinear molecule has $(3N - 6)$ fundamental (normal) modes of vibrating (this excludes overtones and combinations). Thus a molecule such as paracetamol (acetaminophen) with the formula $C_8H_9NO_2$ has $(3 \times 20 - 6) = 54$ fundamental (normal) modes of vibrating. Assigning 54 peaks in an IR spectrum is a daunting task at the very least. Therefore, the total molecular structure of a drug is unlikely to be determined directly from IR spectra information alone.

There are three aspects to identifying a chemical entity. In the first instance, the properties (biological, chemical and spectroscopic) of a drug are assessed and the drug is classified according to its type (e.g. nonsteroidal anti-inflammatory drug, barbiturate, steroid, etc.). The analyte may be a previously characterised compound, in which case a comparison of data from the unknown with reference data, often termed fingerprint identification, confirms the identity of the compound. This may be possible through computer matching of the spectra. The molecular structure of a new chemical entity will most likely need to be determined by NMR spectroscopy, perhaps in combination with MS. However, information such as the existence of specific functional groups or the elimination of putative structures is a great help in processing the NMR information.

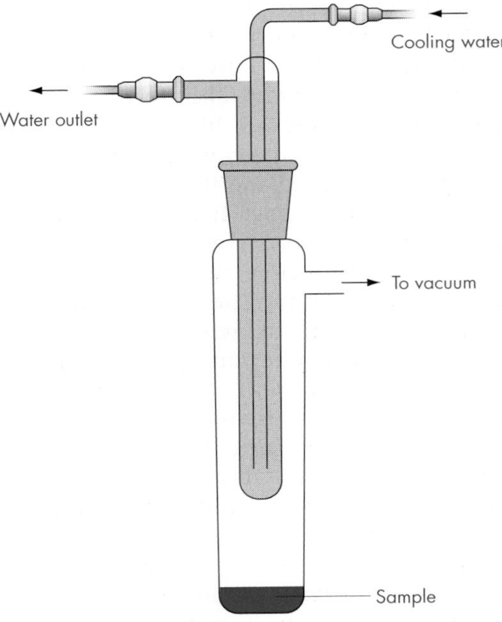

Figure 16.19 Apparatus for microsublimation.

Functional group identification

Table 16.1 lists the important IR vibration frequencies. The precise location of a band often gives an indication of the structural environment of the group (e.g. the C=O group in cyclohexanone and cyclopentanone, the amide bond in an α-helix or β-sheet polypeptide chain). More substantial lists of peak assignments are found in the standard texts on IR spectroscopy (see Further Reading).

Qualitative analysis

Infrared spectra matching and fingerprint identification

In the simplest case, two spectral printouts – one of the reference and the other of the analyte – can be overlaid on a light box and the spectral features related by eye. Overlaying spectra on the computer screen achieves the same objective.

When the spectrum of a substance being examined is compared with a reference spectrum, the positions and relative intensities of the absorption bands of the spectrum of the substance being examined should conform to those of the reference spectrum. When the two spectra are compared, care should be taken to allow for the possibility of differences in resolving power between the instrument on which the reference spectrum was prepared and the instrument used to examine the substance. It is good practice to run a spectrum of a polystyrene film on the same instrument to compare it with that recorded on the reference spectrum. The greatest variations through differences in resolving power are likely to occur in the region between 4000 and 2000 cm^{-1}.

When a chemical reference substance is available, the substance being examined and the chemical reference substance should be prepared by the same procedure before recording the spectra (see later under Polymorphism). The transmission minima in the spectrum obtained with the substance being examined should correspond in position and relative size to those in the spectrum obtained with the reference substance.

In recent years, IR spectral compilations have been created and stored electronically in databases and/or libraries. The spectrum of the analyte is presented to the database and the computer attempts to match the spectrum with one already held in the database. A report is made of the best matches. The computer program lists the most likely hits in order of a closeness of fit. Many spectra compilations (databases) are private collections, held typically by individual pharmaceutical companies; some can be purchased and a few are in the public domain.

The number of compounds for which IR spectra have been measured is now massive. Potentially, the greater the number of spectra in a database, the greater is the probability of making a good match for the unknown sample. However, the probability of making a mismatch is also greater, as more spectra with fine differences are available for comparison. The computer is simply matching 'pictures' by the number of peaks, their positions and their relative intensities. The best the computer fitting can do is to indicate a mathematical similarity. It is important to qualify a computer search:

- a visual overlay of the test compound spectrum and the hit spectrum ensures that the search has not chosen a match that is mathematically acceptable but not chemically acceptable
- knowledge of the class of a compound can help restrict the search to a more refined reference set (database) and can also help in deciding whether the substance given as a best fit is actually likely to be present in a sample
- other properties of the sample and the reference compound should match, such as chromatographic retention times, chemical and colour reactions, where these are available, and functional group assignments
- the computer can only select spectra that are in its library; if the spectrum of the compound under investigation is absent, then it will select those that give the next-best fit
- different forms of the same compound give different IR spectra (different polymorphs, racemate and/or enantiomer, ionisation status, cations and anions).

Some examples of the identification of drugs are given below.

Infrared spectra of amfetamines

The IR spectra of amfetamine base and the hydrochloride have many similarities, but the hydrochloride spectrum shows much finer detail (Fig. 16.20A and B). The IR spectra of the hydrochloride and mandelate salts show differences (Fig. 16.20B and C) because of the absorption of the mandelic acid. However, the spectra of the hydrochloride and sulfate salts (Fig. 16.20B and 16.20D) are similar since they both have inorganic anions. The only major difference is the absorption band caused by the sulfate at 1110 cm^{-1}.

Infrared spectra of barbiturates

Important derivatives of malonylurea (barbituric acid) have two substituents at position 5. Others are also substituted at position 1 and in others the oxygen atom attached to position 2 is replaced by sulfur to form thiobarbiturates (Fig. 16.21).

The barbiturates can be classified chemically into three classes: 5,5-disubstituted barbituric acids, 1,5,5-trisubstituted barbituric acids and 5,5-disubstituted thiobarbituric acids. These classes can be further divided depending on whether the substituents in position 5 are alkyl, alkenyl, aryl or cycloalkenyl. In most common barbiturates, one of the 5-substituents is either ethyl or allyl and the other is either a straight- or branched-chain alkyl or alkenyl group with five or fewer carbon atoms. Some barbiturates are available as sodium salts. The IR spectrum of a barbiturate therefore depends on the class of compound, the nature of the substituents and whether it is the free acid or the sodium salt.

With the exception of phenobarbital and barbituric acid, the free barbiturates do not absorb appreciably above 3300 cm^{-1} (e.g. barbital, Fig. 16.21A), a feature that distinguishes them from the ureides; a weak band of unknown origin sometimes occurs between 3500 and 3400 cm^{-1}. All the barbiturates have two bands which occur near 3200 and 3100 cm^{-1} and are caused by N—H stretching vibrations. In the 5,5-disubstituted compounds, the relative intensities of the two bands are similar, although that at 3100 cm^{-1} is usually slightly less intense. In compounds substituted on the nitrogen atom at position 1, the intensity of the band at 3100 cm^{-1} may be greatly reduced and is often present only as a shoulder on the band at 3200 cm^{-1}, e.g. metharbital. Methylphenobarbital appears to be an exception in that the band at 3100 cm^{-1} is the most intense one in the region. A similar phenomenon occurs with the sodium salts, since here again one of the hydrogen atoms in either position 1 or 3 has been replaced.

A series of up to four medium-to-intense bands occurs in the region 3000–2800 cm^{-1}, and is caused by alkyl C—H stretching vibrations of the substituents in positions 1 and 5. The intensity of the bands gives a very approximate indication of the number of C—H bonds and hence the number of carbon atoms in the chain. This does not appear to apply to the sodium salts, in which the band that occurs at 3000–2950 cm^{-1} is usually increased in intensity, compared to that of the free acid, and becomes the strongest band. Compare, for example, the spectra of barbital (Fig. 16.21A) and barbital sodium (Fig. 16.21B).

The barbiturates have up to three strong bands in the region 1765 to 1670 cm^{-1}, which result from C═O stretching vibrations. Knowledge of the origin of these bands helps us to understand the differences in the spectra of the various types of barbiturate.

In symmetrical molecules, the three bands are all of similar intensity. In asymmetrical molecules, the band at the highest frequency is often less intense than the other two, particularly so when the molecule is substituted in position 1. The sodium salts of the barbiturates have only two bands in this region, since the molecule is no longer symmetrical, and these occur at a lower frequency, between 1700 and 1650 cm^{-1}. In addition, a broad strong band occurs between 1600 and 1550 cm^{-1}; the free barbiturates show practically no absorption in this region. The sodium salts of the thiobarbiturates exhibit only the lowest of the three C═O vibrations in the region 1700–1680 cm^{-1}. They do, however, exhibit the broad, strong band that occurs between 1550 and 1600 cm^{-1}. Therefore, the number, position and intensity of the bands

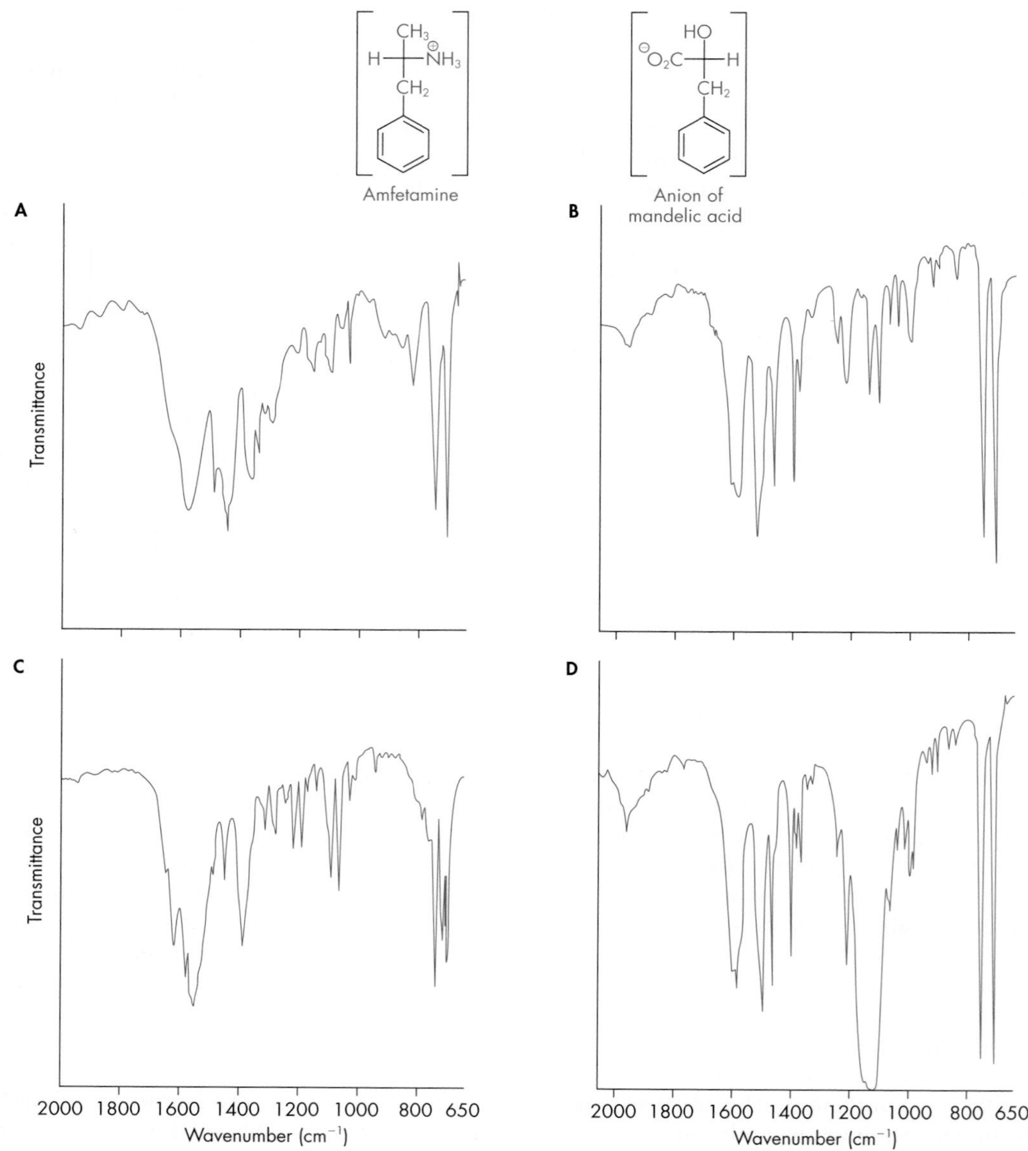

Figure 16.20 IR spectra of (A) amfetamine base, (B) amfetamine hydrochloride, (C) amfetamine mandelate, (D) amfetamine sulfate.

between 1800 and 1500 cm^{-1} give a very good indication of whether the barbiturate is the free acid, the salt or a thiobarbiturate.

Most barbiturates have a number of strong bands between 1460 and 1250 cm^{-1}, and some of these result from C—H deformation and C—N stretching vibrations. The sodium salts of the thiobarbiturates have a broad strong band between 1500 and 1480 cm^{-1}, which is believed to be caused by C—N stretching vibrations of the carbon atom attached to sulfur. This band is not present in the ordinary barbiturates and therefore provides another way to distinguish those that contain sulfur. Many barbiturates

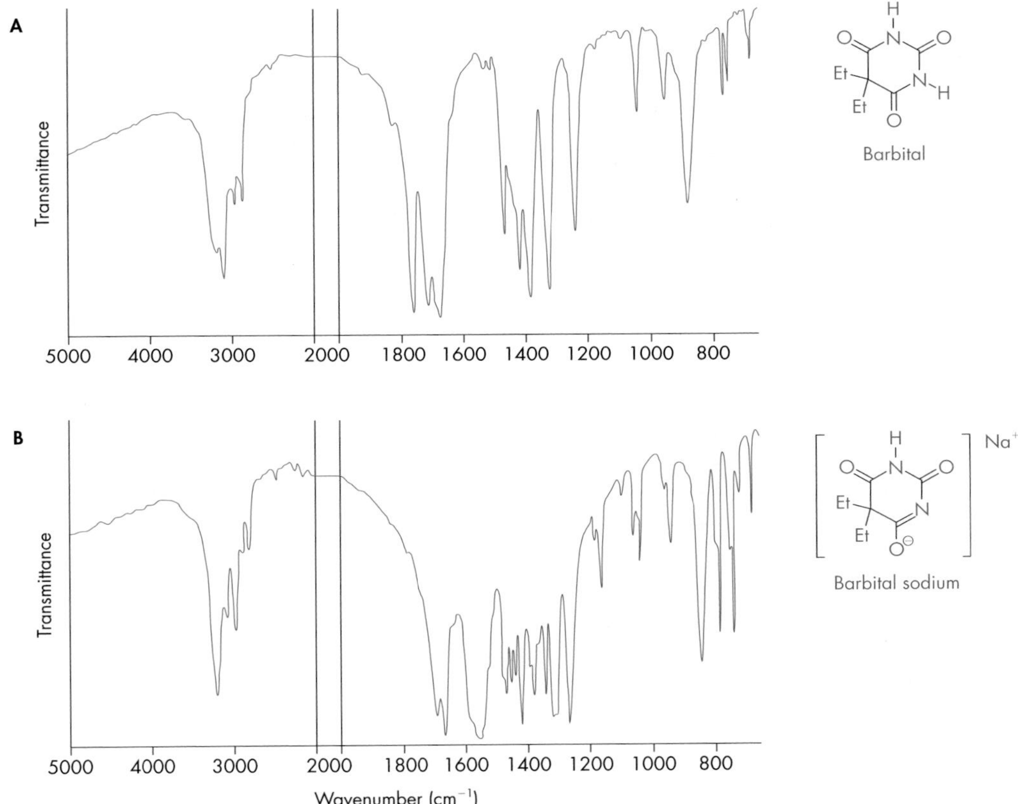

Figure 16.21 IR spectra of (A) barbital and (B) barbital sodium.

exhibit a few weak-to-medium intensity bands in the region 1150–900 cm^{-1}. The 1-substituted barbiturates exhibit a greater number of sharp bands of medium intensity. Those compounds that contain an allyl group exhibit bands at about 1000–960 cm^{-1}, which probably result from C—H deformation vibrations. The sodium salts of the thiobarbiturates show a band of medium intensity between 1020 and 1000 cm^{-1}. Finally, many barbiturates, but not the thiobarbiturates, exhibit a broad band of medium-to-strong intensity between 900 and 800 cm^{-1}.

Infrared spectra of aspirin, Nujol and paracetamol

The spectra of aspirin, Nujol and paracetamol are given in Fig. 16.22, which illustrates the differentiation of N—H, O—H, ester, carboxylic acid and amide groups. In particular, the effect of Nujol on the drug spectra is apparent.

Polymorphism

Many drugs exist in polymorphic forms and have different IR spectra for each different crystalline form. IR spectroscopy can therefore be used to distinguish between different polymorphic forms, to identify them and also to measure quantitatively the proportions of each in a mixture.

If a test compound gives a different spectrum from the corresponding chemical reference substance, and polymorphism is suspected, both should be treated in the same manner so that they crystallise or are produced in the same form. This can often be achieved by dissolving them in a suitable solvent and evaporating to dryness.

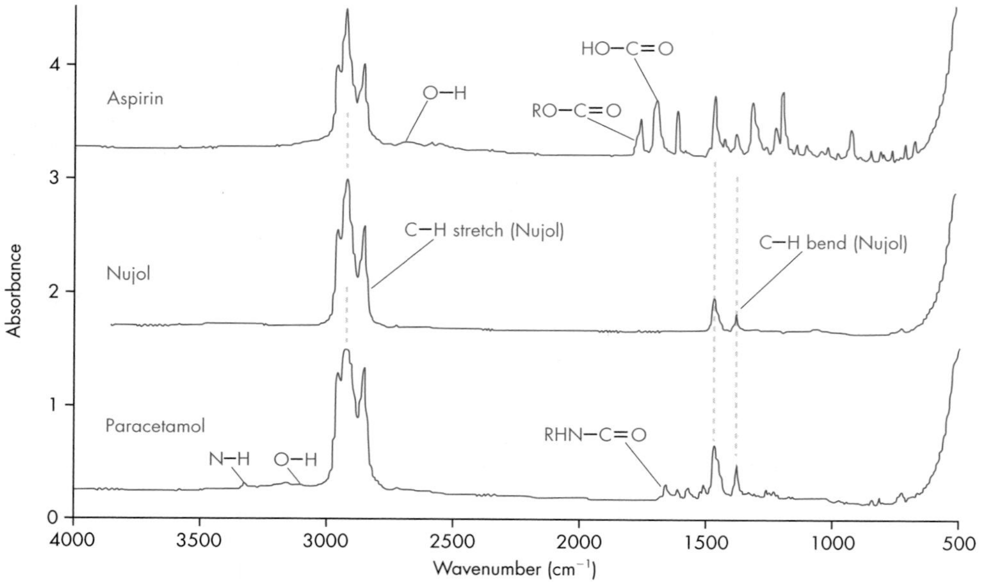

Figure 16.22 The IR spectra of aspirin, Nujol and paracetamol (acetaminophen). The drug spectra were measured as Nujol mulls.

The barbiturates are notable for the extent to which they exhibit polymorphism, including many metastable forms found only in mixtures. Spectral differences between polymorphs are associated with different types of hydrogen bonding, and there is a correlation between hydrogen bond strength and duration of action of the barbiturates on the central nervous system. The crystalline structure of barbiturates can be affected by grinding with an alkali halide or in preparing a mull, but if precautions are taken to ensure reproducibility, the spectra of the barbiturates are sufficiently different to be used for identification purposes.

Interferences

Spurious bands can occur readily in IR spectra, particularly when a biological sample has undergone several purification procedures. Traces of plasticisers, surfactants and oils left on glassware can all give rise to spurious IR bands. A useful list has been compiled by Szymanski (1971), part of which is given in Table 16.2.

Infrared data in monographs

Modern spectral identification by reference to computer databases involves sophisticated chemometric algorithms to compare all the digitised points in a test spectrum with a set of reference spectra. Spectra that are judged to be most similar are said to be a match, which allows the identity of the test spectrum to be established. This type of work requires specialised database reference sets and computer programs, much of which is proprietary and related to the software of the spectrometer being used.

However, it has been shown (Curry *et al.* 1969; Ingle and Mathieson 1976) that an IR spectrum of a particular substance can be retrieved from a collection, with some degree of confidence, by reference to its six major absorption bands. This forms the basis for a system of identification.

Table 16.2 Spurious peaks in IR spectroscopy. (After Szymanski 1971)

Wavenumber (cm^{-1})	Assignment	Comments
3800–2500	H_2O	Bound or unbound water in a molecule can give rise to sharp or broad bands. In alkali halide disks a water band at 3350 cm^{-1} may appear
3300–3000	NH_3^+	Lens tissues
1810–1600	C=O	Impurities that contain the carbonyl group, e.g. phosgene in chloroform, plasticisers
1750–1500	H_2O	Bound or unbound water can give rise to sharp or broad bands
1610–1515	COO^-	Alkali salts (which also have a weaker band at 1425 cm^{-1}) can be produced from alkali halides
1400	NH_3^+	Lens tissues
1265	Si—CH_3	Stopcock grease or silicone oil
1110–1050	Si—O—Si	Glass or hydrolysed Si compounds
730, 720	Polyethylene	Polyethylene laboratory ware
700	Polystyrene	Polystyrene laboratory ware

Quantitative analysis

Concentration of molecular species

FTIR spectrometers are now very stable instruments and, coupled with computer control and data manipulation, should be as easy to operate as UV–visible spectrophotometers. They can operate routinely in the absorbance mode, which is required for concentration determinations. However, relatively high concentrations are required given the restriction of solvent absorption, the need for narrow pathlengths and the low extinction coefficients of vibrations. Assuming Beer's law is obeyed, absolute concentrations can be determined in solution from specific bands in windows of solvent transparency. In the solid state, the relative amounts of two components can be estimated readily from the relative intensities of two specific absorption bands:

$$A_{1\lambda_1} = \varepsilon_{1\lambda_1} c_1 l$$
$$A_{2\lambda_2} = \varepsilon_{2\lambda_2} c_2 l$$
$$\frac{A_{1\lambda_1}}{A_{2\lambda_2}} \propto \frac{c_1}{c_2} \qquad (16.6)$$

where $A_{1\lambda_1}$, $A_{2\lambda_2}$, $\varepsilon_{1\lambda_1}$ and $\varepsilon_{2\lambda_2}$ are, respectively, the absorbances and extinction coefficients of species 1 and 2 at the corresponding wavelengths λ_1 and λ_2. The concentration of species 1 and 2 are c_1 and c_2, and the pathlength is l.

Collections of data

General collections

Compilations of IR spectral data are available in two forms, either as pictures or as digital absorbance/wavenumber in electronic databases. Pictures are available in book or computer form and are suitable for visual inspection. Spectral characteristics can be determined with the aid of a ruler. Electronic databases are available in computer memory for data manipulation and spectral matching. The reader is referred to *Clarke's Analaysis of Drugs and Poisons* (Moffat *et al.* 2004) for a comprehensive listing of sources of IR software and spectral libraries.

Near infrared

(R D Jee)

Overview of NIR

As noted above, the near-infrared (NIR) region extends from about 800 to 2500 nm (or 12 500 to 4000 cm^{-1}). NIR absorbances correspond to overtones and combinations of molecular vibrations that have their fundamentals in the mid IR region of the spectrum. The absorbances produced tend to be weaker than those for the mid IR. This can be put to good advantage in that samples may be measured without any need for sample dilution or preparation. For the qualitative analysis of solid samples, NIR spectra are invariably measured by reflectance (diffuse reflectance). The resultant spectra are considerably more complex to interpret than IR spectra, having many overlapping peaks. Computer algorithms are used to convert NIR reflectance spectra to a simpler form for interpretation with so-called 'second-derivative' spectra obtained (Fig. 16.23). Taking the second derivative of the spectrum largely removes the effects of baseline offsets and baseline slopes which are common in NIR spectra (Fig. 16.24). The positions of the negative peaks in the second-derivative spectrum correspond to the positions of peaks in the original spectrum as can be seen for acetomenaphthone (Fig. 16.23). Peak positions (e.g. the six most intense) can be used as the basis of a method of quantification. The theory of NIR and the techniques used in spectral conversion are beyond the scope of this textbook and the reader is referred to Moffat *et al.* (2004) and to texts in the reference section of this chapter for more detailed discussion. Sampling techniques and the particular advantages offered by NIR compared to mid IR will be discussed here.

The strength of NIR lies in its ability to identify relatively pure samples rapidly or to identify a matrix of nearly fixed composition, such as tablets. Although this analysis could also be done in the mid IR, providing the same information, samples can be analysed by NIR in glass bottles (Fig. 16.25A), something which would not be possible for mid IR. This is because common types of glass such as borosilicate and soda glass are virtually transparent to NIR radiation. The radiation reflected by the sample is measured as a function of wavelength and with respect to the reflectance of a suitable standard, such as a flat disc of a ceramic or Spectralon. Spectralon is a thermoplastic resin with very high diffuse reflection such that at NIR wavelengths it will have >95% reflectance. Spectra are dependent upon the reference chosen and the reproducibility of such standards can be a problem when it comes to transferability of spectra from one instrument to another. This problem has not been completely resolved at present. Fibre-optic probes that can be inserted directly into the sample can be attached to many NIR instruments (Fig. 16.25B). This makes it possible to sample directly from production lines.

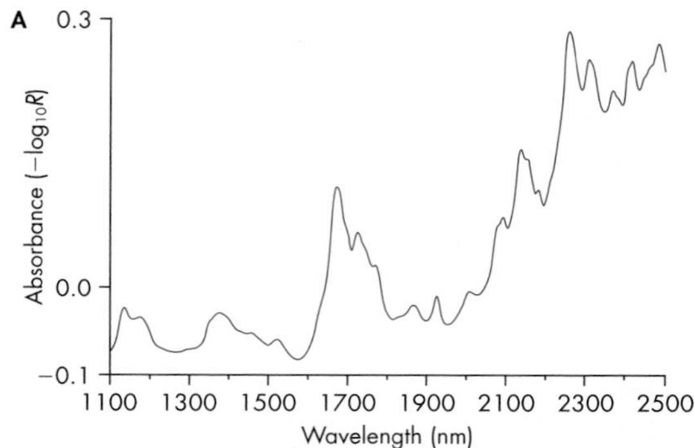

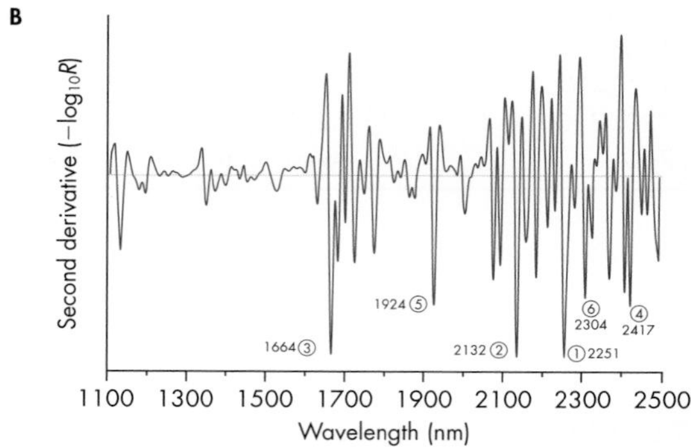

Figure 16.23 (A) Near-infrared spectrum of acetomenaphthone measured by reflectance; (B) second derivative spectrum of (A). Circled numbers indicate the six most intense negative peaks in order of decreasing intensity.

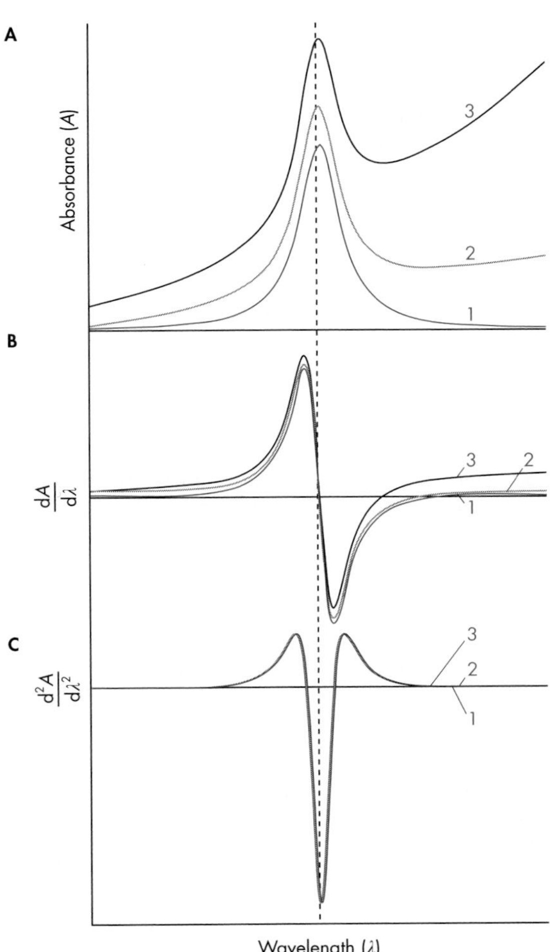

Figure 16.24 Advantages of using second-derivative spectra: (A) original spectra; (B) first-derivative spectra, and (C) second derivative spectra. 1, zero baseline; 2, linear sloping baseline; 3, curved (quadratic) baseline with offset.

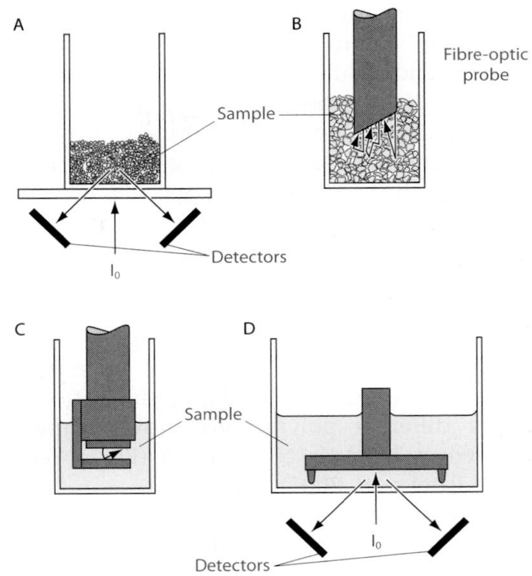

Figure 16.25 Sample presentation methods: (A) sample bottle on sample stage; (B) fibre-optic probe; (C) liquid sample using a fibre-optic probe fitted with transflectance adapter; and (D) liquid sample measured by transflectance.

Sample preparation and presentation

Liquids can be measured using conventional cuvettes or by transflectance, again using a fibre-optic probe fitted with a transflectance tip (Fig. 16.25C), or directly on a sample stage in a cup with a suitable reflector (Fig. 16.25D). For the measurement of powders, it has been recommended that sample bottles should be filled by 'pouring' the powder into the bottle without tapping (Yoon *et al.*, 1998). Tapping causes compaction of the powder and was found to result in poor sample-measurement repeatability. For reflectance measurements, the sample thickness should be such that any further increase in sample thickness has no effect upon the spectrum. Typically, NIR radiation penetrates 1–3 mm into a powdered sample and a sample thickness of >10 mm is recommended to give an effective 'infinite thickness'. For a compact material such as a tablet the reflected radiation will penetrate only 0.1–1 mm. The sample bottle diameter should exceed that of the radiation beam. For many instruments, this means a bottle of diameter of about 10 mm or greater. Samples bottles should be chosen that have smooth bases, otherwise specular reflectance varies from one bottle to the next as well as the orientation on the sample stage. The same type of sample bottle should be used for both test samples and reference materials to minimise differences due to sampling containers.

Sample-measurement repeatability is very dependent upon the nature of the sample. Liquids and solutions are highly reproducible because of the homogeneous nature of the sample. Crystalline powders usually show poor repeatability because of varying specular reflection from the crystal surfaces. Specular reflection distorts the 'absorbance' spectrum and limits the usable photometric range. Identification algorithms can be affected markedly by the crystallinity of samples. Careful crushing of the material to reduce the particle size can help to minimise the effects. Vibrational patterns are affected by differences in the crystal lattice and hence different polymorphs show significant differences in their NIR spectra (Blanco *et al.* 1998; Patel *et al.* 2001).

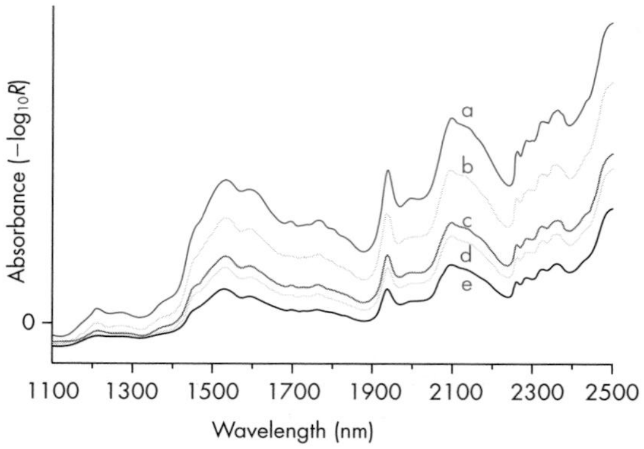

Figure 16.26 Reflectance spectra of lactose monohydrate of varying particle sizes: (a) >150, (b) 93, (c) 63, (d) 45 and (e) 32 μm. Note the characteristic absorption peak due to water at 1900–1940 nm.

As for analysis in the mid IR region, solvents for the preparation of solutions are somewhat limited for NIR analysis. Only carbon tetrachloride and carbon disulfide among the common solvents are transparent throughout the entire NIR region. Methylene chloride, dioxane, heptane, acetonitrile and dimethyl sulfoxide have regions below 2200 nm that can be used.

Water has a particularly strong absorbance spectrum in the NIR region and samples must be protected from uptake or loss of water from or to the atmosphere. The presence of water can be recognised easily by the characteristic absorption peak in the range 1900–1940 nm. The exact peak position depends on the nature of the water – free or water of crystallisation – and the extent of hydrogen bonding. The water peak in the spectrum of lactose monohydrate (Fig. 16.26) can easily be seen.

Intact tablets may be measured as easily as any other sample. A sample bottle that contains tablets randomly packed may be placed on the sample stage or single tablets may be measured directly. The depth of penetration of reflected radiation from compact materials, such as tablets, is limited to only a few tenths of a millimetre. Markings on tablets can affect the spectra and a decision has to be made whether to measure one side or both. With coated tablets it is possible for the reflectance spectrum to be dominated by the coating material, though some radiation will penetrate into the core. Tablets can be crushed and the powder measured in a sample bottle if required.

With grating instruments, spectra commonly exhibit a small anomalous peak known as a Wood's peak at about 1520 nm. The magnitude of the peak is dependent upon the difference in diameters of the sample and reflectance standard used: the greater the difference, the larger the peak (Fig. 16.27). It can be quite pronounced in the spectra of poorly absorbing substances and care is required not to confuse the Wood's peak with peaks from the material. Tablets, which generally have a small diameter, often show a prominent Wood's peak when they are measured by placing them directly on the sample stage.

Interpretation of spectra

Functional groups such as X—H, where X is C, N, O and S, have a small reduced mass and hence high fundamental frequency of vibration and are particularly important for NIR spectroscopy – the first and second overtones appear in the NIR region. Groupings such as C—Cl, C—F, C=O, etc., with high reduced masses are of less importance in NIR spectroscopy as their fundamental frequencies are low and their overtones generally also appear in the mid IR region. For organic

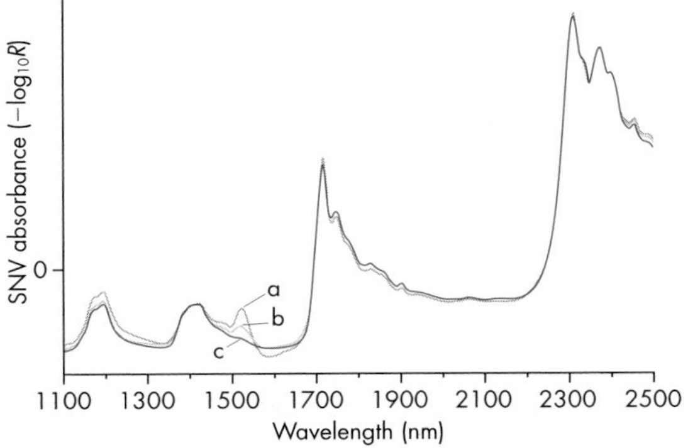

Figure 16.27 Wood's anomaly observed with grating monochromator instruments. Reflectance spectra of poly(vinyl chloride) powder measured in sample bottles of different diameters. Bottle diameter: (a) 8 mm, (b) 15 mm and (c) 25 mm. Reference diameter: 50 mm.

molecules, the C—H bond is the most important and for alkanes its fundamental stretching vibration in the mid IR region at about 2960–2850 cm^{-1} gives rise to first and second overtones at approximately 1700–1730 and 1150–1170 nm in the NIR region. The C—H group stretching and deformation vibrational modes give rise to combination bands in the region 2000–2500 nm. Water is a particularly strong absorber in the NIR region, with the O—H first overtone of the stretching vibration occurring at 1450 nm (second and third overtones at 970 and 760 nm, respectively). Alcohols similarly show absorptions around 1450 nm. A very intense absorption occurs in the region 1900—1940 nm for water and has been assigned to the combination band between the fundamental stretching and deformation vibrations of the O—H bond; in the case of alcohols this vibration occurs at a somewhat longer wavelength. Temperature can have a marked effect on the spectra of compounds with hydrogen bonds. The spectrum of water is particularly sensitive to temperature, with changes in both the intensities and band positions. Similar shifts are observed for different states of adsorbed water.

While characteristic wavelengths, such as those mentioned above, can often be identified readily in the NIR spectrum of a material, the general complexity of NIR spectra precludes any easy interpretation and identifications are based on comparison with reference spectra. Figure 16.28 gives a summary of the positions of some of the more important NIR absorptions. More extensive lists of NIR vibrations are given by Osborne *et al.* (1993) and Burns and Ciurczak (2001).

Problem compounds

Compounds with long aliphatic chains, such as hydrocarbons, stearates and waxes, are difficult to distinguish as the spectrum becomes dominated by the —CH_2 groups. Starches and related compounds, such as maltodextrins, gums and other materials with polysaccharide groupings, are difficult to distinguish from one another reliably. With inorganic compounds, which often have little or no genuine absorbance, care is required that any apparent spectral matching is not from absorbances caused by residual moisture, Wood's peak and/or the sample bottle itself. Mid IR and other spectroscopic techniques are most probably no better for these problem compounds – the extremely good signal-to-noise level in NIR spectra means that often the chemometric classification techniques used in interpreting NIR spectra are able to distinguish more easily between closely related compounds than they can for other spectra.

Detection of counterfeit materials

The ability of NIR spectroscopy to detect both physical and chemical differences between samples means it can be used like fingerprinting. For example, batch-to-batch variation of tablets, or tablets manufactured at different sites, can often be distinguished. Similarly, the detection of counterfeit products is possible (Scafi and Pasquini 2001). Spectra of a representative sample of the genuine product are compared to those of the suspected counterfeit. While spectral comparison methods such as maximum wavelength distance may be used, methods such as Principal Component Analysis (PCA) are often to be preferred (Fig. 16.29).

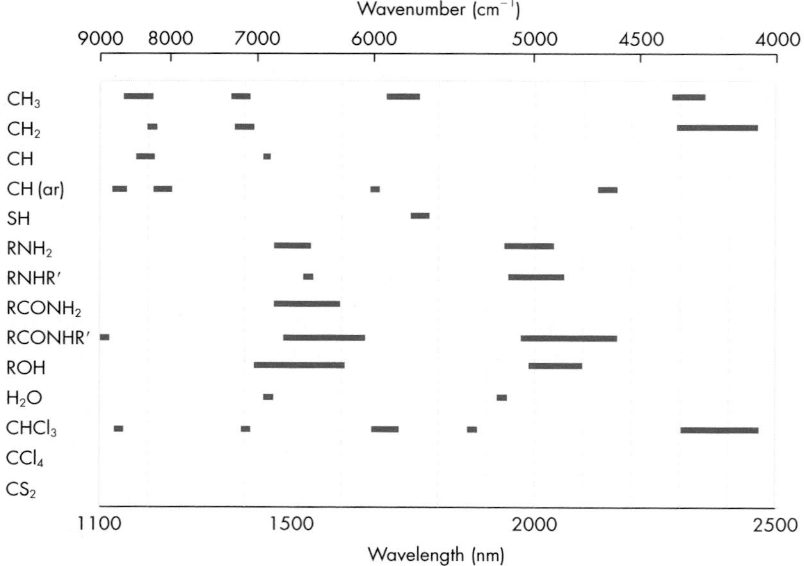

Figure 16.28 Wavelengths of important near-infrared absorbances. Black bars show regions of absorption.

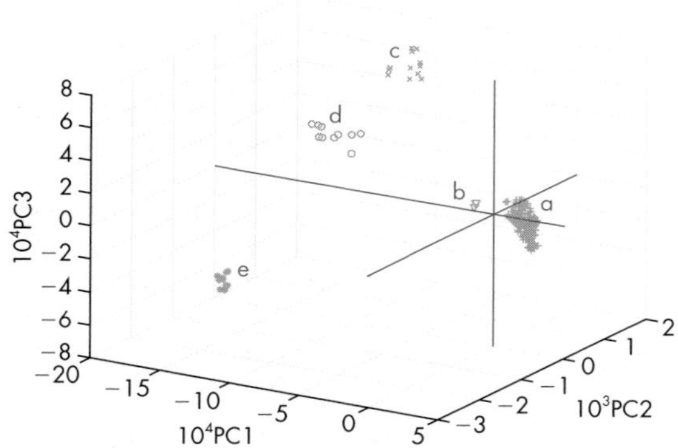

Figure 16.29 Principal components analysis score plot (first three principal components, PC1, PC2 and PC3) illustrating the detection of counterfeit tablets. (a) and (b) genuine product; (c), (d) and (e) counterfeit samples.

Materials and/or products must be handled with care. Tablets and the like often rapidly exchange moisture with the atmosphere and an apparently suspect product might simply have a different moisture content. If moisture differences are not important, then genuine and suspect samples should be allowed to equilibrate to ambient humidity before measurement. When differences in moisture are important, measurements must be made as soon as the samples are opened (e.g. tablets should be measured immediately they are removed from a blister pack).

Quantitative analysis

Quantitative methods of NIR analysis are generally time consuming to set up and not suited to 'one-off' assays. However, once developed, a quantitative assay takes little more than the time to record a sample spectrum. Caution should be exercised by non-experts when setting up quantitative NIR analyses as there are many factors that can influence quantification.

Instrumentation

Instrumentation used for NIR measurements is similar to that used for UV and/or visible absorption spectroscopy and based on fixed wavelengths, scanning or diode array systems. Tungsten-halogen lamps serve as energy sources, while lead sulfide and/or indium gallium arsenide detectors are used. Instruments are typically computer controlled, which enables spectra to be measured in a matter of seconds and saved to disc. As for mid IR instruments, system suitability checks should be performed regularly (daily) to maximise accuracy of data output.

Near-infrared imaging

The coupling of a NIR spectrometer and a scanning microscope allows spectroscopic imaging of surfaces. Not only can small samples be identified, but information about the distribution of different chemical components and their particle size can be obtained. Commercial reflectance NIR microscopy mapping systems with spectral resolution of 4–16 cm^{-1} and spatial resolution of approximately 5–20 μm are available. Typically, a surface area of 1–10 mm^2 of the sample is analysed by recording a spectrum for each 20 μm × 20 μm area of sample, which allows a 'grid' of spectral information to be constructed – this gives many thousands of spectra. Spectral information comes from the top surface layers down to a depth of approximately 30–100 μm and represents 10–100 ng of sample. By using suitable chemometrics, the spectra may be processed to determine the chemical identity at each 'grid' position. Chemical image plots to show the distribution of the various chemical species may then be created for the whole surface. Such information is of value when comparing good and poor tablet blends, distinguishing between genuine and counterfeit materials, etc., and is being used in the development of an NIR-imaging system to assess burn damage in clinical treatment (Sowa *et al.*, 2006). Clarke *et al.* (2001) have described such a system using both NIR and Raman spectroscopic data to give a chemical image of pharmaceutical formulations.

Collections of data

Although NIR spectral libraries are beginning to be available commercially, the libraries that are currently available are nowhere near as extensive as those for the mid IR region.

References

M. Blanco *et al.*, Critical review: near-infrared spectroscopy in the pharmaceutical industry, *Analyst*, 1998, **123**, 135R–150R.

British Pharmacopoeia Commission, *British Pharmacopoeia 2007*, Volume IV, Appendix 11A, A145, London, The Stationery Office, 2007.

D. A. Burns and E. W. Ciurczak (ed.), *Handbook of Near-Infrared Analysis*, 2nd edn, London, Marcel Dekker, 2001.

F. C. Clarke *et al.*, Chemical image fusion. The synergy of FT–NIR and Raman mapping microscopy to enable a more complete visualization of pharmaceutical formulations, *Anal. Chem.*, 2001, **73**, 2213–2220.

A. S. Curry *et al.*, Micro infra-red spectroscopy of gas chromatographic fractions., *J. Chromatogr.*, 1968, **38**, 200–208.

A. S. Curry *et al.*, A simple infrared spectrum retrieval system, *J. Pharm. Pharmacol.*, 1969, **21**, 224–231.

P. H. B. Ingle and D.W. Mathieson, *Pharm. J.*, 1976, **216**, 73.

P. Kubelka and F. Munk, Ein Beitrag zür Optik der Farbanstriche, *Z. Tech. Physic*, 1931, **12**, 593–601.

A. De Leenheer, Coupling of chromatographic techniques with micro-infrared spectrometry for the determination of phenothiazine and related drugs, *J. Chromatogr.*, 1972, **74**, 35–41.

A. C. Moffat *et al.* (eds), *Clarke's Analysis of Drugs and Poisons*, 3rd edn, London, Pharmaceutical Press, 2004.

B. G. Osborne *et al.*, *Practical NIR Spectroscopy with Applications in Food and Beverage Analysis*, 2nd edn, Harlow, Longman Scientific and Technical, 1993.

A. D. Patel *et al.*, Low-level determination of polymorph composition in physical mixtures by near-infrared reflectance spectroscopy, *J. Pharm. Sci.*, 2001, **90**, 360–370.

D. L. Pavia *et al.*, *Introduction to Spectroscopy: Guide for Students of Organic Chemistry*, Philadelphia, Saunders College Publishing/Holt, Rinehart and Winston, 1979.

S. H. F. Scafi and C. Pasquini, Identification of counterfeit drugs using near-infrared spectroscopy, *Analyst*, 2001, **126**, 2218–2224.

M. G. Sowa *et al.*, Classification of burn injuries using near-infrared spectroscopy, *J. Biomed. Opt.*, 2006, **11** (5), 054002.

H. A. Szymanski, *A Systematic Approach to the Interpretation of Infra-red Spectra*, Buffalo, New York, Hertillon Press, 1971.

D. Williams and I. Fleming, *Spectroscopic Methods in Organic Chemistry*, 5th edn, McGraw-Hill Education Europe, 1995.

W. L. Yoon *et al.*, Optimisation of sample presentation for near-infrared spectra of pharmaceutical excipients, *Analyst*, 1998, **123**, 1029–1034.

Further reading

L. J. Bellamy, *Infrared Spectra of Complex Molecules*, London, Chapman and Hall, Vol. I, 3rd edn, 1975; Vol. II, 2nd edn, 1980.

J. Chalmers and P.R. Griffiths, *The Handbook of Vibrational Spectroscopy*, London, Wiley, 2001.

P. R. Griffiths and J. A. De Haseth, *Fourier Transform Infrared Spectrometry*, New York, Wiley, 1986.

K. Nakamoto, *Infrared & Raman Spectra of Inorganic & Co-ordination Compounds*, 5th edn, Vols 1 and 2, New York, Wiley, 1997.

N. P. G. Roeges, *A Guide to the Complete Interpretation of Infrared Spectra of Organic Structures*, New York, Wiley, 1994.

B. Schrader, *Infrared and Raman Spectroscopy, Methods and Applications*, Weinheim, VCH, 1995.

B. C. Smith, *Fundamentals of Fourier Transform Infrared Spectroscopy*, Boca Raton, CRC Press, 1996.

B. C. Smith, *Infrared Spectral Interpretation – A Systematic Approach*, Boca Raton, CRC Press, 1998.

D. Williams and I. Fleming, *Spectroscopic Methods in Organic Chemistry*, 5th edn, London, McGraw-Hill Education Europe, 1995.

J. Workman, Jr. and A. Springsteen, *Applied Spectroscopy, A Compact Reference for Practitioners*, San Diego, Academic Press, 1998.

17

Raman spectroscopy

D E Bugay and P A Martoglio Smith

Introduction and theory 455
Instrumentation 457
Coupled techniques 459
Data processing and presentation of results 459
System suitability tests 460
Sample preparation and sample presentation 461
Interpretation of spectra 462
Qualitative analysis 464
Quantitative analysis 466
Collections of data 467
References 468
Further reading 468

Introduction and theory

Vibrational spectroscopy has been an integral tool for the identification and characterisation of drugs. When one thinks of vibrational spectroscopy, typically infrared (IR) techniques come to mind, not Raman spectroscopy. However, since the late 1980s a renaissance of the Raman technique has occurred, mainly through instrumentation development. These developments have led to unique applications in the pharmaceutical and forensic industries in which drug identification and characterisation are necessary. This chapter presents the theory, instrumentation, sampling techniques and applications of Raman spectroscopy as applied to drugs.

Raman spectroscopy is a form of vibrational spectroscopy that has widespread use in pharmaceutical investigations. Applications include chemical structure elucidation, routine chemical identification and solid-state characterisation, such as polymorphism. Raman spectroscopy is also applicable to drug product characterisation, including solid form analysis of the drug incorporated into the formulation, contaminant analysis, drug–excipient interaction and problem solving. A distinct advantage of pharmaceutical analysis by Raman spectroscopy is the ease of the technique and its broad range of applicability. Analysis can be performed on virtually any type of sample, such as single crystals, bulk materials, slurries, creams, particulates, films, solutions (aqueous and organic), oils, gas-phase samples and on-process streams (the latter through the use of fibre-optic probes). Additionally, Raman spectroscopy is typically nondestructive in nature, and so the material can be recovered for further characterisation. Since Raman spectroscopy measures the vibrational motions associated with a molecule, it is complementary to IR spectroscopy as well as to other characterisation techniques. Finally, under proper sampling conditions, Raman spectroscopy is a quantitative technique.

When a compound is irradiated with monochromatic radiation, the radiation is transmitted, absorbed or scattered by the molecule. As we have seen from the preceding chapters, UV and IR spectroscopy are primarily concerned with absorbed and transmitted radiation. However, it is the scattered radiation that is of interest in Raman spectroscopy. Of the scattered radiation, a majority of the photons are scattered at the same frequency as the incident radiation frequency. This form of scattering has been termed *elastic* or *Rayleigh scattering*. If the scattered radiation is passed into a spectrometer, a strong Rayleigh line is detected at the unmodified frequency of radiation used to excite the sample. Additionally, a very small proportion of photons (about one per million) are scattered at frequencies arrayed above and below the frequency of the Rayleigh line. The *differences* between the incident frequency of radiation and arrayed frequencies correspond to the frequency of molecular vibrations present in the molecules of the sample. These wavelength-shifted frequencies are due to what is termed *inelastic scattering*, and a collection of these wavelength-shifted frequencies is termed a Raman spectrum. The frequencies of molecular vibrations are typically 10^{12} to 10^{14} Hz. A more convenient unit, which is proportional to frequency, is wavenumber (cm^{-1}) since fundamental vibrational modes lie between 3600 and 50 cm^{-1}. For example, a Raman line at $\pm 2980\ cm^{-1}$ may be obtained on either side of the Rayleigh line and thus the sample possesses a vibrational mode at this frequency.

As shown in Figure 17.1, when a molecule is irradiated with monochromatic radiation, a number of different transitions may occur. If the radiation is of sufficient energy, an absorption process may occur that represents an electronic transition ($S_0 \rightarrow S_1$, UV-visible spectroscopy). If a slightly less energetic source is used, the molecule is promoted to a *virtual state*. The virtual state represents a distortion of the electron distribution of a covalent bond within the molecule. After promotion to the virtual state, the molecule immediately relaxes back to the original ground electronic state by emitting a photon. If the molecule relaxes back to the original vibrational state, the emitted photon is of the same frequency as the incident radiation. This represents Rayleigh or elastic scattering. If the molecule relaxes back to a higher vibrational energy state, the emitted photon represents less energy than the incident radiation. The inelastically scattered photon has a longer wavelength (lower frequency) than the incident radiation. This energy transition represents Stokes Raman scattering. Conversely, if the molecule relaxes back to a lower vibrational energy state, the emitted photon represents greater energy than the incident radiation. The inelastically scattered photon has a shorter wavelength (higher frequency) than the incident radiation. This energy transition represents anti-Stokes Raman scattering. Generally, the anti-Stokes lines are less intense than the Stokes lines because these transitions arise from higher vibrational energy levels that will be populated in only a small proportion of molecules, as described by the Boltzmann distribution. Hence, the Stokes portion of the spectrum is generally used.

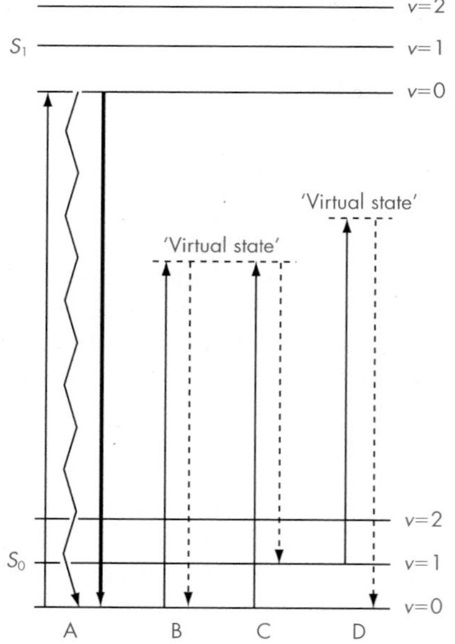

Figure 17.1 Jablonski energy level diagram illustrating possible transitions. Solid lines represent absorption processes and dotted lines represent scattering processes. A, electronic transition with nonradiative decay (heat, zigzag line) or radiative decay (fluorescence, thick line); B, Rayleigh scattering; C, Stokes Raman transition; D, anti-Stokes Raman transition. S_0 is the singlet ground state, S_1 the lowest singlet excited state and *v* represents vibrational energy levels within each electronic state.

A Raman spectrum is normally represented as a plot of Raman scattering intensity (ordinate, *y*-axis) versus wavelength (abscissa, *x*-axis). Normally, the abscissa of the spectrum is labelled as wavenumber shift or Raman shift (cm^{-1}) and the negative sign (for Stokes shift) is omitted (Fig. 17.2). The wavenumber or Raman shift represents the shift in frequency of a photon from the exciting wavelength.

Pharmaceutically and forensically relevant molecules are typically covalently bound organic molecules. The chemical bonds within these molecules comprise an electron cloud. In a Raman experiment, the electromagnetic radiation incident on the molecule consists of oscillating electric and magnetic fields. Interaction of the electromagnetic radiation with the chemical bond causes the electron cloud to oscillate. The oscillation, in turn, causes a photon to be emitted, which is called scattering. In Rayleigh scattering, the energy from the incident electromagnetic radiation causes electron oscillation and the emitted photon is observed at the same frequency. In Raman scattering, an additional energy transition occurs. The polarisability of the electron cloud may change as the position of the atoms that make up the chemical bond changes. In other words, a vibrational mode may cause atoms to be displaced, which in turn affects the polarisability of the electron cloud of the chemical bond. In this case, the incident radiation causes the electron cloud to oscillate, but the electron cloud oscillation is also affected by the change in polarisability caused by a change in the position of the atoms during the molecular vibration. Oscillation causes a photon to be emitted, but the frequency is perturbed by the change in polarisability of the chemical bond. For a vibrational mode to be Raman active, a change in polarisability must take place during the vibration. This is termed the Raman selection rule. Since the polarisability of a chemical bond is dependent upon the atoms making up that bond, as well as atoms in close proximity, Raman spectroscopy is a probe into the chemical or physical structure of a molecule. This is why Raman spectroscopy is an important tool for pharmaceutical analysis.

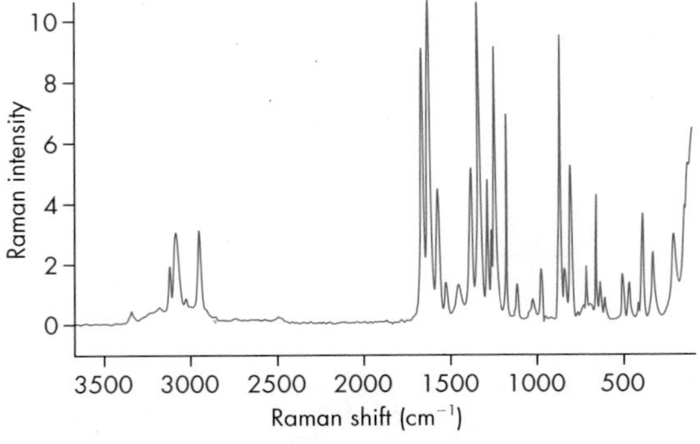

Figure 17.2 FT-Raman spectrum of paracetamol (acetaminophen).

Instrumentation

Although the Raman effect was discovered in 1928, the first commercial Raman instruments did not start to appear until the early 1950s. These instruments did not use laser sources, but used elemental sources and arc lamps. In 1962, laser sources started to become available for Raman instruments and the first commercial laser Raman instruments appeared in 1964 to 1965. The first commercial Fourier transform (FT)-Raman instruments were available from 1988, and by 1989 FT-Raman microscopy was possible.

Dispersive spectrometers

The basic configuration and components of a dispersive spectrometer are shown in Figure 17.3. The source of monochromatic radiation is a laser. Typically, helium–cadmium (325, 354 or 442 nm), air-cooled argon-ion (488 or 514 nm), doubled continuous-wave neodymium–yttrium aluminium garnet (Nd:YAG or Nd:$Y_3Al_5O_{12}$) (532 nm), helium–neon (633 nm), or stabilised diode (785 and 830 nm) lasers are used for dispersive Raman spectrometers. The stability of the emitted radiation from a laser is one of the key attributes of a good spectrometer. Frequency stabilisation of the laser under standard laboratory conditions (slight temperature fluctuations, vibrational effects, etc.) is required. Laser lifetimes and cost are also considerations in the choice of laser to use. One additional but very important consideration for laser selection in dispersive Raman systems is the generation of fluorescence. As stated previously, the Raman signal is fairly weak. For many organic systems, fluorescence may occur depending upon the laser used and, instead of promoting the molecule of interest to a virtual state, an electronic transition occurs with subsequent radiative decay (fluorescence, Fig. 17.1). The fluorescence background signal can be so intense as to mask the Raman scattered photons. Fluorescence is wavelength dependent, so a sample that fluoresces with one laser source may not with another. If fluorescence does not pose a problem, lower-frequency lasers can be used (532, 514 nm) for enhanced sensitivity, as the efficiency of Raman scattering is proportional to $1/(\lambda)^4$, where λ is the wavelength. If fluorescence is a problem when using these high-energy sources, then lower-energy sources, such as those used in FT-based Raman spectroscopy, can be used to minimise the fluorescence affects.

In a dispersive Raman spectrometer, the sample is positioned in the laser beam and the scattering radiation collected in either a 180° backscattering or a 90° right-angle scattering configuration. Subsequently, a laser-line rejection filter is put in place to filter out the Rayleigh scattering. Finally, a detector is positioned in the spectrometer. For dispersive systems, typically a charge-coupled device (CCD) is utilised. Silicon CCD detectors are normally used for Raman spectrometers in which visible wavelength lasers are used. Previously, photomultiplier tubes (PMTs) were used for detection, but since the advent of CCDs and because of their inherently better performance, PMTs are no longer normally used. Unfortunately, CCD detectors are sensitive to cosmic rays, which add artefacts to the spectra; these artefacts can be removed via software methods. All commercial spectrometers are controlled digitally by a computer system.

Interferometric spectrometers

Figure 17.4 displays the configuration of a FT-based Raman spectrometer. Advantages of a FT-Raman spectrometer are wavelength accuracy and the use of a near-IR laser, which typically eliminates fluorescence. In the FT-based system, a neodymium–yttrium laser (1064 nm) is used to irradiate the sample. Examples of Nd:Y lasers include Nd:YAG (neodymium–yttrium aluminium garnate) and Nd:YVO_4 (neodymium–yttrium orthovanadate). Analogously to the dispersive system, the sample is positioned in the laser beam and the scattering radiation collected in either a 180° backscattering or a 90° right-angle scattering configuration. The scattered photons are then passed into an interferometer with laser-line filtering. Detectors of the scattered photons from systems that utilise lasers emitting light with wavelengths greater than 1000 nm are of the single-element type, either

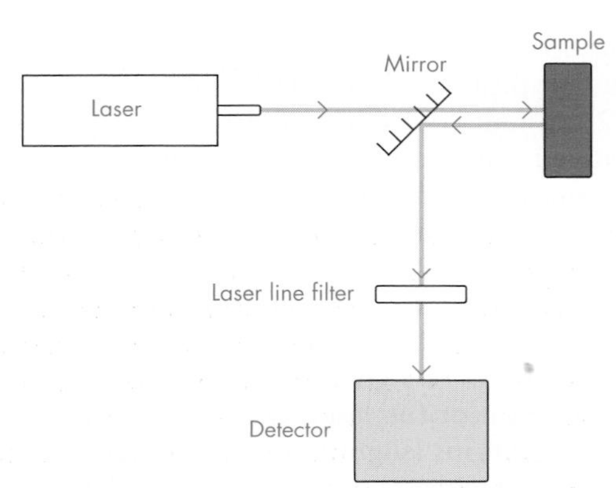

Figure 17.3 A dispersive Raman spectrometer.

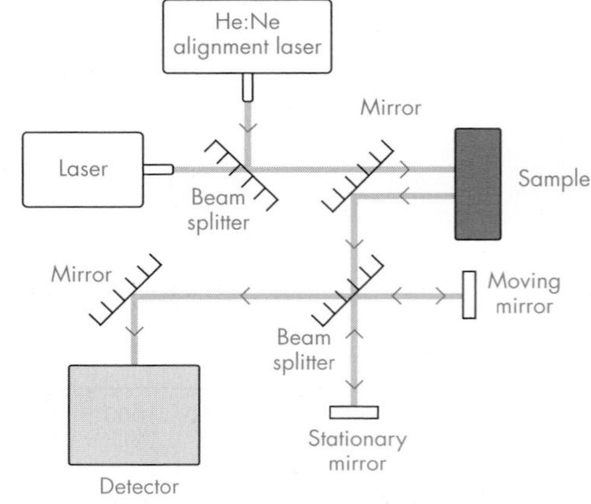

Figure 17.4 A FT-based Raman spectrometer.

high purity p-type germanium (Ge) or indium–gallium–arsenic (InGaAs) detectors. These detectors are noisier than CCDs or PMTs, but do exhibit high quantum efficiencies. Cooling of the Ge detector to 77 K extends the frequency response to 3400 cm^{-1}. Unfortunately, Ge detectors are subject to interference by cosmic rays so artefacts in their output may be generated. However, the number of interferograms containing artefacts from cosmic rays can be reduced utilising software methods.

Fluorescence is minimised by utilising the longer-wavelength Nd:YVO_4 or Nd:YAG laser in a FT-Raman spectrometer. The fluorescence minimisation arises because the longer-wavelength excitation poses a smaller chance of inducing an electronic transition with subsequent fluorescence as the relaxation mechanism.

Coupled techniques

Microscopy

Raman spectra can be acquired on small amounts of material through the use of a Raman microprobe. Utilising the microscope, the Raman-scattered photons are collected in a 180° backscattering configuration that allows the operator to view the sample optically, focus the incident radiation and subsequently collect the Raman spectrum. Most commercial Raman microscope systems utilise confocal microscopy to increase axial resolution (*z*-axis). Confocal points are defined as the point source, the in-focus sample location and the focused image of the sample point. Axial resolution, defined as the distance away from the focal plane in which the Raman intensity from the sample decreases to 50% of the in-focus intensity, can be approximated from the numerical aperture (NA) used in the microscope. When utilising a 0.95 NA objective on a confocal microscope system, the axial resolution is proportional to the square of the NA, in this case 0.9025 μm.

An additional advantage of Raman microscopy is spatial resolution as opposed to axial resolution. The spatial resolution (*x*–*y* plane) is dependent upon the NA of the collecting objective and the wavelength of the laser radiation. Larger NA values and shorter wavelengths provide higher spatial resolution, often down to 1 μm. Since a high intensity of monochromatic radiation from the laser is focused upon a small amount of sample, degradation of the sample by the laser must be monitored. Otherwise, the Raman microprobe is ideal for investigating polymorphism (single crystals), particulate contamination and small amounts of samples. Using an apparatus similar to those used for IR microspectroscopy, variable temperature studies can be performed with a Raman microprobe.

Fibre optics

Fibre optics have been used in Raman spectroscopy since the early 1980s. Solids and liquids can be analysed with an arrangement of optical fibres on the end of a probe. Fibre systems include single-fibre (in which the laser excitation and collected scattered radiation travel along the same fibre), and multifibre (in which laser excitation is transmitted along one (or multiple) fibres, and the scattered radiation is transmitted to the detector along different fibres). The greatest single advantage of the use of fibre optics in Raman spectroscopy is the ability to sample remotely. No longer does the spectrometer have to be brought to the sample or vice versa. Fibre optics can link the spectrometer to the sample, typically over distances of tens of metres. Common applications include monitoring process streams or hazardous reactions.

Data processing and presentation of results

All modern-day dispersive and FT-based Raman spectrometers are controlled through a digital computer that handles instrument control, data collection, data processing and presentation of the spectral results. Utilisation of a FT-Raman spectrometer requires one extra step of data processing that is not needed for dispersive-based Raman spectrometers. In the FT system, the original data are collected on a time scale and subsequently Fourier transformed to obtain a frequency domain spectrum. After this point, data processing for both systems is analogous.

Since the Raman spectrum of a particular sample is represented digitally, various additional processing applications can be performed. Spectral subtraction is one commonly used data-processing technique, as are spectral smoothing, spectral searching and resolution enhancement. Figure 17.5 displays some of these processing techniques on one original data file. Since Raman spectroscopy can be utilised for quantitative measurements, digital representation of the spectrum allows numerous ways to measure the analytical response of an analyte's signal and relate it to concentration. Electronic integration of the peak area, curve fitting of the Raman spectrum and chemometric approaches can be utilised (see Fig. 17.5).

System suitability tests

In a good laboratory practice (GLP) environment, all laboratory instrumentation must be inspected, cleaned and maintained adequately. Additionally, instruments used for the generation, measurement or assessment of data must be tested, calibrated and/or standardised adequately. For GLP requirements, the accuracy of Raman spectrometers needs to be assessed before their use. Typically, where measurements are made using Raman spectroscopy for regulatory purposes, a recognised standard material, distributed by an official agency, should be used for the calibration testing of the spectrometer. The American Society for Testing and Materials (ASTM) has published a guide for Raman shift standards for

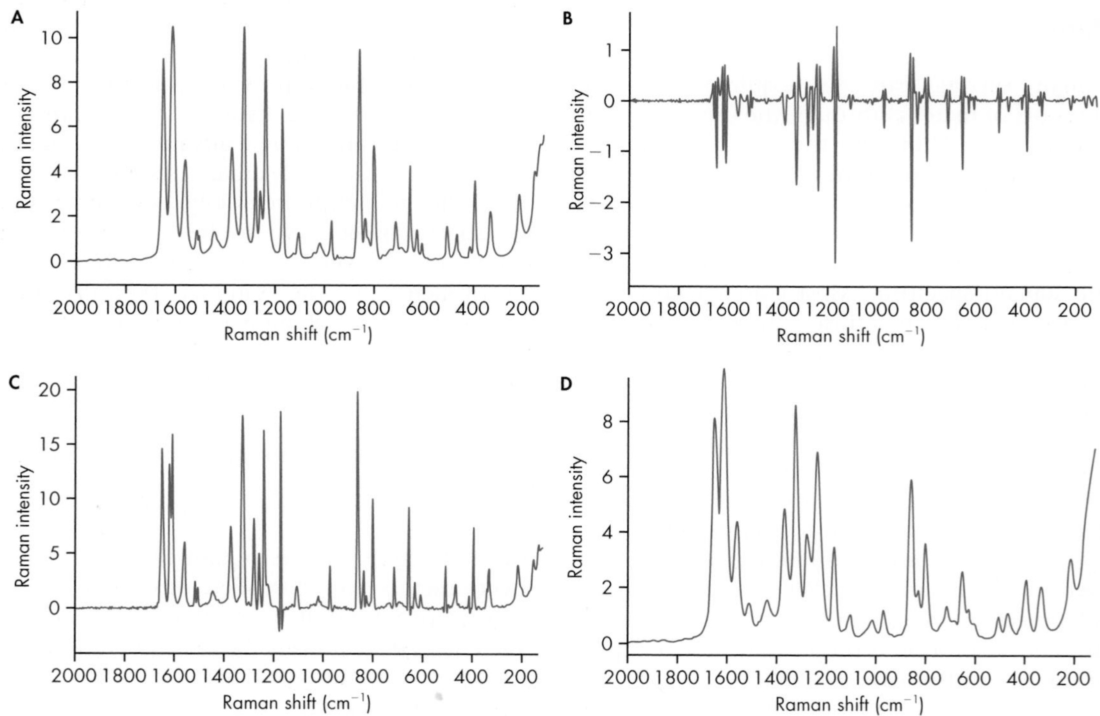

Figure 17.5 Examples of digitally processed spectral files. (A) original Raman spectrum; (B) spectral result after calculating the second derivative of the original Raman spectrum; (C) spectral result after resolution enhancement by Fourier deconvolution of the original Raman spectrum; (D) spectral result after Fourier smoothing the original Raman spectrum by 80%.

spectrometer calibration (ASTM 2007). The spectroscopy community has recognised cyclohexane and sulfur as calibration standards for the frequency scale (cm^{-1}) of Raman spectrometers. The Raman spectra of sulfur and cyclohexane are shown in Fig. 17.6. In many pharmaceutical spectroscopy laboratories, the spectral features of these two compounds are used to calibrate Raman instruments and determine system suitability.

Sample preparation and sample presentation

Sampling techniques for Raman spectroscopy are relatively simple, since the only requirements are that the monochromatic laser beam irradiates the sample of interest and the scattered radiation is focused upon the detector.

Raman spectroscopy may be performed on very small samples (e.g. a few nanograms). Powders do not need to be pressed into disks, the material simply has to be irradiated by the laser beam. Solid samples are often examined in gold-coated or glass sample holders that generally require about 25–50 mg of material. Typically, liquid samples are analysed in quartz or glass cuvettes, which may have mirrored rear surfaces to improve the signal intensity. Glass is a very weak Raman scatterer and so many samples (liquid and solid) can be analysed directly in a bottle or, for example, in a nuclear magnetic resonance (NMR) tube, although fluorescence from some types of glass can be problematic.

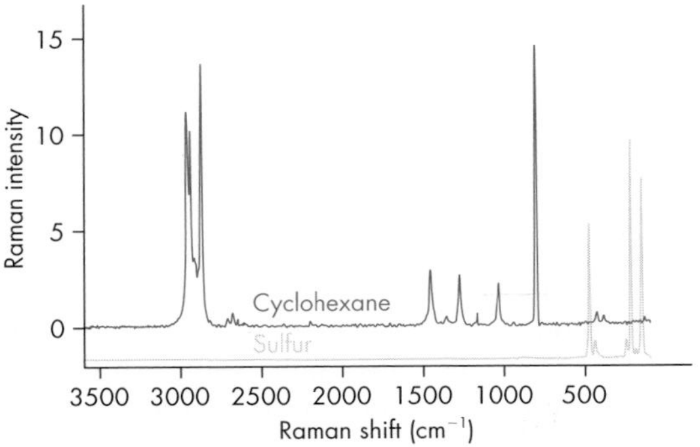

Figure 17.6 FT-Raman spectra of wavelength calibration standards cyclohexane and sulfur.

Water is a good solvent for Raman studies, since the Raman spectrum of water is essentially one broad, weak band at 3500 cm^{-1}. One sample type that may pose a problem is darkly coloured material. Often, these samples absorb excessive heat and burn, which causes sample degradation and spectral degradation. Amorphous materials also have a tendency to absorb heat in the laser beam. To avoid sample burning, it may be necessary to dissipate the heat. This can be accomplished by reducing the laser power or by using an accessory that spins the sample and so avoids irradiation of a single point in the sample. Further reduction of the laser power can also be accomplished through a neutral density filter. Sometimes, the sample can be diluted in KBr to help reduce sample burning.

The complete Stokes Raman spectrum, which covers shifts in the range 100–3500 cm^{-1}, can be obtained and the intensity of Raman scattering is directly proportional to the concentration of the scattering species, an important factor for quantitative analysis. However, the Raman effect is relatively weak and hence the material needs to be present at a concentration of at least about 0.1–0.5% for accurate assessments, whereas IR can be used to detect materials down to a concentration of approximately 0.01%. As noted above, fluorescence can also be problematic in Raman studies, but typically arises from additives in the glass sample tubes or impurities within the sample of interest. Data massaging techniques can sometimes blank out Raman spectral contributions from fluorescent materials. Photobleaching is another way to suppress fluorescence. This technique involves irradiating the sample for a prolonged period of time (seconds to hours) with the laser. During this time the fluorescence may decrease through the destruction of the fluorescing component from the prolonged exposure to the laser irradiation. The spectrum is then acquired after photobleaching is complete. Of course, it is also possible that the laser radiation may change the component of interest. For example, a solvated crystalline material may desolvate with exposure to laser radiation. It is wise to establish sample integrity by comparing spectra acquired with short acquisition times to those acquired with long acquisition times. Additionally, another technique, such as IR spectroscopy or X-ray powder diffraction, could be used to check for sample integrity after Raman analysis.

Variable-temperature studies in Raman spectroscopy provide a wealth of information. A Raman spectrum typically covers a wavelength range that extends beyond the range normally associated with mid-IR spectroscopy (typically 4000–400 cm^{-1}), so information about the lattice vibrations of compounds is readily available. By varying the temperature of a sample, the lattice energies of the compound can be changed, which allows the nature of the crystal lattice to be interpreted. In addition, information similar to that obtained in IR variable-temperature studies (crystal form changes and the nature of solvate association) can be obtained with variable-temperature Raman investigations.

Interpretation of spectra

The number of fundamental vibrational modes of a molecule is equal to the number of degrees of vibrational freedom. For a nonlinear molecule of n atoms, there are $3n - 6$ degrees of vibrational freedom. Hence, there are $3n - 6$ fundamental vibrational modes. The number of degrees of freedom is reduced by 6 for a nonlinear molecule because:

- three coordinates are required to locate the molecule in space
- an additional three coordinates are required to describe the orientation of the molecule in the position based defined by the three coordinates that locate the molecule in space.

For a linear molecule, $3n - 5$ fundamental vibrational modes are possible, since only two degrees of rotational freedom exist. Thus, in a total vibrational analysis of a molecule by complementary IR and Raman techniques, $3n - 6$ or $3n - 5$ vibrational frequencies should be observed. In complex molecules (such as pharmaceuticals), it may not be possible to observe every vibration because of overlap and relative intensity differences.

Regarding spectral interpretation, two of the best textbook sources are *Introduction to Infrared and Raman Spectroscopy* (Colthup *et al.* 1990) and *The Handbook of Infrared and Raman Characteristic Frequencies of Organic Molecules* (Lin-Vien *et al.* 1991). Both of these texts contain chapters dedicated to functional groups (e.g. methyl and methylene groups) and chemical compound types (e.g. ethers, alcohols and phenols). By examining peak location and intensity in Raman spectra, functional groups (and chemical compound type) can be determined. Discussed below are some guidelines on interpretation of a Raman spectrum, but clearly these serve only as general background information. Any complete spectral interpretations should be made with the guidance of one of the reference texts.

Raman spectroscopy provides information about the molecular bonding of a molecule. Certain functional groups give rise to fundamental vibrational modes. For example, the C═C stretch in ethylenes occurs near 1650 cm^{-1}. The C—N stretch (amide III peak) for primary amides occurs between 1430 and 1390 cm^{-1}. A C—S stretch usually appears strongly in the 735 to 590 cm^{-1} region. Many other functional groups give rise to Raman peaks in specific spectral regions. IR bands also occur in the same spectral regions, but because of selection rules, the band intensities differ, often dramatically. As noted above, in the most basic terms, a vibrational mode is Raman active when there is a change in polarisability during the vibration. Conversely, a vibrational mode is IR active when there is a change in the molecular dipole moment during the vibration. Hence, vibrational modes that give rise to strong Raman peaks often give weak IR bands and vice versa. It is this characteristic that provides the description 'complementary' for the use of IR and Raman spectroscopy together to examine the molecular bonds in a compound. Some of the strongest Raman peaks come from functional groups such as C═C, N═N, S—S, C—H, S—H, C≡N, C═S and C—S, which have low polarity and high polarisability. These functional groups tend to occur in rather constant frequency ranges, although some shifts can occur from the influence of other substituents in the molecule. Vibrational modes can be separated into two classes: those in which the molecular bond is stretching and those in which it is bending. It takes a specific amount of energy for these actions to occur. The amount required is dependent on the atoms involved and the strength of the bond. The nature of Raman excitation of a molecule is discussed in the theory section at the beginning of this chapter. The location of the vibrational mode (its peak wavelength position in the spectrum) is related to the frequency of the excitation source (the laser) and the frequency of the scattered light. The equation that defines this relationship is

$$h\upsilon = h\upsilon' + \Delta E_{vib} \quad (17.1)$$

where h is Plank's constant, υ is the excitation frequency, υ' is the scattered light frequency and ΔE_{vib} is the vibrational energy. The vibrational energy is related directly to the strength of the bond and the amount of energy required to make that bond stretch or bend. These actions are elaborated below.

A stretching vibration is the motion a molecular bond undergoes when the two atoms involved in the bond move apart and then contract. The stretch can be a simple contraction–expansion between two atoms, such as the C═C stretch of ethylene. This type of motion occurs as a peak in the Raman spectrum at approximately 1650 cm^{-1}. When three atoms are involved, two types of stretches are possible, symmetric and antisymmetric. Using a methylene group as an example, a symmetric CH_2 stretch occurs when the two hydrogen atoms move apart from the carbon atom at the same time. This type of stretch appears near 2853 cm^{-1}. The antisymmetric CH_2 stretch occurs when one hydrogen atom moves away from the carbon atom while the other hydrogen atom moves closer to the carbon atom. This vibrational mode appears near 2926 cm^{-1}. The symmetric stretches are typically more intense in Raman spectra (greater change in polarisability), whereas the antisymmetric stretches are more intense in IR spectra. When many atoms are involved in the stretching, such as with aromatic rings, the types of stretches become more complicated. For example, a benzene ring monosubstituted with a halogen has 30 vibrational modes. Of these modes, some are strictly stretches, some are bends and some are combinations of both. Perhaps the simplest stretching mode for benzene rings is the ring-breathing mode, in which the 2-, 4- and 6-carbons move outwards. This mode occurs as a very strong Raman peak near 1000 cm^{-1} for mono-, *meta*- and 1,3,5-trisubstituted benzenes. Clearly, many types of stretches can occur.

In a bending vibration, the molecular bond bends instead of stretches. Many types of bends can occur: antisymmetric, symmetric, torsion, scissor, wag, twist and rock. Using a CH_3 group as an example, antisymmetric, symmetric, rock and torsion bends are possible (Fig. 17.7). In the antisymmetric bend, two of the C—H bonds bend towards each other in a pinching motion, while the third bends outwards and away from the pyramid. This mode occurs between 1470 and 1430 cm^{-1}. In the symmetric bend, the three CH bonds all bend inwards, similar to a grasping action. This mode occurs from 1395 to 1365 cm^{-1}. In the CH_3 rock, the three CH bonds all bend in one direction, in a sweeping mode. Finally, the CH_3 torsion involves the three CH bonds all bending in a clockwise direction in a twisting motion. The spectral ranges for these last two vibrational modes are highly variable.

The CH_2 group can bend in slightly different ways (Fig. 17.8). A CH_2 scissor bend occurs when the two hydrogen atoms move towards each other in a scissoring motion. For a CH_2 wag, the two hydrogen atoms are bent towards the carbon atom. If the two hydrogen atoms alternately twist around one another, it is a CH_2 twist. Finally, if the two hydrogen atoms move back and forth, in line with the carbon atom, it is a CH_2 rock. As seen with the CH_3 modes, all of these different types of motions appear in different portions of the spectrum because they

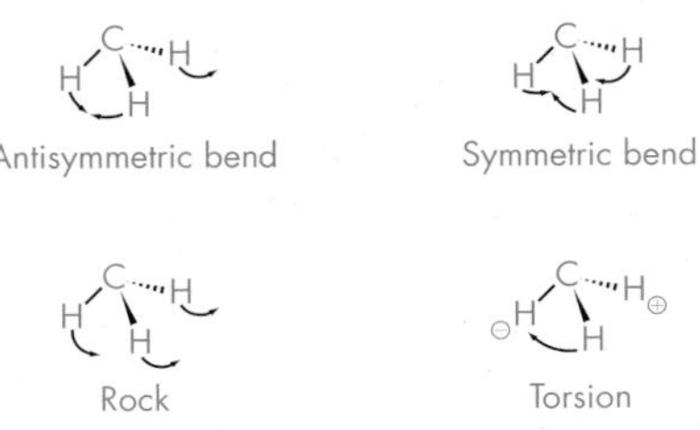

Figure 17.7 Bending vibrational motions associated with CH_3 groups (⊕ represents movement above the plane, ⊖ represents movement below the plane).

each require a different and unique amount of energy to occur. The scissor mode appears near 1465 cm^{-1}. The rocking, wagging and twisting modes are more complicated, falling in the range 1422–719 cm^{-1}. Depending on the substituents in the molecule, each of these modes can be narrowed down to tighter ranges. It is this dependence of certain modes on substituents that gives rise to correlation tables, discussed next.

Although the general location for a certain type of mode, for example a C═C stretch, can be listed, the exact location of the peak varies slightly with the type of molecular substitution present. For example, a vinyl C═C stretch (monoalkyl) occurs from 1650 to 1638 cm^{-1}. A vinylidine C═C stretch (1,1-dialkyl) occurs from 1660 to 1640 cm^{-1}. A *cis*-dialkyl-substituted C═C stretch occurs from 1662 to 1631 cm^{-1}, whereas a *trans*-dialkyl-substituted C═C stretch occurs from 1676 to 1665 cm^{-1}. Finally, trialkyl- and tetraalkyl-substituted C═C stretches appear from 1680 to 1665 cm^{-1}. Some modes are very sensitive to substituents, whereas others appear relatively consistently near a certain wavenumber.

Over the years, many types of compounds have been studied in great detail. When a spectrum of a single compound is interpreted such that every peak or band is assigned to a type of motion, we have a vibrational assignment. Through the examination of many vibrational assignments, it has been possible to draw correlations between types of vibrational modes and types of substituents. The culmination of this work is detailed in correlation tables that an investigator can use to aid in spectral interpretation (Dollish *et al.* 1974; Colthup *et al.* 1990; Lin-Vien *et al.* 1991).

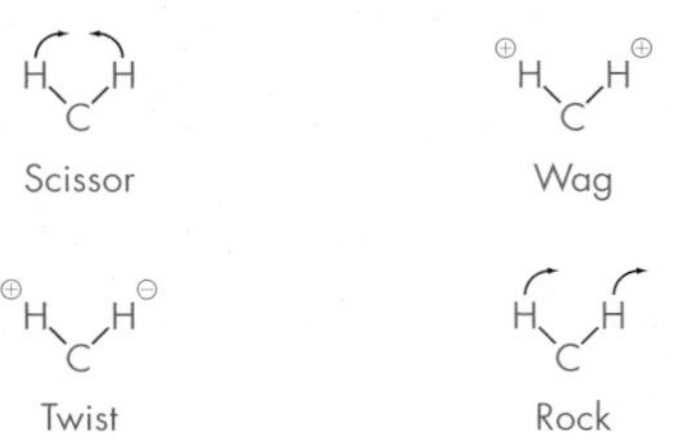

Figure 17.8 Bending vibrational motions associated with CH_2 groups (⊕ represents movement above the plane, ⊖ represents movement below the plane).

The most efficient way to use correlation tables is to look for certain peaks that will quickly narrow down the type of compound. For example, if peaks are found at 3000 cm^{-1} or slightly higher, the compound is aromatic or olefinic. However, if the CH_2 stretches appear below 3000 cm^{-1}, the compound is aliphatic. Once that determination is made, the correlation tables can be consulted to look for other confirmatory modes, such as CH wags for aromatic compounds. This type of process is continued until a compound class can either be verified or discounted.

For complex molecules, it may not be possible to determine the structure from the Raman spectrum alone, or even if the IR spectrum is available as well. Other techniques such as NMR and mass spectrometry provide important information to aid the elucidation of structure.

Qualitative analysis

Chemical identity testing of compounds is one role of the pharmaceutical spectroscopy laboratory. Testing can be accomplished with methods that utilise Raman spectroscopy. A FT-Raman method has been developed to identify the two active components (tegafur and uracil) in formulated capsules (Petty *et al.* 1996). The Raman spectrum of the formulated product displayed a spectral region in which Raman bands unique to uracil and tegafur were observed. The presence of these bands allowed the analyst to confirm that both components were present in the formulated product. In part because of the ease of use and chemical specificity inherent in Raman spectroscopy, it has become an essential chemical and physical identification tool for the pharmaceutical spectroscopist.

Polymorphism (the ability of a molecule to crystallise in different three-dimensional structures) is a very important aspect of the drug-development process. Raman spectroscopy is now being used for the qualitative and quantitative characterisation of polymorphic compounds of pharmaceutical interest. Figure 17.9 displays the Raman spectra of different polymorphs of carbamazepine.

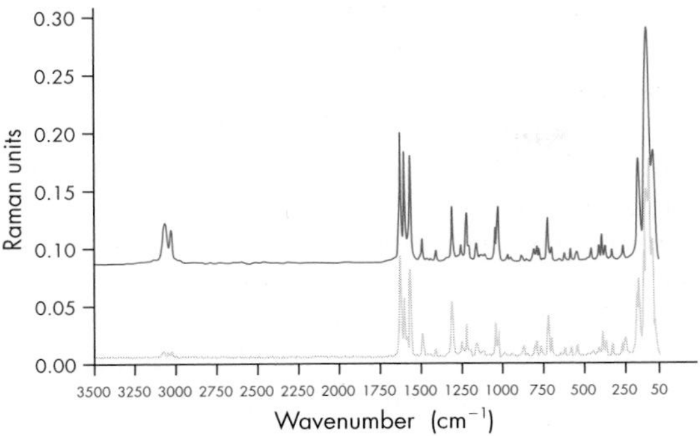

Figure 17.9 FT-Raman spectra of the polymorphs of carbamazepine (top, polymorph I, bottom, polymorph III).

Raman microspectroscopy is well suited for in-situ analysis of contaminants found in pharmaceutical processes. The nondestructive nature of the analysis means that further experiments, such as energy-dispersive X-ray analysis or IR microspectroscopy, may be performed on the same sample. A consideration for contaminant analysis by Raman spectroscopy is the axial and spatial resolution of the technique as compared to that of IR microspectroscopy. In general, IR microspectroscopy is diffraction limited to investigating samples typically larger in size than 5 μm. As discussed earlier, with a 0.95 NA objective, 1 μm spatial resolution can be achieved with a Raman microscope, which enables the analysis of very small amounts of contaminant.

Real-time monitoring of pharmaceutically relevant processes is an exciting application for Raman spectroscopy. This has been utilised to examine synthetic organic reaction schemes to investigate kinetics, as well as to identify non-isolated reaction intermediates. Distinct advantages for Raman spectroscopy in this area are:

- ability to work with aqueous-based systems with little spectral interference from water
- utilisation of a fibre-optic probe for direct and/or remote sampling
- collection of the Raman spectrum directly through the glass vessel with little or no spectral interference
- ability to analyse the spectrum quantitatively.

Other recent applications of real-time process monitoring by Raman spectroscopy include polymorphic interconversion under slurry conditions and crystallisation monitoring (Findlay and Bugay 1998).

Another exciting application of Raman spectroscopy is chemical imaging. By incorporating a programmable, *xyz*-movement stage into a Raman microscope, it is now possible to generate a chemical image of a two-dimensional area of a sample. With the use of a mapping stage, a sample such as a microtomed tablet can be moved in the *x* and *y* directions, obtaining spectra at each step. If the sample requires refocusing at different locations, the *z*-direction can be automated as well. The distance the stage moves in the *x* or *y* direction is called the step size and usually can be as small as 1 μm.

A series of images that demonstrate the dispersion of several excipients in a tablet is displayed in Figure 17.10. This particular area map was obtained with a step size of 4 μm, a sampling spot size of approximately 1 μm and a total sampling area of 87 μm × 52 μm. The time required to collect this map was approximately 26 hours, but not all Raman mapping experiments require this amount of time. For example, if a map is to search for a particular component, the step size need only be on the order of the particle size of that substance. A good approach is to first obtain a larger-area map on the sample with larger step sizes and shorter sampling times per point. Once an area of interest is defined by analysing the data from the first map, a smaller, higher-resolution map can be defined. Also, area maps and imaging have experienced a recent surge in popularity, mainly because of the use of CCD array cameras and liquid crystal tuneable

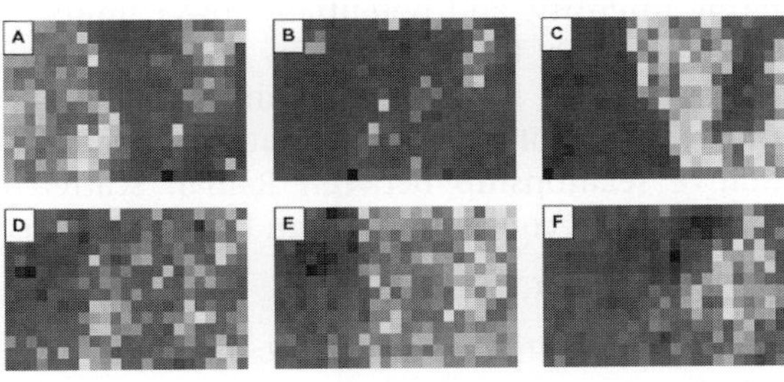

Figure 17.10 Peak area profiles (images) representing: (A) mannitol, (B) aspartame, (C) cellulose, (D) magnesium stearate, (E) corn starch, (F) monoammonium glycyrrhizinate.

filter (LCTF) technology, respectively. These detectors greatly reduce the amount of time required to collect an area map (Zugates and Treado 1999). In one case, the time required to collect an area map decreased by approximately 4 hours upon switching from a CCD camera (>5 hours) to LCTF technology (<1 hour). The mapping technique can also be applied to the Raman examination of samples in 96-well plates and examination of drugs of abuse in forensic science.

Literature references of other mapping applications relative to the pharmaceutical industry include some of the following: solid dispersions of ibuprofen in polyvinylpyrrolidone (Breitenback *et al.* 1999), crystal formation in hormone replacement therapy patches (Armstrong *et al.* 1996), particle size analysis in mixtures (Theophilus and Lancaster 2000) and pharmaceutical matrix determination of dosage formulations (Clarke *et al.* 2000).

Quantitative analysis

The ability to perform quantitative analysis by Raman spectroscopy is a significant advantage of the technique. Through mathematical treatments, it has been shown that the Raman scattering intensity is proportional to the number of molecules being irradiated. The intensity of scattered radiation is also proportional to the intensity of the incident radiation and the fourth power of the difference in frequencies between the laser frequency and the molecular vibrational frequency. Thus, increased Raman scattering intensity, and potentially lower limits of detection, can be achieved by increasing the intensity of the laser radiation and/or increasing the frequency of the laser irradiation. This quantitative relationship between Raman scattered intensity and concentration can be expressed as

$$I_R = (I_L \sigma K)PC \qquad (17.2)$$

where I_R is the measured Raman intensity (photons per second), I_L is the laser intensity (photons per second), σ is the absolute Raman cross-section (cm^2 per molecule), K is the measurement parameters, P is the sample path length (cm) and C is the concentration (molecules per cm^3). The constant K represents measurement parameters such as utilising the same spectrometer (collection optics efficiency), sample positioning and overall efficiency of the Raman spectrometer.

In the past, quantitative analysis was not often performed with Raman spectroscopy because of problems inherent to dispersive systems. When FT-Raman spectrometers became popular, the feasibility of quantitative applications greatly improved.

Although FT-Raman spectroscopy is more applicable to quantitative applications than dispersive Raman spectroscopy, some issues are still of concern. These are mainly with the optimisation of sampling conditions. FT-Raman spectroscopy typically samples a relatively small area (e.g. a 1–2 mm spot) of the total sample. As such, it is important that any spectra collected be truly representative of the bulk sample. For solution studies, homogeneity of the multicomponent samples presented for quantitative analysis is not an issue. Conversely, solid-phase analysis can present significant inhomogeneity issues for quantitative analysis.

Another factor to consider when using Raman spectroscopy quantitatively is that the power output of the Raman laser can vary from day to day, and thereby affect the intensity of spectral peaks. It is advisable to normalise any data before using them in a quantitative manner. One possible method for normalising spectra is to ratio the spectral response of the analyte against a peak response for a non-changing component (e.g. an excipient in a drug product or an internal standard). Alternatively, a ratio can be measured using a peak response of a component that changes in the opposite direction to that of the component being monitored. For example, in a quantitative method used to monitor the amount of crystalline drug substance in the presence of the amorphous form, a crystalline peak response (e.g. peak area or peak height) can be normalised by dividing it by an amorphous peak response.

When developing a quantitative method, it is very important to follow regulatory agency guidelines. Important quantitative issues include:

- system suitability – an overall test of system function
- specificity – the ability of Raman spectroscopy to differentiate the analyte from the matrix
- working range – the concentration range over which the method is validated
- linearity – demonstration of a direct relationship between a measured analytical response and concentration over the working range of the method
- precision – the repeatability with which a number can be represented
- accuracy – degree of conformity of a measurement to a standard or true value
- limit of detection – lowest concentration at which an analyte can be detected
- minimum quantifiable limit – lowest concentration at which an analyte can be quantified with acceptable accuracy and precision
- robustness – demonstration of the reliability of an analysis with respect to deliberate variations in method parameters.

One literature example of quantitative Raman analysis addresses the question of amorphous versus crystalline content of indometacin samples (Taylor and Zografi 1998). The article highlights the quantitative nature of Raman spectroscopy, the need to produce homogeneous calibration and/or validation samples and difficulties associated with collecting a Raman spectrum that is truly representative of the concentration. A linear correlation curve was constructed in which low concentrations of both amorphous and crystalline material could be detected and predicted in mixtures. The authors felt that the largest source of error in the measurements arose from inhomogeneous mixing of the amorphous and crystalline components in the blends. For solid-state analysis, this conclusion illustrates the need for a sampling device that collects a truly representative Raman spectrum of the sample, in this case a mixture.

Chemometrics

In the above literature example of quantitative analysis, a univariate approach (a single-peak response) was used to create the calibration curve or predictive model. Chemometrics represents a multivariate approach to creating a predictive model for quantitative analysis. Chemometrics may be defined as the 'use of statistical and mathematical techniques to make either quantitative or qualitative measurements on chemical data'.

A chemometric approach is useful when there are very few spectroscopic differences between the compounds in a mixture, which is often the case for polymorphic studies. Partial least squares (PLS) and discriminant analysis are examples of two types of chemometric approach that can be taken for quantitative and semi-quantitative work. The reader is referred to Further Reading for further publications regarding chemometrics.

Collections of data

By far the quickest method to identify unknown materials is to search the spectrum against spectral libraries. Often an answer can be found within seconds. However, care must be taken when performing spectral searching.

Computer search programs determine the difference between a sample spectrum and the reference spectra in a library. Several possible algorithms are used to compare spectra, some based on intensity and others based on peak position. Perhaps the most versatile search algorithm is *correlation*, which balances the contributions of both intensity and peak position. This algorithm normally gives the best results and is recommended for most applications.

When a search is performed, a hit list is produced that ranks the reference spectra in order of match quality. Some programs assign a value of 100 to a perfect match, others use zero. In either case, a good hit would obviously be one that is closest to perfection. In the best-case scenario, the top hit (if 100 is perfect) is above 90 and all other hits are significantly lower. In cases of spectral mixtures, however, the best hit may not even be 50. In such cases, the best reference spectra are compared with the sample spectrum to determine whether they could represent a portion of the sample. If so, a spectral subtraction can be performed to remove the reference component from the sample spectrum and the resultant spectral subtraction can be searched again to look for additional components. Often, if strong peaks are being subtracted from one another, regions of over- or under-subtraction will occur, producing derivative-shaped peaks in the subtraction spectrum. In these cases, it may be advantageous to 'blank' these regions before searching for lesser components. The process of spectral searching and subtracting can be repeated until the signal-to-noise ratio of the subtraction spectrum yields unusable results and no more components can be identified.

A number of spectral libraries are available commercially. These include libraries for polymers, pharmaceutical drugs and excipients, and drugs of interest in forensic science including excipients, precursors and metabolites, and libraries covering more general organic and inorganic compounds. Of course, sometimes the most useful libraries are ones that analysts create themselves.

A final note on the use of spectral libraries: the results from a hit list should always be verified by:

- comparing the reference spectrum to the sample spectrum
- ensuring that the reference spectrum is named accurately in the library (no library is completely perfect)
- determining that the suggested hit is a component logically to be expect in that particular sample.

References

C. L. Armstrong *et al.*, Fourier transform Raman microscopic study of drug distribution in a transdermal drug delivery device, *Vib. Spectrosc.*, 1996, **11**, 105–113.

ASTM, *Standard guide for Raman shift standards for spectrometer calibration*, E1840–96(2007), ASTM, 2007.

J. Breitenback *et al.*, Confocal Raman-spectroscopy: analytical approach to solid dispersions and mapping of drugs, *Pharm. Res.*, 1999, **16**, 1109–1113.

F. Clarke *et al.*, Chemical images – the key to pharmaceutical matrix determination, Paper number 601 presented at FACSS, Nashville, TN, 24–28 September, 2000.

N. B. Colthup *et al.*, *Introduction to Infrared and Raman Spectroscopy*, 3rd edn, New York, Academic Press, 1990.

F. R. Dollish *et al.*, *Characteristic Raman Frequencies of Organic Compounds*, New York, Wiley, 1974.

W. P. Findlay and D. E. Bugay, Utilization of Fourier transform Raman spectroscopy for the study of pharmaceutical crystal forms, *J. Pharm. Biomed. Anal.*, 1998, **16**, 921–930.

D. Lin-Vien *et al.*, *The Handbook of Infrared and Raman Characteristic Frequencies of Organic Molecules*, New York, Academic Press, 1991.

C. J. Petty *et al.*, Applications of FT-Raman spectroscopy in the pharmaceutical industry, *Spectroscopy*, 1996, **11**, 41–45.

L. S. Taylor and G. Zografi, The quantitative analysis of crystallinity using FT-Raman spectroscopy, *Pharm. Res.*, 1998, **15**, 755–761.

A. Theophilus and R. Lancaster, Particle size analysis of binary or tertiary mixtures using Raman image analysis, Paper number 600 presented at FACSS, Nashville, TN, 24–28 September, 2000.

C. T. Zugates and P. J. Treado, Raman chemical imaging of pharmaceutical content uniformity, *Int. J. Vib. Spectrosc.*, 1999, **2**, 59–68.

Further reading

K. R. Beebe *et al.*, *Chemometrics: A Practical Guide*, New York, Wiley, 1998.

D. B. Chase and J. F. Rabolt (eds), *Fourier Transform Raman Spectroscopy, From Concept to Experiment*, San Diego, Academic Press, 1994.

N. B. Colthup *et al.*, *Introduction to Infrared and Raman Spectroscopy*, 3rd edn, New York, Academic Press, 1990.

G. Herzberg, *Infrared and Raman Spectra of Polyatomic Molecules*, New York, D. Van Nostrand Co., 1945.

D. Lin-Vien *et al.*, *The Handbook of Infrared and Raman Characteristic Frequencies of Organic Molecules*, New York, Academic Press, 1991.

D. L. Massart *et al.*, *Chemometrics: A Textbook*, 3rd edn, New York, Elsevier Science, 1990.

M. J. Pelletier (ed.), *Analytical Applications of Raman Spectroscopy*, Oxford, Blackwell Science, 1999.

18

Gas chromatography

S Dawling, S Jickells and A Negrusz

Introduction 469
Gas chromatography columns 470
Inlet systems 483
Detector systems 493
Specimen preparation 498
Quantitative determinations 505
Optimising operation conditions to customise applications 506
Specific applications. 508
References 510
Further reading 511

Introduction

Gas chromatography (GC) is applicable to a wide range of compounds of interest to toxicologists, pharmaceutical and industrial chemists, environmentalists and clinicians. Adsorption GC was developed by a German scientist, Fritz Prior, in the late 1940s. In the early 1950s Archer J. P. Martin and Richard L. M. Synge, two scientists from the UK, invented partition chromatography, for which they received the Nobel Prize in chemistry in 1952. This marks a true beginning of GC as a broadly used analytical technique. If a compound has sufficient volatility for its molecules to be in the gas or vapour phase at or below 400°C, and does not decompose at these temperatures, then the compound can probably be analysed by GC.

The separation is performed in a column (containing either a solid or liquid stationary phase) that has a continuous flow of mobile phase passing through it – usually an inert carrier gas, but more recently supercritical fluids (SCFs) have been used for some applications – maintained in a temperature-regulated oven. When a mixture of substances is injected at the inlet, each component partitions between the stationary phase and the gas phase as it is swept towards the detector. Molecules that have greater affinity for the stationary phase spend more time in that phase and consequently take longer to reach the detector. The detector produces a signal proportional to the amount of substance that passes through it, and this signal is processed and fed to an integrator or some other recording device. Each substance that elutes from the column has a characteristic retention time, defined as the time interval from injection to peak detector response. Figure 18.1 shows a schematic of a GC system.

Identification of components was traditionally based primarily on peak retention time, but it is becoming increasingly more reliant on the nature of the response obtained from the detector. The analyst has two main goals: firstly, to make each different compound appear in a discrete band or peak with no overlap (or co-elution) with other components in the mixture, and, secondly, to make these bands uniform in shape and as narrow as possible. This is achieved

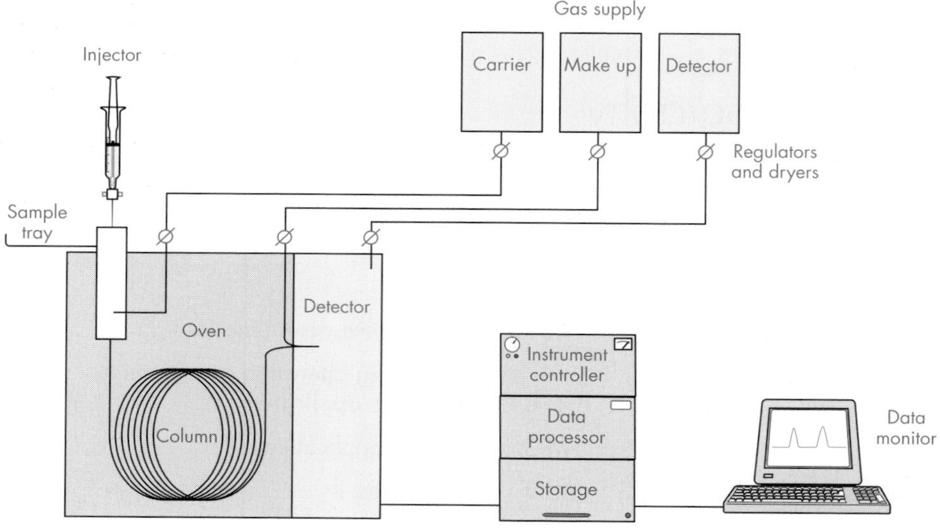

Figure 18.1 A modern GC system.

partly by judicious choice of the column stationary phase and its loading, and partly by optimising the operating conditions of the column. In addition, the method of introducing the sample into the chromatograph, the choice of detector, and chemical modification to improve the volatility of the compounds also contribute to converting a mediocre analysis into a first-class one.

There has been a continuous synergism between enhanced detector performance and column performance, each advance being reciprocally dependent on the other. Initially, high-sensitivity detectors permitted the development of a precise column theory that, in turn, enabled the design of columns that had much higher efficiencies. The improved efficiency of columns resulted in substances eluting from the separation columns as very low volumes compared to the volume of the detectors and dispersion of the substance into that relatively large volume resulted in reduced efficiency. Thus the efficiency of separations became limited by the geometry of the detector, and not by its intrinsic sensitivity. Detector design was modified to incorporate smaller tube dimensions, and the volume of the sensing cell was thereby reduced greatly. The introduction of capillary columns suitable for routine use in GC in the mid-1980s provided much higher resolution efficiencies and smaller peak volumes, which provoked further modifications in detector design. The latest column developments mean that peaks of only a few milliseconds are a real possibility in both GC and liquid chromatography (LC). Since this matches the response time of the current sensor electronics, the ingenuity of the detector design engineers is again being tested.

Gas chromatography columns

Packed columns made of glass or steel contain a stationary phase (see below), either loaded directly into the column if it is a solid at its operating temperature, or coated onto the surface of a solid support if it is liquid at its operating temperature. Thus, the operating principle of GC can be distinguished as either gas–solid chromatography (mainly an adsorptive process by the stationary phase) or gas–liquid chromatography (GLC; mainly partition of the analytes between the mobile and stationary phases), based on the physical characteristics of the stationary phase. Capillary columns, introduced in the early 1980s, have now replaced packed columns for most applications. The original glass columns were fragile and have been superseded by fused-silica capillary columns. Fused silica is high-purity synthetic quartz, with a protective coating of polyimide applied to the outer surface. Since these columns retain their flexibility only as long as the coating remains undamaged, their operating temperature must be maintained below 360°C for standard columns (400°C for high-temperature polyimide coatings). The first capillary columns were 0.2, 0.25 or 0.32 mm internal diameter (i.d.) and between 10 and 50 m long. Subsequently 'megabore' (0.53 mm i.d.), 'minibore' (0.18 mm i.d.) and 'microbore' (0.1 or 0.05 mm i.d.) columns have been developed. When coated with a heat-resistant polymer, these have the advantages of flexibility and strength, and can be threaded with ease through intricate pipework. A single column can be fitted into almost any manufacturer's GC apparatus. Capillary columns provide improved resolution, sensitivity and durability, less bleed with increasing temperatures, and ease of maintenance and repair; they yield reliable and highly reproducible separations, typically over many hundreds or thousands of injections. This has reduced the number of columns required to achieve a satisfactory separation of quite complex mixtures.

The internal surface of the silica is deactivated by a variety of processes that can react silanol groups (Si—OH) on the silica surface with a silane reagent (usually a methyl or phenylmethyl surface is created). For gas–solid capillary chromatography, a fine layer (usually less than 10 μm) of stationary phase particles is adhered to the tubing (porous layer open tubular columns, or PLOT columns). For gas–liquid capillary chromatography, the stationary phase may be coated or covalently bonded directly onto the walls of the column (wall-coated open tubular columns, or WCOT columns) or onto a support (e.g. microcrystals of sodium or barium chloride) bonded to the column wall (support-coated open tubular columns, or SCOT columns). Stainless-steel capillaries are usually reserved for applications that require extremes of temperature, or where the possibility of column breakage cannot be tolerated. Nowadays, the internal surface of metal columns is specially deactivated chemically or by lining with fused silica, which allows for more flexibility and greater durability and reduces the possibility of degradation of analytes which can be catalysed by the presence of metal surfaces.

Both bonding and cross-linking impart enhanced thermal and solvent stability to the stationary phase (often designated 'DB'), and should be used if they are available. For conventional packed column chromatography, however, the stationary phase must first be coated onto the surface of a solid support.

Stationary phases and support materials

Solid stationary phases

In gas–solid chromatography, the stationary phase is an active solid at its operating temperature. A conventional packed column is filled completely by stationary phase particles, but in a capillary column a fine layer (usually less than 10 μm) of particles is adhered by proprietary processes to the inner surface of the tubing, to create a PLOT column. These solid phases may be inorganic materials (e.g. aluminium oxides, molecular sieves, silica gel, or graphitised carbon), or they may be organic polymers such as styrene. Both packed and capillary columns use similar solid-phase materials. Sample compounds undergo a dynamic gas–solid adsorption–desorption process with the stationary phase, and since the particles are porous, size exclusion and shape selectivity processes also occur. The carrier gas (mobile phase) merely serves to sweep towards the detector those solute molecules that are not currently adsorbed. The resultant columns are highly retentive, and separations impossible with liquid phases can be accomplished easily on PLOT columns above ambient temperature. These columns are generally reserved for the separation of low-molecular-weight materials, such as hydrocarbon and sulfur gases, noble and permanent gases, and low boiling solvents. Since PLOT columns occasionally shed particles, their use is not advised with detectors that are affected adversely by the intrusion of particulate matter (the mass spectrometer is particularly vulnerable, as the column interface operates under vacuum).

Graphitised carbon black

Carbopaks are graphitised carbon black, having adsorptive surfaces of up to 100 m^2/g. They are usually modified with a light coating of a polar stationary phase. Difficult separations of the C_1 to C_{10} hydrocarbons can be achieved rapidly. Carbopak C with 0.2% Carbowax 20M has been used to resolve substances abused by 'glue-sniffers'. Carbopak C modified with 0.2% Carbowax 1500 and Carbopak C with 0.8% tetrahydroxyethylenediamine (THEED) are useful for the analysis of ethanol and ethylene glycol, respectively, in blood. Resolution is superior to that obtained with the Porapak and Chromosorb polymers, although the elution order is similar.

Molecular sieves

Activated alumina is unique for its extremely wide pore-diameter range, and is very useful for separating most C_1 to C_4 molecules, separating light hydrocarbon saturates from unsaturates in the C_1 to C_5 range, and separating benzene, toluene and xylenes. Deactivation of alumina with potassium hydroxide reverses the elution of some molecules (acetylene and *n*-butane). Carbosieves are granular carbon molecular sieves that give good separation of C_1 to C_3 hydrocarbons. Carboxen 1006 is useful in resolving formaldehyde, water and methanol, and impurities in ethylene. Zeolites (5A, 13X) give a good general separation of inorganic gases. Carbon dioxide is irreversibly adsorbed below 160°C. Oxygen, nitrogen, carbon monoxide and methane are well separated. These columns have a tendency to adsorb water and carbon dioxide, which results in changes in retention over time.

Polymers

Chromosorb 101–108 and Porapak are divinylbenzene cross-linked polystyrene copolymers. Incorporation of other functional groups, such as acrylonitrile and acrylic esters, into the polymer matrix provides moderately polar to polar surfaces with different pore sizes and surface areas (polarity increases with ascending number or letter). HayeSep phases are polymers of divinylbenzene and ethylene glycol dimethylacrylate. Separations range from free fatty acids to free amines, and small alcohols from methanol to pentanol. Tenax-TA is a porous polymer of 2,6-diphenyl-*p*-phenylene oxide, used both as a chromatographic phase and as a trap for volatile substances prior to analysis. It is also used for high-boiling alcohols, polyethylene glycols (PEGs), phenols, aldehydes, ketones, ethanolamines and chlorinated aromatics.

Liquid stationary phases

In GLC, the stationary phase is a liquid or gum at the normal operating temperature. Components injected into the column are partitioned between the moving (mobile) gas phase and the stationary phase. Molecules that have greater affinity for the stationary phase spend more time immobilised in the column and consequently take longer to reach the detector. The process of immobilisation and subsequent release back into the mobile phase occurs thousands of times during the course of the analysis. The separation of components is dependent, to a large extent, on the chemical nature of the stationary phase. Stationary phases are essentially two types of high-boiling polymers, siloxanes (often incorrectly called silicones) and PEGs. Chiral stationary phases based on cyclodextrins (cyclic glucose chains) have specific applications in the separation of enantiomers and are discussed separately.

Polysiloxanes

Standard polysiloxanes (PSXs) are characterised by their repeating siloxane backbone in which each silicone atom has the potential to attach two functional groups, the type and amount of which distinguish the stationary phase and its properties (Fig. 18.2). The basic PSX is 100% methyl-substituted. When other groups are incorporated into the stationary phase, the amount is indicated as a percentage of the total substituent groups. For example, if 5% of silicon atoms contain two phenyl groups and the remaining 95% of silicon atoms are methyl-substituted, this may be written as (5% diphenyl/95% dimethyl)-PSX, (5% phenyl/95% methyl)-PSX or simply (5% phenyl)-PSX. In some instances, two different groups are present on the same silicon atom, so a (10% cyanopropylphenyl/dimethyl)-PSX contains a total of 5%

cyanopropyl, 5% phenyl and 90% methyl residues (see Fig. 18.2).

While PSXs are generally less polar in nature than PEGs, the substitution of polar residues for a proportion of the methyl groups confers added polarity to the column. Polar phases retain polar compounds more effectively than do nonpolar compounds, and vice versa. The 100% methyl-substituted-PSX is often considered the 'standard' nonpolar phase, and has been used extensively in compilations of retention indices. This column is an ideal choice for starting a new application. However, substitution by *n*-octyl groups (up to 50%) renders the column extremely nonpolar, and similar to squalene. Substitution with up to 5% phenyl groups still furnishes an essentially nonpolar column with improved thermal stability. This phase has also been used for retention index (RI) work and is another good column with which to start a new application. Increasing the phenyl substitution to 20%, 35% or 50% yields columns classed as intermediate in polarity, which predictably retain aromatic compounds relative to aliphatic solutes. All these are available as bonded phases that can be solvent rinsed, are not damaged by organic acids or bases, and can tolerate small injections of water if sufficiently highly loaded, but are sensitive to strong inorganic acids and bases.

Substitution of cyanopropylphenyl groups (typically 6% or 14%) creates an intermediate polarity mixed phase with unique elution relative to simple phenyl substitution, but renders the column more susceptible to damage from oxygen, moisture and mineral acids. 50% substitution is specifically designed to separate *cis*- and *trans*-fatty acid methyl esters (FAMEs). However, even low-level bleeding of the stationary phase produces a high background signal with certain types of detector (nitrogen–phosphorus detector; NPD). Bleeding is the term given to the phenomenon wherein stationary phase degrades during analysis and elutes from the column. Depending on the nature of the stationary phase and the detector used, the degraded material may be detected and can contribute to the detector signal, potentially causing problems with the analysis. More polar columns are produced by substitution of bis-cyanopropyl and cyanopropylphenyl groups (80:20 or 90:10). 100% biscyanopropyl substitution gives the highest polarity of the PSXs. This phase can be operated at both high and low temperatures. To

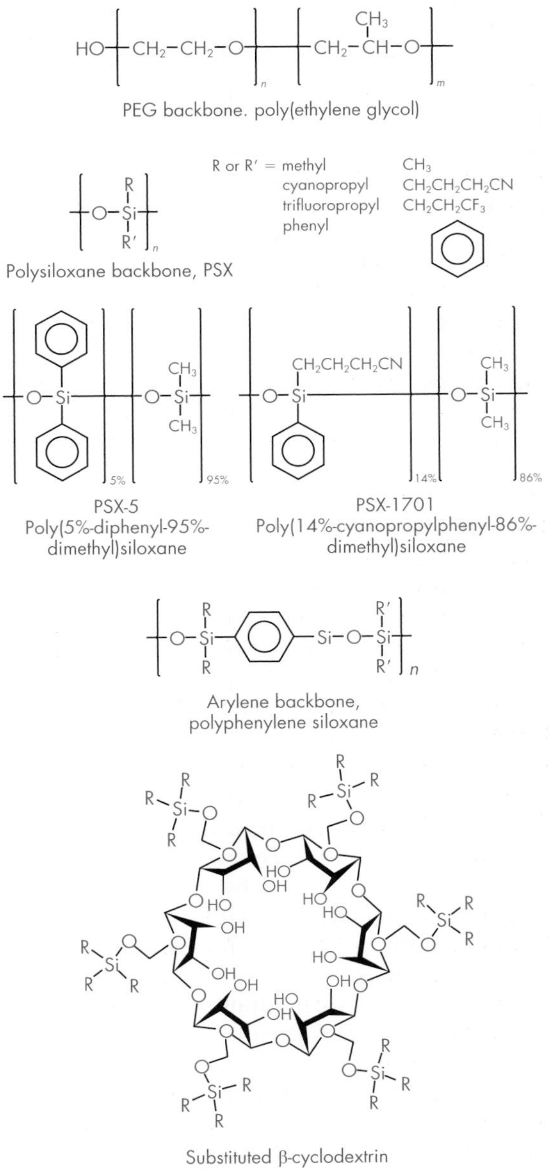

Figure 18.2 Structures of some common capillary GC stationary phases.

date, these are nonbonded columns, and should not therefore be rinsed with solvent. Trifluoropropyl/methyl-PSX is a mid-to-high polarity phase especially suited for otherwise difficult-to-separate positional isomers. Its unique interactions with nitro, halogen, carbonyl and other electronegative groups give it application in the analysis of herbicides and pesticides.

Increasing polarity in general is associated with some negative effects. Polar phases tend to have a narrower operating temperature range (higher minimum, lower maximum), are more prone to bleed at higher temperatures, are more sensitive to moisture and oxygen, and consequently have a shorter life expectancy than nonpolar phases. More recently, low-bleed arylene stationary phases (sometimes designated mass spectrometry or 'ms') have been introduced that have phenyl groups incorporated into the siloxane backbone (see Fig. 18.2). The incorporated phenyl groups confer additional strength to the backbone, which prevents the formation of cyclic fragments and associated 'bleed' at higher temperatures.

Polyethylene glycols

PEGs are widely used polar stationary phases and their general structure is shown in Fig. 18.2.

They are less stable, less robust (especially to oxidative damage) and have lower temperature limits and a shorter life expectancy than polar PSX phases, but they have unique resolving qualities. Acid-modified PEG (also referred to as free fatty acid phase, FFAP) substituted with terephthalic acid is especially useful for separating acidic polar compounds, such as acids, alcohols, acrylates, ketones and nitriles. Nitroterephthalic acid-substituted PEG (e.g. Nukol) is designed for volatile fatty acids and phenols. Both are highly resistant to damage from water-based samples. Base-modified PEG (CAM) is suited to analysis of strongly basic compounds, such as primary amines, that do not chromatograph well on polar PSXs. Since this phase is usually cross-linked rather than covalently bonded, it cannot be used with water or alcohol, but it can be solvent rinsed. New bonded and cross-linked PEG phases are now available to separate free fatty acids and other organic acids. These show superior inertness and can tolerate repeated injections of water, alcohols, aldehydes and acids without the need for acidification treatment.

Chiral phases

Second-generation chiral phases are based on cyclodextrins (toroidal shaped structures formed by α_{1-4} linkages of multiple glucose units). The enzyme cyclodextrin glucosyl transferase is used to cleave partially digested starch, and link the glucose units into three forms, referred to as α, β, and γ, that have six, seven and eight glucose units, respectively. The mouth of the cyclodextrin molecule has a larger circumference than the base and is linked to secondary hydroxyl groups of the C2 and C3 atoms of each glucose unit. The primary hydroxyl groups are located at the base of the torus, on the C6 atoms. The number of glucose units thus determines the cavity size and electrophilic orientation (see Fig. 18.2), and affects the order of the enantiomeric forms. The hydroxyl groups can be functionalised selectively to provide various physical properties and inclusion selectivities. Six different cyclodextrin derivatives are manufactured: permethylated hydroxypropyl (PH), dialkylated (DA), trifluoroacetylated (TA), propionylated (PN), butyrylated (BP) and permethylated (PM). Changes in elution order can be seen between the different derivatives, and also between cyclodextrin cavity sizes. Unlike the cyclodextrins used in high-performance liquid chromatography (HPLC), these phases separate both aromatic and nonaromatic enantiomers of a wide range of chemicals, including saturated alcohols, amines, carboxylic acids, epoxides, diols, lactones, amino alcohols, amino acids, esters, pyrans and furans. Derivatised cyclodextrins are thermally stable, highly crystalline and virtually insoluble in most organic solvents. Chiral phases are fragile, however, and unless chemically bonded or cross-linked, they cannot be washed with solvent or taken to temperatures outside the 0 to 225°C range.

A subsequent development has been the embedding of PM cyclodextrins (usually 10% or 20% by volume) into columns that contain standard liquid stationary phases of intermediate polarity, such as 35% phenyl-PSX. Silyl-substituted cyclodextrins, such as 2,3-di-*O*-

methyl-6-*O*-*t*-butyldimethylsilyl are also available embedded (usually 25–35% by weight) in 20% phenyl-PSX, another intermediate polarity stationary phase. These columns are useful for separating positional isomers (phenols, xylenes, etc.), as well as enantiomers.

Solute–stationary phase interactions

For liquid stationary phases, three major types of interaction between the stationary phase and the solute determine chromatographic elution: dispersion, dipole and hydrogen bonding. The volatility of a substance is the most important factor defining its separation in GC. The more volatile the compound (the lower its boiling point), the more likely it is to be in the mobile phase and so the faster it elutes from the column. Although this holds true for groups of compounds with similar functional groups or within homologous series, it cannot be applied universally. In general, a difference of 30°C in boiling point is sufficient to predict and maintain elution order, but differences of less than 10°C can be overturned by the influence of other interactions.

Table 18.1 shows the contribution of each of these interactions for the common types of liquid stationary phases. It should be remembered that hydrogen-bonding interactions are considerably stronger than dipole–dipole interactions, which are themselves stronger than dispersion interactions. Thus, although the dispersion interaction between the various stationary phases is listed as strong or very strong, and the hydrogen-bonding interactions as weak or moderate, if the analyte has functional groups that can undergo hydrogen bonding with the particular stationary phase employed, the hydrogen-bonding interaction is likely to be stronger than interaction by dispersion, unless the analyte also has a high proportion of groups in its molecular structure that can participate in dispersion interactions, as would be the case for example, for long-chain fatty acids.

Dipole interactions of PEG phases and the cyanopropyl- and trifluoropropyl-substituted PSXs enable these phases to separate solute molecules that have different dipole moments. Such solutes are those with positional isomers of electronegative groups, such as pesticides, halocarbons and many pharmaceuticals.

Functional groups of solutes that exhibit strong hydrogen bonding include alcohols, carboxylic acids and amines. Aldehydes, esters and ketones generally have less effect; hydrocarbons, halocarbons and ethers produce negligible hydrogen bonding. Moderate hydrogen bonding is exhibited by PEGs and cyanopropyl-substituted PSXs, with less marked effects shown by phenyl- and trifluropropyl-substituted PSXs.

Although the amount of separation obtained through dipole interactions or through hydrogen bonding can be difficult to predict, resolution of compounds with smaller differences in dipoles or in hydrogen bonding strengths requires larger percentages of siloxane substitution in order that solute–stationary

Table 18.1 Contribution of different types of interactions to solute separation on GC stationary phases

Functional group	Type of interaction		
	Dispersion	Dipole	Hydrogen bonding
Methyl-PSX	Strong	None	None
Phenyl-PSX	Very strong	None	Weak
Cyanopropyl-PSX	Strong	Very strong	Moderate
Trifluoropropyl-PSX	Strong	Moderate	Weak
PEG	Strong	Strong	Moderate

phase interaction via dispersion forces can be exploited to bring about separation.

McReynolds constants

The retention behaviour of probe compounds has been used traditionally to classify stationary phases in terms of their polarity. Lutz Rohrschneider in 1966 pioneered this type of classification using five probe compounds, followed closely by McReynolds (1970). McReynolds increased the number of probe compounds to ten but the following five compounds are considered as the most important: benzene, butanol, pentan-2-one, nitropropane and pyridine. The retention indices of each of these five reference compounds are measured on the stationary phase being tested, and then compared to those obtained under the same conditions on squalene (a standard nonpolar stationary phase). The differences in the retention indices between the two phases (ΔI) for the five probe compounds are added together to give a constant, known as the *McReynolds constant*, which is used to compare the ability of stationary phases to separate different classes of compounds. Phases that provide McReynolds values of ± 4 can be substituted freely for each other as they should give similar retention and specificity; those differing by ± 10 units generally yield similar separations but may show some greater differences in terms of retention and elution order. Phases with McReynolds values below 100 are considered nonpolar, those above 400 indicate a highly polar phase and values between 100 and 400 indicate intermediate polarity. Table 18.2 shows the McReynolds constants, operating temperature range, the relationship between capillary and packed column nomenclature and example applications for the most popular stationary phases. ΔI values for individual probes indicate the deviation from boiling point order and consequently represent the contribution of forces other than dispersion to elution for that probe. The probes are chosen to represent different functional groups as follows:

- benzene for aromatics and olefins (π-type interactions)
- butan-1-ol for alcohols, nitriles, carboxylic acids and diols (electron-attracting effect)
- pentan-2-one for ketones, ethers, aldehydes, esters, epoxides and dimethylamino derivatives (dipole–dipole effect)
- nitropropane for nitro and nitrile derivatives (electron-donating effect)
- pyridine for bases (nonbonding electron attraction and hydrogen-bonding effects).

Moffat *et al.* (1974a) devised a system to assess the effectiveness of liquid stationary phases by calculating the discriminating power, and examined a number of phases commonly used in toxicology (Moffat *et al.* 1974b). Contrary to popular belief, it was shown that one column could be used to elute all the drugs studied, and that for screening purposes a single column, either SE-30 or OV-17 (100% dimethyl-PSX or 5% phenyl-PSX capillary equivalents), was sufficient for the reliable identification of drugs.

Solid supports for packed columns

As noted above, in packed column GC where the stationary phase is a liquid, it is typically coated onto the surface of a solid support. The raw material for the most commonly used supports is diatomaceous earth, calcined, usually with a flux, then crushed and graded into a number of particle sizes (60–80, 80–100 and 100–120 mesh). Diatomaceous earths are available with a variety of properties and include the Chromosorb series of supports. Chromosorb G has a surface area of about 0.5 m^2/g, and is suitable for low-loaded columns – the amount of stationary phase should not exceed 5% (w/w). Chromosorb W has a larger surface area (1 m^2/g) and accepts higher loadings, but is more fragile. Chromosorb P, obtained from crushed firebrick, accepts loadings up to 35% (w/w) for some phases. Supelcoport is the most inert of the diatomite supports, and can accept 20% (w/w) loadings. Carbopack, Porapak, HayeSep and Tenax-TA (see above) can also be used as solid supports. Table 18.3 shows the maximum suggested coating percentages for the most common solid supports.

Deactivated support materials are nearly always preferred. Deactivation procedures include acid or base washing to remove

Table 18.2 Polarity (McReynolds values) of some common stationary phases, and example applications

Capillary phase[a]	Packed equivalent	Temperature range (min/max) (°C)	McReynolds values[b]					$\Sigma(\Delta I)$	Applications
			x'	y'	z'	u'	s'		
SPB-Octyl	Squalene, Apiezon L	–60/300	3	14	11	12	11	51	Separates by boiling point, polychlorinated biphenyls (PCBs)
*-1	SE30, OV-1, OV-101, SP2100	–60/320	4	58	43	56	38	199	Amines, hydrocarbons, pesticides, PCBs, phenols, sulfur compounds, flavours, fragrances
*-5	SE-52, OV-73	–60/320	19	74	64	93	62	312	Alkaloids, drugs, FAMEs, halogenated compounds, aromatic compounds
*-1301	SE-54, CP-624	–20/280	69	113	111	171	128	592	Aroclors, alcohols, phenols, volatile organic acids
*-35	OV-11	0/300	101	146	151	219	202	728	Aroclors, amines, pesticides, drugs
*-1701	OV-1701	10/280	67	170	153	228	171	789	Aroclors, herbicides, pesticides, trimethylsilyl (TMS) sugars
*-50, *-17	OV-17, SP-2250	30/310	125	175	183	268	220	971	Drugs, glycols, pesticides, steroids
*-210	OV-25	–45/250	178	204	208	305	280	1175	Aldehydes, ketones, organochlorines, organophosphates
*-225	XE-60, OV-210	40/230	146	238	358	468	310	1520	FAMEs, alditol acetates, neutral sterols
*-23	OV-225	40/250	228	369	338	492	386	1813	*cis–trans* FAMEs, stereoisomers
*-wax, *-20M	Carbowax-20M TPA	35/280	305	551	360	562	484	2262	Alcohols, free acids, essential oils, ethers, glycols, solvents, primary amines
*-FFAP	Carbowax-1500 PEG	50/250	340	580	397	602	627	2546	Acids, alcohols, aldehydes, acrylates, nitriles
Nukol	SP-1000, OV-351	60/200	314	569	372	578	504	2337	Alcohols, free acids, essential oils, ethers, glycols, solvents
*-2330	SP-2330	10/250	382	610	506	710	591	2799	*cis–trans* FAMEs, positional isomers
*-2380	–	10/275	402	629	520	744	623	2918	*cis–trans* FAMEs, positional isomers, alditol acetates
*-2340	SP-2340, OV-275	25/250	419	654	541	758	637	3009	*cis–trans* FAMEs, positional isomers
–	DEGS	20/200	496	746	590	837	835	3504	Acids, esters, phenols, terpenoids
–	EGS	100/200	537	787	643	903	889	3759	TMS or methyl sugars, acidic drugs
TCEP	TCEP	10/145	594	857	759	1031	917	4158	Flavours, fragrances, essential oils

Continued

Table 18.2 (*Continued*)

Capillary phase[a]	Packed equivalent	Temperature range (min/max) (°C)	McReynolds values[b]					$\Sigma(\Delta I)$	Applications
			x'	y'	z'	u'	s'		
α-Cyclodextrin in 35% phenyl-PSX		30/240	102	243	142	221	170	878	Enantiomers and isomers
β-Cyclodextrin in 35% phenyl-PSX		30/240	119	264	154	134	187	858	Enantiomers and isomers

[a] * is the proprietary prefix for the phase, for example; * = HP supplied by Hewlett Packard/Agilent; * = DB supplied by J&W; * = CPSil supplied by Chrompack; * = RT supplied by Restek; * = SP supplied by Supelco; * = OV supplied by Ohio Valley. This list is not intended to be exhaustive.

[b] x' = benzene; y' = butan-1-ol; z' = pentan-2-one; u' =1-nitropropane; s' = pyridine.

Table 18.3 Maximum recommended loadings for the most commonly used packed column supports

Phase	Maximum coating (%w/w)
Carbopak B	1–6 non-silicone phase
Carbopak C	0.1–1.0 non-silicone phase
Carbopak F	0.1–1.0 non-silicone phase
Chromosorb G	20 (15 for gums)
Chromosorb P	30 (25 for gums)
Chromosorb T	15 (7 for gums)
Chromosorb W	20
Gas Chrom Q	15
HayeSep Polymers	15 (5 for gums)
Porapak	15 (5 for gums)
Supelcoport	20
Tenax-TA	15 (5 for gums)

impurities and fines, and treatment with a silanising agent that reacts with surface hydroxyl groups to reduce adsorptive effects. Support materials that have the liquid phase chemically bonded to them are available. These offer decreased bleed rates of stationary phase, an advantage when operating a temperature programme or when using a mass spectrometer as the detector.

Installing, conditioning and maintaining columns

Column installation

A GC column is attached at one end to the injector and at the other end to the detector. Attachment is typically via a nut and ferrule, the nut attaching to a screwthread on the injector and detector. As the nut is tightened, the ferrule is compressed and helps produce a gastight fitting.

Glass columns must have straight smooth ends to allow them to fit into unions at the injector and detector using either graphite or Vespel (polyimide) ferrules inside the nuts. Fused-silica capillaries should also have their ends freshly cut after insertion through ferrules, to eliminate blockages. The injector end of the column should be fitted first, adjusting the height of the protrusion above the ferrule into the injector according to the type of inlet being used (this information is supplied by the GC manufacturer for the particular system in use), then tightening the fittings just enough to prevent leakage when tested with a proprietary leak-testing fluid (not soap solution which leaves a residue). The detector end of a packed column can be attached to a bubble-flow meter to ensure adequate flow through the column before connecting the detector end. The detector end of the capillary column may be immersed into a small tube of methanol to ensure adequate flow and the capillary end re-cut and then attached to the detector and checked for leaks. The detector is activated and the column tested at room temperature with an injection of 1 or 2 μL of methane, when a needle-sharp peak should be obtained. When the carrier-gas pressure has been adjusted to give a flow of approximately 20 mL/min of carrier gas for a packed column or 1 to 2 mL/min for a capillary, the column may be heated and a test mixture injected. Commercial columns are invariably supplied with a chromatogram obtained from a test mixture, and it should be possible to obtain a performance equal or close to the supplied chromatogram. Various test mixtures are used, including a mixture of dimethylphenol and dimethylaniline with straight-chain paraffins. Any acidity or alkalinity of the column is apparent by loss of the peak shape of the amine or phenol. The efficiency obtained is a function of the entire chromatographic system. Poor efficiency or peak shape often results from a non-swept volume somewhere in the system.

It may be necessary to add an additional gas supply to the column outlet to ensure that the detector is purged effectively, because most detectors are designed to operate with packed columns and a flow rate of about 30 mL/min, as opposed to the 1 or 2 mL/min delivered by a capillary column (see Fig. 18.1, p. 470). Make-up gas is integral in the design of most modern GC instruments.

Column conditioning

A new column requires conditioning before use to remove volatile impurities that remain after deactivation of the support, and/or the coating and packing processes. The column should be installed in the injector port only, with the detector end disconnected. With the column at room temperature, a low carrier gas pressure (14–35 kPa) should be maintained for half an hour to purge oxygen from the system. The temperature may then be raised by about 1°C/min, to 10°C above the anticipated working temperature or the maximum operating temperature, whichever is less, and the temperature is maintained (2 h for a manufactured capillary, 12 h for a packed column or self-packed capillary). Care must be taken not to exceed the maximum operating temperature. After conditioning, the column is connected to the detector, and a period of further conditioning is carried out if the background signal is excessive. Some phases (e.g. OV-17) are particularly oxygen-sensitive and can be ruined by careless conditioning. A constrictor fitted to the detector end of the column helps prevent back diffusion of oxygen if air or oxygen is supplied to the detector.

Guard columns and retention gaps

A guard column and a retention gap are essentially the same thing, but are installed to serve different purposes. These 1–10 m lengths of fused silica tubing are attached to the front of the chromatography column via a press-snap connector or zero dead-volume union, and then installed into the injector port. The surface of the silica is deactivated to minimise solute interactions, but no stationary phase is added. The tubing diameter should be the same as that of the column, but if different it should, ideally, be of a wider bore.

The function of a guard column is to trap deposits of nonvolatile residues, thereby preventing their contamination of the analytical column. Solutes are not retained by the guard column (since there is no stationary phase) and pass directly onto the column. Portions can be cut periodically from the top of the guard column as deterioration in chromatography requires, without any appreciable loss of resolution from the analytical column.

A retention gap is used to improve peak shape either when poor chromatography is the result of a large injection volume (>2 μL) or when there are solvent–stationary phase polarity mismatches. Greatest improvement is seen in early-eluting peaks, or for solutes with similar polarity to that of the solvent.

Maximum operating temperatures

Maximum operating temperatures for stationary phases are usually quoted assuming isothermal operation with a flame ionisation detector (see Table 18.2). Other detectors may impose different limits, the mass spectrometer being much more susceptible to bleeding of the stationary phase than the thermal conductivity detector. All phases bleed very slightly at high temperatures because of the loss of smaller-sized (and hence lower-boiling) polymer chains, although normally this is not noticeable. Operating temperature has a profound effect on column life, particularly for capillary columns. Loss of stationary phase, or breakdown of the thin film into pools to expose part of the tubing surface, results in serious loss of performance. Additionally, in columns that contain PSX phases with two different functional groups, one group (usually that which confers additional polarity) is preferentially lost. This results in a change of relative separation as well as a loss of resolution. The temperature limit of a column may be determined by the deactivation procedure used in production, rather than by the stationary phase itself. Newer silica columns have a very low metal oxide content, thought to act as a catalyst for the degradation of both sample and stationary phase, and thus enable phases to be run at higher temperatures. Fused-silica capillary columns have a protective external coating of polyimide that is slowly degraded at elevated temperatures (maximum temperature 360°C, but now to 400°C), which can also limit column life. However, separations are usually achieved at much lower temperatures.

Temperature programming

For complex mixtures with components of widely varying retention characteristics, it is often impractical to choose a single column temperature that allows all the components to be resolved. Increasing the column temperature throughout the analysis dramatically reduces the time taken for higher-boiling compounds to elute, and simultaneously improves the sensitivity of the assay, as the peaks are remarkably sharper. If the early-eluting compounds are resolved inadequately, a lower starting temperature or slower initial ramp should be used, taking care to observe the temperature requirements of the type of injector used. All instruments currently manufactured are available with a temperature program option, and a multi-ramp programmer is particularly useful for capillary chromatography. The first ramp can be used during splitless injection (see p. 485) to bring the column rapidly up to the initial chromatography temperature, followed by a slower analytical ramp to perform the separation. One problem with temperature programming is that the back-pressure increases with temperature and reduces the carrier gas flow if a mass-flow controller is not used. For polar stationary phases, the polarity increases with temperature. Column bleed also increases, which results in an increasing baseline. For this reason the column should be well conditioned before use.

Evaluating column performance

Column performance, whether of capillary or packed columns, is made on the basis of efficiency (the narrowness of a peak), the peak shape (whether it tails or fronts) and ability to resolve compounds. This section deals with separation theory, and the reader may find it useful to refer at intervals to Fig. 18.3.

Retention time

Retention time (t_R) is the time taken for a given solute to travel through the column, and is the time assigned to the corresponding peak on the chromatograph. It is a measure of the amount of time the solute spends in the column, and is therefore the sum of time spent in both the stationary and the mobile phases.

Retention time of a non-retained compound or hold-up time (tM)

The retention time t_M is the time taken for a non-retained solute to travel along the column; it represents the transit time for the mobile phase (carrier gas) in the column and is a column-specific parameter, applicable only under the prevailing conditions of gas flow and oven temperature. No other peak can be expected to elute earlier than this time. t_M is obtained by injecting a non-retained compound suitable for the detector system being used (butane or methane for flame ionisation detection (FID) or thermal conductivity detection (TCD); acetonitrile for nitrogen–phosphorus detection (NPD); methylene chloride for electron-capture detection (ECD); vinyl chloride for photoionisation detection (PID) or electrolytic conductivity detection (ELCD)).

Average linear velocity

The average linear velocity ($\bar{\mu}$) represents the average speed of carrier gas through the column, usually expressed in cm/s, and is considered more meaningful than measuring the flow (usually expressed in mL/min) at the column effluent, since flow is dependent on column diameter. This term directly influences solute retention times and column efficiency. Velocity is controlled by altering the column head pressure, and is calculated from the equation:

$$\bar{\mu}(\text{cm/s}) = \frac{L}{t_M} \tag{18.1}$$

where L is the column length (cm), and t_M is the retention time (s) of a non-retained solute.

Retention factor

Retention factor (k) is the ratio of the amount of time a solute spends in the stationary and mobile phases and is calculated from t_R and t_M using the equation:

$$k = \frac{t_R - t_M}{t_M} = \frac{t'_R}{t_M} \tag{18.2}$$

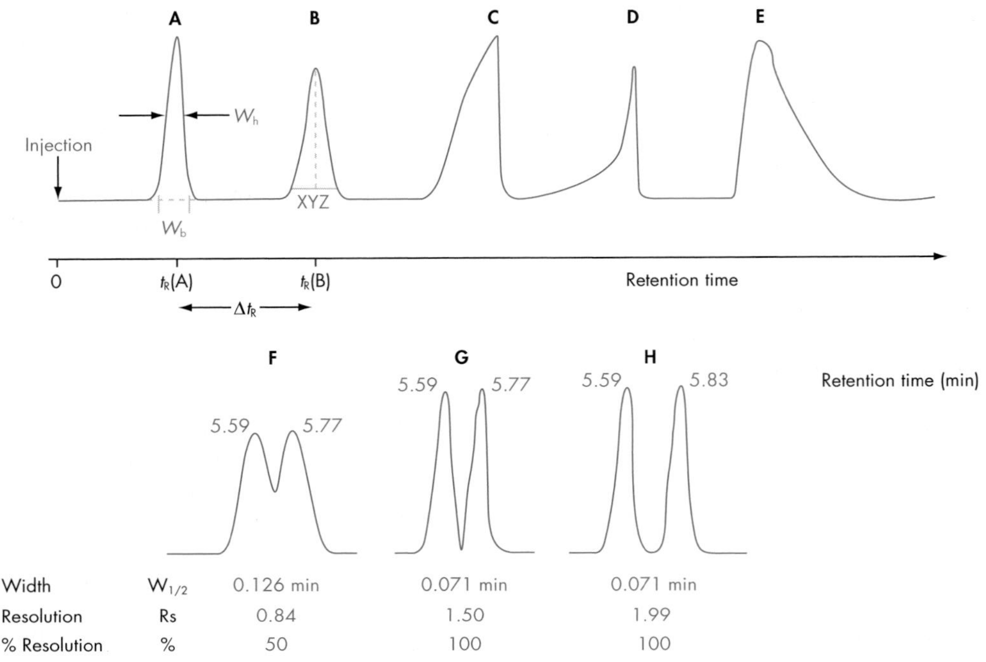

Figure 18.3 A and B are symmetrical peaks that show the measurement of significant parameters. W_b, width at the base of the peak; W_h, width at half peak height; $t_R(A)$ and $t_R(B)$, retention times of peaks A and B, respectively; Δt_R, the difference in retention time between A and B; XYZ, a line drawn at 10% of peak height. Peak C is symptomatic of column overload with solute. Peak D is symptomatic of degradation of a thermally unstable solute. Peak E is symptomatic of adherence to active sites in the injection port or on the column.
Resolution of two compounds: In F and G the peaks of the two compounds have identical retention times (5.59 and 5.77 min, respectively), but in G the peaks are narrower (W_h 0.071 versus 0.126 min, respectively), and are fully resolved (Rs 1.50 versus 0.84, respectively). In H the peak widths of the two compounds are the same as in G, but the retention time of peak B is later (5.83 versus 5.77 min, respectively). Again, the peaks are fully resolved and Rs is larger than in G (Rs = 1.99 versus 1.50).

where t_M is the retention time of a non-retained solute, t_R is the retention time of the solute and t'_R is the adjusted retention time of the solute.

Since all compounds spend an identical time in the mobile phase, k is a measure of retention by the stationary phase. A compound with a retention factor of 4 spends twice as much time in the stationary phase (but not twice as much time on the column) as a compound with a retention factor of 2. Thus, k provides relative rather than absolute information, and is to a large degree independent of the operating conditions.

Separation factor

The separation factor (α) is a measure of the time interval between two peaks. If α equals 1, then the peaks have the same retention time and co-elute. Separation factor is calculated using the equation:

$$\alpha = \frac{k_2}{k_1} \tag{18.3}$$

where k_1 is the retention factor of the first peak, and k_2 the retention factor for the second peak.

The value of α, however, does not indicate whether the peaks are resolved completely from one another. Two peaks may have only 0.01 min between them on one column but still be resolved completely, while on another column they may have 0.1 min between them but not be resolved adequately (refer to Fig. 18.3).

Number of theoretical plates or column efficiency

The theoretical plate is an indirect measure of peak width at a specific retention time. Higher plate numbers indicate greater column efficiency and narrower peaks. The number of plates per metre of column (N) is calculated from either form of equation (18.4):

$$N = 16(t_R/W_b)^2 \quad (18.4a)$$

$$N = 5.54(t_R/W_h)^2 \quad (18.4b)$$

where t_R is the time from injection to peak maximum for the solute, W_b is the peak width at base in units of time and W_h is the peak width at half height in units of time.

Efficiency is a function of the column dimensions (diameter, length, film thickness or loading), the type of carrier gas and its flow, as well as the chemical nature of the solute and the stationary phase.

Peak shape or asymmetry

A well-designed system should give symmetrical peaks, as tailing or fronting adversely affects resolution. Tailing may result from non-swept volume in the system or from component–stationary phase or component–support interactions. Tailing of polar compounds can often be remedied by the use of a more polar stationary phase. Fronting (shark's fin peaks) is usually caused by overloading, particularly with capillary columns, and can be resolved by making a smaller injection, by diluting the sample, or by using a column with a higher stationary phase ratio. Column capacity is the maximum amount of a solute that can be chromatographed successfully without loss of peak shape. Peak fronting caused by thermal decomposition can be reduced by either lowering the injection temperature or using a cold on-column injector system.

Peak shape is usually expressed by the peak asymmetry (A_s). In Fig. 18.3, the peak asymmetry factor for substance B is given by:

$$A_s = \frac{YZ}{XY} \quad (18.5)$$

where a vertical line is drawn through the peak maximum and XYZ is drawn at 10% of the peak height. A symmetrical peak has $A_s = 1$.

Inlet systems

The inlet system provides the means of introducing the specimen into the GC. Obtaining a narrow sample band at the start of the chromatographic process is critical to achieve good resolution, since broad sample bands usually produce broad peaks, especially for analytes that elute early. The choice of injector depends on:

- the characteristics of the specimen or residue
- the quantity and characteristics of the analytes to be separated
- the temperature and nature of the stationary phase and the column.

Solid samples are normally chromatographed by dissolving in a suitable solvent and injecting with a micro-syringe. Liquids can be injected using a micro-syringe, but with sensitive detection systems the sample should be dissolved in a suitable solvent to reduce the sample size and avoid overloading the detector. Gases and vapours may be introduced by injection through the inlet port septum using a gas-tight syringe.

The four main types of GC injectors are megabore direct (or packed column), split, splitless and cold on-column. In reality, split and splitless injection are carried out using the same hardware; the so-called split/splitless injector. Conventional glass syringes of 1–10 μL volume with stainless-steel needles can be used on the packed column, or vaporisation capillary injectors, and the injection is made by piercing a silicone rubber septum. Care must be taken to select septa that have low bleed characteristics at the operating temperature, and those with Teflon backs are most reliable in this respect. Unstable solutes can be decomposed by the high temperature of the injection system, particularly if the system is constructed of metal. For labile substances, cold on-column injection is preferred, but clean extracts must be used to minimise column contamination. The injection system typically utilises a removable liner to minimise contact with metal surfaces. These liners are usually made of glass. They come in various configurations (see Fig. 18.4) and the type used depends on the nature of the sample being analysed, the injector system used and the injection volume. With repeated injection of samples, liners inevitably become contaminated with nonvolatile material. This can cause unwanted interactions with subsequent injection of samples. Hence liners can be removed, cleaned by solvent washing and replaced in the injector.

Megabore direct (or packed column) injection

The packed column is usually inserted such that the top butts directly onto the septum or septum plate, and is housed in a heated port. The sample is injected directly on to the top of the column, and the carrier gas (typically 10–40 mL/min) sweeps the compounds directly along the column. A deactivated glass-wool plug at the top of the column serves as a filter to retain nonvolatile co-injected material, and must be replaced regularly to prevent turbulence or blockage of the carrier gas flow. Packed column inlets (6.3 mm diameter) can usually be modified by insertion of a reducing fitting and glass liner to take megabore capillary (0.53 or 0.45 mm i.d.) columns, but the high flow requirements to sweep the compounds onto the column in a narrow band (4 mL/min minimum) preclude the use of narrower capillaries. One type of injection liner usually has a restriction at the top to prevent backflush and septum contamination (see Fig. 18.4E), to which the top of the column is abutted to reduce interaction of the sample with the steel surface of the injection port. The injection is made directly onto a capillary column (sometimes referred to as hot on-column injection), and it is essential to maintain clean specimens to avoid poor chromatographic performance. The installation of a retention gap (see p. 480) may be useful in this situation. This type of injection is ideally suited to high-boiling compounds, and minimises degradation of thermally labile compounds. An alternative type of liner (flash vaporisation) avoids direct injection onto the capillary by having a second restriction about half way down (Figure 18.4F), to which the top of the column is abutted. This creates a vaporisation chamber above the column into which the injection is made. Chromatography is generally more efficient, since the second taper acts as a concentrating zone for the solutes, and produces a narrow solvent front, which enables analysis of highly volatile compounds. Glass wool should not be inserted into these liners. The injector temperature is usually held about 50°C above the boiling point of the solvent, with the initial column temperature (if a temperature programme is available) some 10°C below the boiling point. Usually, experimentation is needed to balance the injector temperature with the column temperature and carrier gas flow to obtain the most efficient chromatography. This is the simplest capillary injector available and is compatible with most samples. The highest concentration is usually limited by the column capacity, and the smallest amount by the sensitivity of the detector.

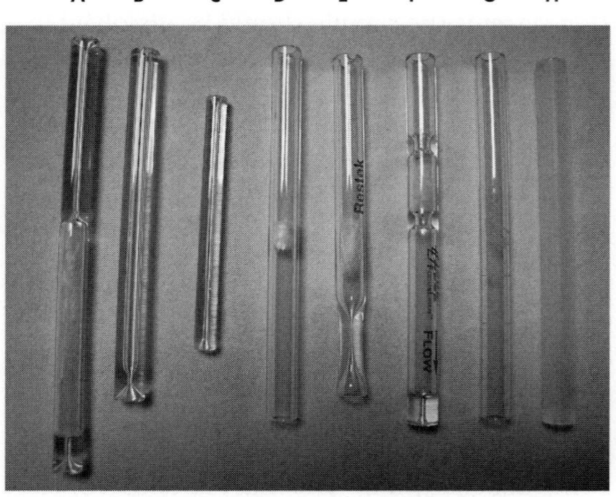

Figure 18.4 Examples of injector liners. Note the different shapes that are available and the fact that glass wool is used in some liners.

Split and splitless injectors

As noted above, modern GC instruments have the split/splitless injector combined in a single injection system (see Figure 18.5).

The split mode of injection is used for more concentrated samples, since only a fraction of the sample actually enters the column. An inlet splitter allows a high flow of carrier gas through the injector while maintaining a low flow (1–4 mL/min) through the column: the excess gas and associated sample components are vented to the atmosphere through the split line (also referred to as the split outlet/split vent). The ratio of these two flows (the split ratio) controls the proportion of the injected sample that reaches the column. The total flow through the injector may be from 10 to 100 mL/min, which gives split ratios of 10:1 to 100:1. The injection of a sample in split mode is shown in Figure 18.6. A good splitter should be linear, that is it should split high- and low-boiling point compounds equally. The function of the splitter is not primarily to reduce sample volume, but rather to ensure that the sample enters the column as a compact plug. Split injections, therefore, produce some of the most efficient chromatographic separations, and allow the use of very narrow capillary columns. A lower split ratio channels a larger fraction of the injected sample down the column and may result in column overload. High split ratios waste large amounts of carrier gas and insufficient analyte may reach the column. The analyst therefore needs to find the optimum split ratio for a particular analysis.

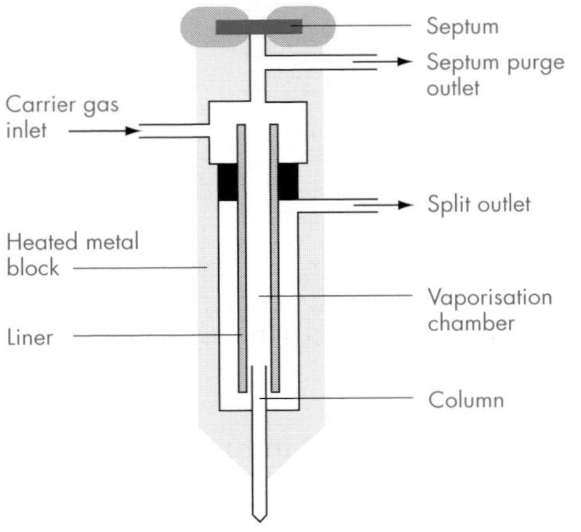

Figure 18.5 Cross section through a split/splitless injector.

In splitless injection, all the carrier gas passes to the column. This is useful for very volatile compounds, for low sample concentrations or for trace analysis. The flow rate in the injector is the same as that in the column (1–4 mL/min), and the only path for the injection to take is into the column, since the split vent is closed. At a fixed time after injection (usually 15–60 s), the injector is purged by opening the split vent to introduce a much larger flow of carrier gas through the injector (typically 20–60 mL/min) and any remaining sample in the injector is discarded through the split vent. Injection of a sample in splitless mode is shown in Figure 18.7

Since the rate of sample transfer onto the column is so slow in splitless mode (because of the low gas flow), peaks are usually somewhat broader than for split injections. Temperature conditions can be adjusted to narrow or focus the sample band at the top of the column. Splitless injections should therefore be made with the initial column temperature at least 10°C below the boiling point of the solvent, and the initial temperature should be held at least until after the purge activation time. Solvent condenses on the front of the column and traps the solute molecules, which focuses the sample into a narrow band (known as the solvent effect) (see Fig. 18.8). Individual solutes with boiling point 150°C above the initial column temperature condense and focus at the top of the column in a process known as cold trapping. Either the solvent effect or cold trapping must occur before efficient chromatography can be obtained.

Some newer chromatographs have the option of a pulsed splitless injection. In this mode, the column head pressure is increased immediately upon injection (typically to 174 kPa) and held there for 30–60 s, before returning to the normal operating pressure. This facilitates band sharpening and, while the process is not guaranteed to increase the fraction of the injection delivered onto the column, sensitivity is often improved because of improved chromatography.

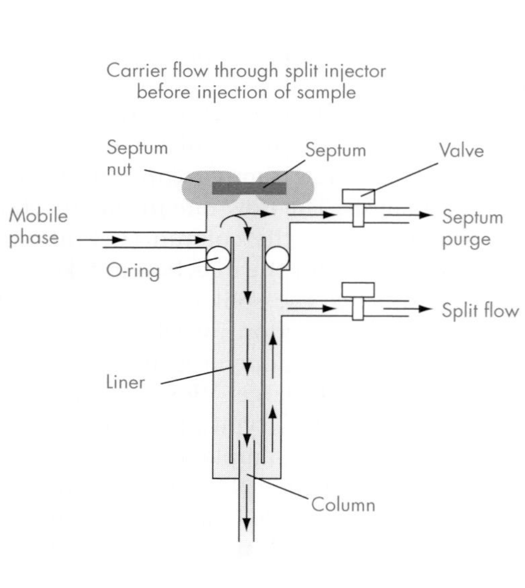

Split injector at point of injection of sample

Septum nut

Septum

Valve

Mobile phase

Septum purge

O-ring

Split flow

Liner

Column

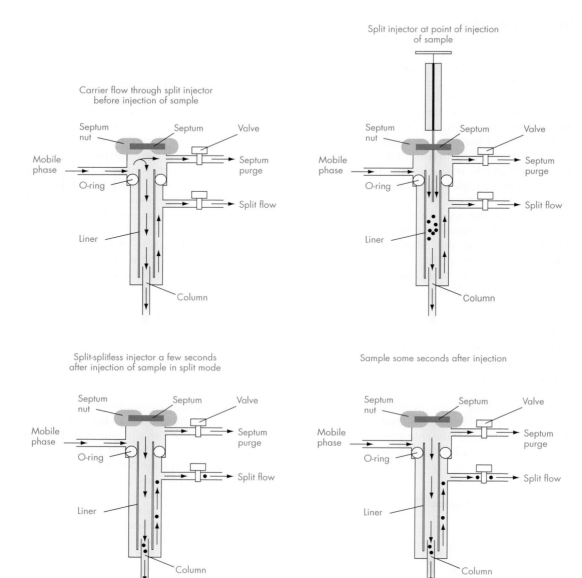

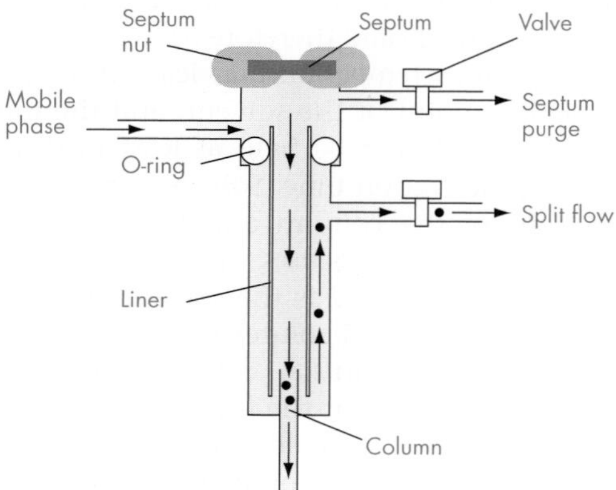

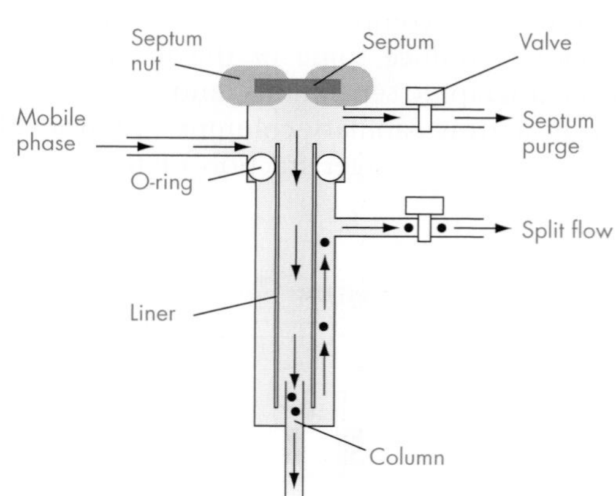

Figure 18.6 Injection of sample in split mode.

Glass liners for split and splitless injectors come in a variety of shapes and volumes (see Fig. 18.4) and it is prudent to start with a straight liner, and to investigate some of those that cause turbulence (e.g. the inverted cup style) later if this is unsatisfactory. A plug of deactivated glass wool in the liner helps prevent the deposition of nonvolatile or particulate material on the column, but may cause some peak discrimination, and for the best results needs to be placed at a consistent position in the liner. Packing splitless injection liners with

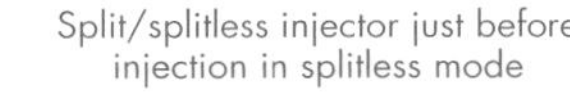

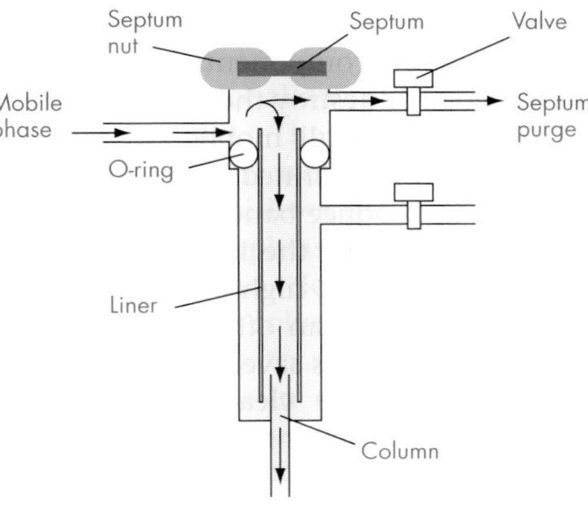

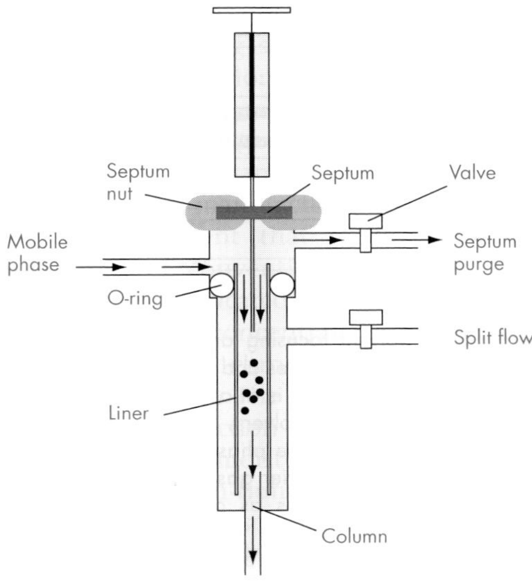

Split/splitless injector a few seconds
after injection in splitless mode

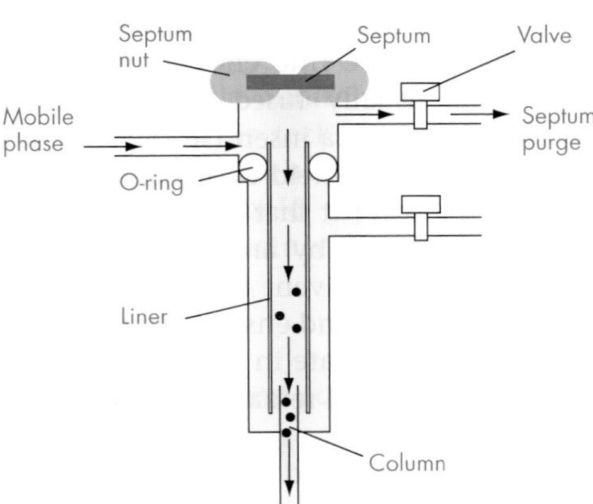

Split/splitless injector after split valve opened
ca 15–60 s after injection in splitless mode

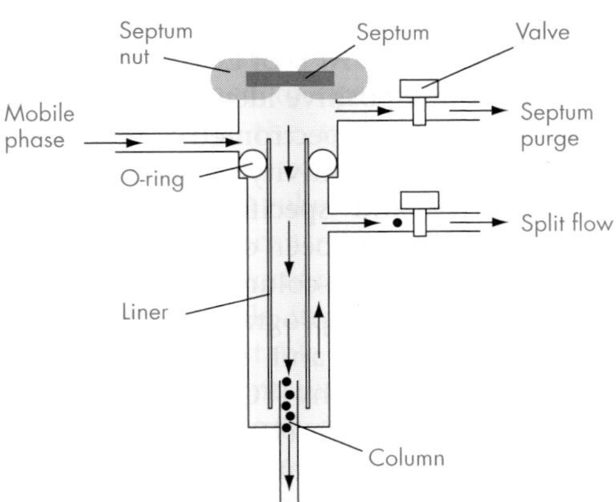

Figure 18.7 Injection of sample in splitless mode.

deactivated glass wool may decrease the chromatographic performance, but this must be weighed against the potential for damage to the stationary phase from the repeated injection of nonvolatile or particulate material.

Large-volume injectors

The analysis of trace amounts of components or contaminants in complex matrices such as foods, beverages, faeces and environmental

and for the determination of anticonvulsant drugs. A solution of the material to be injected is placed on the tip of the glass needle with a syringe. A small flow of carrier gas sweeps the solvent out of the top of the device to waste. The dry residue is then introduced by moving the needle into the heated injection zone of the chromatograph with a magnet. This form of injection can only be used with compounds that do not volatilise with the solvent.

Backflush

Upon vaporisation, the injected sample undergoes considerable expansion, sometimes up to 100 to 1000 times its original volume, which creates a pulse of pressure that often exceeds the column carrier-gas pressure. If the volume of the liner is smaller than the expanded solvent volume (see Table 18.4), some of the sample is propelled out of the injector in a process known as backflush. This can appear as a broad tailing solvent front, since it now takes longer to flush the expanded solvent out of the injector and carrier-gas line. Backflush can also cause injector contamination, since the analytes condense in the cooler carrier-gas line, from where they may bleed continuously into the injector and cause high background or spurious peaks. Carryover or peak ghosting can occur when the next injection backflushes and carries previously condensed compounds back into the vapour phase and onto the column. Backflush can usually be solved by using a smaller injection volume, a less expansive solvent, a lower injector temperature, a liner with an upper restrictor or a faster carrier gas flow. The use of an adjustable septum purge gas (0.5–1 mL/min usually) also decreases the potential for backflush, as components that would normally condense on the cooler septum and travel into the carrier-gas lines are swept away by the septum purge. Too high a purge flow results in loss of highly volatile components. Boiling points and expansion volumes for commonly used injection solvents are presented in Table 18.4

Table 18.4 Boiling points and expansion volumes for commonly used injection solvents

Solvent	Boiling point (°C)	Expansion volume (μL) per μL of solvent[a]
Methylene chloride	40	330
Carbon disulfide	46	355
Acetone	56	290
Methanol	65	525
n-Hexane	69	165
Ethyl acetate	77	215
Acetonitrile	85	405
iso-Octane	99	130
Water	100	1180
Toluene	111	200

[a] Values are given at 250°C and 105 kPa head pressure.

Injector discrimination

Injector discrimination occurs because not all the compounds in the sample vaporise at the same rate. Since the sample remains in the liner for a limited time, this usually results in some loss of higher-boiling solutes, potentially resulting in lower sensitivity for these compounds (see Fig. 18.10). It is particularly notable with split injection or splitless injection with a low purge time. Discrimination can be alleviated by increasing the residence time of the sample within the injector, or by using a higher injector temperature (Fig. 18.10) or smaller injection volume. However, there is usually a compensatory loss in lower-boiling compounds. Discriminating behaviour can usually be managed by making reproducible injections.

Gas pressure and flow control

For accurate and reproducible gas chromatography, either a constant carrier-gas flow or a constant carrier-gas pressure must be maintained. Under isothermal conditions, simple pressure control is adequate for packed or capil-

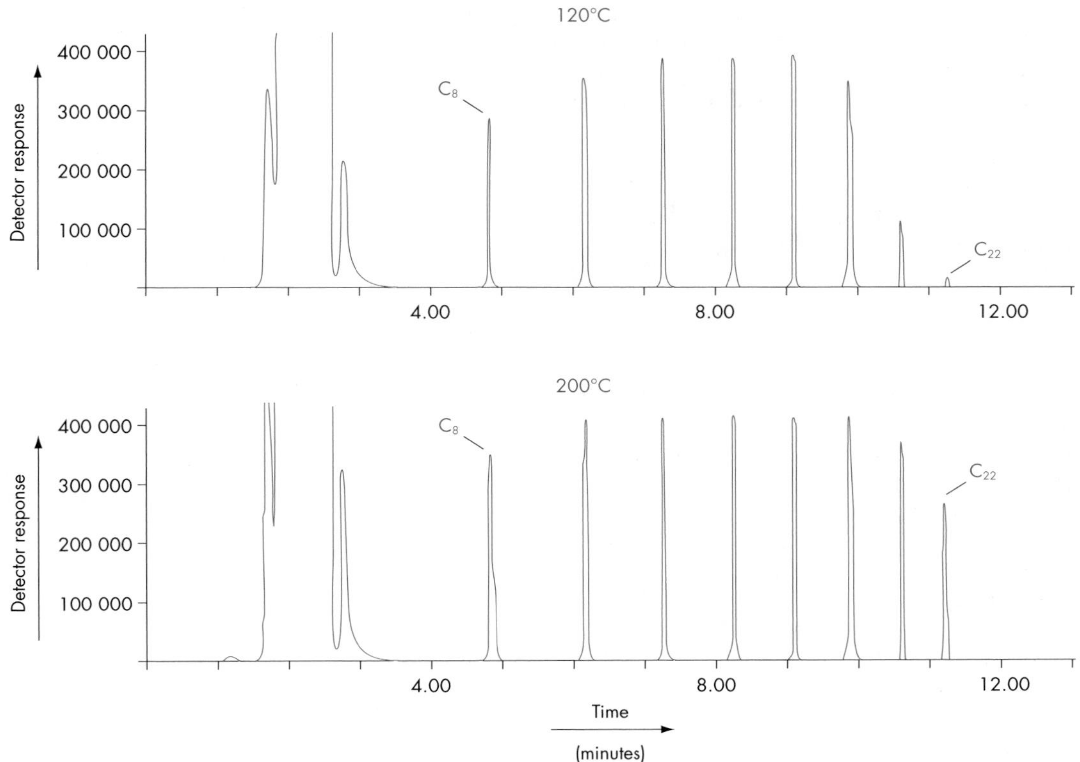

Figure 18.10 Analysis of alkanes, showing discrimination during injection. Injection in splitless mode. Note the lower signal-to-noise ratio for the alkanes with the injector at 120°C. When the injector temperature is raised to 200°C there is improved transfer of alkanes, most notably the higher boiling point alkanes.

lary columns and back pressure can be monitored by a pressure gauge between the flow controller and the injector. A decrease indicates a leaking septum and an increase suggests contamination of the injector liner or the top of the column. Flow control is highly desirable, if not essential, during temperature programming with packed columns and can be used to advantage with capillary columns. The added convenience of a digital (electronic) flow controller may be worthwhile.

Since the carrier gas becomes more viscous in the column as the temperature rises, the gas pressure must be increased as the run progresses to maintain constant velocity (or constant flow) throughout the analysis. Figure 18.11 shows the effects of increasing the column temperature on the carrier gas flow and velocity if the head pressure is held constant during the run. As flow and velocity do not respond identically to increasing temperature (see Fig. 18.11D), late-eluting analytes are recovered more quickly using constant flow than under constant pressure conditions. Furthermore, since column efficiency is a function of the carrier gas velocity (Fig. 18.12), resolution at the end of the chromatogram is improved under constant flow conditions. Switching between conditions of either constant flow or constant pressure can sometimes resolve otherwise co-eluting compounds.

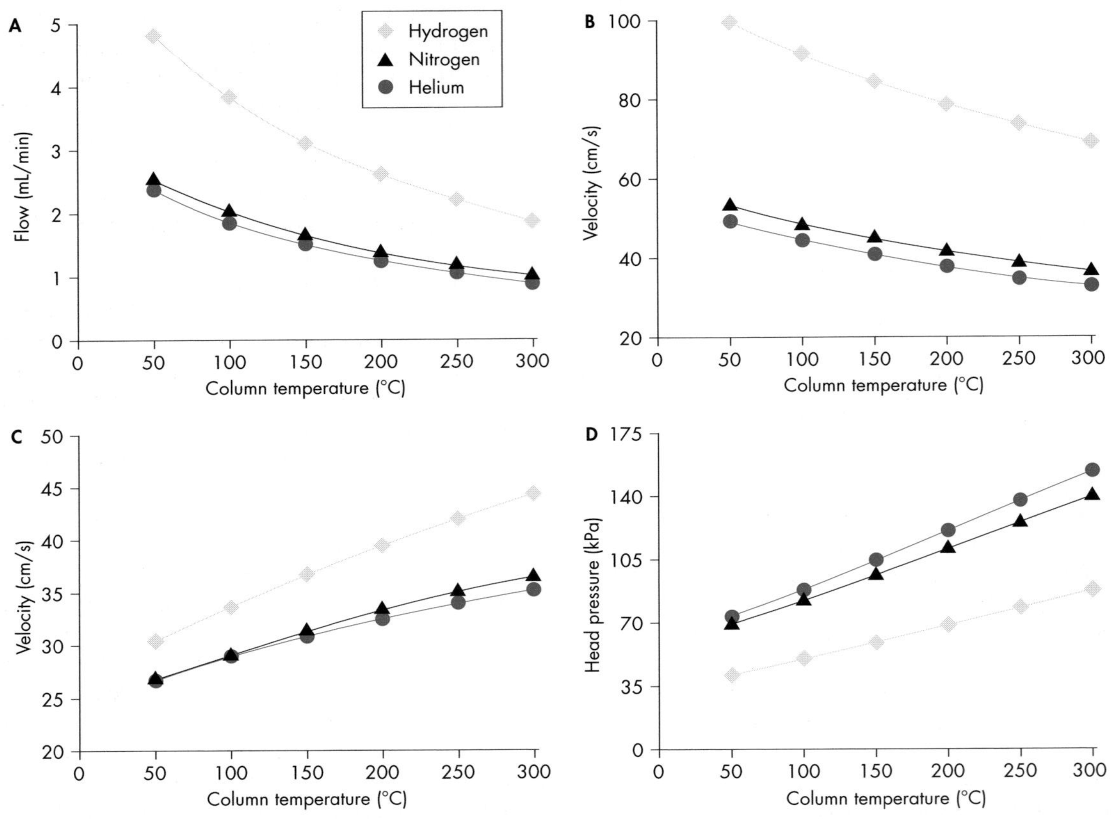

Figure 18.11 Effect of temperature on carrier-gas flow and velocity. (A) and (B) are under conditions of constant carrier-gas head pressure (140 kPa). (A) shows the change in column flow (mL/min) with change in temperature from 50 to 300°C. (B) shows the change in velocity (cm/s) with change in temperature from 50 to 300°C. (C) and (D) are under conditions of constant carrier-gas flow (1 mL/min). (C) shows the change in carrier-gas velocity (cm/s) with change in temperature from 50 to 300°C. (D) shows the change in column head pressure (kPa) with change in temperature from 50 to 300°C. All calculations are for a 25 m column of 0.25 mm i.d. operating at atmospheric pressure.

The way in which carrier-gas velocity affects column efficiency is best demonstrated by reference to the van Deemter curves in Figure 18.12. These demonstrate that the optimum column efficiency (minimum plate height, *H*) occurs at intermediate velocity, and that column efficiency is compromised at both low and very high velocity. A small loss in efficiency for a shorter analysis time is usually tolerated. Curves are shown for the three most common carrier gases (helium, nitrogen and hydrogen). Of the three gases, nitrogen produces the highest efficiency (smallest value for height equivalent of a theoretical plate; HETP) but it can be seen that the chromatography is much less tolerant to changes in nitrogen velocity than to helium. Helium is favoured by most users, as analysis times are half that with nitrogen, with only a slight loss in efficiency. Although hydrogen gives the best dynamic range and shortest analysis times, there are safety issues relating to its use. While the gas used for the carrier gas should always be of the highest purity available, a lower-quality gas can sometimes be used for the makeup or detector, since these do not contribute to column deterioration by oxidation.

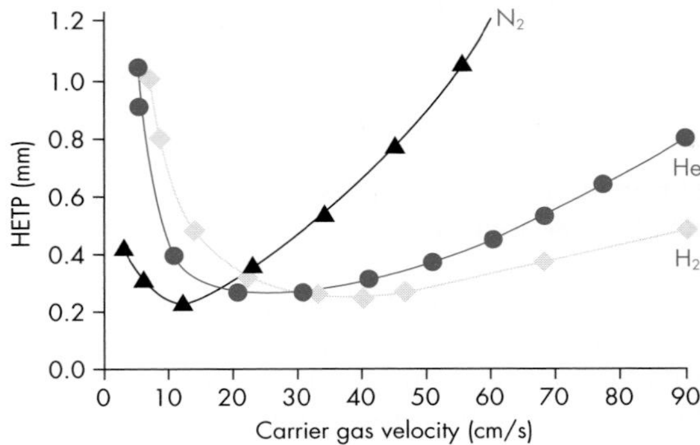

Figure 18.12 Van Deemter plots for a 25 m × 0.25 mm i.d. WCOT OV-101 column (HETP, height equivalent of a theoretical plate).

Regardless of quality, it is advisable always to use a scrubber (to remove oxygen and hydrocarbons) followed by a dryer (to remove water vapour) between the supply and the instrument. Metal trap bodies are recommended, as plastics are permeable to impurities in laboratory air, especially when large amounts of organic solvents are used. Most traps have an indicator to show when they are saturated, and they can be changed without interruption to the gas flow. Stainless steel or copper tubing is recommended for plumbing of all gases, as plastics are permeable to moisture and oxygen, and Teflon, nylon, polyethylene, polypropylene and PVC contain contaminants that degrade gas purity.

Detector systems

The choice of chromatography detector for an application depends on factors such as cost, ease of operation, consumables' supply, sensitivity, selectivity and the linear working range (see later in this section).

Some detectors respond to almost all solutes, while others (selective detectors) respond only to solutes with specific functional groups, atoms or structural configurations. Additional functional groups can often be added to solutes, generally after extraction (see p. 503), to achieve a response from a selective detector and gain additional sensitivity and selectivity. The use of detectors such as the ECD to identify amenable compounds, and the NPD to detect compounds that contain phosphorus and nitrogen, removes many of the extraneous peaks frequently observed when using nonselective detectors, such as the FID. However, these selective detectors have also led to the detection of substances such as plasticisers from blood-collection tubes or transfusion lines, which interfere in many toxicological analyses. Detectors that detect the presence of a solute and also give information about its structure are increasingly popular and MS, Fourier transform infrared spectroscopy and atomic emission spectrometry have been invoked to achieve this goal. Detector sensitivity is measured as signal-to-noise ratio, in which the signal corresponds to the height of the peak, and the noise to the height of the baseline variability. A signal-to-noise ratio of 8 to 10 is considered sufficient to confirm the presence of a peak. Each type of detector has a linear operating range in which the response obtained is directly proportional to the amount of solute that passes through, although this can be modified slightly by the nature of the solute and the chromatographic conditions (mobile phase type and flow, detector temperature). The linear operating range is considered to be exceeded when the incremental response obtained from the detector varies by more than 5% from that expected.

Most detectors (except MS) rely on gas other than the mobile phase (combustion, reagent or purge gas) for their operation. Usually, a total flow of at least 30 mL/min is necessary to sweep the solute molecules physically through the body of the detector at sufficient speed to prevent flow disturbances and produce narrow peaks. Thus, the addition of a 'makeup' gas is invariably required with capillary columns. Recommended gases and their flows for each detector are included in the manufacturer's instruction manuals, and it is important to follow these guidelines (and those on maintenance) to achieve the stated performance.

Here, only the most widely used detectors are considered in detail. Several other types of detectors are available; for a more detailed discussion, the reader is referred to the text by Scott (1996).

Flame ionisation detector (FID)

The FID is the most widely used of all detectors, since it responds to nearly all classes of compound. The effluent from the column is mixed with hydrogen and the mixture burnt at a small jet in a flow of air. A polarising current is applied between the jet and an electrode situated above it (Fig. 18.13).

When a component elutes from the column, it burns in the flame to create ions that carry a current between the electrodes and provide the signal. The background current and noise are both low. Any of the usual carrier gases can be used and minor changes in gas flow are without effect. Sensitivity is moderate (0.1–10 ng), with linearity extending sometimes as high as six orders of magnitude. The response of the FID is dependent on the number of carbon atoms in the molecule, but the response is lowered if oxygen or nitrogen is also present in the molecule. It responds to all organic compounds that contain carbon–hydrogen bonds with the exception of formic acid. Both the sensor design and electronics are simple, and manufacturing cost is therefore low. The FID is easy to clean, and when operating with capillary columns it is virtually maintenance free. With packed columns, however, there is a tendency for a build up of stationary phase bleeding from the column, which must be periodically removed. The insensitivity of the detector to water is a useful feature that allows aqueous solutions to be used.

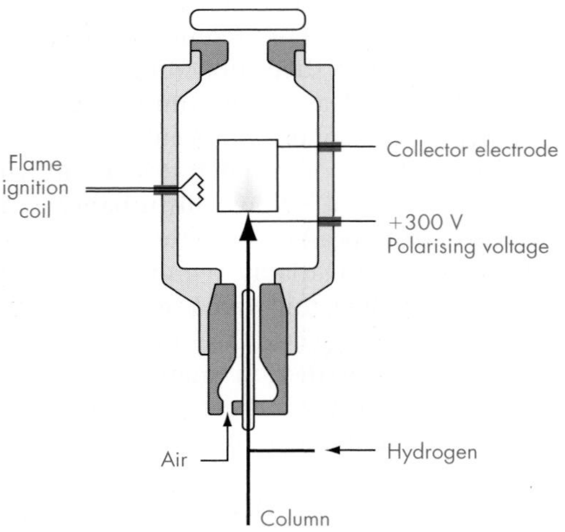

Figure 18.13 Cross-section though a flame ionisation detector.

Nitrogen–phosphorus detector (NPD) or alkali flame ionisation detector

The introduction of alkali metal vapours (usually supplied by an electrically heated bead of rubidium or caesium chloride) into the flame or 'plasma' of an FID confers an enhanced response to compounds containing phosphorus and nitrogen. By adjustment of the plasma gases, the detector can be made virtually specific for phosphorus compounds (e.g. a phosphorus:carbon response ratio of 50 000:1 and a phosphorus: nitrogen response ratio of 100:1). Even when optimised for nitrogen compounds, it retains its response to phosphorus (e.g. a nitrogen:carbon response ratio of 5000:1 and a nitrogen:phosphorus response ratio of 10:1). This detector is particularly useful for drug analysis, since most drugs contain nitrogen, while the solvent and the bulk of the co-extracted material from a biological sample do not. The NPD is ideal to detect pesticides that contain phosphorus, and therefore has wide application in environmental and regulatory analysis (air, soil, water and residues in food) and in clinical and toxicological analysis where pesticide poisoning is suspected. The extreme sensitivity to compounds that contain phosphorus can be further exploited by the preparation of derivatives that contain this element. Sensitivity is excellent (1–10 pg), with a good linear range of up to four or six orders of magnitude. A disadvantage is the need for the supply of three gases and, unlike with the FID, their control is absolutely critical to selectivity. The detecting element (bead) lasts between 1 and 3 months depending on usage. Stationary-phase bleeding from packed columns coats the bead and collector assembly and can be rinsed off using methanol or dilute (0.1 M) sulfuric acid. Most of the early problems that arose from poor reproducibility in bead coating have now been resolved, and the most stable detectors nowadays have a geometry that enables the bead to be located and fixed in its optimal position with relative ease.

Electron-capture detector (ECD)

The early form of this detector consists of a small chamber with a pair of electrodes and a radioactive source, usually ^{63}Ni, placed close to the cathode to ionise the carrier gas. Potential applied to the electrodes produces a steady background current. There is an interaction with the electrons emitted from the ^{63}Ni source with the carrier gas to produce 'low-energy' electrons. These electrons then interact with electronegative solutes (Fig. 18.14). The response of the detector is therefore a loss of signal rather than an increase, as is given by most other detectors. Although the ECD can be polarised from a suitable low-voltage direct-current supply, it is more sensitive when a pulsed power supply is used, and in modern detectors the polarising pulses are modulated to maintain a constant current. A voltage dependent on the modulation frequency is generated as the output signal. Additional carrier gas is necessary, even with packed columns, to obtain a flow of at least 60 mL/min to purge the detector adequately and avoid peak broadening and distortion. Sensitivity can also be improved dramatically by raising the operating temperature of the detector, and decreasing the makeup gas flow.

The ECD is a selective detector with a very high sensitivity to compounds that have a high affinity for electrons; for many compounds, the sensitivity of the ECD often exceeds that of MS, and sometimes even that of the NPD. Compounds that contain a halogen, nitro group or carbonyl group are detected at concentrations of 0.1–10 pg, 1–100 pg and 0.1–1 ng, respectively. This makes it very useful for compounds such as the benzodiazepines or halogenated pesticides and herbicides. Alternatively, the great sensitivity of the detector may be utilised by preparing derivatives with halogenated reagents, such as trifluoroacetic, heptafluorobutyric or pentafluoropropionic (PFP) anhydrides. Linearity (at best only two or three orders of magnitude) is a limiting factor for quantitative analysis. In older models, the addition of a small amount of quench gas, such as methane, improves stability and linearity, and is essential if argon or helium carrier gas is used. Newer models can be operated successfully with helium as both carrier and detector gas. The ECD, because of its high sensitivity, can be contaminated easily: an impure cylinder of gas can damage a detector beyond repair in a matter of only a few hours. The use of electrophilic solvents as dissolution agents for solutes should

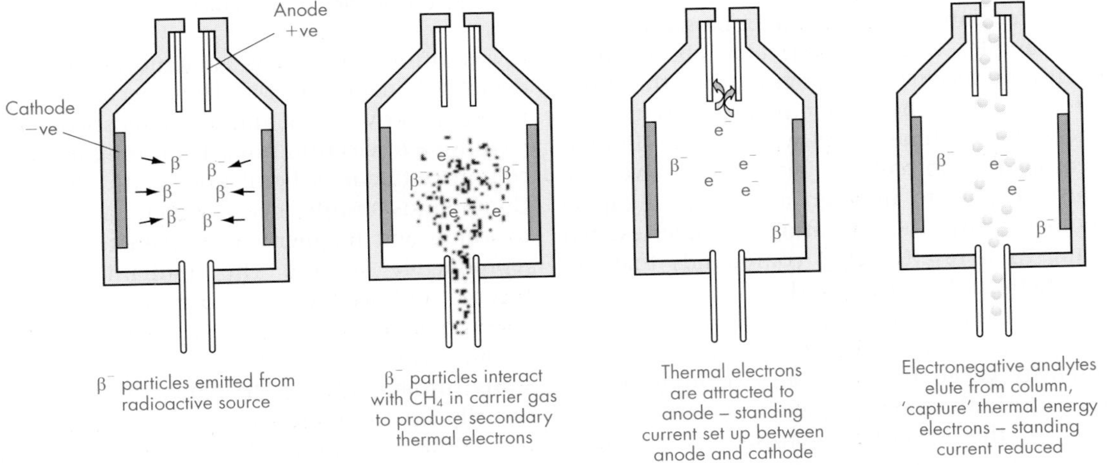
Anode
+ve
Cathode
−ve
β^- particles emitted from radioactive source
β^- particles interact with CH_4 in carrier gas to produce secondary thermal electrons
Thermal electrons are attracted to anode – standing current set up between anode and cathode
Electronegative analytes elute from column, 'capture' thermal energy electrons – standing current reduced

Figure 18.14 Schematic of operation of electron capture detector (ECD), simplified to note the most important principles of how the detector operates.

be avoided. Cleaning is difficult, although some material can be removed by heating the detector to its maximum operating temperature overnight, and the injection of water in 100 μL aliquots through an empty glass column can also help. However, if contamination is avoided, it is virtually maintenance-free. The radioactive source requires special handling procedures that may be subject to regulation. More recently, it has been shown that this detector can work with greater sensitivity and operate over an increased linear range using a helium plasma in place of the radioactive source.

Fourier transform infrared detector (FTIRD)

In the FTIRD, the column effluent is conducted through a light pipe and swept by a scavenging gas into the path of an infrared light beam that has been processed by an interferometer. The interferometer directs the entire source light to a beam splitter, which sends the light in two directions at right angles. One beam takes a fixed pathlength to a stationary mirror, while the other takes a variable pathlength to a computerised moving mirror. The two beams are recombined, and the difference in path lengths creates constructive and deconstructive interference, or an interferogram (see the associated discussion in Chapter 16 on infrared, Fig. 16.6).

The recombined beam is then passed through the sample. Analyte molecules absorb light energy of specific wavelengths from the interferogram, and the sensor reports variation in energy versus time for all wavelengths simultaneously. For molecules to be infrared active they must be able to undergo a change in dipole moment with the transition to their excited state. As a result, many compounds that are symmetrical do not respond.

Fourier transform refers to the mathematical computation that converts the data from an intensity versus time plot into an intensity (% transmission) versus frequency spectrum. Each dip in the spectrum corresponds to light absorbed, and can be interpreted as characteristic of specific functional groups in the molecule. Computer libraries allow for easy and rigorous comparison of spectra and sample identification. FTIR can be fully quantitative, but it is relatively insensitive (10 ng range). Its advantages are that it is nondestructive and it can distinguish between isomers (MS cannot).

Atomic emission detector (AED)

With the AED, carrier gas that elutes from the column delivers solutes into a high-temperature helium plasma, where heat energy is absorbed by the constituent elements. In returning to their ground state, they emit energy as light, the wavelength of which is characteristic for each element. Emitted light is focused by a quartz lens and spherical mirror onto a diffraction grating, and the dispersed light is focused onto a diode array that is continuously scanned (wavelength usually 170–800 nm). Typically, some 15 elements can be monitored simultaneously, and each is plotted against time. The composite chromatogram allows the percentage elemental composition of each peak to be determined. Sensitivity is very good and, although these detectors are complex and expensive to operate, they find use in environmental, nutritional and clinical and toxicological analysis.

Mass spectrometry (MS) detector

A gas chromatograph is an almost ideal inlet device for quadrupole MS. The detector is maintained under vacuum, and in the most common technique of electron impact (EI) ionisation the column effluent is bombarded with electrons. Compounds absorb energy, which causes them to ionise and fragment in a characteristic and reproducible fashion. The resultant ions are focused and accelerated into a mass filter that allows fragments of sequentially increasing mass to enter the detector stepwise. The mass filter scans through the designated range of masses (usually up to about 700 a.m.u.) several times per second. The abundance of each mass at a given scan time produces the mass spectrum, which can be summed and plotted versus time to obtain a total ion chromatogram (TIC). The MS detector can be operated either in full scan mode (collecting all the ions within a given mass range) or selected ion monitoring (SIM) mode, which collects only pre-selected masses characteristic for the compound under study. Sensitivity for the two modes of operation is quite different, 1–10 ng for full scan, increasing to 1–10 pg in SIM because of the dramatic decrease in background noise. The linear range is excellent and often spans five or six orders of magnitude. Recent advances in computer technology, coupled with improved detector design, have revolutionised the use of the MS detector from a research tool to one of routine application. This technique is described in more detail in Chapter 21.

Ion-trap mass spectrometer

In ion-trap mass spectrometers the production of ions in EI or chemical ionisation (CI) mode is achieved in pulses rather than continuously. The fundamental difference is that all the solute ions generated over the entire pulse period are trapped in the detector and are then sequentially ejected in increasing mass number from the trap into the electron multiplier. The addition of helium into the trap (133 mPa) contracts the ion trajectory to the centre of the trap, where it is further focused by the ring electrode to form dense ion packets that are expelled more efficiently than diffuse clouds, and thus greatly improves resolution. The spectral patterns can be quite different from those produced by mass filter spectrometers, and are often characteristic of the conditions under which the instrument is run, which makes comparison difficult between instruments. However, because the ion collection period is longer, the sensitivity of the ion trap in full scan mode is similar to that obtained in SIM on the average mass spectrometer. Furthermore, an improved mass range (sometimes up to several thousand a.m.u.) gives this type of detector many applications, particularly for quantitative trace analysis, and for higher mass components. This technique is described in more detail in Chapter 21.

Dual detector systems

The simultaneous use of a combination of a universal detector (FID) with a specific detector to monitor the effluent of a column can provide useful information about the properties of functional groups and substituents in a molecule. The FID response is roughly dependent on the number of carbon atoms in a molecule and is quite predictable. However, the ECD response varies widely for different compounds, is dependent on the electron-deficient part of the compound, and is difficult to predict. The NPD response of a compound depends to some extent on the number of phosphorus or nitrogen atoms in a molecule, but it also depends on their environment. Thus, by using the FID as a reference, and measuring the ECD or NPD response relative to it, another characteristic for identification is obtained in addition to retention behaviour (see Fig. 18.15).

Dual detector systems can be used in several ways. The column can be split at the detector end and the effluent passed into two different detectors that operate in parallel. This approach allows the most flexibility, since the choice of detectors is wide, and the effluent can be split in proportion to the sensitivity required from each detector. For capillary columns this is accomplished easily with zero dead volume press-fit tee connectors, but it is a more complicated operation for packed columns. Additional makeup gas may be required to ensure a good flow through the detectors, and care should be taken to use tubing of area smaller than or equal to the total area of the analytical column to avoid loss of peak shape through refluxing at the detector. Alternatively, the GC oven houses two completely separate but identically matched columns, each connected to a single detector. This is not an ideal approach, as matching of columns is difficult and has to be checked at frequent intervals. Another approach is to stack the detectors in series, and some manufacturers deliberately provide detectors in identical modules for this purpose. There are limitations to the choice of possible detector combinations, as the first detector must always be a nondestructive detector, such as the ECD, AED or FTIRD.

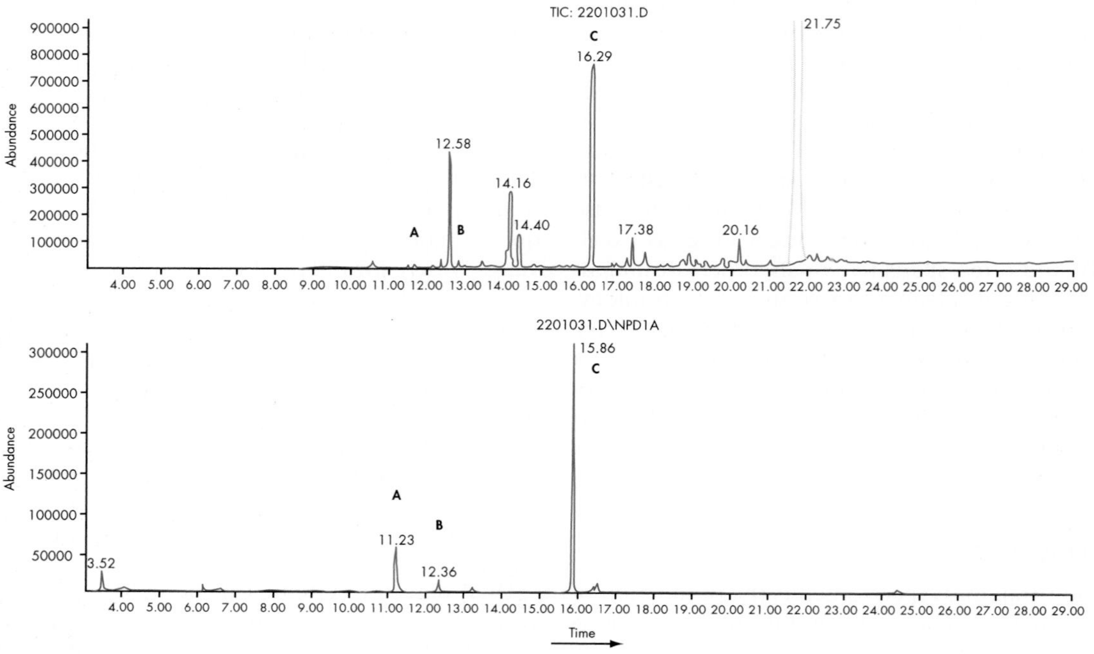

Figure 18.15 Analysis of basic drugs in blood using dual GC-MS and GC-NPD detection. A, caffeine; B, propyphenazone; C, proadifen (used as internal standard for the analysis). *Upper trace:* GC-MS TIC chromatogram. *Lower trace:* GC-NPD chromatogram. Several nitrogen-containing drugs barely detected by GC-MS in scan mode are clearly detected by the NPD detector, indicating the high sensitivity of NPD. The lower chromatographic trace is much simpler, indicating the high specificity offered by NPD detectors. Note: there is a slight difference in retention times between the two columns because columns of different length were used for the analysis. (Reprinted from A. Beat and Werner, Gas chromatography with dual mass spectrometric and nitrogen-phosphorus specific detection: a new and powerful tool for forensic analyses, *Forensic Science International*, 1999, **102**, 11, with permission from Elsevier.)

Specimen preparation

Prior to chromatography, it is usually necessary to isolate the compound(s) of interest from either a biological matrix (plasma, urine, stomach contents, hair and tissue) or some other matrix, such as soil, food and drink, tablets and other drug formulations, air or water. Removal of extraneous material and concentration of the compounds of interest usually take place simultaneously. The high water solubility of some drug metabolites (e.g. glucuronide conjugates) requires chemical conversion to a less polar entity to permit isolation from water-based samples, and a hydrolysis procedure is often used for this purpose.

Hydrolysis

Recovery of conjugated drug metabolites from biological fluids can be increased by hydrolytic cleavage of the conjugate bond prior to extraction. This offers a vast improvement in sensitivity for qualitative analysis, particularly from urine, and is essential to identify drugs (e.g. laxatives) that are excreted almost exclusively as conjugated metabolites. However, reliable quantitative analysis of conjugated metabolites requires that the unconjugated metabolite must first be removed or quantified, and then the total (conjugated plus unconjugated) metabolite be measured after hydrolysis in a subsequent separate procedure. For quantitative work, appropriate standards that contain conjugated metabolites must be carried through the procedure to monitor the efficiency of the hydrolysis step.

Enzymatic hydrolysis

The use of a specific enzyme to cleave chemical bonds is the more specific of the two approaches, but incurs additional cost and time. It also provides cleaner extracts, and therefore prolongs the life of the chromatography column. There are a number of commercial preparations of purified glucuronidases and sulfatases harvested from different species. It is important to pay attention to the pH and temperature optima of the specific enzyme preparation. The best results are achieved by overnight hydrolysis at 37°C (C. Luckie *et al.*, unpublished data); however, temperature-tolerant preparations allow heating up to 60°C, which permits relatively short (2 h) incubation times.

Chemical hydrolysis

This quicker and less expensive approach can provide suitable extracts for chromatography for some analytes, although they are generally more demanding in terms of clean-up procedures. Typically, strong mineral acids or alkalis are used, often with boiling or treatment in a microwave or pressure cooker. Extracts must be neutralised, otherwise the chromatography column deteriorates quickly. Care should be taken to ensure the stability of the analytes to the hydrolysis conditions. Vigorous hydrolysis conditions often yield undesirable by-products or, if several compounds can be hydrolysed to a single entity, preclude accurate identification of the original compound present. For example, both the acid and the enzymatic hydrolysis of benzodiazepines remove glucuronide conjugates, but acid hydrolysis also converts two or three drugs to the same benzophenone compound. Diazepam, temazepam and ketazolam are all converted into 2-methylamino-5-chlorobenzophenone; while this compound has good chromatography characteristics, the approach is unsuitable for those applications (such as forensic analysis) that require absolute identification of the drug ingested.

Isolation and concentration

Protein precipitation

If the analyte is present in blood in high concentration, a simple protein precipitation step often provides a suitable extract, although the possibility of losing significant amounts of analyte with the precipitate must be considered. Mixing with a solution of mercuric chloride or barium sulfate readily precipitates plasma proteins, and centrifugation provides a supernatant for direct injection onto the chromatography column. Use of perchloric or trichloroacetic acids (10%) is not advised, unless the resultant solution is neutralised prior to injection. Dimethylformamide is a good organic precipitation reagent that is well tolerated by most GC stationary phases. Other organic precipitating agents are methanol, acetone and acetonitrile, all of which should be added in the proportion of two volumes to each volume of blood. While the extract is still water-based, most columns with a high stationary-phase loading (5 μm film thickness) can tolerate the injection of 1 μL of water. If the column is not water tolerant, it is possible to evaporate small volumes of the supernatant to dryness for reconstitution in a more suitable solvent. Caution must be exercised for some solutes when evaporating aqueous solutions because volatile components may be lost, e.g. amfetamine and methamfetamine in base form are relatively volatile.

Liquid–liquid extraction

Liquid–liquid extraction is the most frequently used method to isolate and concentrate solutes for GC. The pH of the specimen is adjusted to ensure that the compounds to be extracted are not ionised (basic for bases, acid for acidic compounds). Bearing in mind that some portion of the aqueous acid or base will dissolve in the solvent, the use of strong mineral acids or alkalis is not advised as this adversely affects column performance. Best results are obtained with acidic buffers (phosphate or acetate) and with ammonium hydroxide or basic buffers (borate), using a 5:1 ratio of solvent to specimen. The solvent chosen should be sufficiently polar to partition the compound of interest without co-extracting excessive amounts of polar contaminants. For more water-soluble drugs, such as β-blockers, the addition of 2–10% of a polar solvent (e.g. propan-2-ol or butanol) is helpful, or solid sodium chloride can be added to 'salt out' the analyte. If a derivatisation step is to be carried out subsequently, the use of a solvent compatible with the derivatisation eliminates the need for an evaporation step. Use of solvents with a higher density than the sample (e.g. dichloromethane) can lead to difficulty in isolation of the organic phase. Purification of extracts by back extraction (re-extraction of the analytes from the organic solvent at the opposite pH followed by re-extraction into solvent at the original pH) may be helpful for trace analysis. The use of a small volume of solvent for the final extraction serves as a concentration step without the need for separation and evaporation of the organic phase.

Solid–liquid or solid-phase extraction

Solid-phase extraction (SPE) uses a polypropylene cartridge with a small amount (200 mg to 3 g) of high-capacity (1–20 mL) silica-based packing at the base of the reservoir. On introduction of the sample matrix, the compounds of interest are withheld by the packing. Impurities are then rinsed selectively from the column, and the final elution releases the compound of interest (Fig. 18.16).

Evaporation followed by reconstitution in a suitable solvent provides a clean, concentrated sample ready for analysis by GC. Bonded-phase packings that have been modified by the addition of various functional groups are available. The mechanisms of interaction for the matrix, analytes and packings are similar to those in liquid chromatography (see Chapter 19). Polar stationary phases preferentially retain polar analytes (normal phase) and are eluted with organic solvents, while nonpolar stationary phases preferentially retain nonpolar analytes (reversed phase) and are eluted with aqueous solvents. Ion-pair extraction uses a nonpolar stationary phase and polar analyte, with a counterion added to the sample solution, and allows retention of the (now neutral) analyte by a reversed-phase mechanism. In ion-exchange extraction, the adsorbent surface is modified with ionisable functionalities. Analytes with ionic charges opposite to those on the packing

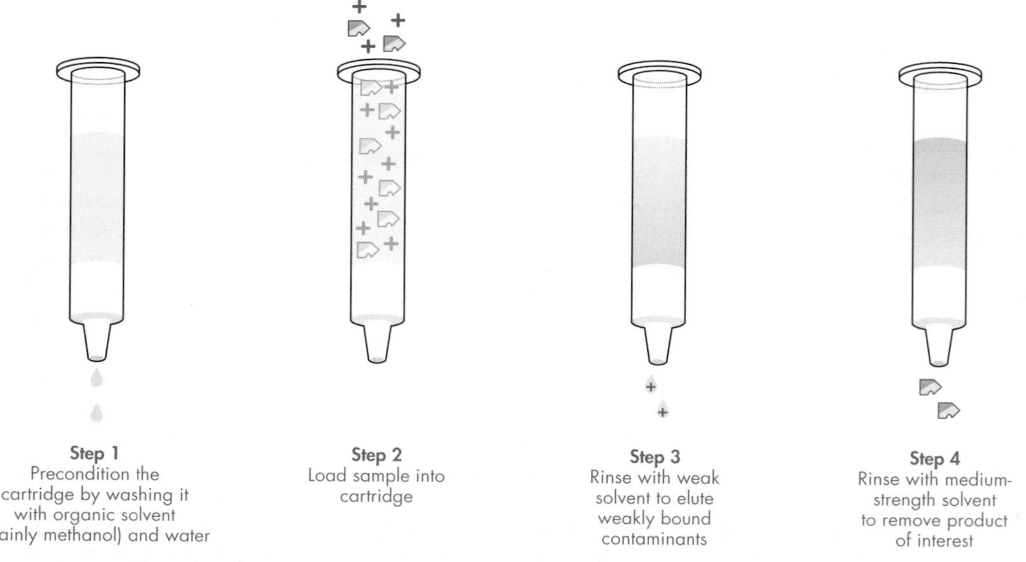
Step 1
Precondition the cartridge by washing it with organic solvent (mainly methanol) and water
Step 2
Load sample into cartridge
Step 3
Rinse with weak solvent to elute weakly bound contaminants
Step 4
Rinse with medium-strength solvent to remove product of interest

Figure 18.16 Steps involved in SPE.

are retained. Solvents that contain counterions of greater strength are used to elute the analytes of interest from the tube.

Solid-phase microextraction

Solid-phase microextraction (SPME) requires no solvents or complicated apparatus and can concentrate volatile and nonvolatile compounds in both liquid and gas samples. The unit consists of a fused-silica fibre attached to a stainless-steel plunger coated with a stationary phase (mixed with solid adsorbents as required). The plunger is inserted through a septum into a vial that contains the sample, and the fibre is exposed by depressing the plunger either into the liquid or the headspace for 20–30 min. The retracted fibre is inserted into the injection port of the GC, and is desorbed when the plunger is depressed (Fig. 18.17).

The unit may be reconditioned and used 50 to 100 times. For field analysis, adsorbed samples can be stored and transported in the needle sealed in a special container for subsequent analysis by GC (or LC). Pesticides recovered from water samples have been shown to be more

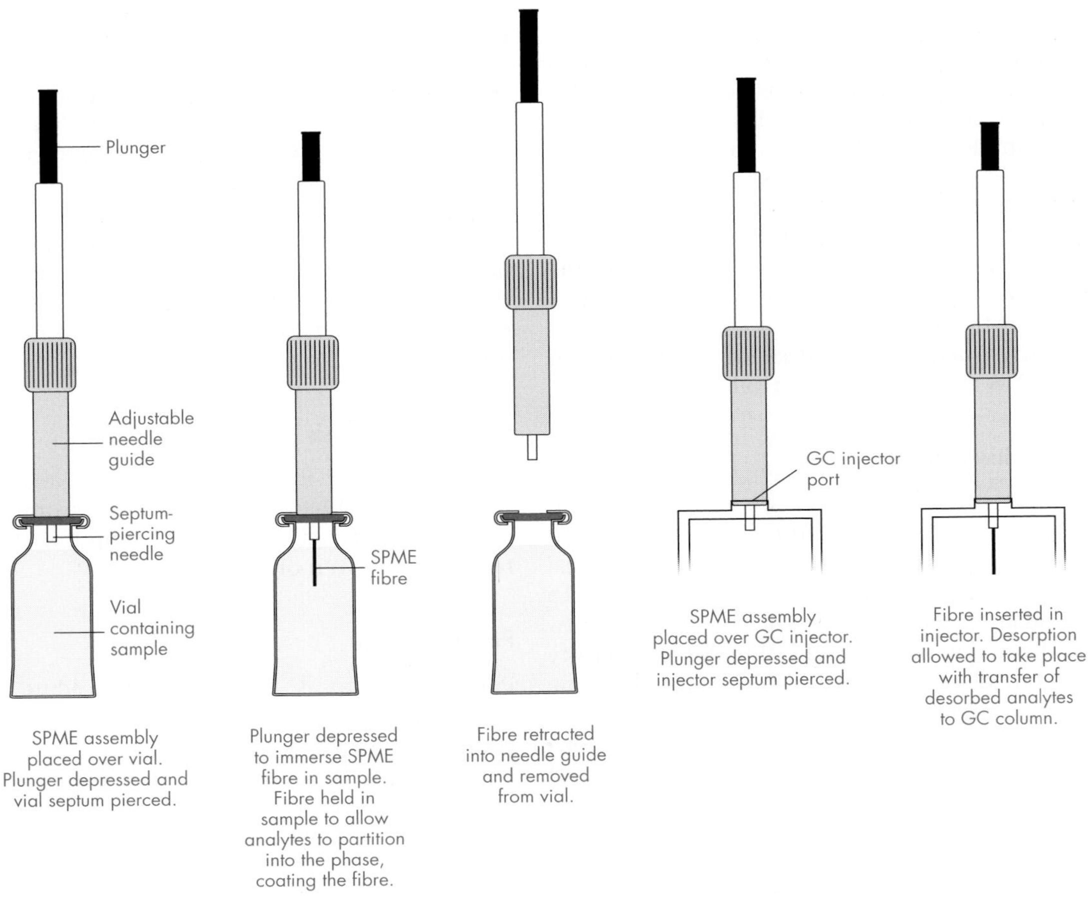
Plunger
Adjustable needle guide
Septum-piercing needle
Vial containing sample
SPME fibre
GC injector port
SPME assembly placed over vial. Plunger depressed and vial septum pierced.
Plunger depressed to immerse SPME fibre in sample. Fibre held in sample to allow analytes to partition into the phase, coating the fibre.
Fibre retracted into needle guide and removed from vial.
SPME assembly placed over GC injector. Plunger depressed and injector septum pierced.
Fibre inserted in injector. Desorption allowed to take place with transfer of desorbed analytes to GC column.

Figure 18.17 Extraction using solid-phase microextraction (SPME). The SPME fibre is coated with a phase similar to the types of stationary phases used in GC. Analytes partition into the phase and hence are extracted from solution. It is also possible to carry out headspace analysis using SPME in which case the fibre is held in the headspace above the sample.

stable when stored in this way than in water. The special small-volume injection liner fits any model of chromatograph, and produces sharper peaks because of the higher linear gas velocity, with little or no backflush. Suitable stationary phases are:

- 100 μm dimethyl-PSX film for low-molecular-weight compounds or volatiles, or a thinner film (7 μm) for higher-weight semivolatile compounds
- 85 μm polyacrylate film for polar compounds
- 65 μm film of dimethyl-PSX–divinyl benzene for volatile alcohols and amines
- for surfactants, 50 μm Carbowax-templated resin
- for trace level volatiles, a 75 μm Carbowax–carboxen phase is suitable.

An alternative approach uses a small magnetic stir bar encapsulated in glass and coated with a layer of dimethyl-PSX. The bar is left to stir in the sample for 30–120 min and then removed and placed in a thermal desorption tube. From there, it is introduced onto the GC as described in the section on thermal desorption injectors (p. 489). Both approaches give similar performance for higher-boiling compounds (>350°C), but SPME is inferior for lower-boiling compounds such as naphthalene and fluorene (b.p. 218 and 298°C, respectively).

Supercritical fluid extraction

A supercritical fluid (SCF) is a substance that is maintained above its critical temperature and pressure, where it exhibits physicochemical properties intermediate between those of a liquid and a gas. Properties of gas-like diffusivity, gas-like viscosity and liquid-like density combined with a pressure-dependent solvating power provided the impetus to apply SCFs to analytical separation. The initial applications most often involved isolation of flavours and contaminant residues from food and soil. These have now been extended to the isolation of drugs from blood and other aqueous-based media by using adsorbents added in-line (such as molecular sieves, diatomaceous earth, silica gel, and so on) to filter proteinaceous material and adsorb water. It is possible, by adding small volumes of co-solvent to the SCF, to extract highly polar solutes with excellent efficiency. In contrast to the conventional extracting solvents, the fluid most often used in supercritical fluid extraction (SFE) – supercritical carbon dioxide – is nonpolluting, nontoxic and relatively inexpensive. Additionally, extractions are carried out quickly at temperatures that avoid degradation of temperature-sensitive analytes and provide clean extracts with extremely high efficiency. Several dedicated SFE analysers are available; each consists of a gas supply, pump and controller used to pressurise the gas, temperature-controlled oven, extraction vessel, internal diameter regulator and collection device. The supply carbon dioxide is compressed to a selected pressure (e.g. 28 000 kPa) and its temperature is adjusted (e.g. 50°C). As the supercritical CO_2 passes through the sample material, the solutes are extracted to an equilibrium solubility level, typically about 10% (w/w). The gaseous solution that leaves the extractor is passed through the pressure reduction valve, where the pressure (and thus the dissolving power) of the CO_2 is reduced. The solutes precipitate in the separator, and the CO_2 is recycled through the system several times until the extraction is completed, when it is vented to waste.

Headspace analysis

This method of isolation is used for analytes with volatility higher than that of the common extraction solvents. A detailed description of the technique is given on p. 311.

Purge and trap

Purge and trap is a powerful procedure for extracting and concentrating volatile organic compounds from soil, sediment, water, food, beverages, etc. It is especially useful for poorly water-soluble compounds and those with boiling points above 200°C. The procedure involves bubbling an inert gas (nitrogen or helium) through an aqueous sample or suspension at ambient temperature, which causes volatile organic compounds to be transferred into the vapour phase. Alternatively, an inert gas is passed across the headspace of the sample and onto the trap. The removal of volatile components from the headspace causes the sample–headspace equilibrium to be perturbed such that further vaporisation of the volatile components occurs, resulting in concentration of sample in the trap. During the purge step, purge gas sweeps the vapour through a trap containing adsorbent materials that retain the volatilised compounds. Water vapour may be removed by dry purging. The trap is rapidly heated to 5–10°C below the desorption temperature. The valve is then switched to join the trap flow to the carrier-gas flow, and the trap heated to its desorption temperature for a fixed time. Adsorbent tubes are usually packed with multiple beds of sorbent materials, each one more active than the preceding one, which allows compounds with a wide range of boiling points and polarities to be analysed simultaneously. During purge, the smaller and more nonpolar solutes are readily carried down the beds, and since the carrier gas passes in the opposite direction during the desorption phase, the larger and more polar compounds do not come into contact with the innermost active beds, from which their release may be difficult to effect.

Thermal desorption

This technique is used extensively for air monitoring in industrial hygiene, environmental air, indoor air or source-emission monitoring and for examination of accelerant residues in arson investigations. Devices may be portable or fixed and of varying size. In some devices the trap is integral whereas in others the trapping device is a removable tube packed with the adsorbent. This tube is then attached to a pump or a syringe for sampling. Air is pumped continuously through the device or adsorbent tube at a fixed rate or, in the case of a syringe attached to the adsorbent tube, drawn up by hand. Components are concentrated onto the adsorbent beds. The arrangement of the beds may be the same as described above for the purge and trap or it may be a single adsorbent. The direction of the flow is simply reversed during desorption. Analysis requires a special interface to the GC. For removable adsorbent tubes, the tube is fitted into a specially designed thermal desorption unit. The adsorbents must have high capacity to remain active during the entire sampling period, and show an acceptable pressure drop during sampling. Ideally, a minimal amount of unwanted analytes should be absorbed, as these will contribute to the background noise.

Tissues and hair

Tissues and hair require treatment prior to drug extraction to break down the biological matrix and enable a good recovery of the drug. For solid tissues, good results are obtained by incubation of a portion of the tissue with a mixture of a collagenase, a protease and a lipase in a buffer of suitable pH. For small amounts of tissues (100 mg), overnight treatment at room temperature suffices, although gentle agitation or occasional mixing speeds up the process. Larger amounts of tissue benefit from mechanical homogenisation prior to incubation. For the analysis of hair, an initial washing to remove residues from cosmetic products or environmental contaminants is recommended, followed by incubation with either caustic alkali (for basic drugs) or mineral acid (for acidic drugs). After adjustment of the pH, drug recovery can proceed by the usual procedures established for the specific compounds under investigation. For additional information see p. Chapters 6, 7 and 8.

Derivative formation

The main reasons derivatisation is performed are:

- to permit analysis of compounds not directly amenable to analysis owing to inadequate volatility or stability
- to improve the analysis by improving chromatographic behaviour or detectability.

To some extent the availability of stable polar stationary phases in capillary columns and the use of temperature programming has negated the requirement for derivatisation, although it is still widely used. Choice of reagent is based on the functional group that requires derivatisation, the presence of other functional groups in the molecule and the reason for performing the reaction. Although the retention characteristics are changed, the order of elution of a series of derivatives will be the same as that for the parent compounds. The preparation of derivatives modifies the functionality of the solute molecule to increase (or sometimes decrease) volatility, and thereby shortens or lengthens the retention time of a substance, or to speed up the analysis. The major derivatisation reactions for GC are silylation, alkylation and acylation.

Silylation is usually used as an abbreviation for trimethylsilylation. Examples of derivatising agents include: *N,O*-bis(trimethylsilyl)trifluoroacetamide (BSTFA); a mixture of BSTFA and trimethylchlorosilane (TMCS); *N*-methyltrimethylsilyltrifluoroacetamide (MSTFA); *N*-methyl-*N*-(*t*-butyldimethylsilyl)trifluoro acetamide (MTBSTFA); and others. Typically derivatives are formed by replacement of active hydrogens from acids, alcohols, thiols, amines, amides, ketones and aldehydes with the trimethylsilyl group.

Alkylation. Typical derivatives are formed by replacement of an active hydrogen (carboxylic acids and phenols) by an aliphatic or aliphatic-aromatic (i.e. benzyl) group. The reagents include 3 M HCl in butanol or *N,N*-dimethylformamide dimethyl acetal.

Acylation is the conversion of compounds that contain active hydrogen (—OH, —SH, and —NH) into esters, thioesters and amides, respectively. Typical derivatising reagents include heptafluoropropionic anhydride (HFPA), pentafluoropropionic anhydride (PFPA), and others. An example of a derivatising reaction is presented in Fig 18.18.

Derivatisation can improve resolution and reduce tailing of polar compounds (hydroxyl, carboxylic acids, hydrazines, primary amines and sulfhydryl groups). For instance, hydroxylated compounds often have long retention times and column adsorption causes tailing, which results in low sensitivity. However, they readily form silyl ethers and these derivatives show excellent chromatography; sensitivity can often be improved by a factor of 10 or more.

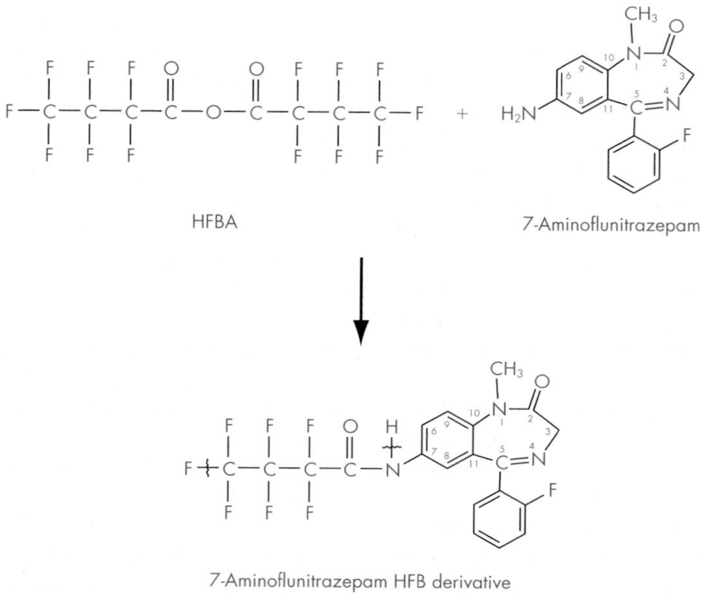

HFBA

7-Aminoflunitrazepam

7-Aminoflunitrazepam HFB derivative

Figure 18.18 Derivatisation of 7-aminoflunitrazepam with heptafluorobutyric anhydride (HFBA).

Derivatisation can also help to remove the substance peak away from interfering material.

Derivatives may also be used to make the molecule amenable to detection by selective detectors (e.g. introducing halogens to the molecule can increase detectability by an electron capture detector, see Fig 18.18), or can be used to improve the fragmentation pattern of the compound in the mass spectrometer.

Derivatisation reactions may be carried out during extraction (e.g. extractive alkylation), on the dry residue after solvent extraction (e.g. silylation), or during injection (e.g. methylation). In choosing a suitable reagent, certain criteria must be used. A good reagent produces stable derivatives without harmful by-products that interact with the analytical column, in a reaction that is almost 100% complete. Poor reagents cause rearrangements or structural alterations during formation, and contribute to loss of sample during reaction. Most manufacturers of derivatising reagents provide information on the potential uses of each product, along with standard operating instructions. Entire texts, such as that by Blau and Halket (1993), are devoted to this topic.

Chiral separations

Chiral compounds can be derivatised to improve their chromatographic characteristics, and the enantiomers separated on a chiral stationary phase. Both enantiomers behave similarly, provided that steric hindrance does not preclude a reaction with one enantiomer. An alternative approach is to use a chiral derivatising reagent which, when reacted with enantiomers, produces diastereoisomers that can then be separated on a conventional stationary phase. As with enantiomers, diastereoisomers still produce similar mass spectra, but they are resolved in time by the chromatography column. This approach is less expensive and also less restrictive, since a dedicated column is not required. Care should be taken to ensure the enantiomeric purity of the derivatising reagent, and to guard against racemisation during the reaction. *n*-Trifluoroacetyl-1-propyl chloride (TPC) in triethylamine and chloroform (or ethyl acetate) is a commonly used chiral reagent that couples with enantiomeric amines. Excess reagent is washed off with 6 M HCl and the organic phase is dried over magnesium sulfate. For chiral alcohols, (1*R*,2*S*,5*R*)-(−)-menthylchloroformate (MCF) reacts well if pyridine is used as a catalyst.

Quantitative determinations

Quantitative work usually requires some form of sample preparation to isolate the drug from the bulk of the sample and some degree of concentration or, more rarely, dilution. These processes inevitably introduce a degree of analytical error. A further problem is caused by the difficulty of reproducibly transferring the same mass of all sample components to the GC column with each injection. To compensate for these errors, it is usual to compare the response of the unknown with the response of an added internal standard. The internal standard should be added as early as possible in the assay process and should have chromatographic properties matching those of the solute as closely as possible, preferably with a longer retention time. It is often possible to obtain unmarketed analogues of drugs, or compounds specially synthesised for use as internal standards (e.g. a methyl addition or a halogen substitution). However, the internal standard usually does not behave exactly as the drug and careful control of variables, such as pH, is necessary. If a derivative is to be prepared, the internal standard should also be amenable to derivatisation. Use of an inappropriate internal standard can seriously affect precision (Dudley 1980). If a mass spectrometer is being used as the detector, then the ideal internal standard is a ^{2}H-substituted (deuterated) analogue of the drug, a number of which are readily available at reasonable cost. Some examples of deuterated internal standards are shown in Figure 18.19. Potential disadvantages of deuterated internal standards include a possibility of chemical exchange and loss of a label. In addition, the presence of too many ^{2}H atoms may alter the chromatographic properties of a labelled compound. The alternative solution is to use compounds labelled with stable isotopes such as ^{13}C. Calibration should include points of higher and lower concentrations than the sample, and quality assurance samples should be included at appropriate concentrations in frequently run assays.

Peak measurement may be by peak height or by the peak area obtained by integration. If the peaks show even a modest degree of tailing, use of peak area usually provides a more accurate quantitative result. A plot of the ratio of peak height (or area) of the drug to internal standard versus concentration is a straight line with most detectors. Care should be taken in the preparation of standards to match the matrix to that of the specimens, and to allow for any associated salt or water of crystallisation in the calculation of the concentration. The best results are obtained when the amount of internal standard used produces a peak response ratio of unity at the mid point of the calibration range.

Optimising operation conditions to customise applications

If sensitivity is an issue, it can be increased by increasing sample size, using a concentration step, derivatisation, injecting a larger sample volume, selecting a different stationary phase and using the detector at a higher sensitivity level.

When attempting a new analysis, it is advisable first to review published literature for a method that can be copied or for a method that involves a similar type of compound and can be adapted. Column manufacturers' catalogues or websites are a useful source of information and invariably show examples of separations performed with their columns, and manufacturers typically have technical departments to offer specific advice. Data on boiling points and RI are also useful indicators, as is consideration of the chemical structure of the substances present in the sample. If the review is not helpful, a start can be made with a standard column, selecting either a 100% methyl-PSX capillary column (25 m with a 0.25 μm film or an OV1-packed column (1.7 m with a 3% loading on 100–120 mesh support) and using standard flow conditions (1–2 mL/min helium for a capillary or 30–60 mL/min for a packed column). The oven temperature should be taken from 80 to 300°C at 10°C/min (or started at 200 or 250°C if only an isothermal oven is available). Lower temperatures may be needed for substances which are relatively volatile. A solution of the compounds of interest in ethanol or methanol should be injected with the injector

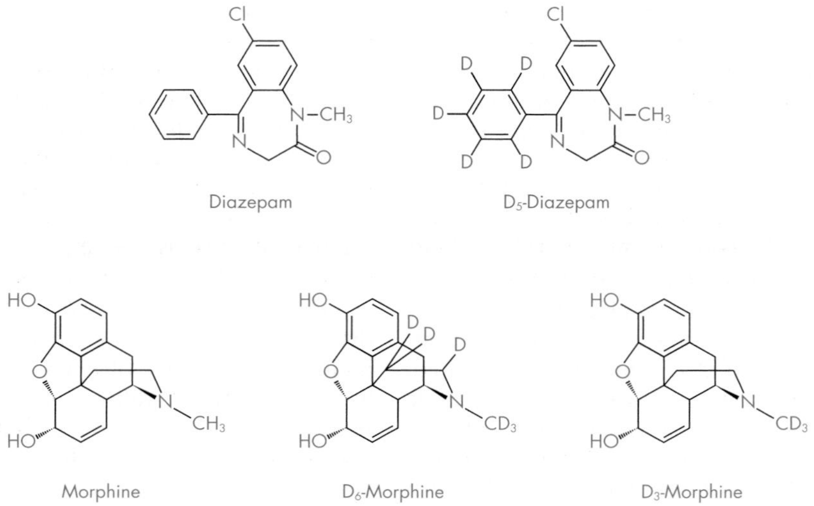

Diazepam

D_5-Diazepam

Morphine

D_6-Morphine

D_3-Morphine

Figure 18.19 Diazepam, morphine and their deuterated analogues.

temperature set at 250°C. If a peak tails, derivatisation or use of a more polar stationary phase should be considered. Fine-tuning is carried out once some peaks have been obtained. Having established the chromatography, the extraction and concentration steps can be determined. Manufacturers' catalogues are again a useful source for both derivatisation and solid-phase extraction procedures.

Good preventative maintenance is essential. The injector (or liner) should be cleaned periodically, and any glass wool changed regularly (approximately every 100 to 1000 injections, depending on the quality of the extracts). For capillary columns, the performance is improved by periodically removing the first 5–10 cm of capillary tubing (a retention gap could be considered for dirty samples), and for packed columns by replacing the glass wool and first few centimetres of packing. It is advisable to monitor performance by selecting certain performance criteria (e.g. a certain response size, running a standard test mix or amount of acceptable separation between two closely eluting components) to indicate when maintenance is required. The manufacturer's instructions for cleaning detectors should be followed.

The presence of traces of contaminants in the carrier gas supply shortens the column life drastically, and also causes detector deterioration. In-line filters (to remove oxygen, hydrocarbons, etc.) and molecular sieves (to remove water vapour) are strongly recommended, and the use of stainless-steel gas tubing minimises further contamination. Carrier-gas flow should be optimised for a particular column and a particular carrier gas. This is most important for capillary columns. Fig. 18.12 shows the relationship between efficiency expressed as the HETP versus carrier-gas velocity (van Deemter plot) for a 25 m by 0.25 mm i.d. WCOT OV-101 column. Modifying the nature of the mobile phase in GC has very little effect compared with that observed with HPLC or thin-layer chromatography (TLC) and, in general, affects efficiency rather than selectivity. Nitrogen gives higher efficiency, but at the expense of longer analysis time, while the less dense, but more hazardous, hydrogen gives slightly lower efficiency, but faster analysis. In practice, nitrogen is usually used for packed columns and helium for capillary columns. Certain detectors impose restrictions on the choice of carrier gas, but an additional supply of gas can be added to the column effluent to purge the detector. Experimenting with higher flow and a lower operating temperature (or vice versa) can give rewarding results for the separation of compounds that elute closely. This effect is particularly noticeable for two compounds that have different polarities, as the retention of the more polar compound is influenced to a greater extent the longer it resides in the column (nonpolar compounds elute in boiling point sequence). Conditions of constant flow improve the efficiency of late-eluting peaks and produce faster chromatography than do constant pressure conditions.

For a particular separation, the lowest temperature compatible with a reasonable analysis time should be used. In general, retention times double with each 20°C decrease in temperature. If the time is excessive, it is generally better to reduce the stationary phase loading or use a shorter column than to increase the column operating temperature. There is a maximum temperature at which a column can be operated and there is also a minimum temperature below which efficiency drops sharply. Manufacturers give the temperature operating ranges for each of their stationary phases (see Table 18.2). For GLC, the stationary phase must be a liquid at the temperature of operation, and if a column is run at too low a temperature to obtain longer retention times the stationary phase may still be in the solid or semi-solid form. When using temperature programming, experimentation with a faster initial ramp followed by a slower subsequent ramp or an isothermal period can help resolve problematic separations.

Efficiency can also be improved by decreasing the column diameter or increasing the column length. The resultant increase in analysis time (particularly if the flow must be reduced to accommodate the increased pressure demand imposed by a narrower column), can usually be offset by using a slightly higher operating temperature (temperature increases affect retention time much more than do increases in gas flow). Reducing the diameter of a capillary column markedly increases efficiency, but the retention time remains constant only as long as the same phase ratio is maintained. Therefore, unless there is a simultaneous reduction in film thickness, retention increases in direct proportion to the phase ratio.

The solvent used for the sample can sometimes produce unexpected derivatives that give different retention times (traces of acetic anhydride that remain in butyl acetate avidly derivatise primary amines at room temperature). An inert nonpolar solvent should be used if possible to minimise the co-extraction of unwanted contaminants. Acetone, other ketones, ethyl acetate and carbon disulfide readily form derivatives with primary amines and should be avoided.

The choice of injector type and injection solvent also plays an important part in the chromatography. A solvent volume should be chosen that does not expand to exceed the capacity of the injector (see Table 18.4), otherwise backflush and irreproducible results are obtained. Split injection significantly reduces the amount of solvent and associated contaminants that enter the column and, although the analyte response is reduced, the improvement in the signal-to-noise ratio often results in enhanced sensitivity.

The use of a selective detector, such as an ECD (with the preparation of a strongly responsive derivative if appropriate), can improve sensitivity typically up to 100-fold. Similarly, switching from full scan to selected-ion monitoring in MS improves the sensitivity, usually by a factor of 10. However, selective detectors should not be used as a substitute for cleaning up of sample extracts, as loading contaminants onto the column affects the chromatography adversely, even if the selective detector does not respond to the compounds. Increasing the detector temperature may also improve sensitivity.

Fronting or splitting of peaks indicates column overload. If the detector sensitivity permits, the best option here is to inject a smaller sample volume (or a more dilute sample), rather than to increase the column loading or diameter, otherwise efficiency is also affected.

If trace levels of solutes are sought in the presence of a preponderant component, a number of stationary phases of differing polarities should be tried. Trace impurities are seen easily if they emerge before the main component of a mixture, while they may be lost completely in the tail if they elute just after the large peak. Early peaks are also sharper and thus, for the same peak area, higher – an effect that can contribute enormously to the successful detection of trace substances.

Specific applications

Amfetamines and other stimulants

Amfetamines are basic drugs that require strongly alkaline conditions to be extracted from aqueous solution. These conditions are too basic to extract the phenolic metabolites, but these can be recovered at pH 8 or 9 and the extracts combined prior to chromatography. For high sensitivity, back extraction into dilute sulfuric acid (0.05 M) is a useful clean-up procedure. When using packed columns, derivatives are almost always required for the primary and secondary amines, since the peaks tail badly. Suitable derivatives are acetyl, trifluoroacetyl, pentafluoropropionate or TMS (see p. 503, Derivative Formation). With capillary columns, derivatives are used most often to improve mass spectral patterns or to modify the separation of compounds that elute closely. For hydroxylated metabolites, derivatisation is invariably required to achieve acceptable chromatography. Care must be taken to avoid drug loss during solvent evaporation, which can be obviated by adding a small amount of concentrated aqueous acid (20 μL of 6 M HCl) to the organic solvent. Unless otherwise stated, GC retention data and mass spectral data are identical for both *d*- and *l*- (+ and −) enantiomers. To differentiate enantiomers (such as *d*- and *l*-methamfetamine or amfetamine), a chiral column or chiral derivatising reagent is required (Cody and Schwarzhoff 1993). At present, all amfetamine- or methamfetamine-producing drugs (aminorex, amfetaminil, clobenorex, ethylamfetamine, fencamine, fenethylline, fenproporex, mefenorex, prenylamine, benzfetamine, dimethylamfetamine, famprofazone, furfenorex) are racemates (with the exception of *l*-selegiline, *l*-methamfetamine and dexamfetamine). Stereoinversion does not occur in humans (Nagai *et al.* 1991). Drugs that are metabolised to amfetamines, but are not themselves classified as such, are also listed

Antidepressants

Antidepressants (tricyclics, selective serotonin reuptake inhibitors (SSRIs), monoamine oxidase inhibitors (MAOIs)) can be extracted readily under mildly basic conditions (pH 10) into many solvents, such as ethyl acetate, hexane, diethyl ether. Less polar solvents, such as hexane, limit the extraction of hydroxylated metabolites. An acidified (0.05 M H_2SO_4) back extraction is a useful clean-up procedure where sensitivity is important. Chromatography of primary and secondary amines is poor on packed columns, but is adequate on well-maintained capillary columns, particularly those of low-medium polarity such as PSX-5. Some authors prefer to chromatograph the secondary amines and hydroxylated metabolites as acetylated derivatives, prepared by heating the dried residue with acetic anhydride and pyridine (3:2, v/v; Maurer and Bickeboeller-Friedrich 2000). Others employ an enzymatic hydrolysis procedure to improve recovery of both parent drug and metabolites, although the additional sensitivity gained is often negated by the increased analytical time in the emergency setting. Acid hydrolysis is quicker, but some relevant compounds are destroyed under these conditions.

Benzodiazepines

The analysis of benzodiazepines in biological specimens is hampered by their high potency and resultant low-plasma concentrations, and by their interconnected metabolic pathways. Several benzodiazepines appear in urine almost exclusively as glucuronide-conjugated metabolites, and these can be hydrolysed with glucuronidase (1000 U glucurase/mL of urine at 60°C for 1–2 h), although some can degrade with prolonged heating. Extraction can be performed at any pH between 3 and 12, but basic extracts (pH 9 to 11) give cleaner chromatograms. The extraction solvent should be moderately polar (ethyl acetate is appropriate), and TMS derivatives form easily in 20–30 min at 60°C using 50% BSTFA with 1% TCMS in acetonitrile. These derivatives markedly improve peak shape and sensitivity. All compounds except 7-aminonitrazepam show electron-capture responses with high sensitivity. However, quantification with ECD is problematic as it has a narrow linear range, and a multiple-point calibration is essential. Alternatively, for most compounds a nitrogen detector (NPD) gives adequate sensitivity with a much-improved linear range, although it is not advisable to make TMS-derivatives if using this detector. MS detection is required to confirm the identity

Hydrolysis of benzodiazepines (preparation of benzophenones)

An aqueous solution (or urine) should be boiled with concentrated hydrochloric acid (1 part to 10 parts urine or solution) for 30–60 min, cooled, and neutralised with solid $KHCO_3$ or the pH adjusted to 8–9 with 10 M KOH. It is then mixed with an equal volume of petroleum ether for 10 min and then centrifuged, and the upper organic phase is evaporated to dryness at 60°C. The reconstituted extract can be used for GC or other analytical procedures such as TLC. Not all benzodiazepines make benzophenones when hydrolysed with acid, and a number of other degradation products are furnished. The α-OH-metabolites of alprazolam, brotizolam and triazolam are partly altered by the elimination of formaldehyde. Hydrolysis products of bis-desethylflurazepam and di-OH-tetrazepam are dehydrated; OH-bromazepam, lorazepam and oxazepam form artefacts by rearrangement; the nor-metabolites of clobazam are cleaved and rearranged to benzimidazole derivatives; tetrazepam, and its two hydroxylated metabolites, are transformed into a pair of *cis*- and *trans*-isomeric hexahydroacridone derivatives.

Since the metabolism of benzodiazepines is complex, assays that convert drugs and metabolites into hydrolysis products are not ideal, since they do not permit unequivocal identification of the parent compound. After acid hydrolysis, care must be taken to ensure that the acid is neutralised prior to extraction or before injecting the solvent onto the chromatograph, otherwise the column deteriorates rapidly.

Narcotic analgesics, opiates and opioids

Many laboratories perform specific assays for opiates for federal or legal purposes; these are generally limited to codeine, morphine and more recently 6-monoacetyl morphine (MAM; Paul *et al.* 1999). However, for clinical purposes a wider range of analytes is desirable and can include codeine, dihydrocodeine, hydrocodone, hydromorphone, oxycodone and oxymorphone. All assays involve a hydrolysis step (acidic or enzymatic; see p. 498 for an evaluation of these) to cleave the glucuronide conjugates, followed by a basic extraction (often using solid phase or acidic back extraction for cleanliness). Derivatisation is possible with a number of reagents (PFP, TMS, TFA or AC derivatives are the most common; Maurer and Pfleger 1984; Chen *et al.* 1990; Grinstead 1991). The derivatising reagent is selected on the basis of personal preference for a desired separation or the formation of unique ions on MS fragmentation. Analysis of hydromorphone, oxycodone and oxymorphone is complicated by the possibility that several structurally different derivatives will form in non-reproducible proportions from the tautomerisation of the enol and keto forms. However, these compounds can be stabilised in their keto forms by incubating with hydroxylamine or methoxyamine–pyridine, and then yield only a single derivatised oxime product (Broussard *et al.* 1997; Meatherall 1999).

Non-amfetamine stimulants and hallucinogens

Non-amfetamine stimulants and hallucinogens have a variety of clinical and toxic actions. Extraction of cocaine is straightforward under basic conditions, and most metabolites, except benzoylecgonine, can be detected in the clinical setting without derivatisation. For regulated testing, quantification of benzoylecgonine is required, and most laboratories use TMS as the derivatising reagent.

For analysis of cannabis metabolites, hydrolysis of conjugates with 10 M potassium hydroxide is usually performed on urine prior to weakly acidic extraction (pH 6.5); TMS is the derivative of choice. Phencylidine (PCP) analysis is complicated by the low concentration present, although extraction is straightforward and derivatisation is only required for metabolite measurement (Nakahara *et al.* 1997). Chromatographic confirmation of lysergide (LSD) is hampered by the low concentrations and acidic nature of the metabolites, which necessitates both derivatisation (TMS) and tandem MS (Nelson and Foltz 1992).

References

K. Blau and J. Halket (eds), *Handbook of Derivatives for Chromatography*, 2nd edn, New York, Wiley, 1993.

L. A. Broussard *et al.*, Simultaneous identification and quantitation of codeine, morphine, hydrocodone, and hydomorphone in urine as trimethylsilyl and oxime derivatives by gas chromatography–mass spectrometry, *Clin. Chem.*, 1997, **43**, 1029–1032.

B. H. Chen *et al.*, Comparison of derivatives for determination of codeine and morphine by gas chromatography/mass spectrometry, *J. Anal. Chem.*, 1990, **14**, 12–17.

J. T. Cody and R. Schwarzhoff, Interpretation of methamfetamine and amfetamine enantiomer data, *J. Anal. Toxicol.*, 1993, **17**, 321–326.

K. H. Dudley, Trace organic sample handling, in *Methodological Surveys Sub-series (A)*, E. Reid (ed.), Chichester, Ellis Horwood, 1980, p. 336.

G. F. Grinstead, A closer look at acetyl and pentafluoropropionyl derivatives for quantitative analysis of morphine and codeine by gas chromatography/mass spectrometry, *J Anal. Toxicol.*, 1991, **15**, 293–298.

H. H. Maurer and J. Bickeboeller-Friedrich, Screening procedure for detection of antidepressants of the selective serotonin reuptake inhibitor type and their metabolites in urine as part of a modified systematic toxicological analysis procedure using gas chromatography–mass spectrometry, *J. Anal. Toxicol.*, 2000, **24**, 340–347.

H. H. Maurer and K. Pfleger, Screening procedure for the detection of opioids, other potent analgesics and their metabolites in urine using a computerized gas chromatographic–mass spectrometric technique, *Fresenius Z. Anal. Chem.*, 1984, **317**, 42–52.

W. O. McReynolds, Characterization of some liquid phases, *J. Chromatogr. Sci.*, 1970, **8**, 685–691.

R. Meatherall, GC-MS confirmation of codeine, morphine, 6-acetylmorphine, hydrocodone, hydromorphone, oxycodone, and oxymorphone in urine, *J. Anal. Toxicol.*, 1999, **23**, 177–186.

A. C. Moffat *et al.*, Optimum use of paper, thin-layer and gas–liquid chromatography for the identification of basic drugs. I. Determination of effectiveness for a series of chromatographic systems, *J. Chromatogr.*, 1974a, **90**, 1–7.

A. C. Moffat *et al.*, Optimum use of paper, thin-layer and gas–liquid chromatography for the identification of basic drugs. III. Gas–liquid chromatography, *J. Chromatogr.*, 1974b, **90**, 19–33.

T. Nagai and S. Kamiyama, Simultaneous HPLC analysis of optical isomers of methamfetamine and its metabolites, and stereoselective metabolism of racemic methamfetamine in rat urine, *J. Anal. Toxicol.*, 1991, **15**, 299–304.

Y. Nakahara *et al.*, Hair analysis for drugs of abuse. XVII. Simultaneous detection of PCP, PCHP, and PCPdiol in human hair for confirmation of PCP use, *J. Anal. Toxicol.*, 1997, **21**, 356–362.

C. Nelson and R. L. Foltz, Determination of lysergic acid diethylamine (LSD), iso-LSD, and *N*-demethyl-LSD in body fluids by gas chromatography/tandem mass spectrometry, *Anal. Chem.*, 1992, **64**, 1578–1585.

B. D. Paul *et al.*, A practical approach to determining cutoff concentrations for opiate testing with simultaneous detection of codeine, morphine, and 6-acetylmorphine in urine, *Clin. Chem.*, 1999, **45**, 510–519.

R. P. W. Scott, *Chromatographic Detectors – Design, Function, and Operation*, Chromatographic Science Series, Vol. 73, J. Cazes (ed.), New York, Marcel Dekker, 1996.

Further reading

K. Blau and J. Halket (eds), *Handbook of Derivatives for Chromatography*, 2nd edn, New York, Wiley, 1993.

K. Grob, *Split and Splitless Injection in Capillary Gas Chromatography*, Heidelberg, Hüthig, 1993.

K. Grob, *On-Column Injection in Capillary Gas Chromatography*, Heidelberg, Hüthig, 1993.

H. H. Hill and D. G. McMinn (eds), *Detectors for Capillary Chromatography*, New York, Wiley, 1992.

W. Jennings *et al.*, *Analytical Gas Chromatography*, 2nd edn, London, Academic Press, 1997.

K. Jinno, *Chromatographic Separations Based on Molecular Recognition*, New York, Wiley, 1997.

D. Rood, *A Practical Guide to the Care, Maintenance, and Troubleshooting of Capillary Gas Chromatographic Systems*, 2nd edn, Heidelberg, Hüthig, 1995.

R. P. W. Scott, *Chromatographic Detectors – Design, Function, and Operation*, Chromatographic Science Series, Vol. 73, J. Cazes (ed.), New York, Marcel Dekker, 1996.

D. Stevenson and I. D. Wilson (eds), *Sample Preparation for Biomedical and Environmental Analysis*, New York, Plenum Press, 1994.

19

High-performance liquid chromatography

T Kupiec, M Slawson, F Pragst and M Herzler

Introduction 513
Practical aspects of HPLC theory 514
Hardware 515
Columns 522
Maintenance 525
Separation techniques 526
Quantitative analysis 528
Validation 530
New emerging trends 530
Systems for drug analysis 531
Selection of chromatographic systems . . 533
Analysis of drugs in pharmaceutical preparations 533
Analysis of drugs in biological fluids and tissues 534
References 536
Further reading 536

Introduction

The ability to separate and analyse complex samples is integral to the biological and medical sciences. Classic column chromatography has evolved over the years, with chromatographic innovations introduced at intervals of roughly a decade. These techniques offered major improvements in speed, resolving power, detection, quantification, convenience and applicability to new sample types. The most notable of these modifications was high-performance liquid chromatography (HPLC). Modern HPLC techniques became available in 1969; however, they were not widely accepted in the pharmaceutical industry until several years later. Once HPLC systems capable of quantitative analysis became commercially available, their usefulness in pharmaceutical analysis was fully appreciated.

By the 1990s, HPLC had begun an explosive growth that made it the most popular analytical method judged according to sales of instruments and also scientific importance. Its present popularity results from its convenient separation of a wide range of sample types, exceptional resolving power, speed and nanomolar detection levels. It is presently used in pharmaceutical research and development

- to purify synthetic or natural products
- to characterise metabolites
- to assay active ingredients, impurities, degradation products and in dissolution assays
- in pharmacodynamic and pharmacokinetic studies.

Improvements made in HPLC in recent years include:

- changes in packing material, such as smaller particle size, new packing and column materials

- high-speed separation
- micro-HPLC, automation and computer-assisted optimisation
- improvements in detection methods, including the so-called hyphenated detection systems.

These innovations will be discussed in the appropriate sections of this chapter.

Practical aspects of HPLC theory

The practical application of HPLC is aided by an awareness of the concepts of chromatographic theory, in particular the measurement of chromatographic retention and the factors that influence resolution.

Chromatographic principles

The retention of a drug with a given packing material and eluent can be expressed as a retention time or retention volume, but both of these are dependent on flow rate, column length and column diameter. The retention is best described as a column capacity ratio (k), which is independent of these factors. The column capacity ratio of a compound (A) is defined by equation (19.1):

$$k_A = \frac{V_A - V_m}{V_m} = \frac{t_A - t_m}{t_m} \qquad (19.1)$$

where V_A is the elution volume of A and V_m (in some texts denoted by V_0) is the elution volume of a non-retained compound (i.e. void volume). At constant flow rate, retention times (t_A and t_m, referred to in some texts as t_0) can be used instead of retention volumes. The injection of a solvent or salt solution can be used to measure V_0, but the solute used should always be recorded along with reported k data. The importance of selecting suitable solutes for the measurement of V_0 has been discussed (Wells and Clark 1981).

It is sometimes convenient to express retention data relative to a known internal standard (B). The ratio of retention times (t_A/t_B) can be used, but the ratio of adjusted retention times, $(t_A - t_0)/(t_B - t_0)$, is better when data need to be transferred between different chromatographs (Ettre 1980).

Resolution is the parameter that describes the separation power of the complete chromatographic system relative to the particular components of the mixture. By convention, resolution (R) is expressed as the ratio of the distance between two peak maxima ($V_{R,2} - V_{R,1}$) to the mean value of the peak width ($[W_1+W_2]/2$) at the baseline (equation 19.2):

$$R = \frac{2(V_{R,2} - V_{R,1})}{W_1 + W_2} \qquad (19.2)$$

If we approximate peaks by symmetric triangles, then if R is equal to or more than 1.5, the components are completely separated. If R is less than 1.5, the components overlap.

Sensitivity in chromatographic analysis is a measure of the smallest detectable level of a component in a chromatographic separation and is dependent on the signal-to-noise ratio in a given detector. Sensitivity can be increased by derivatisation of the compound of interest, optimisation of chromatographic system or miniaturisation of the system. The limit of detection is normally taken as 3 times the signal-to-noise (S/N) ratio and the limit of quantification as 10 times the S/N ratio.

Chromatographic mechanisms

The systems used in chromatography are often described as belonging to one of four mechanistic types: adsorption, partition, ion exchange and size exclusion. *Adsorption chromatography* arises from interactions between solutes and the surface of the solid stationary phase. Generally, the eluents used for adsorption chromatography are less polar than the stationary phases and such systems are described as 'normal phase'. *Partition chromatography* involves a liquid stationary phase that is immiscible with the eluent and coated onto, or more usually covalently bonded to, an inert support. Partition systems can be normal-phase (stationary phase more polar than eluent) or reversed-phase chromatography, referred to as RPC (stationary phase less polar than eluent). *Ion-exchange chromatography* involves a solid stationary phase with anionic or cationic groups on the surface to which solute molecules of opposite charge are attracted. *Size-exclusion chromatography* involves a stationary phase with controlled pore size. Solutes are separated according to their molecular size, with the large molecules unable to enter the pores elute first. However, this concept of four separation modes is an over-simplification. In reality, there are no distinct boundaries and several different mechanisms often operate simultaneously.

Other types of chromatographic separation have been described. *Ion-pair chromatography* is an alternative to ion-exchange chromatography. It involves the addition of an organic ionic substance to the mobile phase, which forms an ion pair with the sample component of opposite charge. This allows a reversed-phase system to be used to separate ionic compounds. *Chiral chromatography* is a method used to separate enantiomers, which can be achieved by various means. In one case, the mobile phase is chiral and the stationary phase is nonchiral. In another, the liquid stationary phase is chiral with the mobile phase nonchiral or, finally, the solid stationary phase may be chiral with a nonchiral mobile phase.

Hardware

HPLC instrumentation includes a pump, injector, column, detector and recorder or data system (Fig. 19.1). The heart of the system is the column in which separation occurs. Since the stationary phase is composed of micrometre-size porous particles, a high-pressure pump is required to move the mobile phase through the column. The chromatographic process begins by injecting the solute onto the top of the column. Separation of components occurs as the analytes and mobile phase are pumped through the column. Eventually, each component elutes from the column and is registered as a peak on the recorder. Detection of the eluting components is important; this can be either selective or universal, depending upon the detector used. The response of the detector to each component is displayed on a chart recorder or computer screen and is known as a chromatogram. Computers, integrators and other data-processing equipment are frequently used to collect, store and analyse the chromatographic data.

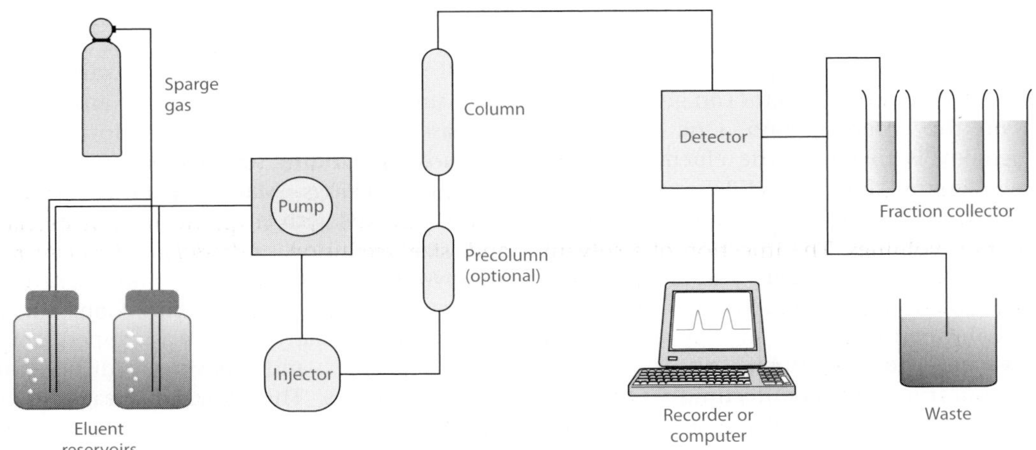

Figure 19.1 A typical HPLC system.

Mobile phase reservoir and eluent preparation

The most common type of solvent reservoir is a glass bottle. Most of the manufacturers supply these bottles with special caps, Teflon tubing and filters to connect to the pump inlet and to the sparge gas (helium) used to remove dissolved air.

The quality of solvents, inorganic salts (or volatile organic acids for LC-MS) used in eluent (mobile phase) preparation is an important consideration. Soluble impurities can give noisy baselines and spurious peaks or can build up on the surface of the packing material, eventually changing chromatographic retention. Furthermore, the eluate may need to be collected for further experimentation and all contamination must be avoided. In addition, particulate matter should be removed from the mobile phase, otherwise pump filters, frits and tubing can become blocked.

A wide range of HPLC-grade solvents are now available commercially that are free from particulate matter, have low residues on evaporation and have guaranteed upper limits of UV-absorbing and fluorescent impurities. However, if a detector is not to be operated at its maximum sensitivity, analytical grade solvents may be used. A general rule of thumb is to use the highest purity of solvent that is available and practicable depending on the particular application.

Air dissolved in the mobile phase can lead to problems. The formation of a bubble in a pump head usually reduces or stops eluent flow, while bubbles formed in the detector can give spurious peaks on the chromatogram. One commonly used remedy is to de-gas the eluent using an in-line vacuum chamber. HPLC solvents are pumped from the reservoirs into a vacuum chamber in line with the HPLC eluent flow. This method ensures continuous and efficient de-gassing of the mobile phase. Vacuum de-gassing can also be performed off line by applying a weak vacuum to the mobile phase reservoir while sonicating. Off-line techniques do not offer the advantage of continuous de-gassing throughout the analysis. Eluents can also be de-gassed by purging with helium, which has a very low solubility and drives the air out. This technique can be performed on line, and can be controlled by the HPLC system, or off line. Care must always be taken when de-gassing eluents that contain volatile components to avoid changing the composition.

It is convenient to prepare eluents as volume plus volume mixtures of solvents (i.e. the volume of each solvent is measured separately and then mixed). Volume changes can occur when solvents are mixed (e.g. methanol and water show a contraction in volume), which must be remembered if the volume of only one solvent is measured and the second solvent is added to make up to volume (v/v).

True pH values can only be measured in aqueous solutions and any measurements made with a pH meter in aqueous–organic solvents should be described as 'apparent pH'. In general, the apparent pH of a buffer solution rises as the proportion of organic solvent in the aqueous mixture increases. When an eluent is prepared it is usually best to dissolve the required buffer salts in water at the appropriate concentrations, adjust the pH and then mix this solution (v/v) with the organic solvents.

Pumps

High-pressure pumps are needed to force solvents through packed stationary phase beds. Smaller bed particles (e.g. 3 μm) require higher pressures. There are many advantages to using smaller particles, but they may not be essential for all separations. The most important advantages are higher resolution, faster analyses and increased sample load capacity. However, only the most demanding separations require the use of 3 μm packings. Many separation problems can be resolved with larger particle packings (e.g. 5 μm) that require less pressure.

Flow-rate stability is another important pump feature that distinguishes pumps. Constant-flow systems are generally of two basic types: reciprocating piston and positive displacement (syringe) pumps. The basic advantage of both systems is that they produce highly repeatable elution volumes from run to run, regardless of viscosity, up to the pressure limit of the pump. Although syringe-type pumps have a pressure capability of up to 540 000 kPa (78 000 psi), they have a limited ability to form mobile phase gradients. Reciprocating piston pumps can maintain a liquid flow for an indefinite length of time, while a syringe pump needs to be refilled after the syringe volume has been displaced. Dual-headed reciprocating piston pumps provide more reproducible and pulse-free delivery of solvent, which reduces detector noise and enables more reliable integration of peak area. Reciprocating pumps now dominate the HPLC market and are even useful for micro-HPLC applications, as they can maintain a constant flow at flow rates in μL/min ranges.

An additional pump feature found on the more elaborate pumps is external electronic control. Although it adds to the expense of the pump, external electronic control is a very desirable feature when automation or electronically controlled mobile phase gradients are to be run. Alternatively, this becomes unnecessary when using isocratic methods. The degree of flow control also varies with pump expense. More expensive pumps include such state-of-the-art technology as electronic feedback and multiheaded configurations.

Modern pumps have the following parameters:

- flow-rate range, 0.01–10 mL/min
- flow-rate stability, not more than 1% (short term)
- for size exclusion chromatography, flow-rate stability should be <0.2%
- maximum pressure, up to 34 500 kPa (5000 psi).

Injectors

An injector for an HPLC system should provide injection of the liquid sample within the range 0.1–100 μL of volume with high reproducibility and under high pressure (up to 27 600 kPa). The injector should also minimise disturbances to the flow of the mobile phase and produce minimum band broadening. Sample introduction can be accomplished in various ways. The injection valve has, in most cases, replaced syringe injection. Valve injection offers rapid, reproducible and essentially operator-independent delivery of a wide range of sample volumes. The most common valve is a six-port Rheodyne valve in which the sample fills an external stainless-steel loop. A clockwise turn of the valve rotor places the sample-filled loop into the mobile phase stream, which deposits the sample onto the top of the column. These valves can be operated manually or actuated via computer-automated systems. One minor disadvantage of valve injection is that the sample loop must be changed to obtain various sample volumes. However, this is a simple procedure that requires only a few minutes. Automatic sampling devices are incorporated in more sophisticated HPLC systems. These autosamplers have a piston-metering syringe-type pump to suck the preset sample volume into a line and transfer it to a sample loop of adequate size in a standard six-port valve. Most autosamplers are computer controlled and can serve as the master controller for the whole system.

In HPLC, liquid samples may be injected directly and solid samples need only be dissolved in an appropriate solvent. The solvent need not be the mobile phase, but frequently it is wise to choose the mobile phase to avoid detector interference, column-component interference, loss in efficiency, or all of these. It is always best to remove particles from the sample by filtration or centrifugation, since continuous injections of particulate material eventually cause blockage of injection devices or columns.

Sample sizes may vary widely. The availability of highly sensitive detectors frequently allows the use of small sample injection volumes that yield the highest column performance.

Thermostats

It often is advantageous to run ion-exchange, size-exclusion and reversed-phase columns above room temperature and to control precisely the temperature of liquid–liquid columns. Therefore, column thermostats are a desirable feature in modern HPLC instruments. Temperature variation within the HPLC column should generally be held within ±0.2°C. Maintenance of a constant temperature is especially important in quantitative analysis, since changes in temperature can seriously affect peak-size measurement.

It is often important to be able to work at higher temperatures for size-exclusion chromatography of some synthetic polymers because of solubility problems. High-velocity circulating air baths, which usually consist of high-velocity air blowers plus electronically controlled thermostats, are the most convenient for HPLC. Alternatively, HPLC columns can be jacketed and the temperature controlled by contact heaters or by circulating fluid from a constant-temperature bath. This latter approach is practical for routine analyses, but is less convenient when columns must be changed frequently.

Column switches

These valve devices are used to divert the flow from one column to another within a single HPLC system. Column-switching techniques can be used during method development when several columns are to be evaluated for their efficiency, retention, etc. More recently, the use of column switching has been employed in the on-line analysis of biological matrices. Raw plasma or other liquid sample matrix is injected directly onto the first column. Chromatographic conditions are optimised such that interfering substances are eluted from the column while the analytes of interest are retained. The column switch then diverts the eluent that contains the analytes of interest from the 'clean-up column' onto the analytical column, which then separates the analytes of interest for quantification or characterisation. Another use of column switches is in gradient chromatography for which high throughput is essential. The first column is switched off-line to re-equilibrate to initial conditions, while the second column is brought on-line for the next injection. This conserves valuable analysis time that would otherwise be wasted waiting for the column to re-equilibrate. The most up-to-date information on the use of column switching can be found by searching the current literature.

Detectors

Optical detectors are now frequently used in HPLC systems. These detectors pass a beam of light through the flowing column effluent as it passes through a flow-cell. Flow-cells are available in preparative, analytical and micro-analytical sizes The variations in light intensity, caused by ultraviolet (UV) absorption, fluorescence emission or change in refractive index (depending on the type of detector used) from the sample components that pass through the cell, are monitored as changes in the output voltage. These voltage changes are recorded and fed into an integrator or computer to provide retention time and peak-area data. Further details on UV-visible and fluorescence detectors can be found in Chapter 15. Most applications in drug analysis use detectors that respond to the absorption of UV radiation (or visible light) by the solute as it passes through the flow-cell. Absorption changes are proportional to concentration, following the Beer–Lambert law. Flow-cells generally have pathlengths of 5–10 mm with volumes between 5 and 10 μL. These detectors give good sensitivities with many compounds, are not affected by slight fluctuations in flow rate and temperature, and are nondestructive, which allows solutes to be collected and analysed further if desired.

The simplest detectors are of the fixed-wavelength type and usually contain low-pressure mercury lamps that have an intense emission line at 254 nm. Some instruments offer conversion kits that allow the energy at 254 nm to excite a suitable phosphor to give a new detection wavelength (e.g. 280 nm). Variable-wavelength detectors have a deuterium lamp with a continuous emission from 180 to 400 nm and use a manually operated diffraction grating to select the required wavelength. Tungsten lamps (400–700 nm) are used for the visible region.

Many organic compounds absorb at 254 nm and hence a fixed-wavelength detector has many uses. However, a variable-wavelength detector can be invaluable to increase the sensitivity of detection by using the wavelength of maximum absorption. This is particularly useful when analysing proteins that absorb at 280 nm, or peptides that are detected commonly at 215 nm. Using a variable-wavelength detector can also increase the selectivity of detection by enhancing the peak of interest relative to interfering peaks.

Eluents must have sufficient transparency at the selected detection wavelength. Buffer salts can also limit transparency. The spectra of some drugs change with pH, and the sensitivity and selectivity of an assay can sometimes be controlled by changing the eluent pH. The influence of such changes on the chromatography must also be considered.

Other detection systems commonly used include diode array, refractive index (RI), fluorescence (FL), electrochemical (EC) and mass spectrometry (MS). Infrared (IR) and nuclear magnetic resonance (NMR) spectrometers may also be used as detectors.

Photodiode array detection

The photodiode array detector (DAD) is an advanced type of UV detector. Depending on the wavelength, a tungsten lamp and a deuterium lamp are used as light sources. The polychromatic light beam is focused on a flow-cell (volume 8–13 μL) and subsequently dispersed by a holographic grating or quartz prism (see Fig. 15.7, p. 401). The spectral light then reaches a chip that contains 100–1000 light-sensitive diodes arranged side by side. Each diode only registers a well-defined fraction of the information and in this way all wavelengths are measured at the same time. Note that although having more diodes in an array increases the resolution of UV spectra, it lowers the absolute sensitivity since less radiation is absorbed by each individual diode. The wavelength resolution of up-to-date detectors is of the order of 1 nm per diode, with a wavelength accuracy of better than ± 1 nm and a sensitivity below 10^{-4} absorbency units. All operations of the detector are controlled by a computer: correction of fluctuations of the lamp energy, collection of signals (I_λ) from all the diodes, storage of the data of the mobile phase ($I_{0\lambda}$, measured at the start of the chromatogram) and calculation of the absorbance according to the Beer–Lambert law from I_λ to $I_{0\lambda}$. The number of spectra recorded per second can be chosen from between 0.1 and 10; usually one spectrum per second is optimal with respect to chromatographic resolution and noise. At the end of the run, a three-dimensional spectrochromatogram (absorbance as a function of wavelength and time) (see Fig. 15.2, p. 395) is stored on the computer and can be evaluated qualitatively and quantitatively. A detailed description of the operation of DAD is given in Huber and George (1993).

DAD offers several advantages. Knowledge of the spectra of compounds of interest enables interfering peaks to be eliminated such that an accurate quantification of peaks of interest can be achieved despite less than optimal resolution. Simultaneous detection at two wavelengths allows calculation of an absorbance ratio. If this ratio is not constant across a peak, the peak is not pure, regardless of its appearance. An additional advantage of DAD is the subtraction of a reference wavelength. This reduces baseline drift during gradient elution. HPLC-DAD systems linked to libraries of UV spectra are particularly useful in clinical and forensic toxicology in screening for drugs in biological samples and their use in this context is described in detail later (F. Pragst and M. Herzler, personal observations).

Refractive index detection

The RI detector is a universal detector, in that changes in RI (either positive or negative) that arise from the presence of a compound in the eluent are recorded. However, it is also the least-sensitive detector (as little as 1/100 as sensitive as UV detection). RI detectors may be used for excipients such as sugars in pharmaceuticals. Many factors influence RI, such as temperature, eluent composition and pressure, and must be controlled during separation. The chromatography is best implemented using a thermostatically controlled cabinet and high-quality pump to minimise pressure fluctuations.

Fluorescence detection

In FL detectors, the solute is excited with UV radiation and emits radiation at a longer wavelength. Most detectors allow the selection of both excitation and emission wavelengths. There are only a few drugs and natural compounds that have strong natural fluorescence (e.g. ergot alkaloids), but many drug derivatives are fluorescent. FL detection can offer great selectivity, since excitation and emission wavelengths as well as retention time can be used to identify drugs. It is necessary to choose eluents carefully when using FL detection. The eluent must neither fluoresce nor absorb at the chosen wavelengths. It is also necessary to consider the pH of the system, because some drugs show fluorescence only in certain ionic forms.

Electrochemical detection

EC detectors measure the current that results from the electrolytic oxidation or reduction of analytes at the surface of an electrode. These detectors are quite sensitive (down to 10^{-15} mole) and also quite selective. Two types of detector are available. The coulometric detector has a large electrode surface at which the electrochemical reaction is taken to completion. The amperometric detector has a small electrode with a low degree of conversion. Despite the difference in conversion rate, in practice these two types have approximately the same sensitivity. Eluents for EC detection must be electrically conductive. This is accomplished by the addition of inert electrolytes to the mobile phase. EC detection is most easily used in the oxidative mode, as use in the reductive mode requires the removal of dissolved oxygen from the eluent.

Hyphenated techniques

The development of the so-called hyphenated techniques has improved the ability to separate and identify multiple entities within a mixture. These techniques include LC-MS, LC-MS/MS, LC-IR and LC-NMR. These techniques usually involve chromatographic separation followed by peak identification with a traditional detector such as UV, combined with further identification of the compound with the MS, IR or NMR spectrometer.

Mass spectrometry as a detection system for HPLC has gained wide popularity, and advances in data systems and the simplification of the user interface have facilitated its implementation. The most common types of mass spectrometers used in conjunction with HPLC are quadrupoles and ion traps. Tandem mass spectrometers (also called triple quadrupoles) are also commonly available and are widely used in the pharmaceutical industry for the quantitative analysis of trace concentrations of drug molecules. Further information on LC-MS can be found on p. 568.

The process of mass analysis is essentially the same as in any other mass spectrometric analysis that utilises quadrupole or ion-trap technology. The unique challenge to interfacing HPLC equipment to a mass spectrometer is the need to convert a liquid-phase eluent into a gas phase suitable for mass spectral analysis. Modern mass spectrometers commonly utilise a technique known as atmospheric pressure ionisation (API) to accomplish this. API can be subdivided into electrospray (ion spray) ionisation (ESI) and atmospheric pressure chemical ionisation (APCI). Each technique has its own advantages. ESI is particularly useful for the analysis of a wide variety of compounds, especially proteins and peptides. APCI is also very well suited for the analysis of a large variety of compounds, particularly less polar organic molecules. Both techniques are very rugged and well suited to pharmaceutical and toxicological analysis.

An important consideration when using API is the need for volatile mobile-phase modifiers in the chromatographic separation. Acetic acid and formic acid are commonly used as acidic modifiers. Ammonium formate and ammonium acetate salts can also be used when more pH control is required for the separation. Organic modifiers are most often methanol or acetonitrile. One very important issue that must be considered when developing a method using API (electrospray, in particular) is the phenomenon of ion suppression. Co-eluting contaminants compete with the analyte of interest for ionisation, which results in a loss of signal for the analyte of interest. This can be very problematic if extremely small quantities of analyte are to be measured (as is often the case when MS is being used). Additional sample clean-up or adjustment of the chromatography to prevent co-elution of the contaminant is often necessary to correct this problem.

LC-MS/MS is commonly used in the pharmaceutical industry and in forensic science to analyse trace concentrations of drug and/or metabolite. MS/MS offers the advantage of increased signal-to-noise ratio, which in turn lowers the limits of detection and quantification easily into the sub-nanogram per mL range. MS/MS is also a very useful technique in the qualitative identification of previously unidentified metabolites of drugs, which thus makes MS/MS a very powerful technique in research laboratories. MS/MS as a high-throughput analytical technique is now used routinely in the pharmaceutical industry.

LC-IR has proved to be an effective method for detection of degradation products in pharmaceuticals. IR provides spectral information that can be used for compound identification or structural analysis. The IR spectra obtained after HPLC separation and IR analysis can be compared with the thousands of spectra available in spectral libraries to identify compounds, metabolites and degradation products. An advantage of IR spectroscopy is its ability to identify different isomeric forms of a compound based on the different spectra that result from alternative locations of a functional group on the compound. Unlike MS, IR is a nondestructive technique in which the original compound is deposited on a plate as pure, dry crystals and can be collected afterwards if desired.

LC-NMR is also growing in popularity for the identification of various components in natural products and other disciplines. Although a relatively new hyphenated system, LC-NMR has several applications on the horizon. The miniaturisation of the system and the possibility of measuring picomole amounts of material are both areas currently attracting considerable attention. Also, in the future LC-NMR systems will be interfaced with other detectors, such as Fourier transform IR and mass spectrometers. This will provide a wide range of possibilities for further applications, which could include the analysis of mixtures of polymer additives and the ability to identify unknowns without first having to isolate them in a pure form.

Data systems

Since the detector signal is electronic, the use of modern data-acquisition techniques can aid in the signal analysis. In addition, some systems can store data in a retrievable form for highly sophisticated computer analysis at a later time.

The main goal in using electronic data systems is to increase accuracy and precision in analysis, while reducing operator attention. There are several types of data systems, each of which differ in terms of available features. In routine analysis, where no automation (in terms of data management or process control) is needed, a pre-programmed computing integrator may be sufficient. If higher control levels are desired, a more intelligent device is necessary, such as a data station or minicomputer. The advantages of intelligent processors in chromatographs are found in several areas. Firstly, additional automation options become easier to implement. Secondly, complex data analysis becomes more feasible. The analysis options include such features as run-parameter optimisation and deconvolution (i.e. resolution) of overlapping peaks. Finally, software safeguards can be designed to reduce accidental misuse of the system. For example, the controller can be set to limit the rate of solvent switching. This acts to extend column life by reducing thermal and chemical shocks. In general, these stand-alone, user-programmable systems are becoming less expensive and increasingly practical.

Other more advanced features can also be applied to a chromatographic system. Features such as computer-controlled automatic injectors and multi-pump gradient controllers can be found on most modern HPLC instruments. They save much time and effort for the chromatographer and the additional initial expenditure is recouped rapidly through efficiency gains.

Sample fraction collectors are also available and can prove exceedingly beneficial where post-column fractions need to be collected for additional experiments.

Columns

Typical HPLC columns are 3, 5, 10, 15 and 25 cm in length and are filled with extremely small-diameter (3, 5 or 10 μm) particles. The columns may be made of stainless steel, glass-lined stainless steel or polyetheretherketone (PEEK). The internal diameter of the columns is usually 4.0 or 4.6 mm for traditional detection systems (UV, FL, etc.); this is considered the best compromise between sample capacity, mobile phase consumption, speed and resolution. However, if pure substances are to be collected (preparative scale), larger-diameter columns may be needed. Smaller-diameter columns (2.1 mm or less) are often used when HPLC is coupled with MS. The smaller-diameter columns also have the advantage of consuming less solvent because of their lower optimal flow rates. HPLC systems sold today can often be plumbed with narrower tubing diameters to take advantage of the benefits of these smaller column diameters.

Packed capillary microcolumns are also gaining wider use when interfacing the HPLC to a mass spectrometer and extremely low flow rates (nL/min) are needed to maximise sensitivity for the analysis of proteins and peptides.

Packing of the column tubing with small-diameter particles requires high skill and specialised equipment. For this reason, it is generally recommended that all but the most experienced chromatographers purchase pre-packed columns, since it is difficult to match the high performance of professionally packed HPLC columns without a large investment in time and equipment.

In general, HPLC columns are fairly durable and one can expect a long service life unless they are used in some manner that is intrinsically destructive, such as with highly acidic or basic eluents, or with continual injections of 'dirty' biological or crude samples. It is wise to inject some test mixture (under fixed conditions) into a column when it is new and to retain the chromatogram. If questionable results are obtained later, the test mixture can be injected again under specified conditions. The two chromatograms are compared to establish whether or not the column is still useful.

Column dimensions

The description of column dimensions and assignment of a category to that size varies greatly depending on the reference consulted. The following categories were suggested by Rozing *et al.* (2001), and may be more stratified than other categories.

Preparative

Preparative columns are generally of larger bore than analytical columns. Some have inner diameters as large as 100 mm and may have lengths of up to 600 mm. These columns are usually packed with materials of larger particle size that may range from 10 to 50 μm. The flow rate used with these columns normally exceeds 5 mL/min.

Normal bore

The normal bore for an analytical column can range from 3.9 mm to 5.0 mm inner diameter, but the most common is 4.6 mm. This diameter is the best compromise between sample capacity, mobile phase consumption, speed and resolution. The normal flow rate for this type of column is 1.0–5 mL/min.

Minibore

A minibore or narrow-bore column has an inner diameter of 2.1–3.9 mm. The flow rate for this column size ranges from 500 to 1500 μL/min.

Microbore

Microbore columns have a 1.0–2.1 mm inner diameter and have flow rates of 100–500 μL/min. These small columns save solvent, are popular when HPLC is interfaced with MS, and provide increased sensitivity in situations of limited sample mass.

Capillary
Capillary columns have inner diameters of 50 μm to 1.0 mm and have a typical flow rate of 0.2–100 μL/min. So-called 'nanobore' columns usually fall into the lower end of this size range. The inner surface of these very narrow columns must be extremely smooth. Since this is difficult to obtain with stainless-steel columns, many of these columns are glass-lined stainless steel. Fused-silica columns also fall into this category.

Packing materials

Silica-based packing materials

Silica ($SiO_2 \cdot xH_2O$) is the most widely used substance for the manufacture of packing materials. It consists of a network of siloxane linkages (Si—O—Si) in a rigid three-dimensional structure that contains interconnecting pores. The size of the pores and the concentration of silanol groups (Si—OH) which line the pores, can be controlled in the manufacturing process. Thus, a wide range of commercial products are available with surface areas that range from 100 to 800 m^2/g and average pore sizes from 4 to 33 nm.

Spherical packing materials are now the only types being introduced for analytical HPLC. Irregular shaped materials are still being used to pack preparative columns. The silanol groups on the surface of silica give it a polar character, which is exploited in adsorption chromatography using organic eluents. Silanol groups are also slightly acidic and hence basic compounds are adsorbed particularly strongly. Unmodified silicas can thus be used with aqueous eluents for the chromatography of basic drugs.

Silica can be altered drastically by reaction with organochlorosilanes or organoalkoxysilanes to give Si—O—Si—R linkages with the surface. The attachment of hydrocarbon chains to silica produces a nonpolar surface suitable for reversed-phase chromatography in which mixtures of water and organic solvents are used as eluents. The most popular material is octadecyl silica (ODS), which contains C_{18} chains, but materials with C_1, C_2, C_4, C_6, C_8 and C_{22} chains are also available. The latest silica-based bonded phase to be introduced is a long C_{30} phase, which has 24% carbon coverage, making it one of the most retentive phases available.

During manufacture, phases covalently bonded to silica gel may be reacted with a small monofunctional silane (e.g. trimethylchlorosilane) to further reduce the number of silanol groups that remain on the surface. This is referred to as endcapping. Recent advances in column technology include multiple reactant endcapping, use of type B (high-purity, low-trace-metal, low-acidity) silica and encapsulating the surface with a polymeric phase. These silicas are often referred to as 'base-deactivated' and are especially useful in reversed-phase chromatography in the pH range 4–8 when many basic compounds are partially ionised. Variations in elution order on different commercial packing materials of the same type (e.g. ODS) are often attributed to differences in surface coverage and the presence of residual silanol groups. For this reason it must not be assumed that a method developed with one manufacturer's ODS column can necessarily be transferred easily to the ODS column of another manufacturer.

Speciality silicas

A vast range of materials have intermediate surface polarities that arise from the bonding to silica of organic compounds that contain groups such as phenyl, cyano, nitro, amino, fluoro, sulfono and diols. There are also miscellaneous chemical moieties bound to silica, as well as polymeric packings, designed to purify specific compounds.

Phenyl
Propylphenylsilane ligands attached to the silica gel show weak dipole-induced dipole interactions with polar analytes. Usually this type of bonded phase is used for group separations of complex mixtures. Newer phases have phenyl backbones that allow π–π (stacking) interactions. These are recommended for peptide mapping applications. Amino-compounds show some specific interactions with phenyl-modified adsorbents.

Cyano
A cyano-modified surface is very slightly polar. Columns with this phase are useful for fast separations of mixtures that consist of very different components. These mixtures may show a very broad range of retention times on the usual columns.

Cyano-columns can be used in both normal- and reversed-phase modes of HPLC.

Amino
Amino-phases are weak anion-exchangers. This type of column is mainly used in normal-phase mode, especially for protein separation and also the selective retention of aromatic compounds.

Fluoro
A newer type of silica packing has fluorinated surfaces. This phase is generally more hydrophilic than phases with hydrocarbons of similar chain length. It has increased retention and unique selectivity for halogenated organic compounds and lipophilic compounds.

Sulfono
Sulfonic functional groups separate compounds on the basis of hydrophobic interactions. These packing materials allow the isocratic separation of mixtures that normally require gradient elution.

Diols
Diols are slightly polar adsorbents for normal-phase separations. These are useful to separate complex mixtures of compounds with different polarities that usually have a strong retention on unmodified silica.

Miscellaneous
Cyclodextrins, amylose, avidin, ristocetin, nitrophenylethyl, carbamate, ester, diphenylethyldiamine and Pirkle-type functional groups are all bound to silica packing material to enable enantiomeric separations. These columns are often referred to as chiral columns. Strong ion-exchangers are also available, in which sulfonic acid groups or quaternary ammonium groups are bonded to silica. These packing materials are useful to separate proteins. There are also proprietary functional groups added to silica packing materials for a variety of uses. These include petrochemical analysis, environmental analysis, detection of DNA adducts, purification of double-stranded DNA, separation of cationic polymers and separation of nitro-aromatic explosives.

For size-exclusion chromatography, a special type of silica is available that has a narrow range of pore diameters. Size-exclusion chromatography can be complicated by adsorption, but this can be reduced by treating the surface with trimethylchlorosilane.

pH range
The useful pH range for silica-based columns is 2–8, since siloxane linkages are cleaved below pH 2 while silica may dissolve at pH values above 8. However, the pH range may be extended above 8 if a pre-column packed with microparticulate silica is included between the pump and injector to saturate the eluent before it enters the analytical column.

Zirconia packing materials

Zirconia is a metal oxide that is more chemically and thermally stable than silica. It can be used for separations conducted at temperatures as high as 200°C and is unaffected by changes in ionic strength or organic content of the mobile phase. Zirconia packings have a wider pH range and are especially useful for basic separations at pH 10 or higher, where silica gel starts to dissolve. Zirconia can be used for reversed-phase chromatography and is extremely stable and efficient through surface modification with polymer or carbon coatings. Other chemical modifications of zirconia produce packing materials suitable for normal-phase or ion-exchange chromatography.

Polymer-based packing materials

Several packing materials based on organic polymers are available. For example, unmodified styrene–divinylbenzene co-polymers have a hydrophobic character and can be used for reversed-phase chromatography. Although they traditionally give lower column efficiencies than ODS, this situation has been improved greatly. Polymeric materials are best when separation conditions require a mobile phase that can go beyond the upper pH limits of silica gel (usually pH 6.5–7), as they have the advantage of being stable over a wide pH range. Polymeric materials also provide different selectivity and retention characteristics to silica-based reversed-phase packings. They also avoid problems associated with residual silanol groups (e.g. peak tailing). Ion-exchange materials of the styrene–divinylbenzene type are also available in which sulfonic acids, carboxylic acids or quaternary ammonium groups are incorporated in the polymeric matrix.

Monolithic columns

Monoliths are chromatographic columns that are cast as continuous homogeneous phases rather than packed as individual particles, creating porous rods of polymerised silica that are mechanically stable. Monolithic phases have flow-through pores with macroporosity (~2 μm) and mesopores, which are diffusive pores with an average pore diameter that can be controlled. To create the column, a silica gel polymer is formed, which, after ageing, is dried into the form of a straight rod of highly porous silica with the bimodal pore structure. The rod is then encased (or clad) in a PEEK cover, ensuring that there is absolutely no void space between the silica and PEEK material. The pore structure yields a very large internal surface area and ensures high-quality separations. In addition, the high porosity of the column means very high flow rates can be used with lower pressures. This enables separations in a fraction of the time needed when using a column with conventional packing materials.

A polymeric monolithic column has been introduced. It contains a poly(glycidylmethacrylate–ethylene glycol–dimethacrylate) co-polymer that has functional groups added to make various types of stationary phases.

Maintenance

An effective maintenance programme is essential to keep an HPLC system in proper working order. The maintenance programme should include preventive, periodical and necessary repairs of the HPLC system. This programme is essential to ensure that all of the components of the system are in proper working condition. In this section, the general maintenance of columns, pumps, injection valves and detectors is discussed. For information on the functions and uses of these components, refer to the earlier sections of this chapter.

It is always recommended that the maintenance guidelines provided with the system should be consulted to ensure compliance with the manufacturer's suggestions. This guide should be used whenever maintenance is required.

Columns

The column is an essential key to good chromatography and its maintenance ensures proper functionality of the HPLC system. High back pressures, poor resolution, nonuniform peak symmetry and decreasing retention times are several signs that may indicate the column is in need of repair or is failing.

Column degradation is inevitable, but a column's life can be prolonged if it is maintained properly. Flushing a column with a mobile phase of high elution strength after sample runs is essential. When a column is not in use, it should be capped to prevent it from drying out. Particulate samples should be filtered and, when possible, a guard column should be utilised. Column regeneration can instil some life into a column, but preventive maintenance is the vital key to prevent premature degradation.

Pumps

The pump forces the mobile phase through the HPLC system. A steady pump pressure is needed to ensure reproducibility and accuracy. Inability to build pressure, high pressures or leakage may indicate that the pump is not functioning correctly.

Pumps are typically known to be robust, but adequate maintenance must be performed to maintain that characteristic. Good maintenance practice includes replacing components, such as inlet check valves, outlet check valves, frits, pump seals and piston rods, on a routine schedule, based on the amount of usage. Proper maintenance of the pump system minimises downtime.

Injection valves

Injection valves play the role of directing injected volumes into the mobile phase, where they then travel onto the column. Proper valve function is a necessity to ensure reproducibility between injections. The symptoms of injection valve failure are low pump pressure, leakage or inadequate inert gas pressure to the switch valve.

The seals of the injection valve may eventually falter, after numerous injections. Replacement of these seals is necessary to maintain system reproducibility with respect to injections made.

Detectors

Detector maintenance is generally performed as needed. Baseline drift, erratic baseline and decreasing response may be indicators of a failing detector.

A malfunctioning or contaminated flow cell can also cause baseline drift. The cell should be flushed regularly with water to remove salts when using mobile phases of high salt concentration. An organic mobile phase of high elution strength should be used to remove any organic residue that may remain in the cell. An erratic baseline can occur because of an air bubble in the flow cell. Increasing the flow rate may push the bubble out of the cell. Ensure that mobile phases are suitably degassed to minimise the possibility of air bubbles in the detector cell (see the earlier section on Mobile phase reservoir and eluent preparation, p. 516). Decreasing response when using a UV-visible or fluorescence detector can also result from a decrease in lamp intensity. Most modern UV-visible and fluorescence detectors have some form of inbuilt mechanism for monitoring lamp lifetime and indicate when the lamp needs replacing.

Separation techniques

Isocratic

When the mobile-phase composition does not change throughout the course of the run, it is said to be *isocratic*. A mixed mobile phase can be delivered at a constant ratio by the pumps themselves or the solvent mixture can be prepared prior to analysis and pumped through a single reservoir. This is the simplest technique and should be the method of first choice when developing a separation.

Gradient elution

HPLC can be performed with changes in composition over time (gradient elution). The elution strength of the eluent is increased during the gradient run by changing polarity, pH or ionic strength. In RP-HPLC, the norm is to increase the percentage of organic modifier in the eluent relative to the aqueous component. Gradient elution can be a powerful tool for separation of mixtures of compounds with widely different retention. A direct comparison can be drawn with temperature programming in gas chromatography (see Chapter 18).

Eluent gradients are usually generated by combining the pressurised flows from two pumps and changing their individual flow rates with an electronic controller or data system, while maintaining the overall flow rate constant. Alternatively, a single pump with a low sweep volume can be used in combination with a proportioning valve, which controls the ratio of two liquids that enter the pump from two liquid reservoirs. Equipment and data systems that allow the gradient to take almost any conceivable form (e.g. step gradients, concave and convex gradient curves) are commonly available. The gradient can be programmed to return the system to the original eluent composition for the next analysis.

While most, if not all, commercially available pumps are capable of performing reliable gradient elutions, there are some potential difficulties. The technique can be very time consuming, as the column must be reconditioned with the initial eluent between runs. This drawback can be overcome by using a column-switching apparatus (see Column switches, p. 518). In addition, drifting of the detector response and the appearance of spurious peaks that arise from solvent impurities may occur. While isocratic elution is usually favoured over gradients for simplicity, gradient elution can be a very important and useful technique in the separation of complex mixtures.

The more recent use of 'fast gradient' separation has enabled the implementation of high-throughput analysis in laboratories with a high sample load.

Derivatisation

Derivatisation involves a chemical reaction that alters the molecular structure of the analyte of interest to improve detection and/or chromatography. In HPLC, derivatisation of a drug is usually unnecessary to achieve satisfactory chromatography. This applies to compounds of all polarities and molecular weights and is an important advantage of HPLC over GC. Derivatisation is used to enhance the sensitivity and selectivity of detection when available detectors are not satisfactory for the underivatised compounds. Both UV-absorbing and fluorescent derivatives have been used widely. UV derivatisation reagents include *N*-succinimidyl-*p*-nitrophenylacetate (SNPA), phenylhydrazine and 3,5-dinitrobenzoyl chloride (DNBC), while fluorescent derivatives can be formed with reagents such as dansyl chloride (DNS-Cl), 4-bromomethyl-7-methoxycoumarin (BMC) and fluorescamine. The characteristics of a good derivative in HPLC are similar to those in GC (stability, low background, convenience, and so on).

Derivative formation can be carried out before the sample is injected on to the column (pre-column) or by on-line chemical reactions between the column outlet and the detector. Such post-column reactions generally involve the addition of reagents to the eluent. With pre-column derivatisation there are no restrictions on reaction conditions (e.g. solvent, temperature) and a large excess of reagent can be used, as this can be separated from the derivatives during the chromatography. The major drawback of pre-column reactions is the need to obtain reproducible yields for accurate quantification, which is best achieved when the reactions proceed to completion. Furthermore, it is important that the products of pre-column derivatisation reactions be characterised fully. With post-column derivatisation, the reaction is well controlled by the flow rates of eluate and reagents, temperature, etc. Hence, it is less necessary for the reaction to proceed to completion or even for the chemistry to be understood as the system is calibrated by the injection of known quantities of the reference standards. A much more detailed discussion can be found in Snyder *et al.* (1997).

Chiral separation

Separation of compounds by chiral chromatography began in the early 1980s. At that time, the separation of enantiomeric compounds was one of the most challenging problems in chromatography. However, subsequently more than 100 chiral columns have been made available. These columns are based on several different approaches to solve the many enantiomeric separation problems. Chiral columns are used in a variety of different applications that range from pharmacokinetic and pharmacodynamic studies to measuring enantiomeric impurity of amino acids.

Chiral stationary phases (CSPs) are designed to separate optical isomers. The use of these columns provides an efficient and economical way to separate optical isomers by HPLC. CSPs are used for both resolving optical isomers to determine enantiomeric purity and for isolating enantiomerically pure compounds. Figure 19.2 shows the separation of enantiomers of flurbiprofen. This separation was performed at 15°C to improve selectivity.

The columns can be classified according to class or according to origin. The class category is based on the structural properties of the chiral selector. The category is made up of five different column types (macrocyclic, polymeric, π–π associations, ligand exchange, miscellaneous) and hybrids. The macrocyclic chiral columns have had the largest impact on analytical enantiomeric separations. The origin category separates columns according to their source and classifies them into three types (naturally occurring, semisynthetic and synthetic chiral selectors).

High-speed/high-temperature HPLC

The speed of a chromatographic method directly affects the economy and operating cost of the separation. High-speed HPLC is accomplished by using short microbore columns packed with small particles (3 μm). In addition, the use of higher temperatures increases the speed of HPLC separations through the 5- to 10-fold decrease in eluent viscosity upon an increase of the eluent temperature from 25 to 200°C. High-speed/high-temperature HPLC is not universally useful because of several limitations. Silica-based stationary phases are unstable in aqueous media at temperatures above 50 to 60°C. Also, some detectors are not able to tolerate high temperatures.

Quantitative analysis

The quantification methods incorporated in HPLC derive mostly from GC methods. The basic theory for quantification involves the measurement of peak height or peak area. To determine the concentration of a compound, the peak area or height is plotted against the concentration of the substance (Fig. 19.3). For peaks that are well resolved, both peak height and peak area should be proportional to the concentration. When establishing HPLC methods, the concentration range over which the calibration is linear should be established. Any deviation from linearity should be investigated and corrected. Three different calibration methods, each with its own benefits and limitations, can be employed in quantitative analysis: external standard, internal standard and the standard addition method.

External standard

The external standard method is the simplest of the three methods. The accuracy of the method

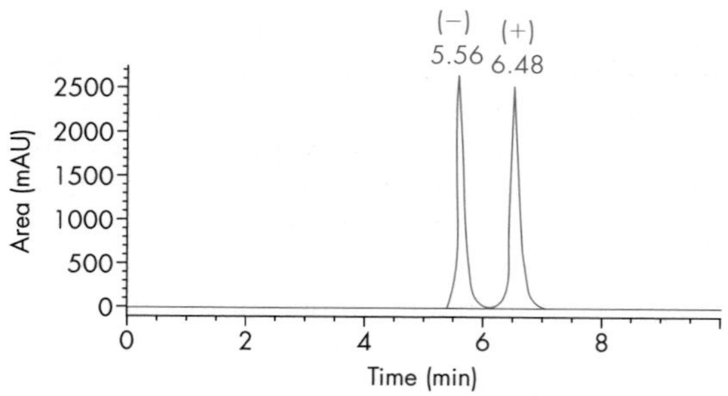

Figure 19.2 Chiral separation of the (+) and (−) enantiomers of flurbiprofen. Enantiomers were separated on a CHIRALPAKbAD-RHTM column using methanol–0.1% trifluoroacetic acid (TFA) as the mobile phase.

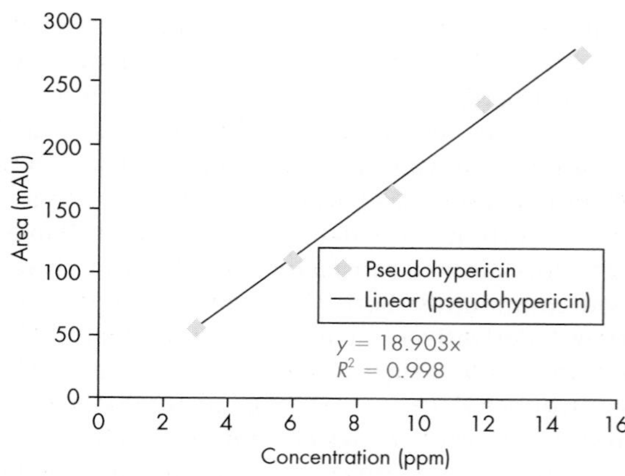

Figure 19.3 Example of a calibration curve for pseudohypericin.

is dependent on the reproducibility of the injection of the sample volume. For this method, a standard solution of known concentration of the compound of interest is prepared. A fixed amount, which should be similar in concentration to the unknown, is injected. Peak height or area is plotted against the concentration for each compound. The plot should be linear and go through the origin. The concentration of the unknown is then determined according to equation (19.3):

$$\text{Conc}_{\text{unknown}} = \left(\frac{\text{Area}_{\text{unknown}}}{\text{Area}_{\text{known}}}\right) \times \text{Conc}_{\text{known}} \qquad (19.3)$$

The calibrator concentrations should cover the range of the likely concentration in the unknown sample. Only concentrations read within the highest and lowest calibration levels are acceptable. Concentrations read from an extrapolated regression line may not be accurate. This applies to all of the quantification methods.

Internal standard

Although each method is effective, the internal standard method tends to yield the most accurate and precise results. In this method, an equal amount of an internal standard, a component that is not present in the sample, is added to both the sample and standard solutions. The internal standard selected should be chemically similar to the analyte, have a retention time close to that of the analyte and derivatise in a similar way to the analyte (where derivatisation is used). For biological samples, the internal standard should extract similarly to the analyte without significant bias toward the internal standard or the analyte. Additionally, it is important to ensure that the internal standard is stable and that it does not interfere with any of the sample components. The internal standard should be added before any preparation of the sample so that extraction efficiency can be evaluated. Quantification is achieved by using ratios of peak area or height (PAR) of the component to the internal standard (equation 19.4):

$$\text{Conc}_{\text{unknown}} = \text{PAR}_{\text{unknown}}/\text{PAR}_{\text{known}} \times \text{Conc}_{\text{known}} \qquad (19.4)$$

Standard addition method

The third approach for quantification is the standard addition method. This is especially useful when there is a problem with interference from the sample matrix, since it cancels out these effects. If sufficient sample is available, the sample is divided into several portions. A known and increasing amount of analyte is added to several portions (akin to standards spiked into the sample matrix, while one portion is retained with no analyte added. The unspiked sample and spiked samples are then analysed. A calibration line is plotted of concentration versus detector response. The calibration line is back-extrapolated to the *x*-axis and the concentration of analyte in the unspiked sample is determined (Fig. 19.4). Where sample mass or volume is limited, and where the detector response is known to be linear with concentration, the sample is divided into two portions, so that a known amount of the analyte (a spike) can be added to one portion. These two samples, the original and the original-plus-spike, are then analysed. The sample with the spike shows a larger analytical response than the original

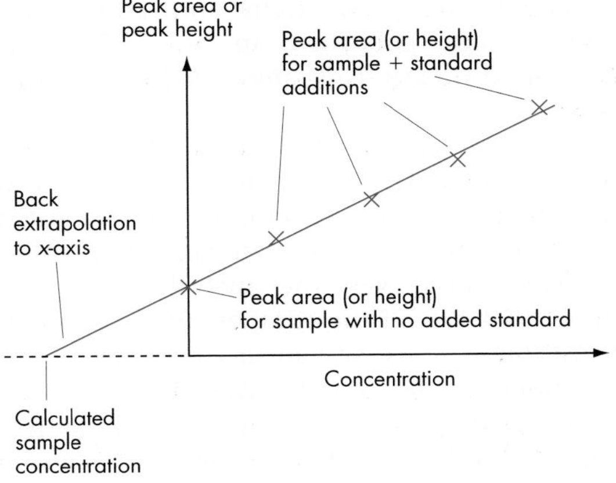

Figure 19.4 Calibration plot for standard addition where replicate portions of the sample are spiked with a known and increasing mass of analyte. The calibration plot is back-extrapolated to the *x*-axis and the concentration of analyte in the sample is determined.

sample because of the additional amount of analyte added to it. The difference in analytical response between the spiked and unspiked samples results from the amount of analyte in the spike. This provides a calibration point to determine the analyte concentration in the original sample. Equation (19.5) is used for this method:

$$\text{Amount}_{\text{unknown}} = \frac{\text{Amount}_{\text{spiked}}(\text{Area}_{\text{unspiked}})}{\text{Area}_{\text{spiked}} - \text{Area}_{\text{unspiked}}} \quad (19.5)$$

The standard addition method has drawbacks if only a small volume of sample is available. Internal standards can be used as part of the standard addition method, with a suitable internal standard added to the unspiked and spiked samples. Peak area ratio is then substituted for peak area in the calibration line or in equation (19.5).

Validation

It is important to use a validated HPLC method when carrying out analyses. Typical analytical characteristics evaluated in an HPLC validation may include precision, accuracy, specificity, limit of detection, limit of quantification, linearity and range. Some appropriate suggestions for LC validation for postmortem and body fluids samples are published in the *SOFT/AAFS Forensic Toxicology Laboratory Guidelines* (http://www.soft-tox.org).

System suitability tests evaluate the function of the overall HPLC system. This includes all parts that make up a system, such as the instrument, reagents, packing material, details of the procedure and even the analyst. These tests imply that the all the components of a system constitute a single system in which the overall function can be tested. These tests are very valuable and have been accepted in general application because reliable and reproducible chromatographic results are based on a wide range of specific parameters.

Most laboratories have a standard operating procedure that outlines the specifications of running a systems suitability test. For example, in pharmaceutical analysis at least five replicate injections should be made of a single solution that contains 100% of the expected active and excipient ingredient levels. The peak response is measured and the standard deviation of that response should not exceed the limit set by the testing monograph or 2%, whichever of the two is the lowest. Using the USP method, the tailing factors of the analytes should be determined. The values should not exceed 2.0. Peak-to-peak resolutions are also determined by using the USP calculations and the value should not be lower than 1.5. The system test should be used to ensure the quality of the data and of the analysis.

New emerging trends

On-line sample preparation

The preparation of samples typically demands a large amount of time, work and cost in an analytical laboratory. The innovation of on-line sample preparation makes the process more efficient and reduces the cost. On-line sample preparation techniques usually involve direct elution of the extract from a solid-phase extraction (SPE) cartridge into the system by the mobile phase. The on-line method gives superior analytical results and can be automated fully. Another benefit is that the sample preparation is reliable, reproducible and robust. This sample preparation method is also discussed in Column switches, p. 518.

Rapid screening

The need for high throughput in a laboratory environment is ever increasing. The use of short (2 mm), highly efficient analytical columns, rapid gradients and column-switching apparatus in HPLC systems is helping to facilitate this. Sample turnaround time can often be reduced to a few minutes or less in highly automated and optimised systems. Other information on this topic is given earlier in this chapter in relation to gradient elution and column switching.

Systems for drug analysis

Eluent systems

A large number of eluent and/or packing material combinations have been used for drug analysis. However, currently most are performed on silica or one of the hydrocarbon-bonded silicas (usually ODS). Other types of packing are employed when these conventional materials fail. The majority of drug analyses can be carried out with the four types of system described next.

Silica with nonpolar eluents

With silica normal-phase systems the principal mechanism is adsorption chromatography. Separation is controlled by the competition between solute molecules and molecules of the mobile phase for the adsorption sites on the silica surface. Polar groups are attracted most strongly to these sites and hence polar compounds are retained more strongly than nonpolar ones. Retention can be decreased by increasing the polarity of the eluent.

Adsorption energies of numerous solvents on alumina (ε° values are given in Table 19.1) have been measured and this scale can be used as a good guide to the elution strengths of eluents on silica as well as alumina (Snyder 1968).

Table 19.1 ε° values for numerous solvents on alumina (Snyder 1968)

Solvent	ε°
Pentane	0.00
Hexane	0.01
Isooctane	0.01
Cyclohexane	0.04
Toluene	0.29
1-Chlorobutane	0.30
Ether	0.38
Chloroform	0.40
Methylene chloride	0.42
Tetrahydrofuran	0.45
Acetone	0.56
Ethyl acetate	0.58
Diethylamine	0.63
Acetonitrile	0.65
Isopropyl alcohol	0.82
Ethanol	0.88
Methanol	0.95
Acetic acid	large
Water	large

Mixtures of solvents can be employed to give elution strengths between those of the pure solvents. Furthermore, different solvent mixtures that have the same ε° value often give different separations of a group of compounds.

Water is strongly bound to silica and thus the water content of the eluent must be controlled strictly to maintain constant activity of the silica surface and hence reproducible retention times. This is most critical when the eluent is of very low polarity. However, because anhydrous systems are difficult to maintain, a low concentration of water can be used in the eluent, sufficient to deactivate the most active sites without deactivating the whole surface. Typical water concentrations range from 0.01% to 0.2% (v/v). The most satisfactory method used to prepare a solvent of known water content is to mix anhydrous and water-saturated solvents in known proportions. Anhydrous hydrocarbon or halohydrocarbon solvents can be prepared by passing them through a bed of activated silica or alumina (200 μm) in a glass column. The problems associated with the control of water concentration mean that commonly alcohols, such as methanol (0.01–0.5% v/v), are employed to moderate the silica surface (Engelhardt 1977).

Silica with polar eluents

Several systems have been described that involve the use of silica with eluents of moderate-to-high polarity that contain alcohols and/or water as major components. With such eluents, adsorption chromatography is most probably not the principal mechanism. The mechanisms are poorly understood, which makes the prediction of retention behaviour difficult; nevertheless, many of these systems are very useful for drug analysis.

An eluent that consists of methanol–ammonium nitrate buffer (90:10) is suitable for a wide range of basic drugs (e.g. amfetamines and opiates). Retention can be controlled by changes to the pH, ionic strength or methanol : water ratio, or by the addition of other organic solvents such as methylene chloride. With these alkaline eluents the silica surface must bear a negative charge and the principal mechanism is probably cation exchange.

Benzodiazepines can be chromatographed with methanolic eluents that contain perchloric acid (typically 0.001 M). Retention can be modified by the addition of other organic solvents (e.g. ether) or by changes in the acid concentration.

Both acidic and basic drugs can be chromatographed on silica using aqueous methanolic eluents that contain cetyltrimethylammonium bromide (Hansen 1981). Hydrophobic quaternary ammonium ions are strongly adsorbed on silica to give a dynamically coated stationary phase. Retention may be controlled by varying the concentration or nature of the quaternary ammonium ion, changing the ionic strength or pH of the buffer or changing the concentration or nature of the organic component.

ODS with polar eluents

Eluents for reversed-phase chromatography on ODS are usually mixtures of methanol or acetonitrile (often referred to as organic modifiers) with an aqueous buffer solution. Retention is controlled mainly by the hydrophobic interactions between the drugs and the alkyl chains on the stationary phase packing material. Retention increases as the analytes decrease in polarity (i.e. polar species are eluted first). Hence, the elution time is increased by increasing the polarity of the eluent (i.e. increasing the water content). Nonpolar substances can be highly retained in mobile phases containing a high percentage of buffer due to the hydrophobic effect. Nonpolar analytes have low water solubility and hence partition preferentially into the nonpolar phases used in RP-HPLC. Elution is favoured by increasing the percentage of organic modifier. Where mixtures of polar and nonpolar analytes are to be analysed, gradient HPLC is performed, with the percentage of organic modifier typically increased during the analysis. The pH of the eluent and the pK_a of the drug are also important, since non-ionised species show greater retention. Thus, acids show an increase in retention as the pH is reduced while bases show a decrease. It is important to use a buffer of sufficient capacity to cope with any injected sample size, otherwise tailing peaks can arise from changes in ionic form during chromatography. Phosphate buffers (0.05–0.2 M) are widely used as they have a good pH range and low UV absorbance. Caution should be exercised in LC-MS analysis because the commonly used ionisation techniques such as electrospray ionisation and atmospheric pressure chemical ionisation are not compatible with non-volatile buffers.

Drugs that contain basic nitrogen atoms sometimes show poor efficiencies and give tailing peaks caused by interactions with residual silanol groups on the packing material. This can often be improved by the addition of an amine or quaternary ammonium compound to the eluent, which competes with the analytes for adsorption sites on the silica. Amines of small molecular weight (e.g. diethylamine) can be used as part of the buffer system. Alternatively, low concentrations (0.001 M) of long-chain hydrophobic modifiers (e.g. *N,N*-dimethyloctylamine) can be added to eluents together with conventional buffers. As noted previously, endcapped ODS phases are available and judicious choice of these can overcome the problems of peak tailing.

Other hydrocarbon-bonded packing materials can be used in reversed-phase chromatography. A decrease in retention is associated with a decrease in the alkyl chain length.

ODS with polar eluents that contain hydrophobic cations or anions

Drugs that bear positive or negative charges are retained poorly in reversed-phase systems. If the pH of the eluent cannot be changed to convert the drug into its non-ionised form, a hydrophobic ion of opposite charge can be added to form a neutral ion pair and increase retention. Hence, for a basic drug an acidic eluent is chosen and a hydrophobic anion added. This technique is referred to as reversed-phase ion-pair chromatography.

The sodium salts of alkylsulfonic acids (RSO_3^- Na^+, where R = pentyl, hexyl, heptyl or octyl) are used widely as ion-pair reagents for basic drugs, while quaternary ammonium compounds (e.g. tetrabutylammonium salts) are used for acidic drugs. Ion-pair reagents are generally added to eluents in the concentration range 0.001–0.005 M, and within this range an increase in concentration leads to an increase in retention. When detergents such as sodium lauryl sulfate or cetyltrimethylammonium bromide are used as the ion-pair reagents, the method is sometimes referred to as 'soap chromatography'. With these salts, ions build up on the surface of the packing material and produce a stationary phase, which behaves like an ion-exchanger. This type of mechanism has been described as 'dynamic ion-exchange' and probably also occurs with less hydrophobic ion-pair reagents. It is virtually impossible to remove an ion-pair reagent completely from a hydrocarbon-bonded phase, and such columns should not, therefore, be re-used with other reversed-phase eluents.

Selection of chromatographic systems

Many different combinations of packing material and eluent may be suitable for the analysis of a particular compound or group of compounds and the final choice can be influenced by many factors. The time required to develop a new system can be shortened if it is possible to predict the way in which changes in eluent composition influence chromatographic retention. Systems that use hydrocarbon-bonded phases are particularly attractive from this viewpoint as a large range of parameters can be adjusted (pH, organic solvent, ionic strength, ion-pair reagents) with largely foreseeable consequences. Predictions for silica are generally less reliable. Silica is good for separating drugs that belong to different chemical classes, while hydrocarbon-bonded silicas are preferred for separations of drugs with closely related structures (e.g. barbiturates).

Most of the endogenous materials in biological extracts that can interfere with the analysis of a drug are fairly polar. In reversed-phase systems this material generally elutes before the drug and can obscure the drug peak. In these circumstances, reversed-phase ion-pair chromatography can be valuable to increase selectively the retention of the drug relative to the interfering peaks. Normal-phase systems that use silica do not generally suffer from this problem, as most of the endogenous material usually elutes after the drug. However, these slow-eluting compounds can lead to a noisy baseline or may remain adsorbed to the packing material and thus eventually lead to a loss in column performance. As a result of the difficulties that can arise using silica, most LC separations these days are carried out by RP-HPLC.

The vast majority of compounds are separated using a silica-based column with C_{18} bonded stationary phase. Fine-tuning of the separation can be made by selecting a column with a shorter bonded phase, such as C_8 (see Fig. 19.5).

Specially endcapped columns designed to minimise the tailing common with nitrogen-containing weak bases are available. These are often marketed as a 'basic' column (e.g. Metachem's MetaSil Basic). Problems can occur when alkyl phases are used with a very high concentration of aqueous mobile phases (95–100%) because the hydrophobic alkyl chains tend to 'collapse' such that the surface area available for interaction is vastly reduced (Fig. 19.5A). There are specially endcapped columns designed to withstand extremely high concentrations of aqueous mobile phase (95–100%). These columns are endcapped with a hydrophilic moiety that ensures proper 'wetting' of the silica to prevent bonded-phase collapse (Fig. 19.5B). The columns are typically marketed as 'AQ' for aqueous (e.g. YMC's ODS-AQ).

Analysis of drugs in pharmaceutical preparations

HPLC has found widespread use for the quantitative analysis of drugs in preparations of pharmaceutical and illicit manufacture. Drug concentrations are generally high enough to allow dissolution of the sample (tablet, powder, ointment, etc.) in a suitable solvent followed by injection. UV, visible, FL, RI or mass spectrometric detection methods are used often. These

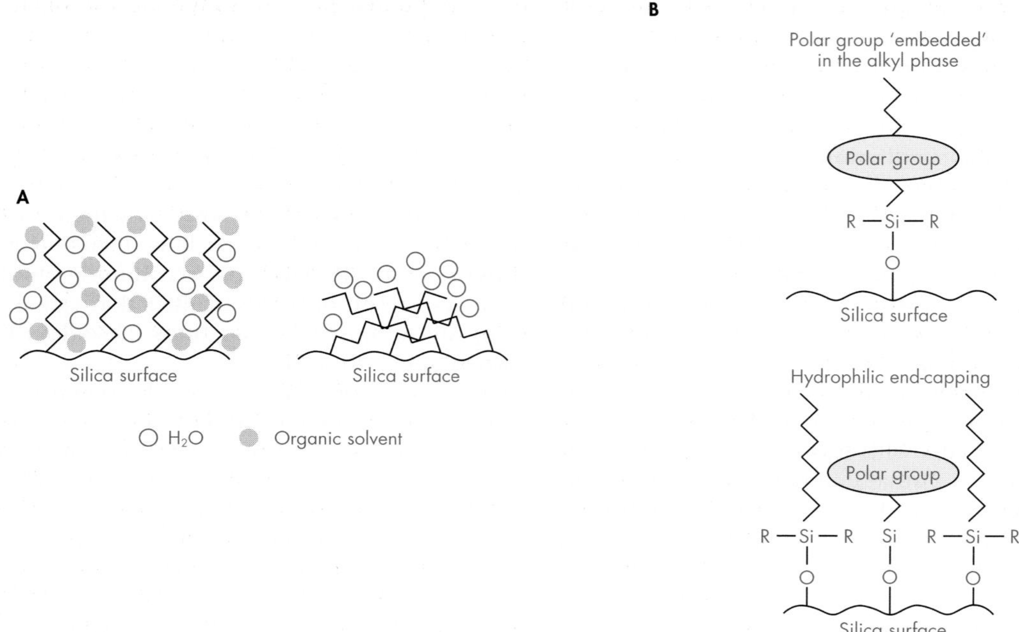

Figure 19.5 (A) Alkyl phase in eluent with organic modifier. Note how the alkyl chains 'stand out' from the silica surface and are readily available to analytes in the mobile phase. In 100% aqueous eluent the alkyl chains collapse in on one another such that the area for analyte–stationary phase interaction is much reduced. (B) Introduction of a hydrophilic moiety in the stationary phase to prevent bonded-phase collapse. The polar group can be embedded in the alkyl phase or endcapped.

techniques are well-suited to provide specific data as to the chemical composition of the sample in question (e.g. a UV spectrum, mass spectrum, etc.).

Within the pharmaceutical industry, HPLC is used at various stages of drug development, such as the optimisation of synthetic reactions and stability testing. Furthermore, it is used extensively for quality control during production to monitor the purity of drugs and excipients. HPLC systems can be automated easily (including injection and data handling), which allows large numbers of samples to be analysed rapidly and economically. HPLC is particularly valuable for the analysis of drugs that are polar (e.g. aspirin), thermally unstable (e.g. benzodiazepines) or present in oil-based formulations for which analysis by GC can be very difficult. Similarly, HPLC can be used for the forensic analysis of illicit preparations to aid the identification of an unknown drug by the measurement of retention times and UV spectra and comparison with spectral libraries. Furthermore, as the technique can be nondestructive, depending on the detection system used, the eluted compounds can be collected for further analysis.

Analysis of drugs in biological fluids and tissues

Several factors determine the ability of HPLC to detect a drug among the endogenous compounds present in biological material. Clearly, selective detection of the drug relative to the endogenous material is advantageous. In addition, the stationary phase and/or mobile phase can be altered to separate the drug peak from interfering peaks (e.g. using ion-pair reagents). Finally, the sample may be extracted before HPLC to concentrate the drug relative to the endogenous material.

The chromatographic system and detector should always be chosen to minimise the time needed for sample preparation. The complexity of the sample preparation procedure is controlled by several factors, which include the nature of the sample (urine, blood, liver, etc.), the condition of the sample, and the concentration of the drug. Interference from endogenous compounds is most acute when drug concentrations are low (e.g. therapeutic drug monitoring), so more extensive sample preparation and more sensitive and specific detectors are often required. Such assays can be very susceptible to changes in the condition of the sample (e.g. a method developed for fresh blood may not be satisfactory for urine or hair samples), which can present severe difficulties in forensic toxicology. Thus, methods should be tested and validated with the most difficult samples that may be encountered. In contrast, the analysis of biological samples that contain high drug concentrations (e.g. fatal drug overdose) by HPLC may require much less sample preparation and is less susceptible to changes in sample condition.

Sample preparation for HPLC is essentially the same as for other methods of drug analysis. A drug that is physically trapped within solid tissue (e.g. liver), or chemically bound to the surface of proteins, must be released; then the protein is precipitated to leave the drug in aqueous solution. The protein may be degraded by strong acids or enzymes, precipitated by various chemicals (e.g. tungstic acid, ammonium sulfate) or removed by ultrafiltration. Some drugs are destroyed by protein degradation methods, while ultrafiltration and precipitation can lead to drug losses through protein binding. No single procedure works well for all drugs and the method should be selected to give the maximum recovery of the drug being analysed, with validation of the method to ensure that it is fit for purpose.

When drug concentrations are high (typically μg/mL) and systems with polar mobile phases are used, the direct injection of deproteinised solutions may be acceptable. Proteins must be removed to protect the column from irreversible contamination. A rapid procedure is to mix the biological fluid with at least two volumes of methanol or acetonitrile, centrifuge to remove the precipitated protein, evaporate the organic supernatant and reconstitute the sample in a volume of mobile phase. Urine can be treated similarly to guard against the precipitation of salts on the column. Great care and consideration should be taken when injecting minimally prepared biological samples onto a HPLC system. Particulates are more likely to become trapped in the system plumbing and a more rapid degradation of column performance may be observed from contaminant build-up on the head of the column. To help maximise column performance and lifetime, it is good policy to use a guard column between the injector and analytical column. This is packed with the same material as the analytical column and replaced at frequent intervals. The configuration of guard columns ranges from easily replaceable and relatively inexpensive frit-like filters and/or cartridges to shorter versions of the analytical column itself. All are designed to protect the analytical column by acting as a trap for components that would otherwise irreversibly bind to the analytical column, and thus decrease the useable life of the column.

Extraction of drugs and other analytes away from endogenous materials prior to analysis is a common procedure for all types of biological samples. This may also entail a concentration step, which increases the sensitivity of the method. Solvent extraction remains the most popular approach, as many factors can be modified to optimise the extraction. These modifications include changing the polarity of the organic solvent and the pH and ionic strength of the aqueous phase and the use of ion-pairing agents. It is generally recommended that the collected organic phase be evaporated to dryness and the residue dissolved in a suitable solvent, typically something greater than or equal to the polarity and composition of the initial mobile phase, before injection. Care must be taken that volatile drugs are not lost by evaporation and that lipid material in the residue does not prevent the drug from dissolving in the new solvent.

Although there is a move to use minimal sample preparation with HPLC, caution must be exercised with LC-MS because interferents in the sample can cause ion suppression, which is not always easy to recognise.

Solid phase extraction (SPE) columns are also widely used to extract drugs from biological samples. The column is washed with suitable solvents to remove endogenous material before the drug is removed by passing through a solvent of higher elution strength. Such columns are usually attached to extraction manifolds utilising either positive or negative pressure to draw the liquids through the sorbent beds. Extraction selectivity can be controlled by adjustments to the biological fluid before extraction (e.g. pH, ionic strength) and the choice of washing solvents. Most, if not all, manufacturers of SPE columns offer methods and columns optimised for a particular drug class and/or matrix. As less traditional biological matrices are used for drug analysis (e.g., sweat, hair, oral fluids), some modifications of the sample preparation scheme are needed. Hair requires solubilisation prior to extraction; oral fluids and sweat may need to be isolated from their respective collection devices. Consideration of the pH and solubility may be necessary prior to sample preparation, but in general the principles in place for the extraction of blood, urine, etc., apply to these alternative matrices. Some important issues unique to these matrices are:

- sample volume is typically much less than blood or urine
- the amount of drug extracted from a particular matrix may be much less than from traditional matrices, so that much more sensitive detectors (e.g. MS or MS/MS) are required.

References

H. Engelhardt, The role of moderators in liquid-solid-chromatography, *J. Chromatogr. Sci.*, 1977, **15**, 380–384.

L. S. Ettre, *J. Chromatogr.*, 1980, **198**, 229–234.

S. H. Hansen, *J. Chromatogr.*, 1981, **209**, 203–210.

S. Huber and A. George (eds), *Applications of Diode-array Detection in HPLC*, Chromatographic Science Series 62, New York, Marcel Dekker, 1993.

G. Rozing *et al.*, A system and columns for capillary HPLC, *Am. Lab.*, May 2001, 26–38.

L. R. Snyder, *Principles of Adsorption Chromatography*, New York, Marcel Dekker, 1968, pp. 194–195.

L. R. Snyder *et al.*, *Practical HPLC Method Development*, New York, Wiley, 1997.

M. J. M. Wells and C. R. Clark, *Anal. Chem.*, 1981, **53**, 1341–1345.

Further reading

D. Armstrong and B. Zhang, Chiral stationary phases for high-performance liquid chromatography, *Anal. Chem.*, 2001, **73**, 557A–561A.

J. Ayrton *et al.*, Use of generic fast gradient liquid chromatography–tandem mass spectroscopy in quantitative bioanalysis, *J. Chromatogr. B*, 1998, **709**, 243–254.

S. C. Bobzin *et al.*, LC-NMR: a new tool to expedite the dereplication and identification of natural products, *J. Ind. Microbiol. Biotechnol.*, 2000, **25**, 342–345.

T. Fornstedt and G. Guiochon, Nonlinear effects in LC and chiral LC, *Anal. Chem.*, 2001, **73**, 609A–617A.

V. C. X. Gao *et al.*, Column switching in high-performance liquid chromatography with tandem mass spectrometric detection for high-throughput preclinical pharmacokinetic studies, *J. Chromatogr. A*, 1998, **828**, 141–148.

R. J. Hamilton and P. Sewell, *Introduction to High-performance Liquid Chromatography*, 2nd edn, London, Chapman & Hall, 1977.

K. Heinig and F. Bucheli, Application of column-switching liquid chromatography–tandem mass spectrometry for the determination of pharmaceutical compounds in tissue samples, *J. Chromatogr. B*, 2002, **769**, 9–26.

J. Henion *et al.*, Sample preparation for LC-MS-MS: Analyzing biological and environmental samples, *Anal. Chem.*, 1998, **70**, 650A–656A.

R. P. Hicks, Recent advances in NMR: expanding its role in rational drug design, *Curr. Med. Chem*, 2001, **8**, 627–650.

D. Johns, Resolving isomers on HPLC columns with chiral stationary phases, *Am. Lab.*, Jan. 1987, 72–76.

H. T. Karnes and M. A. Sarkar, Enantiomeric resolution of drug compounds by liquid chromatography, *Pharm. Res.*, 1987, **4**, 285–292.

G. Lunn and N. R. Schmitt, *HPLC Methods for Pharmaceutical Analysis*, New York, Wiley, Vol. 1, 1997; Vols 2–4, 2000.

R. E. Majors, New chromatography columns and accessories at the 1997 Pittsburgh Conference Part 1, *LC–GC*, 1997, **15**, 220–237.

R. E. Majors, New chromatography columns and accessories at the 1998 Pittsburgh Conference Part 1, *LC–GC*, 1998, **16**, 228–244.

R. E. Majors, New chromatography columns and accessories at the 1999 Pittsburgh Conference Part 1, *LC–GC*, 1999, **17**, 212–220.

R. E. Majors, New chromatography columns and accessories at the 2000 Pittsburgh Conference Part 1, *LC–GC*, 2000, **18**, 262–285.

V. R. Meyer, *Practical High-performance Liquid Chromatography*, 2nd edn, New York, Wiley, 1979.

S. X. Peng *et al.*, Direct determination of stability of protease inhibitors in plasma by HPLC with automated column-switching, *J. Pharm. Biomed. Anal.*, 1999, **25**, 343–349.

R. S. Plumb *et al.*, The application of fast gradient capillary liquid chromatography–mass spectrometry to the analysis of pharmaceuticals in biofluids, *Rapid Commun. Mass Spectrom.*, 1999, **13**, 865–872.

C. Schüfer *et al.*, HPLC columns: The next great leap forward, Part 1, *Am. Lab.*, Feb. 2001, 40–41.

C. Schüfer *et al.*, HPLC columns: The next great leap forward, Part 2, *Am. Lab.*, Apr. 2001, 25–26.

C. F. Simpson, *Practical High-performance Liquid Chromatography*, London, Heyden and Son Ltd, 1976.

L. R. Snyder, HPLC past and present, *Anal. Chem.*, 2000, **72**, 412A–420A.

N. Tanaka *et al.*, Monolithic LC columns, *Anal. Chem.*, 2001, **72**, 420A–429A.

T. Wehr, Configuring HPLC systems for LC-MS, *LC–GC*, 2000, **18**, 406–416.

I. Wilson *et al.*, 2000. Analytical chemistry: advancing hyphenated chromatographic systems, *Anal. Chem.*, 2000, **71**, 534A–542A.

J. L. Wolfender *et al.*, The potential of LC–NMR in phytochemical analysis, *Phytochem. Anal.*, 2001, **12**, 2–22.

L. Y. Yang *et al.*, Applications of new liquid chromatography–tandem mass spectrometry technologies for drug development support, *J. Chromatogr. A*, 2001, **926**, 43–55.

20

Capillary electrophoresis for drug analysis

D Perrett

Background to capillary electrophoresis 539
Theoretical outline 540
Modes of capillary electrophoresis. 543
Instrumentation for capillary electrophoresis 545
Method development and optimisation 548
Analytical methods 550
General applications to drug assays . . . 554
Conclusions and future directions. 556
References 556
Further reading 556

Background to capillary electrophoresis

Traditional electrophoretic methodologies, although they used simple and reliable equipment, were always limited by their low resolution of analytes, low throughput, the need to visualise the separated bands and the qualitative nature of the results. They were, in fact, the electrophoretic equivalent of thin-layer chromatography (TLC) and, like TLC, fell from favour with the uptake of high-performance liquid chromatography (HPLC) during the 1970s.

Since 1981 a new 'form' of separation science, namely capillary electrophoresis (CE) has become accepted as both a research and a routine technique for the analysis of a wide variety of analytes, including drugs. Modern capillary electroseparation was introduced by Jorgenson and Lukacs (1981) and was developed rapidly by many other groups of separation scientists. By 1987 the first commercial instrument for performing CE had been introduced. CE now occupies a complementary role to HPLC in analysis, and by 2005 some 2500 assays for drugs had been produced, many of which are unique to CE.

The seminal publication of Jorgenson and Lukacs (1981) is usually taken as the origin of modern CE. A period of rapid development from about 1987 to 1997 was followed by a period of acceptance of the technology. Following this period, many of the HPLC companies that originally entered the field either abandoned commercialisation of CE systems or concentrated on building dedicated systems for techniques such as deoxyribonucleic acid (DNA) analysis or nanotechnologies. Today only two major instrument companies market general-purpose systems, although a number of smaller companies are also active in the field.

Theoretical outline

The basic principles behind CE differ little from those of traditional electrophoresis in that the separation of two or more charged analytes (ionic compounds) or particles results from their different mobilities (i.e. speed plus direction of movement) when placed in a conducting medium under the influence of an applied direct current (d.c.) electric field. In electrophoresis the movement is towards the electrode of opposite charge to that of the ion or charged particle. Cations, being positively charged ions, move towards the negative electrode (the cathode). Anions are negatively charged and therefore move to the positive electrode (the anode). Importantly, neutral species do not move under the influence of the electric field, although they may diffuse from the load position or be carried by electro-osmotic flow.

At its simplest, the speed of migration in an electric field of any ion or compound that carries an overall charge at a given pH is considered to be the vector sum of a driving force (the electrical potential) and any resistant forces. In simple solution, ions move freely towards the opposite electrode and the product of the charge on the ion and the applied voltage (V) gives the electric force (F_{ef}) experienced by the charged species. The potential gradient down which the ion moves is given by the electric field strength (E).

$$\text{Electric field strength } (E) = \frac{\text{Applied voltage}}{\text{Distance between electrodes}} = \frac{V}{d} \tag{20.1}$$

$$\text{Applied field } (F_{ef}) = qE \tag{20.2}$$

where q is the total charge on the ion.

However, even a simple ion can be considered as a particle, so this movement is opposed by a frictional drag (F_{fr}) given by Stokes' law:

$$\text{Friction } (F_{fr}) = 6\pi r v \eta \tag{20.3}$$

where η is the viscosity of the medium, r is the 'radius' of the molecule and v is the velocity.

When a voltage is applied there is a rapid acceleration of all the ionic species and equilibrium is achieved in a few microseconds, at which point the following equilibrium conditions apply:

$$F_{ef} = F_{fr} \tag{20.4}$$

Therefore,

$$qE = 6\pi r v \eta \tag{20.5}$$

So the velocity is given by

$$v = \frac{\text{distance moved}}{\text{time taken}} = \frac{qE}{6\pi r v \eta} \tag{20.6}$$

Electrophoretic mobility (μ) is defined as the average velocity with which an ion moves under unit applied electric field under defined conditions:

$$\mu = \frac{\text{Average migration velocity}}{\text{Electric field strength}} = \frac{v}{E} \tag{20.7}$$

Substituting for v from equation (20.3):

$$\mu = \frac{q}{6\pi r \eta} \tag{20.8}$$

Mobility can therefore be interpreted as proportional to a charge-to-size ratio for a charged molecule in a given buffer at a set pH. The units of μ are cm/s divided by volts/cm, that is $cm^2\ V^{-1}\ s^{-1}$. The magnitude of μ for typical small ions is of the order of $10^{-6}\ cm^2\ V^{-1}\ s^{-1}$ (e.g. μ is $-5 \times 10^{-5}\ cm^2\ V^{-1}\ s^{-1}$ for a typical anionic sulfonamide, such as sulfacetamide). Note that differences in the sign of the mobility lead to different directions of movement in traditional electrophoresis.

The above theoretical description, well established by the 1950s, clearly showed that faster analyses should be achieved by using high voltages. However, the limitations to electrophoretic separations brought about by convectional mixing caused by the heating effect of the current were also appreciated. This Joule heating seriously limited the speed of separation, since it restricted the voltages that could be used. For macromolecular separations the use of anti-convective gels such as polyacrylamide became, and has remained, the standard approach, but to limit the heat generated, voltages are still low (~200–500 V) and runtimes correspondingly long (3–18 h).

Jorgenson and Lukacs (1981), although not the first to attempt to overcome the problem of Joule heating, demonstrated a very simple solution. They showed that the rate of cooling could be increased substantially by increasing the surface-to-volume ratio of the electrophoresis buffer. This could be done readily using small-bore capillaries, with which the Joule heating was shown to be dissipated efficiently to give very high-resolution separations. The increased rate of cooling dramatically lowered the deterioration in peak efficiency and resolution caused by Joule heating. Although Jorgenson originally worked with glass capillaries, these were soon replaced by silica capillaries. In addition, this new format could use the significant electro-osmotic flow (EOF) of the background electrolyte (BGE) in the capillary to separate cations, anions and uncharged molecules simultaneously, with all analytes usually going towards the cathode at which a single online detector is placed.

Most surfaces, including silica, acquire an intrinsic charge when wetted (Fig. 20.1) and attach a layer of solvent when under the influence of an electric field. This causes a movement of liquid towards one of the electrodes (i.e. electro-osmosis). In traditional electrophoresis, electro-osmosis is usually detrimental, but in CE it can be of major benefit.

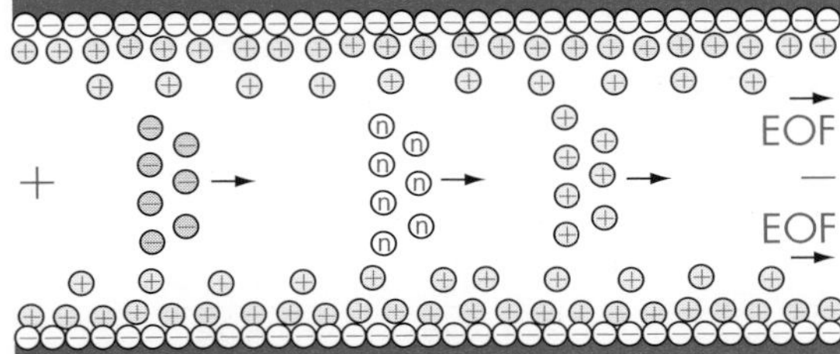

Figure 20.1 Formation of a double layer at the surface of silica capillary.

The mobility of the bulk liquid (μ_{EOF}) is given by

$$\mu_{EOF} = \frac{\varepsilon E \zeta}{4\pi\eta} \tag{20.9}$$

where ε is the dielectric constant of the solution and ζ is the zeta potential of the surface.

For silica capillaries, the charge on the surface results from ionisation of the silanol groups. The pK_a of silanol groups of silica is variable but is about 4.5.

Zeta potential is given by

$$\zeta = \frac{4\pi\delta e}{\varepsilon} \tag{20.10}$$

where δ is the thickness of the double layer and e is the total excess charge per unit of area.

The zeta potential is an inverse function of the square root of the total molarity of BGE (the Debye–Hückel equation), and therefore the EOF decreases as the square root of molarity. Since EOF is generated at the capillary wall, its flow profile is flat rather than parabolic as in pumped flows. This effect contributes to the efficiency of CE.

The addition to the BGE of reagents that can bind to the surface silanols, such as cationic detergents like tetradecyltrimethyl ammonium bromide (TTAB), can reverse the direction of the EOF. This is beneficial in the analysis of anions such as nitrate and nitrite, but it is essential to saturate all the silanols prior to establishing the separation.

Mobility in capillary electrophoresis

On an electropherogram the mobility (μ) of an analyte is calculated from its migration time (t) and the length of the analytical section of the capillary, which is normally less than the total length down which the applied potential is dropped:

$$\mu = \frac{\text{Velocity}}{\text{Potential gradient}} = \frac{(l/t)}{(V/L)} \tag{20.11}$$

where l is the length to detection window and L is the total capillary length.

Separation depends on differences in mobility for the analytes, but μ is the sum of the mobility of the analyte, μ_a, and the EOF, μ_{EOF}, and is called the apparent mobility (μ_{app}).

$$\mu_{app} = \mu_a + \mu_{EOF} \tag{20.12}$$

(The sign of μ is important.)

Peak efficiency

Jorgenson also developed a simple theoretical understanding of this new separation mode. The separation efficiency of CE is expressed in terms similar to those used in chromatography that are familiar to chromatographers. For a Gaussian peak – this is more likely in CE than HPLC – the number of theoretical plates (N) for a peak migrating at time t is given by

$$N = (l/\sigma)^2 \text{or } [5.54\,(t/w_{1/2})^2] \tag{20.13}$$

where σ is the standard deviation of the peak and $w_{1/2}$ is the width of the peak at half height.

In a capillary the only major contribution to zone dispersion is the time-dependent longitudinal diffusion. This can be characterised by Einstein's equation for diffusion in liquids:

$$\sigma^2 = 2Dt \tag{20.14}$$

where D is the diffusion coefficient for the analyte. Substituting for time and combining this equation with that for mobility:

$$\sigma^2 = \frac{2DLl}{V\mu_{app}} \tag{20.15}$$

Combining this equation with that for efficiency:

$$N = \mu_{app}\frac{lV}{2DL} \tag{20.16}$$

If the length to the detector and total length are similar, which is the usual case in CE, this equation can be further simplified to

$$N = \mu_{app}\frac{V}{2D} \tag{20.17}$$

From these equations it is apparent that in CE peak efficiency, measured as N, increases linearly with the applied voltage. So the higher the voltage, the faster the separation and the narrower the peaks. A high pH, and therefore high μ_{EOF}, is also advantageous to high efficiency. Analytes with a high mobility are separated efficiently and those analytes with low diffusion coefficients, such as proteins, should have high separation efficiencies.

Typical diffusion coefficients in water at room temperature are given in Table 20.1.

The generic Giddings' resolution equation (R_s) as expressed in electrophoretic terms,

$$R_s = \frac{\sqrt{N}}{4}(\Delta\mu/\mu_{av}) \tag{20.18}$$

can now be rewritten as

$$R_s = \frac{1}{4}\sqrt{\left(\frac{\mu_{av} + \mu_{EOF}}{2D}V\right)}\left(\frac{\Delta\mu}{\mu_{av} + \mu_{EOF}}\right) \tag{20.19}$$

From this equation two findings are apparent:

- although peak efficiency increases linearly with voltage, resolution requires a 4-fold increase in voltage to double resolution
- infinite resolution is possible when μ_{EOF} is equal in magnitude, but opposite in direction, to μ_a.

Since Jorgenson originally derived these formulae, a number of variations have appeared

Table 20.1 Typical diffusion coefficients in water at room temperature

Molecule	Molecular weight	D (10^{-9} m^2 s^{-1})
H^+	1	9.31
Na^+	23	1.68
Glycine	75	1.055
Sucrose	342	0.45
Albumin	66 000	0.059
Collagen (Type 1)	345 000	0.069

that include corrections for sample injection size, Joule heating variations across the capillary, etc. However, his formulae still offer a reasonable approximation to the experimental observations. A number of reviews on the theory of CE have been published (Mosher *et al.* 1992; Poppe 1998, Bartle and Myers, 2001).

Modes of capillary electrophoresis

Capillary electrophoresis is recognised generally as the description appropriate for the whole field of separation science based on electromigration techniques. With the increasing number of variants on the basic technique, more specific definitions are now required, although no International Union of Pure and Applied Chemistry (IUPAC) definitions had been agreed by the time of writing. The following working definitions are the author's own.

Capillary zone electrophoresis (CZE), in which ionic species are separated according to their mobility and polarity in aqueous solution, is the most frequently used option in CE. CZE does not necessarily require aqueous electrolytes and nonaqueous background electrolytes (NACE) such as acetonitrile can be used, provided the current can be carried by a suitable soluble electrolyte such as ammonium acetate. CZE does not separate neutral compounds, although they do move towards the detector, travelling with the EOF front. A subtype of CZE is capillary ion analysis (CIA), which is used to determine simple ionic species in aqueous solution rapidly and usually employs indirect detection. CZE is illustrated by the separation of members of the sulfonamide family shown in Figure 20.2.

Other forms of capillary electrophoresis might be entitled interaction CE (ICE), in which the analytes' mobilities are modified by the presence of additives in the BGE that cause:

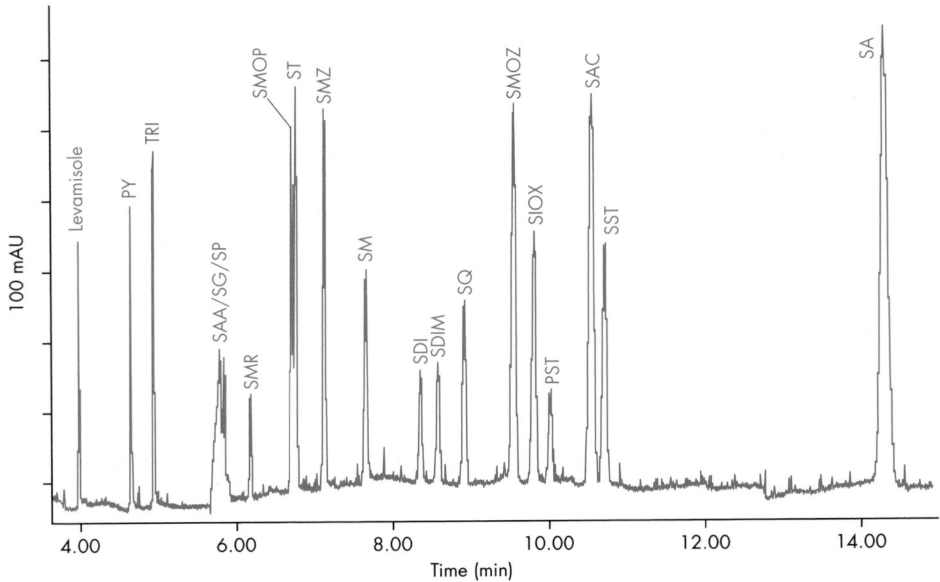

Figure 20.2 Capillary zone electrophoresis separation of sulfonamides. Separation of twenty compounds, 17 sulfonamides, levamisole, trimethoprim, and pyrimethamine (all 50 μM); separation with 30 mM sodium dihydrogen phosphate/10 mM sodium tetraborate pH 6.75, 15 kV, HD 1.8 s at 50 mbar; hydrodynamic injection, 60(47) × 50 μm, 200 nm. Key: PST, phthalsulfathiazole; PY, pyrimethamine; SA, sulfanilic acid; SAA, sulfanilamide; SAC, sulfacetamide; SDI, sulfadiazine; SDIM, sulfadimethoxine; SG, sulfaguanidine; SIOX, sulfaisoxazole; SM, sulfameter; SMOP, sulfamethoxypyridine; SMOZ, sulfamethoxaxole; SMR, sulfamerazine; SMZ, sulfamethazine; SP, sulfapyridine; SQ, sulfaquinoxaline; SST, succinyl-sulfathiazole; ST, sulfathiozole; and TRI, trimethoprim.

- complexation, for example metals and amino acids or borate in the case of sugars
- inclusion into chemical additives such as cyclodextrins.

A similar mechanism is involved in affinity CE (ACE), in which biospecific interactions occur, usually with macromolecules. Chiral separations by CE can be obtained using either ICE or ACE methods. A long-established form of ICE is micellar electrokinetic capillary chromatography (MEKC), often also called MECC. This separation mode, introduced in 1984 by Terabe *et al.*, allows the separation of neutral molecules by differential partitioning into migrating charged micelles formed from suitable detergents incorporated into the background CE electrolyte. MEKC is considered to offer an intermediate mechanism between electrophoresis and reversed-phase chromatography in that the hydrophobicity of the analyte can be a dominant factor in the final separation. As well as surfactants, other additives (such as cyclodextrins) can be included in the MEKC electrolyte to enhance separations. MEKC does not prevent the simultaneous separation of charged species in the samples, a factor of some importance in drug analyses, since an uncharged drug often gives rise to charged metabolites. MEKC is illustrated in Figure 20.3, in which the metabolism of ibuprofen is being monitored. A more recent, but related, development is microemulsion electrokinetic capillary chromatography (MEEKC), in which a charged surfactant-based microemulsion is formed in the BGE to produce the hydrophobic pseudo-chromatographic phase.

Other early forms of electrophoresis, such as isoelectric focusing (IEF) and isotachophoresis (ITP), can also be performed in capillary format, known as capillary isoelectric focusing (cIEF) and capillary isotachophoresis (cITP). In cIEF the order of the final separation is according to the isoelectric points of the analytes when they migrate in a pH gradient formed in the capillary using ampholytes. Although IEF is a standard methodology in gel electrophoresis and offers a

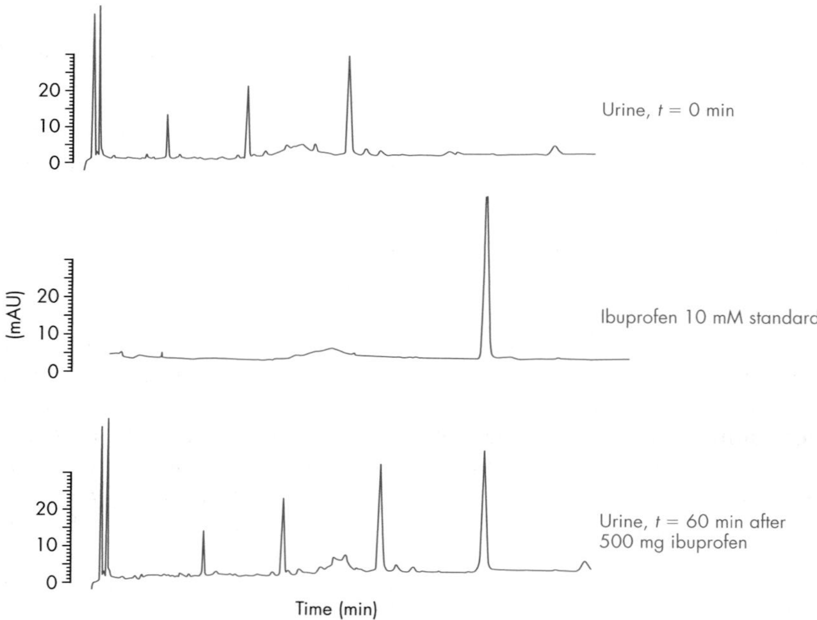

Figure 20.3 MEKC (micellar electrokinetic capillary chromatography) separation of ibuprofen and its metabolites in urine. Conditions: HP3D system; capillary, silica, 47(38.5) cm × 50 μm; buffer, 25 mM sodium tetraborate pH 9.5 that contains 75 mM sodium dodecyl sulfate (SDS) and 6.2 mM sulfated-β-cyclodextrin; sample, normal pooled urine (dilute 1 + 1) or standard; load, HD 2 s at 50 mbar; voltage, 22 kV; temperature, 25°C; detection, 195–300 nm (195 nm shown).

high resolution of proteins, it has been used relatively little in CE because of the high background absorbance of the ampholytes. In cITP, the separation occurs in an electrolyte system composed of two buffers with widely different mobilities that encompass the mobilities of the analytes. At equilibrium, adjacent zones must migrate with equal velocities, which can be achieved only if all the bands contain ions at the same concentration, and therefore cITP can be used to concentrate dilute samples prior to CZE and has proved useful in combination with mass spectrometry (MS).

Another separation mode, capillary sieving electrophoresis (CSE), involves the electromigration of macromolecules through a sieving medium to generate a separation based on molecular size. Initially, the medium was a porous semi-solid gel, as in slab gel electrophoresis, and the mode was termed capillary gel electrophoresis (CGE). The filling of capillaries with gels has now been supplanted by the use of replaceable entangled viscous polymer solutions, such as 0.5% w/v hydroxyethylcellulose. It may be necessary to minimise electro-osmosis for maximum resolution. CSE is now commonplace in a number of commercial DNA sequencers.

A recent development is capillary electrochromatography (CEC), in which EOF is used to drive eluent through a capillary that contains a stationary phase. The stationary phase may be HPLC phases mechanically packed into the capillary, open-tubular capillaries with a phase chemically bonded to the capillary wall, or porous monolithic beds of a phase chemically formed in the capillary. In HPLC the flow resistance afforded by the particle size and narrow-bore columns limits column efficiencies, but CEC does not suffer from flow-generated back-pressures and can therefore use narrow capillaries packed with submicrometre particles.

Comparison with other analytical separation methods

For many analyses, CE is a complementary technique to HPLC. However, it can offer a number of advantages. It can analyse very small samples; in fact, many CE runs can be made from as little as 10 μL of sample and still leave sufficient sample for a HPLC injection. It is less sensitive than HPLC, but it can be used to detect at wavelengths below those normally used in liquid chromatography (LC; e.g. <200 nm). CE can be used with a wider range of analytes, since anions, cations and neutrals can all be assayed in one CE run, especially when using MEKC. Compared with HPLC, it can be applied readily to a wider range of analytes, from ions to macromolecules. Chiral CE is much simpler and cheaper to investigate than chiral HPLC. The capital costs of the instruments are equivalent for both systems, but CE is significantly cheaper to run and does not require the disposal of large quantities of organic solvent.

Instrumentation for capillary electrophoresis

Jorgenson's experimental work led to the development of a new type of instrument for analytical separations that was very similar in its operation to HPLC. Most major HPLC instrument manufacturers had, by the end of the 1980s, introduced CE systems of various degrees of sophistication. There was also considerable hype that CE was going to replace HPLC for analytical separations. This has certainly not been the case, although the number of papers in the chromatographic journals in which CE is used for analysis continues to grow. However, it is not now envisaged that it will rival HPLC.

CE is characterised by its ability to resolve rapidly the components of usually complex aqueous samples using applied d.c. voltages with field strengths up to 1 kV/cm to give a very high resolution ($N > 250\,000$) and measures >10 nL of sample with analytical precision. To maintain efficiency, detection (UV, including diode-array detection, and/or fluorescence) is nearly always on-line (i.e. across a window burnt into the polyimide coating of the silica capillary). Detection at the end of the capillary can be achieved using electrochemical detectors or, more importantly, MS.

A typical CE instrument consists of a capillary, detector, a high-voltage power source and a recording device (Fig. 20.4). The capillary used is made of fused silica and externally coated with a thin layer of polyimide that prevents surface hydration, so making the capillary flexible. The capillary is usually about 375 μm outside diameter and 10–150 μm internal diameter (i.d.), with 50 and 75 μm the more usual. There is no typical or required capillary length for CE, although in commercial instruments there are minimum lengths that can be used, usually dependent on the position of the detector. Clearly, the combination of aqueous salt solutions and very high voltages means that instruments must be designed with appropriate safety features. It must not be possible to gain access, particularly to the anodic vial, when high voltages are being applied.

Modern commercial instruments are sophisticated computer-controlled instruments capable of unattended reliable operation with capacities of some 100 samples. The capillary temperature must be well controlled to minimise Joule heating and optimise migration-time reproducibility. Detection is usually by diode array, although other detection options are on offer. The Royal Society of Chemistry has published a checklist to aid in the selection of CE instruments (Greenfield *et al.* 2000).

Power supplies and electrodes

All systems require a power supply able to generate stable voltages up to 30 kV d.c. at up to 300 mA. The standard maximum is 30 kV because voltages much above that cause shorting within the system. The system should be able to operate both in normal mode and in reversed-potential mode, in which the detector end of the capillary becomes the positive electrode. Reversed polarity is useful both for CIA and when using short-end injection. The voltage must be regulated carefully and controls that either cut off the power or reduce the wattage if the current limits are exceeded must be included in the software. It is often advantageous to be able to ramp the voltage to the operational voltage over a short period (e.g. 10 seconds at the start of the run). The voltage is conducted via high-voltage cables to the electrodes, which are either simple platinum wires or platinum tubes of about 1 mm bore.

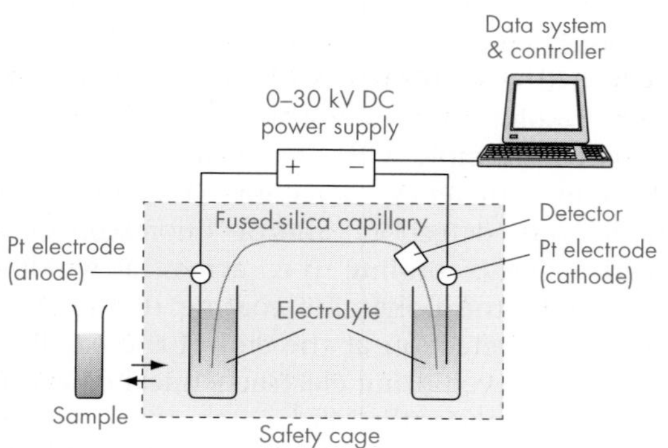

Figure 20.4 A capillary electrophoresis system.

Capillaries

CE capillaries can be obtained from instrument manufacturers with a pre-prepared detection window or made in the laboratory from polyimide-coated fused-silica capillary. The capillary must be mounted in the CE instrument's specially designed holder and loaded into the thermostatted capillary compartment of the instrument. In some instruments the ends of the capillary are guided by the cassette through the centre of the platinum electrodes into the electrolyte. In others the capillary merely sits next to a solid electrode wire. To allow detection, a small section of polyimide coating has to be removed, which makes a weak point in the capillary.

Although a basic concept in CE is that efficient cooling is generated by the capillary format, in practice additional cooling is built into commercial instruments. Capillaries are cooled either by a forced stream of cooled air or by immersion in a cooling liquid. Use of a cooling liquid has been shown to be more efficient than forced air, but in practice there is no difference in performance between the two methods.

Samples and sample injection

As in all analytical methods, correct sample preparation and treatment is essential. Since the capillary internal diameter is small, samples for CE should be free from particulate matter and care should taken to avoid formation of precipitates.

As in HPLC, the sample to be analysed is placed in a small vial, typically a 1.5 mL HPLC vial, in the sample holder of the CE system. Polypropylene vials can often be used in CE since samples are usually in aqueous solution. Micro insert vials are often used, since commonly only nanolitres are injected from very small (<10 μL) samples. In most systems the vials are capped to reduce evaporation, which can be significant when only small volumes of sample are to be used. The cathodic and anodic electrolyte solutions are also usually held in 1.5 mL vials. The sample racks in some instruments are thermostatted to reduce sample evaporation by cooling or heated to enable reactions such as enzyme digestions to take place.

Most instruments offer two means of injection. Hydrodynamic (HD) injection is the most widely used. The injection end of the capillary is moved into the sample vial and either a controlled pressure (e.g. 50 mbar) is applied to the sample or a vacuum is applied to the other end of the capillary for a few seconds. In this way a few nanolitres of sample enter the capillary. The amount injected is given by Poiseuille's law (see, e.g., http://en.wikipedia.org/wiki/Poiseuille's_law). In HD injection there is no sample bias. In electrokinetic (EK) injection, the injection end of the capillary is moved into the sample vial and analytes are migrated into the capillary under a transient high voltage (e.g. 5 kV for 5 s). EK injection biases the sample injection towards the most electrophoretically mobile species, so it can be used to analyse samples in difficult matrices such as pharmaceutical syrups as well as oligonucleotides in DNA analysis.

Detectors

Although many detectors have been proposed for CE, few are commercially available. The standard detector supplied with commercial instruments is a UV-visible spectrophotometric detector, most often a diode-array detector (DAD). The light from the lamp is focused via suitable optics through a window formed in the capillary. Since the Beer–Lambert law governs detection sensitivity, the micrometre-long paths within the capillary mean that optical detection in CE is sensitivity-limited by this very reduced pathlength. Various attempts to overcome this limitation have been developed, which include capillaries with bubbles at the detection site and two forms of Z-cell. One design places a bend in the capillary, but this is fragile. The second uses a cell, rather like an HPLC flow cell, coupled to the capillary and gives a light path of 1 mm, but it is difficult to align this micro plumbing. However, an advantage of silica is that very low UV wavelengths can be used. It is common practice to detect at 200 nm, or even as low as 185 nm. At such wavelengths a very large number of compounds exhibit significant UV absorbance, although selectivity of detection can be compromised. A confusion can arise because only very small volumes of samples are analysed in CE, typically 1–20 nL. This means that the mass sensitivity of CE (i.e. the numbers of molecules detected) is very low, whereas the concentration sensitivity is usually much higher. A modern UV-visible detector for CE operating with clean buffers should be capable of better than 10 milli-absorbance units full-scale sensitivity with 1–2% baseline noise.

Although papers have been published proposing several types of electrochemical detectors, there is no commercially available model for CE.

A fluorescence detector based on the designs for HPLC that offers a wide range of excitation wavelengths is also available. At least two manufacturers produce laser-induced fluorescence (LIF) detectors, but the choice of excitation wavelengths is limited. Only commercial laser wavelengths are available (e.g. 325 nm from a helium–cadmium laser and 488 nm from an argon laser) and there is no readily available UV laser. With the best systems a few hundreds of molecules can be measured, which corresponds to picomole detection limits. Pre-, on- and post-capillary reaction schemes have been developed successfully to derivatise analytes with fluorescent reagents. Most of the derivatisation reagents used with HPLC have been used with CE, especially so with derivatives, such as dansyl chloride, for primary amines. Unfortunately, most derivatives react with the charged groups on analytes, which renders them less suitable for CZE. For this reason, MEKC is usually required.

MS is being increasingly used with CE. Samples can be measured off-line if fraction collection on the CE column is possible or by collecting a continuous trace of sample on a film. This type of output has been used with matrix-assisted laser desorption ionisation–time of flight mass spectrometry (MALDI-TOF-MS). Direct interfacing with MS, especially electrospray, is most common. Most commercial systems can be linked either via commercial or laboratory-constructed interfaces to mass spectrometers. It is often necessary both to add make-up solvent and sometimes to degrade the sharpness of the CE peak to ensure it is not missed during the scan cycle of the MS. Although simple volatile CE buffers, such as formate and acetate, are MS compatible, not all CE electrolytes systems are compatible. In particular, MEKC buffers and cyclodextrin additives should not be sprayed directly into most MS systems.

Indirect detection is often used with CE when it is necessary to detect a non-UV-absorbing species, such as inorganic ions. Indirect detection works by the displacement of a UV-absorbing, fluorescent or electroactive BGE component by the analyte. This leads to reduction of a high background signal level. Important parameters are the background signal noise level, stability and the efficiency of displacement of the detected compound by the analyte.

Some idea of the relative sensitivities of CE detectors towards favoured analytes, expressed both in terms of mass and concentration limit of detection (LOD) is given in Table 20.2. However, the rule of thumb is that CE detection is 10 times less sensitive than that of HPLC.

Automation and data output

In modern CE instruments, autosampler technology has improved injection reproducibility, and capillary and sample cooling has improved migration-time reproducibility. Instruments can run unattended, run samples in a pre-programmed order, and allow combinations of washes and buffers to be used during analysis. Different methods can be programmed to run sequentially to analyse the same samples for different analytes or completely unrelated samples. Most instruments allow all the instrument parameters mentioned in this chapter and some instruments allow full control of both detection and data collection, which makes the whole system self-contained. Data analysis is the same as for HPLC systems.

Data acquisition rate and response time

The narrow peaks inherent in CE necessitate the use of faster detector rise times than is normal in HPLC, and therefore data acquisition rates for CE should be >25 Hz. Response time is adjustable on most detectors and is the time it takes for a detector to change for 10% to 90% of its range. Narrow peaks can be misrepresented if slow response times are used, and very narrow peaks may even be missed. In addition, a high-mobility analyte may give a non-Gaussian peak shape, which produces poor quantitative data when low data collection rates are used. The higher data collection rates give a better representation of the true peak shape.

An unusual requirement in CE is the need to work with spatial area rather than the simple integrated area. This is because the area of a peak is dependent on its apparent mobility (i.e. later migrating components move through the detector more slowly than earlier peaks and so record a larger peak area for the same amount of analyte). This is simply corrected for by dividing the measured area by the migration time to give the spatial area. The calculation of spatial area must be included in the integration software used for CE. It is spatial area that should be used in quantitative calculations.

Method development and optimisation

The starting point for developing a CE separation is to first study the literature. There are over 15 000 published CE articles, of which some

Table 20.2 Relative sensitivity of CE detection systems towards appropriate compounds

Detection mode	LOD (moles injected)	LOD (mol/L)	Commercial availability	Comments
UV/visible	10^{-13}–10^{-16}	10^{-3}–10^{-8}	Yes; DAD supplied with the major instruments	At <200 nm almost a universal detector; sensitivity limited by capillary ID
Fluorescence	10^{-15}–10^{-17}	10^{-5}–10^{-9}	Yes – stand-alone add-on	Limited to fluorescent compounds and derivatives; xenon-lamp-based
Laser-induced fluorescence	10^{-18}–10^{-22}	10^{-10}–10^{-16}	Yes	Very sensitive, but restricted to situations in which the wavelength of lasers matched the excitation wavelength of the analyte
Amperometric	10^{-18}–10^{-20}	10^{-5}–10^{-11}	No	Limited to electroactive species
Conductivity	10^{-15}–10^{-16}	10^{-4}–10^{-8}	Yes, but not currently manufactured	Universal towards ions, but lacks sensitivity
Mass spectrometry	10^{-15}–10^{-17}	10^{-8}–10^{-10}	Interfaces available from both CE and MS companies	Universal detection, but CE modes limited
Indirect UV	10^{-10}–10^{-12}	10^{-2}–10^{-5}	Yes, with UV detector	Universal for ions, but lacks sensitivity
Indirect fluorescence	10^{-15}–10^{-17}	10^{-5}–10^{-6}	Yes, but requires fluorescent detector	Universal for ions, but lacks sensitivity

DAD, diode array detector.

500 describe drug analyses in biofluids or other biological matrices. If there is no publication on the compound(s) in question, but some basic physicochemical data that include pK_a values are known, then migration by CZE is amenable to simple modelling from first principles. The various modelling approaches range from the calculation of the change in the degree of ionisation with pH using the Henderson–Hasselbalch equation, possibly corrected for molecular size, performed in a standard spreadsheet, to commercial computer simulations. In CZE, compounds are best resolved in a buffer with a pH that is mid-way between their respective pK_a values. A plot of pH against mobility clearly shows this and enables the selection of the optimum pH for the BGE.

Generic systems for drug assays

Its high resolving power means that a limited number of simple CE electrolyte systems can be used to separate a large number of diverse drug types. A number of authors have developed generic approaches to CE separations. MEKC, especially when modified by the addition of sulfated-β-cyclodextrin, was developed by the author's laboratory as a powerful generic methodology especially applicable to biological fluid analyses (Alfazema *et al.* 2000). Table 20.3, based on the methods used in the author's laboratory, summarises these generic systems.

Analytical methods

Quantification and validation

The ultimate goal of any analysis is the identification and, if required, quantification of the analytes in the given sample. Confidence in the results obtained requires a full validation of the assays, and this is no different for CE assays.

Identification can be achieved in a variety of ways:

- matching of migration and/or retention times with standard compounds. This can suffer from matrix effects with real samples, so ideally real samples should be spiked with standard compounds
- matching of relative migration times or mobilities to internal standards or the use of capacity factors and/or retention time in MEKC
- the use of detectors that provide qualitative data, such as DADs and mass spectrometers
- the use of enzymatic and/or chemical derivatisation to modify and/or remove peaks from the electropherograms
- fraction collection and subsequent use of MS, nuclear magnetic resonance, etc., to provide qualitative and structural data.

Quantitative measurements are the same for CE as for HPLC and gas chromatography (GC) in that peak areas or heights should be determined using an integration method. One difference, though, is the need with CE to use spatial areas to correct for velocity differences in the detector (see p. 548). External or internal standardisation or standard addition can be used. Although CE offers higher resolution than HPLC, there is still a possibility of peaks not being resolved, but if a DAD detector is used then peak purity can usually be determined automatically.

Validation is an important aspect of any separation assay (see p. 612). Limit of detection (LOD) is defined as the smallest measured amount from which it is possible to deduce the presence of the analyte with reasonable certainty; in CE this is calculated as the apparent content that corresponds to three times the peak-to-peak baseline noise. Repeatability is defined as the closeness of agreement between n mutually independent tests obtained under identical conditions, where n is typically 10 sequential tests. The measure of this is the relative standard deviation (RSD), also known as coefficient of variation (CV) and is the ratio of the standard deviation to the mean value. The injection repeatability of commercial CE instrumentation is excellent, about 1% RSD. Linearity is best determined using corrected peak areas because the linear range of peak heights is shorter through band broadening and mobility matching effects in CE. Overall assay reproducibility in CE, particularly for drug assays in biofluids, should not be significantly different from that in HPLC (i.e. 5–10%).

Samples and sample preparation

Sample preparation depends on the drug and matrix to be analysed and ranges from none to procedures that are as extensive as those required for other separation techniques. The degree of preparation depends on the matrix, the analyte(s) and their concentration, the detection mode to be employed and the required selectivity and sensitivity. The first 'obvious' statement is that the analyte(s) must be in solution, preferably in an aqueous buffer, to be analysed by CE. An analyte soluble only in organic solvents and injected from such a solution can precipitate in the electrolyte and possibly block the capillary, although injection from organic solvents can also generate useful stacking effects.

In CE, sample preparation methods should fulfil at least one but preferably more of the following requirements:

- enhance analyte selectivity and concentration
- stabilise the analyte(s)
- control the composition of the final sample, especially with respect to pH
- enhance sample loading via stacking
- remove matrix components, such as protein that can change the EOF

Table 20.3 Suggested generic CE buffer systems for drugs and their metabolites

Generic buffer	Composition	pH	CE conditions			Analytes	Comments
			Mode	Typical voltage (kV)	Temperature (°C)		
A	25 mM sodium phosphate	2.8	CZE	25–30	25	Water-soluble basic analytes, peptides	A standard system for peptides, but can be used for other cations
B	20 mM sodium tetraborate	9.2	CZE	20–25	25	Water-soluble acidic compounds	
C	25 mM sodium tetraborate plus 75 mM SDS	9.2	MEKC	15–25	20	Readily soluble and poorly water soluble, charged and neutral analytes, endogenous compounds	Optimised for urine; useful for unextracted assay of drug in serum
D	10 mM sodium tetraborate plus 2 mM TTAB + 5 mM sodium chromate	9.0	CIA	25–30	20	Water-soluble anions	A standard system used with indirect UV
E	10 mM sodium tetraborate plus 2 mM TTAB + 5 mM imidazole	9.0	CIA	25–30	25	Water-soluble organic and inorganic cations	A standard system used with indirect UV
F	25 mM sodium tetraborate plus 75 mM SDS plus 6.25 mM sulfated β-cyclodextrin	9.2	CD-modified MEKC	18–22	25	Readily soluble and poorly water-soluble, charged and neutral analytes, endogenous compounds	Optimised for urine; useful for unextracted serum assay of drugs
G	Methanol plus acetonitrile (50:50) plus ammonium acetate (1 mM)		Non-aqueous CZE	20–30	25	Nonpolar analytes	
H	Heptane (0.8% v/v) plus butan-1-ol (6.6% v/v) plus 3.3% w/v SDS in 25 mM sodium tetraborate	9.2	MEEKC	20	30	Charged and neutral analytes; endogenous compounds	A useful alternative to MEKC

- free analyte(s) bound onto proteins
- remove particulate material that could block the capillary
- give high recovery of the analyte(s)
- avoid excessive dilution
- work with the very small amounts of sample required in CE (<20 nL).

Methods without extraction for drugs in biofluids

For a protein-free biofluid, such as urine, the minimum preparation usually necessary is to filter the sample through a 0.45 μm membrane, or if volumes are very limited, centrifuge at about 13 000*g* to remove any particulates present. For some CZE assays this minimal approach can cause changes in migration times because of the variable salt molarity in some samples, such as urine. These variations can often be overcome by using one or more of the following approaches:

- diluting all samples approximately 10-fold with water or, better, a 1 + 9 dilution of the running buffer with deionised water, since this also controls sample pH
- injecting less sample
- changing to another injection mode
- diluting to a constant salt concentration
- increasing the molarity of the running electrolyte within the current constraints of the instrument.

If these fail to control migration-time variation, an MEKC-based assay should be tried. It is our experience that sodium dodecyl sulfate (SDS)-based MEKC is more robust with respect to sample matrix. This robustness of MEKC is such that drugs in plasma, serum and other protein-containing fluids can be assayed without any sample preparation. This approach, introduced by Nakagawa *et al.* (1988), relies on the ability of SDS to solubilise proteins, which prevents them adsorbing to the capillary surface and gives the proteins an overall negative charge, so further retarding their electrophoretic migration. At the same time, an MEKC separation of the analyte is developed. Choosing a selective detection wavelength can further enhance the utility of this approach. A representation of this for ibuprofen in serum is shown in Figure 20.5. Between the broad protein peak and the neutral peak there is a zone in which it is possible to separate and quantify analyte peaks.

Ultrafiltration gives minimal matrix disruption and is very suitable for CE. A 10 kDa cut-off ultrafilter gives 20–50 μL of protein-free filtrate from 500 μL of serum in 10–20 min when centrifuged at about 13 000*g*. The low sample yield is not a problem for CE analysis. Only free analytes of molecular weight below the cut-off are in the filtrate and recoveries can be very variable.

Extraction-based capillary electrophoresis methods

Off-line sample pre-concentration methods prior to CE, such as freeze-drying, liquid–liquid extraction and solid-phase extraction (SPE), as for HPLC, can achieve most of the effects listed above. The most important reason to use such techniques is to remove proteins. Protein-free extracts of serum prepared by most standard methods (e.g. acid precipitation or precipitation with organic solvents) are suitable for both CZE and MEKC. The important aspects are to avoid excessive dilution and interference of the precipitant with the electrophoresis. The final extract must not affect the electrophoresis by being too acidic or too alkaline compared to the separation buffer. Such differences in pH and/or molarity can cause major variations in migration times in CZE. Traces of solvents that remain from liquid–liquid or SPE extracts may disturb MEKC separations.

Unfortunately, trichloroacetic acid, the most efficient protein precipitant, leaves interference peaks that absorb in the short-wavelength UV. Therefore, when using CE below 220 nm, perchloric acid followed by neutralisation with potassium hydroxide or potassium carbonate and removal of the resultant precipitate is the recommended acid precipitant.

Another method of sample concentration in the capillary is sample stacking, which is achieved by dissolving the sample in a buffer more dilute than the running electrolyte. The

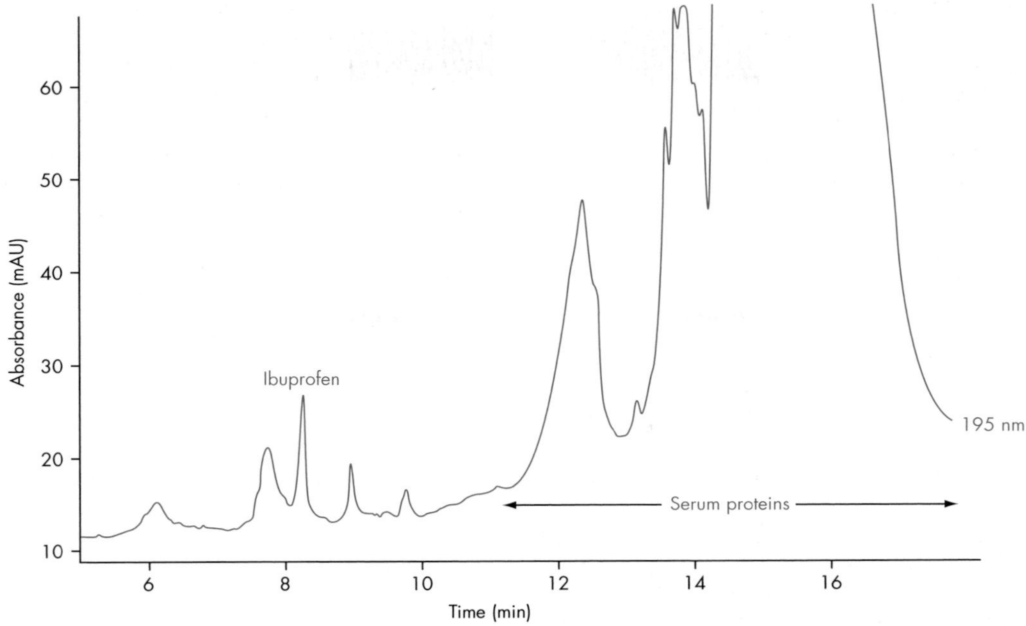

Figure 20.5 The use of MEKC to determine ibuprofen in neat serum. Conditions: HP3D system; capillary, silica 47(38.5) cm × 50 μm; buffer, 25 mM sodium tetraborate pH 9.5 that contains 75 mM SDS and 6.2 mM sulfated-β-cyclodextrin; sample, normal serum post 500 mg ibuprofen diluted 1 + 5 with water; load, HD 2 s at 50 mbar; voltage, 22 kV; temperature, 25°C; detection, 195–300 nm (195 nm shown).

sample is hydrodynamically injected, but when the voltage is applied the electric field strength is greater in the dilute sample than in the running electrolyte. Since electrophoretic velocity is proportional to field strength, the analyte ions move rapidly towards the cathode, but when they reach the higher concentration running electrolyte the field strength drops rapidly and they stack against this boundary in a narrow zone. This suggests that the sample is best dissolved in water, but unfortunately peak narrowing is countered by peak broadening because of mixing in the sample zone and poor solute buffering. The optimal sample buffer concentration for stacking is about one-tenth that of the electrolyte. Although stacking can be used to narrow the final peak width, it is still not advisable to increase the initial sample plug length beyond 1% of the capillary length. A popular and simple extraction method for drugs in CE assays is to extract the plasma and/or serum with acetonitrile and then inject relatively large amounts of the extract, which leads to a degree of sample stacking that enhances sensitivity.

When modifying clean-up methods such as SPE for CE, the aim should be to produce a 10-fold more concentrated final extract. This is often as simple as re-dissolving in only 10% of the suggested final volume. The low injection volumes required by CE, even with dilute analytes, mean it is possible to work with much smaller amounts of final sample and/or extract, provided there is sufficient for the sample injection vial in the instrument. It is routine for CE to use vial inserts of samples when as little as 5 mL suffices for many injections.

Automated SPE has become the method of choice for sample preparation prior to HPLC. A number of attempts have been made to automate SPE for use with CE, but these have not yet proved popular. These and related techniques, such as immuno-extraction, have been reviewed by Veraart *et al.* (1999) and Gilar *et al.* (2001).

General applications to drug assays

Clearly, CE is very good for separating charged species, whether small molecules or macromolecules. It is necessary to operate in MEKC mode to separate more neutral molecules, such as many drugs. There are now over 8000 publications that describe thousands of separations by CE. Charged and neutral compounds are all separated easily, but there are too many examples in the literature to even attempt to describe them here; the following section attempts to offer some concise summaries.

Drugs in formulations

A number of workers have demonstrated that CE can be used readily to analyse drugs in formulations. In such situations the limited sensitivity of CE is usually no problem, since suitable dilutions can be prepared. EK injection can minimise problems caused by viscous solutions and particulates from crushed tablets. Care must be taken when using HD injection and viscous solutions, since differences in viscosity between sample and standard solution can lead to differences in the amount of sample injected and thereby to quantification errors.

Drugs in biofluids

CE has proved valuable for the analysis of drugs and their charged metabolites, such as glucuronide and sulfate conjugates. At present CE separations tend to be of high efficiency but are relatively slow, and drug assays are no exception. Time saving can be achieved by the reduction in sample preparation that can be afforded by the selectivity of CE, both with regard to sample loading and system selectivity. Another advantage is that CE is able to work at short UV-wavelengths (i.e. $<$210 nm), which enables the detection of drugs without obvious chromophores.

Assays for drugs in biofluids that use CE are, in general, either for drugs taken in relatively high doses (e.g. paracetamol (acetaminophen) or aspirin) or where sample extract clean-up is employed to increase the final analyte concentration. The majority of assays of this type use a common simple MEKC separation (e.g. 10 mM borate, pH 9 with 50 mM SDS at 30 kV in 50 μm capillaries). To obtain additional pharmacological information from drug assays in biofluids it is necessary to link CE with MS. Pharmacogenetics has become an important area of drug metabolism and therapy in which MEKC is used to probe differences in the metabolism of drugs, such as caffeine, between individuals. Most drug assays are relatively slow (e.g. 10–15 min). With current commercial CE equipment samples must be analysed in series, so the throughput of samples is perhaps 80–100 per day. This is well below the throughput achievable with enzyme-linked immunosorbent assay (ELISA), for example. Much faster analyses of drugs by CE are possible by actively cooling short capillaries or by using short-end injection (see below) and minimising sample preparation. Recently a drug analysis system with multiple parallel capillaries has been introduced.

Fast assays by capillary electrophoresis

CE can generate a large number of theoretical plates rapidly (e.g. in 1 min a CZE separation can produce more plates than a typical 15 cm HPLC column). Short capillaries are needed to fully utilise such capabilities. On some instruments short capillaries of $<$25 cm can be used by bypassing parts of the capillary cassette, while on others very short paths are achievable by running the system in reverse (i.e. using what is normally the cathode end as the injection (anode) end). This is often referred to as short-end injection. When working with the high potential gradients used in such rapid analyses it is necessary to avoid too much Joule heating. This may be achieved by reducing the applied voltage, which can defeat the goal of the rapid system. It is beneficial, if the instrument allows, for the capillary to be held at a sub-ambient temperature and so actively cool the capillary. Using such techniques, the analysis time for some assays may be reduced to less than 1 min per sample. Figure 20.6 shows such a short-end injection applied to the separation of normal human urine by MEKC for which the total analysis time was less than 3 min. Combining such rapid analyses with CE's abilities to work with minimal sample preparation could mean that sample throughput and ease of analysis rival that of ELISAs.

Assay of chiral drugs in biofluids

CE has proved to be an adaptable method to determine enantiomeric drug purity and is widely used for this purpose in the pharmaceutical industry. Many types of electrolyte additives can be employed to resolve enantiomers; these range from proteins to chiral surfactants. However, the most commonly employed method is to include native cyclodextrins in the electrolyte. Native β-cyclodextrin (CD) is the most commonly employed, since its internal cavity matches well the largest number of drug molecules. More recently, chemically modified cyclodextrins, especially the sulfated derivatives of β-CD have been shown to give separations of chiral compounds with spectacular resolution between the enantiomers. As a starting point for developing enantiomeric separation methods, a 25 mM phosphate pH buffer (~ pH 2.5) with highly sulfated-β-CD, hydroxypropyl-β-CD, heptakis-(2,6-*O*-dimethyl)-β-CD or heptakis-(2,3,6-*O*-trimethyl)-β-CD has been shown to form a BGE combination capable of resolving over 90% of the chiral drug compounds.

Although most commonly used with standard preparations of drugs for quality-control purposes, chiral CE has also been used to study enantiomeric metabolism in humans and other species. A variety of drug classes have been resolved chirally and quantified in samples that range from urine to hair extracts.

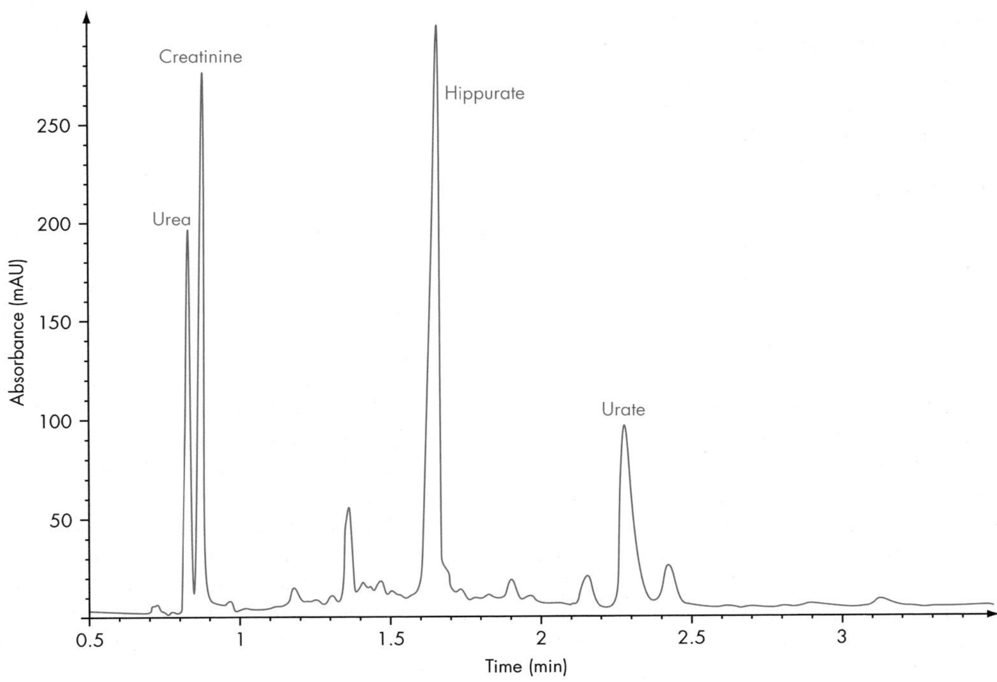

Figure 20.6 Rapid CE analyses. A short-end injection employed for the separation of normal human urine by MEKC. Conditions: HP3D system; capillary, silica 47(38.5) cm × 50 μm; buffer, 25 mM sodium tetraborate pH 9.5 that contains 175 mM SDS; sample, normal pooled urine (diluted 1 + 1); load, HD 1 s at 50 mbar; voltage, (−)20 kV; temperature, 25°C; detection, 195–300 nm (195 nm shown).

Conclusions and future directions

In comparison with HPLC, CE achieves better resolution than both isocratic and gradient HPLC using simpler instrumentation. CE is not a preparative technique, although it has been used as a micro-preparative system to isolate very small amounts of protein for sequencing. It is less sensitive than HPLC by about an order of magnitude. There is little difference in terms of quantitative data and analytical precision. Sample preparation probably needs to be better controlled and understood than it does for HPLC. At present, CE instrumentation is more expensive than that for HPLC, although running costs are considerably lower. CE uses considerably less sample and reagents than does HPLC. Waste disposal problems are reduced considerably. The high resolving power of CE means that a relatively simple CE system can resolve as many peaks as a gradient HPLC system in a shorter time, with greater throughput and lower running costs. Today, therefore, CE is a very complementary technique to other separation methods.

CE has found a role in many laboratories and offers useful complementary separations to HPLC and is clearly an established technique with a long-term future in the separation of pharmaceuticals, in both simple preparations and biofluids. Future developments in pharmaceutical analysis may see miniaturisation developing even further, with the commercialisation of the experimental systems for chemical analysis on a chip (Lab-on-Chip), since such devices are already available for macromolecules such as DNA.

References

L. N. Alfazema *et al.*, Optimised separation of endogenous urinary metabolites using cyclodextrin-modified micellar electrokinetic capillary chromatography, *Electrophoresis*, 2000, **21**, 2503–2508.

K. D. Bartle and P. Myers, Theory of capillary electrochromatography, *J. Chromatogr. A*, 2001, **916**, 3–23.

M. Gilar *et al.*, Advances in sample preparation in electromigration, chromatographic and mass spectrometric separation methods, *J. Chromatogr. A*, 2001, **909**, 111–135.

S. Greenfield *et al.*, Evaluation of analytical instrumentation. Part XII. Instrumentation for capillary electrophoresis, *Analyst*, 2000, **125**, 361–366.

J. W. Jorgenson and K. D. Lukacs, Zone electrophoresis in open-tubular glass capillaries, *Anal. Chem.*, 1981, **53**, 1298–1302.

R. A. Mosher *et al.*, *The Dynamics of Electrophoresis*, Berlin, VCH, 1992.

T. Nakagawa *et al.*, Separation and determination of cefpiramide in plasma by electrokinetic chromatography with micellar solution and an open tubular-fused silica capillary. *Chem. Pharm. Bull.*, 1988, **36**, 1622–1625.

H. Poppe, Theory of capillary zone electrophoresis, in *Advances in Chromatography*, P. R. Brown and E. Grushka (eds), New York, Marcel Dekker, 1998, pp. 233–300.

S. Terabe *et al.*, Electrokinetic separations with micellar solutions and open-tubular capillaries. *Anal. Chem.*, 1984, **56**, 111–113.

J. R. Veraart *et al.*, Coupling of biological sample handling and capillary electrophoresis, *J. Chromatogr. A*, 1999, **856**, 483–514.

Further reading

K. D. Altria, *Analysis of Pharmaceuticals by Capillary Electrophoresis*, Wiesbaden, Vieweg, 1998.

D. R. Baker, *Capillary Electrophoresis*, New York, Wiley Interscience, 1995.

P. Camilleri, *Capillary Electrophoresis: Theory and Practice*, 2nd edn, Boca Raton, CRC Press, 1997.

J. P. Landers (ed.), *Handbook of Capillary Electrophoresis*, Boca Raton, CRC Press, 1994.

R. Weinberger, *Practical Capillary Electrophoresis*, 2nd edn, New York, Academic Press, 2000.

R. Weinberger and R. Lombardi, *Method Development, Optimisation and Troubleshooting for High Performance Capillary Electrophoresis*, Needham Heights, Simon & Schuster, 1997.

21

Mass spectrometry

D Watson, S Jickells and A Negrusz

Introduction 557
Theory 559
Instrumentation 563
Coupled techniques 568
Data processing. 572
System suitability tests 573
Sample preparation and presentation 574
Data interpretation. 574
Mass spectrometry in qualitative analysis 579
Identification of drug metabolites. 582
Some applications of mass spectrometry in quantitative analysis. 583
Collections of data 584
References 585

Introduction

The development of the mass spectrometer has revolutionised analytical chemistry, providing an exceedingly powerful detection technique which, when combined with chromatographic separation, provides the analyst with an exceedingly sensitive and specific tool for both qualitative and quantitative analysis. Although it is still relatively expensive compared with UV-visible, flame ionisation and electron capture detectors, the benefits offered by mass spectrometry (MS) have made the mass spectrometer one of the most commonly used detectors in analytical toxicology.

A mass spectrometer works by generating charged molecules or molecular fragments either in a high vacuum or immediately before the sample enters the high-vacuum region. Once the molecules are charged and in the gas phase, they can be manipulated by the application of either electric or magnetic fields to enable the determination of their relative molecular mass (RMM) and the RMM of any fragments produced by the molecules breaking up during ionisation.

As shown in Figure 21.1, in its very simplest form, a mass spectrometer can be considered to consist of means of

- introducing the sample into the mass spectrometer
- ionising the sample molecules
- separating ionised molecules according to their mass
- detecting and quantifying the separated ions
- recording and plotting and manipulating data.

MS instruments typically maintain vacuums of about 10^{-6} mmHg, since ionised molecules have to be generated in the gas phase to allow their manipulation using magnetic or electrostatic fields.

The field of MS is complicated in terms of terminology because of the flexibility offered

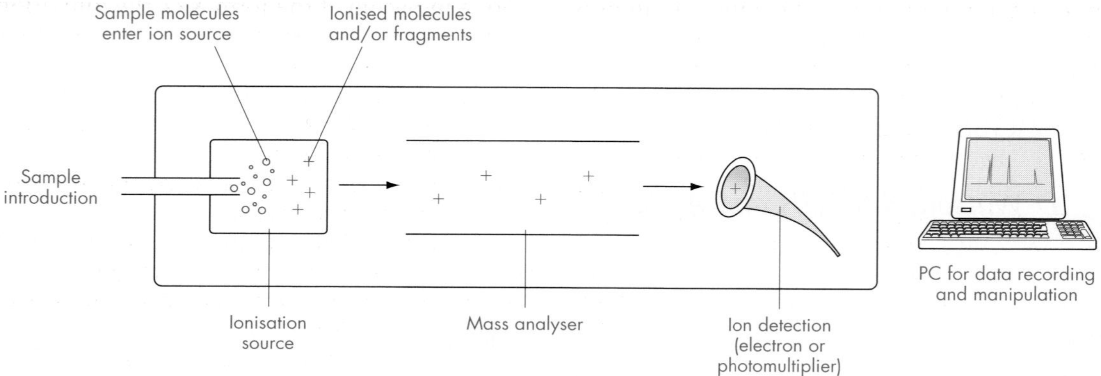

Figure 21.1 Generalised schematic of a mass spectrometer showing the typical component parts. Note that the orientation of components and the actual components may vary for some types of mass spectrometers.

by MS instrumentation. There are various mechanisms available for ionisation and for separating ions according to their mass. Techniques available for ionisation include:

- election impact (EI) ionisation
- chemical ionisation (CI)
- electrospray ionisation (ESI)
- atmospheric-pressure chemical ionisation (APCI)
- fast-atom bombardment (FAB)
- matrix-assisted laser desorption ionisation (MALDI).

As we will see later in this chapter, some of these ionisation techniques are used in association with specific chromatographic techniques or with other sample introduction techniques.

Several different 'mass analysers' are also available for separating ions according to mass. Examples include:

- (linear) quadrupole
- ion trap
- time of flight (TOF)
- magnetic sector.

Different mass analysers can be combined with different ionisation techniques and it is this flexibility which makes MS such a powerful technique.

Until relatively recently, most mass spectrometers used electron impact to ionise molecules, with samples in the vapour phase being bombarded with high energy-electrons. This permitted gas chromatography (GC) to be coupled to MS (GC-MS), enabling the combination of a powerful chromatographic separation technique with an equally powerful identification technique. GC-MS rapidly became established as the premier analytical tool in forensic toxicology. EI ionisation cannot be used to ionise analytes in the liquid phase and this restricted the direct coupling of high-performance liquid chromatography (HPLC) and MS. Considerable research in this area over the past three to four decades has led to the development of techniques that can ionise molecules from liquid streams and the direct coupling of HPLC and capillary electrophoresis (CE) to MS. Liquid chromatography–mass spectrometry (LC-MS) is rapidly expanding in the field of forensic toxicology analysis, enabling the analysis of polar drugs (which were not readily amenable to GC-MS analysis without derivatisation), thermally labile analytes and high-molecular-weight substances that cannot be analysed by GC. The particular advantage of techniques such as GC-MS, LC-MS and CE-MS lies in their ability to identify unknown substances or to confirm the presumptive presence of a compound. These techniques are typically used to analyse organic molecules.

Elemental analysis, particularly the trace analysis of metallic elements, is also required in toxicology. Such elements require a different approach for ionisation. The most commonly applied ionisation mechanism utilises an inductively coupled plasma (ICP). ICP-MS is described in further detail on p. 572 at the end of the section on coupled techniques.

A number of useful introductory texts that describe mass spectrometers and mass spectral interpretation are available (Williams and Fleming 1980; McLafferty and Turecek 1993; Davis and Frearson 1994; Chapman 1995; Watson 1997; Lee 1998; Smith and Busch 1999; Ardrey 2003).

Theory

Ionisation

As noted above, the original method for producing ionisation, which is still used for routine MS analyses (particularly for GC-MS), is to bombard the analyte with electrons produced by a rhenium or tungsten filament. The electrons, with an energy most commonly of 70 eV, are accelerated towards a positive target. The analyte, in vapour form, is introduced into the instrument between the filament and the target. Since the electrons used to promote ionisation are of much higher energy than the strength of the bonds within the analyte (which are of the order 4–7 eV), extensive fragmentation of the analyte usually occurs.

For a molecule of the form XYZ the ionisation reactions of the type shown in Scheme 21.1 may occur with EI ionisation.

Ionisation reactions resulting in negative ions are relatively rare with EI ionisation but can occur for electronegative substances and can give high sensitivity to analysis in so-called negative-ion analysis mode.

The extensive fragmentation of molecules that occurs with EI ionisation typically gives rise to the production of a relatively large number of fragment ions. The fragmentation pattern is characteristic for a particular substance (and for very closely related substances). The data system can be interrogated to plot the mass-to-charge ratio of the fragment ions detected for a substance versus the abundance of the ions. The resultant plot is referred to as a mass spectrum (e.g. see Fig. 21.4).

Ionisation mechanisms such as CI, ESI, FAB and MALDI impart less energy to the sample molecules. As a result, there is generally no fragmentation or restricted fragmentation. Typically the molecular ion, or $[M+H]^+$ ion, is formed along with just a few fragment ions. Thus the mass spectra formed from these so-called softer ionisation techniques are less characteristic than EI mass spectra and not so amenable for identifying the compound using computerised mass spectral library searching.

Ions formed in the ion source (the region where ionisation takes place) are transferred out of the source by means of a series of

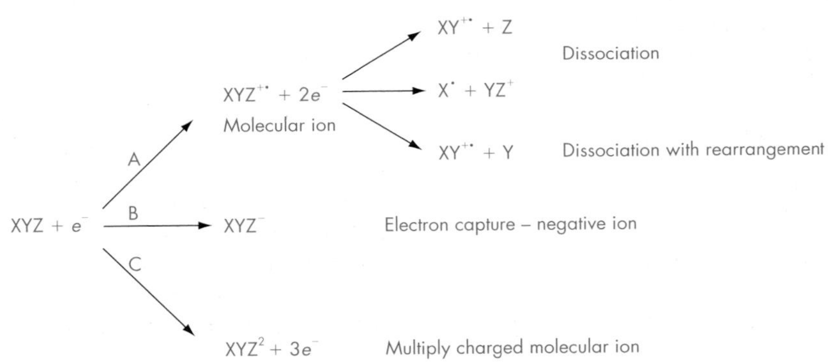

Scheme 21.1 Electron impact ionisation showing: (A) formation of molecular ion and 'fragment' ions; (B) electron capture; (C) formation of multiply charged molecular ion.

electrically charged plates into the mass analyser region.

Separation of ions

As already noted, several different types of mass analyser are available. However, the end result is generally the same: separation according to the ratio of the mass of the ion (m) to the charge on the ion (z), i.e. the mass-to-charge ratio (m/z).

Ion detection

In most modern mass spectrometers, ions are detected by an electron multiplier or photomultiplier. The number of analyte molecules ionised in the source is estimated to be a very low percentage of the total number in the source available for ionisation. Also, in some types of mass analyser, the percentage of ionised molecules which exit the analyser is lower than the percentage entering. Thus the total number of ions reaching the detector is relatively low compared with the number of sample molecules introduced into the mass spectrometer and the signal has to be amplified to provide quantifiable data. Electron multiplier and photomultiplier detectors amplify the signal from the ions striking the detector.

Data analysis

Because MS analysis results in a large volume of data which can be manipulated in a variety of ways to provide data useful to analysts, all modern MS instruments are now linked to computers, typically with sophisticated software for data analysis.

Some useful rules for evaluating mass spectra

One of the most important pieces of information obtained from MS analysis is the mass spectrum of a compound. In the early days of mass spectrometry, before commercial libraries of mass spectra were compiled, mass spectroscopists identified unknown compounds from interpretation of mass spectra. With the advent of commercially available mass spectral libraries, many containing spectra of hundreds of thousands of compounds, together with the commercial availability of a wide range of organic compounds, direct interpretation of mass spectra for substance identification is becoming less common. However, the analyst using MS should have sufficient knowledge to be certain that the mass spectrum they obtain does correspond to the substance that they claim. Interpretation of mass spectra is beyond the scope of this book and the reader is referred to texts such as Lee (1998), McLafferty (1993), Smith and Busch (1999) for further information on this topic, but information on the possible significance of the RMM of a compound and on isotope patterns can be useful.

Relative molecular masses and elemental composition

The nitrogen rule

Most RMMs of analytes are even numbers, unless the molecule contains a nitrogen atom. Compounds that contain a single nitrogen atom have odd-number RMMs, two nitrogen atoms in a structure produce an even RMM, three an odd RMM and so on. Other elements (e.g. boron) can produce odd-number RMMs, but nitrogen is the most common element within the structures of drug molecules.

Isotopes

Some of the elements commonly found in drug molecules exist as isotopes. Because the mass spectrometer can separate ions of different mass, the isotopes of these elements contribute to the mass spectrum and can provide useful information either about the elements that may be present or the number of atoms of the element that may be present in a molecule. Table 21.1 summarises the isotope abundances of some elements. Chlorine and bromine have abundant isotopes and the presence of ^{35}Cl and ^{37}Cl or ^{79}Br

Table 21.1 Abundances of isotopes commonly found in drug molecules

Isotope	Relative atomic mass	Natural abundance (%)
^{1}H	1.0078	99.985
^{2}H	2.014	0.015
^{12}C	12.000 000	98.9
^{13}C	13.003	1.1
^{14}N	14.003	99.64
^{15}N	15.0001	0.36
^{16}O	15.995	99.8
^{17}O	16.999	0.04
^{18}O	17.999	0.2
^{19}F	18.998	100
^{28}Si	27.977	92.2
^{29}Si	28.977	4.7
^{30}Si	29.974	3.1
^{31}P	30.974	100
^{32}S	31.972	95
^{33}S	32.971	0.8
^{34}S	33.968	4.2
^{35}Cl	34.969	75.8
^{37}Cl	36.966	24.2
^{79}Br	78.918	50.5
^{81}Br	80.916	49.5
^{127}I	126.904	100

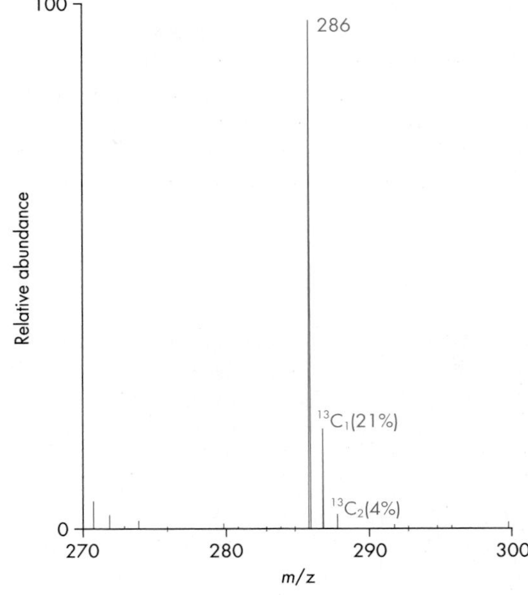

Figure 21.2 Molecular ion of androstenedione with associated isotope peaks.

and ^{81}Br produces characteristic 3:1 or 1:1 molecular ion patterns, respectively. These isotope patterns are very distinctive and are particularly so if a molecule contains more than one chlorine or bromine atom. The ^{13}C isotope has quite a high abundance, 1.1% of the abundance of the ^{12}C isotope. For instance, androstenedione has a molecular ion at *m/z* 286 (Fig. 21.2) and, since the molecule contains 19 carbon atoms, it has an isotope peak at *m/z* 287, which is about 21% ($19 \times 1.1\%$) of the ion at *m/z* 286, which is the probability of the occurrence of one ^{13}C atom in its structure. By the same logic, there is an ion at *m/z* 288, which is about 4% of the *m/z* 286 ion and results from two ^{13}C atoms in androstenedione. Androstenedione also contains 26 hydrogen atoms, so its mass will be higher by about 0.2 atomic mass units (a.m.u.) from its nominal mass, based on hydrogen having an exact mass of 1.0078 (Table 21.2). These two effects have to be taken into account when dealing with molecules of very high RMM, such as proteins. The deviation of the mass of hydrogen from unity makes a significant difference to the exact mass of a protein, and the abundance of ^{13}C in protein molecules makes the isotope patterns of protein spectra complex. The ^{15}N isotope and the ^{34}S isotope also add to the complexity of the isotope pattern of protein spectra. Often, the average mass of a molecule is quoted. This is not an accurate mass, but rather an average of the contribution of all the isotopes towards its mass. Thus, HCl has an average mass of 36.5, since it contains 75% of ^{35}Cl and 25% of ^{37}Cl.

The technique of gas chromatography–combustion–isotope ratio MS (GC-IRMS) (see Chapter 3) to evaluate the content of ^{13}C or ^{15}N has potential for forensic toxicology. GC-IRMS is now being applied for the differentiation of endogenous and exogenous testosterone in sports drug testing.

Table 21.2 Masses relative to ^{12}C having a mass of exactly 12

Species	Exact mass
^{1}H	1.00782
^{14}N	14.0031
^{16}O	15.9949
CO	27.9949
$CH_2{=}CH_2$	28.0313
N_2	28.0061

Accurate mass measurement

Some types of mass spectrometer can measure the mass of a compound with high precision. Historically, magnetic sector instruments were used for this purpose, but other types of MS instruments have been developed with this capability, including TOF instruments. Using such instruments, the mass of a molecule can be measured to several decimal places. Based on the convention that the carbon-12 isotope (^{12}C) has an exact mass of 12, the atoms of other elements do not have exactly integral masses, as seen in Table 21.1. Thus, a high-resolution mass spectrometer would be able to distinguish between CO, $CH_2{=}CH_2$ and N_2, which all have a rounded mass of 28 a.m.u. The difference in mass between $CH_2{=}CH_2$ and N_2 is 0.0252 a.m.u., which relative to a mass of 28 is 900 parts per million (ppm; 1 ppm relative to 28 = 0.000028). To carry out accurate mass measurements, the instrument has to be calibrated. This is done using one or more standard substances covering the mass range of interest.

Figure 21.3 shows the mass spectrum of chloroquine phosphate obtained using FAB ionisation. FAB is a soft ionisation technique, so that the spectrum is quite simple and the molecular ion for chloroquine (+H) is seen at m/z 320 for the chlorine-35 isotope and m/z 322 for the chlorine-37 isotope. A feature of FAB is that matrix peaks are usually also present in the spectrum. Two clear peaks can be seen at m/z 277 and m/z 369. These result from the formation of cluster ions from the glycerol matrix in which the sample is dissolved. These two peaks, and other glycerol cluster ions, have a known elemental composition/exact mass ratio and can be used to calibrate the mass axis of the instrument with high precision, so that an elemental composition for the two molecular ions of chloroquine can be obtained. Other commonly used calibrants are perfluorokerosene (PFK) and perfluorotributylamine (PFTBA), which are volatile, and polyethylene glycol and Ultramark (used in calibrating the masses of high-molecular-weight compounds). The EI mass spectrum of PFTBA is shown in Fig. 21.4. PFTBA ionises to produce a number of fragment ions with good abundance and spanning a relatively wide mass range. This makes it a good substance for calibrating mass spectrometers to ensure the accuracy of mass measurement.

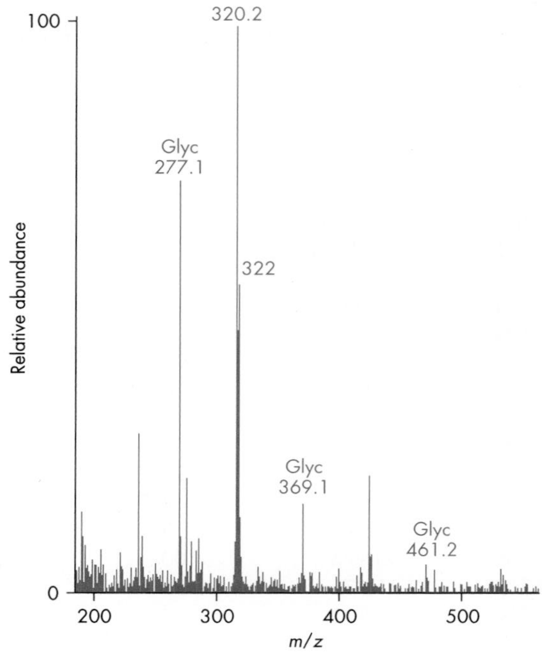

Figure 21.3 Fast-atom bombardment mass spectrum of chloroquine in a glycerol matrix.

Resolution

Resolution (R) is defined as follows:

$$R = m/\Delta m \quad (21.1)$$

where m is the mass of the ion and Δm is the smallest mass increment that can be differenti-

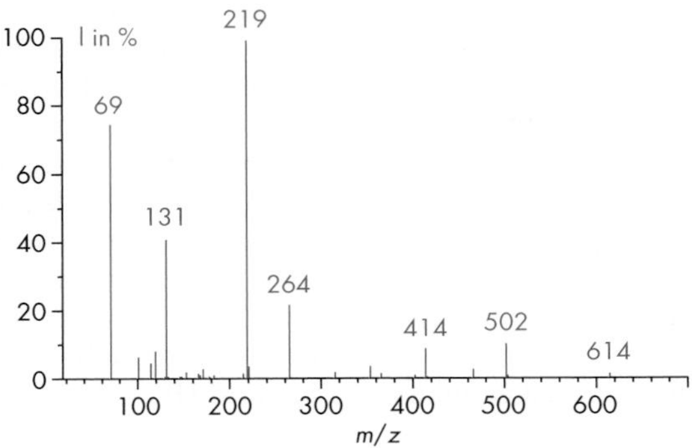

Figure 21.4 Electron-impact ionisation mass spectrum of PFTBA.

ated from *m* by the mass spectrometer. It is therefore a measure of the ability of the mass spectrometer to differentiate between ions of similar mass.

Unit resolution implies that two masses differing by one mass unit are completely separated (0% peak/valley ratio); for example, if *m/z* 100 is separated completely from *m/z* 101 or, as shown in Fig. 21.5A, *m/z* 505 is separated from *m/z* 506. Instruments with high mass accuracy such as magnetic sector and TOF instruments can effect resolution of up to 20 000 at 50% peak/valley, that is they can resolve masses of 20 000 and 20 001, so there is a valley of 50% of the peak height between them.

Greater resolution can be achieved by narrowing the slits in the instrument, allowing ions of a specified mass only to pass through the analyser. However, the greater the restriction on the mass, the fewer ions of that absolute mass

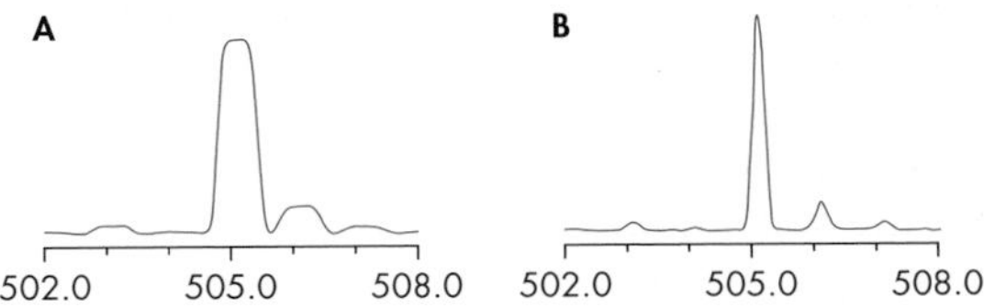

Figure 21.5 (A) Showing unit resolution. The ion at *m/z* 505 is just resolved from the ^{13}C isotope ion at *m/z* 506. (B) Showing resolution of approximately 1000. The *m/z* 505 ion is clearly resolved from the *m/z* 506 ion due to the higher resolution offered by the MS instrument used for this analysis.

that pass through the analyser, resulting in lower sensitivity, dependant on the resolution of the instrument. High-resolution instruments offer the advantage of high sensitivity and specificity. The mass analyser can be operated to permit only ions corresponding to the specific mass of the analyte(s) of interest, effectively 'filtering out' ions of all other masses such that they are not detected. This means that only the analytes of interest are detected (assuming they are present), i.e. specificity is high, and also reduces the background noise resulting in increased sensitivity. High-resolution instruments are more expensive than low-resolution ones and this cost has to be weighed against the advantages offered.

Instrumentation

A prominent feature of MS is the range of instrumentation available, a range that is still rapidly expanding. Mass spectrometer instruments are generally referred to by names that refer to the methodology used to separate the ions according to their mass-to-charge ratio. However, it must be remembered that ion production must take place before mass analysis. As mentioned in the introductory section, a variety of ionisation techniques are available in MS. It is generally possible to use virtually any ionisation technique with any type of mass analyser, although there are some limitations for certain combinations. The discussions of instrumentation that follow do not include a discussion of compatible ionisation techniques. EI ionisation has already been discussed. Ionisation techniques compatible with liquid chromatography are discussed on p. 568.

Magnetic sector instruments

Magnetic sector instruments were one of the first types of mass spectrometers to be developed. They are still available but, to a large extent, they have been superseded by ion trap and quadrupole instruments which offer similar performance, typically at lower cost. A magnetic sector mass spectrometer is illustrated in Fig. 21.6.

In magnetic sector mass spectrometers the ions are separated by application of an electrostatic field followed by a magnetic one, or the reverse in so-called reverse-geometry instruments.

In a straight-geometry magnetic sector mass spectrometer the ions generated in the source are pushed out of the source by a repeller potential, which has the same charge as the ions. These ions are then accelerated and focused into a beam using a series of electrostatic lenses, which can be tuned to give optimum sensitivity. As the ions leave the ion source they have a range of kinetic energies because they were formed at different points in the source. The kinetic energies of the ions are focused into a narrow range using an electrostatic field applied at right angles to their direction of travel. As a result they take a circular path through the electrostatic analyser. Only ions with a narrow range of velocities then pass through the slit separating the ion source from the magnetic analyser. The width of the slits in the instrument can be varied to control its resolving power (see above). Once the ion beam has been focused, the ions are then separated in the magnetic analyser according to equation (21.2) where B is the magnetic field strength, r is the radius of the path through the magnet and V is the accelerating velocity.

$$\frac{m}{z} = \frac{B^2 r^2}{2V} \tag{21.2}$$

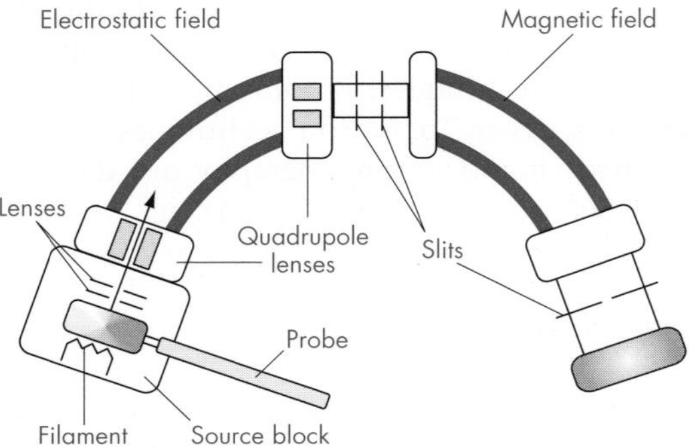

Figure 21.6 Schematic diagram of a double-focusing magnetic sector mass spectrometer.

By varying the magnetic field B, ions with a range of mass/charge (m/z) values can be collected and detected using either an electron multiplier or photomultiplier. A typical sweep time for the magnetic field across a mass range of 50–800 a.m.u. would be 1 s, but faster speeds are required if high-resolution chromatography is being used. Quadrupole and ion trap instruments typically offer a more rapid sweep (or scan) time making them more amenable for hyphenated capillary GC-MS and HPLC-MS.

It is also possible to vary the potential of the electrostatic field and keep B constant. In this case, the mass range is limited by the range of kinetic energies of the ions generated in the source and scans may be only over a mass range of 5–10% of the mass of the ion being measured.

Magnetic sector instruments are still widely used to determine the elemental compositions of ions because they offer high mass resolution and accurate mass determination although, as noted above, other MS instruments are now available which offer these capabilities at lower cost. Software programs are available that can be used to generate molecular formulae corresponding to a particular mass. If the mass of a compound can be determined accurately by MS, the possible molecular formula corresponding to that mass can be obtained and then chemical structures corresponding to the molecular formulae can be generated. There are many situations in analytical chemistry in which one does not know the identity of substance(s) in a sample. If one carries out a GC-MS analysis and detect peaks but cannot determine the identity of the substances from mass spectral library searches, this can pose problems, particularly in forensic toxicology where one may be trying to determine the cause of death. The ability to generate chemical structures from accurate mass data may help identify potential substances. The analyst can then obtain a standard of the substance and analyse on the system, checking for match in retention time and, ideally, match in mass spectrum.

For MS that follows chromatographic separation, other methods of ion separation are generally preferred on the basis of the cost relative to magnetic sector instruments.

Quadrupole instruments

For many years, quadrupoles were the only alternative to magnetic sector instruments. Quadrupole instruments have largely superseded magnetic sector instruments for routine MS analysis due to their considerably lower cost and superior sensitivity. The term quadrupole as used here refers to a linear quadrupole, as opposed to an ion trap, although it is recognised that the ion trap is a form of quadrupole.

In a quadrupole mass spectrometer, the mass analyser is formed from four rods arranged in a parallel and opposite arrangement (see Fig. 21.7). Two varying electrostatic fields, one direct current (d.c.) and one at varying radiofrequency, are applied at right angles to each other via the four rods of the quadrupole. This creates a resonance frequency for each *m/z* value in a mass spectrum. Thus at any particular combination of d.c. and radiofrequency, only ions of a corresponding *m/z* transit the quadrupole and reach the detector. The full mass range is scanned by varying the resonant frequency of the quadrupole such that ions of sequential *m/z* transit the analyser. This is referred to as scan mode. It is also possible to operate the quadrupole so that ions of a specified *m/z* only can transit the analyser. This is known as selected-ion monitoring (SIM) mode. SIM mode is used where the identity of the analytes of interest is known. Two, or perhaps three, ions which are characteristic for the analyte under investigation are selected to be monitored. The instrument then sets the combination of d.c. and radiofrequency voltages to sequentially permit the specified ions to transit the quadrupole. Operation in SIM mode offers increased sensitivity and selectivity compared to scan mode. However, it should be remembered that the MS monitors only the specified ions in SIM mode and hence will not detect substances not possessing these ions in their mass spectra. This aspect should not be overlooked, particularly in situations where limited information is available about analytes that might be present in a sample. In such situations, if sensitivity is not an issue, an analysis in scan mode may help identify unknown analytes.

Most 'bench-top' (relatively small size and low-cost) quadrupole MS instruments give only unit mass resolution. However, these instruments are generally adequate for most types of analysis required in forensic toxicology and, until the advent of LC-MS instruments, have been the workhorse instruments in most toxicology laboratories.

Ion-trap instruments

Ion traps are a relatively recent development. The ion trap is a modification of the quadrupole

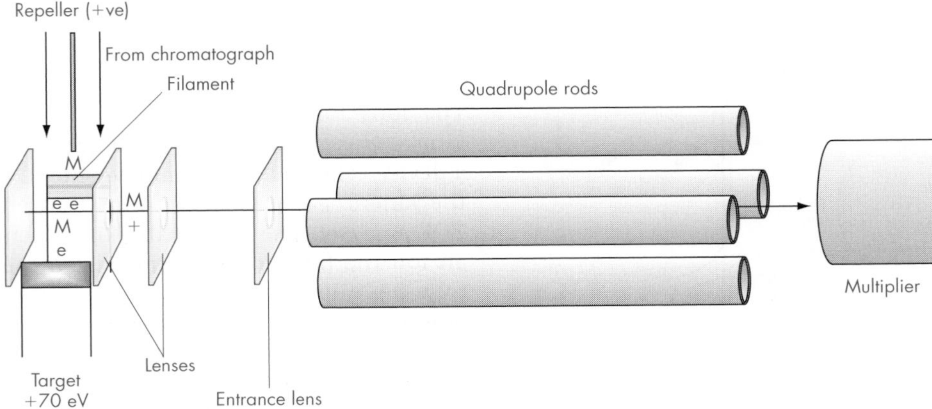

Figure 21.7 Schematic diagram of a quadrupole mass spectrometer.

mass analyser and is compatible with most types of ionisation. The analyte is ionised using one of the available methods and the ions are transferred into the trap in which they are then confined by application of a radiofrequency voltage to the circular electrode (Fig. 21.8). The energy of the ions in the trap is quenched by helium, which is introduced into the trap to give a pressure of about 1 mmHg, so that the ions focus near the centre of the trap (i.e. their centrifugal energy is reduced). The ions can then be mass-selectively ejected from the trap by increasing a radiofrequency potential applied to the endcap electrodes (which also have a d.c. potential applied to them). On ejection, ions are detected by the electron multiplier or photomultiplier tube. The power of the technique resides in the amount of control that can be exerted on the ions in the trap. The ions can be confined within the trap and excited by changing the radiofrequency potential applied to the ring electrode so that their kinetic energy increases and they fragment more extensively through collision with the helium atoms in the trap. Selectivity can be introduced by ejecting all ions apart from, for instance, the molecular ion of the analyte of interest. The analyte is thus freed from any interfering peaks in the background and can be subjected to additional fragmentation by changing the radiofrequency potential of the trap. This technique provides a low-cost alternative to tandem MS (see bp. 567). Ion trap instruments, like quadrupole systems, are commonly used in forensic toxicology because of their relatively low cost.

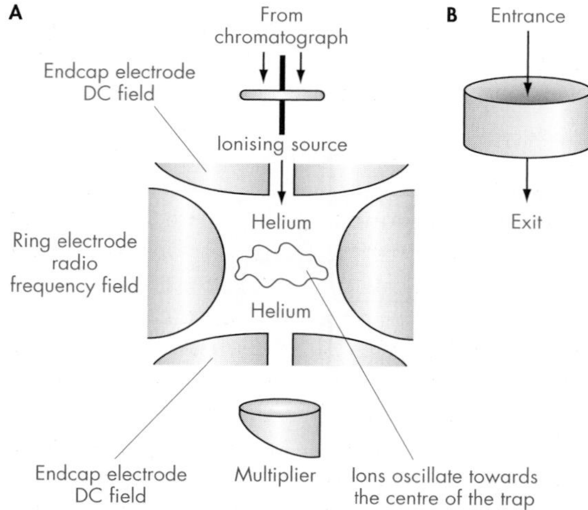

Figure 21.8 (A) Ion-trap MS. (B) View of the trap from outside.

Time-of-flight instruments

The principle of TOF instruments is simply that the larger an ion, the longer it will take for it to travel from the ionisation region to the detector of a mass spectrometer after acceleration through a given electric field. Hence ions formed in the ion source are accelerated in an electric field and then allowed to pass across free vacuum until they reach the detector. Ions reach the detector in order of increasing *m/z*. Because the technique relies on the time taken between ionisation and detection, the period during which the ions leave the ion source has to be well defined. All TOF mass spectrometers consist of three major components: pulsed or continuous ion source (EI ionisation, ESI, MALDI), linear flight tube or a reflectron mass analyser, and a time-to-digital converter (TDC) or a fast analog-to-digital converter (ADC) detector. MALDI uses short pulses of laser energy focused on the sample dissolved in a matrix that absorbs ultraviolet (UV) light. Alternatively, ESI (see p. 568) may be used in conjunction with a gating mechanism that allows ions to enter the separation field for only a very short period of time. The ions formed in the source have varying kinetic energies and, to avoid broad mass peaks, a device called a reflectron may be used to focus the kinetic energies of the ions that enter the TOF analyser. The greater the kinetic energy of an ion the further it penetrates into the reflectron, and thus the faster ions are retarded by the reflectron, which allows the slower ions to catch up. Improvements in reflectron focusing and gating mechanisms have enabled TOF to become capable of accurate mass measurement. TOF is a very good technique for the analysis of high-RMM compounds such as proteins, and MALDI-TOF instruments are used widely in proteomics.

Ion cyclotron resonance mass spectrometer

This instrument operates in a similar way to an ion trap. The ions are formed and introduced into a trap where they orbit within a circular magnetic field. As they circulate within the trap they pass close to two opposing electrode plates and thus induce a small alternating electric current within the circuit attached to the two plates. The amplitude of this current is proportional to the number of ions in the trap and its frequency is the same as the cyclotron frequency of the ions. The ions are thus detected without colliding with the detector via the current (the image current) that they induce. The ions in the trap can be excited by application of a radiofrequency pulse of radiation, which boosts the image current, which in turn falls off as the ions return to their unexcited state. The fall-off in the current can yield frequency information by the use of Fourier transformation, which leads to the construction of a mass spectrum. This process is analogous to Fourier-transform nuclear magnetic resonance (FT-NMR) spectroscopy, and can yield extremely high-resolution mass measurement, about ten times greater than the best performance of a magnetic sector instrument. The resolving power of this type of instrument is good enough to allow the accurate mass measurement of proteins. Ion cyclotron instruments are not often encountered in forensic toxicology laboratories owing to their cost, which is considerably higher than that of benchtop GC-MS systems, LC-MS systems and even magnetic sector instruments.

Tandem mass spectrometry

The most common form of tandem MS started with three quadrupole mass spectrometers linked together, but it can be carried out at a lower cost using ion-trap instruments. It is the most powerful mass spectrometric technique because it enables analytes to be separated rapidly by using a mass spectrometer rather than chromatography. In a triple-quadrupole instrument, the three quadrupoles are linked in series (Fig. 21.9). MS 1 and MS 2 separate ions in the usual way, both quadrupoles being operable in scan or SIM mode. No *m/z* separation takes place in the second quadrupole (MS 2). Instead, ions are allowed to collide with atoms of a heavy gas, typically a noble gas such as argon. This process is referred to as collision-induced dissociation (CID). There are other techniques available to induce dissociation, but the important aspect is that dissociation in MS 2 results in additional fragmentation. There are several ways of operating a tandem quadrupole MS system. One of the most common ways is to allow ions of selected *m/z* only to transfer sequentially through MS 1 to MS 2. Each 'precursor' ion undergoes dissociation in MS 2 to produce 'product' ions. The product ions are then scanned in MS 3 to produce a product ion spectrum. This is called product ion scanning or product ion analysis and is, effectively, a SIM-SCAN analysis. Alternatively, MS 3 can be operated to allow one or two characteristic product ion(s) only to pass to the detector (effectively a SIM-SIM analysis). This is called selected-reaction monitoring (SRM). This offers high sensitivity as both MS 1 and MS 3 act as filters to remove ions from the system which are not of interest. In precursor ion scanning (or precursor ion analysis), MS 1 is operated to scan while MS 3 is operated to allow a single *m/z* ion to reach the detector (SCAN-SIM). The product ion selected to transit MS 3 is normally one which represents a fragment typical for a group of compounds of interest. Common neutral loss scanning can be used to provide structural information about analytes. In this mode, both MS 1

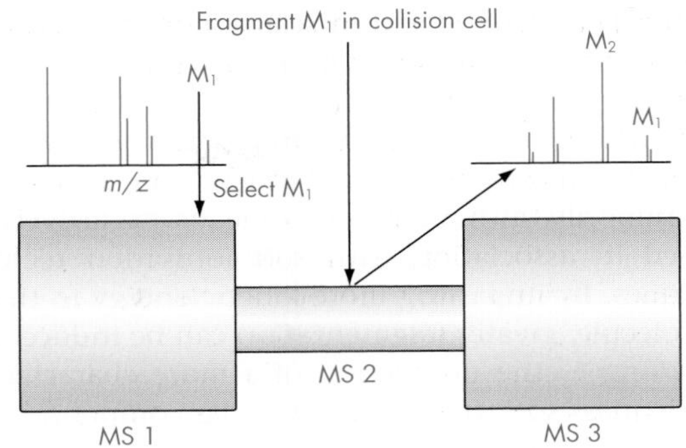

Figure 21.9 Schematic diagram of a tandem mass spectrometer.

and MS 3 are operated in scan mode but with a fixed mass offset in MS 3 characteristic for the neutral loss fragment. Only compounds producing the specific neutral loss fragment in MS 2 will be detected. Tandem MS is most commonly, although by no means exclusively, used in association with soft ionisation techniques. By imparting more kinetic energy to the molecule, greater fragmentation can be induced, leading to the production of a more characteristic mass spectrum for a particular compound.

Coupled techniques

Introduction

The most powerful mass spectrometric techniques involve the coupling of separation techniques with mass spectrometers. The development of ionisation techniques is linked intimately to the development of coupled techniques. Thus, in the majority of applications the ionisation technique has been developed and refined in conjunction with a separation technique. This is particularly true of the ionisation techniques used in conjunction with liquid chromatography (LC).

Gas chromatography–mass spectrometry

When capillary GC columns are used, the GC-MS interface is very simple and no special interface design is required. The GC effluent is simply introduced into the ionisation source. Although many analyses are now carried out by LC-MS, GC-MS is still important for many drug analyses. GC-MS is generally carried out in the positive-ion mode but can be operated in negative-ion mode. In the negative-ion mode, it is probably the most sensitive analytical technique available for analytes that are strongly electron capturing. The main areas of application for GC-MS in forensic toxicology are the identification and quantification of drugs and their metabolites in blood, urine, hair, etc. Many narcotics can be analysed by GC-MS with a high degree of selectivity, as can other abused drugs such as anabolic steroids. An advantage of GC-MS is that electron-impact (EI) spectra can be obtained which are correlated readily with library spectra that have been built up over many years. EI mass spectra are information rich compared with spectra resulting from soft ionisation techniques, which makes it possible to do 'fingerprint' type matching of EI spectra using commercial mass spectral libraries. The disadvantage of GC-MS is that more sample preparation is required than with LC-MS techniques.

Liquid chromatographic interfaces with mass spectrometers

The interfacing of a liquid chromatograph to a mass spectrometer proved much more difficult than for a gas chromatograph, since each mole of solvent produces 22.4 litres of solvent vapour even at atmospheric pressure. This solvent has to be removed before the sample enters the mass analyser which operates under vacuum. The technique has made huge advances in the past ten to twenty years and many types of interface are available, the most successful of which are the electrospray and atmospheric pressure ionisation sources (Neissen 1998).

Electrospray ionisation mass spectrometry and atmospheric pressure chemical ionisation mass spectrometry

ESI (Snyder 1996; Cole 1997) and APCI are the most widely used interfaces between liquid chromatography and mass spectrometers. In ESI the eluent from the LC is sprayed in solution into the source via a needle held at a high potential of 3–5 kV. The formation of an aerosol from the sample is assisted by a flow of heated nitrogen, which enters the instrument along a direction co-axial with the needle. The sample enters the instrument through a narrow orifice in a metal cone, which leads to a chamber at an intermediate level of vacuum; it then passes through a second orifice into a high-vacuum region. Figure 21.10 illustrates the production of the electrospray. At the tip of the capillary, positive ions are separated from their negative counterions,

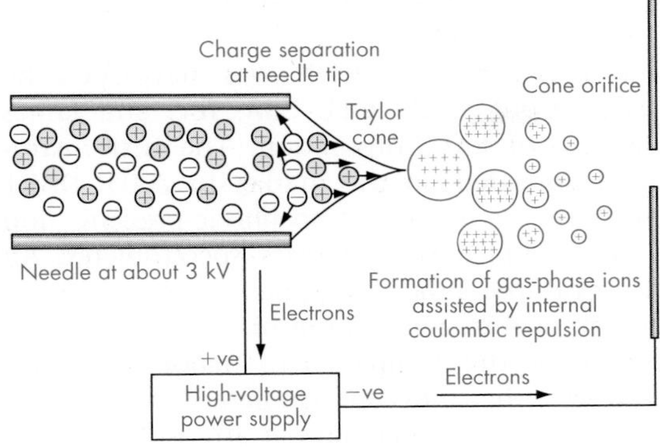

Figure 21.10 The electrospray process.

which are pulled towards the capillary. The isolated positive ions generated are repelled by the capillary. This force breaks up the surface tension of the liquid in which the sample is dissolved, to generate a cone (Taylor cone) that breaks up into charged droplets. This process is charge dependent and, since the analyte is usually of low concentration, electrolytes must also be in the liquid at a minimum concentration of 10^{-5} M to assist in promoting ESI. Once the sample has formed into charged droplets, the excess of positive charges in the droplets produces repulsion, which causes the droplets to break up further. This is assisted by evaporation of solvent from the droplets, which increases their charge and thus further promotes their break up. At the final stage, the analyte is believed to abstract one or more protons from the solvent (or donate a proton if a negative ion is formed) to give a positively charged gas-phase ion. If analytes can be protonated at multiple sites, they will carry several charges. Thus, a protein of molecular weight 10 000 a.m.u. that carries 10 charges appears to the mass analyser to have a mass of 1000 a.m.u. Figure 21.11 shows the electrospray mass spectrum of porcine insulin. The charge on a given ion may be obtained from two adjacent ions in the mass spectrum according to the formula:

$$n = \frac{M_A - 1}{M_A - M_B} \tag{21.3}$$

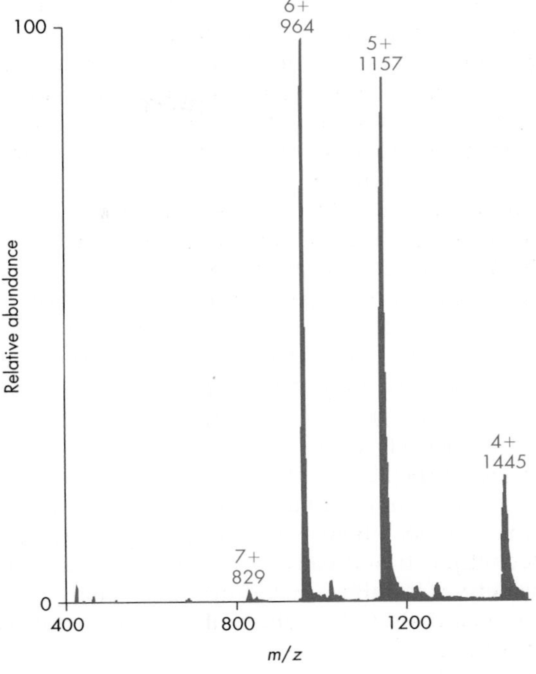

Figure 21.11 Electrospray mass spectrum of porcine insulin.

where n is the charge on M_B, and M_A and M_B are the masses of adjacent ions with M_A the higher in mass. Thus, for the spectrum of porcine insulin shown in Figure 21.11,

$$n = \frac{1157 - 1}{1157 - 964} = \frac{1156}{193} = 5.99 \tag{21.4}$$

Thus the charge on the ion (M_B) at m/z 964 is 6+, giving a relative molecular mass of 5784 for hexaprotonated porcine insulin. Insulin has six basic centres and, in this case, the predominant ion is that with all six centres protonated. Protonation of all the basic centres of a protein does not always occur.

To carry out APCI, the instrument used for ESI simply has to be reconfigured to introduce a corona discharge pin at the point where the stream of solvent that contains the analyte enters the instrument. Although APCI is carried out on the same instrument as ESI, it is quite a different process. It does not depend on the production of ions by evaporation, but rather it uses chemical species to promote the ionisation process in a manner analogous to the production of ions under positive ion chemical ionisation (PICI) conditions. In this case the reagent ions that promote the ionisation include N_2^+ and H_3O^+. APCI tends to be less sensitive than ESI, but it is useful for molecules that will not ionise readily (e.g. neutral drugs such as steroids).

An interesting variant of ESI is desorption electrospray ionisation (DESI) (Cooks *et al.* 2006). In DESI, a solution, typically of solvent plus water and possibly with other reagents to promote ionisation, is sprayed through a charged capillary at an angle onto the sample surface which is positioned close to the inlet of the mass spectrometer (Fig. 21.12). Ionisation takes place at or near the sample surface and the ions are drawn into the MS which is under vacuum. The DESI technique has already been applied to a wide variety of samples including direct analysis of urine and also the analysis of drugs in sweat by directing the spray at the fingertip of a volunteer who had taken a pharmaceutical drug. The advantage of DESI is the simplicity of sample handling.

Direct analysis in real time (DART)

The concept of DART™ was developed by Robert Cody from JOEL USA, Inc. and James Laramee of EAI Corporation. The first instrument appeared on the market in 2005. DART itself refers to an atmospheric-pressure ion source coupled with a mass spectrometer. An electrical potential is applied to gas such as helium or nitrogen to form plasma which interacts with the sample. The major difference between other mass spectrometers and DART is that the sample inlet stays at atmospheric pressure, so the samples such as tablets, powders, plant materials, gases, liquids, clothing, etc., can be directly held in front of the so-called sample cone of the DART system (Figure 21.13). As a result, the ions are formed immediately and they are subsequently directed to the mass spectrometer for immediate analysis. The masses detected are recorded. Liquid samples can be analysed by dipping an object into the liquid and placing it in the instrument. Vapours are introduced directly into the DART gas stream. The most important advantages of DART technology include there being no need for solvents,

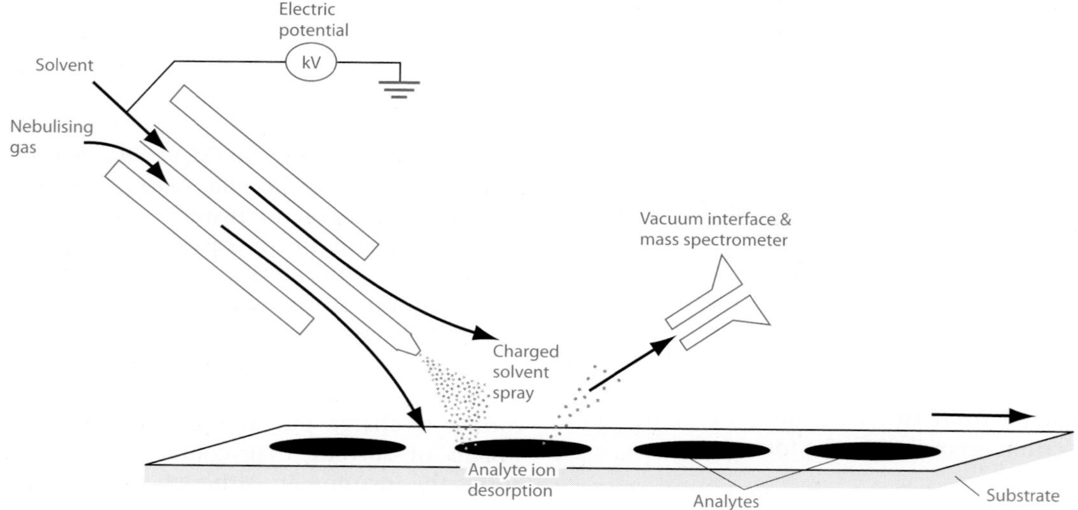

Figure 21.12 Schematic of DESI analysis.

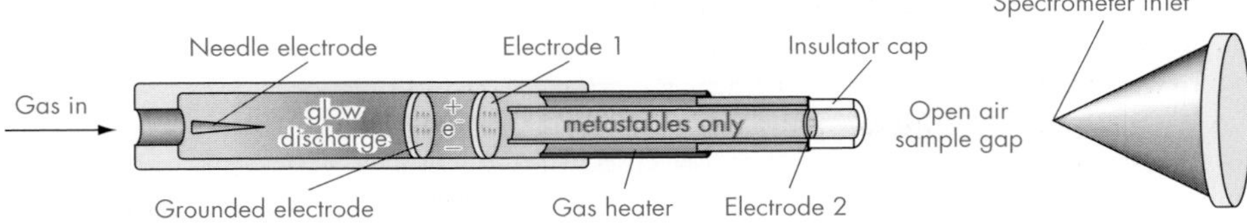

Figure 21.13 DART ion source.

fast and immediate response, no sample preparation, easy analysis of non-volatile chemicals: and high resolution.

Fast-atom bombardment mass spectrometry

Fast-atom bombardment (FAB) MS is a popular technique for direct insertion-probe MS, but it is also available as a LC-MS interface. Before the popularisation of ESI, FAB was the major technique for the ionisation of large molecules. FAB ionisation was also used as the basis for the only thin-layer chromatography–MS interface developed, but this interface was not really popularised. Now the application of FAB is confined largely to promoting the ionisation of molecules to determine their elemental composition, as illustrated for chloroquine in Figure 21.3.

Capillary electrophoresis–mass spectrometry

The preferred mode of ionisation for interfacing a capillary electrophoresis (CE) instrument with a mass spectrometer is ESI. The technique has been improved by the development of a method to introduce a sheath flow of mobile phase, which augments the nanolitre per minute flows through the CE column to form a stable electrospray. The CE interface is one of the most recent developments in MS and it is expected to have a wide range of applications in obtaining impurity profiles of both conventional synthetic drugs and biotechnological drugs.

Inductively coupled plasma-mass spectrometry

ICP-MS is used for analysis of elements, typically with an atomic mass of 7–250 a.m.u. While it can be coupled to chromatographic techniques such as GC, HPLC and CE for speciation analysis, in the toxicology laboratory it is most often used as a standalone instrument. ICP-MS instruments offer high sensitivity and the great advantage, compared to instruments such as graphite furnace atomic absorption spectrophotometry (GFAAS) and AAS, of multi-element analysis. This latter aspect has made ICP-MS the instrument of choice in busy toxicology laboratories.

As for all mass spectrometers, the instrument consists of a means of sample introduction, an ionisation source, mass analyser, ion detector and data system (Fig. 21.14). The ionisation source consists of a torch, typically made from quartz, surrounded by a copper coil attached to a radiofrequency generator. The radiofrequency energy passing through the coils produces an electromagnetic field. Argon gas at relatively high flow is fed through the torch which is held at a high temperature (7000–10 000 K). A high-voltage spark is introduced into the hot argon gas, producing free electrons. These electrons move in the oscillating electromagnetic field and collide with the argon gas to produce Ar^+ ions. Ultimately, a stable high-temperature plasma is established consisting of Ar^+ ions, electrons and neutral argon atoms. Samples are introduced into the plasma via a nebuliser. Desolvation takes place to give solid particles which vaporise in the hot plasma. Collision of the gaseous sample with electrons and argon ions results in

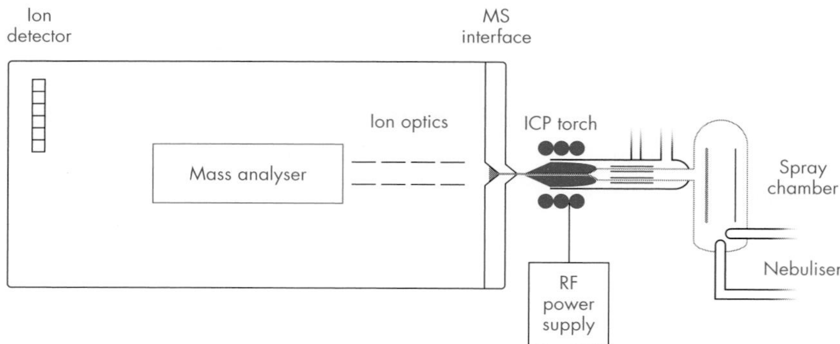

Figure 21.14 Schematic of an ICP-MS system.

ionisation of elements in the sample. Ions are then filtered through a series of cones and ion-focusing lenses before they pass into the mass analyser. This can be a quadrupole, mass sector or TOF device. Mass sector analysers offer high sensitivity and high resolution but low scan rates and high cost compared to quadrupole systems. Quadrupole analysers typically have only unit resolution which can give rise to problems in separating certain elements from background interferences. For example, $^{40}Ar^{16}O$ is formed in the plasma. This cannot be readily separated from ^{56}Fe. Modern ICP-MS instruments may incorporate a reaction/collision cell ahead of the mass analyser. This is typically a multipole (quadrupole, hexapole or octapole) with only radiofrequency applied (no d.c. voltage is applied). The radiofrequency focuses the ions. A stream of gas, typically helium or hydrogen or, in some instruments, methane or ammonia, is fed in. Collision with the gas results in the removal of interferences from argon species produced in the plasma.

Data processing

Considerations with regard to processing data obtained from mass spectrometers overlap those involved in the processing of chromatographic data obtained using other types of detector.

The plot of the sum of the ion current detected versus time obtained from GC-MS or LC-MS analysis is referred to as a total ion current (TIC) chromatogram (because it is generated from a plot of total ion current versus time). Although this looks similar to the type of chromatogram obtained from, for example GC-FID analysis, because it is a sum of all ions reaching the detector, it is possible to display the underlying data in a number of formats. The difficulties of peaks that are not fully resolved in TIC chromatograms can often be circumvented by interrogating the MS data system to plot the chromatographic traces of selected ions that are characteristic of the compound of interest. For example, in the chromatogram shown in Figure 21.15, the peaks for testosterone, estradiol and estradione partially overlap. However, it is possible to extract the molecular ions for each individual compound. Figure 21.15 shows the extracted ion traces for the molecular ions of the three analytes with very little interference between them. However, interference is not necessarily completely eliminated: the testosterone peak produces some response in the selected-ion trace for estrone since *m/z* 270 occurs in the mass spectrum of testosterone through the loss of water from its molecular ion at *m/z* 288.

The use of extracted ion traces is common in LC-MS data processing used for the screening of drug metabolites. The background produced by ions derived from the LC solvent in LC-MS mode

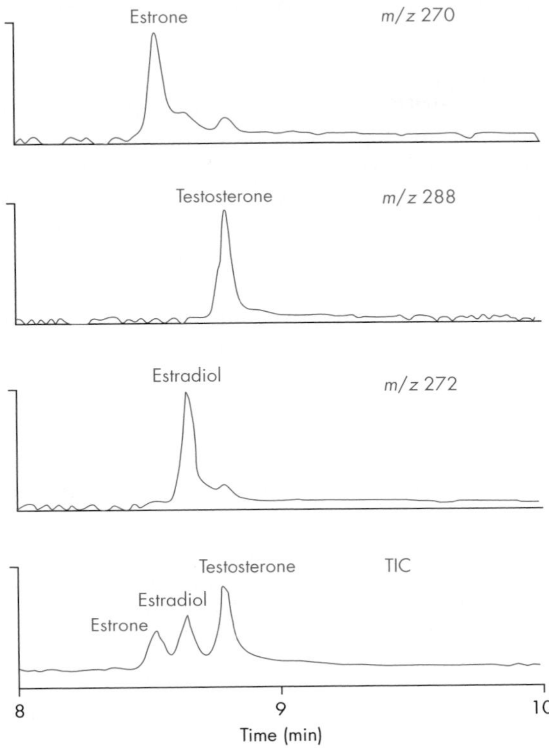

Figure 21.15 GC-MS trace of a mixture of estradiol, estrone and testosterone showing extracted ion traces for their molecular ions and the total ion current.

means that when metabolites are present in only low amounts the molecular ions of potential metabolites can be predicted and used to generate extracted ion traces to check for their presence. However, chromatograms such as these do not show the same sensitivity as does single-ion monitoring.

Data processing in the generation of accurate mass data is a little more complex since the mass spectrum of the compound of interest has to be calibrated against a standard, which is typically introduced into the mass spectrometer at the same time as the sample. For example, three of the calibrant ions are picked manually by the operator and the computer can construct a calibration curve based on the known masses of all the major calibrant ions (see Fig. 21.3).

System suitability tests

Chromatographic tests

Chromatographic systems interfaced with mass spectrometers are subjected to the same system suitability tests as used in conjunction with other types of chromatographic detectors described in preceding chapters.

Calibration of the mass axis

A test of fundamental importance in MS is to calibrate the mass axis of the mass spectrometer with a suitable tuning compound or mixture. If the mass axis is not calibrated correctly then mass spectra obtained will be in error and give rise to incorrect interpretations of the data. In GC-MS systems the most popular tuning compound is PFTBA (Fig. 21.4). The use of a fluorinated tuning compound has two advantages. On the carbon-12 scale of relative atomic mass, fluorine is very close to its nominal mass of 19, whereas the mass of hydrogen is considerably greater than its nominal mass of unity. Secondly, since PFTBA is electron capturing, it can be used to tune in the negative-ion chemical ionisation (NICI) mode. In the electron-impact mode, PFTBA produces a number of abundant ions below a mass of *m/z* 219 and weaker ions above this value. Tuning should be carried out on a minimum of three ions that cover the mass range of interest. Typically, the ions at *m/z* 69, 219 and 502 generated by PFTBA are used to calibrate the mass axis in EI ionisation mode. These ions are used also to determine resolution between masses. There is always a trade-off between resolution and sensitivity, and if the mass window is narrowed to reduce peak width, sensitivity is lost. The PFTBA ions at *m/z* 69, 219 and 414, and at 452, 595 and 633 are suitable for instrument tuning in PICI and NICI, respectively. Instruments can either be automatically or manually tuned, although automated tuning is more common on modern instruments. With quadrupole mass spectrometers and other low-resolution instruments, such as ion traps, the ions used in tuning are assigned masses to the nearest whole number. When high-resolution calibration is being carried out, masses of four or five decimal places are assigned to calibration ions; thus, for instance, the CF_3^+ ion at *m/z* 69 would be assigned its exact mass of *m/z* 68.9952. All the major ions in the spectrum of PFTBA would be used to carry out a high-resolution calibration, and thus enable accurate mass assignment.

In LC-MS the tuning mixtures used are less well defined than those used in GC-MS, and generally laboratories and manufacturers develop their own. Typical examples include valine, tri-tyrosine and hexatyrosine, which provide ions at *m/z* 118, 508 and 997, respectively, in the positive ESI mode. To determine proteins in positive ESI mode, the instrument may be tuned to the known average masses of the multiply charged ions derived from horse myoglobin, which gives ions at *m/z* 848.5, 1060.4, 1211.8, 1413.5 and 1696. In the negative ESI mode, polyethylene glycols may be used for tuning or a mixture of flavonoids, quercetin, quercitrin and rutin in the range *m/z* 300–610. Polyethylene glycols are used for calibration in ESI mode and they are also used to calibrate TOF instruments.

Sensitivity checks

There is no specific test for checking the sensitivity of a mass spectrometer. The ion counts provided by the tuning compound provide an indication of sensitivity, but beyond that the usual checks are of the sensitivity of the system when interfaced with chromatography. Manufacturers usually have their own favourite compounds for assessing sensitivity, such as methyl stearate to assess EI sensitivity in GC-MS mode, or octafluoronaphthalene to assess NICI sensitivity in GC-MS mode. However, these particular analytes are not typical of the average drug molecule, for which chromatographic factors contribute to the overall sensitivity. Sensitivity checks are usually carried out by diluting the compound of interest until it is no longer detectable by the particular system being used.

Sample preparation and presentation

The preparation of samples for GC-MS and LC-MS analysis does not differ from the types of preparation that would be carried out prior to any chromatographic method, that is extraction to remove interferences by the sample matrix as far as possible. Some extra considerations apply, for instance in GC-MS mode, as very often derivative formation may be necessary. For example, trimethylsilyl derivatives provide fairly abundant $[M-15]^+$ ions, which may be useful. Also, fluoroacylated derivatives may be prepared so that the sample is suitable for analysis in the negative-ion mode. The presence of nonvolatile salts in samples may also interfere in LC-MS in the ESI or APCI mode, since the nonvolatile salt will elute from the column and deposit on the cone, and so reduce instrument sensitivity quite rapidly. The cone can be continually washed to remove buffer salts, but despite this, sensitivity tends to fall quite rapidly with time. The use of nonvolatile buffers should be avoided for LC-MS.

Data interpretation

Introduction

The interpretation of a mass spectrum (Williams and Fleming 1980; McLafferty and Turecek 1993; Davis and Frearson 1994; Chapman 1995; Watson 1997; Lee 1998; Smith and Busch 1999) is intimately bound up with the type of ionisation used to generate the mass spectrum. With EI–MS, the fragmentation patterns for molecules are generally quite complex. Under other types of ionisation, fragmentation is less extensive and more predictable.

Electron-impact mass spectrometry

EI ionisation uses high-energy electrons at 70 eV, which produce extensive fragmentation of the bonds within the analyte. It is still very commonly used in standard chemical composi-

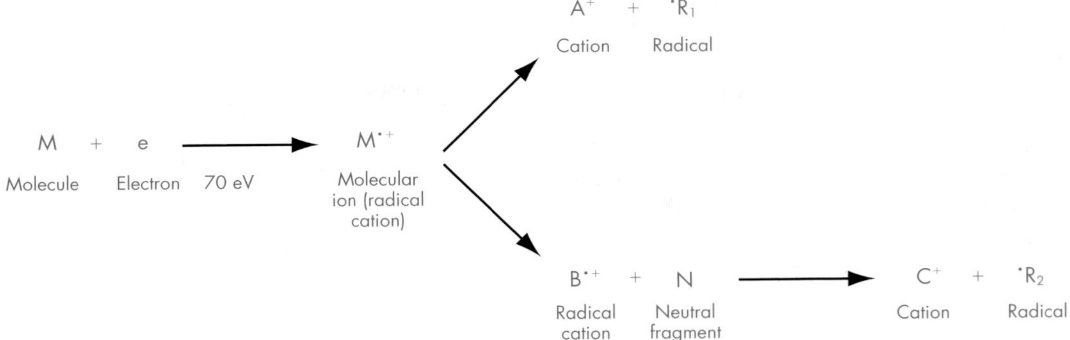

Figure 21.16 Electron-impact ionisation.

tion analyses, but is not as readily applicable if the molecule being analysed is very nonvolatile or unstable.

Figure 21.16 shows a generalised scheme for decomposition of a molecule under EI conditions:

- $M^{\cdot+}$ represents the molecular ion that bears one positive charge, since it has lost one electron, and the unpaired electron that results from the loss of one electron (represented by a dot).
- $M^{\cdot+}$ may lose a radical that, in a straightforward fragmentation not involving rearrangement, can be produced by the breaking of any single bond in the molecule. The radical removes the unpaired electron from the molecule to leave behind a cation A^+.
- This cation (A^+) can lose any number of neutral fragments, such as H_2O or CO_2, but no further radicals.
- The same process can occur in a different order, with a neutral fragment (H_2O, CO_2, etc.) being lost to produce the radical cation $B^{\cdot+}$; since this ion still has an unpaired electron, it can lose a radical to produce C^+, which can thereafter only lose neutral fragments.

An EI spectrum is shown for heroin in Fig. 21.17 and the fragmentation pathways that give rise to the spectrum are shown in Fig. 21.18. The molecular ion can be seen at *m/z* 369 (and therefore, according to the nitrogen rule, must contain a nitrogen atom) and the fragments at *m/z* 327 and 310 correspond to ions B and A in Fig. 21.16. The ion at *m/z* 268 corresponds to ion C in Fig. 21.16, and can also be derived via loss of acetate from ion B. The ion at *m/z* 284 results from the loss of two neutral fragments. As with many molecules, the simply explained losses occur only within about 100 a.m.u. of the molecular ion, and below *m/z* 268 the fragment ions are derived from complex rearrangements of the structure of the molecule. An advantage of EI is that the complex fragmentation pattern produced can be used as a fingerprint to identify the molecule, for instance to confirm the identity of traces of heroin in a forensic sample or the identity of an anabolic steroid in a urine sample. Thus, with EI spectra there is plenty of scope to identify an unknown via interpretation. Table 21.3 shows some of the common losses

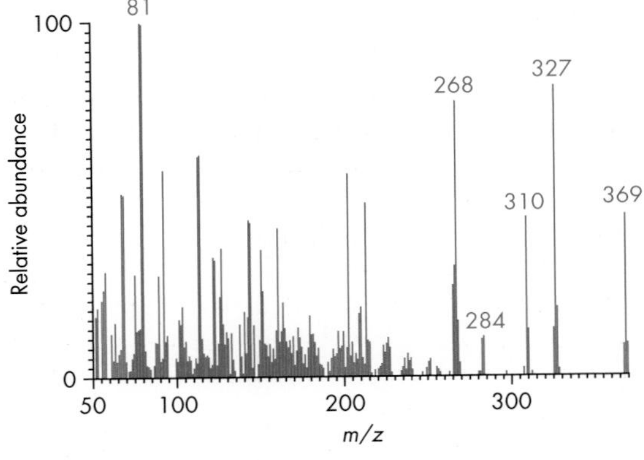

Figure 21.17 Electron-impact mass spectrum of heroin.

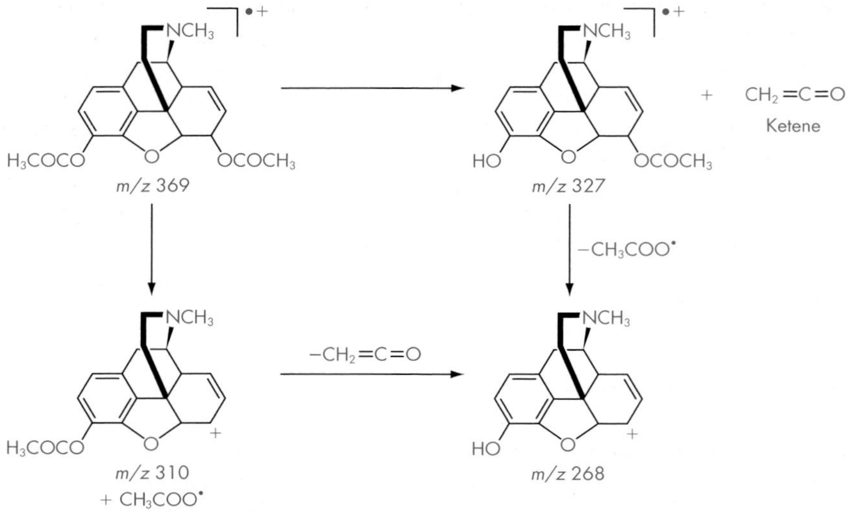

Figure 21.18 Fragmentation pathways that produce some of the ions in the EI spectrum of heroin.

Table 21.3 Some common losses from a molecular ion

Loss a.m.u.	Radicals and/or neutral fragments lost	Interpretation
1	$H^{\bullet}$	Often major ion in amines and aldehydes
15	$CH_3^{\bullet}$	Most readily lost from quaternary carbon
17	$OH^{\bullet}$ or NH_3	
18	H_2O	Readily lost from secondary or tertiary alcohols
19/20	$F^{\bullet}/HF$	Fluorides
28	CO	Ketone or acid
29	$C_2H_5^{\bullet}$	
30	CH_2O	Aromatic methyl ether
31	$CH_3O^{\bullet}$	Methyl ester/methoxime
31	CH_3NH_2	Secondary amine
32	CH_3OH	Methyl ester
33	$H_2O + CH_3$	
35/36	$Cl^{\bullet}/HCl$	Chloride
42	$CH_2=C=O$	Ketene
43	$C_3H_7^{\bullet}$	Readily lost if isopropyl group present
43	$CH_3CO^{\bullet}$	Methyl ketone or acetate
43	$CO + CH_3^{\bullet}$	
44	CO_2	Ester
45	$CO_2H^{\bullet}$	Carboxylic acid
46	$CO + H_2O$	
57	$C_4H_9^{\bullet}$	
60	CH_3COOH	Acetate
73	$(CH_3)_3Si^{\bullet}$	Trimethylsilyl ether
90	$(CH_3)_3SiOH$	Trimethylsilyl ether

from molecular ions that may be used in the interpretation of an EI mass spectrum.

The fragmentation patterns of large molecules may be difficult to interpret. For instance, steroid molecules give particularly complex patterns. Most of the ions in the EI mass spectrum of hydrocortisone (Fig. 21.19) arise from rearrangements of the structure that involve migrations of hydrogen atoms. These types of spectra give a characteristic fingerprint and the base peak ion (most abundant ion) at *m/z* 123 occurs in many steroids. However, it may vary in mass from one hydrogen atom higher to one lower than 123. The base peak in the mass spectrum of testosterone occurs at *m/z* 124, even though it has exactly the same A and B rings as hydrocortisone. However, the mass spectrum of prednisolone, which has an additional unit of unsaturation in the A ring, is consistent with hydrocortisone and yields a base peak ion at *m/z* 121.

In many drug molecules, the use of EI results in a low abundance of the molecular ion. Thus chloroquine under EI conditions gives less than 1% abundance of molecular ion (*m/z* 319) (Fig. 21.20) and its mass spectrum is dominated by an alpha cleavage fragment, which arises as shown in Figure 21.21. Caution therefore needs to be exercised when examining EI mass spectra. It should not automatically be assumed that the ion of highest mass (excluding the isotope ion) is the molecular ion.

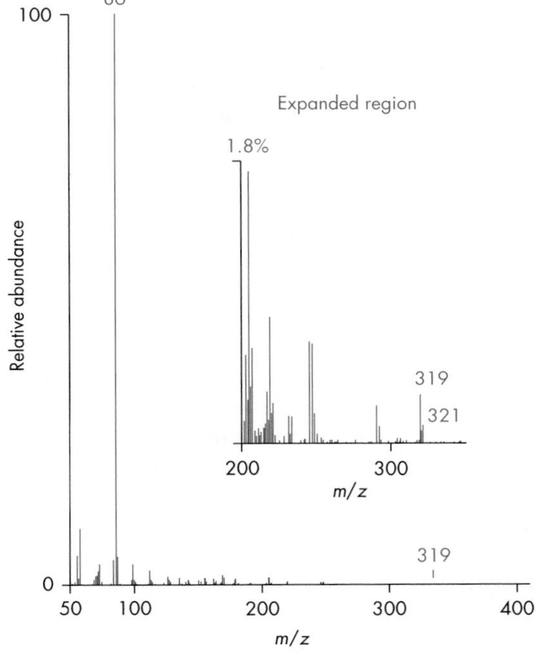

Figure 21.20 Electron-impact mass spectrum of chloroquine.

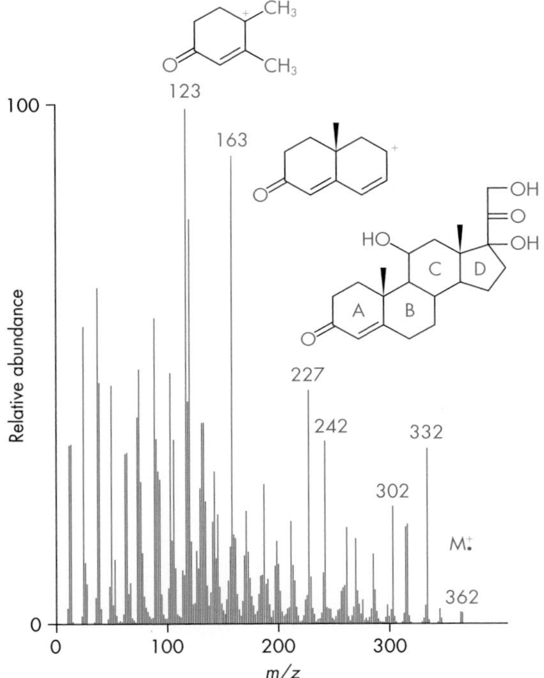

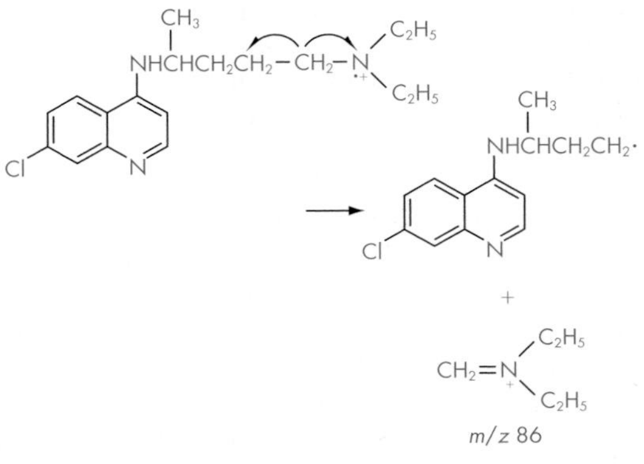

Figure 21.19 Electron-impact mass spectrum of hydrocortisone.

Figure 21.21 Alpha homolytic cleavage of chloroquine.

The spectra of heroin, hydrocortisone and chloroquine illustrate the three most common types of spectra observed in drug molecules. The spectra of heroin and hydrocortisone are most useful, since they are complex, provide a fingerprint and are more open to interpretation than simple spectra such as the spectrum of chloroquine. Other dominant fragmentation modes exist, such as the formation of a tropylium ion, which occurs in benzyl compounds, but these are not as common as those mentioned above and are discussed elsewhere (Williams and Fleming 1980; McLafferty and Turecek 1993; Davis and Frearson 1994; Chapman 1995; Watson 1997; Lee 1998).

If more information is required about the relative molecular mass of a drug that fragments easily under EI conditions, such as chloroquine, softer ionisation techniques should be used.

Positive-ion chemical ionisation

PICI can be carried out with a number of reagent gases (methane, isobutene and ammonia are most commonly used), and it is most applicable in GC-MS. The gas is introduced into the source of the mass spectrometer continuously during the analysis and the source configuration is changed so that the gas is contained within a small chamber within the source. Gas is introduced to give a source pressure of about 1 mmHg and bombarded with electrons produced by the same filament as used for EI ionisation at energies of about 200 eV. The electrons cause the reagent gas to ionise and further ions are produced through the gas reacting with itself. In the case of methane, three major reagent ions are produced, namely CH_5^+ (*m/z* 17), $C_2H_5^+$ (*m/z* 29) and C_3H_5 (*m/z* 41). These reagent ions can either transfer a proton to the analyte, thus ionising it, or combine with it to produce adduct ions.

When chloroquine is ionised under PICI conditions the spectrum shown in Fig. 21.22 is produced, which can be compared with the EI spectrum in Fig. 21.20. It can be seen that with chemical ionisation, the molecular mass of the substance is far easier to determine than using EI. In the PICI spectrum the $[M+H]^+$ ion is the base peak and ions seen at *m/z* 348 and *m/z* 360 are from the addition of *m/z* 29 and *m/z* 41 reagent ions to chloroquine. There is also an ion at *m/z* 284, which is caused by ionisation via abstraction of the chlorine atom from chloroquine by the reagent ions. PICI is not commonly used in chromatographic analyses, since it is usually of low efficiency, but it can sometimes be a useful method to help identify impurities in drugs; it is also a useful way to generate an abundant molecular ion for elemental composition determination when using high-resolution MS.

Negative-ion chemical ionisation

NICI spectra are generated in the same way as PICI spectra, except that the instrument is set to focus and detect negative ions. Most negative-ion spectra are not true chemical ionisation spectra, but are rather electron-capture spectra. Molecules that contain electronegative and/or electron-rich groups, such as halogens, oxygens or conjugated double bond systems, have a high affinity for electrons and thus capture the low-energy electrons produced by collision with methane. Thus, NICI is only suitable for mol-

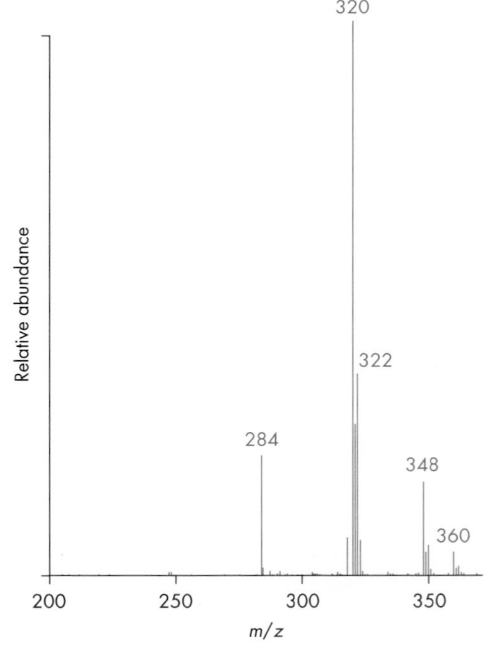

Figure 21.22 Positive-ion chemical ionisation spectrum of chloroquine.

ecules that contain electron-capturing groups, but for this type of molecule it is an extremely efficient and selective mode of ionisation resulting in high sensitivity. The NICI spectrum of chloroquine is shown in Fig. 21.23. As in PICI, the spectrum is dominated by the molecular ion, in this case at *m/z* 319.

When operating in chemical ionisation mode, tuning can be carried out using PFTBA (as used for tuning in EI mode). Some instrument manufacturers recommend perfluoro-5,8-dimethyl-3,6,9-trioxidodecane (PFDTD) for tuning where CI is carried out.

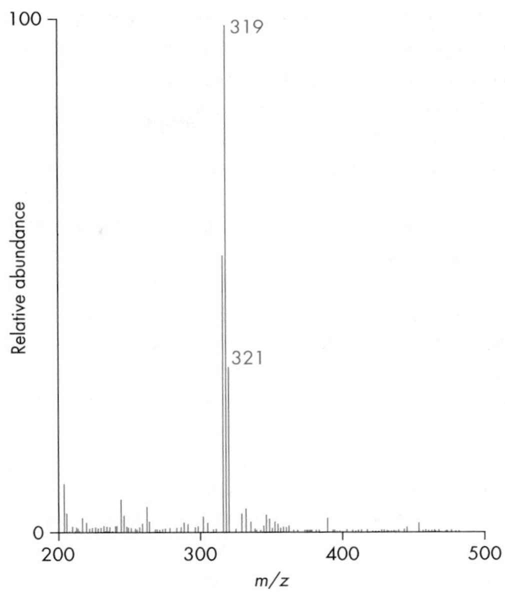

Figure 21.23 Negative-ion chemical ionisation spectrum of chloroquine.

Mass spectrometry in qualitative analysis

Some applications of GC-MS in qualitative analysis

Identification via library matching

Figure 21.24A shows the chromatogram obtained from the analysis of a sample of rosemary oil by

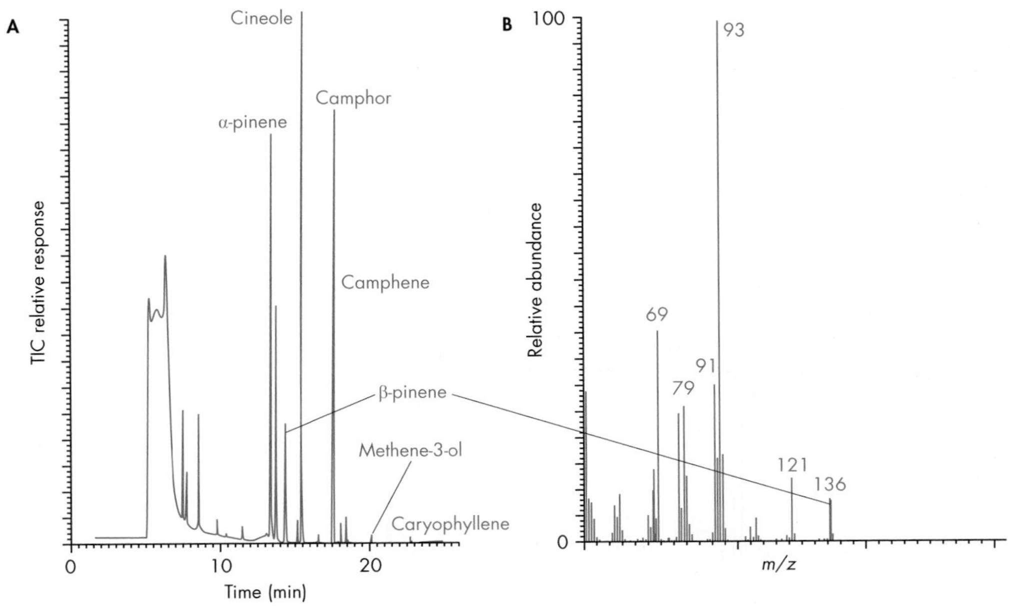

Figure 21.24 (A) Total ion current (TIC) chromatogram of rosemary oil by GC-MS. Conditions: ZB-1 column (60 m × 0.32 mm i.d. × 0.5 μm film); head pressure 130 kPa; programmed at 50°C (1 min), 5°C/min to 80°C, then 10°C/min to 270°C. (B) The mass spectrum of the peak at 14.37 min (β-pinene).

GC-MS. The mass spectrum shown in Figure 21.24B is for the peak at 14.37 min. This spectrum was computer-matched against the NIST library spectrum and gave two match figures of 932 and 941. Spectra are matched with the library and a correlation coefficient is obtained indicative of the closeness of match. Any match of between 900 and 1000 is regarded as excellent but must still be confirmed by visual comparison of mass spectra (see Electron-impact libraries, p. 584). The higher second-match figure in this case was obtained by matching the library spectrum to the unknown, omitting any peaks in the unknown that did not occur in the library spectrum, which is why the correlation number is slightly higher.

GC-MS is useful in the identification of unknown residual solvents and library search matches are very useful for identifying these types of materials. Even though solvents are relatively simple molecules, there is quite a wide range of possibilities when an unknown is picked up, so library matching is very useful in such cases. In addition to solvents, many manufacturing intermediates have a relatively low molecular weight and are volatile and thus suitable for GC-MS analysis.

While library searching can be exceedingly useful to identify substances, the identity should be considered presumptive unless additional information is available to confirm identification. Ideally, a standard of the substance should be obtained from a verified source and analysed alongside the original sample to verify a match in retention time and mass spectrum.

Impurity profiling

The US Food and Drug Administration now requires that impurities of greater than 0.1% be identified in pharmaceuticals. Such impurities can arise either from the manufacturing process or from degradation of the drug. Figure 21.25 shows a GC-MS trace for a commercial sample of the β-blocker oxprenolol. The compound contains three major impurities, one of which is resolved poorly from the very large peak obtained for the drug. The manufacture of β-blockers is by fairly standard routes, which helps the identification of manufacturing impurities.

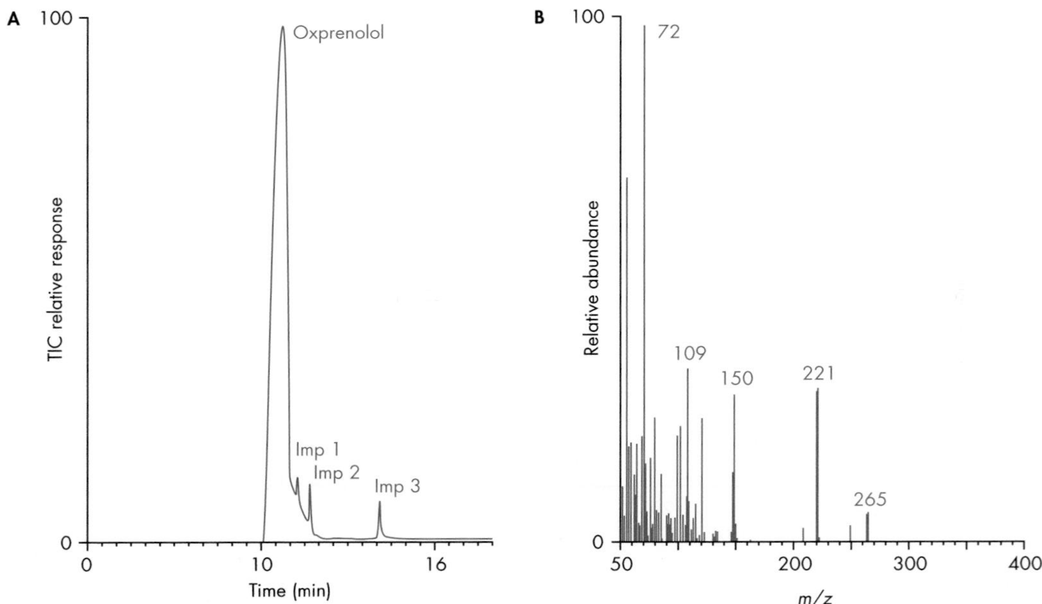

Figure 21.25 (A) GC-MS TIC trace of commercial sample of oxprenolol and (B) the EI mass spectrum of oxprenolol.

The mass spectrum of oxprenolol is shown in Fig. 21.25B. Under EI conditions it gives a relatively weak molecular ion at *m/z* 265 and the spectrum is dominated by the fragment that arises from alpha homolytic cleavage next to the amine in the side-chain, which is typical of many amines (as in chloroquine).

Let us take, as an example, the impurity peak 3. The EI spectrum of this impurity (Fig. 21.26) shows only two major ions at *m/z* 158 and *m/z* 72. Its GC retention time is longer than that of oxprenolol and, on the nonpolar GC column used, this suggests that the impurity has a higher molecular weight than oxprenolol. Under PICI conditions, the base peak of the mass spectrum of the impurity is an ion at *m/z* 308; the ion at 158 is still present but is much weaker. Taking into account the final step in the synthetic route to oxprenolol, the product possibly arises from the presence of a small amount of diisopropylamine in the isopropylamine used in the final step of the synthesis. Impurities 1 and 2 are isomers of oxprenolol; impurity 1 could arise via opening of the epoxide ring in the final step of the synthesis to form a primary alcohol, but both might also arise from isomers of the dihydroxybenzene present in the starting material for the synthesis.

Application of LC-MS in qualitative analysis

Determination of a degradation product from salmon calcitonin by ESI with triple quadrupole tandem MS

With the advent of biotechnologically produced pharmaceutical products, LC-MS (Neissen 1998) has come into its own as a quality control method. The complexity of proteins means that quality control by any other method is very difficult.

Salmon calcitonin (SC) is a single-chain 32-amino-acid polypeptide that is active in humans and is used to treat osteoporosis. The potency and duration of action of the drug depend on eight residues at the N-terminus, the formation of a S–S bridge between cysteine residues at positions 1 and 7, and the presence of a proline residue at the C-terminus. SC is formulated in aqueous solution for injection and thus is susceptible to degradation with time. Examination of a 2-year-old ampoule by LC-MS revealed an impurity peak in the LC-MS chromatogram of a few per cent running before the SC (Silvestro and Savu 1996). Figure 21.27 shows the mass spectrum of the impurity and the mass spectrum of SC, which gives a doubly charged molecular

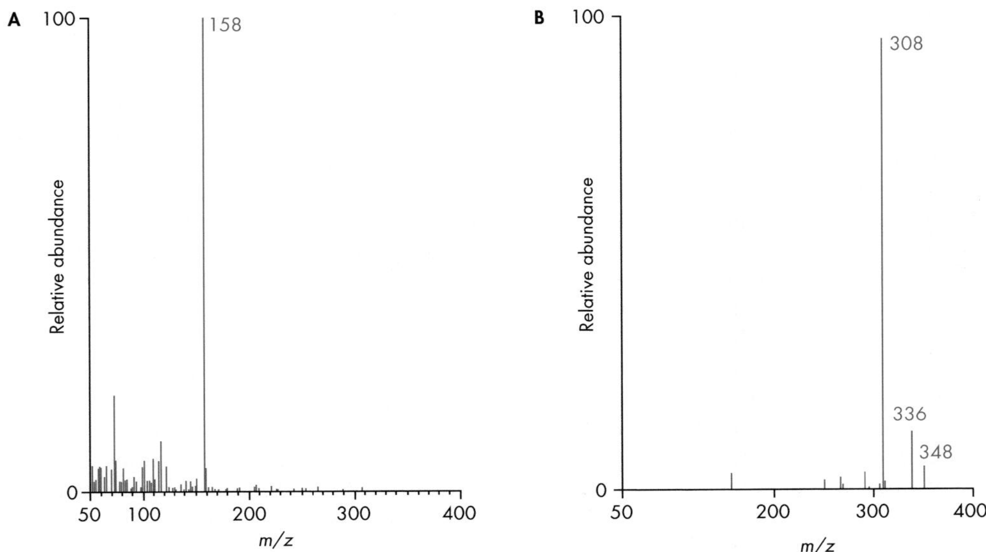

Figure 21.26 (A) EI and (B) PICI spectra of impurity 3 in Figure 21.25.

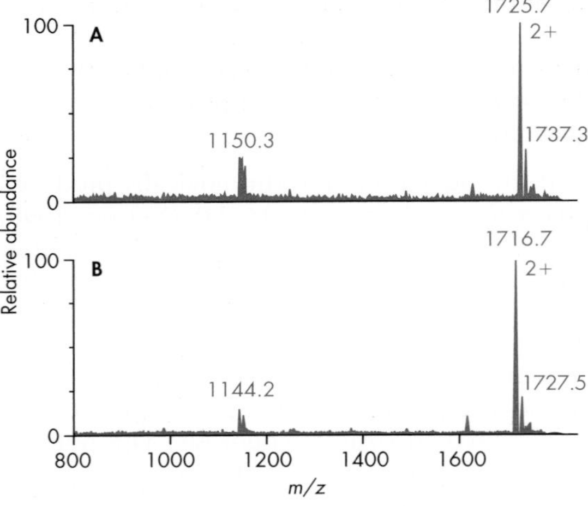

Figure 21.27 EI mass spectra of (A) a degradant of calcitonin formed upon storage in aqueous solution and (B) calcitonin.

ion at 1716 a.m.u. with which is associated a small ion at 1727 a.m.u. from the addition of sodium (23/2) to the molecular ion. The impurity gives a doubly charged molecular ion at m/z 1725, which differs from SC by 9 a.m.u. and suggests the addition of water to the molecule. To find the position of the modification, the SC impurity was isolated and treated with trypsin, which selectively cleaves polypeptides next to arginine and lysine residues. SC is expected to produce seven fragments from trypsin treatment. The impurity produced a similar pattern of degradants to SC. One of the fragments produced by the impurity, which corresponded to the 1–18 fragment in SC, gave a single-charge molecular ion, which indicated a difference of 18 a.m.u. from the corresponding SC fragment. It was possible to induce fragmentation of this ion by changing the cone voltage, and the series of ions produced when compared with those derived from SC suggested that hydrolysis of the S–S bridge between residues 1 and 7 had occurred. Storage of the SC in ampoules filled with an inert gas minimised the formation of this degradant. This illustrates the power of MS. Very few, if any, other techniques would have the sensitivity to identify the degradation product without significant sample preparation to isolate the product.

Identification of drug metabolites

Metabolism is an important component in the drug discovery and development process, and LC-MS has an important role in identifying drug metabolites (Oliveira and Watson 2000). The pathways of phase 1 and phase 2 drug metabolisms are well known, and it is possible to derive useful information even from a single-quadrupole instrument by using extracted-ion chromatograms to search for predicted metabolites. For example, formation of a monoglucuronide of a drug results in a shift of 176 a.m.u. from the molecular ion of the parent. However, the process of searching for metabolites is easier if tandem MS is available. The preferred mode of metabolite profiling in the preliminary analysis of metabolites is to use product-ion scanning. The predicted ion for a metabolite is selected by the first quadrupole and subjected to fragmentation in the collision cell, and the fragments are analysed by the third quadrupole. This enables acquisition of clean metabolite spectra that are free from any interfering solvent background. If a quantitative analysis is required, selected-reaction monitoring may be carried out, in which a critical transition is monitored. For example, the transition produced by loss of a glucuronide moiety from a glucuronide metabolite might be monitored if it gives a very specific response for that particular metabolite. Constant neutral-loss scanning is especially useful for searching for a particular class of metabolite, since it can readily detect metabolites resulting from both phase 1 and phase 2 metabolisms. For example, glucuronide metabolites for which the loss of the glucuronide moiety (−177 a.m.u.) is a major fragmentation pathway might be monitored. If the masses of the metabolites fall in a range (e.g. between 400 a.m.u. and 700 a.m.u.), the first quadrupole is set to scan between 400 and 700 a.m.u. and the second quadrupole to scan in the range (400 − 177) a.m.u. to (700 − 177) a.m.u. In this way, any metabolites that are, for example, methylated or undergo additional hydroxylation followed by glucuronidation are picked out, as well as simple glucuronides.

Ion-trap instruments can also be used to good effect in drug-metabolism studies and have approximately ten times the sensitivity of triple-sector quadrupole instruments when used to examine full-scan spectra. This is advantageous in the first phase of metabolite identification when the metabolites are unknown. Another advantage of trap instruments is that fragmentation of selected ions can be carried out several times with all the ions, apart from the molecular ion of the metabolite of interest, being ejected from the trap before the next fragmentation. This process produces clean spectra for the metabolite.

Some applications of mass spectrometry in quantitative analysis

Mass spectrometric detectors are able to carry out precise and accurate quantification of analytes. However, it is generally necessary to use an internal standard in analyses, since the instrumentation is more subject to sensitivity fluctuations than are simpler detectors such as the UV–visible detectors used in HPLC analyses. The selection of an internal standard has to be made carefully so that its mass spectrometric behaviour is reproducible and closely similar to that of the analyte. The internal standards labelled with stable isotopes (described below) are ideal, since they mimic the analyte very closely, but often a close structural analogue of the analyte will suffice.

The most common application of MS to quantitative analysis of biomedical samples is in the quantitative determination of drugs and their metabolites in biological fluids and tissues. The advantage of MS in this area is that its selectivity means it is less subject to interference by other compounds extracted from the biological matrix along with the compound of interest. The greatest accuracy in such analyses is afforded by using as internal standards analogues of the compound being measured that are labelled with stable isotopes. An isotopomeric internal standard of a drug co-elutes with it from a chromatographic column (sometimes deuterated compounds elute very slightly earlier than the unlabelled compound) and should have an almost identical response factor. Figure 21.28 shows the NICI mass spectra of the trimethylsilyl oxime derivative of prednisolone and its tetradeuterated analogue. The deuterated analogue of prednisolone can be used as an internal standard in the determination of prednisolone in a biological matrix. On the basis of the mass spectra shown, the ions at *m/z* 457 and 472 are monitored for prednisolone and those at *m/z* 461 and 476 for the tetradeuterated internal standard.

Since isotopomeric internal standards co-elute with the analyte, they aid in the recovery of the analyte from the chromatographic system (carrier effect). Figure 21.29 shows a selected-ion chromatogram of prednisolone methyl oxime/trimethylsilyl (MO/TMS) derivative (Knapp 1990) (monitored as the sum of the ions *m/z* 457 and 472; see Fig. 21.28), which was extracted from aqueous humour after addition of 10 ng of tetradeuterated prednisolone (the MO/TMS derivative was monitored as the sum of the ions *m/z* 461 and 476; see Fig. 21.28); the analysis was carried out using GC-MS. Similar types of approaches can be taken in LC-MS analysis.

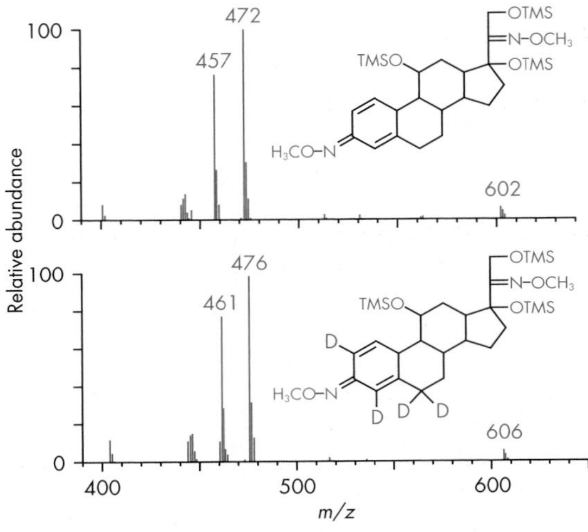

Figure 21.28 NICI spectra of trimethylsilyl prednisolone oxime and its tetradeuterated isotopomer.

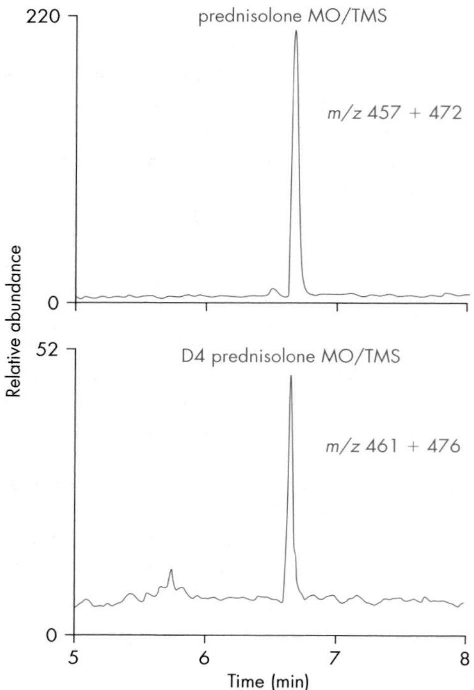

Figure 21.29 Prednisolone extracted from aqueous humour in comparison with tetradeuterated (D_4) prednisolone (10 ng) added as an internal standard (both as their trimethylsilyl oximes).

Collections of data

Electron-impact libraries

The most comprehensive collections of mass spectral data are based on EI mass spectra that have been acquired over many years and are used most commonly in conjunction with GC-MS analysis. The most popular libraries are the NIST library (details from www.hdscience.com), which contains the mass spectra of over 190 000 compounds, and the Wiley Registry of Mass Spectral Data, which contains 390 000 reference spectra. The MS data system is interrogated to plot the mass spectrum corresponding to a chromatographic peak of interest and then the mass spectrum is automatically searched against mass spectral databases stored on the data system. Alternatively, the mass spectrum of a molecule in the library may be called up using its CAS number, its name or its relative molecular mass and compared with the sample spectrum. Commercial libraries use peak-based matching to compare the mass spectrum of an unknown against the library spectrum. Spectra are matched in a manner analogous to the way two UV spectra are matched, except in this case the *m/z* values and the relative intensities of the ions of library spectrum and the unknown are matched. To simplify matching, a threshold can be set to eliminate, for example, ions of less than 1% intensity from the mass spectra being compared. A perfect match to a library spectrum has a value of 1000 and a value above 900 is regarded as a good match; a poor match has a value below 600. Regardless of the match value, a visual comparison of mass spectra should always be made. In particular, an inspection should be made to check that all ions which are abundant in the library spectrum are present in the sample spectrum and that the relative abundance of the ions in the sample spectrum have a reasonable correspondence with those in the library spectrum. An exact correspondence of relative abundance of all ions is unlikely because the library spectrum will probably have been generated on a different instrument. Nevertheless, a marked difference in the relative abundance of ions should flag a note of caution in accepting the identification without at least obtaining a sample of the substance (assuming this is possible) from a guaranteed source and analysing it. If the original analysis involved a hyphenated chromatographic separation, a concurrence in retention time together with a matching mass spectrum may be the clinching factor for confirming identity. If there is a relatively abundant ion in the library spectrum which is not present in the sample spectrum, this should also flag a note of caution regarding the putative match. The presence of one or more abundant ions in the sample spectrum which are not present in the library spectrum may indicate a non-match or the presence of a co-eluting substance. Interrogation of the baseline either side of the peak of interest and/or plotting the mass spectrum repeatedly across the width of the peak may shed light on the origin of these additional ions.

Libraries associated with LC-MS ionisation methods

Mass spectra obtained under the ionisation conditions used in LC-MS, such as electrospray, show little fragmentation, and the established libraries of EI spectra are of little use in searching such spectra. The use of tandem techniques increases the degree of fragmentation of molecules, but these do not reproduce exactly the EI spectrum of a molecule. Extensive libraries such as exist for EI, are not available for LC-MS but limited libraries are now becoming available (Halket *et al.* 2005).

Comprehensive databases based on MALDI-TOF or electrospray–ion trap spectra have been built up in the field of proteomics (James 2000; Kinter and Sherman 2000). The databases built up from MALDI-TOF data have been in operation for longer than those based on ion-trap data. The standard approach used in conjunction with MALDI-TOF is to separate proteins by gel electrophoresis, and thus obtain an approximate p*I* value (the pH of the isoelectric point of the protein), which can also be used in identification. The protein is cut from the gel, a proteolytic digest (most often using trypsin) is carried out, and the peptide fragments generated are analysed using MALDI-TOF. The pattern of peptides obtained can be matched against one of a number of databases using a linking program, such as Protein-Prospector. The linking program searches one of the large protein-sequence databases, such as SwissProt, for the proteins that contain amino acid sequences most closely matching those of the unknown. Additional information can be obtained by varying the laser power during the ionisation step or by post-source decay using the reflector to produce additional fragmentation of the peptides in the digest, and this information can be used to further refine the database search. A similar process is used for the ion-trap instruments using ESI. In this case the peptide digest can be separated by HPLC prior to its introduction into the mass spectrometer. A program such as TurboSEQUEST can be used to search protein sequence databases and MS/MS spectra can be obtained from the peptides in the digest to refine the search.

References

R. E. Ardrey, *Liquid Chromatography – Mass Spectrometry: An Introduction*, Chichester, Wiley, 2003.

J. R. Chapman, *Practical Organic Mass Spectrometry*, Chichester, Wiley, 1995.

R. B. Cole (ed.), *Electrospray Ionisation Mass Spectrometry*, Chichester, Wiley, 1997.

R. G. Cooks *et al.*, Ambient mass spectrometry, *Science*, 2006, **311**, 1566–1570.

R. Davis and M. Frearson, *Mass Spectrometry*, Chichester, Wiley, 1994.

J. M. Halket *et al.*, Chemical derivatization and mass spectral libraries in metabolic profiling by GC/MS and LC/MS/MS, *J. Exp. Bot.*, 2005, **56**, 219–243.

P. James (ed.), *Proteome Research: Mass Spectrometry*, Berlin, Springer-Verlag, 2000.

M. Kinter and N. E. Sherman, *Protein Sequencing and Identification Using Tandem Mass Spectrometry*, Chichester, Wiley, 2000.

D. R. Knapp, Chemical derivatisation for mass spectrometry, *Methods Enzymol.*, 1990, **193**, 314–329.

T. A. Lee, *A Beginner's Guide to Mass Spectral Interpretation*, Chichester, Wiley, 1998.

F. W. McLafferty and F. Turecek, *Interpretation of Mass Spectra*, New York, University Science Books, 1993.

W. M. A. Neissen (ed.), *Liquid Chromatography–Mass Spectrometry*, New York, Marcel Dekker, 1998.

E. J. Oliveira and D. G. Watson, Liquid chromatography–mass spectrometry in the study of the metabolism of drugs and other xenobiotics, *Biomed. Chromatogr.*, 2000, **14**, 351–372.

L. Silvestro and S. R. Savu, High performance liquid chromatography/tandem mass spectrometry identification of salmon calcitonin degradation products in aqueous solution preparations, *Rapid Commun. Mass Spectrom.*, 1996, **10**, 151–156.

R. M. Smith and K. L. Busch, *Understanding Mass Spectra*, Chichester, Wiley, 1999.

A. P. Snyder (ed.), *Biochemical and Biotechnological Applications of Electrospray Ionisation Mass Spectrometry*, Washington DC, American Chemical Society, 1996.

J. T. Watson, *Introduction to Mass Spectrometry*, Philadelphia, Lippincott Williams and Wilkins, 1997.

D. H. Williams and I. Fleming, *Spectroscopic Methods in Organic Chemistry*, London, McGraw-Hill, 1980.

22

Emerging techniques

M Sanchez-Felix

Introduction 587
Emerging techniques 587
Conclusion 602
References 603
Useful websites 605

Introduction

This chapter is devoted to analytical techniques not included in the previous chapters and categorised as 'emerging', to mean that they have future potential to scientists in various application areas. Attempts have been made to avoid highly specialised techniques with limited applications, but, as will be clear to the reader, the chapter content cannot hope to incorporate all emerging techniques. Some of the techniques included here are well established and used routinely in various industries but are included here because they are still rapidly developing and may have applications in other sectors. Established or 'older' techniques are also included because technological advances have overcome past limitations and opened up new scope. In addition to techniques, overviews of scientific areas such as genomics, pharmacogenetics and proteomics are included to provide an insight into these rapidly developing areas. Furthermore, these areas have given rise to a revolution in new techniques, computer tools and decision-making processes. The overall objective of this chapter is to provide the reader with an overview of the advances in techniques and science, highlighting their advantages and disadvantages.

In the area of forensic science, use of any new technique must be validated before it is employed in forensic science casework and the results are subsequently given in evidence in court. This is to ensure that the prosecution, defence and court are satisfied that the evidence presented in court is reliable and that the methods have been shown to work. In the USA, there is a requirement for formal validation of methods and techniques before the evidence is admissible, whereas in the UK it is sufficient to demonstrate that they pass the ordinary tests of relevance and reliability. For example, the Forensic Science Service (FSS) in the UK demonstrates that all new methods and techniques are fit for their specified purpose; these are authorised by its Chief Scientist before they are introduced into casework for use in criminal or civil proceedings, or offered as commercial services.

Emerging techniques

New multiwavelength ultraviolet spectrophotometric method

Ultraviolet (UV) detection is commonly used as part of high-performance liquid chromatography

(HPLC) to detect compounds in various sectors. UV spectrophotometric methods are also used to quantify drugs in dosage forms (Fujita *et al.* 1993; Issa and Amin 1994; Revanasiddappa *et al.* 1999), although this is becoming less common because they are believed to lack the specificity and level of automation required for today's applications. In this section, a fresh look at what UV has to offer is made thanks to advances in the use of fibre optics and the power of modern computers.

This method is generally dependent upon Beer's law for calculation of the concentration of the compound, as described in Chapter 15. To use this technique, the molar absorption coefficient of the compound is required, which may be determined by relatively straightforward means for non-ionisable compounds or when the other components present do not interfere. However, this approach has considerable restrictions in the case of ionisable compounds because the absorbance varies, as different species can exist in solution depending upon the pH and the ionic strength.

Consider, for example, labetalol, which is a diprotic compound and can exist as three different species in solution, as illustrated in Figure 22.1. The resultant spectrum at certain pH values can therefore be a combination of these species' spectra. To overcome this problem, solutions are buffered at a suitable pH value to ensure that only one species is present at any one time. The determination of the molar absorption coefficients of all the species can be deduced. However, the manual titration procedure employed is rather tedious and time-consuming (Albert and Serjeant 1984). In addition, the ionic strength may vary between experiments, which may lead to a shift in the dissociation constant (pK_a value) and accuracy of results.

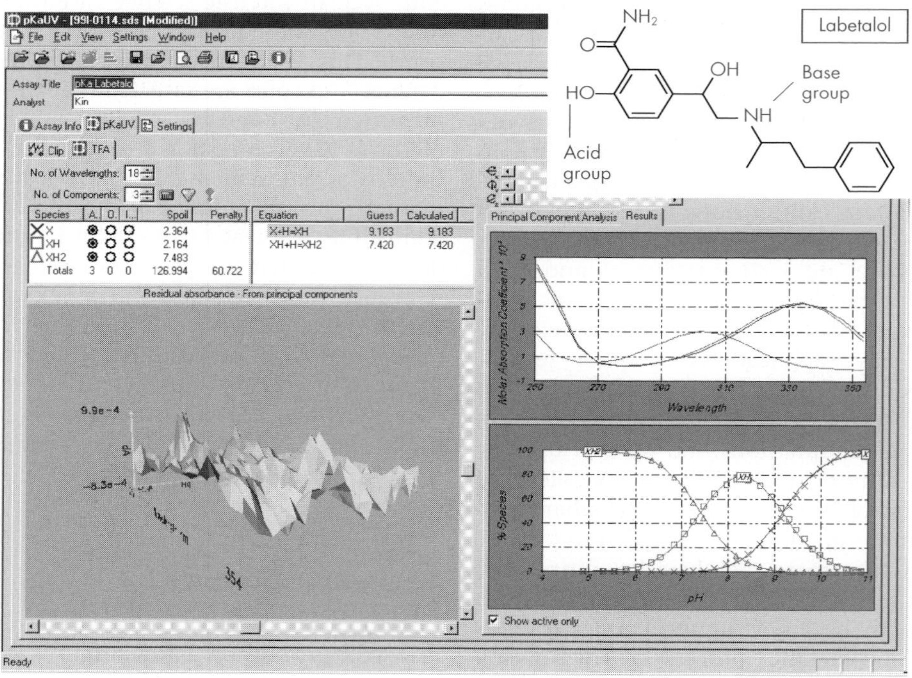

Figure 22.1 Software output for labetalol (top right) using D-PAS. Middle right: deconvoluted spectra of different species of labetalol. Bottom right: distribution of species in solution across the pH range. Bottom left: residual absorbance from principal components and for good fit to the model should show an error below $\times 10^{-3}$. Top left: boxes show model for systems. (Courtesy of Sirius Analytical Instruments.)

A UV multiwavelength spectrophotometric technique, termed Dip-Probe Spectroscopy (or D-PAS), has been developed to measure pK_a values. Figure 22.2 shows the commercially available instrument, which consists of a fibre-optic dip probe, a UV light source and a photodiode-array detector in conjunction with a commercially available titrator to capture the absorption spectra automatically in the course of a pH-metric titration. This technique has been validated extensively and shown to deduce pK_a values with high accuracy (Allen *et al.* 1998; Hadley *et al.* 1999; Mitchell *et al.* 1999; Tam and Takacs-Novak 1999).

The real power of the technique is the use of target factor analysis (TFA) to deduce the pK_a from the spectral data generated and also the molar absorption coefficients of the various species of a compound (Hendriksen *et al.* 2001). The software is extremely flexible, since it is designed for the discovery environment in which each compound has a different number of pK_a values (e.g. 1 to 10 pK_a values per compound) or for multicomponent systems (i.e. salts).

An example of a pH versus spectral plot for labetalol is shown in Figure 22.3. Figure 22.1 shows the data output – the distribution of species, pK_a values and deconvoluted spectral profiles of the various species of labetalol. Also shown in Figure 22.1 is the residual absorbance for the principal components (i.e. species in solution) across the pH versus absorbance range. This is the difference between the real and predicted data for the model proposed. If large peaks appear in this plot, the model is not correct and it indicates whether too many or too few pK_a values have been defined. A spoil value is also generated that provides an overall indication of the error for the complete model. In a way, these two features mean that the program is self-validating for every sample run, which is extremely important when less than 1 mg is available for the assay.

When the pK_a values and the molar absorption coefficients of all the species of a compound in solution are known, it is possible to determine the concentration and spectral profile of a compound in solution at any pH. Furthermore, the software is extremely flexible and has the potential to be used to deconvolute multicomponent systems or to be adapted for reaction monitoring by replacing pH with time. The potential applications include identification, reaction and process monitoring, protein folding and quantitative measurements. Disadvantages of this technique are that the compound must have a chromophore and the event must give rise to a change in the chromophore. Furthermore the compound must be soluble and in solution during the experiment. Sensitivity may also be an issue.

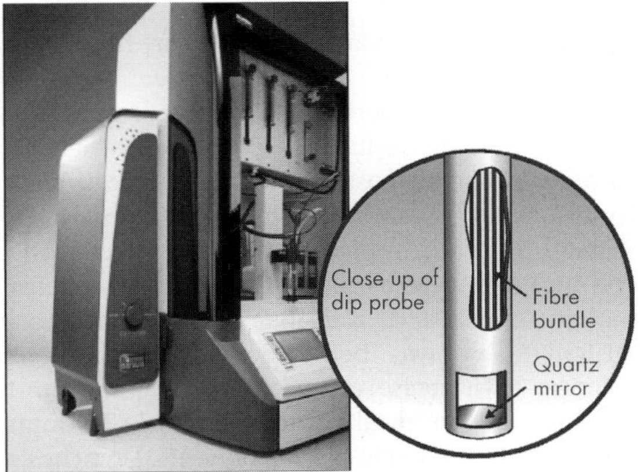

Figure 22.2 The UV multiwavelength spectrophotometric technique termed Dip-Probe spectroscopy. It is currently used to determine dissociation constants of compounds, but has other potential applications. (Courtesy of Sirius Analytical Instruments.)

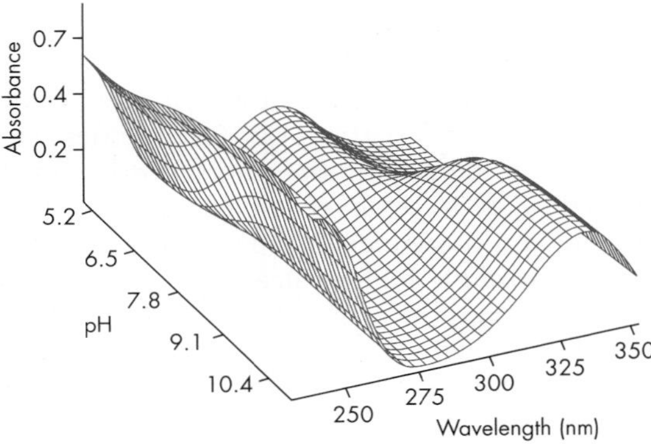

Figure 22.3 Spectral versus pH output from the D-PAS instrument used to determine the pK_a of labetalol. (Courtesy of Sirius Analytical Instruments.)

The multiwavelength UV technique described above has resulted in the evolution of a new instrument called ProfilerSGA. This instrument takes samples directly from stock solutions in a 96-well plate and dilutes them to the appropriate concentration. Each of these solutions is injected directly into a pH gradient stream, mixed and passed through a quartz flow cell, to generate multiwavelength UV spectra for the compounds over a linear pH range 2 to 12. This instrument has been designed for high-throughput discovery screening and is able to determine the pK_a of a compound in 2 min compared to 20 min for the D-PAS instrument.

Clearly, the option of placing the probe directly into processes for reaction monitoring is a further potential application. TFA is an interesting software tool, which has the potential to be used to deconvolute data from other techniques and applications areas. Its strengths are its ease of use, flexibility for different model systems and self-validation.

High-throughput screening

One of the major advances that has taken place over the past ten years is the strategic implementation of high-throughput screening (HTS), mainly by the research divisions of pharmaceutical and biotechnology companies. HTS is often defined as the rate at which compounds can be screened, which is typically between 100 to 1000 data points per day. More recently, 'ultra high-throughput screening' (uHTS) techniques have been described (Hill 1998; Ram 1999), which have the ability to produce 100 000 data points per day. Most of the HTS laboratories are involved in identifying the interaction of small molecules with a target molecule, usually a protein, and consequently the tools available are targeted towards biological assays. This should not discourage the application of HTS in new sectors, although HTS has distinct advantages and disadvantages that may limit its potential in a previously unapplied area. Among the major disadvantages are:

- The costs of implementation. These can be considerable and require expertise to effect successfully. Data-management systems (e.g. storage, retrieval, integration of data and interpretation) also contribute greatly to the costs.
- Poor suitability towards non-robust procedures.
- Inappropriate for data that require interpretation. The quantity of data generated by HTS can be so considerable that human interpretation of it becomes the bottleneck. However, new software tools are overcoming this issue
- sample handling. Samples have to be in solution for the screens to work. Reagents can be in solid state, but a liquid has to be added for the reaction to take place. There is potential to think laterally here and use a solid sample as well as the reagents in solution. Attempts to develop solid handling systems have been unsuccessful to date.
- Stability and solubility. As indicated, samples are generally in solution to enable dispensing via a robotic system. Unfortunately, solution stability can be a problem. A further issue is the solubility of compounds in water or buffers required for the assays; to overcome this, many compounds are prepared in dimethyl sulfoxide (DMSO) and assays are designed so that the final concentration of DMSO is approximately 10%. Solubility and stability pre-screens are often conducted as part of the process to identify compounds that would give false results.

Despite these disadvantages, HTS has the virtue that it is suited to 'screen-intensive' areas in which large numbers of repetitive assays are required and the reduction of volume is needed to reduce reagent costs. HTS can be traced back to the early 1990s with the development of 96-well microtitre plates, which replaced the common test tube as the receptacle of choice for biological assays. At a similar time, combinatorial chemistry was being developed and was offering to increase productivity of compound synthesis. Both resulted in a major paradigm shift from knowledge-based sequential synthesis and testing to parallel synthesis and testing of multiple compounds. This has led to a significant reduction in the cycle time for discovery projects and increases in productivity. However, the initial optimism that it would completely replace the traditional methods and skills was ill-founded; most companies have modified their processes to incorporate these new technologies to complement the sequential synthesis and testing techniques performed upstream and on the candidates identified from HTS.

Information technology (IT) associated with computational chemistry also developed rapidly during the evolution of HTS. This is no surprise, as computational tools were required to store the large quantities of data, and rapidly search and retrieve this data so that it could be used to make structural relationship correlations. Two early problems encountered were:

- how to process and make decisions from the data generated
- how to deal effectively with the number and nature of new targets (projects) investigated by the sponsoring company.

These problems have been overcome by the most significant change, new business processes. All of the successful companies have developed business processes that map the assays used at each stage, as well as the decisions made and, more importantly, the criteria set for the compound to progress to the next phase (i.e. set of tests) to reduce the amount of human intervention. IT tools are now available that enable much faster decisions to be made by presenting information in simple formats, e.g. intuitive colours, symbols and pictures (Ladd 2000). One of the more interesting approaches is the use of traffic-light reporting, in which the values from screens have coloured backgrounds of red, orange or green. Green indicates that the value is above the set criteria (for example, the test shows that the compound is active for that test), orange indicates that it is borderline and red that it fails. Using this approach, multiple results for different compounds can be screened visually, so enabling a quick and simple trend analysis to be carried out.

One important consideration is the nature of drug discovery, by which unwanted compounds are screened out at the same time as new compounds are designed using the information obtained. As the discovery process progresses, the tests being performed become less automated, require more material and take more time. The net effect is that they become more expensive; hence there is a need to screen out and develop an understanding of the chemistry that makes a compound reactive at the site of action. Thus the throughput of the screen is only one way that a company may obtain an economically competitive edge. The rapidity with which multiple rounds of testing takes place, the quality of the structure–activity relationship (SAR) deduced from the assay, the novelty of the assay technology (giving access to unique targets), the sophistication of the data analysis and the ability to mine data from previous screens are all areas in which companies can gain an advantage.

Currently, the industrial sectors that are adopting HTS are those that function similarly to the pharmaceutical discovery process; for example, the chemical catalyst sector, in which there is a need to use SARs to design and synthesise new catalysts. The drivers here are speed and the necessity to screen out compounds to select those that should be optimised. HTS is beginning to make inroads into other sectors, such as clinical and forensic testing, absorption–distribution–metabolism–excretion studies, toxicology, genomics and proteomics areas. In these instances, the driver is the number of samples requiring the same assay. Those who have to deal with large quantities of samples should take a close look at what HTS has to offer.

Assays for HTS were originally used to screen libraries of compounds in solution and were consequently designed to utilise the smallest amount of compound possible, as the synthesis is often rate-limiting and costly. In addition, the assay should be configured to use the smallest number of steps or reagent additions so as to maximise throughput and minimise costs. Two different categories of assays are used – 'homogeneous' and 'heterogeneous'. In the case of homogeneous assays, all reagents are in the same phase and the instrument takes a measurement when a steady-state reading is obtained; readings for kinetic measurements are taken over a defined period. Heterogeneous assays require a phase separation which removes the free from the bound compound. This type of assay is more difficult to perform and is common for the older types of assay. A short description of the consumables, instrumentation and some of the assays is given below.

One of the most important considerations to be made when carrying out HTS is the plate format. The lowest density and most common format is the 96-well plate with a typical volume capacity of 200 μL per well, although larger volumes are available. Gaining in popularity is the 384-well microtitre plate, with a typical volume capacity of 100 μL per well. Various advantages can be gained by moving from 96 to 384 wells, namely, smaller quantities of compound and reagent and also a higher throughput per day. In the area of uHTS a 3456-well microtitre plate format has been developed recently (Fig. 22.4) for a system that can run 100 000 to 200 000 assays per day in volumes of 2 μL per assay. The system uses handling robotics modified from those used in the semiconductor industry, with automation capable of accurately transferring 2–20 nL of solution into the assay well at a rate in excess of 100 000 compounds per day. Other companies have reported working with even higher densities, such as 6500 (Schullek 1998) and 9600 assays per plate (Oldenburg 1998).

Novel technologies are being reported that provide even higher capacities than those described above. For example, Biotrove Inc. has developed a technology called 'Living Chip' that consists of 3.3 inch × 5 inch (8.38 cm × 12.70 cm) square chips containing up to 10 000 × 50 nL hydrophilic wells bored entirely through the plates; the plate surface itself is hydrophobic to prevent cross-contamination. Samples can be applied in two different ways:

1. By dunking in a solution that contains the sample.
2. By stacking a number of the chips and drawing syringes that contain each reagent through the aligned through-holes. This technique offers an interesting new approach, in which the samples can be pre-dispensed into one chip and reagents in others. Since the plates have neither a top nor a bottom, reactions can be set up by stacking the plates in the appropriate order so that the samples mix through the exposed menisci.

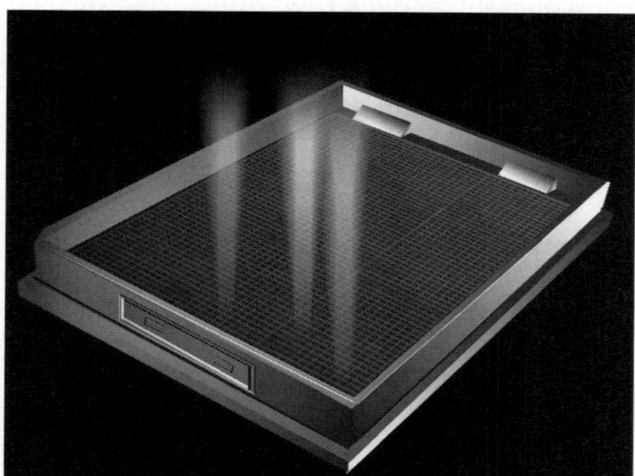

Figure 22.4 A 3456-well plate. (Courtesy of Aurora Biosciences Corp.)

Diversa Corp. has announced a technology called GigaMatrix that can screen up to one billion clones per day. It has a microplate that contains 100 000 wells, each of 250 nL capacity. This system is currently being developed for enzyme and small-molecule discovery programmes.

A considerable number of instrument manufacturers provide all the key hardware components required for an HTS system. Some manufacturers also provide a fully integrated system that includes the compound library stores, robotics, sampling management systems (e.g. bar coding), scanners and databases for the storage of data. Both approaches have their advantages and disadvantages. Essentially, any procedure that can be performed routinely by a scientist can be replicated by HTS (Fig. 22.5). Examples of items that can be incorporated into HTS include:

- plate-handling robot that can dispense the reagents and samples in solution
- shakers
- both heated and cooled blocks
- centrifuges
- plate stackers
- thermocyclers (for DNA polymerase chain reactions (PCRs))
- vacuum manifolds (for membrane filtration)
- extraction blocks (for DNA, solid-phase extraction and proteins)
- plate readers (e.g. spectrometers, UV, fluorescence).

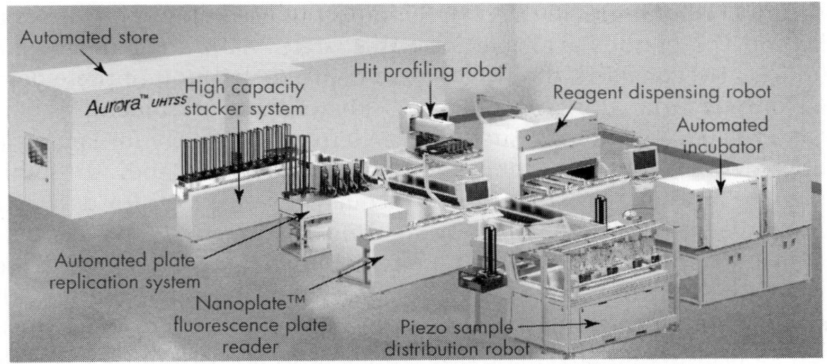

Figure 22.5 Aurora-integrated ultra-high-throughput systems. (Courtesy of Aurora Biosciences Corp.)

Assays that have been developed are aimed predominantly at the study of the interaction of small molecules with proteins and therefore require both sensitivity and selectivity. A short description is given below of a number of assays that have proved especially amenable to HTS.

Radioligand binding

The technique used is the scintillation proximity assay developed by Bosworth and Towers (1989). This relies on β-emitting radioisotopes detected by means of a scintillant that converts the energy of the β-particle into light. In this assay system, the target protein is captured onto the bead (containing scintillant). The radiolabelled drug molecules that bind to the target protein activate the scintillant, while those in free solution are too distant to do so. Radioactive detection methods are very reliable and are still the method of choice for determining the interaction of small molecules with a protein-binding site. However, the technique can only be used if a high-affinity ligand for the site has already been identified, and its sensitivity means that it is not ideal for microtitre plate formats greater than 384.

Fluorescence techniques

Several fluorescence techniques are used for HTS and have evolved because of the obvious benefits this technique has to offer. Considerable advances in a variety of speciality fluorescence techniques have been made in recent years, offering the potential of single-molecule detection and *in vitro* imaging in cells: Basché *et al.* (1997) give an overview. Naturally, the sensitivity and selectivity offered have been exploited in HTS. Three techniques are used to determine the interaction of two molecules in a variety of different ways, including time-resolved fluorescence (Hemmila 1990), fluorescence resonance energy transfer (Hemmila and Webb 1997) and fluorescence polarisation (see examples in Fig. 22.6).

A publication by Begg (2000) entitled 'HTS – where next?' provides a valuable insight into the

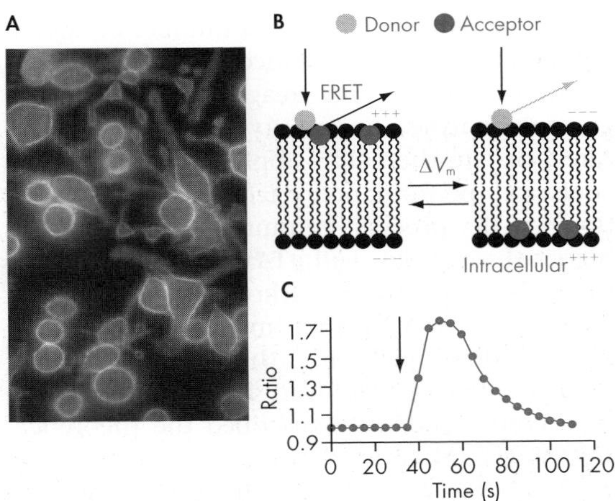

Figure 22.6 Example of (A) membrane voltage sensors in cells using (B) fluorescence resonance energy transfer (FRET) to (C) monitor changes in membrane potential induced by modulation of ion channels by test compounds. (Courtesy of Aurora Biosciences Corp.)

challenges that face HTS laboratories in the pharmaceutical sector and the options available for its future progression. He considers the drivers from increasing output and the virtues of either moving towards new technology, such as 'lab-on-a-chip' approaches (see next section) or restructuring along the lines of a task-orientated production facility (called drug discovery factory facilities). Either way, HTS is still evolving rapidly and its adoption into other 'screen-intensive' areas of genotyping, forensics and toxicology is likely to lead to new advances.

Micro total-analysis systems and chip-based microsystems

One of the objectives of a number of manufacturers and academic groups in recent years has been to develop micro total-analysis systems (μTASs), also called by many the 'laboratory on a chip'. As the name implies, these systems are designed with the potential ability to perform a complete chemical analysis on a single integrated microchip. In principle, they offer a complete analytical system that allows all or combinations of the processes, such as sample introduction, sample pre-treatment, reaction, product separation, product detection and finally product isolation.

Such systems would offer a number of advantages that may include reduced fabrication costs, reduced sample and reagent consumption, greener analysis, portability offering point-of-care or in-the-field applications, superior analytical performance, facile process integration, facile process automation and, finally, higher throughput. Full μTASs are currently not available commercially, although various groups have demonstrated that manufacturing techniques developed in the microelectronic industry can be deployed for laboratory-scale prototyping and have described the theoretical advantages (Manz *et al.* 1991; Martynova *et al.* 1997; Duffy *et al.* 1998; Bessoth *et al.* 1999).

The following sections summarise the two categories of microsystem device that have evolved, namely microarrays and microfluidics. These microsystems are developments towards μTAS devices and have made an immeasurable impact in the fields of genomics and proteomics (see later). Manz and Sanders (2000) provide an in-depth description of these devices.

Microarrays (or biochips) have become the preferred technology for large-scale gene expression, genotyping and, to some extent, DNA sequencing (see later for descriptions and applications). Aitman (2001) discusses the way in which microarrays have started to affect clinical practice and research, and how the role of these devices is likely to develop in the future. Microarrays consist of thousands of fragments of DNA (short chains of oligonucleotides, complete genes, or other DNA) immobilised at a specific point to a chemically modified glass slide or other substrate to form spots. In the case of genotyping, before the sample DNA can be applied to the microarray, it must be isolated, the fragments of DNA of interest replicated using PCR (to obtain quantities required for detection), and finally labelled with a fluorescent tag (see Figs 22.7 and 22.8). This is applied to the microarray, in which the replicated fragments of the DNA molecule from the sample bind to a complementary DNA molecule on the microarray (i.e. by Watson–Crick base pairing). This process is referred to as hybridisation (see later). The unbound sample DNA (or RNA) is washed off to leave the hybridised DNA only. A digitised image of the hybridised microarray is then created on scanners and the image is analysed using software that determines on which spot fluorescence is associated with gene expression or single-nucleotide polymorphism (SNP).

Clearly, a microarray is not a μTAS device, as considerable pre-treatment is conducted before the application of the sample onto the slide. However, the advantage of microarrays is that they allow a large number of reactions to occur within a very small area without the need for huge amounts of material or robotics. The high spot density of such systems when using photolithography techniques means that, in the case of gene expression profiling, up to 15 000 genes can be measured on a single slide. To put a perspective on the performance gains obtained, researchers are now able to generate large quantities of data in a few hours that a decade ago would have taken them years to achieve. Readers

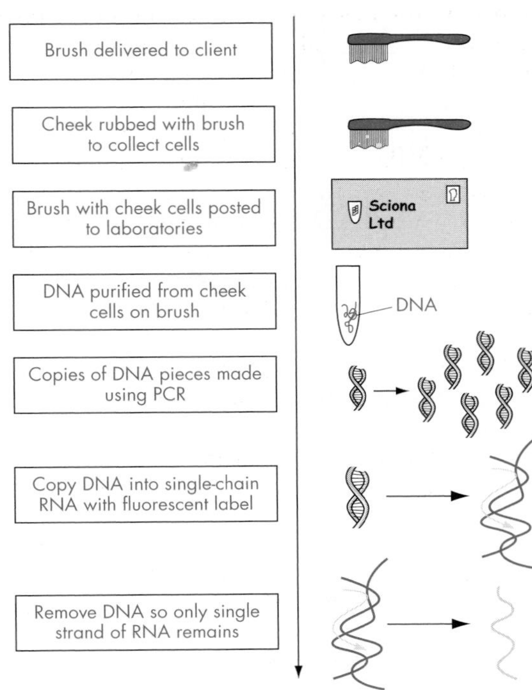
Brush delivered to client
Cheek rubbed with brush to collect cells
Brush with cheek cells posted to laboratories
Sciona Ltd
DNA purified from cheek cells on brush
DNA
Copies of DNA pieces made using PCR
Copy DNA into single-chain RNA with fluorescent label
Remove DNA so only single strand of RNA remains

Figure 22.7 Steps required to prepare DNA for microarrays. (Courtesy of Sciona Ltd.)

wishing to obtain a more in-depth knowledge of microarrays are recommended to key reviews by Lockhart (2000), Chipping Forecast (1999) and a book by Schena (2000).

The technology for producing spotted microarrays is widely available, and these devices are produced in scores of biomedical research laboratories. Production and use of custom arrays are now within the grasp of any molecular biology laboratory and, once the DNA has been prepared, the costs are low. The disadvantage of this technique is that consistency of spotting and reliable annotation of the DNA on the microarray is hard to achieve. The technology available for proteomics using microarrays is still in its infancy but has much to offer (Manz and Sanders 2000). A website providing reviews on the commercially available systems can be found at www.gene-chips.com.

Microfluidic systems differ from the previously described microarrays in that the sample can be transported within miniature channels. Table 22.1 illustrates some of the applications for these devices. They are able to perform reactions, separations and analysis within a single micro device, thus making these devices a step closer to μTAS. Figures 22.9 and 22.10 show components from the commercially available microfluidic system from Nanogen. This system combines microfluidics and electronics to analyse DNA, RNA and proteins quickly and accurately.

A cursory comparison of microarrays and microfluidic devices would highlight that the former are suited to systems in which many thousands of results need to be generated from one sample. The benefits offered by this type of device are speed and the relatively low cost of analysis. In the latter system, the opposite may be said to be true on first appearances; namely, the ability to run many samples and generate one type of result per sample. However, the concept of multicomponent microfluidic systems has already been demonstrated to open up the possibility of designing devices that can provide more than one type of analysis or result simultaneously. Furthermore, since microfluidics offers a possible approach to the potential benefits of μTAS, these devices are more suited to applications in other sectors (e.g. continuous sampling, reactions, separation and detection). Note, though, that this review has limited its focus to the genomic and proteomic areas to demonstrate the advances made in these devices.

As with any new technique, there are a number of problems with the devices described. These include loading of the sample onto the devices, designing re-useable devices, and detection limits. The concluding comments of Manz and Sanders (2000) seem most appropriate, that 'commercial developments will undoubtedly catalyse solutions to many of these problems'.

Genomics and proteomics

These are exciting times for researchers and organisations within the areas of genomics and proteomics, because of the speed at which developments in our understanding have occurred. Also the emerging technologies in these areas have direct applications in drug discovery and the potential to revolutionise healthcare, bringing about a new form of therapy based on

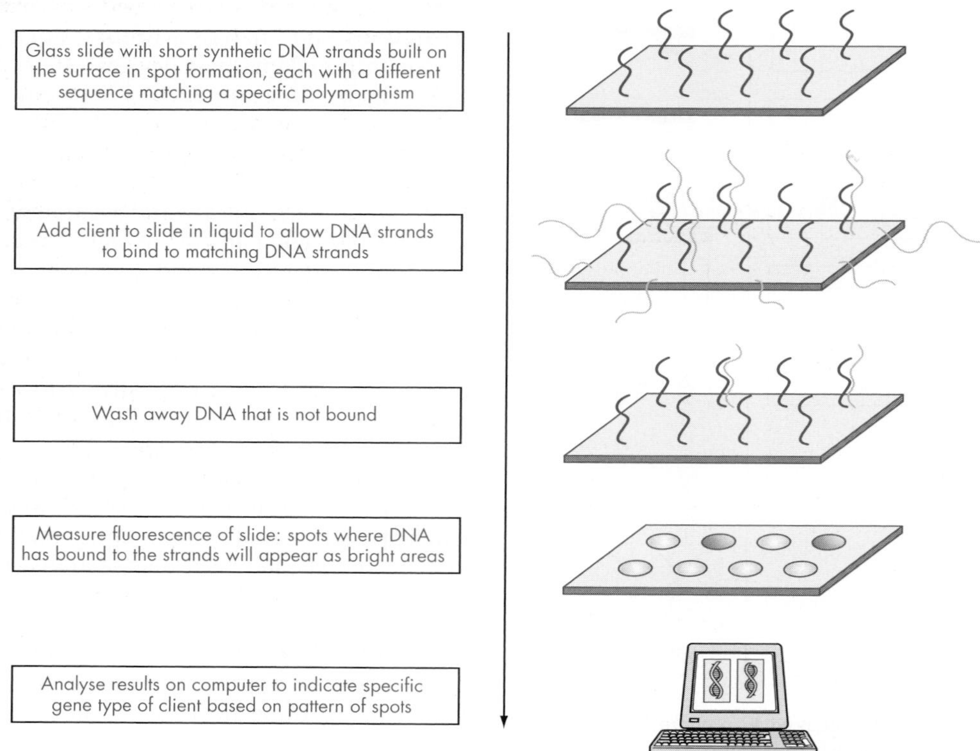
Glass slide with short synthetic DNA strands built on the surface in spot formation, each with a different sequence matching a specific polymorphism
Add client to slide in liquid to allow DNA strands to bind to matching DNA strands
Wash away DNA that is not bound
Measure fluorescence of slide: spots where DNA has bound to the strands will appear as bright areas
Analyse results on computer to indicate specific gene type of client based on pattern of spots

Figure 22.8 Process required for DNA analysis using microarray. (Courtesy of Sciona Ltd.)

the in-depth knowledge of patients' genetic make-up. The catalyst for this was the completion of the draft sequence of the human genome (International Human Genome Sequencing Consortium 2001; Venter *et al.* 2001).

Genomics is the study of the organism's entire genome. It basically deals with issues such as techniques of sequencing, genome mapping, data storage, bioinformatic analysis, etc. A gene is a sequence of different combinations of the four nucleotide bases and may be composed of thousands of bases. An individual gene occupies a specific place or locus on the DNA strand on a chromosome and is always found on the same type of chromosome. The current estimation is that there are between 30 000 and 40 000 genes in all the human chromosomes. It is your genes that provide the specific codes for the formation of your body's proteins, the type of protein that is made and what it will be used for within your body.

Proteomics is the study of the entire collection of proteins produced by a particular cell type. This includes determining the number, level and turnover of all expressed proteins, their sequence and the post-translational modifications to the sequence, and protein–protein and protein–other molecule interactions within the cell. It is now known that there is a poor correlation between the level of gene expression (i.e. messenger RNA production) and the abundance of the corresponding steady-state proteins. Furthermore, the initial theory that one gene is responsible for the generation of a single protein has been found to be incorrect. Our current knowledge indicates that a single gene may be responsible for a number of possible proteins, through alternative splicing or post-translational modifications. Consequently, the estimated number of potential human proteins lies between 1 million and 100 million.

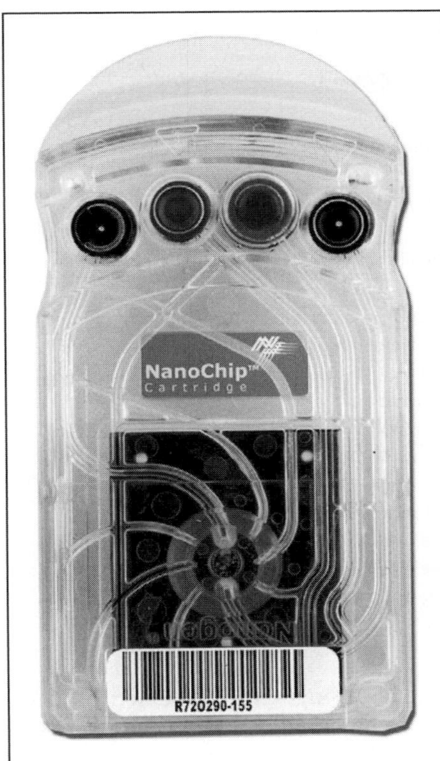

Figure 22.9 The NanoChip Cartridge, which is used with a NanoChip Molecular Biology Workstation. Electrical charges guide DNA samples down microfluidic channels to the NanoChip Microelectronic Array (see Fig. 22.10), which enables the precise identification of active genes. (Courtesy of Nanogen.)

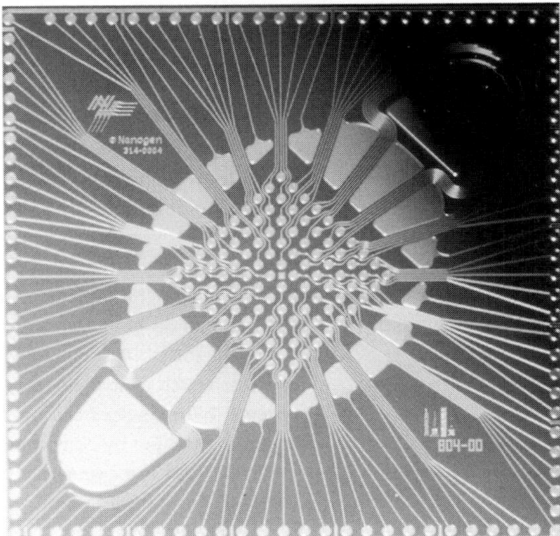

Figure 22.10 NanoChip Microelectronic Array, which is the inner component of the NanoChip Cartridge (see Fig. 22.9). This is a 100–site electronically powered microarray fluidic device. DNA and RNA are moved and concentrated by controlling the current at each test site. (Courtesy of Nanogen.)

The relationship between genomics and proteomics is shown in Figure 22.11, and unravelling the complex interaction of genes and proteins will eventually enable us to understand and predict the molecular bases of disease. Developments in these fields have already had considerable impact on the pharmaceutical industry and, in particular, the discovery organisations (Kahn 2000; Powell 2000; Wells and Feger 2000). Of greater impact is how genomic and proteomic data will be used in healthcare for individuals. Peakman and Arlington (2000) discuss the promise of pharmacogenetics and pharmacogenomics and how these have the potential to reduce the number of drug-adverse events, which have been reported to be the fourth to sixth leading cause of death in the USA (Lazarou *et al.* 1998). They also describe how these two disciplines may lead to new techniques that select the correct treatment for an individual. This is possible by establishing the SNP profile of an individual (referred to as genotyping), influencing proteins that affect absorption, distribution and metabolism of some drugs, and also the proteins related to the disease. This information would be combined with that for the drugs available to select the best drug and dosage. Peakman and Arlington (2000) go on to say that in the next ten years every patient could carry a swipe card that contains details of his or her genomic data. The doctor would use this card to select not only the best treatment for the illness but also the patient's susceptibility to disease.

Forensic toxicologists also need to have an appreciation of genetic toxicology to interpret blood and tissue drug concentrations accurately in cases of suspected drug toxicity. Knowledge of whether an individual is a fast or slow metaboliser of a drug may well assist in linking a

Table 22.1 Areas of applications published on the microfluidic systems (adapted from Manz *et al.* 2000)

Application	Comment	Reference or company
PCR	Device used for replication of DNA fragments with ability for multiple PCR reactions to occur simultaneously. Advantage offered is speed of analysis; 5-fold improvements versus conventional PCR instruments have been reported.	Kopp *et al.* (1998a, 1998b)
DNA fragment sizing and concentration determination	Commercial microfluidic DNA chips are available using polyacrylamide gel CE to separate different length DNA fragments for DNA sequencing. Run times can be as low as 90 s, which is considerably faster than conventional systems. New devices are being developed that enable higher throughput by combining arrays of microfluidic chips.	Caliper Technologies Corporation Agilent Technologies Aclara Biosciences Mathies *et al.* (1998)
Immunoassays	Immunoassays are commonly used to determine protein presence and concentration. The publications that report this application have used modified electrophoresis microchips. Analysis time of 90 s has been reported.	Koutny *et al.* (1996) Von Heeren *et al.* (1996) Chiem and Harrison (1997) Cheng *et al.* (1998)
Protein and peptide analysis	A number of publications have reported the analysis of proteins and peptides using microfluidic systems interfaced to electrospray MS. The advantage conferred is increased throughput.	Xu *et al.* (1998) Figeys *et al.* (1998) Xue *et al.* (1997) Li *et al.* (1999)

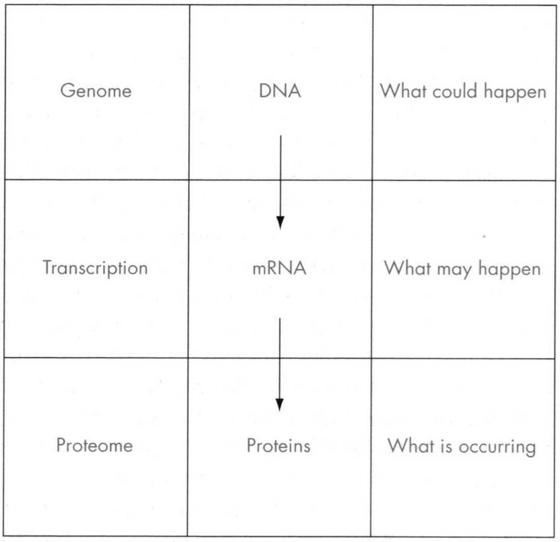

Genome	DNA	What could happen
Transcription	mRNA	What may happen
Proteome	Proteins	What is occurring

Figure 22.11 Relationship of genomics to proteomics.

blood concentration to an acute dose of a drug. Also, the presence or absence of receptors for a drug in an individual will greatly affect that individual's response to the drug. In the near future, it will be possible from simple gene-chip tests to determine an individual's polymorphic profile of drug-metabolising enzymes (such as the P450 cytochromes, which oxidise drugs). Such tests could well become part of forensic toxicologists' everyday work.

Considerable progress in high-throughput genotyping (i.e. SNP analysis) has occurred in recent years and a review by Shi (2001) describes some of the techniques available. These techniques fall into various subgroups summarised in Table 22.2. In fact, the number of companies and techniques for SNP analysis appearing on the market is increasing almost on a weekly basis. It is not possible to include all the techniques available in this area, some of which are hybrid techniques that combine two or more of the features shown in Table 22.2. Despite recent progress in high-throughput genotyping, the obstacles that will have to be overcome in the areas of technical, data-analysis and cost levels are formidable. The good news is that the techniques developed in this field may have benefits for other sectors of science. Furthermore, the energised environment combined with large potential profits means that there is still a great deal in store with regard to advances in genotyping techniques.

Table 22.2 Examples of different types of SNP techniques available (adapted from Shi 2001)

Category	Technique
Gel electrophoresis-based methods (requiring PCR step)	Restriction fragment length polymorphism Muliplex PCR Oligonucleotide ligation assay Mini sequencing
Fluorescence dye-based methods (requiring PCR step)	Oligonucleotide ligation assays Pyrosequencing Single-base extension with fluorescence detection Homogeneous solution hybridisation, such as TaqMan and Becon genotyping
Other techniques	Rolling circle amplification[a] Invader assay[a] DNA microchips Mass spectroscopy genotyping

[a] Techniques not requiring a PCR step.

Techniques currently used in the area of proteomics are limited to two-dimensional gel electrophoresis (Gorg *et al.* 2000) and mass spectrometry techniques using either matrix assisted laser desorption ionisation (MALDI) or electrospray ionisation (ESI) (Yates 1998; Snyder 2000; Mann *et al.* 2001). Another technique which has a high-throughput ability but is currently in its infancy is protein microarrays (Kiplinger 2001). The following paragraphs describe some of the current techniques, their limitations, and developments in this evolving field.

The most important aspect of proteomics is that it is a different paradigm from conventional reductionistic scientific investigations, which typically focus on a single gene or protein. Proteomics research asks what protein levels or activities change between two experimental conditions (e.g. diseased and normal cell protein levels). This is simply because there are estimated to be one million proteins and advances in technology allow us to look for differences using automated processes.

Two-dimensional gel electrophoresis is currently the most popular technique: it actually consists of a number of steps in which cellular proteins are first isolated from cells or tissue. This is followed by a process of enrichment of the fraction of interest using biochemical and/or chromatographic methods (e.g. organelle, affinity complex). The cellular proteins are separated on an acrylamide gel matrix along a pH gradient, allowing each protein to migrate in the gel to its isoelectric point. This initial resolution on the gel is followed by a second separation (perpendicular to the first) on the same gel, according to relative molecular mass, which results in a two-dimensional display of proteins that can be visualised and quantified crudely by protein-staining methods or radioisotope detection.

Following separation and quantification, the proteins of interest must be isolated from the gel matrix before they can be subjected to further analysis. This isolation can be accomplished using automated robotic systems to punch out 'spots' from the gel and eluting the contained protein, or using an alternative technology in which the separated proteins can be transferred via an electric current to a supporting membrane. Isolated proteins from the gel or membrane are proteolysed with trypsin to yield peptide fragments that range from 10 to 20 amino acid residues in size. The mass of the resultant peptides can be determined accurately by mass spectrometry, discussed in more detail later. A fingerprint of the peptide mass-to-charge (m/z) ratios can be characteristic of a protein, which allows its identification by comparison with calculated m/z ratios derived from each potential protein sequence in the databases being searched. This method is known as peptide mass fingerprinting. An alternative technique, known as uninterpreted MS/MS (or MS^2) matching, which involves gas-phase fragmentation of peptide ions using MS/MS, enables the conclusive identification of a specific peptide through matching the experimentally derived fragment ion masses with those calculated for all peptides of the same size in the database (Patterson 2000). The advantages of this approach are that it allows matching of peptides to small regions of a translated genomic sequence without the need to assemble full-length transcripts, and it can be used to distinguish reliably proteins that differ in mass by amounts too small to be measured by conventional MS.

Two-dimensional electrophoresis has a number of significant limitations, which include poor resolution of proteins at extremes of isoelectric points and relative molecular mass, the fact that membrane proteins tend to be under-represented, difficulty of automation and poor reproducibility of gels.

Recently, a new approach known as 'complex mixture analysis' has been introduced, which takes advantage of multidimensional chromatography and a new generation of mass spectrometers (McCormack *et al.* 1997; Patterson *et al.* 2000). In this, complex mixtures are subjected to proteolysis with trypsin (i.e. enzymatic digestion), the resultant peptides are separated via liquid chromatography, and the eluent is fed directly to a mass spectrometer. This method is designed to identify as many components as possible, and is commonly known as 'profiling' (Spahr *et al.* 2001; Washburn *et al.* 2001). A technique called isotope-coded affinity tagging (ICAT) has evolved from the above and is used to compare protein quantities in normal and diseased tissue (Gygi *et al.* 1999). These new techniques are claimed to have a number of advantages over the traditional two-dimensional gel method and seem to be gaining in popularity.

MS is the preferred detection method for peptides and proteins. This is mainly because of sensitivity, and also the advances in computer algorithms that are able to use MS data to identify the gene coding for the peptide and automate a number of complex operations without operator intervention. The two ionisation techniques preferred for peptides and proteins are MALDI or ESI. In the MALDI technique, the ionisation process results from firing a laser at the sample, which is co-crystallised with an organic matrix of low molecular weight. ESI is triggered by spraying a solution through a charged needle. The ions generated are measured in a mass analyser, of which the ion-trap and time-of-flight modes are the most commonly used. Considerable advances are likely to occur in high-throughput protein analysis and it is worth keeping an eye on the developments in this area.

Microdialysis for clinical monitoring

Microdialysis is an *in vivo* sampling technique that enables collection, separation and characterisation of biological samples and analytes. It is used extensively in drug-discovery animal experiments to measure endogenous substances (such as neurotransmitters and their metabolites), as well as exogenous therapeutic agents in various tissue systems (Ungerstedt 1991; Chaurasia 1999). In recent years, the focus of microdialysis applications has changed from animal to human clinical studies (Denoray *et al.*, 1998; Foster and Roberts 2000; Muller 2000; Verbeeck 2000; Siddique and Shuaib 2001). However, because of lack of commercially available devices the use of this technique is restricted to specialist clinical groups. This section describes the general aspects of the techniques and looks at a microdialysis devices under development for human use.

Microdialysis is an *in vivo* sampling technique based on the passive diffusion of substances across a semipermeable dialysis membrane. The sampling device is inserted into the blood vessel (or tissue of interest) and a minute stream (e.g. 2 μL/min) of sterile saline solution is passed down one channel and up through another, which causes passive diffusion of substances from the environment it is in, without unduly altering it. This enables continuous monitoring over an extended period of time without loss of fluid from the patient or animal. In the case of drug-concentration monitoring in plasma (during a clinical trial), this provides considerable advantages, as the conventional approach of withdrawing blood samples at given intervals may overlook events relating to drug concentration (Fig. 22.12). Thus, microdialysis offers considerable advantages for pharmacokinetic and pharmacodynamic studies.

Probe Scientific Ltd developed a microdialysis device designed for human use that was entered into clinical testing. It is designed to increase the safety and tolerance of the procedure over prolonged periods. Figure 22.13 shows the device and a standard blood catheter. The process involves inserting the catheter into a forearm vein, followed by insertion of the device through the lumen of the catheter and securing it using the cap that fits onto the catheter Luer-lock port. The distal portion of the device protrudes beyond the end of the catheter, thus coming into contact with the patient's blood. Essentially, the device contains a miniaturised haemodialysis cartridge that protrudes into the patient's blood vessel. A minute stream of saline solution passes through the device, which allows the diffusion of substances from the blood in the standard manner.

O'Connell *et al.* (1996) reported results for an initial prototype used to study the pharmacokinetics of levodopa therapy in the treatment of Parkinson's disease. This showed excellent tolerance of the device by the eight patients, as well as acceptable dialysate concentrations for levodopa with respects to the plasma content. Subsequent modifications have resulted in higher recoveries using this device. The microdialysate that emerges from the outlet line of the device can be assayed at-point or on-line for the rapid determination of blood chemistry. This includes most substances with low molecular weight, such as drugs and their metabolites. Also of interest is the possibility of concurrently monitoring surrogate endpoint markers of the disease process and/or indices of drug efficacy, such as electrolytes, sugars, by-products of metabolism, amino acids, vitamins, trophic factors, hormones, cardiac markers, polypeptides, and drugs and metabolites. This is currently an area of great interest both as a means to accelerate the clinical-evaluation phase of drug development and because of the obvious safety benefits to volunteers and patients taking part in these trials.

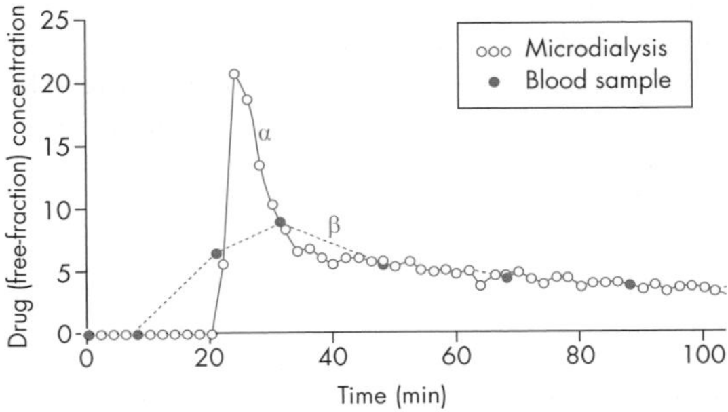

Figure 22.12 Illustration of benefits of continuous monitoring offered by microdialysis compared with conventional sampling of blood at defined intervals. (Courtesy of Probe Scientific Ltd.

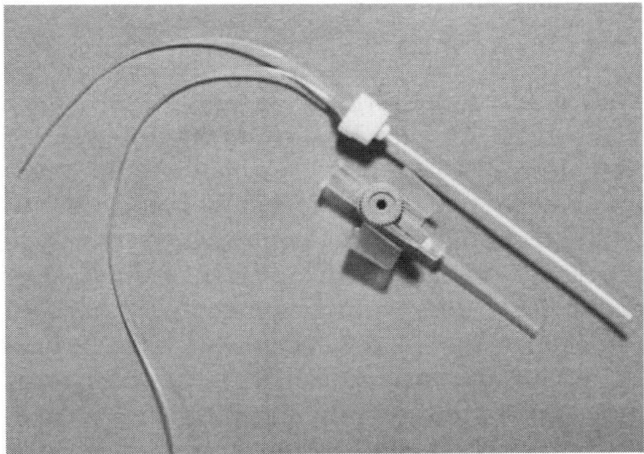

Figure 22.13 The μEye microdialysis device (above) and a standard blood catheter (below). (Courtesy of Probe Scientific Ltd.)

An additional advantage of the technique is that the membrane excludes cells and large molecules, such as large proteins (>20 kDa), which enables the direct assay onto biosensors, capillary eletrophoresis, HPLC and MS systems (with desalting if sensitivity is an issue) or the use of some of the techniques discussed in this chapter. There is considerable scope for the future in this area, as this arrangement would provide continuous and automated point-of-care blood-chemistry monitoring. Such a system would enable clinicians to make informed decisions during clinical trials or at point-of-care with monitoring systems.

Conclusion

Lord ('Solly') Zuckerman wrote in *The Sunday Times* in 1973: 'We live as we live because of the decisions, however explicit or however undefined, that were taken yesterday about which technological developments to encourage to satisfy man's enduring urge for an ever better life.' These words are included to remind the reader that the selection of a technique should be based upon which is the best technique to solve the particular problem or need. Unfortunately, in the author's experience, such decisions are more often based on which techniques we are familiar with and therefore, not surprisingly, can result in failure or the wastage of resources. It is therefore not unusual to find senior management reluctant to implement new techniques. This can lead to stagnation and loss of any competitive advantages, which results in a company or even a government-run laboratory losing business to others. It is hoped that this chapter identifies some new options available that may address the reader's needs.

Table 22.3 summarises some additional new techniques that could not be presented in detail within this chapter.

Table 22.3 New techniques in which developments have occurred and applications

Technique	Company and/or application	References
Magnetic resonance imaging (MRI)	Endoscan Ltd is developing MRI-compatible flexible endoscopes; applications include imaging of gastrointestinal mucosal disease	Furness (2001)
Atomic force microscopy	Applications include: chemical force microscopy, force mapping of biomolecules, protein–protein interaction, dimerisation, antibody–antigen interaction, bond rupture	Viani *et al.* (1999) Xia *et al.* (1996) Anczykowski *et al.* (1999) Lee *et al.* (1994) Leckband (2000)
Cell-based biosensors	Applications include use of whole cell sensors for:	Racek (1995)
	toxicity	Evans *et al.* (1998)
	environmental monitoring	Cardosi and Haggett (1997)
	in vitro and *in vivo* monitoring	
Surface-enhanced resonance Raman scattering	Applications include: DNA and SNP analysis, single molecule detection	Graham *et al.* (2000)
Single molecule spectroscopy	Applications include ability to detect and manipulate single molecules in chemical and biological analysis, e.g.	Ishijima and Yanagida (2001)
	conformational changes of proteins, DNA and RNA	Kelley *et al.* (2001)
	diffusion across lipid membranes	
	catalytic turnover rates of individual enzymes	
	live-cell imaging and individual molecules in solution or bound to surfaces	
Modulated temperature differential scanning calorimetry (DSC)	Study of solid state chemistry	Craig and Royall (1998)

References

T. J. Aitman, DNA microarrays in medical practice, *Br. Med. J.*, 2001, **323**, 611–615.

A. Albert and E. P. Serjeant, *The Determination of Ionization Constants*, 3rd edn, London, Chapman and Hall, 1984.

R. I. Allen *et al.*, Multiwavelength spectrophotometric determination of acid dissociation constants of ionizable drugs, *J. Pharm. Biomed. Anal.*, 1998, **17**, 699–712.

B. Anczykowski *et al.*, How to measure energy dissipation in dynamic mode atomic force microscopy, *Appl. Surf. Sci.*, 1999, **140**, 376–382.

M. Begg, *Drug Discov. World*, 2000, **2**, 25–30.

T. Basché; *et al.*, *Single-molecule Optical Detection, Imaging and Spectroscopy*, New York, VCH, 1997.

F. G. Bessoth *et al.*, Microstructure for efficient continuous flow mixing, *Anal. Commun.*, 1999, **36**, 213–215.

N. Bosworth and P. Towers, Scintillating proximity assay, *Nature*, 1989, **341**, 167–168.

M. Cardosi and B. G. D. Haggett, Biosensor devices, in *Sensor Systems for Environmental Monitoring*, M. Campbell (ed.), London, Blackie Academic and Professional, 1997, pp. 210–267.

C. S. Chaurasia, In vivo microdialysis sampling: theory and applications, *Biomed. Chromatogr.*, 1999, **13**, 317–332.

S. B. Cheng *et al.*, in *Micro Total Analysis Systems*, D. J. Harrison and A. Van Berg (eds), Dordrecht, Kluwer, 1998, p. 157.

N. Chiem and D. J. Harrison, Microchip-based capillary electrophoresis for immunoassays: analysis of monoclonal antibodies and theophylline, *Anal. Chem.*, 1997, **69**, 373–378.

Chipping Forecast, The Chipping forecast, *Nat. Genet.*, 1999, **21** (Suppl. 1), 1–60.

D. Q. M. Craig and P. G. Royall, The use of modulated temperature DSC for the study of pharmaceutical systems: potential uses and limitations, *Pharm. Res.*, 1998, **15**, 1152–1153.

L. Denoray *et al.*, Assessment of pharmacodynamic and pharmacokinetic characteristics of drugs using microdialysis sampling and capillary elecrophoresis, *Electrophoresis*, 1998, **19**, 2841–2847.

D. C. Duffy *et al.*, Rapid prototyping of microfluidics systems in poly(dimethylsiloxane), *Anal. Chem.*, 1998, **70**, 4974–4984.

M. R. Evans *et al.*, Biosensors for the measurement of toxicity of wastewaters to activated sludge, *Pesticide Sci.*, 1998, **54**, 447–452.

D. Figeys *et al.*, An integrated microfluidics–tandem mass spectrometry system for automated protein analysis, *Anal. Chem.*, 1998, **70**, 3728–3734.

K. A. Foster and M. S. Roberts, Experimental methods for studying drug uptake in the head and brain, *Curr. Drug Metab.*, 2000, **1**, 333–356.

Y. Fujita *et al.*, *Bunseki Kagaku*, 1993, **42**, T1–T5.

J. Furness, *Med. Device Technol.*, 2001, Sept, 20.

D. Graham *et al.*, Detection and identification of labeled DNA by surface enhanced resonance Raman scattering, *Biopolymers (Biospectrosc.)*, 2000, **57**, 85–91.

A. Gorg *et al.*, The current state of two-dimensional electrophoresis with immobilized pH gradients, *Electrophoresis*, 2000, **21**, 1037–1053.

S. P. Gygi *et al.*, Quantitative analysis of complex protein mixtures using isotope-coded affinity tags, *Nat. Biotechnol.*, 1999, **17**, 994–999.

M. Hadley *et al.*, Multiwavelength spectrophotometric determination of acid dissociation constants, Part IV. Water insoluble pyridine derivatives, *Talanta*, 1999, **49**, 539–546.

I. Hemmila, *Applications of Fluorescence in Immunoassays*, New York, Wiley-Interscience, 1990.

I. Hemmila I. and S. Webb, Time-resolved fluorometry: an overview of the labels and core technologies for drug screening applications, *Drug Discov. Today*, 1997, **2**, 373–381.

B. A. Hendriksen *et al.*, A new multiwavelength spectroscopic method for the determination of the molar absorption coefficients of ionisable drugs, *Spectrosc. Lett.*, 2001, **35**, 9–19.

D. Hill, *Drug Discov. Dev.*, 1998, **1**, 92–129.

International Human Genome Sequencing Consortium, Initial sequencing and analysis of the human genome, *Nature*, 2001, **409**, 860–921.

A. Ishijima and T. Yanagida, Single molecule nanobioscience, *Trends Biochem. Sci.*, 2001, **26**, 438–444.

Y. M. Issa and S. A. Amin, Spectrophotometric microdetermination of sulfamethoxiazole and trimethoprim using Alizarin and Quinalizarin, *Anal. Lett.*, 1994, **27**, 1147–1158.

S. D. Kahn, *Drug Discov. World*, 2000, **2**, 49–54.

A. M. Kelley *et al.*, Chemical physics. Single-molecule spectroscopy comes of age, *Science*, 2001, **292**, 1671–1672.

J. P. Kiplinger, Protein arrays: new technologies for the proteomics era, *Drug Discov. World*, 2001, **2**, 40–46.

M. U. Kopp *et al.*, in *Micro Total Analysis Systems*, D. J. Harrison and A. Van Berg (eds), Dordrecht, Kluwer, 1998a, p. 7.

M. U. Kopp *et al.*, Chemical amplification: continuous-flow PCR on a chip, *Science*, 1998b, **280**, 1046.

L. B. Koutny *et al.*, Microchip electrophoretic immunoassay for serum cortisol, *Anal Chem.*, 1996, **68**, 18–22.

B. Ladd, Intuitive data analysis: the next generation, *Modern Drug Discov.*, 2000, **Jan./Feb.**, 46–54.

J. Lazarou *et al.*, Incidence of adverse drug reactions in hospitalized patients: a meta-analysis of prospective studies, *J. Am. Med. Assoc.*, 1998, **279**, 1200–1205.

D. Leckband, Measuring the forces that control protein interactions, *Annu. Rev. Biophys. Biomol. Struct.*, 2000, **29**, 1–26.

G.U. Lee *et al.*, Direct measurement of the forces between complementary strands of DNA, *Science*, 1994, **266**, 771–773.

J. Li *et al.*, Integration of microfabricated devices to capillary electrophoresis–electrospray mass spectrometry using a low dead volume connection: application to rapid analyses of proteolytic digests, *Anal. Chem.*, 1999, **71**, 3036–3045.

D. J. Lockhart and E. A. Winzeler, Genomics, gene expression and DNA arrays, *Nature*, 2000, **405**, 827–836.

M. Mann *et al.*, Analysis of proteins and proteomes by mass spectrometry, *Annu. Rev. Biochem.*, 2001, **70**, 437–473.

A. Manz and G. H. W. Sanders, Chip based microsystems for genomic and proteomic analysis, *Trends Anal. Chem.*, 2000, **19**, 364–378.

A. Manz *et al.*, Micromachining of monocrystalline silicon and glass for chemical analysis systems – a look into next century's technology or just a fashionable craze? *Trends Anal. Chem.*, 1991, **10**, 144–149.

L. Martynova *et al.*, Fabrication of plastic microfluid channels by imprinting methods, *Anal. Chem.*, 1997, **69**, 4783–4789.

R. Mathies *et al.*, in *Micro Total Analysis Systems*, D. J. Harrison and A. Van Berg (eds), Dordrecht, Kluwer, 1998, p. 1.

A. L. McCormack *et al.*, Direct analysis and identification of proteins in mixtures by LC/MS/MS and databases searching at the low-femtomole level, *Anal. Chem.*, 1997, **69**, 767–776.

R. C. Mitchell *et al.*, Multiwavelength-spectrophotometric determination of acid dissociation constants: Part III. Resolution of multi-protic ionization systems, *J. Pharm. Biomed. Anal.*, 1999, **20**, 289–295.

M. Muller, Microdialysis in clinical drug delivery studies, *Adv. Drug Deliv. Rev.*, 2000, **45**, 255–269.

M. T. O'Connell *et al.*, Clinical drug monitoring by microdialysis: application to levodopa therapy in Parkinson's disease, *Br. J. Clin. Pharmacol.*, 1996, **42**, 765–769.

K. Oldenburg, *J. Biomol. Screen.*, 1998, **3**, 55–62.

S. D. Patterson, Proteomics: the industrialization of protein chemistry, *Curr Opin. Biotechnol.*, 2000, **11**, 413–418.

S. D. Patterson *et al.*, Mass spectrometric identification of proteins released from mitrochrondria undergoing permeability transition, *Cell Death Diff.*, 2000, **7**, 137–144.

T. Peakman and S. Arlington, *Drug Discov. World*, 2000, **2**, 35–40.

K. Powell, *Drug Discov. World*, 2000, **1**, 25–30.

J. Racek, *Cell-based Biosensors*, Lancaster, Technomic, 1995.

P. Ram, *Drug Discov. Today*, 1999, **4**, 401–410.

H. D. Revanasiddappa *et al.*, Spectrophotometric method for the determination of ritodrine hydrochloride and amoxicillin, *Anal. Sci.*, 1999, **15**, 661–664.

M. Schena, *Microarray Biochip Technology*, Westborough, Eaton, 2000.

K. M. Schullek, A high-density screening format for encoded combinatorial libraries: assay miniaturization and its applications to enzymatic reactions, *Anal. Biochem.*, 1998, **146**, 20–29.

M. M. Shi, Enabling large-scale pharmacogenetic studies by high-throughput mutation detection and genotyping technologies, *Clin. Chem.*, 2001, **47**, 167–172.

M. M. Siddique and A. Shuaib, *Methods*, 2001, **223**, 83–94.

A. P. Snyder, *Interpreting Protein Mass Spectra: A Comprehensive Resource*, Oxford, Oxford University Press, 2000.

C. S. Spahr *et al.*, Automated LC–LC–MS–MS platform using binary ion-exchange and gradient reversed-phase chromatography for improved proteomic analyses, *J. Chromatogr. B*, 2001, **752**, 281–291.

K. Y. Tam and K. Takacs-Novak, Multiwavelength spectrophotometric determination of acid dissociation constants: Part II. First derivative vs target factor analysis, *Pharm. Res.*, 1999, **16**, 374–381.

U. Ungerstedt, Microdialysis – principles and applications for studies in animal and man, *J. Int. Med.*, 1991, **230**, 365–373.

M. B. Viani *et al.*, Small cantilevers for force spectroscopy of single molecules, *J. Appl. Phys.*, 1999, **86**, 2258–2262.

R. K. Verbeeck, Blood microdialysis in pharmacokinetics and drug metabolism studies, *Adv. Drug Deliv. Rev.*, 2000, **45**, 217–228.

F. Von Heeren *et al.*, *Anal. Chem.*, 1996, **68**, 2044.

M. P. Washburn *et al.*, Large-scale analysis of the yeast proteome by multidimensional protein identification technology, *Nat. Biotechnol.*, 2001, **19**, 242–247.

T. Wells and G. Feger, *Drug Discov. World*, 2000, **2**, 16–21.

Y. N. Xia *et al.*, Pattern transfer: self-assembled monolayers as ultrathin resists, *Microelectron. Eng.*, 1996, **32**, 255.

J. C. Venter *et al.*, The sequence of the human genome, *Science*, 2001, **291**, 1304–1351.

N. Xu *et al.*, A microfabricated dialysis device for sample cleanup in electrospray ionization mass spectrometry, *Anal. Chem.*, 1998, **70**, 3553–3556.

Q. Xue *et al.*, Multichannel microchip electrospray mass spectrometry, *Anal. Chem.*, 1997, **69**, 426–430.

J. R. Yates, Mass spectrometry and the age of the proteome, *J. Mass Spectrom.*, 1998, **33**, 1–19.

Useful websites

Government and regulatory affairs

Europe

EMEA: www.emea.eu.int/

Eudralex – Rules Governing Medicinal Products: www.emea.eu.int/index/indexh1.htm

European National Agencies – Index: www.heads.medagencies.org

International

ICH Homepage: www.ich.org

OECD EHS homepage: www.oecd.org/ehs/

OECD Good Laboratory Practice: www.oecd.org/ehs/glp.htm

World Health Organization: www.who.org/

USA

Electronic Orange Book – Approved Drug Products: www.fda.gov/cder/ob/

US Environmental Protection Agency: www.epa.gov/epahome/index.html

US Food and Drug Administration: www.fda.gov/

US GPO Official Documents: www.access.gpo.gov/so_docs/

United States cGMP: www.fda.gov/cder/dmpg/index.htm

UK

DoH Guidance for Business: www.open.gov.uk/doh/busguide.htm#lab_prac

Houses of Parliament Home Page: www.parliament.uk/

UK Government Information Service – Index: www.open.gov.uk/

UK Official Documents home page: www.official-documents.co.uk

UK Medicines and Healthcare Products Agency: www.mca.gov.uk

United Kingdom GLP Monitoring Authority: www.open.gov.uk/doh/busguide/goodlab/glpbioh.htm

Others sites and addresses

Centre for Process Analytics and Control Technology: www.ncl.ac.uk/cpact/

Pharmaceutical Analytical Sciences Group (PASG): www.pasg.org.uk

Specialised Organic Chemical Sector Association, Kings Buildings, Smith, Square, London, SW1P 3JJ, UK.

The New Technology Forum: www.rpsgb.org.uk/science/

United Kingdom Accreditation Service (UKAS): www.ukas.com

UK Analytical Partnership (UKAP): www.chemsoc.org.uk/networks/ukap

Web sites of companies referred to in the chapter

Aurora Biosciences corporation: www.aurorabio.com

Biotrove Inc: www.biotrove.com

Diversa Corp: www.diversa.com

Hamilton GB Ltd: www.hamiltongb.co.uk

Malvern Instruments Ltd: www.malvern.co.uk

Nanogen Inc: www.nanogen.com

Probe Scientific Ltd: www.probe-sci.co.uk

Process Analytical & Automation: www.paa.co.uk

Sirius Analytical Instruments Ltd: www.Sirius-Analytical.com

Ultrasonic Sciences Ltd: www.ultrasonic-sciences.co.uk

23

Quality control and assessment

R K Bramley, D G Bullock and J R Garcia

Introduction 607
Quality assurance terminology 608
Quality systems 609
Customer requirement and/or specification 609
Procedures for sample selection, collection, preservation, packaging, identification, storage and transport 610
Validation of new methods 612
Measurement uncertainty 614
Equipment maintenance and calibration . . 615
Evaluation of materials and reagents . . . 615
Sample and data handling in the laboratory 616
Sample disposal 616
Protocols for sample preparation, analyte recovery and analysis. 616
In-process performance monitoring 616
Assessment, interpretation and reporting of results 618
External quality assessment arrangements 618
Corrective actions for noncompliance . . . 619
Management of laboratory facilities. . . . 620
Avoidance of contamination 620
Competence standards, training programme and monitoring arrangements for the analyst. 620
Assessment and accreditation 620
References 622
Further reading 622

Introduction

It is important in many applications to have reliable, interchangeable data on the recovery, identification and quantification of drugs. The most critical fields include forensic toxicology, drugs of abuse, workplace drug testing, drug abuse in sport, clinical toxicology, therapeutic drug monitoring, and drugs in research and development.

In the pharmaceutical industry, quality control and assessment (QC&A) is required to monitor production and assess the quality, safety and efficacy of its products. In clinical analysis, QC&A is vital to the quality and safety of patient care, to diagnosis, management and control of therapy for the individual patient, and for research and public health purposes. For toxicologists and pathologists, QC&A helps to distinguish between therapeutic and overdose levels and to determine the cause of death. In law enforcement, it is used to provide information to link drugs offences, to identify drug distribution networks and to provide evidence of possession or misuse for the courts. It plays a major role in analyses for drink- and drug-driving offences. It is also essential for monitoring individuals on drug rehabilitation programmes, for workplace testing of employees in certain occupations and for determining whether drug abuse in sports is taking place.

To produce reliable and interchangeable data, analytical laboratories have to employ competent analysts and use validated methods. These analysts need appropriate accommodation and environmental conditions in which to work and access to all the equipment and other materials required to carry out their analyses safely and to an acceptable standard. They must also have systems that monitor and maintain the quality of their results and establish the accuracy and associated uncertainty of their measurements, and they should participate in relevant external quality assessment (EQA; interlaboratory proficiency testing) exercises (ISO/IEC 1997).

These requirements all fall within the ambit of the quality-assurance programme to which laboratories must work if they seek accreditation to national or international quality standards or to protocols relevant to the field of drugs testing. Various national and international bodies have been set up to deal with quality-assurance issues. These include the International Organization for Standardization (ISO) and the International Electrotechnical Commission (IEC). These organisations publish standards which are updated regularly. The Organisation for Economic Co-operation and Development (OECD) has working groups and publishes guides on good laboratory practice (GLP) (OECD 1992). The US Department of Health and Human Services has published *Mandatory Health and Human Services Guidelines for Federal Workplace Drug Testing Programs* (DHHS 1994)

Quality assurance terminology

Quality is the totality of features and characteristics of a product or service that bear on its ability to satisfy stated or implied needs. It is its fitness for the purpose or use specified by the customer. It is determined by the competence of the people who produce the product or provide the service, the facilities available to them and the processes and procedures they employ.

Quality assurance (QA) is a global term to describe those means of ensuring that the results and interpretations issued by a laboratory are dependable and sufficiently unbiased and precise to allow decisions to be taken with confidence. It is a management tool concerned with the prevention of quality problems through planned and systematic activities. These include the establishment of a documented *quality system* that sets out the organisational structure, responsibilities, procedures, processes and resources to implement quality management; assessment of the adequacy of this quality system, audit of its operation and review of the system itself.

Quality control (QC) is that aspect of QA concerned with the practical activities and techniques employed to achieve and maintain the product or service quality. It thus also involves monitoring the processes and procedures used and the identification and elimination of causes of quality problems so that the requirements of the customer are met continually. The aim of QC is to ensure compliance with the quality specification and to provide economic effectiveness by eliminating causes of unsatisfactory performance at the relevant stages of the operation.

Internal audit is a process of critical review of the laboratory's processes. It is conducted by quality managers and experienced laboratory staff. Audits usually aim to monitor the accuracy, timeliness and cost of work and compliance with the quality management system, and to identify for action areas where errors can occur.

External audit involves customers or other stakeholders in the evaluation of the quality and usefulness of the laboratory's services. It facilitates comparison of methods, working practices, costs and workload between laboratories (testing sites), and forms part of the cyclic process of setting standards, examining compliance and re-examining the standards.

External quality assessment (EQA) is a way to benchmark the performance of one laboratory against that of other testing sites by comparing the results of their analyses of an identical specimen with each other's results and with the 'correct' answer. It allows laboratories to identify areas for improvement and best practice.

Assessment is the process by which an independent accrediting body inspects and evaluates the operation of an organisation that produces the product or provides the service against a relevant national or international quality standard. The factors considered vary from one standard to another, but may include the management structure, the numbers, qualifications and training of staff, the facilities available, the methods and processes adopted, the QA and QC arrangements, documentation, reporting procedures, communications within the laboratory and with users, safety and participation in EQA schemes (EQASs). In essence, the accrediting body has to ensure that the organisation's quality system is sufficiently comprehensive for the operation being assessed and that the organisation consistently does what the quality system says it should. If the assessment is satisfactory the organisation may be *accredited* for the particular operation.

Accreditation is thus one way to demonstrate the quality of an organisation's products or services to its customers. Accreditation may be voluntary or may be linked to a formal system of licensing, whereby only accredited laboratories are legally entitled to practise (or to receive payment for their services).

Quality systems

The quality system should address all stages of an operation that could affect the reliability of the end result and the monitoring of performance, so that timely corrective action can be taken where necessary. It requires specification, determination and documentation of the following:

- customer requirement/specification
- procedures for sample selection, collection, preservation, packaging, identification, storage and transport
- protocol for the validation of new methods
- measurement uncertainty
- equipment maintenance and calibration routines
- evaluation of materials and reagents
- sample and data handling in the laboratory
- sample disposal
- protocols for sample preparation, analyte recovery and analysis
- requirements for in-process performance monitoring
- assessment, interpretation and reporting of results
- EQA arrangements
- corrective actions to be taken for noncompliance
- management of laboratory facilities
- avoidance of contamination
- competence standards, training programme and monitoring arrangements for the analyst.

Customer requirement and/or specification

Analysts can be most effective if they are consulted about the nature of the problem that the customer (and end user of the data, if different) seeks to address rather than simply being asked to carry out specific analyses, as this allows them to agree the approach that is fit for purpose in the particular circumstances. This includes consideration of the order in which analyses and other examinations should be carried out and requirements for such parameters as the specificity, accuracy and precision of the analysis. The degree of consultation will depend on the knowledge and experience of the analyst, with more experienced staff taking a greater role in this aspect. If interpretation and assessment of the results are part of the service provided, the customer needs to provide sufficient information to facilitate this. Analysts also need to be informed of any constraints on the fee the customer is prepared to pay for the analysis and when the results are needed.

Where analyses are of a routine nature, the customer requirement and specifications are best included in a contract between the customer and analyst. In less routine circumstances, these need to be established for each request. The use of standard submission forms helps ensure that all the necessary information is provided.

An increasing number of investigations using 'desktop' analysers or single-use devices (e.g. to detect drugs of abuse in individuals in treatment centres, in the workplace or at the roadside) are now being considered for use at peripheral sites. Such field-testing (point-of-care testing) technology is apparently simple to use, but it has to be used correctly and must be capable of producing results of the right quality. It is thus essential to examine critically the circumstances in which it is planned to be used and to agree with the customer whether it is an appropriate approach: laboratory professionals must be involved in such decisions.

Procedures for sample selection, collection, preservation, packaging, identification, storage and transport

Selection

Ideally, the entire item of interest is made available for examination. In most circumstances, however, this is not possible and only a portion of the item can be provided, so it is important to ensure that the correct sample is obtained in the right way by competent personnel.

A variety of sampling protocols from which meaningful statistical inferences can be drawn are available: which is used depends on the size of the whole material involved, its characteristics, access and location, and the sampling objective. These protocols include random sampling, systematic sampling, stratified sampling and sequential sampling.

The objective is that the results for the analytical sample can be considered as representative of the entire population or subject from which the sample originated. This primarily involves consideration of any inhomogeneity in the material being sampled. For illicit drugs seizures and biological specimens, inhomogeneity can result from segregation or separation of the sample matrix, and from variable analyte content and distribution in the population. In drugs manufacture it can arise from periodicity in continuous processes. It can be reduced by good mixing, small particle size and taking large samples, or by repeated sampling in small increments in continuous processes.

Where drugs are encountered as discrete packages, tablets or capsules, large numbers may be available, so it would be impracticable to consider analysing them all. The issue is then to select a meaningful composite sample to obtain a result representative of the whole, to estimate either the proportion that contains drugs or the quantity of drug present. The customer or the analyst can carry out this selection, but it should only be undertaken by agreement between the two. A common approach is to select not fewer than 10 samples to form the composite if the number of packages, tablets or capsules is less than 100, and to take a number of samples equal to the square root of the total if there are more than 100. In postmortem toxicology, drugs may be distributed unevenly between tissues, or even within one particular tissue, and may also undergo redistribution after death. Careful consideration with respect to sampling and subsequent interpretation of results is therefore required (see Chapter 7 for more in-depth discussion).

Collection

Samples should be collected in such a way as to avoid both loss of analyte and the introduction of contaminating substances that could interfere with the analysis and interpretation of the analytical results. The provision and use of quality-assured sampling kits, sampling materials and collection protocols is helpful in this respect, as is a comprehensive standard operating procedures (SOPs) policy.

For forensic purposes, it is often a requirement not only to identify what is present in a sample but also to compare this with the results from another sample, to establish that they came from the same source. It is thus vital that such samples should not come into direct contact with one another and that steps are taken to ensure no secondary transfer of material occurs, for example via the person taking the samples or the sampling equipment.

It may be necessary in some circumstances (e.g. obtaining samples of urine for workplace drugs testing or from patients in addiction clinics) for the collection process to be supervised, to remove the risk of substitution or adulteration and thus false negative or false positive results (see Chapter 5).

Preservation

Analytes and the sample matrix itself can, in some circumstances, deteriorate prior to analysis and subsequently interfere with analysis and the interpretation of the results, unless precautions are taken to avoid this. It is important that the analyst is made aware if any preservative has been added so that the level present, and thus its effectiveness, can be determined, if necessary, and an appropriate analytical protocol can be used in which the preservative does not interfere. In some areas, such as analysis for ethanol, different preservative concentrations may be needed for clinical and for forensic applications.

Packaging

The choice of sample container depends on its intended purpose and should be prescribed by the analyst. Special considerations are required to avoid loss of analyte or leakage of sample where volatile and liquid materials are involved. Additional packaging requirements may also need to be specified to protect sample containers against damage during transport to the laboratory for examination or to comply with regulations that apply when body fluids are involved. It is also important that packaging is selected that does not give rise to transfer of substances that might cause problems in the analysis. For forensic purposes, samples must also be sealed in such a way that any evidence of tampering would be evident.

Identification

It is essential that sample containers and any intermediate containers used to carry the sample be labelled in sufficient detail to remove any doubt about the sample origin. It is necessary to have documentation as to who took the sample, where it came from and when and how it was obtained. A unique identification number that accompanies the sample at all stages is a valuable safeguard. Transposition errors in clinical analysis can prove harmful or even fatal to the patient. In cases of drug abuse in sports, workplace drug testing and drink- and drug-driving cases, any mix up in samples could have serious consequences for a person's employment. In the legal context, it must also be possible to demonstrate the chain of evidence through a record of who had possession of the sample, what they did with it and when.

Storage

If the sample cannot be analysed immediately, it must be stored at an appropriate temperature in a safe and suitable environment, accessible only to authorised staff, so as to ensure its security and integrity. In some circumstances, these considerations may also have to be applied to the transport and continued storage of samples after analysis.

Transport

Transport is normally the responsibility of the customer, but there will be constraints on what can be transported or posted legally. Where drugs are involved, even in the smallest quantities, transportation across national frontiers is a criminal offence without appropriate import/export licences. Temperature and other environmental factors may also need to be controlled.

The chain of custody of samples should be maintained throughout transport. This is particularly important in cases where the outcome of testing may be disputed in court. Any weak link in the chain of custody may result in the test result being rejected.

Validation of new methods

Analytical method development can vary between laboratories but it typically includes the following steps:

- Ensure that the compound can be detected by the chosen instrumentation in a suitable solvent and appropriate analytical conditions (UV wavelength, selected ions in MS, etc.).
- Adjust chromatographic conditions for optimal peak shape, run time, separation between compounds and/or metabolites and a chosen internal standard.
- Determine the limit of detection (LOD) and limit of quantitation (LOQ) of the analytical procedure.
- Ensure that any endogenous compounds or contaminants do not interfere with the assay.
- Determine the recovery of the test compound by extraction of appropriate spiked biological samples. The type of extraction will be determined by the chemical properties of the candidate compound.
- Determine the stability of the compound in a given biological sample by spiking naive (analyte-free) specimens and analysing them over time. Stability of the extracts is determined by storing them under specified conditions and analysing them over a certain period of time.
- Prepare standard stock solution which will be used to prepare a standard curve, and control stock solution for preparation of control working solutions.
- Prepare calibration curves and appropriate control solutions for compounds under investigation and for each specimen/matrix type, determine range and linearity of standard curve.
- Determine method validation parameters.
- Establish the accuracy and precision of the method.
- Assess the ruggedness (robustness) of the method.
- Prepare a standard operating procedure (SOP).

Analytical methods should be characterised and documented fully, and their reliability in the specified area of application demonstrated before they are brought into use. Such method-validation ensures that methods are under statistical control and are fit for their intended purpose. Validation should cover all stages through sample selection and preparation, analyte recovery, calibration of equipment, the analysis protocol and the assessment, interpretation and reporting of results.

Validation of methods for the quantitative analysis of drugs involves determining, as a minimum, their selectivity, limit of detection, limit of quantification, linearity, working range, accuracy, precision and ruggedness under the conditions and with the typical sample matrices that will be met in practice. For qualitative analysis, usually only the selectivity, limit of detection and robustness (ruggedness) are important. Where there is a predefined threshold concentration for reported results, the accuracy and precision should be determined at the threshold level. For methods that are to be used by more than one laboratory, each laboratory should verify the method, and the interlaboratory variation should be determined. These data should be used to define how the performance of the method is to be monitored through QC and to specify what performance is fit for purpose. If it is necessary to compare the results with those from other methods, the compatibility of data from the different methods should also form part of the validation.

Any subsequent change at any stage of the method, or in the sample matrix or concentration range, will require re-validation of the method. The extent and requirements of re-validation will depend on what changes have been made.

When a laboratory adopts an already validated method, it should demonstrate that the performance characteristics it can achieve are fit for the intended purpose of the method. Particularly important in this respect are selectivity (if the sample matrix is different), limit of detection, accuracy and precision.

In addition to analytical validation, it may also be necessary to carry out clinical validation. This requires:

- determination of expected concentrations
- differences associated with age, sex or other factors
- cut-off values to classify results as 'normal' or 'abnormal', or as decision points in screening
- clinical sensitivity ('positivity in users')
- clinical specificity ('negativity in non-users').

Selectivity

Selectivity is the extent to which the method can determine particular analytes in a complex mixture without interference from the other components of the mixture. A method that is perfectly selective for a particular analyte or group of analytes is said to be specific. Selectivity is usually concentration dependent and is determined by adding materials that might be encountered in test samples to the analyte of interest and studying their impact (e.g. cross-reactivity in immunological methods; overlapping chromatography peaks; masking of colour reactions), both individually and in the presence of other potentially interfering substances ('influence quantities').

Limit of detection

The limit of detection is the lowest content of analyte that can be distinguished from background noise and measured with reasonable statistical certainty. It is estimated from the analysis of blank specimens and a study of the signal-to-noise (S/N) ratio, with a minimum ratio of 3:1 being widely accepted. In some areas of testing a S/N ratio of 5:1 is specified for LOD.

Limit of quantification

The lower limit of quantification is the amount equal to or greater than the lowest concentration point on the calibration curve that can be measured with an acceptable level of accuracy and precision. A S/N ratio of 5:1 is widely accepted for the LOQ but in some areas a value of 10:1 is specified.

Linearity

Linearity is a measure of the ability of the method to elicit test results that are directly, or by means of well-defined mathematical transformations, proportional to the concentration of analytes within samples within a given range. Normally, a linear relationship is anticipated for chromatographic analyses. Sometimes the relationship is not linear but follows, for example, a quadratic or other defined mathematical relationship. Ideally, the reason for nonlinearity should be identified and corrected such that a linear relationship is established. This is not always possible and, provided the relationship follows a well-defined mathematical transformation, is reproducible and gives acceptable accuracy and precision, this may be acceptable for QA purposes.

Working range

The working range is the concentration interval within which acceptable accuracy and precision can be achieved.

Accuracy (lack of bias)

Accuracy (also referred to as trueness) is a measure of the ability of the method to provide the true result. For quantitative tests, it is the closeness of agreement between the true value and the value obtained by applying the test procedure a number of times. It is affected by systematic and random errors (see above) and is usually expressed as a percentage. An acceptable variation of ±20% at the lowest calibration point and ±15 % for higher concentrations is often acceptable for biological specimens. Ideally, bias is assessed using samples spiked at three different concentration levels at least (low, medium and high) with certified reference materials (CRMs) or reference standards from an authoritative organisation or reputable commercial supplier.

Accuracy can be easily calculated using the expression:

$$\frac{\text{Mean measured concentration} - \text{Theoretical concentration}}{\text{Theoretical concentration}} \times 100\% \quad (23.1)$$

Precision

Precision is the closeness of agreement (degree of scatter) between independent test results obtained under prescribed conditions. It depends on analyte concentration and the distribution of random errors, and is often measured under repeatable (same analyst, same day, same instrument, same materials) and reproducible (any variation from these) conditions. Normally, it is expressed in terms of the coefficient of variation (CV), or relative standard deviation (RSD), of the test results. An acceptable CV of 20% at the lowest calibration point and 15% for higher concentrations is usually acceptable. The acceptance criteria may be widened in circumstances in which matrix effects may be significant (e.g. analysis of autopsy samples), or tightened where better reliability is required.

Robustness

A method is robust, or rugged, if it can withstand small uncontrolled or unintentional changes in the operating conditions or environment, such as those likely to arise in different laboratories or over time. Robustness/Ruggedness is best determined by systematically varying the most important experimental parameters within set limits of tolerance and studying the effects on the results. With efficient experimental planning, this requires approximately the same number of experiments as the number of factors to be varied.

Analyte recovery

Analyte recovery is measured from the detector response obtained from a known amount of analyte added to the matrix prior to extraction compared with the detector response for the same quantity of pure standard. It is calculated correctly as (final − initial)/added, expressed as a percentage, and should be determined at low, medium and high concentrations. Recovery can also be influenced by interfering substances ('influence quantities').

Method comparison

In analytical chemistry, instances arise when a laboratory may wish to compare the results of two different methods. For example, if a laboratory has previously used a GC-MS method for a particular analysis but then develops an LC-MS method as a replacement, the laboratory will want to confirm that the LC-MS method produces the same result before adopting it for testing purposes. The comparison of two methods should be carried out using a suitable statistical procedure to test whether there are significant differences between them. The t-test provides a simple check on accuracy and the F-test on precision. The data sets should also be compared by orthogonal or robust (e.g. Deming) regression analysis for proportional and constant deviations. A minimum of 20 data points is recommended for these purposes.

Measurement uncertainty

It is rare, if not impossible, to develop an analytical method which would give the same, true result on repeated analysis of a sample. There is always some variability associated with the result. This is known as measurement uncertainty and it is made up of contributions from sample selection, sample preservation/transport, sample preparation, sample analysis and data evaluation. Those from sample selection have been discussed above. During sample preparation, the uncertainty may arise from preferential selection, because of the different hardness of particles when crushing the sample, for example, or through incomplete dissolution or through density separation during the attempted homogenisation of liquids. It may also result from the loss of sample material or analyte by adsorption or degradation, interference or contamination, or chemical changes in the material composition through oxidation or various other factors. Analytical measurement errors can be caused, for example, by breakdown of the analyte in the process, incomplete reaction processes, instrumental errors or maladjustments, poor calibration or matrix effects. Data evaluation errors can result from the use of incorrect or incomplete algorithms and the response can be additive, multiplicative or nonlinear.

The errors that affect analytical measurements are of four types:

- random errors, which are manifested as a spread of results of repeat determinations to higher and lower values around a mean for the sample and determine the reproducibility or precision of the measurements
- systematic errors, which displace the results of measurement to higher or lower values and whose existence and magnitude characterise the trueness of the measurement
- outliers, which are random errors of such large deviation that they would distort the mean if they were not eliminated
- gross errors, which are caused by human mistakes, or instrumental or mathematical problems, and may have either a random or systematic character.

A comprehensive guide to analytical uncertainty is available via EURACHEM/CITAC (see EURACHEM/CITAC 1998, 2000, 2001).

Random errors are a fundamental characteristic of the design of the processes and analytical method chosen. They can be minimised, but not eliminated, and are usually characterised in terms of a confidence interval in an assumed normal distribution of results about the mean value. If this is determined simply by repeat measurement in the analytical method, the confidence interval represents only the error of the result caused by measurement. If the total error of the procedure is to be reflected in the confidence interval, parallel samples have to be selected and taken through the whole process.

Systematic errors can only be recognised if results fall outside the random error confidence interval on one side of the mean, but they can be eliminated once their cause is known. They are best identified by analysis of certified reference materials (where these are available), by comparison with results from independent validated methods or by EQA. The observed mean result is said to be correct if its confidence interval includes the true value.

Gross errors and outliers are usually, but not always, easy to identify and correct if other aspects of QC are working effectively.

Equipment maintenance and calibration

All equipment should be maintained and calibrated according to the manufacturer's recommendations and laboratory requirements. This may include ensuring traceability to calibration reference materials (e.g. for mass and volume measurements).

Evaluation of materials and reagents

The choice of reagents requires considerable thought and coordination, and may be cost-effective in that it reduces duplication of effort and prevents repetition of expensive mistakes. Reagents should be selected according to rational criteria, which might include cost of purchase and revenue consequences. Unfortunately, the initial evaluation cannot guarantee the continuing quality of subsequent batches of materials and reagents, and some system of continual monitoring (e.g. batch-acceptance testing) may be needed. Ongoing evaluation is particularly important for 'kit' methods and for point-of-care testing systems.

Sample and data handling in the laboratory

The principles outlined in the section on Procedures above must also be applied in the laboratory to ensure the identity, integrity and security of material submitted for examination and analysis and, where appropriate, the maintenance of records for chain-of-evidence purposes. Care must also be exercised when critical observations are made, calculations are performed and data are transcribed, to ensure that the results are recorded correctly and attributed to the right sample. It is best practice to use standard forms to facilitate these processes, and to demonstrate that these records have been checked independently (e.g. by double-entry systems), where appropriate. The use of automated processes under the control of laboratory information management systems (LIMS) reduces the risks significantly.

Sample disposal

There must be a clear policy in place for the disposal of materials on completion of examination and analysis. In some instances, this involves returning what remains of the samples to the customer, subject or legal custodian. In other cases, the samples need to be destroyed safely, immediately or after a specified time period, and statutory requirements may have to be observed in doing this. However, in no circumstances should anything be disposed of without the consent of the customer or other relevant authority, and records should be maintained of what has been disposed of and what has been retained.

Protocols for sample preparation, analyte recovery and analysis

All procedures must be documented appropriately, and the use of written standard operating procedures (SOPs) is both highly recommended and normally essential to satisfy accreditation requirements. Once a method is accepted as validated, the SOP should be available for the analysts to use. Adherence to SOPs helps avoid unintended 'drift' in the procedures used and thus continued relevance of the method-validation data. Internal audit is needed to monitor adherence. The cover page of a SOP document should include the following elements: a title and indication of the SOP's position in the entire Quality Manual, the purpose of the SOP, the effective date of an SOP, the edition number, and a statement that this edition replaces an earlier SOP, distribution of the SOP, the signature of the author of the SOP, and the signature of the person(s) authorising the SOP.

In-process performance monitoring

Internal quality control (IQC) assesses, in real time, whether performance is sufficiently similar to the individual laboratory's own previous performance for the results to be reported. It helps control reproducibility (precision) and facilitates continuity of service over time. Most IQC procedures employ analysis of a control material and comparison of the results obtained on this with preset limits of acceptability, which thus allows unsatisfactory sets of results to be identified and corrected before release to the customer.

For qualitative testing, it is important to include characterised positive and negative control materials with each batch of analyses. In both qualitative and quantitative analysis, it is essential that these control samples be taken through as much of the process as is possible, otherwise errors may go undetected. Sample collection may represent a major source of variation which it is not possible to control using IQC measures and so must be minimised through careful training and supervision procedures.

Some IQC procedures can be simple and inexpensive to implement, and include:

- recording lot numbers of all reagents, calibrants and controls used, with particular attention when reagent and/or calibrant lots change

- recording and monitoring instrument readings (e.g. absorbance for the calibration material) as a check on reagent and instrumental drift
- recording and monitoring assay properties (e.g. nonspecific binding and signal for zero and highest standards in immunoassays) as a check on drift
- analysis of one or more samples (at different concentrations) from the previous analytical batch, as a check on assay stability (provided that the samples are stable for the intervening period).

These procedures do not require sophisticated statistical techniques or expensive materials, but can provide invaluable information on assay performance.

Replication

The validity of results is sometimes checked by repeating the analysis of a proportion of the samples. This can be achieved in a variety of ways, such as by:

- the laboratory itself carrying out the repeat analyses, either openly or blindly
- comparison of results obtained by the laboratory with those from samples submitted independently to reference laboratories
- selecting an appropriate percentage of samples reported as negative and as positive by the laboratory and re-examining these in a reference laboratory.

Statistical monitoring of performance

Most in-process performance monitoring procedures rely on introducing control samples into each batch of analyses. These samples must be stable and of known, reproducible composition, and the results obtained on them must be able to reflect the assay's performance with test samples. Graphical or statistical analyses can then be applied to the results to confirm whether or not the analytical process is 'in control' and thus whether or not the results can be reported. It is important that different materials are used for the calibration and in-process performance monitoring functions, otherwise the monitoring will not be effective.

The number of control samples included in each batch processed depends on the size of the batch and its homogeneity. For the routine analysis of large numbers of samples of a similar type it is common to have 5–10% as controls, with a minimum of two per batch. For smaller, inhomogeneous batches this level may need to be increased to 25% or even more.

Shewhart QC charts are plots of measurements on the control samples over time in relation to the assigned value for the analyte, with upper and lower warning limits related to the customer requirement or the expected standard deviation (SD) when the process is under control. These charts can be used to plot single values of measurements, means, medians, blank values, SDs, ranges, etc. Decision-making on whether to accept a batch of results or to take corrective action is facilitated if horizontal lines are drawn at the target value and at 2 SD and 3 SD above and below this value. If the analysis is in control, the results are scattered randomly above and below the assigned value, with a distribution such that only 5% are more than 2 SD from this value and only 1% more than 3 SD from it. Bias causes a shift to higher or lower values, while loss of precision yields a wider scatter of results. A result of more than 2 SD should act as a warning to investigate the method to avoid future problems, and a result of more than 3 SD should prompt rejection of the batch and investigation of the problem before repetition of the analyses.

More complex and effective control rules have been formulated, with validation of their power to reject unsatisfactory batches and accept satisfactory batches. The so-called 'Westgard rules' are based on the analysis of two controls in each batch (usually one with 'normal' and one with 'abnormal' values). If both results fall within 2 SD of the target value (the 'warning' limit) the batch is accepted, but otherwise the remaining rules are evaluated in turn and the batch is rejected if any fail. If none fail, the batch is accepted but the situation should be investigated before the next batch is analysed.

Where automated systems incorporate IQC software, this should be reviewed to confirm its appropriateness to the application.

Cusum control charts provide an alternative sensitive method of identifying when processes are out of control by displaying cumulative deviations from the assigned value.

Materials for internal quality control and external quality assessment

The materials used as controls for IQC or EQA purposes must be selected to behave in the analyses as similarly as possible to routine samples. They must also be homogeneous, stable, safe, available in sufficient quantity and affordable.

Many QC materials are obtained from commercial sources and are produced in large quantities to specified quality standards. However, these standards may not always cover the properties of interest and care still has to be taken to ensure that they are fit for the particular analysis required. For example, materials may be guaranteed to be 95% pure, but the impurities may not be specified; these impurities could interfere with the analysis required. Also, biological materials may be stabilised by lyophilisation and their behaviour may therefore not mimic that of the test samples (e.g. lack of commutability and 'matrix effects'). It is therefore essential when using commercial materials to be aware of their often limited range of suitability (sometimes to one system only) and to test their suitability. It is good practice to use third-party controls (i.e. from a different manufacturer from those of the reagents and instrument used).

An alternative is to prepare the QC materials locally. However, the reproducibility of preparation and homogeneity of such materials is sometimes difficult to achieve, and where a biological fluid matrix is involved, the addition of pure analyte may not produce a control sample directly comparable with a routine sample. In some circumstances, it may be possible to obviate this by obtaining samples from volunteer donors (e.g. serum or urine known to contain the analyte of interest) and to use these singly or pooled to achieve the concentration levels required. However, both ethical and safety issues need to be considered in this approach. CRMs are the best materials to use but are often available for a limited range of analytes, matrices and concentrations.

Assessment, interpretation and reporting of results

Once analytical results are obtained, the analyst needs to be certain of their validity. This involves checking that the results of the in-process performance monitoring fall within the limits of acceptance and that the test results can be demonstrated to relate to the appropriate sample. The effects of transposition or transcription errors can often be severe.

It is also advisable to apply a common-sense test of plausibility to the results in the circumstances known about the sample or against previous experience of samples of the same type or from the same source. Specimen source (e.g. femoral or cardiac blood *post mortem*) and sampling time may also be relevant. An 'unusual' result may not be wrong, but usually merits further investigation.

A standard report format is very helpful to the customer (data user) and results should be reported in appropriate units, preferably written out in full to avoid confusion (e.g. between mg/L and μg/L: milligrams per litre versus micrograms per litre), with appropriate reference data or information to assist the customer understand their significance. This may, for example, be a reference to legislation, production criteria, published details in the scientific literature, or the expected values for clinical investigations. It may also be a requirement to indicate the measurement uncertainty.

External quality assessment arrangements

EQA addresses differences between testing sites for comparability of results over geography. It usually involves the analysis of identical samples at many laboratories and comparison of the results with one another and with the 'correct' answer. The process is necessarily retrospective.

Purpose of external quality assessment

EQA is concerned primarily with the assessment of an individual laboratory's performance and is one means for the laboratory to identify areas for improvement. This is only truly possible, however, if the EQA samples have been processed in the same way as routine samples.

It is essential that the EQA scheme provider respects the confidentiality of the laboratory's performance data, but EQA can give information on:

- overall interlaboratory standard of performance and best practice
- influence of variations in analytical procedures (e.g. methods, reagents, instruments and calibration)
- quality of the samples provided.

Such information can be useful to participants (e.g. in identifying more reliable procedures and encouraging adoption of best practice).

Participation in an EQA scheme should thus be seen as essential to the maintenance of professional standards and a requirement for accreditation. Results should not be used to 'police' or license laboratories, and the level of confidentiality of data must be agreed between the scheme and participant laboratories.

Selection of an external quality assessment scheme

Where alternative EQA schemes are available, laboratories may need to make a choice between them, though participation in more than one can provide complementary information. To gain value for money, EQA cost should be secondary to quality, and should be considered relative to reagent and equipment costs. Factors to be taken into account when making the selection include:

- scheme design validity, especially sample appropriateness and concentration range, report and scoring quality
- independence from manufacturing and marketing interests
- scheme service and responsiveness, including turnaround time and response to enquiries
- reputation and previous experience
- accreditation status
- cost (value for money).

Corrective actions for noncompliance

Learning from errors through improvement and corrective actions is an important element of any QA regime. Such changes need to be documented, reinforced through staff training and audited post-implementation to ensure they are effective.

If issues related to sample identity or integrity are identified, the problem is likely to be caused by poor sample collection or identification, data transposition, sample handling errors or contamination, and changes to the process should be introduced to prevent recurrence.

Where issues are indicated through the statistical monitoring of performance, the nature of the problem depends on whether it has resulted in the analysis becoming imprecise (random errors) or biased (systematic errors). Loss of precision can be contributed to by:

- specimen inhomogeneity (uneven particle size, poor mixing, clots, etc.)
- inconsistent amounts of sample or reagents being taken
- instability in the instrumentation employed or the analysis conditions.

Possible causes of bias include:

- incorrect sample or reagent volumes being used routinely
- deterioration of calibration material
- incorrect settings on the instrumentation
- incorrect analysis conditions
- systematic calculation errors.

Management of laboratory facilities

Laboratory facilities should be adequate for the work to be carried out. Equipment, glassware and other requirements should be available, and kept clean, well-maintained and in good working order. It is essential that sufficient spare parts for equipment be available, with expertise in maintenance, to permit the full and appropriate use of all equipment. A log should be maintained for each instrument, with any maintenance to the instrument noted in the log with the date, what work was carried out and the name and signature of the person carrying out the work.

Management must be good, in that all resources (personnel, equipment, facilities, raw materials such as blood, and finance) are used appropriately and effectively to the customer's benefit. Procedures used must be not only reliable but also fully documented: documentation applies as much to QC measures and managerial procedures as it does to the analytical methods themselves. A designated quality manager is normally essential (see Assessment and Accreditation, below).

Avoidance of contamination

Where the laboratory deals with both trace amounts of material (e.g. illicit drugs on balance pans or other paraphernalia) and bulk drugs, it is essential prior to analysis to separate spatially or temporally those activities that may result in contamination. Ideally, analysis involving trace amounts of material and bulk drugs should be carried out in separate areas to prevent or minimise contamination. However, it is recognised that in some laboratories this is not possible. It is important for QA purposes to have effective cleaning regimes in place before, between and after the examination of separate samples, and to control and monitor the environment carefully (clothing, benches, equipment, etc.) in the trace analysis laboratory.

Competence standards, training programme and monitoring arrangements for the analyst

Staff in analytical laboratories should demonstrably be competent to do the range of work for which they are employed. This requires a code of ethics to which the individual must conform, clearly stated expected standards of performance and behaviour, a programme of training to help the individual attain those standards, and a mechanism in place to assess independently that they are working to the standards in the workplace. Training itself does not guarantee competence, so the assessment stage is vitally important. As soon as possible, the individual should be formally certified as competent by an appropriate authority and the scope of his or her competence should be recorded. Any extensions to scope should require the individual to go through the same process for the new area of work, and his or her competence should be reassessed regularly through task-related performance monitoring and participation in internal and external proficiency-testing programmes.

Assessment and accreditation

Quality standards and protocols for analytical laboratories

The main quality standards and protocols used in the analytical sector are those published by ISO and ISO/IEC and the reader should consult their website (http://www.iso.org/iso/home.htm) for more information about the latest publications. Because of its importance both in terms of finances and public safety, QA is a rapidly developing field and standards are updated regularly. No attempt is made here to discuss each and every current standard relating to QA matters because information is likely to be outdated fairly rapidly.

Good Laboratory Practice and Compliance Monitoring

The Good Laboratory Practice and Compliance Monitoring guidance (GLP) evolved through the Organisation for Economic Development and Cooperation (OECD) in response to the need to regulate the design, conduct and reporting of studies carried out in support of the licensing of pharmaceuticals and other chemicals for human or animal use. It is recommended for the setting up and maintenance of a laboratory QA system; compliance with its principles is applied mainly to analytical chemical laboratories concerned with genetic, clinical, pharmacological, toxicological and other biochemical studies, in particular where laboratory animals are used. Its main function is to enable licensing authorities to reconstruct research studies exactly, to internationally recognised standards.

There is no conflict between GLP and ISO/IEC 17025 (at the time of writing the latest ISO standard for general requirements for the competence of testing and calibration laboratories), and the GLP regulations can be considered as complementary to the general criteria for specialised chemical laboratories. However, on its own, GLP does not provide an assurance of fitness for purpose.

Quality standards and protocols for toxicology and drugs testing laboratories

Specific guidelines have also been produced in some areas of drugs testing:

- Mandatory (HHS) Guidelines for Federal Workplace Drug Testing Programs (DHHS 2004)
- SOFT/AAFS Forensic Toxicology Laboratory Guidelines (SOFT/AAFS 2006)
- UK Laboratory Guidelines for Legally Defensible Workplace Drug Testing (2001)
- World Anti-Doping Agency (WADA) International Standard for Testing (2003).

Mandatory Guidelines for Federal Workplace Drug Testing Programs

These guidelines were developed by the Department of Health and Human Services (DHHS) in the USA and contain comprehensive standards for point-of-collection testing and laboratory testing for drugs in the workplace. They were first published in the Federal Register in 1988 (CFR 1988) and then revised in 1994 (DHHS 1994). The most recent proposed revisions of the guidelines were issued in 2004. The DHHS also developed the National Laboratory Certification Program to certify compliance with the standards by laboratories that test specimens collected for the federal agency drug-testing programmes. The National Laboratory Certification Program includes a requirement to participate in a performance-testing programme that includes blind sample submissions.

SOFT/AAFS Forensic Toxicology Laboratory Guidelines (2006)

The Society of Forensic Toxicologists (SOFT) and the Toxicology Section of the American Academy of Forensic Sciences (AAFS) first produced these guidelines in 1991 and they have been revised several times since. They cover both postmortem forensic toxicology and human performance forensic toxicology, with the exclusion of forensic urine drugs testing (which is covered by the DHHS Guidelines and College of American Pathologists Accreditation Program), and provide detailed guidance for laboratory practices. They also originally contained a checklist for self-evaluation and preparation for accreditation, but this was removed when it was adopted by the American Board of Forensic Toxicology as the basis of their Forensic Toxicology Accreditation Program in 1996.

UK Laboratory Guidelines for Legally Defensible Workplace Drugs Testing (2001)

These guidelines have adopted the general principles established internationally and represent an overview of best practice in the UK. They are also now being used as the basis for new European guidelines for best practice. They focus on urine specimens, but are equally applicable in principle to all specimen types.

World Anti-Doping Agency International Standard for Testing

The World Anti Doping Agency (WADA), the governing body set up to control doping in sports, publish various standards and associated documents for testing laboratories in order to ensure that their results are fit for purpose. Their website (www.wada-ama.org) should be consulted for the latest version of these documents.

The accreditation process

A laboratory that seeks accreditation must first develop a documented quality management system in a form that addresses all the requirements of the relevant quality standard for the range of activities it wishes to be included in its scope of accreditation. Assessors from the accrediting body review this and may make a pre-assessment visit to the laboratory to help identify areas that still need to be addressed. Once the necessary follow-up actions have been completed, the assessors return to carry out the formal assessment. Any further deficiencies in the quality management system and any perceived noncompliances of practice in relation to the documented quality management system are brought to the laboratory's attention. If the laboratory responds satisfactorily within the specified timescale, accreditation is awarded. The awarding body carries out regular surveillance visits to monitor continued compliance with the standard, and there is normally a process for formal re-accreditation after a few years.

References

CFR 1988, Code of Federal Regulations (CFR), see http://origin.www.gpoaccess.gov/cfr/.

DHHS, *Mandatory Guidelines for Federal Workplace Drug Testing Programs*, Rockville, Division of Workplace Programs, Department of Health and Human Services, 1994, www.SAMHSA.org.

EURACHEM, *The Fitness for Purpose of Analytical Methods, A Laboratory Guide to Method Validation and Related Topics*, EURACHEM, 1998, www.eurachem.ul.pt/.

EURACHEM/CITAC, *Quantifying Uncertainty in Analytical Measurement*, EURACHEM/CITAC, 2000, www.eurachem.ul.pt/.

EURACHEM/CITAC, *Guide to Quality in Analytical Chemistry – An Aid to Accreditation*, EURACHEM/CITAC, 2002, www.eurachem.ul.pt/.

ISO/IEC, ISO/IEC Guide 43–1, *Proficiency Testing by Interlaboratory Comparisons – Part 1: Development and Operation of Laboratory Proficiency Testing*, Geneva, International Organization for Standardization, 1997.

ISO/IEC, ISO/IEC 17025, *General Requirements for the Competence of Testing and Calibration Laboratories*, Geneva, International Organization for Standardization, 2005.

OECD, *Good Laboratory Practice and Compliance Monitoring*, Paris, OECD, 1992.

SOFT/AAFS, Forensic Toxicology Laboratory Guidelines, Mesa, SOFT/AAFS, 2000, www.soft-tox.org.

UK Laboratory Guidelines for Legally Defensible Workplace Drug Testing 2001, http://ltg.uk.net/ or www.wdtforum.org.uk.

WADA International Standard for Testing, 2003, World Anti-Doping Agency (WADA), www.wada-ama.org/

Further reading

N. T. Crosby and I. Patel, *General Principles of Good Sampling Practice*, Cambridge, The Royal Society of Chemistry, 1995.

DHHS, National Laboratory Certification Program, Division of Workplace Programs, Rockville, Department of Health and Human Services, 1998.

H. Gunzler, *Accreditation and Quality Assurance in Analytical Chemistry*, Berlin, Springer Verlag, 1994.

ISO, ISO 9000, *Quality Management Systems*, Geneva, International Organization for Standardization, 1994.

ISO, ISO 9000:2000, *Quality Management Systems*, Geneva, International Organization for Standardization, 2000.

ISO, EN ISO 15189:2007, *Medical Laboratories – Particular Requirements for Quality and Competence*, Geneva,

International Organization for Standardization, 2007.

S. L. Jeffcoate, *Efficiency and Effectiveness in the Endocrine Laboratory*, London, Academic Press, 1981.

Office for Official Publications of the European Union, Rules governing medicinal products in the European Union, www.emea.eu.int/htms/human/qrd/qrdguide.htm. (Note: different volumes published in different years).

C. P. Price, A. St John and J. M. Hicks (eds), *Point of Care Testing*, 2nd edn, Washington DC, American Association for Clinical Chemistry, 2004.

Subcommittee on Analytical Goals in Clinical Chemistry of the World Association of Societies of Pathology, Analytical goals in clinical chemistry: their relationship to medical care, *Am. J. Clin. Pathol.*, 1979, **71**, 624–630.

UNDCP, *Guidelines for Validation of Analytical Methodology and Calibration of Equipment used for Testing of Illicit Drugs in Seized Materials and Biological Specimens*, UNDCP/United Nations Office on Drugs and Crime (in preparation).

J. O. Westgard *et al.*, A multi-rule Shewhart chart for quality control in clinical chemistry, *Clin. Chem.*, 1981, **27**, 493–501.

WHO, *External Quality Assessment of Health Laboratories, EURO Reports & Studies 6*, Copenhagen, WHO Regional Office for Europe, 1981.

amatoxins 119
America, horseracing policies 266, 270
American Academy of Forensic Sciences
committee on DFSA 290
SOFT/AAFS Forensic Toxicology Laboratory Guidelines (2006) 621
American Society for Testing and Materials, on Raman spectrometry standards 460–1
amfetamines 44–5, *238*
analysis 70–1
in clandestine laboratories 68
colour test reagents *342*
control status *45*
cross-reactivities of immunoassays 382
derivative spectrophotometry 407, *408*
driving under the influence 304
gas chromatography *62*, 508–9
hair *158*, 160
infrared spectra 443, *444*
Leuckart reaction 44–5, *46*
Marquis reagent test 61, 70, 75
metabolism 25–6
N-substituted *57*
saliva 172, 178
sports, reporting rates *268*
tablet patterns 65
thin-layer chromatography 69
urine pH on excretion 22
workplace drug testing
cut-off values 137, 138, *139*, *142*, *143*
interpretation of results 147–8
amides, insecticides *92*
amino acids with sulfhydryl groups, drug trapping in hair 155
7-aminoclonazepam 295
hair 161
7-aminoflunitrazepam 290
derivatisation *504*
hair 161
saliva 179
aminophylline
DFSA cases *293*
workplace drug testing 140
aminopropylsiloxane layers, TLC 348, *349*
aminosilanes, HPLC 524
amiodarone, half-life 251
amitriptyline *238*
metabolism 27
metabolites 23, 40
postmortem redistribution 208
urine levels for DFSA cases *292*
ammonia, TLC systems using *362*, *365*, *366*
ammonium molybdate test 95
amnesia, clonazepam 295–6
amniotic fluid 258
amobarbital *238*
saliva 178
urine levels for DFSA cases *292*
workplace drug testing *139*
amperometric detectors
capillary electrophoresis *549*
HPLC 520
amphibians 128
amphoteric drugs, extraction 201
amphotericin A, limit test 405
'amyl' nitrite 82
anabolic agents 52–3, *54*
analysis 75
control status *45*
counterfeit tablets 326, *327*
detection 274, 276, 278–9
in food supplements 269
hair 161
horseracing 270
Misuse of Drugs Act (1996) 324
prohibited in sports *265*
thin-layer chromatography 69
anaerobic bioconversion 23
anaesthetic agents
necropsy samples 84
volatile *81*
pharmacokinetics *87*
analgesics, driving and *302*
analyte recovery 614
androstenedione
in food supplements 269
as prohormone 52
angel dust *see* phencyclidine
angiotensin-converting enzyme inhibitors, metabolism 35
anhydroecgonine methyl ester (AEME) 26
hair 160
oral deposition 168
saliva 177
anhydrous solvents, HPLC 531
anilides, insecticides *92*
animals, antisera from 379
anion-exchange cartridges, solid-phase extraction 275
anions 7, 101–2, 111–16
anodic stripping voltammetry (ASV) 110
antacids, aluminium 102
antagonism, drug interactions 30, 58
antemortem specimens 198
anterograde amnesia, clonazepam 295–6
anti-Stokes Raman scattering 456
antibiotics, bioassay 252
antibodies
dilution curves 379–80
gold-labelled, lateral flow methods 385–6
monoclonal 379
production for immunoassays 377–8
saliva tests 171–2
see also microplate antibody capture
antibody-capture systems, enzyme immunoassays 382–4
anticholinesterases *see* cholinesterase inhibitors
anticircular thin-layer chromatography 352
anticoagulants
blood samples for volatile substances 84
coumarins *92*, 100–1
anticonvulsants 233
adverse effect of TDM 250
brain death 222
driving and *302*
poisoning emergencies *228*
saliva 178–9
antidepressants 231
driving and *302*
gas chromatography 509
metabolism 27
see also tricyclic antidepressants
antidotes 222–3
antiepileptic drugs *see* anticonvulsants
antihistamines, driving and *302*
antimony 103
analysis methods *102*
antipsychotic drugs 231
driving and *302*
metabolism 27–8
antisera
antibody dilution curves 379–80
polyclonal 379
antivenoms 125
snakebites 128–9
apparent mobility, capillary electrophoresis 542
arachnids 125
area mapping of tablets, Raman spectroscopy 465–6
areas under curves
calculation of bioavailability 15–16
drug concentrations 252
arsenic 103–4, *238*
analysis methods *102*
Gutzeit test 110
tests 2
artefacts
alkali halide disc IR spectroscopy 436
clinical toxicology 236
infrared spectroscopy 446, *447*
Raman spectroscopy 458
arthropods 125
arylene stationary phases, gas chromatography 474
ascorbic acid, QED Saliva Alcohol Test 174
Aspergillus spp., toxins 118
aspirators, saliva collection 170
aspirin (acetylsalicylic acid) 233, *238*
infrared spectrum 445, *446*
urine pH on excretion 21
assessment of competence 609, 620
see also quality control and assessment
Association of Racing Commissioners International (ARCI), classification of drugs 270
asymmetry, gas chromatography peaks 483
atmospheric pressure chemical ionisation 520, 568, 569
atmospheric pressure ionisation (API) 520–1
atomic absorption spectrophotometry (AAS) 110
atomic emission detectors, gas chromatography 496
atomic force microscopy *602*
atomisers, TLC 350–1
reagents 357
atrazine *91*, 99
attenuated total reflectance, infrared spectroscopy 437–8
audit 608
automation 9
capillary electrophoresis 548
gas chromatography 489
HPLC 517, 521–2
immunoassays 388

solid-phase extraction 276
spectrophotometry 400–1
thin-layer chromatography 351
development chambers 355, *356*
autopsy *see* necropsy; postmortem toxicology
auxochromes 396
average linear velocity, gas chromatography 481
average masses, mass spectrometry 561
Avitar collector 169
axial resolution, Raman microscopy 459
azathioprine, metabolism 35

'B' samples, doping cases 271
back-calculation, ethanol measurements 314–15, *316*
'back-end' steps, automated immunoassays 388
back-extraction 201
backflush, gas chromatography 490
bacteria
blood ethanol samples 310
glucose 6-phosphate dehydrogenase from 387
on postmortem morphine concentrations 213
toxins 116–17
volatile substances from 89
ballistic analysis 65, 75, 326
barbital *238*, *445*
barbiturates *238*
colour test reagents *342*
control status *45*
difference spectrophotometry 406
fluorescence spectrophotometry 417
hyperchromic effect 409
infrared spectra 443–5, 446
metabolism 31
saliva 178–9
spectrophotometry, pH 398
workplace drug testing *138*, *139*
barium *102*, 104
base-deactivated silicas, HPLC 523
base-modified polyethylene glycols, for gas chromatography 474
baseline drift
fluorescence spectrophotometry 418
HPLC 526
basic drugs
colour tests 340
driving and 320
extraction 200, 201
horse urine 275
HPLC 532–3
separation from acidic and neutral drugs 361–4
Basic Tests for Drugs (WHO) 336
bathochromic effect, difference spectrophotometry 405–6
bathochromic shift, spectrophotometry 408–9
bead coating, nitrogen-phosphorus detectors 494
Beer–Lambert law 397, 410–11
Beer's law 397, 413, 423
bending vibrations, Raman spectroscopy 463–4
benzene *87*
benzene rings, vibrations 463
benzfetamine
amfetamines from 26
cross-reactivities of immunoassays 382
benzimidazoles *92*
benzocaine, computer-aided infrared spectroscopy 428
benzodiazepines 53–4, 75, 231
anaerobic bioconversion 23
brain death 222
colour test reagent *342*
control status *45*
in disease states 33
drug-facilitated sexual assault
incidence 288
urine levels *291*
elderly people 33
gas chromatography 509
hair 161
HPLC 532
hydrolysis 499, 509–10
in utero exposure 257
metabolism 24–5
poisoning emergencies *228*
postmortem 213
saliva 179
thin-layer chromatography 69
vitreous humour 195
workplace drug testing *138*, *139*, 140
benzoylecgonine 26
postmortem 212
saliva 176–7
workplace drug testing *138*, *139*
alternative specimens *143*
passive exposure to cocaine 149
benzphetamine 148, *238*
1-benzylpiperazine 56
Berlin blue 109
beryllium *102*, 104, 115
beta-blockers
impurity profiling 580–1
poisoning emergencies *228*
prohibited in sports *265*
sports prohibited in 264
beverages, ethanol content *317*
bezoars, drug overdoses 196
bias 614
bicarbonate, amfetamine abuse 22
bile 17
morphine in 38
postmortem toxicology 196
ethanol 211
sample quantities *192*
bilirubin, Gilbert syndrome 32
binders, thin-layer chromatography 346
binding, irreversible 249
bioassay, antibiotics 252
bioavailability 15–16, 37
biochemistry, poisoning 224, *227*
biochips (microarrays) 594–5, *596*
biofluids
capillary electrophoresis 552, 554, 555
HPLC 534–6
see also specific types
biosensors, cells *602*
bipyridylium reduction products, quaternary ammonium compounds 100
bis-cyanopropyl substitution, polysiloxanes for GC 473
bismuth *102*, 105, *238*
bis(trimethylsilyl)testosterone derivatisation 279
bis(trimethylsilyl)trifluoroacetamide–trimethylchlorosilane, GHB derivatisation 76
black-body radiation 426
blank samples, colour tests 340–1
'bleeding', gas chromatography 473–4
Blighia sapida 122
blockage of cartridges, SPE of horse urine 275
blood
postmortem redistribution into 208
ethanol 211
samples
for anions 114–15
antemortem 198
clinical toxicology 224
contamination, anion poisoning 115, 116
cyanide poisoning 112
driving impairment 319
see also blood concentrations, alcohol
haemolysis 18
headspace gas chromatography 89
heterogeneous immunoassays 382
HPLC 534–6
postmortem toxicology 191, *192*, 194, 213
sports 271, 272
volatile substances 83–4
see also biofluids
blood–brain barrier 248
blood concentrations 17–18
alcohol (BAC)
conversion factor from breath-alcohol results 317
driving 301, 309–10
impairment *vs 308*
legislation 305
validity of tests 34
postmortem 35
volatile substances 90
blood flow
on drug clearance 19
see also plasma flow
blood pressure, poisoning *225*
body content, drugs 40
body water 17
boiling points, solvents *490*
boldenone 52, *54*
boldione 52
borates 111
Bordeaux mixture 106
botulinum toxins 116, 117
Bouguer's law 396
bowel contents, time after substance administration 38
box jellyfish 124
brain
postmortem toxicology 197, 213–14
see also blood–brain barrier
brain death 222
Bratton-Marshall reagent *358*
breath-alcohol tests 175, 308, 310–12
athletes 273
legislation 305, 314
retrograde extrapolation *316*
volatile substances and 83, 312
Widmark's equation 317, *318*

brevetoxin 123, *124*
'bridge' molecules, antibody production for immunoassays 378
British Pharmacopoeia, resolution of IR spectrometers 429–30
brodifacoum 100, *101*, *239*
bromadiolone 100, *101*, *239*
bromide 111, *239*
brompheniramine, urine levels for DFSA cases *292*
bubbles, HPLC 516
buccal absorption of substances 15, 168
  saliva concentrations 173
budesonide, sports, reporting rates *268*
buffers
  capillary electrophoresis *551*
  drug extraction 201
bufotenine 128
buprenorphine 235, *239*
burning, Raman spectroscopy 461
butalbital, workplace drug testing *139*
butane 82, *87*
1,4-butanediol *291*, 293, *294*
n-butanol, TLC systems using *362*

cadmium *102*, 105, *239*
caffeine 235, *239*
  gas chromatography *498*
  horseracing 269
calcium antagonists, poisoning emergencies *228*
calibration
  cross-reactivities of immunoassays 381
  HPLC 528–30
  immunoassays 376, *377*, 389–90
  mass spectrometry 562, 573
  postmortem toxicology 204–5
  spectrophotometry 401–2, 410
    fluorescence 415–16
    infrared 429–31
  statistical 617
  thin-layer chromatography 356
  for volatile substance analysis 86
Camic Datamaster, breath-alcohol test 312
Canada
  Compendium of Pharmaceutical Specialties 332
  horseracing policy 266, 270
cannabidiol, hair 161
cannabinoid receptors 48
cannabinoids 45–8
  oral deposition 168
  saliva 172, 173, 179
  see also carboxy-tetrahydro-cannabinol; tetrahydro-cannabinol
cannabinol 47, *48*
  derivatives and, control status *45*
  hair 161
cannabis 45–8
  activation by liver 16
  analysis 71
  control status *45*
  driving and 303
  estimating time after administration 38–9
  gas chromatography 72, 510
  hair *158*, 160–1
  pregnancy, use rates 257
  saliva 179–80
  sports, reporting rates *268*
  thin-layer chromatography 69
  workplace drug testing 139
    cut-off values 137, 138, *139*, *142*, *143*
    positives from inhalation 149
cannabis resin 46, 71, 72
Cannabis sativa 45–6, *47*, *48*, 71–2
capillaries, capillary electrophoresis 546
capillary columns
  gas chromatography 470–1
    confirmatory testing in doping 277
    maintenance 507
    volatile substances 85
  HPLC 523
capillary electrochromatography (CEC) 545
capillary electrophoresis 539–56
  in combinations 9
  instrumentation 545–8
  mass spectrometry with 9, 548, *549*, 571
capillary ion analysis 543
capillary sieving electrophoresis (CSE) 545
capillary zone electrophoresis (CZE) 159, 543, 549
capsules 67, 323, 327–8
  in stomach contents 196
carbamates *91*, *92*, 98, 231–2
carbamazepine, saliva 178, 179
carbanilates *92*
carbon, isotope ratios, regions of origin of seized drugs 65
carbon-13, mass spectrometry 560–1
carbon-14, radioimmunoassay 384
carbon dioxide, supercritical fluid extraction 502
  drugs in hair 158
carbon monoxide 233–4, *239*
  forensic identification 203
  as metabolite *88*
  poisoning emergencies *228*
  postmortem toxicology 198
carbon tetrachloride *239*
  pharmacokinetics *87*
  spectrophotometry 399
carbonyl stretch, infrared absorption 423
Carbopaks, gas chromatography 472
carbosieves 472
Carboxen 1006 472
carboxyhaemoglobin 234
carboxylic acids, insecticides *92*
carboxy-tetrahydrocannabinol (THCA)
  DFSA, urine levels *291*
  sports *266*
  workplace drug testing
    alternative specimens *143*
    immunoassay 140
carisoprodol, DFSA, urine levels *293*
carrier gases, flow control 490–3, 507
carrier proteins, immunoassays 378
cartridges
  anion- and cation-exchange, solid-phase extraction 275
  immunoassays 385
case investigation 5–7
cassettes, saliva immunochro-matography 171–2
castor oil 121
catalogues, gas chromatography techniques 506
catalyst discovery, high-throughput screening 591
catechols, from amfetamines 26
Catha edulis 55–6
cathine, sports *266*
cathinone, analogues 56
cation-exchange cartridges, solid-phase extraction 275
CE-MS (capillary electrophoresis with mass spectrometry) 9, 548, *549*, 571
CEDIA assay 387
  workplace drug testing 140
cells
  biosensors *602*
  infrared spectroscopy 432
  spectrophotometry 402–4, 416
cellulose layers, TLC 348
central nervous system
  depressants
    on driving 301–3, 306, 320
    see also sedatives
  stimulants *see* stimulants
centrifugal force
  radioimmunoassay, separation step 384–5
  thin-layer chromatography 352, 371
certified reference materials (CRMs) 64–5, 618
  postmortem toxicology 206
cetyltrimethylammonium bromide, HPLC eluents 532
CFR Part 40, DOT Code of Federal Regulations, on workplace drug testing 136
chain of custody of samples 3, 7
  transport 612
  workplace drug testing 145–6
charcoal
  activated 16, 223
    'gut dialysis' 223
    stomach contents 196
    theophylline poisoning 234
  dextran-coated, radioimmunoassay separation step 385
charge-coupled devices (CCD), Raman spectroscopy 458
chat (khat) 55–6, 69, 76
chelating agents, fluorescence 413
chemical hydrolysis 499
chemiluminescence immunoassays 385
chemistry, forensic 323–33
chemometrics 467
Chen's reagent, khat 76
chest, stomach contents in 208, 211
Chicago, study of drug-facilitated sexual assault 289
children
  drug metabolism 32–3
  ethanol 230
  lead on development 107
  poisoning 220
    criminal 223
    salicylates 233
Chinese herbal products, identification 332
'Chinese heroin' 49–50
chirality *see* stereoselective analysis

Chironex fleckeri 124
chlorates 111
chlorbutol 82
chlordiazepoxide *239*
  DFSA, urine levels *291*
  metabolism 24
  saliva 179
chlorinated hydrocarbons, insecticides *92*, 98–9
chlorinated phenoxy acids *92*, 99
chlorobutane, drug extraction 201
chloroform *239*
  infrared spectroscopy 432
  pharmacokinetics *87*
  spectrophotometry 399
  TLC systems using *362*, *365*
chloroform–acetone TLC system, pesticides *367*
chlorophenoxyacetic acids 232, *239*
m-chlorophenylpiperazine 56
chloroquine *239*
  blood *vs* plasma concentrations 18
  electron-impact ionisation 577, *578*
  poisoning emergencies *228*
  positive-ion chemical ionisation 578
chlorpromazine, metabolism 23, 27–8
chocolate drops 329–30
cholinesterase inhibitors 231–2
  pesticide poisoning cases 97
  poisoning emergencies *228*
cholinesterases 98
  organophosphorus poisoning 222–3
choppers, double-beam spectrometers 425
Christensen effect 433
chromatography 9, 514–15
  adsorption chromatography 514, 531
  affinity chromatography, antisera 379
  driving impairment, drug screening 319
  hair 159
  limits of detection 205
  reversed-phase ion-pair chromatography 532–3
  saliva test confirmation 172
  screening 229–30
  for spectrophotometry 395
  spray reagents 341–3
  therapeutic drug monitoring 252–3
  see also specific types
chromophores 396
Chromosorb 101–108 472
Chromosorb G, W and P 476
chronic toxicity 82
chronic *vs* acute drug abuse, hair sampling 163
chrysanthemic acid 99
ciclosporin, pharmacodynamic monitoring 255
cicutoxin 121
cigarette lighter refills *81*, 82
ciguatoxins 126
cimetidine *239*
  drug interactions and 30
  scombroid poisoning 127
circular thin-layer chromatography 352
citrate sample tubes 8
citrates, oral fluid collection 166
clandestine laboratories 68
classifications
  drugs and poisons 7–8, 270
  pesticides 95
'clean-up columns', HPLC 518
cleaning
  electron-capture detectors 496
  spectrophotometer cells 403
clearance 19–20
  extracorporeal elimination procedures 237
clenbuterol
  horseracing, test sensitivity 270
  sports, reporting rates *268*
clinical toxicology 219–37
  colour tests 336
  containers found 80, 197
  drug interactions 36–7
  forensic toxicology and 1–2, 223
  non-drug poisoning 79–134
  organophosphorus compounds 97–8
    cholinesterase measurement 222–3
  pesticides, case numbers by country *93–4*
  samples *6*, 224–7
ClinRep collection device, saliva opiates 176
clobenzorex, amfetamines from 26
clonazepam 231, *239*, 295–6
  hair samples 161
  urine levels for DFSA cases *291*
cloned enzyme donor immunoassay *see* CEDIA assay
clonidine, urine levels for DFSA cases *293*
Clostridium spp., toxins 116–17
clozapine, metabolism 28
Cnidaria 124
coated tablets 326
cobalt nitrate, colour test for GHB 76
cobalt thiocyanate test 72
cobras 128
coca leaves, isotope ratio mass spectrometry 65, *66*
coca teas 149
cocaethylene 26
  hair specimens 157
  saliva 177
cocaine 48–9, *240*
  analysis 72–4
  antemortem specimens 198
  colour test reagents *342*
  control status *45*
  doping in sports 273
  driving and 304
  drug-facilitated sexual assault cases *293*
  gas chromatography *62*, 510
  geography of origins *66*
  gestational exposure 164
  hair 157, *158*, 160
  in utero exposure 256, 257
  meconium 258
    false positives 259
  metabolism 26
  nasal swabs and 197
  oral deposition 168
  poisoning emergencies *228*
  postmortem toxicology 212–13
  pregnancy, use rates 257
  saliva 167–8, 176–8
  sweat *182*
  thin-layer chromatography 69
  vitreous humour 194
  workplace drug testing *139*
    cut-off values 137, 138, *139*, *143*
    positive from passive exposure 149
  see also 'crack cocaine'
codeine *240*
  hair samples in abuse 160
  metabolism 29
    enzyme deficiency 31
  oral deposition 168
  saliva 176
  sports, reporting rates *268*
  urine levels for DFSA cases *292*
  workplace drug testing *138*, 139, 147, 148
    alternative specimens *143*
coefficient of variation 614
  see also relative standard deviation
Coelenterata 124
cold on-column injection, gas chromatography 488–9
cold trapping, gas chromatography 485, *488*
collection of samples
  hair 156
  oral fluid 166, 168–70, 176
  quality control 610–11
  sports 272
  stomach contents 196
  workplace drug testing 145–6
collision-induced dissociation, tandem mass spectrometry 567
colloidal gold, saliva testing 171–2
colorimetry
  instruments 399
  metal compounds 110
  thallium 110–11
colour, flunitrazepam 290
colour of skin, poisoning cases *226*
colour reactions, spectrophotometry 394
colour tests 7, 8–9, 335–43
  anabolic steroids 75
  cannabinoids 71
  cocaine 72
  gamma-hydroxybutyric acid 76
  heroin 74
  lysergic acid 74
  methylenedioxymethylamfetamine 75
  nitrate poisoning 113
  pesticides 95–6
  Psilocybe mushrooms 76
  reagents 341–3
  seized drugs 60–1
  solid dosage forms 332
column capacity ratio 514
column liquid chromatography *see* high-performance liquid chromatography
column switches, HPLC 518
columns
  gas chromatography 470–83
    conditioning 479–80
    efficiency 483, 492
    evaluating performance 481–3
    installation 479
    maintenance 507
    see also capillary columns; porous layer open tubular columns
  HPLC 515, 522–5
    maintenance 525

columns (*continued*)
  see also guard columns
  for solid phase extraction 536
coma, clinical toxicology 222
combustion isotope ratio mass spectrometry (CIRMS)
  doping in sports 277, 279
  gas chromatography with 561
    GHB in drug-facilitated sexual assault 297
combustion products, hydrogen cyanide 112
common neutral loss scanning, tandem mass spectrometry 567
community pharmacists, role in solid dose identification 330
comparison
  cannabis resin blocks 72
  LSD paper squares 74–5
  of methods 614
  seized drugs 65
compartments, body water 17
Compendium of Pharmaceutical Specialties 332
competence standards 620
competitive immunoassays 375
complex mixture analysis 600
compliance testing 248–50
compressed tablets 325–6
computer models, in TLC systems 370
computers
  diode-array detector control 519
  fluorescence spectrophotometry 416
  high-throughput screening 591
  infrared spectroscopy 428, 430–1, 442
  Raman spectroscopy 459–60
  see also data processing
concentration methods
  samples for capillary electrophoresis 552–3
  samples for HPLC 535
concentration ratios, drugs and metabolites 39, 40
  routes of administration 41
concentration–time curves 14, 20
  chronic dosing on 22
  volatile substances 86
concentrations
  areas under curves 252
  athletes, drugs 264, *266*
  blood *vs* plasma 17–18, 213
  dose estimation from 39–41
    hair analysis 162–3
  doses *vs* 214
  driving limits 306, 309–10, 313
  effects *vs* 34–6
  fluorescence quenching 414
  infrared spectroscopy 433
  Raman spectroscopy 466
  in saliva 167–8, 172–3
  stomach contents 196
  therapeutic 36, 207–8, 216, 237, *238*
  therapeutic effects *vs* 247, 248
  at time zero 40
  total amounts *vs* 236
  toxic 36–8, 237, *238*
  volatile substances 90
    metabolites *88–9*
  see also plasma concentrations; tissues, drug concentrations; *specific substances*
concordance testing 248–50
conditioning, gas chromatography columns 479–80
confectionery, resembling drugs 324, 329–30
confidence intervals 615
confidentiality, external quality assessment and 619
confirmation testing
  doping in sports 277–81
  driving under the influence 320
  drug-facilitated sexual assault, samples 296
  after immunoassays 382
  meconium 260
  on-site saliva testing 172
  solid dosage form identification 332
  workplace drug testing
    cut-off values 138–9, *143*
    GC-MS 140–1
confocal microscopy, Raman spectroscopy 459
congener alcohols 89
coniine 121
conjugates, hydrolysis 200–1
conjugation
  drugs in urine 273
  pesticides, GC-MS 96
  see also haptenisation
constant-flow systems, HPLC 516
constant neutral-loss scanning, identification of metabolites 582
containers
  blood samples
    anion poisoning 115
    cyanide poisoning 112
    gels 115, 116, 224
    volatile substances 83–4
  found in poisoning incidents 80, 197
  samples 8
contamination
  by aluminium 110
  anion poisoning, samples for 115, 116
  avoidance 620
  gas chromatography 507
  hair samples 156–7
  pharmaceutical processes, Raman spectroscopy 465
  thin-layer chromatography, removal 350
  volatile substance samples 83, 84
continuous development, thin-layer chromatography 352
contraband, solid dosage form identification 331
contraceptives, ethynyl steroids, thin-layer chromatography 347
control status, drugs listed *45*
controlled substances 43
  gamma-hydroxybutyric acid as 290
controls 616, 617
  lateral flow immunoassays 386
  postmortem toxicology 206
  see also blank samples
cooled tubes, infrared spectroscopy with gas chromatography 440
cooling, capillary electrophoresis 541, 546
copolymeric solid-phase extraction 275
copper *102*, 105–6
Coppinox 329
cores, slow-release products 329
coroners, postmortem toxicology samples and 192
correction fluids *81*
corrective actions, quality assurance 619
correlation, Raman spectroscopy 467
  tables 464
correlation coefficients, linearity of spectrophotometry 411
cosmetic treatments, on hair samples 157
cotinine, labelled with horseradish peroxidase 380
coulometry 159, 520
coumarin anticoagulants *92*, 100–1
coumatetralyl 100, *101*
counterfeit tablets 326–7
  near infrared spectroscopy 451–2
coupled techniques (hyphenated techniques) 9, 520–1, 558
  mass spectrometry 568–72
courts, evidence on drink-driving 313–14
covalent bonds, Raman spectroscopy 456, 457
Cozart RapiScan saliva-sampling device 169, 171
'crack cocaine' 48, *49*, 67
  vs cocaine as salt 72, *73*
  pregnancy 257
'crash' phase, stimulants 304
creatine, abuse in sports 264
creatinine
  clearance 20
  deceptive specimens for workplace drug testing 144–5, 149–50
criminal poisoning, clinical toxicology 223
cross-reactivity of immunoassays 205, 378, 379
  'designer' drugs 140
  quantitative 380–2
Crotalidae 128
crushing, samples for infrared spectroscopy 433–4
crystal *see* phencyclidine
crystals, near infrared spectroscopy 450
cups, intraoral 170
Curie point pyrolyser 85
curve fitting, immunoassays 390
customer requirements 609–10
customs
  colour tests 336
  solid dosage form identification 331
Cusum control charts 618
cut-off values for drugs
  hair 158
  saliva 167–8
  workplace drug testing 137, 138–9
    alternative specimens *142*, *143*, 181
cut-off wavelengths, solvents 398
'cutting' *see* adulterants
cyanide 111–12, *240*
  colour test reagents *342*
  as metabolite *88*
  postmortem toxicology 198
  sample handling 115
cyanopropylphenyl substitution, polysiloxanes for gas chromatography 473, 474

cyanosilanes, HPLC 524
cyclobenzaprine, DFSA *293*
cyclodextrins *473*, 474–5, 555
cyclohexane
  Raman spectra 461
  on spectrophotometry 398, 409
cyclohexane–toluene–diethylamine TLC system *363*, *365*
cyclooxygenase inhibitors 233
cyclotrons *see* ion cyclotron resonance mass spectrometers
cyfluthrine 99
CYP2D6, polymorphisms 256
cypermethrin 99
cystolithic hairs, *Cannabis sativa* 46, 71–2
cytochrome P450 enzymes 23
  IID6 deficiency 215
  drug interactions and 30
  induction and paracetamol poisoning 232
  ketamine metabolism 294
  pharmacogenetics 31, 255–6

2,4-D (herbicide) 99
danger, clandestine laboratories 68
darbepoietin 269, 280
DART (direct analysis in real time) 570
data acquisition rates, capillary electrophoresis 548
data processing
  fluorescence spectrophotometry 416–17
  HPLC 521–2
  infrared spectroscopy 428
  interferometric spectro-photometers, Raman spectroscopy 459–60
  mass spectrometry 572–3
  see also computers
data resolution, infrared spectroscopy 430–1
  HPLC with 441
databases
  drug profiling 65–7
  infrared spectra 442, 446, 447
  mass spectrometry 583–5
  Raman spectroscopy 467–8
  R_F value searches 360–4
  solid dosage form identification 331–2
  spectrophotometry 419
date rape *see* drug-facilitated sexual assault
de-gassing, HPLC 516
deactivation
  gas chromatography columns 471
  gas chromatography supports 476–9
death
  brain death 222
  cocaine 212–13
  'glue-sniffing' 82
  suspicious 4
death sentence, quantification of seized drugs for 64
Debye–Hückel equation 541
decomposition, postmortem toxicology samples and 193, 207
deconjugation, pesticides, GC-MS 96
decontamination, hair samples 156–7
deconvolution
  fluorescence spectrophotometry 416
  multiwavelength UV spectrophotometry 589
  Raman spectroscopy *460*
defence, samples for, doping cases 271
definitions
  deceptive specimens for workplace drug testing 144–5
  drugs of abuse 43
  forensic toxicology 1–2
  poisons 2
  sexual assault 287, 288
  volatile substance abuse 80
deglucuronidation *see* hydrolysis
degradation, salmon calcitonin 581–2
degreasing agents *81*
degrees of vibrational freedom 462
Δ_9-tetrahydrocannabinol *see* tetrahydro-cannabinol
demixing, solvent systems in TLC 368
denaturation, postmortem toxicology samples 207
densitograms 359
deoxynivalenol (DON) 118
Department of Health and Human Services, guidelines on workplace drug testing *see* HHS Guidelines
Department of Transport, alcohol tests 175
Department of Transport Code of Federal Regulations *CFR Part 40*, on workplace drug testing 136
dependence, volatile substances 82
derivatisation
  anabolic steroids 75, 276
  benzodiazepines, gas chromatography 509
  bis(trimethylsilyl)testosterone 279
  capillary electrophoresis 547–8
  domoic acid 124
  gas chromatography 503–5
  HPLC 415, 527
  for immunoassay specificity 378
  opiates, gas chromatography 510
  spectrophotometry 394
  thin-layer chromatography 357–8
  volatile substances 85
derivatised samples, amfetamines 70
derivative spectrophotometry 406–7, *408*
desalkyl metabolites, tricyclic antidepressants 27
desferrioxamine 222–3
'designer drugs' 56, *57*, 77
  cross-reactivity of immunoassays 140
desipramine, postmortem redistribution *209*
desmethyldiazepam *see* nordiazepam
desorption electrospray ionisation (DESI) 570
detection 8, 9
  limit of (LOD) 205–6, 613
    capillary electrophoresis 550
detection windows *see* surveillance windows
detectors
  capillary electrophoresis 545, 547–8, *548*
  gas chromatography 470, 493–8
  HPLC 518–21
    maintenance 526
  mass spectrometry 560
  see also specific types
detergents, ion-pair chromatography 533
deuterated solvents, infrared spectroscopy 433
deuterated triglycine sulfate, detectors 425
deuterium, standards 204, 505
deuterium-labelled cocaine, study on hair samples 160
development, thin-layer chromatography 352–5
  chambers 354–5, 356
  choice of method 364–71
  preparative 371
dextran-coated charcoal, separation step, radioimmunoassay 385
dextropropoxyphene 29, *245*
DFSA *see* drug-facilitated sexual assault
diabetes mellitus
  acetone 212
  postmortem toxicology, ethanol 211
dialysis
  aluminium toxicity 102, 103
  copper toxicity 106
  efficiency for elimination 236–7
  for poisoning 223
diamond anvil, infrared spectroscopy 433–4
diamorphine *see* heroin
diastereoisomers, gas chromatography 505
diatomaceous earths 476
diazepam *240*
  brain death 222
  counterfeit tablets 326
  drug-facilitated sexual assault *291*
  metabolites 23
    concentration ratios, routes of administration 41
  overdose, metabolic profile 40
  saliva 179
dichloromethane 233
2,4-dichlorophenoxyacetic acid (2,4-D) 232
diene products, quaternary ammonium compounds 100
dietary supplements, sports 269
difenacoum 100, *101*
difference spectrophotometry 405–6
differential spectrophotometers, carbon monoxide poisoning 234
diffuse reflectance, infrared spectroscopy 437
diffusion
  Einstein's equation 542
  postmortem redistribution 208
  into saliva 167
  into stomach 17, 196
diffusion coefficients, capillary electrophoresis 542
digestion *see* enzyme digestion
digital imaging, lateral flow immunoassays 386
digital processing, fluorescence spectrophotometry 416–17
digitoxin, blood : plasma ratios 213
digoxin 235, *240*
  blood : plasma ratios 213
  pharmacokinetics 252

fluorescence spectrophotometry (*continued*)
  sample management 416
fluorescent labels, immunoassays 385
fluoride 112, *241*
  on cocaine 198, 212
fluoride oxalate sample tubes 8
fluorine atom 573
fluorocarbons *81–2*
fluorograms 417
4-fluoro-7-nitro-2,1,3-benzoxadiazole, domoic acid derivatisation 124
fluorosilanes, HPLC 524
fluoxetine, metabolism *27*
fluphenazine, oral 41
fly agaric 119
Food and Drug Administration (FDA), immunoassays, workplace drug testing 140
forced diuresis 223
forensic chemistry 323–33
forensic identification 202–3
Forensic Science Service (FSS) 587
forensic toxicology 1–11
  clinical toxicology and 1–2, 223
formulations *see* pharmaceuticals
Fourier transform infrared detectors (FTIRD) 496
Fourier transform infrared spectroscopy 63–4
  gas chromatography with (GC-FTIR) 63, 440
    volatile substances 85
  instruments *see* interferometric spectrophotometers
  microscopy of hair 159
Fourier transform Raman spectroscopy 458–60
  quantification 466
Fourier transformation, ion cyclotron resonance mass spectrometers 567
FPIA *see* fluorescence polarisation immunoassay
FPN (reagent), TLC *358*
fractional clearance 20
free drug levels 251, 253–4
freezing, saliva samples 170
friction, electrophoresis 540
'front-end' steps, automated immunoassays 388
fronting, gas chromatography peaks 483, 508
frustum, PRISMA model of solvent systems in TLC 369–70
Frye hearings (USA) 314
fuel cells, breath-alcohol tests 312
fuel gases
  analysis 85–6
  cigarette lighter refills *81*, 82
  see also LPG
Fugu 127
Fujiwara test 337
functional group identification, Raman spectroscopy 462
functionalised polymers, solid-phase extraction 275
fundamental modes, molecular vibration 422
fungi, toxins 117–20
fungicides *92*
furfuraldehyde test 95
furocoumarins 121–2
furosemide *242*
  horseracing 266, 279–80
  volume of distribution 19
fused-silica cells, spectrophotometry 402
fused-silica columns, gas chromatography 471

β-galactosidase, *E. coli*, in CEDIA assay 387
gambierol 126
gamma-aminobutyric acid (GABA) 53–4
gamma-butyrolactone (GBL) 55, *294*
  conversion to GHB 75–6
  DFSA 293
    analysis 297
    street names and *291*
gamma-hydroxybutyric acid (GHB) 55, *242*
  analysis 75–6
  control status *45*
  DFSA 55, 290, *291*, 293–4, 297
  hair sampling 163
gamma-OH *see* gamma-hydroxybutyric acid
gas chromatography 61, *62*, 68–9, 469–511
  cannabis 72, 510
  choice of techniques 506–7
  in combinations 9
    see also specific combinations below
  combustion isotope ratio mass spectrometry with 561
    GHB in drug-facilitated sexual assault 297
  doping in sports 276
  ethanol 310, *311*
  forensic identification and 203
  Fourier transform infrared spectroscopy with (GC-FTIR) 63, 440
    volatile substances 85
  hair 159, 503
    mass spectrometry with 154, 158, 159
  infrared spectroscopy with 439–40
  limits of detection 205
  mass spectrometry with (GC-MS) 61, 67, 472, 480, 488, 558, 568
    anabolic steroids, horseracing 279
    detectors 496–7
    doping in sports 267, 276, 279
    forensic identification with 202
    hair 154, 158, 159
    after immunoassays 382
    library matching 579–81
    pesticides 96
    positive-ion chemical ionisation 577–8
    quantification 203
    saliva, confirmation testing 172
    total ion current chromatograms 572
    volatile substances 85
    workplace drug testing 140–1, 148
  quantification 64, 505–6
  screening 199
  therapeutic drug monitoring 253
  see also capillary columns, gas chromatography; headspace gas chromatography
gas–liquid chromatography 229
  psychotropic drugs 231
gas-phase derivatisation, thin-layer chromatography 357
gas pressure, gas chromatography 490–3
gaseous substances 7
  infrared spectroscopy 432
gasoline *see* petrol
gastric contents *see* stomach contents
gastrointestinal tract
  absorption via 14–15
    reduction 223
  metabolic reactions in 23
  poisoning on *225*
gel electrophoresis *599*, 600
gels, blood sample containers 115, 116, 224
'general unknown' approach, postmortem toxicology 199
genes 596
genomics 595–600
genotyping 596–7
  high-throughput 598
geography
  cocaine origins *66*
  pesticide poisonings *93–4*
germanium detectors, Raman spectroscopy 459
gestational exposure to drugs of abuse 164, 219, 256–60
giant hogweed 121–2
Giddings' resolution equation 542
GigaMatrix technology 592
gila monsters 128
Gilbert syndrome 32
glandular hairs, *Cannabis sativa* leaves 46, 71–2
glass bottles
  near infrared spectroscopy 448
  Raman spectroscopy 461
  solvent reservoirs for HPLC 516
glass cells, spectrophotometry 402
glass wool, injector liners, gas chromatography 486–7
glomerular filtration 21
glucose 6-phosphate dehydrogenase
  deficiency 113
  enzyme multiplied immunoassay technique 386
β-glucuronidase-sulfatase 235
glucuronidation 23
  morphine 23
  pharmacogenetics 32
glucuronides
  benzodiazepines 231
  ethanol 212, 317
  hydrolysis 200–1
glucuronosyltransferases (UGT1, UGT2), pharmacogenetics 32
glucuronyl transferase 23
glutamate, antagonism by phencyclidine 58
glutaric acid, hypoglycin poisoning 122
glutathione S-transferases, pharmacogenetics 32
glycols 230
gold, colloidal, saliva testing 171–2
gold-labelled antibodies, lateral flow methods 385–6

good laboratory practice (GLP) 621
Raman spectrometers 460
spectrophotometers 402, 404
gradient development, TLC 352–3
gradient elution, HPLC 526–7
gradient-thickness layers, preparative TLC 371
graphitised carbon black 472
gratings, scanning spectrofluorimeters 414
greyhounds, urine sampling 271, 272
growth hormone (GH), sports 280–1
guard columns
gas chromatography 480
HPLC 535
guidelines
quality standards 620–2
workplace drug testing 135, 137
see also HHS Guidelines
'gut dialysis' 223
Gutzeit test 110
gynaecomastia, androstenedione 52

haematocrit, sports 272
haematology, poisoning *227*
haemodialysis *see* dialysis
haemolysis, samples 18
haemoperfusion, efficiency 236–7
haemorrhage, from snakebite 128
haemostatic toxins 128
hair 8, 153–65
arsenic 104
DFSA victims 296
drug incorporation 155–6
gas chromatography 159, 503
mass spectrometry with 154, 158, 159
growth 154
sports 273
stability of drugs in 156
sweat *vs*, drug testing *182*
thallium 109
therapeutic drug monitoring 250
types 154–5
workplace drug testing 142, *144*
half-lives 20–1
concentrations at time zero 40
estimation of original dose 39
number to steady state 251
volatile substances 86
hallucinogenic mushrooms 119–20
hallucinogens, driving and 304–5
haloperidol, metabolism 28
halothane, pharmacokinetics *87*
haptenisation 378
hash oil 47
hashish *48*
HayeSep phases, gas chromatography 472
hazard (World Health Organization), pesticides 95
hCG (human chorionic gonadotropin) *268*, 269, 280
headspace gas chromatography
ethanol 310, *311*
heroin 74
purge and trap 503
volatile substances 84, 85, 89
headspace sampling 7
headspace solid-phase microextraction 85

heart, poisoning *225*
heart blood 194
postmortem redistribution into 208
sample quantities *192*
heat denaturation, samples 207
helium, for gas chromatography 492
hemlock 121
hemp, plants for production 46
Henderson–Hasselbalch equation, saliva 167–8
herbal cannabis 45
herbal products, identification 332
herbicides *92*
heroin (diamorphine) 49–50
analysis 74
control status *45*
electron-impact ionisation 575, *576*, 578
hair samples *158*, 160
in utero exposure 257
Marquis reagent test 61
metabolism 29, 35
metabolites 23
oral deposition 168
postmortem redistribution 210
saliva 175
sweat *182*
syringes at scene 197
thin-layer chromatography 69
time after administration 38
heterocyclic compounds, insecticides *92*
heterogeneous immunoassays 376, 382–6
alternative samples 389
hexanal 89
hexane *81–2*
partitioning, sample extracts 202
TLC 369
hexane–acetone TLC system, pesticides *367*
hexane–methanol extraction, anabolic steroids 52
hexobarbital, saliva 178
HHS Guidelines 136–43
proposed changes (2004) 141–3
high-performance liquid chromatography 61–3, 69, 513–37
cannabis 72
capillary electrophoresis *vs* 545
in combinations 9, 520–1
fluorescence spectrophotometry with 414–15
hair 159
infrared spectroscopy with 440–1, 521
ion-interaction HPLC, *Amanita* mushroom alkaloids 119
mass spectrometry with (LC-MS) 9, 520, 558, 568–70, 581–2
data processing 572, 573
doping in sports 276–7, 281
libraries 584–5
pesticides 97
quantification 203
tuning mixtures 573
pesticides 97
phases used in capillary electrochromatography 545
quantification 64
amfetamines 71

reagents 341–3
screening 199, 229–30
solvent effects 409
for spectrophotometry 395
speed 530
tandem electrospray mass spectrometry with
ciguatoxin 126
doping in sports 276–7
therapeutic drug monitoring 253
thin-layer chromatography *vs* 345–6
see also tandem mass spectrometry
high-performance thin-layer chromatography 344, 345
high-speed/high-temperature HPLC 528
high-throughput genotyping 598
high-throughput screening (HTS) 590–4
Hillory J. Farias and Samantha Reid Date-Rape Drug Prohibition Act (2000) 290
hippurate, as metabolite *88*
histamine, scombroid poisoning 127
histidine, analysis for 127
historical aspects 2
capillary electrophoresis 539
concentrations *vs* therapeutic effects 247
DFSA 289–90
doping in sport 263
drugs of abuse 43
immunoassays 377
solid dosage forms 323–4
thin-layer chromatography *345*
workplace drug testing 136
history of drug abuse, hair analysis 162, 163–4
hogweed, giant 121–2
hold-up time (t_M), gas chromatography 481
holocyclotoxins 125
homogeneous immunoassays 376, 386–8
non-isotopic 253
homogenisation
postmortem toxicology samples 200
samples of seized drugs 60
horizontal chambers, TLC development 354–5
horizontal gaze nystagmus 306, *309*
hormones, prohibited in sports *265*
horseracing, doping 264–7, 269–70
anabolic steroids 278–9
criteria for confirmatory testing 277–8
furosemide 266, 279–80
growth hormone 280–1
hair samples 273
historical aspects 263
screening 273–6
urine sampling 271, 272
horseradish peroxidase
cotinine labelling 380
substrate reagents 384
hospital pharmacists, role in solid dose identification 330
hospital toxicology *see* clinical toxicology
HPLC *see* high-performance liquid chromatography
human chorionic gonadotropin (hCG) *268*, 269, 280

hybridisation 594
hybridoma cells, monoclonal antibodies from 379
hydride-generation systems 110
hydrocarbons *81*
hydrochloric acid
cannabis analysis 71
solubilisation of drugs in hair 157
TLC systems using *366*
hydrocodone *242*
metabolism, enzyme deficiency 31
workplace drug testing *139*
hydrocortisone
electron-impact ionisation 578
ultraviolet *vs* infrared spectra 424
hydrodynamic injection, capillary electrophoresis 547
hydrogen, for gas chromatography 507
hydrogen-bonding interactions, gas chromatography 475–6
hydrogen cyanide 111–12
hydrogen phosphide 100, 113–14
hydrogen sulfide 114
hydrolysis
benzodiazepines 499, 509–10
drugs in hair 157
for gas chromatography 498–9
before GC-MS 382
glucuronides 200–1
urine
doping in sports 273
drugs of abuse 235
hydromorphone *242*
saliva 175
workplace drug testing *139*
α-hydroxyalprazolam, workplace drug testing *139*
α-hydroxybutyric acid (AHB) 297
β-hydroxybutyric acid (BHB) 297
para-hydroxycocaine, saliva 177
4-hydroxy-3-methoxymethamfetamine (HMMA), saliva 178
9α-hydroxyprogesterone, HPLC and spectrophotometry *395*
Hymenoptera 125
hyperchromic effect 409
hypergeometric distribution, seized drug sampling 60
hyphenated techniques *see* coupled techniques
hypochlorites 112–13
hypochromic effect 409
hypoglycaemia 197
children, ethanol 230
hypoglycin 122

iatrogenic intoxications 221, 223
ibotenic acid 119
ichthyosarcotoxism *see* fish
ICP-MS *see* inductively coupled plasma mass spectrometry
IDENTIDEX (database) 332
identification of routes of administration 41
identification of samples 611
identification of substances 8
capillary electrophoresis 550
for courts 202–3
GC-MS 579–80
infrared spectroscopy 441–2
metabolites 582
Raman spectroscopy 464–6
solid dosage forms 323–33
see also systematic toxicological identification
illicit tablets 323, 325
compressed 325–6
drug analysis 533–4
see also 'ecstasy' tablets
image analysers, scanning densitometry 359
imaging
digital, lateral flow immunoassays 386
magnetic resonance
endoscopy with *602*
see also nuclear magnetic resonance spectroscopy
near infrared 453
Raman spectroscopy 465
imipramine *242*
metabolism 27
postmortem redistribution *209*
Immulite system (DPC) 385
immunisation
programmes for antibody production 380
snakebites 129
immuno-chromatographic assays 385–6
immunoassays 7, 61, 375–91
clinical toxicology, screening 227–9
doping in sports 277
driving impairment 319–20
drugs in hair 158–9
microfluidics *598*
roadside test strips 308
saliva 171
specificity 9, 380–2
therapeutic drug monitoring 252–3, 377
workplace drug testing 140
see also cross-reactivity of immunoassays; fluorescence polarisation immunoassay; radioimmunoassay
immunochromatography, saliva 171–2
immunoglobulins 377
immunosuppressive drugs, pharmacodynamic monitoring 255
impairment, psychomotor *see* drivers/driving; psychomotor impairment
imports, parallel 324
impressions on tablets 51, *52*, 65
impurities
amfetamines 71
cocaine 72
GC-MS, profiling 580–1
heroin 74
internal standards 618
see also adulterants
in-house reference materials 206
in-process performance monitoring 616–18
in utero exposure to drugs of abuse 164, 219, 256–60
incremental multiple development, TLC 353
incubation periods, microplate antibody capture 383, 384
indecent assault 287
see also drug-facilitated sexual assault
indicators, TLC 346, 357
indirect detection, capillary electrophoresis 548, *549*
indole alkaloids, hallucinogenic mushrooms 120
indometacin, Raman spectroscopy 467
induction of metabolism, drug interactions 31
inductively coupled plasma emission spectrometry (ICP-AES) 110
inductively coupled plasma mass spectrometry (ICP-MS) 110, 558–9, 571–2
borates 111
industrial accidents, sampling for anions 115
inelastic scattering 456
inertial spray mass spectroscopy 85
information sources, clinical toxicology 237
information technology *see* computers
infrared absorption, breath-alcohol tests 312
infrared microscopy, hair 159
infrared spectroscopy 421–54
cocaine 72, *73*
data processing 428
HPLC with 440–1, 521
Raman spectroscopy with 462
see also Fourier transform infrared spectroscopy
inhomogeneity, samples 610
injection sites
enzymatic digestion of samples 200
postmortem toxicology 197
injections, absorption of substances 15
injector discrimination, gas chromatography 490, *491*
injectors
capillary electrophoresis 547
see also short-end injection
gas chromatography 483–90, 508
HPLC 517, 526
inlet systems
gas chromatography 483–93
see also injectors
inorganic oxide layers, TLC 350
insect stings 125
insecticides *92*
see also pesticides
inspections, laboratories for workplace drug testing 141
insulin
electrospray ionisation 569
syringes at scene 197
insulin-like growth factor 1 (IGF-1) 280–1
interaction capillary electrophoresis 543–4
Intercept saliva-sampling device 169
interferometric spectrophotometers 426–7
calibration 429–30
Raman spectroscopy 458–60
scan speeds 431
interindividual pharmacodynamic variability 248, 249
internal audit 608
internal quality control 616–18
internal standards 618

calibration of HPLC 529
gas chromatography 505
mass spectrometry 583
postmortem toxicology 204
quantification of seized drugs 64
thin-layer chromatography 359
International Agreement on Breeding, Racing and Wagering (IABRW) 264–6
International Conference on Harmonisation (ICH), validation of spectrophotometry 411
International Laboratory Accreditation Co-operation (ILAC) 278
International Standards, World Anti-Doping Agency (WADA) 271, 622
Internet, pharmacy trading 324
interpretation of findings
colour tests 340
ethanol 313–14
mass spectrometry 574–8
postmortem toxicology 207–16
quality control 618
spectrophotometry 407–11
workplace drug testing 147–8
Intoximeter 312
intramuscular injections 15
intraoral cups 170
intravenous infusions, postmortem redistribution from 209
invertebrates 122–5
involuntary ingestion of drugs, DFSA victims 289
iodine-125, radioimmunoassay 384
iodine vapour method, TLC 357
ion cyclotron resonance mass spectrometers 567
ion-exchange, dynamic 533
ion-exchange chromatography 515
ion-exchange extraction, gas chromatography 500
ion-interaction HPLC, *Amanita* mushroom alkaloids 119
ion-pair chromatography, reversed-phase 532–3
ion-pair extraction 515
doping in sports 274
gas chromatography 500
ion ratios, GC-MS 141
ion suppression 521
therapeutic drug monitoring 252
ion-trap mass spectrometers 497, 565–6
identification of metabolites 582
ionisation
fluorescence spectrophotometry 417
mass spectrometry 558, 559, 562, 566
iproniazid, metabolite 23
iron 106, *242*
analysis methods *102*
poisoning emergencies *228*
ISO standards 620, 621
dope testing 278
isocratic technique, HPLC 526
isoelectric focusing method
capillary electrophoresis (cIEF) 544–5
erythropoietin 280
isomers
amfetamines 45, 70–1
gamma-hydroxybutyric acid 297
methamfetamine 148
see also stereoselective analysis
isoniazid *242*
acetylation 34
poisoning emergencies *228*
isooctyl esters, chlorinated phenoxy acids 99
isopropanol, postmortem toxicology 212
isotachophoresis, capillary (cITP) 544, 545
isotope(s)
GC-MS 141
mass spectrometry 560–1
internal standards 583
thin-layer chromatography 359
isotope-coded affinity tagging (ICAT) 600
isotope ratio mass spectrometry
doping in sports 277
regions of origin of seized drugs 65, *66*
isoxsuprine, horseracing 269
itai-itai disease 105

Jamaican vomiting sickness 122
Japan, cadmium poisoning 105
jellyfish 124
Joule heating 540–1

Keeler Weed *see* phencyclidine
ketamine, DFSA *293*, 294–5
ketosis 89
khat 55–6, 69, 76
kidney
clearance 20
excretion 21–2
postmortem toxicology 197
kidney disease
metabolism of benzodiazepines 25
from non-steroidal anti-inflammatory drugs 233
pharmacokinetics 33
from poisoning *225*
from snakebite 128
KIMS assay 388
workplace drug testing 140
kits, immunoassays 253, 389
Kubelka–Munk transformations 437

labelling
packages, anabolic steroids 52
postmortem toxicology samples 192, 194
labetalol, UV spectra 588, 589
laboratories
clandestine 68
clinical toxicology 220
horseracing, criteria for confirmatory testing 277–8
management of facilities 620
postmortem toxicology 191, 192
proficiency testing 206
quality control and assessment 608, 616–22
accreditation 278, 609, 622
proficiency testing 206
volatile substance analysis 83
workplace drug testing 137, 141
'laboratory on a chip' 594
Lambert's law 396
large-volume injectors, gas chromatography 487–8
laser-induced fluorescence detectors, capillary electrophoresis 547–8, *549*
lasers, Raman spectroscopy 457–8
lateral flow methods, immunoassays 385–6
latex particles, immunoassays 388
lathyrism 122
α-latrotoxins 125
lead *102*, 106–7, *242*
leak testing, gas chromatography columns 479
Legally Defensible Workplace Drugs Testing, UK Laboratory Guidelines for (2001) 621–2
legislation
alcohol, drugs and driving 4, 305–6, 314
drug-facilitated sexual assault (USA) 289–90
drugs of abuse 44
solid dose identification 324
lethal concentrations of substances 36
Leuckart reaction 44–5, *46*
libraries
LC-MS 584–5
proteomics 585
spectra for GC-MS of pesticides 96
see also databases
library matching, identification of substances by GC-MS 579–80
lidocaine (lignocaine) *242*, *268*, 269
lifestyle drugs 324
light
percentage transmittance 397, 423
wavelengths 396
see also absorbance
light pipes, infrared spectroscopy 432
limit of detection (LOD) 205–6, 613
capillary electrophoresis 550
limit of quantification 613
linear development, TLC 352
linearity 613
fluorescence spectrophotometry 418
spectrophotometry 410–11
liners, gas chromatography injection systems 484, 485–7
Lion Intoxilyzer 312
lipophilicity, drugs in saliva 171
liquid(s)
infrared spectroscopy 432–3
seized drugs 58, 68
volatile, analysis 85–6
liquid chromatography
with diode-array detector (LC-DAD) 401
see also high-performance liquid chromatography; tandem mass spectrometry
liquid crystal tuneable filter technology, tablet mapping 465–6
liquid ecstasy *see* gamma-hydroxybutyric acid
liquid-filled capsules 328
liquid/liquid extraction
for gas chromatography 499–500
pesticide GC-MS 96
postmortem toxicology samples 201
screening for sports doping 274

liquid paraffin
  fluorescence-quenching technique, TLC 358
  mulls 434–5
liquid petroleum gas (LPG) *81–2*
  deaths 82
liquid stationary phases
  gas chromatography 472–6
  HPLC 514–15
list lengths, TLC screening 360–1
lithium *102*, 107–8, *242*, 252
  poisoning emergencies *228*
  therapeutic drug monitoring 251–2
lithium tantalite detectors 426
liver
  activation of drugs 16
  drug concentrations 39
    routes of administration and 41
  metabolism in 23
  poisoning *227*
    paracetamol 232
  postmortem toxicology 195, 213–14
    ethanol 212
    sample quantities *192*
liver disease
  copper 105–6
  metabolism of benzodiazepines 25
  pharmacokinetics 33
'Living Chip' technology 592
logging, postmortem toxicology samples 192
Logo Index 332
logos on tablets 51, *52*, 65
logs for instruments 620
lorazepam, DFSA cases *291*
LPG (liquid petroleum gas) *81–2*
  deaths 82
LSD *see* lysergide
luminol, chemiluminescence immunoassays 385
lungs
  absorption of substances 15
  beryllium 104, 115
luteinising hormone 279
lychee fruit seeds, hypoglycin 122
lysergic acid 51
  analysis 74–5
  thin-layer chromatography 69
lysergide 50–1, *243*
  control status *45*
  dosage forms 325, 329
  gas chromatography 510
  paper squares 51, 74, 329, *330*
  workplace drug testing 139–40

M&Ms (chocolate drops) 329–30
M1 (tramadol metabolite) 29
mackerel, scombroid poisoning 127
magnetic beads, separation step, radioimmunoassay 385
magnetic resonance imaging
  endoscopy with *602*
  see also nuclear magnetic resonance spectroscopy
magnetic sector mass spectrometers 563–4
maintenance of apparatus
  gas chromatography 507
  HPLC 525–6
maitotoxin 126
Mandatory Guidelines for Drug Testing of Federal Employees (HHS) 136
Mandatory Guidelines for Federal Workplace Drug Testing Programs 621
Mandelin reagent *358*
manufacturers, role in solid dose identification 330
mapping, tablets, Raman spectroscopy 465–6
marijuana *see* cannabis
Marquis reagent, TLC *358*
Marquis reagent test 61, 336, 337–9
  amfetamines 61, 70, 75
  methylenedioxymethylamfetamine 75
  opiates 61, 74
masking agents, prohibited in sports *265*
masks, alkali halide discs 435
mass analysers 558
mass axis, calibration 573
mass sector analysers 572
mass spectra 559, 560
mass spectrometry 61, 557–85
  amfetamines 70
  capillary electrophoresis with 9, 548, *549*, 571
  complex mixture analysis 600
  doping in sports 277
  inductively coupled plasma emission spectrometry 110
  therapeutic drug monitoring 253
  see also under gas chromatography; high-performance liquid chromatography; isotope ratio mass spectrometry
masses, tissue, postmortem 214
maternal drug abuse *see in utero* exposure
matrix assisted laser desorption ionisation (MALDI) 566
  MS libraries based on 585
  proteomics 600
matrix effects
  immunoassays 389
  postmortem toxicology samples 207
Maxalt melts 329
maximum residue limits, drug testing for horseracing 267
McReynolds constants, gas chromatography 476, *477–8*
mean list length, TLC screening 360–1
measurement uncertainty 614–15
meconium 227, 256, 257–60
medical review officers, workplace drug testing 146–7
medication counts 215
mefenorex, amfetamines from 26
Megabore direct injection, gas chromatography 484
melanin, drug trapping in hair 155, 162
melts 329
membrane immuno-bead assay, ciguatoxin 126
meprobamate, DFSA *293*
Merck Tox Screening System 361
mercury 108, *243*
  analysis methods *102*
  selenium, protection 109
mescaline 58
metabolism of substances 13, 22–9
  anabolic steroids 279
  drug interactions 30–1
  ethanol 300–1
  in liver 16, 23
  postmortem toxicology 215
  tolerance 37
metabolites 22–3, 35–6
  active 249
  benzodiazepines 24, 33
  concentration ratios with drugs 39, 40
    routes of administration 41
  cross-reactions of immunoassays 381–2
  detection in DFSA 32
  doping in sports 273
  fetus 258
  LC-MS to identify 582
  toxicity 33–4
  volatile substances 86–9
metals (and metal compounds) 7, 101–11
  fungicides *92*
  mass spectrometry 558–9
  tests for 234
metaraminol, sensitivity of analytical methods, horseracing 270
methadone *243*
  accumulation 22
  colour test reagents *342*
  metabolism 29
  saliva 176
  workplace drug testing *139*
    cut-off values *138*
methaemoglobin, poisoning emergencies *228*
methamfetamine 45, *243*
  'artefact' 138–9
  in clandestine laboratories 68
  DFSA cases *293*
  hair 160
  in utero exposure 256, 257
  isomers 148
  Leuckart reaction *46*
  Marquis reagent test 61
  saliva 178
  workplace drug testing 138–9
    with alternative specimens *143*
    assay 140
    oral fluid 142
    reporting rule 147–8
    sweat 142
methandienone, sports, reporting rates *268*
methanol 212, 230, *243*
  eluents for HPLC 531–2
  as metabolite *88*
  poisoning emergencies *228*
  TLC systems using *362*, *363*, *365*, *366*
methaqualone *243*
  renal excretion 21
  workplace drug testing *138*, *139*
methcathinone, analogues 56
methenolone, sports, reporting rates *268*
methotrexate, poisoning emergencies *228*
8-methoxypsoralen 122
methyl bromide 111
N-methyl-D-aspartate receptors

antagonism by phencyclidine 58
ketamine on *294*
methyl mercury 108
methyl salicylate 233
methylation, pharmacogenetics 32
N-methylbis(trifluoroacetamide) (MBTFA) 70
methylchloroformate (MCF) 505
methylchlorophenoxyacetic acid (MCPA) 232
methylene (CH_2 group), molecular vibration 422, 463–4
methylenedioxyamfetamine (MDA) *52*
poisoning emergencies *228*
saliva 178
urine levels for DFSA cases *293*
workplace drug testing 137, 138
alternative specimens *143*
immunoassays 140
methylenedioxyethylamfetamine (MDEA) *52*
workplace drug testing 137, 138, 140
methylenedioxymethylamfetamine (MDMA) 51–2, *243*
analysis 75
control status *45*
hair *158*, 160
metabolism 25–6
poisoning emergencies *228*
saliva 178
thin-layer chromatography 69
workplace drug testing 137, 138, 139
alternative specimens *143*
immunoassays 140
methylephedrine, sports *266*
N-methyl-1-(3,4-methylenedioxphenyl)-2-butanamine (MDBD), saliva 178
2-methylphenol, as metabolite *88*, 90
4-methylumbelliferyl phosphate, fluorescence immunoassays 385
Metropolitan Police (UK), 'Early evidence kits' 297
micellar electrokinetic capillary chromatography (MEKC; MECC) 544, 549–50, 552, 554
Michaelis–Menten kinetics 39
micro-cells, infrared spectroscopy 432
micro total-analysis systems (mTASs) 594
microarrays 594–5, *596*
microbore columns, HPLC 522
microcapillaries, TLC 351
microdialysis 600–1
microdiscs, alkali halide 435
microdots, LSD 325
microemulsion electrokinetic capillary chromatography (MEEKC) 544
microfluidics 595, *598*
microparticle methods, immunoassays 388
microplate antibody capture 382–4
automated systems 388
microscopy
Cannabis sativa 71–2
hair 159
near infrared imaging 453
Raman spectroscopy 459, 465
microsomal enzymes 23
microsublimation 441
microtitre plates 592
midazolam *243*
brain death 222
glucuronide 231
minibore columns, HPLC 522
Minimata disease 108
miosis, opiate saliva concentration time course 175
mislabelling, anabolic steroids 52
Mitsubishi logo *52*, 65
mixed-mode cartridges, solid-phase extraction 275
mobility (electrophoretic) 540, 541–2
molar absorption coefficients 397, 588
see also hyperchromic effect
molar extinction coefficients 423
molecular fluorescence 411–12
molecular sieves 472
molecular vibration 421–3, 462–4
molecules, virtual states 456
molluscicides *92*
molluscs 122–4
monitoring *see* therapeutic drug monitoring
monoacetylmorphine (MAM)
hair 160
saliva 175
vitreous humour 194
workplace drug testing *138*, 139, 148
alternative specimens *143*
oral fluid 142
sweat 142
monoamine oxidase inhibitors, drug interactions 30
monoamine transmission, ketamine on *294*
monochromators
infrared spectrometers 425
scanning spectrofluorimeters 414
spectrophotometers 399
monoclonal antibodies, immunoassays 379
monoene products, quaternary ammonium compounds 100
monolithic columns, HPLC 525
morphine *243*
analogues, metabolism 28–9
in bile 38
extraction from postmortem toxicology samples 201
glucuronidation 23
hair 153–5, 160
haptenisation 378
hydrolysis of glucuronide 200
liver : blood ratios 41
postmortem 213
redistribution 210
saliva 175
sports *266*
workplace drug testing *138*, 139
alternative specimens *143*
mortality, flunitrazepam 290
Morton–Stubbs method, spectrophotometry 394, 404–5
moulded tablets 325
mouth alcohol 311, 313
'moving needle' injectors, gas chromatography 489–90
trans,trans-muconate, as metabolite *88*
mucoproteins, saliva 168
mulls 434–5
multi-eluate approach, solid-phase extraction 275
multidrug resistance genes 31
multiple development, TLC 352, 353
chambers 355, *356*
multipoint calibration 204
multisectional analysis, hair 162
multiwavelength UV spectrophotometry 587–90
Munchausen's syndrome by proxy 223
murder, volatile substances and 83
muscimol 119
muscle function, poisoning *225*
muscle relaxants, driving and *302*
mushrooms
hallucinogenic 119–20
Psilocybe 56, 76, 120
mycotoxins 117–20

NADPH-methaemoglobin reductase deficiency 113
nandrolone
horses 278
reporting rates in sports *267*, *268*
nanobore columns, HPLC 523
NanoChip Cartridge and Microelectronic Array *596*
nasal swabs, postmortem toxicology 197
National Institute on Drug Abuse (NIDA)
Guidelines 136
survey of drug use in pregnancy 257
National Laboratory Certification Program (NLCP) 141, 621
National Pregnancy and Health Survey, drug use in pregnancy 257
near infrared imaging 453
near infrared spectroscopy 448–53
necropsy
samples for volatile substances 84
see also postmortem toxicology
negative chemical ionisation, hair
benzodiazepines 161
cannabis 160–1
negative-ion analysis mode, mass spectrometry 559
negative-ion chemical ionisation (NICI) 578, *579*
nematocides *92*
nematocysts 124
neonates
drug metabolism 32–3
hair analysis 164
meconium 227, 256, 257–60
tetanus mortality 117
withdrawal symptoms 256
neurological signs, poisoning *225*
neurotransmitters, ketamine on 294
neutral drugs
driving under the influence 320
extraction 200, 202
horse urine 275
separation from basic and acidic drugs 361–4
nicotinamide–adenine dinucleotide, enzyme multiplied immunoassay technique 386
nicotine, gestational exposure 164
NIDA *see* National Institute on Drug Abuse

ninhydrin, TLC *358*
nitrates 113
nitrazepam, saliva 179
nitrites 82, 113
  analysis 89
  deceptive specimens for workplace drug testing 145
  as metabolite *88*
nitrogen, for gas chromatography 492, 507
nitrogen isotope ratios, regions of origin of seized drugs 65
nitrogen–phosphorus detectors (NPD), gas chromatography 199, 494, 497
nitrogen rule 560
nitrophenols 99
nitroterephthalic acid-substituted polyethylene glycols 474
nitrous oxide
  pharmacokinetics *87*
  thermal conductivity detection 84
nomenclature, pesticides 90
non-conditioned SPE, horse urine 275
non-steroidal anti-inflammatory drugs 232, 233, 266, 269
19-norandrosterone *266*
norclozapine 28
norcocaine
  hair specimens 157
  metabolites 26
  saliva 177
nordiazepam *240, 242, 243, 244, 245*
  saliva 179
  urine levels for DFSA cases *291*
  workplace drug testing *139*
normal phase chromatography 514, 515
11-nor-Δ^9-THC carboxylic acid (THC-COOH)
  estimating time after substance administration 38–9
  hair 160
Norway, drink and driving 305
nose swabs, postmortem toxicology 197
nuclear magnetic resonance spectroscopy 9–10, 64
  HPLC with 521
Nujol
  infrared spectrum 445, *446*
  see also liquid paraffin
nutrients, abuse in sports 264, 269

observed collections, workplace drug testing 146
occupation
  aluminium exposure 103
  copper toxicity 106
  place of 7
ochratoxin-A 118
octadecyl silica (ODS) 523, 532–3
octanol-water coefficients 18
odour test, cocaine 72
odours
  hydrogen sulfide 114
  poisoned patients *226*
  scene of crime 5–7
okadaic acid 123
olanzapine *244*
  metabolism 28
    enzyme deficiency 31
Olympic Games (ancient), substance abuse 263
on-line sample preparation, HPLC 518, 530
On-Site Saliva Alcohol Assay 175
on-site testing, saliva 171–2
  ethanol 174–5
opiates
  abuse 43
  antibody production 378
  gas chromatography 510
  hair 160
  in utero exposure 256, 257
  Marquis reagent test 61, 74
  metabolism 28–9
  poisoning emergencies *228*
  presumptive results 9
  prohibited in sports *265*
  saliva 175–6
  tolerance 36
  workplace drug testing 137, 138, 139, *142, 143*, 148
opioid receptors, heroin action 50
opium 49
  alkaloids 'cutting' heroin 50
optical immunoassays 376
optical isomers
  separation by HPLC 527–8
  see also stereoselective analysis
optimisation for polar compounds, TLC systems 370
oral administration
  absorption via 14–15, 37
  bioavailability 16
  metabolite concentration ratios 41
  volumes of distribution 18
oral deposition of drugs 168
oral fluid 8, 165–81
  driving impairment 317, 319
  ethanol 313
  workplace drug testing 142, *144*
  see also saliva
OraSure system, saliva samples 170
organic non-volatile substances 7
organic silanes 523
organophosphorus compounds 90, *92*, 97–8, 231–2
  cholinesterase measurement 222–3
  screening tests 95
  structures *91*
  thin-layer chromatography 96
osmol gap, serum, alcohols 230
osmolality of serum *228*
  alcohols 230
ouch-ouch disease 105
out-of-competition sampling, anabolic steroids 279
outliers (random errors) 615
overdosage 231
  abuse *vs* 44
  brain death after 222
  mixed 236
  pharmacokinetics 40–1
  postmortem redistribution 210
  stomach contents and 196
overtones
  molecular vibration 422
  near infrared spectroscopy 448
oxalate 113
  as metabolite *88*
  see also fluoride oxalate sample tubes
β-*N*-oxalylamino-L-alanine (BOAA) 122
oxazepam 231, *244*
  urine levels for DFSA cases *291*
  workplace drug testing *139*
oxidants, QED Saliva Alcohol Test 174
oxidative metabolism 24–9
oxidising agents, alkali halide disc IR spectroscopy 436
2-oxo-3-hydroxy LSD, workplace drug testing 140
oxprenolol, impurity profiling 580–1
oxycodone 235, *244*
  metabolism 29
    enzyme deficiency 31

P-glycoprotein 31
packaging of samples 611
packing materials *see* stationary phases
pain, chronic, drugs prescribed for 301–3
paint stripper *81*
paint thinners *81*
paper squares, lysergide 51, 74, 329, *330*
paracetamol 232–3, *244*
  gas chromatography of heroin 74
  infrared spectrum 441, *446*
  poisoning emergencies *228*
  toxicity 32, 33–4
parallel imports 324
paraquat 99–100, 232, *244*
  gastrointestinal absorption 15
  poisoning emergencies *228*
parathion, toxic metabolite 33
parotid gland, saliva from 166
  ethanol 173
partition chromatography 514–15
partition coefficients, volatile substances 86, *87*
partitioning, sample extracts 202
passive exposure
  hair false positives 156
  marijuana smoke, saliva negative 180
  workplace drug test positives from 148–9
patches
  sweat patches 181–3
  see also transdermal dosage forms
PCP *see* phencyclidine
peak efficiency, capillary electrophoresis 542–3
peak shape
  gas chromatography 483, 506, 508
  GC-MS, workplace drug testing 141
  spatial peak area, capillary electrophoresis detectors 548
penises, false 272
pentobarbital *244, 246*
  brain death 222
  liver : blood ratios 41
  saliva 178
  workplace drug testing *139*
peptide hormones, sports 280–1
  drugs prohibited *265, 269*
peptide mass fingerprinting 600
'per se' concentration limits, driving and 306, 313
percentage transmittance (light) 397
  infrared 423
perfluorotributylamine (PFTBA), calibration of mass spectrometers 562, 573
performance-enhancing drugs, hair 161, 164–5

performance monitoring, in-process 616–18
performance testing *see* proficiency testing
periodate, 'methamfetamine artefact' prevention 139
peripheral blood, postmortem toxicology, sample quantities *192*
peritoneal dialysis 223
permethrin 99
pesticides 7, 90–101
  containers 80
  hair 162
  nitrogen–phosphorus detectors 494
  systematic toxicological identification 364
    systems *367*
pethidine, metabolism 29
petrol *81–2*
  abuse rates 82
PFTBA (perfluorotributylamine), calibration of mass spectrometers 562, 573
pH
  deceptive specimens for workplace drug testing 145
  fluorescence spectrophotometry 417
  HPLC
    eluents 516, 519, 532
    packing materials 524
  saliva 167, 168
    collection on 170
  spectrophotometry 398, 409–10
  thin-layer chromatography 341–3
  urine 21–2
    therapeutic altering 223
phage display 379
phallotoxins 119–20
pharmaceutical manufacturers, role in solid dose identification 330
pharmaceuticals
  drug analysis 533–4, 554
  impurity profiling 580–1
  sample size 610
pharmacists, role in solid dose identification 330
pharmacodynamics 13, 248
  interindividual variability 248, 249
  monitoring 255–6
pharmacogenetics 31–2, 215, 255–6
  N-acetyltransferases 34
pharmacogenomics 255
pharmacokinetics 13–22, 34–42, 248
  clinical toxicology 236
  clonazepam 295
  digoxin 252
  ethanol, saliva 173
  liver and kidney disease on 33
  postmortem 36, 194, 208–14
  postmortem toxicology 214–15
  software packages 237
  volatile substances 86, *87*, *88*
pharmacological response, drug concentrations *vs* 35
Phases I and II, metabolism 23
phenacetin, toxic metabolite 33
phencyclidine (PCP) 56–8, *245*
  colour test reagents *342*
  control status *45*
  DFSA, urine levels *293*
  gas chromatography 510
  saliva 180–1
  workplace drug testing 137, 138, *142*, 147
    alternative specimens *143*
    GC-MS 141
phenethylamines 56, *57*
  see also methylenedioxymethylamfetamine
phenobarbital *245*
  saliva 178, 179
  spectrophotometry, pH 398
  tolerance 37
  workplace drug testing *139*
phenols
  colour test reagents *342*
  fluorescence spectrophotometry 417
  spectra 398
phenothiazines
  colour test reagents *343*
  metabolism 27–8
  urine, postmortem 195
phenoxy acids
  substituted 99
  see also chlorinated phenoxy acids
phenyl groups, silica-based materials for HPLC 523
phenyl substitution, polysiloxanes for gas chromatography 473
phenylbutazone *245*
  overdose, metabolites 40
phenylpropanolamine *245*
  sports, reporting rates *268*
phenytoin *245*
  doses *vs* concentrations 37
  saliva 178
pholcodine, saliva 176
phosphate buffers, HPLC 532
phosphate washes, hair specimens 156
phosphides *92*, 100, 113–14
phosphine 100, 113–14
phosphors, up-converting, saliva testing 172
phosphorus, detectors for gas chromatography 494
phosphorus test 95
photobleaching, Raman spectroscopy 461
photodiodes 400
  see also diode-array detectors
photons, energy levels 395–6
phycotoxins 122
Physalia physalis 124
physical examination, seized drugs 58–9
physical signs
  drivers under the influence 306, 318–19
  poisoning 224, *225*
pills 324
pink disease 108
piperazines 56, *245*
pipettes 199
  automated immunoassays 388
pit vipers 128
placenta 258
Planck's equation 421
plants, products 120–2
plasma concentrations 17–18
  blood concentrations *vs* 213
  clinical toxicology 224
  dose *vs* 214
  ethanol 310
  saliva concentrations *vs* 167–8
  therapeutic drug monitoring 250–1
  validity of tests 35
plasma esterases 23
plasma flow, to kidneys 21
plastics, volatile substances and 83
plates
  high-throughput screening 592
  thin-layer chromatography 346–9
  preparative 371
  see also microplate antibody capture
platinic chloride *358*
point-of-care testing *see* field tests; roadside testing; workplace drug testing
point-of-collection testing *see* on-site testing
poison hemlock 121
poisoning *see* clinical toxicology
poisons, definition 2
polar compounds, optimisation, TLC systems 370
polar eluents, HPLC 531–2
polar phases, polysiloxanes for gas chromatography 473–4
polarisability, Raman spectroscopy 457, 462
polarity
  gas chromatography 476
  HPLC 532
police
  colour tests 336
  'Early evidence kits' 297
  solid dosage form identification 331
Polo Mints, 'holes' 324
polyclonal antisera 379
polyethylene glycols, for gas chromatography *473*, 474
polyimide coatings
  gas chromatography columns 471
  heat on 480
polymer(s)
  functionalised, solid-phase extraction 275
  for gas chromatography 472
polymer-based packing materials, HPLC 524–5
polymerase chain reaction, microfluidics *598*
polymorphism (molecular)
  infrared spectroscopy and 445–6
  Raman spectroscopy and 464, *465*
polymorphisms (genetic) 255–6
  cytochrome P450 enzymes 31
polysiloxanes, for gas chromatography 472–4
poppy-seed ingestion 148, 163, 176
Porapak, gas chromatography 472
porous layer open tubular columns (PLOT columns), gas chromatography 471–2
  volatile substances 85
Portuguese man-of-war 124
positive-ion chemical ionisation (PICI) 577–8
postmortem redistribution of substances 36, 194, 208–14
postmortem toxicology 191–217
  analysis of samples 198–207
  ethanol 317

postmortem toxicology (*continued*)
gamma-hydroxybutyric acid 297
interpretation of results 207–16
limited specimen volume 207
postmortem validity, blood concentrations 35
potassium bromide, discs for infrared spectroscopy 435
potassium chlorate 111
potassium ferric hexacyanoferrate 109
potassium permanganate, TLC *358*
powders
near infrared spectroscopy 449, 450
seized drugs 58, 67
power supplies, capillary electrophoresis 546
pre-equilibration, TLC *355*
preadsorbent zones, TLC 351
preparative 371
precision 614
precursor ion scanning, tandem mass spectrometry 567
prednisolone
electron-impact ionisation 577
quantification by mass spectrometry 583
pregnancy, drugs of abuse 164, 219, 256–60
preparative columns, HPLC 522
preparative thin-layer chromatography 371–2
prescriptions, workplace drug testing and 147
preservation of samples
quality control 611
saliva 170–1
preservatives, volatile substances as 84
presses, alkali halide discs 435
pressure, gas chromatography 490–3
presumptive results 9
pretreatments of layers, TLC 350
primidone, metabolite 23
principal components analysis, near infrared spectroscopy 451, *452*
printing, on capsules 327
see also logos on tablets
PRISMA model, solvent systems in TLC 369–70
prisons, solid dosage form identification 331
pro-drugs 16
procainamide, renal excretion 21
procaine, horseracing 269
product ion scanning, tandem mass spectrometry 567
metabolite identification 582
proficiency testing
GC-MS for workplace drug testing 141
postmortem toxicology 206
ProfilerSGA 590
profiling 65–7
amfetamines 71
cocaine 72–4
'ecstasy' tablets 75
heroin 50, 74
impurities 580–1
progesterone, HPLC and spectrophotometry *395*
Prohibited List, drugs in sport 264
prohormones
anabolic steroids 52
in food supplements 269
promethazine *245*
three-dimensional graphics, fluorescence spectrophotometry 417
propane *81–2*, *87*
propanediol, spacer-bonded, TLC 348, *349*
propoxyphene
chirality 254
colour test reagents *343*
workplace drug testing *138*, *139*
propylphenazone, gas chromatography *498*
propylphenylsilanes, HPLC 523
protein(s), saliva 168
protein binding 18, 250–1
on volumes of distribution 17
protein hormones *see* peptide hormones
protein precipitation 199–200, 499, 535, 552
proteomics 596–600
MALDI-TOF libraries 585
protocols, driver testing 320
protonation, electrospray ionisation 569
Prussian blue 109
pseudo-endogenous compounds, doping in sports 269, 279
pseudoephedrine *245*
sports, reporting rates *268*
workplace drug testing 138–9, 147
psilocin, control status *45*
Psilocybe mushrooms 56, 76, 120
psilocybe syndrome 120
psilocybine
control status *45*
thin-layer chromatography 69
psoralens 121–2
psychomotor impairment
benzodiazepines, saliva concentrations and 179
ethanol 301, 305
signs 306, 318–19
testing 305, 306–8, *309*
see also drivers/driving
psychosis
ketamine 294
stimulants 304
puffer fish 126–7
tetrodotoxin 116, 126–7
pulse heating, analysis of volatile substances 85
pulsed splitless injection, gas chromatography 485
pumps, HPLC 516–17, 526
pupils
drugs on 307
poisoning cases *225*
purge and trap 85, 489, 502–3
purity
reagents 4
seized drugs 64
putrefaction
postmortem toxicology samples and 207
volatile substances from 89
pyrethrins 99
pyrethroids *92*, 99
pyroelectric IR detectors 425, 426–7
qat (khat) 55–6, 69, 76
QED Saliva Alcohol Test 174
quadrupole mass spectrometers 565
inductively-coupled mass spectrometry 572
tandem mass spectrometry 567
see also triple quadrupole mass spectrometry
quality 608
standards of 620–2
quality assurance 608
breath-alcohol tests 311–12
hair testing 165
pesticide testing 97
postmortem toxicology 206
quality control and assessment 607–23
clinical toxicology 224
immunoassays 389–90
postmortem toxicology 206
quality systems 609
quantification (of substances) 8
amfetamines 71
breath-alcohol tests 312
cannabinoids 72
capillary electrophoresis 550
clinical toxicology 221
cocaine 72–4
gas chromatography 64, 505–6
HPLC 528–30
immunoassays 390
infrared spectroscopy 447
limit of 613
LSD 74
mass spectrometry 583
methylenedioxymethylamfetamine 75
near infrared spectroscopy 452
pesticides 97
postmortem toxicology 203–5
Raman spectroscopy 466–7
seized drugs 64–5
spectrophotometry 410–11
fluorescence spectrophotometry 418
thin-layer chromatography 355–6
validation 206, 612
volatile substances 85–6, 90
quantum efficiency 413
quartz cells, spectrophotometry 402
quartz columns, gas chromatography 471
quaternary ammonium compounds *92*, 99–100
quenching, fluorescence 413–14
self-quenching 418
technique, thin-layer chromatography 356, 357–8

Racing Medication and Testing Consortium (RMTC) 266
radioimmunoassay 375–6, 377, 384–5
anabolic steroids, horseracing 279
driving impairment, drug screening 320
hair 153–4, 159
radioisotopes, TLC 359
radioligand binding, high-throughput screening 593
railroad accident, cannabis use 136
Raman scattering 457
surface-enhanced *602*

Raman selection rule 457
Raman spectroscopy 455–68
random errors 615
rape 287–8
  see also drug-facilitated sexual assault
Rapid Methods for Drugs of Abuse (UN) 336
RapiScan saliva-sampling device 169, 171
ratio mode operation, fluorescence spectrophotometry 418
rattlesnakes 128
Rayleigh scattering 456, 457
re-tests, workplace drug testing 147
reabsorption, by saliva ducts 167
reaction/collision cells, inductively coupled plasma mass spectrometry 572
reagent strip tests, saliva, ethanol 174
reagents
  capillary electrophoresis 541
  colour tests 341–3
  for derivatisation 504, 505
  evaluation of 615
  purity 4
  thin-layer chromatography 357, *358*
    infrared spectroscopy and 439
    preparative 372
  see also substrate reagents
receptors, on drug effect 248
reciprocating pumps, HPLC 517
recombinant human erythropoietin (rhEPO), horses 281
recommended maximum detection limits, drugs used in DFSA *291–3*
recovery, of analyte 614
rectal route
  bioavailability 16
  drug absorption 15
red blood cells
    acetylcholinesterase 98
    drug uptake 17–18
reference standards
  dope testing 278
  in-house 206
  spectrophotometry 410
  see also certified reference materials; standards
reference substances, colour tests 341
reference tables, postmortem toxicology and 215–16
reflectance
  infrared spectroscopy 436–8
  measurement, TLC 356
refractive index detectors, HPLC 519–20
Reinsch test 110
relative density, deceptive specimens for workplace drug testing 144–5, 149–50
relative molecular masses 560–1
relative standard deviation
  capillary electrophoresis 550
  see also coefficient of variation
relaxation, molecules 411–12
renal failure, midazolam glucuronide 231
repeatability, capillary electrophoresis 550
replication 617
  ethanol measurements 314
reporting
  clinical toxicology 237
  quality control of 618
  traffic-light 591
reporting thresholds, drugs in sport 264
representative, samples as being 610
reptiles 128–9
requisitions, with postmortem toxicology samples 191–2, *193*
resolution
  capillary electrophoresis 542
  chromatography 514
  mass spectrometry 561–3
  Raman microscopy 459
  spectrophotometers 402, 429–30
  see also data resolution
respiratory rate, poisoning *225*
response time, capillary electrophoresis detectors 548
results, quality control 618
retardation (R_F value), TLC 345, 360
retention factor, gas chromatography 481–2
retention gaps, gas chromatography 480, 488–9
retention indices, gas chromatography 476
retention maps, TLC 370
retention times
  t_A and t_0 514
  t_R and t_M, gas chromatography 481, 507
retrograde extrapolation, ethanol measurements 314–15, *316*
reversed-optics mode, diode-array detectors 400
reversed-phase chromatography 515
reversed-phase ion-pair chromatography 532–3
reversed-phase thin-layer chromatography 347–8, 368, 369, 370
  infrared spectroscopy and 439
reversible derivatisation reactions, TLC 357
R_F value (retardation), TLC 345, 360
rhodamine, testing for pesticides 96
rhomboid prisms, ATR in IR spectroscopy 437–8
ricin 121
right-angle geometry, single-beam fluorimeters 414
risperidone, metabolism 28
  enzyme deficiency 31
rizatriptan, melts 329
road traffic accidents 4
  see also windshield washer fluid
roadside testing for substances 166, 168, 307–8
  evidential testing *vs* 313
robustness 614
robustotoxin 125
Roche Abuscreen Online system *see* KIMS assay
rodenticides *92*
Rohypnol *see* flunitrazepam
'Roofies' 296
routes of administration 14
  identifying 41
ruggedness 614

salbutamol *246*
  sports *266*
    reporting rates *267*, *268*
salicylates 233
  colour test reagents *343*
  poisoning emergencies *228*
saliva 8, 165, 166–7
  clinical toxicology 227
  ethanol 173–5, 313
    cocaine abuse and 177
  glands 166–7
  roadside tests 308
  sports 272
  therapeutic drug monitoring 251
  see also oral fluid
SalivaSac (BioQuant) 170
Salivette (collector) 168, *169*
salmon calcitonin 581–2
salts, colour tests 340
SAMHSA Guidelines 136
samples 8–10
  for anions 114–16
  blood *see* blood, samples
  capillary electrophoresis 546–7, 550–2
  clinical toxicology *6*, 224–7
  concentration methods 535, 552–3
  DFSA cases 296–7
  documentation 5, *6*
  doping in sports 271–3
  driving impairment 317–19
  fluorescence spectrophotometry 416
  gas chromatography 498–501
  haemolysis 18
  hair *see* hair
  HPLC 534–6
    on-line preparation 518, 530
  information with 5, *6*
  infrared spectroscopy, crushing 433–4
  mass spectrometry 574
  near infrared spectroscopy 449–50
  partitioning of extracts 202
  pesticides 96–7
  poisoning or doping *6*
  postmortem toxicology 191–8, 198–207
  quality control and 610–12, 616
  seized drugs 59–60
  spectrophotometry
    infrared 431–41
    presentation 402–4
    Raman 461–2
  therapeutic drug monitoring 250–1
  thin-layer chromatography
    application 350–1
    preparative 371
  volatile substances 83–4
  workplace drug testing
    alternative to urine 141–2, *143*
    collection 145–6
  see also adulteration of samples; alternative specimens; chain of custody of samples
sandwich chambers, TLC development 354
saturable enzyme systems 215
saturable kinetics, elimination 37
saxitoxins 122–3
scan mode, GC-MS, doping in sports 276
scan speeds
  dispersive IR spectrometers 431
  double-beam spectrophotometers 400

scanning densitometers, TLC 359
scanning microscopes, near infrared imaging 453
scanning spectrofluorimeters 414
scatter
  infrared spectroscopy on solids 433, 436–7
  Raman spectroscopy 456
  Rayleigh scattering 456, 457
  single-beam fluorimeters 414
  Stokes Raman scattering 456, 461
  see also Raman scattering
scene of incident 5–7
  items found 197
scene residues, sampling for anions 115
scheduled substances *see* controlled substances
scintillation proximity assay 593
scombroid poisoning 126, 127
scorpions 125
Scott-Ham, M., and F.C. Burton, on DFSA drugs 296
Scott test 72
screening 9
  clinical toxicology 221, 227–30
  DFSA victims 289, 296
  doping in sports 273–6
  driving impairment 319–20
  drugs of abuse 235
  hair 158–9
  high-throughput (HTS) 590–4
  meconium 258–60
  metal compounds 110
  persons for substances 2, 7–8
  pesticides 95
  poisoning 79
  postmortem toxicology 198, 199
  saliva 171
  samples of seized drugs 60–1
  thin-layer chromatography 360–1
  see also systematic toxicological identification
seafood
  arsenic 104
  shellfish 122–4
  see also fish
sealing bands, capsules 328
secobarbital *246*
  saliva 178
  workplace drug testing *139*
second-derivatives, near infrared spectroscopy 448, *449*
sectional analysis, hair 162
security, urine sampling 271
sedatives
  doping in sports 273–4
  driving and *302*
  see also central nervous system, depressants; drug-facilitated sexual assault
seized drugs
  analysis 58–68
  tablets 325
selected-ion monitoring 565
  GC-MS 203, 497, 508
    doping in sports 276
selected-reaction monitoring, tandem mass spectrometry 567
selective serotonin reuptake inhibitors (SSRI) 231
  metabolism *27*
selectivity 613
selectivity point, three-co-ordinate, PRISMA model of TLC 370
selegiline, metabolism 26, 148
selenium *102*, 108–9
self-poisoning 1
self-quenching, fluorescence 418
semiconductors, infrared detectors 426–7
sensitivity 5
  chromatography 514
  for DFSA drugs 296
  dope tests 267, 270
  electron-capture detectors 495
  fluorescence spectrophotometry 417
  gas chromatography 506
  mass spectrometry 574
separation factor (α), gas chromatography 482–3
separation steps
  immunoassays
    automated 388
    heterogeneous 382
  radioimmunoassay 384–5
sertraline, metabolism *27*
serum
  clinical toxicology 224
  ethanol 310
  osmolality *228*
    alcohols 230
sexual assault 287–8
  see also drug-facilitated sexual assault
shellfish 122–4
Shewhart QC charts 617
Shiga toxins 117
shipments, drug seizures 60
short-end injection, capillary electrophoresis 554, 555
'shy bladder syndrome', workplace drug testing 146
sieves, molecular 472
sieving media, capillary sieving electrophoresis 545
signal-to-noise ratios 613
  gas chromatography 493
silica
  capillary electrophoresis 541
  see also fused-silica cells; fused-silica columns
silica-based materials, for HPLC 523–4, 531–3
silica gel, TLC 346–7, 368
silver chloride, cones for infrared spectroscopy 435–6
silver nitrate, testing for pesticides 96
silyl derivatives
  gas chromatography 504
  GHB 76
single-beam fluorimeters 414
single-beam spectrometers, infrared 425
single-beam spectrophotometers 399
single molecule spectroscopy *602*
single-nucleotide polymorphisms (SNP), investigation techniques 598, *599*
size-exclusion chromatography 515
skin
  poisoning cases *225*, *226*
  salicylate poisoning via 233
slit scanning densitometers, TLC 359
slow-release products *see* sustained-release products
small intestine, absorption via 14
'smart drugs' 235
Smarties 329–30
smoking
  oral deposition of drugs 168, 171
  saliva concentrations, cocaine 177–8
  saliva negative, marijuana (passive exposure) 180
  tobacco
    cadmium 105
    pregnancy 257
snakes 128–9
snorting, saliva concentrations 173
'soap chromatography' 533
Society of Forensic Toxicologists (USA)
  SOFT/AAFS Laboratory Guidelines (2006) 621
  subcommittees on DFSA 290
sodium, reabsorption from saliva 167
sodium bromide, TLC systems using *362*
sodium chlorate 111
sodium chloride, infrared spectroscopy cells 432
sodium dithionate test 95, 234
sodium dodecyl sulfate, MECC 552
sodium hydroxide
  drug extraction 201
  solubilisation of drugs in hair 157
    opiates and 160
sodium oxybate *see* gamma-hydroxybutyric acid
sodium salts, barbiturates, infrared spectra 443–4, 445
SOFT/AAFS Forensic Toxicology Laboratory Guidelines (2006) 621
software packages, pharmacokinetics 237
solid(s), infrared spectroscopy 433–4
  scatter 433, 436–7
solid dosage forms, identification 323–33
solid injection, gas chromatography 489–90
solid-phase extraction
  capillary electrophoresis 553
  gas chromatography 489, 500–1
  for HPLC 536
  pesticide GC-MS 96
  postmortem toxicology samples 202
  saliva samples 170–1
    cannabinoids 180
  screening for sports doping 274–6
solid-phase microextraction
  cannabinoids 180
  gas chromatography 489, 501–2
  headspace 85
solid stationary phases 514
  gas chromatography 471–2
solubilisation, drugs in hair 157–8, 160
solvent effects
  gas chromatography 485
  spectrophotometry 397–8, 409–10
solvents
  abuse *see* volatile substances, abuse
  adsorption energies on alumina 531
  boiling points and expansion volumes *490*
  cocaine manufacture 72
  fluorescence spectrophotometry 416
  gas chromatography 508

HPLC 516
infrared spectroscopy 433
near infrared spectroscopy 450
pesticide products 95
spectrophotometry 404
TLC 61, 361–71
see also eluents
Somotomax *see* gamma-hydroxybutyric acid
spacer-bonded propanediol, TLC 348, *349*
spatial peak area, capillary electrophoresis detectors 548
specific absorbance 397, 410
specificity
breath-alcohol tests 312
fluorescence spectrophotometry 417
immunoassays 9, 380–2
immunogens 378
spectra
excitation spectra 416
GC-MS of pesticides, libraries 96
mass spectra 559, 560
phenols 398
wavelength 396
see also absorption spectra; infrared spectroscopy; Raman spectroscopy
Spectralon 448
spectrophotometry 393–420
carboxyhaemoglobin 234
instruments 399–402
performance checks 401–2
multicomponent systems 405
single component systems 404–5
see also specific types
spectroscopy 9
see also specific types
specular reflectance, infrared spectroscopy 437
speed
capillary electrophoresis 554–5
HPLC 530
see also scan speeds
spiders 125
spleen, postmortem toxicology 197
split and splitless injectors, gas chromatography 485–7
large-volume 488
sport, drug abuse *see* doping
spot tests, seized drugs 60–1
spray-on techniques, TLC 350–1
reagents 357
spray reagents
chromatography 341–3
preparative TLC 372
square root method, seized drug sampling 59, 60
stacking, capillary electrophoresis 552–3
stains, analysis for poisons 5
stand on one leg test *309*
standard addition method 204–5
calibration of HPLC 529–30
standard deviation, system mean, TLC screening 360
standard operating procedures (SOPs) 616
clinical toxicology 224
standards 618
carbon monoxide 234
dope testing 278
ethanol measurement 310
fluorescence spectrophotometry 418
quantification of seized drugs 64
thin-layer chromatography 360
see also internal standards; reference standards
standards (ISO) 620, 621
dope testing 278
standards (of quality) 620–2
stanozolol, sports, reporting rates *268*
statements by witnesses, checking 5
stationary phases 514
gas chromatography 471–6
interactions with solutes 475–6
HPLC 514–15, 523–4, 531–3
particle size 516
solid-phase microextraction 502
thin-layer chromatography 9, 346–9
selection 368
statistical monitoring of performance 617–18
steady state
drug concentrations 22
therapeutic drug monitoring 251
step gradients, TLC 353
stereoselective analysis (chiral separation) 254, 515
capillary electrophoresis 544, 555
gas chromatography 85, 474–5, 505
HPLC 524, 527–8
steroids
colour test reagents *343*
see also anabolic agents; ethynyl steroids
stimulants
driving and 303–4, 320
gas chromatography 508–9
horseracing 270
metabolism 25–6
prohibited in sports *265*
stimulation of saliva secretion 166, 167, 170, 176
stings
arthropods 125
fish spines 128
jellyfish 124
stir bars, solid-phase microextraction 502
Stokes' law, electrophoresis 540
Stokes Raman scattering 456, 461
Stokes shift 385, 412
stomach
drugs absorbed from 15
drugs diffused into 17, 196
stomach contents
anion poisoning 115
clinical toxicology 226–7
estimating time after substance administration 38
postmortem redistribution from 208
ethanol 211
postmortem toxicology 195–6
sample quantities *192*
starch granules 325
thin-layer chromatography 229
stonefish 127–8
storage of samples
postmortem toxicology 192
quality control 611
strategic profiling 65
stray-light effects, spectrophotometry 397
infrared 426, 429
instrument assessment 402
street drugs, Marquis test 337
street-level deals, cannabis resin 72
street names
drugs used in DFSA *291*
flunitrazepam 290
gamma-hydroxybutyric acid 293
ketamine 294
stretching vibrations, Raman spectroscopy 462–3
strychnine, poisoning emergencies *228*
styrene–divinylbenzene co-polymers, HPLC 524–5
subclavian blood, postmortem toxicology 194
sublingual absorption of substances 15, 168
saliva concentrations 173
Substance Abuse and Mental Health Services Administration Guidelines 136
substituted phenoxy acids 99
substituted ureas *92*
substitution, specimens for workplace drug testing 143–5, 147, 149–50
substrate reagents, microplate antibody capture 384
subtilisin Carlsberg 200
subtraction, Raman spectra 468
sugar-coated chocolate drops 329–30
sugar-coated tablets 326
suicide
attempted 1
compliance testing and 250
see also overdosage
sulfation, pharmacogenetics 32
sulfhydryl groups
amino acids with, drug trapping in hair 155
drugs for paracetamol toxicity 33–4
sulfide 114
sulfonamides
capillary zone electrophoresis *543*
colour test reagents *343*
sulfonosilanes, HPLC 524
sulfur, Raman spectra 461
Supelcoport 476
supercritical fluid extraction
drugs in hair 158
gas chromatography 502
supports, gas chromatography columns 476–9
surface-enhanced Raman scattering *602*
surveillance windows
hair 154, 164
saliva 166
urine 195
sustained-release products 329
salicylate preparations 233
swallowing, by fetus 258
sweat 181–3
passage of drugs into hair 155
workplace drug testing 142, *144*
sweat glands 181, *182*
sweat patches 181–3
Sweden, drink and driving 305
sweeteners 330
sweets, resembling drugs 324, 329–30

switching
columns, HPLC 518
solvents, HPLC 521
urine samples 271–2
isoelectric focusing method to detect 280
switching blocks, gas chromatography 489
sycamore seeds, hypoglycin 122
synthesis *see specific substances*
syringes, found on scene 197
system maps, thin-layer chromatography 370
system mean standard deviation, TLC screening 360
system suitability tests
HPLC 530
mass spectrometry 573–4
systematic errors 615
systematic toxicological identification
pesticides 364
systems *367*
procedure (STIP) 229
thin-layer chromatography 361–4
see also screening

t-test 614
tablets 323–7
analysis 67
comparisons 65
methylenedioxymethylamfetamine 51, 52
see also 'ecstasy' tablets
near infrared spectroscopy 449, 450
Raman spectroscopy 465
in stomach contents 196
tactical profiling, seized drugs 65
tailing, gas chromatography peaks 483
tandem electrospray mass spectrometry, HPLC and
ciguatoxin 126
doping in sports 276–7
tandem mass spectrometry (MS/MS) 567
electrospray ionisation with 581–2
liquid chromatography with 521
doping in sports 276–7
horses 267
therapeutic drug monitoring 253
see also triple quadrupole mass spectrometry
uninterpreted matching 600
workplace drug testing 140–1
target factor analysis, UV spectrophotometry 589, 590
target ranges, therapeutic ranges *vs* 254
targeted testing, postmortem toxicology 199
tartar emetic 103
Taylor cones 569
teas, coca 149
technical false positives 156
teething gels, salicylate poisoning 233
tegafur, Raman spectroscopy 464
temazepam *246*
liquid-filled capsules 328
urine levels for DFSA cases *291*
workplace drug testing *139*
temperature
capillary electrophoresis 554
fluorescence spectrophotometry 416
gas chromatography 480–1, 507
on flow 491, *492*
injectors 484
HPLC 517–18, 528
temperature (body), poisoning *225*
Tenax-TA, gas chromatography 472
terbutaline *246*
sports, reporting rates *268*
test strips
ethanol 313
roadside, immunoassays 308
testosterone
CIRMS 277
detection 279
electron-impact ionisation 575
reporting rates *267*, *268*
testosterone/epitestosterone ratio 266, 277, 279
tetanus toxin 116–17
tetrahydrocannabinol (THC) 47, *48*
activation by liver 16
blood *vs* plasma concentrations 18, 213
content in cannabis resin 72
estimating time after substance administration 38–9
hair 160, 161
hydroxylation 23
saliva 173, 179, 180
volume of distribution 18
workplace drug testing *138*
alternative specimens *143*
immunoassay 140
see also carboxy-tetrahydrocannabinol
tetramethylbenzidine (TMB) 384
Tetraodontiformes, tetrodotoxin 127
1,2,4,5-tetrazine, absorption spectra 394
tetrodotoxin 116, 126–7
textbooks, Raman spectroscopy 462
thallium 109, *246*
analysis methods *102*
colorimetry 110–11
poisoning emergencies *228*
thallium halides, disc IR spectroscopy 436
theophylline 234–5, *246*
poisoning emergencies *228*
therapeutic drug monitoring 251
theoretical plates
capillary electrophoresis 542
gas chromatography 483
therapeutic concentrations of drugs 36, 207–8, 216, 237, *238*, 254
therapeutic doses, drugs in 5
therapeutic drug monitoring 219, 237–56
immunoassays 252–3, 377
measurement techniques 252–4
thermal conductivity detection (TCD), nitrous oxide 84
thermal desorption, gas chromatography 489, 503
thermostats, HPLC 517–18
thin films, infrared spectroscopy 436
thin-layer chromatography 9, 61, 69, 229, 335, 343–73
basic tests 336
colour test reagents 341–3
detection 355–60
hair 159
infrared spectroscopy with 438–9
pesticides 96
preparative 371–2
sample application 350–1
screening for sports doping 274
technique 350–61
thiobarbiturates, infrared spectra 443–4
thiocarbamates *92*
thiopental, brain death 222
thioridazine, metabolism 28
three-co-ordinate selectivity point, PRISMA model of TLC 370
three-dimensional graphics, fluorescence spectrophotometry 417
thresholds, drugs in sport 264, 266, 267, 278
ticks 125
TICTAC (database) 331–2
Tillman reagent *358*
time after substance administration 38–9
hair uptake 155
time constants, infrared spectrometers 431
time-of-flight mass spectrometers 566
tissue : plasma concentration 17
tissue masses, postmortem 214
tissues
drug concentrations 35
gas chromatography 503
postmortem 212, 213–14
see also specific organs
ratios 39
routes of administration and 41
HPLC 534–6
titres, drugs for immunoassay 380
TLC *see* thin-layer chromatography
toads 128
tobacco smoke
cadmium 105
pregnancy 257
tolerance to drugs 36, 37–8
toluene
abuse 43
blood concentrations 90
deaths 82
hexanal and 89
pharmacokinetics *87*
toluene–acetone–ethanol–25% ammonia TLC system *366*
toluene–acetone TLC system, pesticides *367*
tolurates, as metabolites *89*
total ion current chromatograms 572
Tox-Elut cartridges 275
toxic concentrations of substances 36–8, 237, *238*
ToxiLab TLC system 229, 364
toxins 116–29
trace levels, gas chromatography 508
track optimisation, scanning densitometry 359
trade names
clonazepam 295
drugs used in DFSA *291–3*
traffic-light reporting 591
training 620
tramadol, metabolism 29
transdermal dosage forms 328
postmortem redistribution from 209

transition electric dipole moments 423–4
transmittance 397, 423
transport of samples, quality control 611–12
transposition errors 611
traps
  gas chromatography 493, 503
  see also ion cyclotron resonance mass spectrometers; ion-trap mass spectrometers
triazines *92*, 99
triazolam *247*
  urine levels for DFSA cases *291*
trichloroacetate, as metabolite *89*
1,1-trichloroethane, pharmacokinetics *87*
2,2,2-trichloroethanol, as metabolite *89*
trichloroethylene, pharmacokinetics *87*
2,4,5-trichlorophenoxyacetic acid (2,4,5-T) 232
trichomes, *Cannabis sativa* leaves 46, 71–2
trichothecenes 118
tricyclic antidepressants 231
  metabolism 27
  poisoning 223
    emergencies *228*
  postmortem, liver and urine 195
  postmortem redistribution 208
  vitreous humour 195
trifluoroacetate, as metabolite *89*
trifluoroacetic anhydride (TFAA) derivatives 70
n-trifluoroacetyl-1-propyl chloride (TPC) 505
trifluoropropyl/methyl-PSX 474
triglycine sulfate, deuterated, detectors 425
triple quadrupole mass spectrometry, liquid chromatography with (LC-MS/MS) 229–30
tritium, radioimmunoassay 384
Triton X-100, fluorescence-quenching technique, TLC 358
trough concentrations 251
trueness 613–14
tryptamines *57*
tubules, kidneys 21
tuna, scombroid poisoning 127
twin-trough chambers, TLC development 354, *355*
two-dimensional gel electrophoresis *599*, 600
two-dimensional TLC 353–4
two-point bracketing, fluorescence spectrophotometry 418

ultra-high-throughput screening 590, *593*
ultrafiltrates
  capillary electrophoresis 552
  free drug levels 251, 253–4
ultraviolet indicators, TLC 346
ultraviolet light
  HPLC, detectors 199, 229
  TLC, detection technique 356
  wavelengths 396
ultraviolet light test, lysergic acid 74
ultraviolet spectra, infrared spectra *vs* 424
ultraviolet spectrophotometry 393–9
  multiwavelength 587–90
Umbelliferae 121–2
uncertainty estimates, ethanol measurements 314
uncertainty of measurement 614–15
unidimensional multiple development, TLC 352
uninterpreted MS/MS matching 600
unit resolution, mass spectrometry 563
United Kingdom
  ethanol concentrations for driving 305, 314
  workplace drug testing 135
    Laboratory Guidelines (2001) 621–2
United States of America
  DFSA
    definitions 287
    legislation 289–90
  ethanol concentrations for driving 305, 314
  horseracing policy 266, 270
  solid dosage form databases 332
  workplace drug testing 135–51
UniTox system 361–4, *366*
units, wavelength 396
up-converting phosphors, saliva testing 172
Up-Link Rapid Detection system, saliva test 172
uracils *92*
  Raman spectroscopy 464
urine
  adulteration of samples 143–5, 146, 149, 390
  aluminium reference value 103
  anion poisoning 115
  benzodiazepines 25
  capillary electrophoresis 552
  clinical toxicology 226
  conjugates of drugs 273
  DFSA victims 296
    recommended maximum detection limits *291–3*
  driving impairment and 318–19
  drugs of abuse 235
  estimating time after substance administration 38
  ethanol 312–13
  vs hair for testing 163
  horse 275
  limitations for dose calculation 22
  neonates 256
  pH 21–2
    therapeutic altering 223
  postmortem toxicology 195
    ethanol 211
    sample quantities *192*
  sports and drugs *266*, 271–3
  sweat *vs 182*
  therapeutic drug monitoring 250
  validity of tests 34–5
  workplace drug testing 142, 145–6
    'dilute specimen' 144, 149–50
  see also biofluids

vacuum de-gassing, HPLC 516
validation 612–14
  capillary electrophoresis 550
  emerging techniques 587
  HPLC 530
  postmortem toxicology methods 205–6
  spectrophotometry 411
validity
  analytical tests 34–5
  specimens for workplace drug testing 145
valproate, DFSA cases *293*
valve injectors, HPLC 517, 526
van Deemter curves 492, *493*, 507
Van Urk reagent
  lysergic acid 74
  thin-layer chromatography *358*
vapour phase, absorption spectra 394
vapour pressures, volatile substances *87*
variability, interindividual pharmacodynamic 248, 249
variable temperature studies, Raman spectroscopy 462
variable-wavelength detectors, HPLC 518–19
vasodilators, volatile *81*
vegetable materials, seized 67
venepuncture 224
venlafaxine, metabolism *27*
venoms
  arthropods 125
  Cnidaria 124
verotoxin 117
versutoxin 125
vertebrates 126–9
vertex posterior, hair collection 156
veterinary practice, drugs in 267
veterinary products 329
vials, capillary electrophoresis 547
vibration, molecular 421–3, 462–4
Vicks Inhaler 148
Vierordt method, overlapping absorption spectra 405
vipers 128
virotoxins 119
virtual states, molecules 456
viscous samples 199
visible light, wavelengths 396
visible spectrophotometry 393–9
vitamin(s), abuse in sports 264
vitamin A, spectrophotometry 405
vitreous humour, postmortem 194–5
  ethanol 211
  sample quantities *192*
volatile substances 7, 80–90
  abuse 43, 80, 82, 83, 230
  antemortem specimens 198
  breath-alcohol tests 83, 312
  postmortem toxicology 212
  screening 229
volatiles interfaces, gas chromatography 489
volatilisation 84
voltage, capillary electrophoresis 546
volume changes, solvent mixing 516
volumes of distribution 17, 18–19
  clearance and 20
  ethanol 19, 211, 315–16
  listed *16*
  postmortem toxicology 214
voluntary use of drugs, DFSA 288–9
VTEC (verotoxin-producing *E. coli*) 117

walk and turn test *309*

wall-coated open tubular (WCOT) columns 471
warfarin 100, *101*, *247*
washing, hair specimens 156
water
  alkali halide disc IR spectroscopy 436
  HPLC 531
  near infrared spectroscopy 450, 451, 452
  Raman spectroscopy 461
  spectrophotometry 399
    solvent effects 398
  TLC
    detection technique 357
    removal from plates 350
    systems using *366*, 369
water compartments, body 17
water hemlock 121
water intoxication 222
water supplies, arsenic poisoning 104
water wettable layers, TLC 348
wavelength(s)
  solvents 398
  spectra 396
  spectrophotometry calibration 401, *402*
wavenumbers
  infrared 421
    instrument calibration 429
    molecular vibration 422
  percentage transmittance *vs* 423
  spectra 396
weeverfish 128
well water, arsenic poisoning 104
Westgard rules 617
whipped cream dispensers *81*
whole-bowel irrigation 223
Widmark's equation 315–17, *318*
Wilson's disease 105
windshield washer fluid, methanol 212
withdrawal phase, stimulants 304, 320
withdrawal symptoms, neonates 256
women, androstenedione abuse 52
Wood's peak, near infrared spectroscopy 450
working range 613
workplace drug testing 2, 135–51
  deceptive specimens 149–50
  Mandatory Guidelines for 621
  saliva 181
    ethanol 175
    phencyclidine, cut-offs 181
  solid dosage form identification 330–1
  UK Laboratory Guidelines (2001) 621–2
World Anti-Doping Agency (WADA) 264
  on 'B' samples 271
  Code 264
  International Standard for Testing 622
  laboratory accreditation 278
World Health Organization
  pesticides 95
  terminology on substance abuse 44
wrapping materials, seized drugs 59

XAD-2 resin, screening for sports doping 274
xanthines, horseracing 270
xenon lines, performance checks for spectrophotometry 415
xylene *81–2*
  abuse 43
  pharmacokinetics *87*

zearalenone 118
zeolites 472
zero-order elimination 20–1
  ethanol 39
zeta potential, capillary electrophoresis 541
zidovudine, metabolism 35
Zimmerman test 75
zinc protoporphyrin (ZPP) 107
zinc selenide, ATR in IR spectroscopy 437–8
zirconia packing materials, HPLC 524
zolpidem 231, *247*
  urine levels for DFSA cases *293*
zopiclone 231, *247*
Zuckerman, S. (Lord), quoted 602